# DIAGNOSTIC IMAGING

## An Algorithmic Approach

*Edited by*

*Ronald L. Eisenberg,* M.D.
PROFESSOR AND CHAIRMAN
DEPARTMENT OF RADIOLOGY
LOUISIANA STATE UNIVERSITY SCHOOL OF MEDICINE
SHREVEPORT, LOUISIANA

*With 77 Contributors*

# DIAGNOSTIC IMAGING

## An Algorithmic Approach

**J. B. Lippincott Company** Philadelphia
London Mexico City New York
St. Louis São Paulo Sydney

Sponsoring Editor: Delois Patterson
Manuscript Editor: Margaret E. Maxwell
Indexer: Alexandra Weir
Design Coordinator: Caren Erlichman
Production Manager: Carol A. Florence
Production Coordinator: Barney Fernandes
Compositor: Circle Graphics
Printer/Binder: Halliday Lithograph



2 3 4 5 6

Library of Congress Cataloging-in-Publication Data

Diagnostic imaging.

Includes bibliographies and index.
1. Diagnostic imaging—Problems, exercises, etc.
2. Algorithms. I. Eisenberg, Ronald L. [DNLM: 1. Algorithms. 2. Radiography—Problems. 3. Radionuclide Imaging—problems. WN 18 D536]
RC78.7.D53D523 1987 616.07′57 87-3013
ISBN 0-397-58300-1

The authors and publisher have exerted every effort to ensure that drug selection and dosage set forth in this text are in accord with current recommendations and practice at the time of publication. However, in view of ongoing research, changes in government regulations, and the constant flow of information relating to drug therapy and drug reactions, the reader is urged to check the package insert for each drug for any change in indications and dosage and for added warnings and precautions. This is particularly important when the recommended agent is a new or infrequently employed drug.

To Zina, Avlana, and Cherina

# Contributors

**John R. Amberg, M.D.** Professor of Radiology, University of California, San Diego, California

**Dixie J. Anderson, M.D.** Associate Professor of Radiology, Mallinckrodt Institute of Radiology, Washington University School of Medicine; Associate Radiologist, Barnes Hospital, St. Louis, Missouri

**Joseph C. Anderson, M.D.** Associate Professor of Radiology, University of Nebraska College of Medicine, University of Nebraska Medical Center, Omaha, Nebraska

**Richard E. Appen, M.D.** Clinical Associate Professor of Ophthalmology, University of Wisconsin Center for Health Sciences, Madison, Wisconsin

**Gary J. Becker, M.D.** Professor of Radiology, Indiana University School of Medicine; Chief, Vascular Radiology, Indiana University Hospital, Indianapolis, Indiana

**John C. Brown, M.D.** Director, Arthritis and Rehabilitation Center, White Memorial Hospital, Los Angeles, California

**Stephen R. Bunker, M.D.** Assistant Clinical Professor of Radiology, University of California, San Francisco; Chief, Department of Nuclear Medicine, Children's Hospital, San Francisco, California

**Barbara A. Carroll, M.D.** Associate Professor of Radiology, Duke University School of Medicine, Durham, North Carolina

**Ronald A. Castellino, M.D.** Professor of Radiology, Stanford University School of Medicine; Acting Chairman, Department of Diagnostic Radiology and Nuclear Medicine, Stanford University Hospital, Stanford, California

**Neil I. Chafetz, M.D.** Associate Professor of Radiology, University of California, San Francisco, California

**Alan J. Davidson, M.D.** Professor of Radiology, Uniformed Services University of the Health Sciences, Bethesda, Maryland; Distinguished Scientist, Department of Radiologic Pathology, Armed Forces Institute of Pathology, Washington, DC

**Robert L. DeLaPaz, M.D.** Assistant Professor of Radiology, Stanford University Medical Center, Stanford, California

**Barbara E. Demas, M.D.** Assistant Professor of Radiology, Cornell Medical College; Assistant Attending Roentgenologist, Memorial Sloan-Kettering Cancer Center, New York, New York

**Leo F. Drolshagen, M.D.** Fellow in Radiology, Vanderbilt University Medical Center, Nashville, Tennessee

**Beth S. Edeiken–Monroe, M.D.** Assistant Professor of Radiology, The University of Texas Medical School, Houston; Chief of Diagnosis, and Assistant, Emergency Radiology, Hermann Hospital, Houston, Texas

**David S. Feigin, M.D.** Associate Professor of Radiology, and Attending Radiologist, University of California, San Diego; Assistant Chief of Radiology, Veterans Administration Medical Center, La Jolla, California

**Madeleine R. Fisher, M.D.** Assistant Professor of Radiology, Northwestern University Medical School; Director, Magnetic Resonance, Northwestern Memorial Hospital, Chicago, Illinois

**Arthur C. Fleischer, M.D.** Associate Professor of Radiology, and Assistant Professor of Obstetrics and Gynecology; Chief, Ultrasound Section, Vanderbilt University Medical Center, Nashville, Tennessee

**D. M. Forrester, M.D.** Associate Professor of Radiology, Medicine, and Orthopedic Surgery, University of Southern California; Chief of Bone and Joint Radiology, LAC-USC Medical Center, Los Angeles, California

**Patrick C. Freeny, M.D.** Associate Clinical Professor of Radiology, University of Washington School of Medicine; The Mason Clinic, Seattle, Washington

**William E. Fulcher, M.D.** Attending Radiologist, Capitol Hill Hospital, Washington, DC

**Linda D. Gillam, M.D.** Assistant Professor of Medicine, University of Connecticut; Attending Cardiologist, John Dempsey Hospital and Newington Veterans Administration Medical Center, Farmington, Connecticut

**Vishan L. Giyanani, M.D.** Associate Professor of Radiology, Louisiana State University School of Medicine; Head, Divisions of Ultrasound and Computed Tomography, Louisiana State University Medical Center, Shreveport, Louisiana

**J. David Godwin, M.D.** Associate Professor of Radiology, University of Washington School of Medicine, Seattle, Washington

**Gretchen A. W. Gooding, M.D.** Professor of Radiology, University of California, San Francisco; Chief, Department of Ultrasonography, and Chief, Department of Radiology, Veterans Administration Medical Center, San Francisco, California

**Richard M. Gore, M.D.** Associate Professor of Radiology, Northwestern University Medical School; Chief, Section of Gastrointestinal Radiology, and Co-Director, Body Computed Tomography, Northwestern Memorial Hospital, Chicago, Illinois

**David B. Hackney, M.D.** Assistant Professor of Radiology, University of Pennsylvania School of Medicine, Hospital of the University of Pennsylvania, Philadelphia, Pennsylvania

**Peter F. Hahn, M.D., Ph.D.** Instructor in Radiology, Harvard Medical School; Assistant in Radiology, Massachusetts General Hospital, Boston, Massachusetts

**Robert A. Halvorsen, M.D.** Associate Professor of Radiology, Durham Veterans Administration Hospital, Duke University Medical Center, Durham, North Carolina

**Roger K. Harned, M.D.** Professor of Radiology, University of Nebraska College of Medicine, University of Nebraska Medical Center, Omaha, Nebraska

**John H. Harris, Jr., M.D., D.Sc.** Professor and Chairman, Department of Radiology, The University of Texas Medical School, Houston; Chairman, Department of Diagnostic Radiology, and Chief, Section of Emergency Radiology, Hermann Hospital, Houston, Texas

**Marcus W. Hedgcock, M.D.** Assistant Professor of Radiology, University of California, San Francisco; Chief, Uroradiology, Veterans Administration Hospital, San Francisco, California

**Charles B. Higgins, M.D.** Professor of Radiology, and Chief, Magnetic Resonance Imaging, University of California, San Francisco, California

**Robert W. Holden, M.D.** Professor of Radiology, Indiana University School of Medicine; Chief of Radiology, Wishard Memorial Hospital, Indianapolis, Indiana

**Jefferson O. Janes, M.D.** Associate Clinical Professor of Radiology, University of California, Davis; Chief, Diagnostic Imaging, Sierra Nevada Memorial Hospital, Grass Valley, California

**Bao-shan Jing, M.D.** Professor of Radiology, The University of Texas Medical School, Houston; Radiologist, Department of Diagnostic Radiology, M. D. Anderson Hospital, Houston, Texas

**Peter Julien, M.D.** Assistant Clinical Professor of Radiology, University of California, Los Angeles; Attending Staff Radiologist, Cedars-Sinai Medical Center, Los Angeles, California

**Donald R. Kirks, M.D.** Professor of Radiology and Pediatrics, University of Cincinnati College of Medicine; Director, Department of Radiology, Children's Hospital Medical Center, Cincinnati, Ohio

**Rajendra Kumar, M.D.** Associate Professor of Radiology, and Director, Genitourinary and Musculoskeletal Divisions, University of Texas Medical Branch, Galveston, Texas

**Faye C. Laing, M.D.** Professor of Radiology, University of California, San Francisco; Chief, Ultrasound Section, San Francisco General Hospital, San Francisco, California

**Erich K. Lang, M.D., M.S.** Professor and Chairman, Department of Radiology, Louisiana State University Medical Center; Director, Department of Radiology, Charity Hospital, New Orleans, Louisiana

**John C. Leonidas, M.D.** Professor of Radiology, State University of New York, Stony Brook; Chief of Pediatric Radiology, Schneider Children's Hospital, New Hyde Park, New York

**Marvin M. Lindell, Jr., M.D.** Associate Professor of Radiology, The University of Texas Health Science Center, Houston; Radiologist, Division of Inpatient Diagnostic Radiology, The University of Texas System Cancer Center, M. D. Anderson Hospital and Tumor Institute, Houston, Texas

**Martin J. Lipton, M.D.** Professor of Radiology and Medicine, and Chief, Cardiovascular Section, University of California, San Francisco, California

**John T. Mail, M.D.** Assistant Professor of Radiology, Indiana University School of Medicine, Indianapolis, Indiana

**Jay C. Mall, M.D.** Associate Clinical Professor of Radiology, University of California; Attending Radiologist, Children's Hospital, San Francisco, California

**Stephen I. Marglin, M.D.** Associate Professor of Radiology, University of Washington School of Medicine; University Hospital, Seattle, Washington

**Alexander R. Margulis, M.D.** Professor and Chairman, Department of Radiology, University of California, San Francisco, California

**William M. Marks, M.D.** Clinical Assistant Professor of Radiology, University of Washington; The Mason Clinic, Seattle, Washington

**Matthew A. Mauro, M.D.** Associate Professor of Radiology, University of North Carolina; Department of Radiology, North Carolina Memorial Hospital, Chapel Hill, North Carolina

**Gordon K. McLean, M.D.** Associate Professor of Radiology, University of Pennsylvania School of Medicine; Chief, Angiography/Interventional Radiology Section, Hospital of the University of Pennsylvania, Philadelphia, Pennsylvania

**David F. Merten** Professor of Radiology, Section Director for Pediatric Radiology, University of North Carolina School of Medicine, Chapel Hill, North Carolina

**Peter C. Meyers, M.D.** Associate Professor of Radiology, Louisiana State University Medical Center; Head, Division of Diagnostic and Gastrointestinal Radiology, University Hospital, Shreveport, Louisiana

**Stephen W. Miller, M.D.** Associate Professor of Radiology, Harvard Medical School; Radiologist, Massachusetts General Hospital, Boston, Massachusetts

**Clark H. Millikan, M.D.** Professor of Neurology, University of Miami School of Medicine, Miami, Florida

**Harold A. Mitty, M.D.** Professor of Radiology, The Mount Sinai School of Medicine of the City University of New York; Attending Radiologist, The Mount Sinai Hospital, New York, New York

**Joanne E. Mortimer, M.D.** Assistant Professor, Division of Medical Oncology, University of Washington School of Medicine, Seattle, Washington

**James A. Nelson, M.D.** Professor of Radiology, University of Washington School of Medicine, Seattle, Washington

**Carl-Olof Ovenfors, M.D., Ph.D.** Professor of Radiological Sciences, University of California, Los Angeles; Chief Radiologist, Chest Section, University of California Medical Center, Los Angeles, California

**L. Alden Parker, M.D.** Assistant Professor of Radiology, University of North Carolina School of Medicine, Chapel Hill, North Carolina

**Barry D. Pressman, M.D., F.A.C.R.** Chief, Section of Neuroradiology and Head and Neck Radiology, Cedars-Sinai Medical Center; Clinical Assistant Professor of Radiology, University of California, Los Angeles, California

**Bharat Raval, M.D.** Associate Professor of Radiology, University of Texas Medical Center, Houston; Chief, Computed Body Tomography, Hermann Hospital, Houston, Texas

**Matthew D. Rifkin, M.D.** Professor of Radiology and Urology, Jefferson Medical College, Thomas Jefferson University; Staff Radiologist, Department of Radiology, Thomas Jefferson University Hospital, Philadelphia, Pennsylvania

**Stuart S. Sagel, M.D.** Professor of Radiology, Washington University School of Medicine; Director, Chest Radiology, and Co-Director, Computed Body Tomography, Mallinckrodt Institute of Radiology, Barnes and Affiliated Hospitals, St. Louis, Missouri

**Carl M. Sandler, M.D.** Associate Professor of Radiology, The University of Texas Medical Center at Houston; Chief, Section of Uroradiology, Hermann Hospital, Houston, Texas

**Donald E. Schwarten, M.D.** Chief, Cardiovascular Laboratories, St. Vincent's Hospital and Health Center, Indianapolis, Indiana

**Max I. Shaff, M.B., Ch.B.** Associate Professor of Radiology, Vanderbilt University School of Medicine; Chief, Computed Tomography Section, Vanderbilt University Medical Center, Nashville, Tennessee

**Edward T. Stewart, M.D.** Professor of Radiology, Medical College of Wisconsin; Chief, Department of Radiology, Milwaukee County Medical Complex, Milwaukee, Wisconsin

**Charles M. Strother, M.D.** Professor of Radiology and Neurology, University of Wisconsin Center for Health Sciences, Madison, Wisconsin

**Ruedi F. Thoeni, M.D.** Associate Professor of Radiology, University of California, San Francisco, California

**William M. Thompson, M.D.** Professor and Chairman, Department of Radiology, University of Minnesota Hospital and Clinic, Minneapolis, Minnesota

**Robert L. Vogelzang, M.D.** Assistant Professor of Radiology, Northwestern University Medical School; Director of Angiography and Interventional Radiology, Northwestern Memorial Hospital, Chicago, Illinois

**Leonard A. Wald, M.D.** Radiology Associates of Westport, Westport, Connecticut

**W. Richard Webb, M.D.** Associate Professor of Radiology, University of California, San Francisco, California

**Susan M. Williams, M.D.** Associate Professor of Radiology, University of Nebraska College of Medicine, University of Nebraska Medical Center, Omaha, Nebraska

**Mary J. Wood, M.D.** Associate Professor of Radiology, Louisiana State University; Chief, Division of Nuclear Medicine, Louisiana State University Medical Center Hospital, Shreveport, Louisiana

**Isabel C. Yoder, M.D.** Assistant Professor of Radiology, Harvard Medical School; Radiologist, Uroradiology Section, Department of Radiology, Massachusetts General Hospital, Boston, Massachusetts

# Preface

The radiologist and referring physician are frequently faced with the problem of determining the best radiographic approach toward documenting a specific diagnosis and establishing a reasonable differential diagnosis for a set of clinical findings. Similarly, these physicians are often faced with a specific radiographic finding and must then decide the most efficacious way in which to reach the precise clinical diagnosis from among a large differential. With the rapid introduction and increasing availability of new radiographic modalities, there is the temptation to perform large numbers of examinations before drawing a conclusion about the likely diagnosis. This approach, however, is inefficient, extremely expensive, and unfair to the patient because it subjects him to unnecessary discomfort and risk. Therefore, it is essential to determine rational diagnostic pathways for reaching definitive diagnoses in the most efficient and cost-effective way.

In this volume, I have chosen 47 clinical and radiographic problems with a multiplicity of possible diagnostic approaches. For each problem a differential diagnosis is presented, followed by a discussion of the available diagnostic modalities. This includes the sensitivity and specificity of various imaging procedures, their advantages and disadvantages, complications, and relative cost. At the conclusion of each chapter, there is a graphic depiction of the algorithm that the author(s) recommends as the most logical and efficient approach to the problem.

I am well aware that certain clinical and radiographic problems may give rise to different, equally valid approaches to the diagnosis. My goal has been to present one well-reasoned diagnostic pathway for each problem to serve as a guide to practicing radiologists and referring physicians. It is my hope that this book will stimulate all radiologists to develop algorithmic approaches for a multitude of specific problems and to continually update these in the light of clinical research and future technological developments.

*Ronald L. Eisenberg, M.D.*

# Acknowledgments

I wish to thank Betty DiGrazia for her expert assistance in typing the manuscript and the Department of Medical Communications at the Louisiana State University School of Medicine in Shreveport for preparing the algorithmic drawings. I also greatly appreciate the unceasing encouragement and support of the staff at the J. B. Lippincott Company.

# Contents

## Part Six CANCER STAGING AND DETECTION OF METASTASES



## Part Seven MISCELLANEOUS

# Introduction to the Algorithmic Approach to Radiology

*Ruedi F. Thoeni*
*Alexander R. Margulis*

Radiologic technology has undergone unprecedented explosive growth and expansion during the last 15 years. There has been progress in an amazingly large number of areas, and the pace of technologic advance still seems to be accelerating.

Spectacular advances in conventional radiographic equipment have included brighter image intensifiers, better resolution of images, multiformatting cameras, excellent image quality, and computerized generators. Angiographic equipment with biplane fluoroscopy is so versatile that the time needed to perform procedures has been significantly shortened, resulting in increased safety for patients. Digital subtraction angiography, particularly with selective intra-arterial injection, has made arteriography safer because less contrast material is injected and more economical because the number of films needed is reduced (Fig. I-1). X-ray tubes have smaller focal spots with greater load capacity of their anodes, allowing for sharper detail and better magnification than in the past.

Ultrasound also has made tremendous advances, both in the gray-scale B mode and in the real-time mode (Fig. I-2). In most institutions, oral cholecystography has been completely replaced by ultrasonography. Doppler ultrasound is used now for many different applications, including atherosclerotic disease, renal transplant rejection, and venous deficiency. Rectal transducers have been developed that promise more accurate evaluation of the prostate and rectum. The female organs are better visualized with the new intravaginal transducers and without the discomfort of a distended bladder. Transducers for intraoperative use have been developed that provide valuable information for the surgeon during renal and cerebral operations. Furthermore, special ultrasonographic transducers today permit easy performance of biopsies because of exact localization of a mass and the needle tip. Ultrasonographic biopsies, where applicable, are faster and less costly to perform than those under computed tomographic guidance. However, the most dramatic development in ultrasound is its use for the detection and surgical correction of fetal abnormalities *in utero*. The many different applications, the speed of examinations, and the general availability and low cost have made ultrasound one of the most frequently used modalities, particularly in those

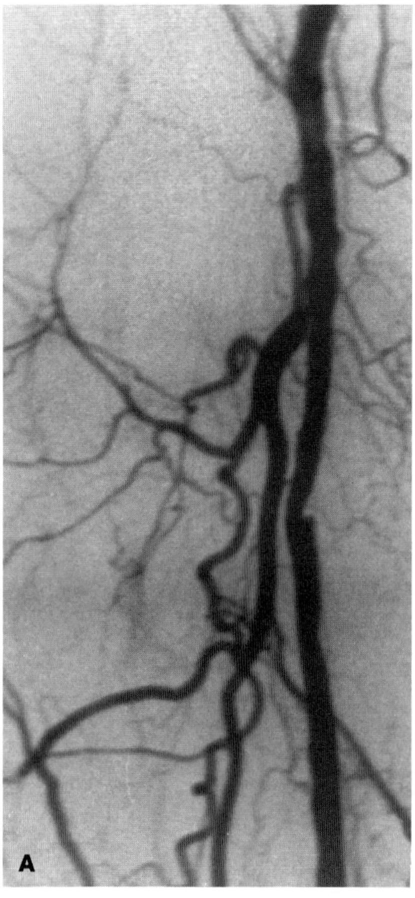

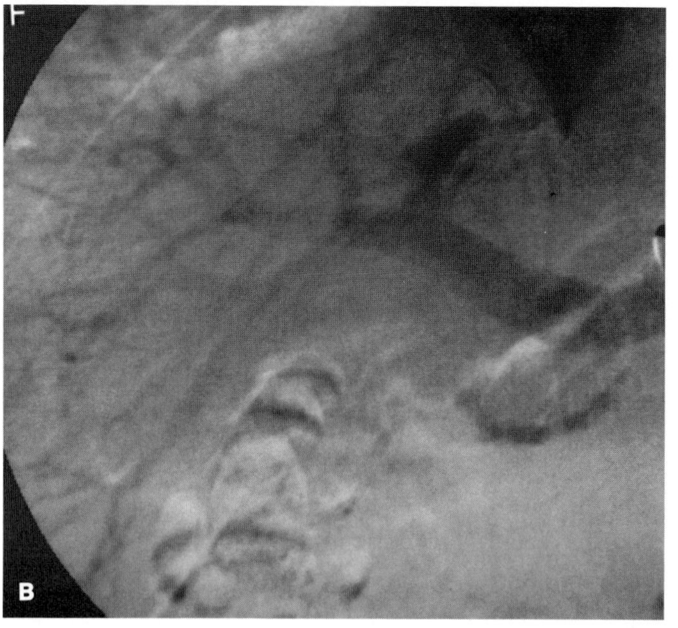

**Figure I-1.** **(A)** Digital femoral arteriogram shows atherosclerotic disease in the deep and superficial femoral arteries. There is no disturbance by bony or soft-tissue densities. **(B)** In the venous phase, the digital selective arteriogram of the celiac axis shows the portal vein to great advantage.

countries where computed tomography (CT) and magnetic resonance imaging (MRI) are not readily available.

Computed tomography has, in the short period of about 10 years, totally revolutionized the diagnostic approach in neurology (Fig. I-3), abdominal surgery, and oncology. It is one of the accepted diagnostic modalities for the study of ischemic heart disease and for diseases involving the spinal column. Dynamic CT is replacing aortography and laryngography, and cine CT is used in place of cardiac angiography (Fig. I-4). Computed tomography has also made possible the preoperative staging of carcinoma of the esophagus, stomach, and rectum (Figs. I-5 and I-6); the detection of recurrent tumors; and the biopsy of primary and metastatic malignancies. The improved tissue-density discrimination, as compared with conventional radiography, the high resolution, the thin-slice tomography, and the increase in speed of scanning that finally has led to real-time or cine CT have rendered this modality one of the most attractive and versatile imaging techniques available. Improvements such as electrocardiogram gating and reformatting in multiple planes, as well as the instantaneous reconstruction of images, have allowed this modality to become an invaluable tool, not only for imaging but also for CT-guided biopsies. In many areas, CT has completely changed the algorithmic approach to a variety of diseases.

Since 1982, MRI has become a clinical diagnostic modality that is progressing rapidly and changing many diagnostic workups. It is rapidly replacing CT in the study of the central nervous system, the musculoskeletal system, and the pelvis (Fig. I-7). Magnetic resonance imaging can distinguish between nodes and vessels in the

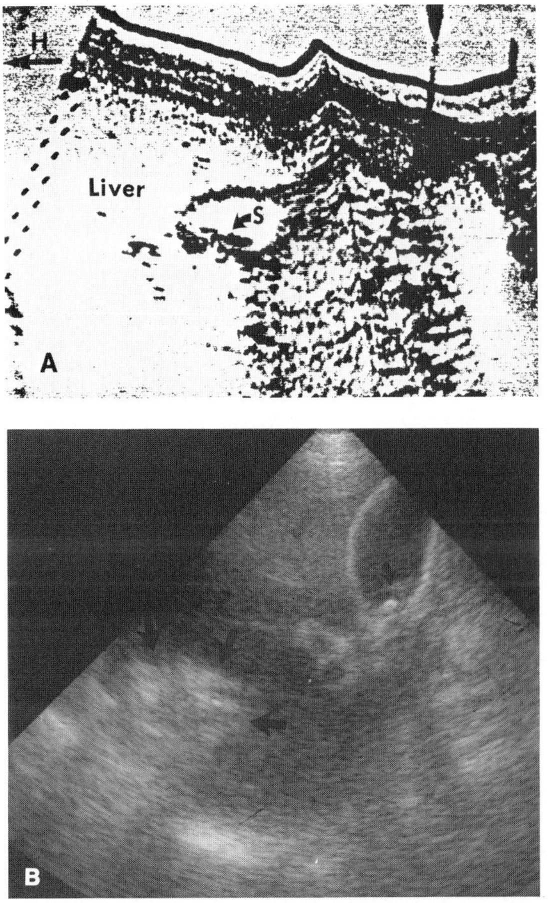


**Figure I-2. (A)** Right parasagittal ultrasound using bistable technique. The gallbladder contains high-amplitude echoes consistent with gallstones (*S*). **(B)** Real-time image in the area of the right upper quadrant shows a thickened gallbladder wall and cholelithiasis (*curved arrow*). An area of high echogenicity with a central region of low echogenicity (*arrows*) seen in the posterior portion of the liver proved to be a liver abscess.

retroperitoneum without the need for intravenous contrast material (Fig. I-8). It has become the method of choice in the staging of mediastinal and abdominal malignancies, and it is becoming the primary imaging method in the evaluation of cardiac and thoracic vascular disease (Fig. I-9). Further improvement of MRI techniques and the use of paramagnetic contrast materials may broaden the diagnostic capabilities of this modality in the near future.

One of the most effective new radiographic technologies that has reduced costs and improved the quality of life for many patients is interventional radiology. Balloon dilatation of stenosed arteries, occlusion of arteriovenous malformations or aneurysms, drainage of abscesses, removal of gallstones, stenting of occluded bile ducts, and percutaneous external drainage have dramatically changed the therapeutic and palliative approach in many instances. Cooperation between different specialties provides even more striking results, such as from the conjoined efforts of endoscopy and interventional radiology in treating patients with biliary obstruction. While such interventional procedures are highly dependent on operator skill and sophisticated equipment, they have markedly reduced the cost of treatment by averting surgical intervention in selected patients. The savings from angioplasty are particularly advantageous.

The explosive growth and spectacular advances in radiologic imaging have occurred at a time when society is concerned about the costs of modern science and technology outpacing the benefits. The nations of the developed and developing world are starting to realize that the world's resources are not endless. Better medicine, better distribution of health care, and the new concept of the right to the best medical and surgical care for everyone have escalated medical costs to more than $387.4 billion in the United States alone in 1984. In terms of percentage of the gross national product (GNP), expenditures for health care in the United States have risen from 5.9% of the GNP in 1965 to 10.6% in 1984.

Hospital care consumes approximately 46% of the total health budget in the United States, and that share appears to be increasing. Between 1972 and 1984, basic hospital room costs and total costs per day increased at an alarming fourfold rate at the University of California at San Francisco (UCSF) hospitals. Equipment prices have increased astronomically. The single-phase generator that cost $18,000 in 1965 now must be replaced by a three-phase unit costing $125,000. The price of cardiovascular special procedure rooms and radiographic–fluoroscopic units has increased 400% to 600% during the same period. Computed tomography scanners in particular

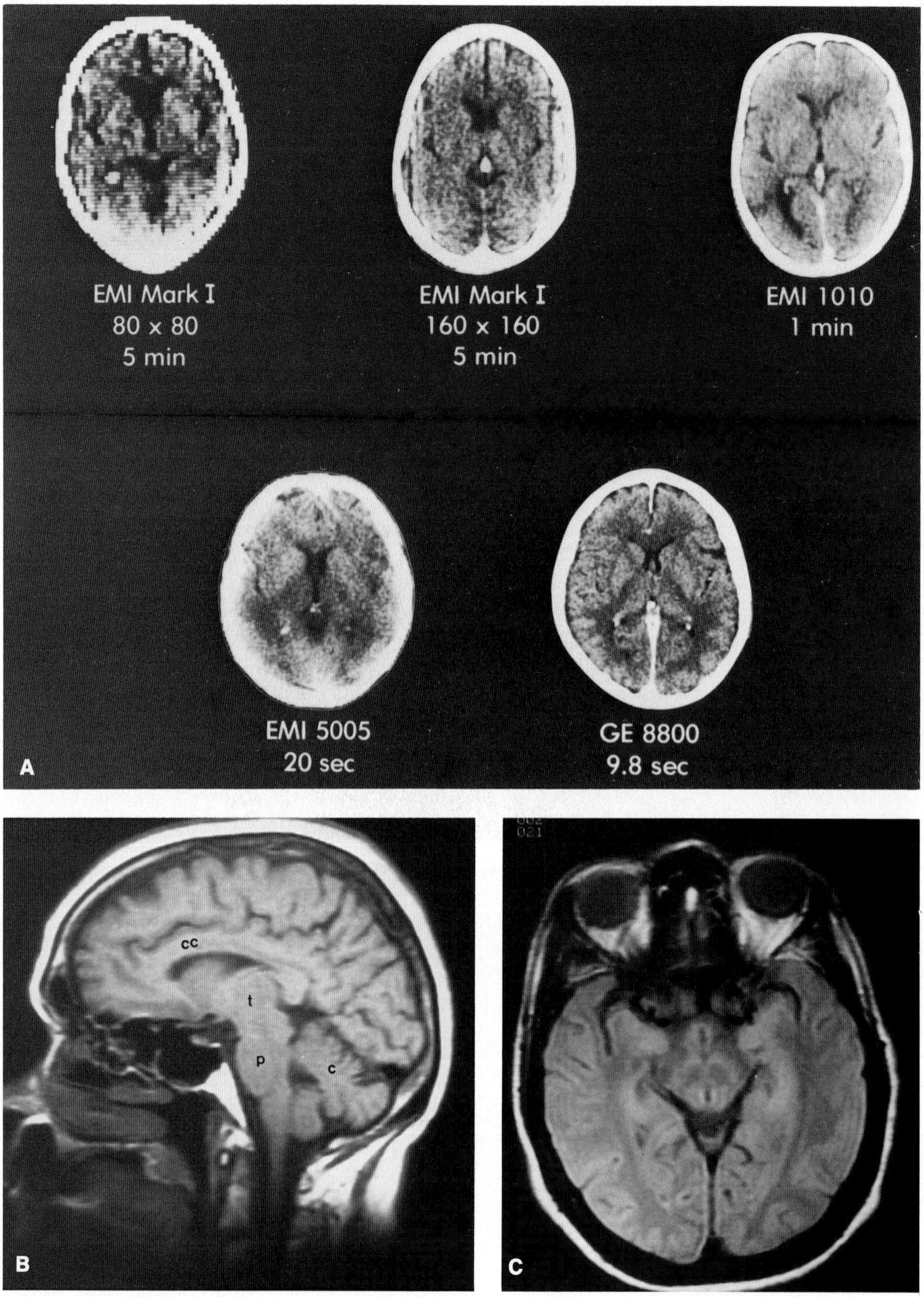


**Figure I-3.** **(A)** Five CT brain scans through the same level of midbrain in five different patients (*A,* 1974; *B,* 1976; *C,* 1977; *D,* 1978; and *E,* 1980). The difference in quality is apparent. **(B)** Midsagittal MRI (TR, 600 msec, TE, 20 msec) of the brain shows the area of the brain stem particularly well (*cc,* corpus callosum; *t,* thalamus; *p,* pons; *c,* cerebellum). **(C)** Axial MRI of the brain demonstrates excellent distinction between gray and white matter. (*A,* Margulis AR: Radiologic imaging: Changing costs, greater benefits. AJR 136:657–665, 1981)

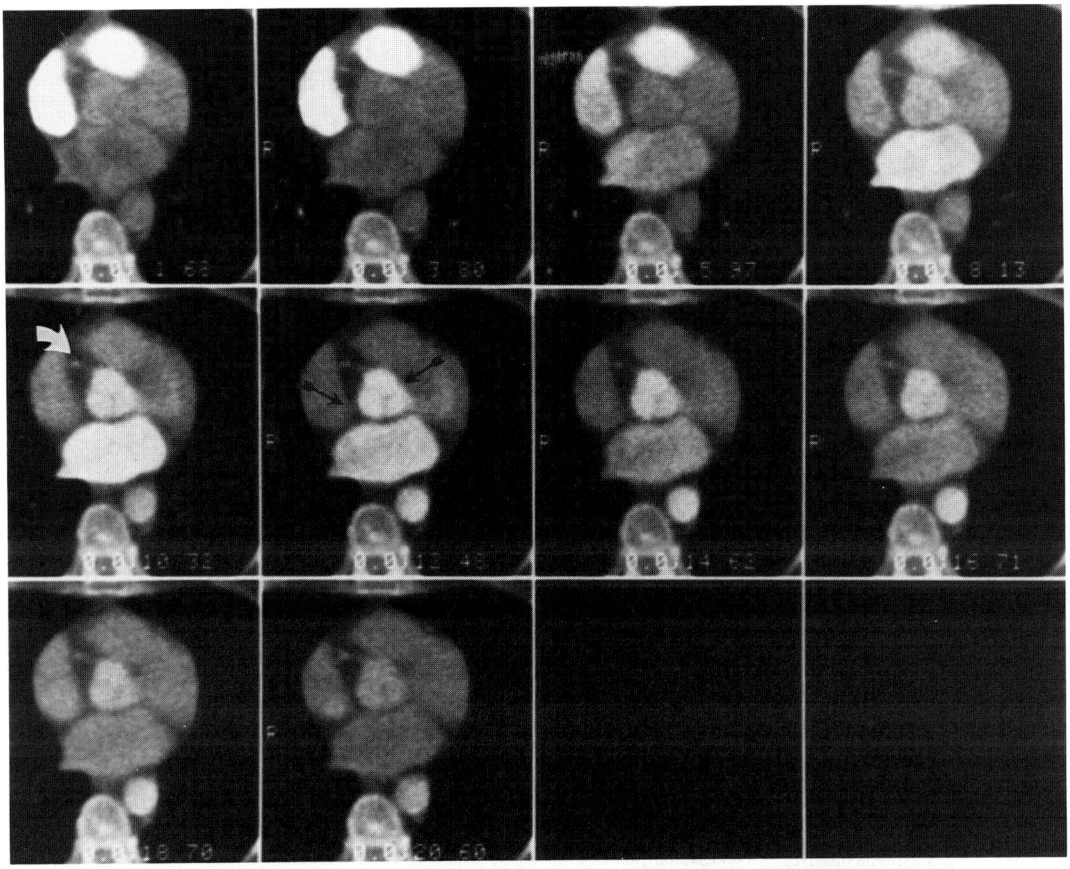

**Figure I-4.** Dynamic sequence of ultrafast 8-mm thick CT images is illustrated following a 25-ml peripheral intravenous injection of contrast agent. Note contrast enhancement of the right atrium and right ventricular outflow tract on the first three upper images, followed by progressive enhancement of the left atrium (in top right and two left images in the middle row). The aortic valve with its three leaflets (*arrows*) can be identified as well as the right coronary artery (*curved arrow*), which contains calcium (see precontrast scans in upper row).

have drawn the ire of critics of the high costs of medical care. The increased costs of CT units from about $300,000 in 1974 to nearly $1 million in 1980 have attracted the attention of many health planners. The ability of the million-dollar scanner to render an accurate diagnosis, to perform many more functions, and to give considerably more information than its relatively primitive forerunners has been ignored for a long time. Today, we are aware that significant reduction in the cost of health care has been made possible because of many of these newer but more expensive machines. Equipment generally has become more sophisticated and more versatile; however, in some areas the cost of certain equipment options has even decreased because of technologic advances. A good example of cost reduction of equipment is the replacement of cine equipment (costing more than $70,000) on fluoroscopy units by excellent videotape capability, which can be obtained for as little as $15,000. Such changes are most noticeable in the purchasing costs for new CT scanners and soon will also become evident for MRI scanners. Computed tomographic scanners of excellent quality are available today for as little as $350,000, and MRI equipment that originally cost as much as $2 million can be obtained for $1.5 million. Mag-

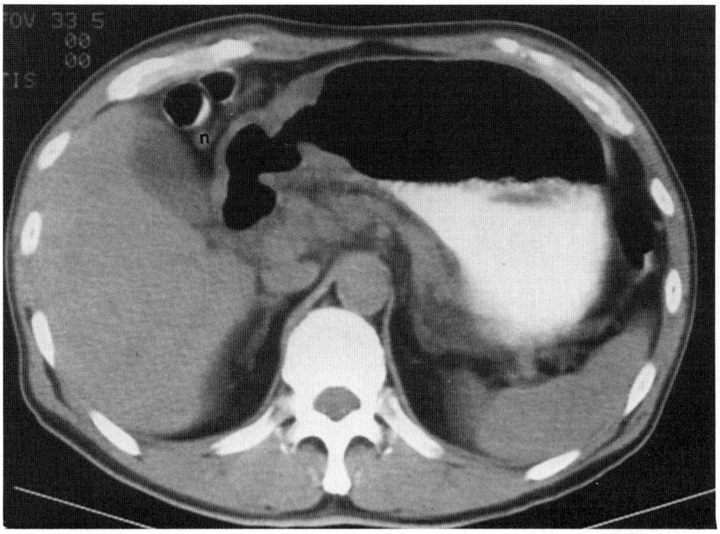

**Figure I-5.** Transaxial CT image through the area of the stomach shows nodular thickening of the antrum and duodenum and one small lymph node (*n*) in a patient with gastric lymphoma.

netic resonance imaging scanners that cost below $1 million will be available in 1987.

At University of California, San Francisco hospitals, CT studies represent approximately 5% of the total number of radiologic procedures but close to 13% of the total departmental operational expenses. Magnetic resonance imaging is starting to absorb a similar proportion of the operational expenditures for even fewer studies. It is absolutely essential to attempt to reduce costs, but this must never be accomplished by sacrificing the quality of medical care.

The major problem in cutting the cost of medical care is the fact that many clinicians are unable to keep up with the latest developments and the large array of sophisticated modalities in the rapidly expanding field of diagnostic radiology, and they often order procedures that are not indicated or are redundant. Therefore, it is essential for cost reduction that diagnostic procedures 1) be streamlined, 2) follow a logical order, 3) be as noninvasive as possible, and 4) be performed on an outpatient basis prior to hospitalization whenever possible. Many hospitals throughout the nation are developing algorithms (critical diagnostic pathways) for the logical investigation of patients presenting with specific symptoms and signs. These algorithms must be flexible and must relate to locally available equip-

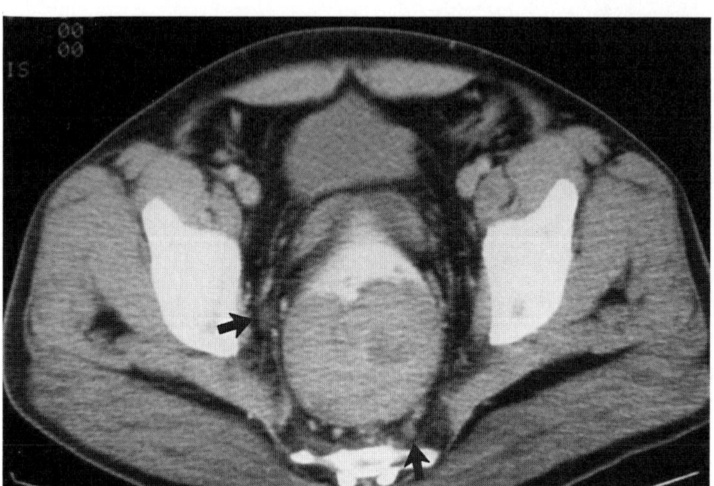

**Figure I-6.** Transaxial CT image of the male pelvis shows a large posterior rectal mass with two small nodes (*arrows*) in the perirectal space.

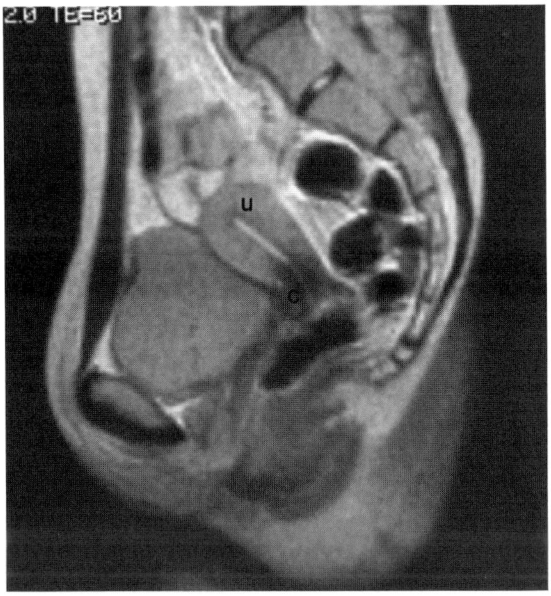


**Figure I-7.** Sagittal MRI of the female pelvis (TR, 2000 msec; TE, 60 msec). The uterus (*u*) and cervix (*c*) are well demonstrated. The uterine stroma appears as an intermediate-intensity signal. The endometrium is seen as a high-intensity signal area surrounded by the well-vascularized low-density signal region of the junctional zone.

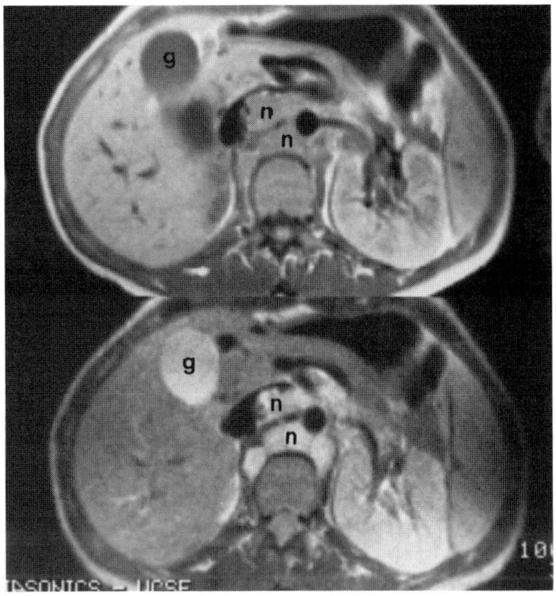


**Figure I-8.** Transverse MR images of the mid-abdomen (TR, 1000 msec; TE, 30 msec [*upper image*]; TR, 2000 msec; TE, 60 msec [*lower image*]) in a patient with lymphoma. Enlarged pericaval and periaortic nodes (*n*) enhance on T2-weighted images (*lower image*) and displace the inferior vena cava and aorta anteriorly. The gallbladder (*GB*) is shown as a low-intensity structure on T1-weighted sequences and as a high-intensity region on T2-weighted images.

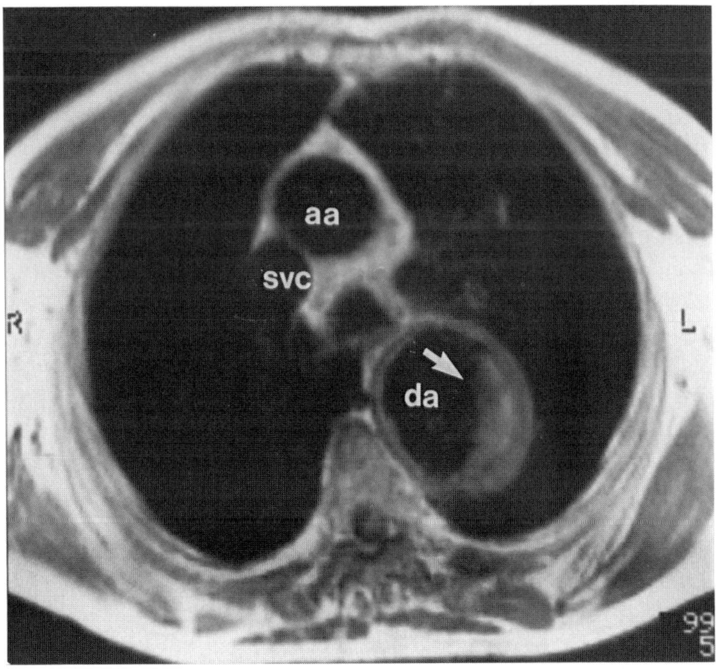


**Figure I-9.** Transverse MRI of the chest (gated; TE, 30 msec). With the help of cardiac gating, MR images in the chest show sharp margins. An aortic aneurysm with large clot (*arrow*) can be demonstrated without the use of intravenous contrast material due to the absence of MR signals in vessels with rapidly flowing blood. (*da,* descending aorta; *aa,* ascending aorta; *svc,* superior vena cava)

**Table I-1** Radiologic Diagnostic Workup of Jaundice (All data at 1987 costs)

| 1975 | | | 1987 | | |
|---|---|---|---|---|---|
| Examination | Hospital Days | Cost | Examination | Hospital Days | Cost |
| Plain abdominal radiograph | — | $101 | Ultrasound | — | $230 |
| Intravenous cholangiogram | 1 | $204 | Computed tomography | — | $869 |
| Upper gastrointestinal and small bowel series | — | $299 | Percutaneous transhepatic cholangiogram | — | $329 |
| Arteriogram | 1 | $1,411 | (or ERCP) | — | ($415) |
| Barium enema | 2 | $298 | | | |
| Hypotonic duodenogram | 1 | $330 | TOTAL: | — | $1,428 |
| Radionuclide scan | — | $360 | (if ERCP) | — | ($1,514) |
| Percutaneous transhepatic cholangiogram | 1 | $329 | | | |
| (ERCP—optional) | (1) | ($415) | | | |
| | 6 | $3,332 | | | |
| | (7) | ($3,747) | | | |
| 6 days at $465 = | | $2,790 | | | |
| (7 days at $465) = | | ($3,255) | | | |
| TOTAL: | | $6,122 | | | |
| (if ERCP) | | ($6,587) | | | |

ment as well as physician expertise. However, algorithms need to be reviewed and updated at frequent intervals by radiologists, internists, and surgeons. Such a flexible approach to algorithms will result in better and earlier diagnoses, will reduce the lengths of hospital stays, and will diminish the indications for hospital admissions.

Several currently available diagnostic algorithms can illustrate the ability of this approach to reduce expenditures and invasiveness. For ease of comparison, the costs in the following tables are all expressed in terms of 1987 prices. Using the modern algorithmic approach to the diagnosis of obstructive jaundice, large savings in cost (Table I-1) and radiation exposure (Table I-2) can be achieved. In the case of obstructive jaundice, over $4,000 can be saved. Similarly, a patient presenting today with a mass in the region of the liver would undergo a few tests performed with sophisticated equipment that result in a precise histologic diagnosis obtained through a radiologically guided biopsy. When compared with the 1975 approach, the new logical diagnostic pathway results in savings of almost $5,000 (Table I-3), or $4,000 if MRI is used; in either case, there is a marked reduction in radiation exposure (Table I-4).

The diagnostic approach to the patient with suspected lymphoma now consists of a chest radiograph and CT examination of the chest and abdomen. Occasionally, CT of the pelvis also is obtained. All the previous tests (including upper gastrointestinal and small bowel series, barium enemas, radionuclide scans, lymphangiograms, and excretory urograms) are no longer required unless the primary lesion is suspected within the gastrointestinal tract or clinical evidence suggests that the gastrointestinal tract also is involved. Lymphangiograms are performed only if CT fails to show the presence of retroperitoneal masses in suspected Hodgkin's disease; in most instances, MRI can resolve the diagnostic dilemma. Further studies are needed to establish the exact role of MRI in the evaluation of patients with suspected lymphoma. Again, this streamlined approach is far less costly (Table

**Table I-2** Radiation Skin Dose for Radiologic Diagnostic Workup of Jaundice

| 1975 | | 1987 | |
|---|---|---|---|
| Examination | Skin Dose (r) | Examination | Skin Dose (r) |
| Plain abdominal radiograph | 0.5 | Computed tomography | 2.0 |
| Intravenous cholangiogram | 2.5 | Percutaneous transhepatic cholangiogram | 16.0 |
| Upper gastrointestinal series and small bowel series | 8.5 | TOTAL: | 18.0 r |
| Arteriogram | 20.0 | | |
| Barium enema | 8.0 | | |
| Percutaneous transhepatic cholangiogram | 16.0 | | |
| (ERCP—optional) | (5.0) | | |
| TOTAL: | 55.0 r<br>(60.0 r) | | |

I-5). Similarly, the radiologic diagnostic workup of aortic aneurysm now includes only plain chest films and MRI of chest or, if MRI is not available, plain chest films and chest CT. This leads to a threefold cost reduction compared with the diagnostic approach used in 1975 (Table I-6).

The development of logical diagnostic pathways requires close cooperation between radiologists and their clinical colleagues. It is important that they be accepted through discussion and education rather than unilaterally imposed. As with tumor boards and utilization committees, this approach not only results in efficient and accurate diagnoses but also in shortened hospital stays, considerable financial savings, and less patient suffering.

**Table I-3** Radiologic Diagnostic Workup of Liver Mass (All data at 1987 costs)

| 1975 | | | 1987 | | |
|---|---|---|---|---|---|
| Examination | Hospital Days | Cost | Examination | Hospital Days | Cost |
| Plain abdominal radiograph | — | $101 | Ultrasound | — | $230 |
| Intravenous cholangiogram | 1 | $204 | Computed tomography | — | $869 |
| Excretory urogram | — | $216 | (MRI) | — | ($770) |
| Arteriogram | 1 | $1,411 | Biopsy | — | $166 |
| Upper gastrointestinal series | | $299 | | | |
| and small bowel series | 1 | $299 | TOTAL: | | $1,265 |
| Barium enema | 2 | $298 | (if MRI used) | — | ($2,035) |
| ERCP | 1 | $415 | | | |
| Radionuclide liver scan | — | $360 | | | |
| | 6 | $3,304 | | | |
| 6 days at $465 = | | $2,790 | | | |
| TOTAL: | | $6,094 | | | |

**Table I-4** Radiation Skin Dose for Radiologic Diagnostic Workup of Liver Mass

| 1975 | | 1987 | |
|---|---|---|---|
| Examination | Skin Dose (r) | Examination | Skin Dose (r) |
| Plain abdominal radiograph | 0.5 | Ultrasound | 0 |
| Intravenous cholangiogram | 2.0 | Computed tomography | 2.0 |
| Excretory urogram | 2.5 | | |
| Arteriogram | 20.0 | TOTAL: | 2.0 r |
| Upper gastrointestinal series and small bowel series | 8.5 | | |
| Barium enema | 8.0 | | |
| ERCP | 5.0 | | |
| TOTAL: | 46.5 r | | |

**Table I-5** Radiologic Diagnostic Workup of Lymphoma (All data at 1987 costs)

| 1975 | | | 1987 | | |
|---|---|---|---|---|---|
| Examination | Hospital Days | Cost | Examination | Hospital Days | Cost |
| Chest radiograph | — | $98 | Chest radiograph | — | $86 |
| Upper gastrointestinal and small bowel series | 1 | $299 | CT (chest and abdomen) | — | $1,663 |
| Barium enema | 2 | $298 | (CT of pelvis) | — | ($794) |
| Radionuclide scan | — | $586 | TOTAL: | — | $1,749 |
| Lymphangiogram | 2 | $1,061 | (if CT of pelvis) | — | ($2,543) |
| Excretory urogram | — | $216 | | | |
| | 5 | $2,558 | | | |
| | 5 days at $465 = | $2,325 | | | |
| | TOTAL: | $4,883 | | | |

**Table I-6** Radiologic Diagnostic Workup of Aortic Aneurysm (All data at 1987 costs)

| 1975 | | | 1987 | | |
|---|---|---|---|---|---|
| Examination | Hospital Days | Cost | Examination | Hospital Days | Cost |
| Chest radiograph | — | $98 | Chest radiograph | — | $98 |
| Plain abdominal radiograph | — | $136 | MRI | — | $770 |
| Aortogram | 2 | $1,196 | (if not available, CT) | — | ($869) |
| | 2 | $1,430 | TOTAL: | — | $868 |
| | 2 days at $465 = | $930 | (if CT used) | — | ($967) |
| | TOTAL: | $2,360 | | | |

As new modalities such as digital radiography and MRI appear on the scene and become of practical clinical value, algorithms will have to be modified to include these new techniques. Flexibility in attitudes, cooperation between radiologists and clinicians, and a willingness to learn and keep up with advances are essential not only to properly diagnose patients but also to preserve the ability of society to pay for health care. Only with such an approach can we justify the use of very expensive and sophisticated equipment, which, even though producing costly examinations, leads to overall reduction of costs by providing information that previously could only be obtained by a multitude of different examinations.

## Bibliography


Alfidi RJ, Haaga JR, El Yousef SJ et al: Preliminary experimental results in humans and animals with a superconducting, whole-body, nuclear magnetic resonance scanner. Radiology 143:175–181, 1982

Brasch RC: Contrast media. In Margulis AR, Higgins CB, Kaufman L, Crooks LE (eds): Clinical Magnetic Resonance Imaging. San Francisco, Radiology Research and Education Foundation, pp 291–302, 1983

Brundage BH, Lipton M, Herfkens RJ et al: Detection of patent coronary bypass grafts by computed tomography. A preliminary report. Circulation 61:826–831, 1980

Chinn D, Filly RA: Ultrasound diagnosis of fetal GU tract anomalies. Urol Radiol 4:115–123, 1982

Cooperberg PL, Pon MS, Wong P et al: Real-time high resolution ultrasound in the detection of biliary calculi. Radiology 131:789–790, 1979

Crooks L, Arakawa M, Hoenninger J et al: Nuclear magnetic resonance whole-body imager operating at 3.5 K gauss. Radiology 143:169–174, 1982

Crooks L, Hoenninger J, Arakawa M et al: Tomography of hydrogen with nuclear magnetic resonance. Radiology 136:701–706, 1980

Doubilet PM, Abrams HL: The cost of underutilization: Percutaneous transluminal angioplasty for peripheral vascular disease. N Engl J Med 310:95–102, 1984

DuBoulay GH, Radue EW: Comparison of computerized tomography with other neuroradiological examination methods. Neuroradiology 16: 474–476, 1978

Godwin JD, Herfkens RL, Skioldebrand CG et al: Evaluation of dissections and aneurysms of the thoracic aorta by conventional and dynamic CT scanning. Radiology 136:125–133, 1980

Higgins CB: New horizons in cardiac imaging. Radiology 156:577–588, 1985

Higgins CB: Overview of MR of the heart. AJR 146:907–918, 1986

Holland GN, Hawkes RC, Moore WS: Nuclear magnetic resonance (NMR) tomography of the brain: Coronal and sagittal sections. J Comput Assist Tomogr 4:429–433, 1980

Houk TL, Kruger RA, Mistretta CA et al: Real-time digital D-edge subtraction fluoroscopy. Invest Radiol 14:270–278, 1979

Hricak H: MRI in the female pelvis. AJR 146: 1115–1122, 1986

Hricak H, Dooms GC, McNeal JG et al: MR imaging of the prostate gland: Normal anatomy. AJR 148:51–58, 1987

Johnson ML, Dunne MG, Mack LA et al: Evaluation of fetal intracranial anatomy by static and real-time ultrasound. J Clin Ultrasound 8:311–318, 1980

Krook PM, Allen FH, Bush WH et al: Comparison of real-time cholecystosonography and oral cholecystography. Radiology 135:145–148, 1980

Kruger RA, Mistretta CA, Houk T et al: Computerized fluoroscopy in real-time for noninvasive visualization of the cardiovascular system. Radiology 130:49–57, 1979

Lauterbur PC: Image formation by induced local interactions: Examples of employing nuclear magnetic resonance. Nature 242:190–191, 1978

Lee KR, Levine E, Moffat RE et al: Computed tomographic staging of malignant gastric neoplasms. Radiology 133:151–155, 1979

Levitt RG, Geisse GG, Sagel SS et al: Complementary use of ultrasound and computed tomography in studies of the pancreas and kidney. Radiology 126:149–152, 1978

Lipton MJ, Brundage BH, Doherty PW et al: Contrast medium-enhanced computed tomography for evaluating ischemic heart disease. Cardiovasc Med 4:1219–1229, 1979

Margulis AR: Editorial: Radiology and the algorithm approach to medicine. West J Med 122:58–61, 1978

Margulis AR: Integrated approach to radiologic imaging. In Moss AA, Goldberg HI (eds): Computed Tomography, Ultrasound, and X-ray: An Integrated Approach. University of California San Francisco, Masson Publishers, 1979

Newton DR, Witz S, Norman D: Economic impact of

CT scanning on the evaluation of pituitary adenomas. Am J Neuroradiol 4:57–60, 1983

Ovitt T, Capp MP, Christenson P et al: Development of a digital video subtraction system for intravenous angiography. SPIE Recent & Future Developments in Medical Imaging II 206:73, 1979

Ring EJ, McLean MD (eds): Interventional Radiology: Principles and Techniques. Boston, Little, Brown & Co, 1981

Shaffer KA, Haughton VM, Wilson CR: High resolution computed tomography of the temporal bone. Radiology 134:409–414, 1980

Showstack JA, Stone MH, Schroeder SA: The role of changing clinical practices in the rising costs of hospital care. N Engl J Med 313:1201–1206, 1985

Snow JH, Goldstein HM, Wallace S: Comparison of scintigraphy, sonography, and computed tomography in the evaluation of hepatic neoplasms. AJR 132:915–918, 1979

Stephens DH, Sheedy PF, Hattery RR et al: Computed tomography of the liver. AJR 128:579–590, 1977

Waldo DR, Lazenby HE: Health spending trends in the 1980s: Adjusting to financial incentives. Health Care Financing Review, vols III and IV, 1985

Whalen JP: Radiology of the abdomen: Impact of new imaging methods. Caldwell Lecture. AJR 133:585–618, 1979

Wittenberg J, Fineberg HV, Black EB et al: Clinical efficacy of computed body tomography. AJR 131:5–14, 1978

Williams AL, Haughton VM, Syversten A: Computed tomography in the diagnosis of herniated nucleus pulposus. Radiology 135:95–99, 1980

# PART ONE

# Chest

# Chapter 1

# Solitary Pulmonary Nodule

*W. Richard Webb*

A solitary nodule is detected on one or two of every 1000 chest radiographs. The differential diagnosis of a solitary pulmonary nodule is extensive. The radiographic diagnosis, however, is primarily directed at differentiating benign from malignant nodules, because malignant nodules are generally treated by surgical excision whereas benign ones are not.

In the patient with a solitary pulmonary nodule suspected of being malignant, radiographic procedures are also useful for staging the tumor and detecting local metastases (to the chest wall, pleura, or mediastinum) prior to therapy. The presence of such metastases usually precludes curative surgery and indicates the need for radiotherapy or chemotherapy rather than for a fruitless operation.

## THE SOLITARY NODULE

There is much disagreement among radiologists and surgeons as to what constitutes a "solitary pulmonary nodule." In keeping with the majority opinion, this chapter defines a solitary pulmonary nodule as fulfilling the following criteria:

1. The lesion is visible on a standard chest radiograph, in either posteroanterior or lateral projection.
2. The lesion is reasonably well defined or circumscribed and is round, oval, or lobular.
3. The lesion is surrounded by air-containing lung but may be in contact with the pleura.
4. Although size criteria for a "nodule" are somewhat arbitrary, it must be large enough to be clearly defined (approximately 5 mm). Very large lesions (more than 6 cm) generally are not included in this category.

## CLINICAL EVALUATION

Only 3% to 5% of solitary pulmonary nodules are malignant. Certain clinical features, however, may increase or decrease the likelihood of cancer.

In patients younger than 30 years of age, the incidence of bronchogenic carcinoma is so low that a solitary pulmonary nodule generally should be followed radiographically without any further evaluation. However, in some patients in this age group, needle biopsy or computed tomographic (CT) nodule densitometry is occasionally performed to further decrease the likelihood of lung cancer.

At the other end of the spectrum, in more than half of patients older than 50 years, a solitary pulmonary nodule represents cancer. Sex is also a significant variable, with cancer being more common in men than in women. However, the incidence of lung cancer in women is increasing rapidly.

Approximately 90% of patients with bronchogenic carcinoma have symptoms, primarily either cough or hemoptysis. A solitary pulmonary nodule is more likely to be a cancer when symptoms are present than when they are absent. However, symptoms are not specific and do not allow a reliable diagnosis. Indeed, a majority of symptomatic patients with a solitary pulmonary nodule have a benign lesion.

### Sputum Cytology

Sputum cytology should be carried out in all patients with a solitary pulmonary nodule in whom cancer is considered a possibility. If cytologic findings are positive, staging procedures should be performed to aid in determining operability.

False-positive sputum cytology is rare (0.7%–3%), and a positive sputum cytology is the most reliable preoperative method (except biopsy) for diagnosing a pulmonary malignancy. False-negative cytology is far more common, occurring in 10% to 30% of all patients with lung cancer and in up to 60% of those with peripheral malignancies. Thus, negative cytologic findings do not preclude the presence of a malignant lesion.

### Bronchoscopy

Bronchoscopy with biopsy, bronchial brushing, or bronchial washing is sometimes diagnostic in patients with central solitary nodules. However, in patients with peripheral nodules, needle biopsy has a higher yield and is usually preferred.

### Mediastinoscopy

Mediastinoscopy with biopsy yields positive results in 23% to 50% of patients with bronchogenic carcinoma, thus reflecting the incidence of mediastinal lymph node metastases with this tumor. The frequency of positive mediastinoscopy is highest with central or undifferentiated carcinomas (40%–75%) and is lowest with peripheral squamous cell tumors (20%–30%). Mediastinoscopy may also be helpful in assessing patients with tuberculosis, but the procedure is of little value in the diagnosis of benign pulmonary nodules.

Mediastinoscopy with biopsy is a reasonably accurate method for diagnosing mediastinal metastases from bronchogenic carcinoma prior to thoracotomy. However, not all mediastinal lymph nodes involved by tumor in patients with lung cancer are accessible to a standard transcervical mediastinoscopy. Using this technique, pretracheal lymph nodes and nodes anterior to the carina or right main bronchus usually can be biopsied. However, posterior or subcarinal nodes, nodes in the aorticopulmonary window, and anterior mediastinal nodes are not routinely sampled. Thus, a false-negative mediastinoscopy occurs in approximately 5% to 25% of cases.

Complications of mediastinoscopy are uncommon (3%–4%) and usually are not serious. Hemorrhage, usually venous, occurs in 1% and may require thoracotomy for control. Transient or permanent injury to the left recurrent laryngeal nerve can also occur.

Mediastinal lymph nodes are also sometimes biopsied using a transbronchoscopic (Wang) needle.

## DIAGNOSTIC EVALUATION

### *DIAGNOSTIC MODALITIES*

1. Plain chest radiography
2. Conventional tomography
3. Computed tomography
4. Bronchography
5. Angiography
6. Radionuclide tumor localization
7. Aspiration lung biopsy

## Plain Chest Radiography

A large number of criteria have been reported to be of some value in differentiating benign from malignant solitary pulmonary nodules on plain chest radiographs. These include size, shape, contour, edge definition, location, the presence or absence of satellite lesions, doubling time, and cavitation (Fig. 1-1). However, these criteria rarely allow the radiologist to confidently make a specific diagnosis of benignancy versus malignancy. Even attempts to use computers to aid in diagnosis have not resulted in more than 90% accuracy. Although an accuracy rate of 90% is quite good in a statistical sense, the individual patient with a solitary pulmonary nodule cannot be properly managed with this degree of uncertainty.

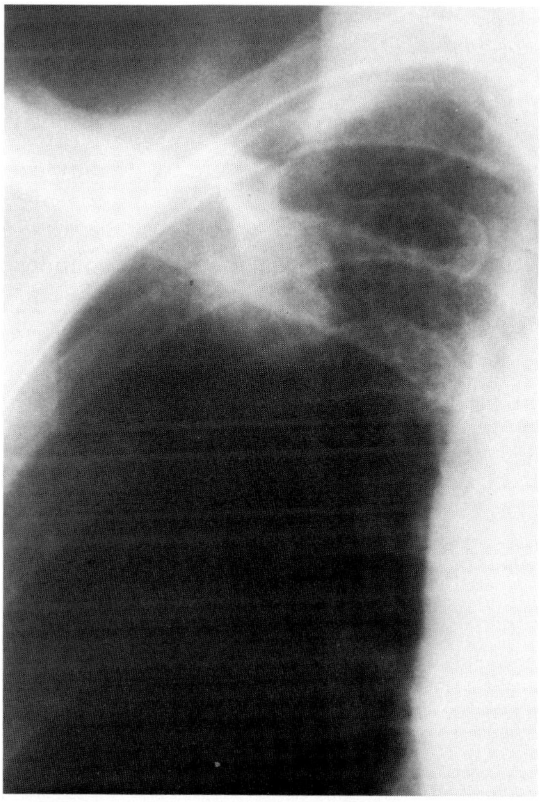

**Figure 1-1.** Solitary nodule in the right apex of a 61-year-old man. The poor definition of the lesion suggests that it is malignant. Other characteristics of a nodule suggesting malignancy are a diameter greater than 2 cm, lobulation, and cavitation. The presence of calcification or satellite lesions often means that a nodule is benign.

However, two radiographic features—dense or central calcification and absence of growth—may be used to diagnose a solitary pulmonary nodule as benign. In patients with either finding, a solitary pulmonary nodule can be followed with sequential chest radiographs without need for other imaging procedures.

Dense central, laminated, or diffuse calcification virtually excludes malignancy (Fig. 1-2). Calcification in a solitary pulmonary nodule is usually best visualized on low-kilovoltage radiographs. Fluoroscopy can be of value in demonstrating the calcification to better advantage. A bronchogenic carcinoma (scar carcinoma) may incorporate an adjacent calcified granuloma and result in a mass with calcification. In such cases, however, the calcification is usually eccentric rather than central (Fig. 1-3). Although bronchogenic carcinomas themselves may occasionally calcify, this calcification is often stippled and frequently is not detectable radiographically. In a study of 72 patients with malignant solitary pulmonary nodules, 10 had calcification visible on radiographs of the resected specimen, although only one had calcification detectable on standard chest radiographs. In the same study, 67 of 135 benign lesions (mostly granulomas and hamartomas) contained calcifications on specimen radiographs; in 46, these calcifications were also visible on standard chest radiographs. Metastatic malignant tumors (particularly osteogenic sarcoma, chondrosarcoma, and thyroid carcinoma) may show stippled or homogeneous calcification. In general, patients with solitary nodules that show central, laminated, or diffuse calcification only require chest radiographs at 6-month intervals for 2 years to demonstrate the stability of the lesion.

The growth rate of a solitary pulmonary nodule (doubling time) has been used to determine its likelihood of being malignant. A pulmonary nodule that doubles in volume in less than 1 month or in more than 18 months usually is benign. However, the overlapping growth rates of benign and malignant lesions, particularly among rapidly growing nodules, makes the

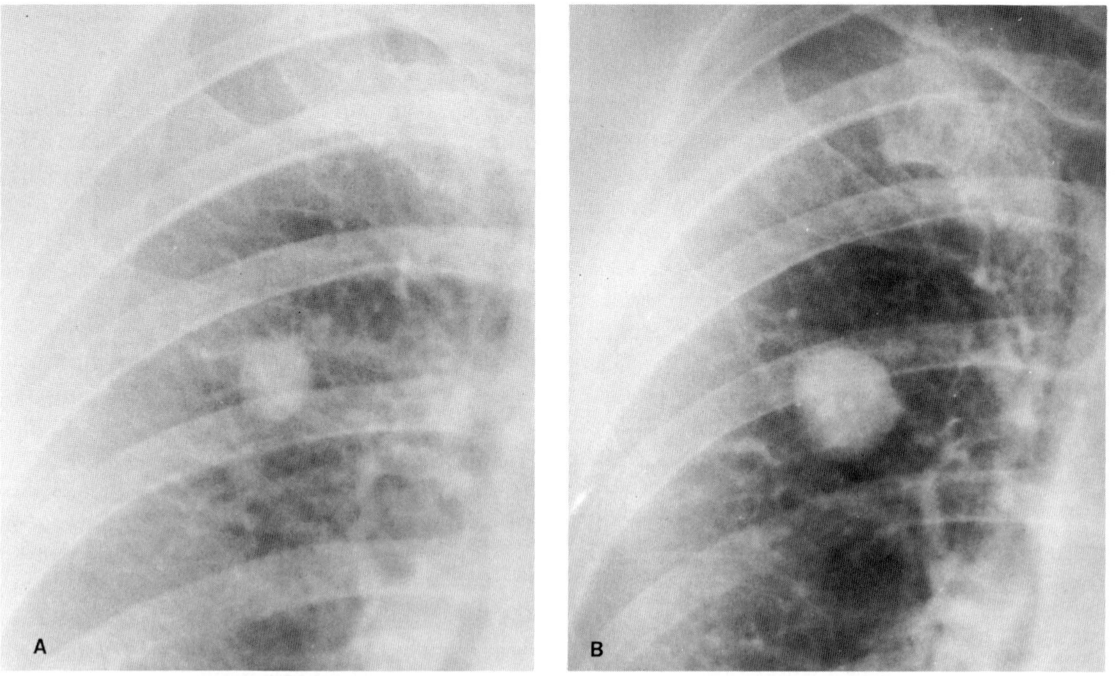

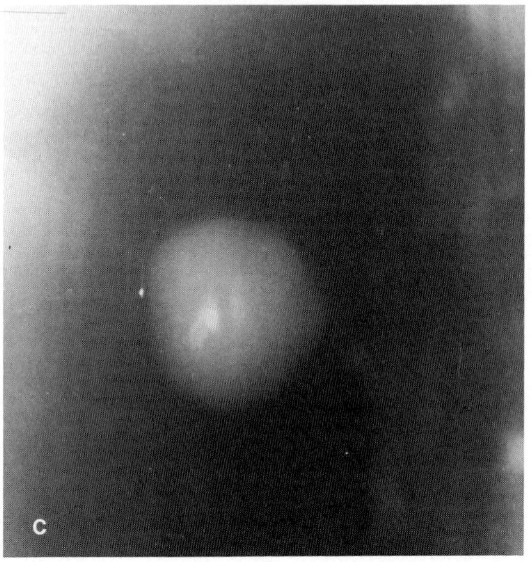

**Figure 1-2.** Solitary nodule in the right upper lobe of a 55-year-old man. **(A)** The nodule is sharply defined. **(B)** Three years later, the nodule has doubled in diameter, representing an eightfold increase in volume and three doublings. Thus, the doubling time of this nodule is 1 year—within the malignant range. **(C)** Plain tomogram reveals two dense central calcifications also visible on the plain film. At surgery, this lesion was found to be a benign hamartoma.

use of doubling time hazardous as an absolute indicator of benignancy (see Fig. 1-2). Nevertheless, it is generally agreed that a solitary pulmonary nodule that does not grow over a 2-year period is benign and does not require resection. Only rare exceptions to this rule have been reported. Therefore, a vigorous search for old films must be the first step in the evaluation of a noncalcified solitary pulmonary nodule. If films that are 2 or more years old show the pulmonary nodule to be unchanged, only routine follow-up radiographs at yearly intervals are required.

If no old films are available, or if prior films are not old enough, the diagnostic approach is based on the patient's age and the plain radiographic appearance of the lesion. If the patient is

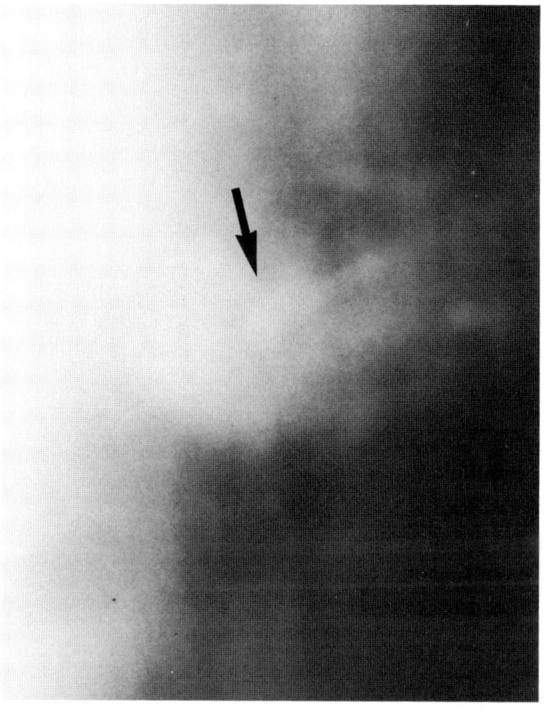

**Figure 1-3.** Solitary nodule with eccentric calcification (*arrow*). At surgery, this nodule was found to be a squamous cell carcinoma incorporating a calcified granuloma.

less than 30 years of age and the pulmonary nodule appears benign (small, round, sharply defined), follow-up with standard chest radiographs is generally sufficient. However, if the patient is older or has a history of an extrathoracic tumor, or if the lesion does not appear benign (large, irregular, ill-defined), further diagnostic procedures must be performed. Occasionally, an acute process (*e.g.,* pulmonary embolism, focal pneumonia) can present as a nodular density on plain chest radiographs. If the patient has acute symptoms, a follow-up radiograph in 1 to 2 weeks often shows a decrease in the size of a nodule, indicating its benign nature. In some asymptomatic patients, repeat radiographs obtained as a follow-up study or prior to lung biopsy show a similar decrease in size. However, as a general rule, it is not advisable to obtain follow-up radiographs in asymptomatic patients, hoping that a nodule will decrease in size. Indeed, in some patients with cancer, a pulmonary nodule may become less well-defined as it grows and thus may appear smaller on chest radiographs.

## Conventional Tomography

Until recently, plain film tomography was often the second step in the radiographic evaluation of a solitary pulmonary nodule. This technique was used to demonstrate calcification not visible on plain films, to further define the characteristics of the lesion, to show additional nodules, and to aid in the detection of hilar or mediastinal metastases associated with the parenchymal lesion.

In current radiologic practice, however, CT has been shown to be more accurate than conventional tomography for the diagnosis of multiple lung nodules and hilar or mediastinal adenopathy. Although conventional tomography can still be quite valuable for detecting calcification of a nodule (see Fig. 1-2), CT can also detect nodule calcification and is undoubtedly more accurate if correct techniques are employed.

## Computed Tomography

Computed tomography may be used for several purposes in evaluating the patient with a solitary pulmonary nodule. To some degree, all of these uses remain controversial.

### Detection of Mediastinal Lymph Node Enlargement

Computed tomography can accurately demonstrate enlargement of mediastinal lymph nodes. In the patient with a solitary pulmonary nodule, enlarged lymph nodes can reflect metastases from bronchogenic carcinoma and thus affect the resectability of the nodule (Fig. 1-4). Therefore, CT could be of value not only for diagnosis but also for planning subsequent treatment.

The importance of CT for detecting mediastinal lymph node enlargement in a patient with a solitary pulmonary nodule has been questioned on several grounds. It has been argued that CT should not effectively govern therapy in the patient with lung cancer, because it is not suffi-

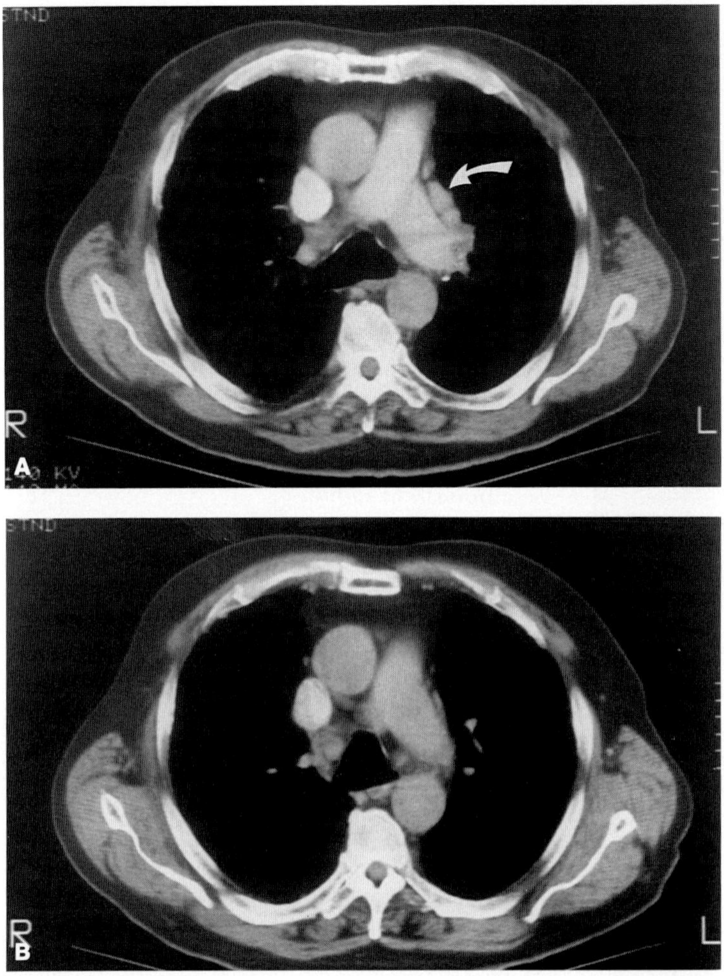


**Figure 1-4.** **(A** and **B)** CT scans in a patient with a solitary nodule show mediastinal lymph nodes, which are both enlarged (*arrow*) and normal. These nodes reflect silicosis, and the solitary nodule was a granuloma.

ciently accurate in predicting whether mediastinal lymph nodes are involved by tumor. The sensitivity and specificity of CT for the diagnosis of mediastinal lymph node metastases vary in different reported series, at least partially because of differences in the criteria used to distinguish benign from malignant nodes and in the methods of node biopsy or sampling performed for comparison with CT. Although most studies report predictive values of positive (large nodes) and negative (normal-sized nodes) CT scans as approximately 80% and 90%, respectively, other studies have shown substantially lower predictive values. Therefore, it is clear that in the patient with a solitary nodule suspected of being lung cancer, a large lymph node cannot be assumed to represent metastatic disease, and thus the lung nodule cannot be assumed to represent a neoplasm. Needle biopsy of the lung mass is necessary to prove that it is a carcinoma, and node biopsy (by needle aspiration or at mediastinoscopy) is required before an attempt at curative thoracotomy is made. It should be noted that CT can be helpful in localizing enlarged lymph nodes so that the surgeon can plan mediastinoscopy accordingly. In addition, CT-guided biopsy of enlarged nodes can be performed by the radiologist.

Because mediastinal lymph node metastases are uncommon in patients with T1 tumors (peripheral nodule, 3 cm or less in diameter), some reports have suggested that CT does not provide useful information and may even be confusing. Conversely, some reports describe patients with

T1 nodules who have CT-diagnosed mediastinal lymph node metastases.

Some surgeons do not regard the presence of mediastinal lymph node metastases (with the exception of subcarinal nodes, contralateral nodes, or high mediastinal nodes) as a contraindication to surgery for the patient with a solitary pulmonary nodule. Several studies have indicated that mediastinal lymph node resection, combined with radiotherapy, can result in 5-year survival rates of more than 20%. If this is the case, the CT detection of mediastinal lymph node metastases may not have any bearing on whether surgery is performed. Other surgeons, however, do not subscribe to this view. In addition, since high mediastinal nodes, contralateral mediastinal nodes, subcarinal nodes, and extranodal mediastinal spread are contraindications to surgery, CT could be important in delineating those patients who are not suitable candidates for operative therapy. It is important to note that the role of CT in the preoperative evaluation of a patient with a solitary pulmonary nodule varies greatly depending on the surgeon's approach. An aggressive surgeon, who performs extensive lymph node dissections, will rely less on CT and lymph node biopsy (needle biopsy or mediastinoscopy) than will a more conservative surgeon, who prefers not to operate on patients with evidence of spread to mediastinal lymph nodes.

### CT Nodule Densitometry

An initial study by Siegelman and colleagues suggested that nodule calcification (indicating benignancy) that was invisible on plain radiographs or conventional tomography might be detectable as an area of high attenuation on CT scans using thin collimation. In a study of solitary pulmonary nodules that appeared uncalcified on conventional tomography, all 58 primary and metastatic nodules had attenuation values less than 164 Hounsfield units (HU), while 60% of benign nodules had higher attenuation values. Other studies have shown that there is considerable variation in nodule density measurements obtained with different scanners for nodules of different sizes and in different locations, and in patients of different size and chest wall thickness.

One approach to the problem of accurate CT nodule densitometry has been the development of an anthropomorphic phantom for use in chest CT. This phantom can simulate the shape, dimensions, and density of thoracic structures in most patients. Cylinders of various diameters, made of plastic to correspond to a density of 164 HU on Siegelman's scanner, serve as the reference density for solitary pulmonary nodules. After a patient with a solitary nodule is studied using thin collimation, the phantom is put together to simulate the same slice level, chest wall thickness, nodule location, and nodule size. The phantom is then scanned using the CT technique identical to that used in scanning the patient (Fig. 1-5). The density of pixels in the patient's nodule and in the phantom nodule are compared. If the pixels in the patient's lung nodules are denser than those in the phantom nodule, calcium is considered to be present. In this way, the phantom is assumed to provide a measurement of density that is independent of equipment-related or patient-related variations. However, because lung carcinomas can contain some calcium, not all nodules shown to contain pixels denser than those of the reference standard can be labeled benign. A diagnosis of benignancy requires that the dense pixels must be diffuse or central within the nodule, must account for 10% or more of the cross-sectional area, and must be visible on more than one scan. In addition, the nodule must be less than 2 cm in size and must be lobulated or smooth rather than spiculated.

In a cooperative study of the use of a phantom in the diagnosis of 298 pulmonary nodules, all but one of 69 nodules determined to contain significant calcification were benign. Of the remaining nodules without significant calcification, more than 75% proved to be malignant. Some current scanners appear to be better densitometers and less susceptible to variations in CT number measurement than those scanners that prompted the invention of this phantom.

Thin-section (1.5 mm) technique is required when using CT for the diagnosis of nodule calcification. Calcium that can easily be detected on thin-section CT may sometimes be invisible with

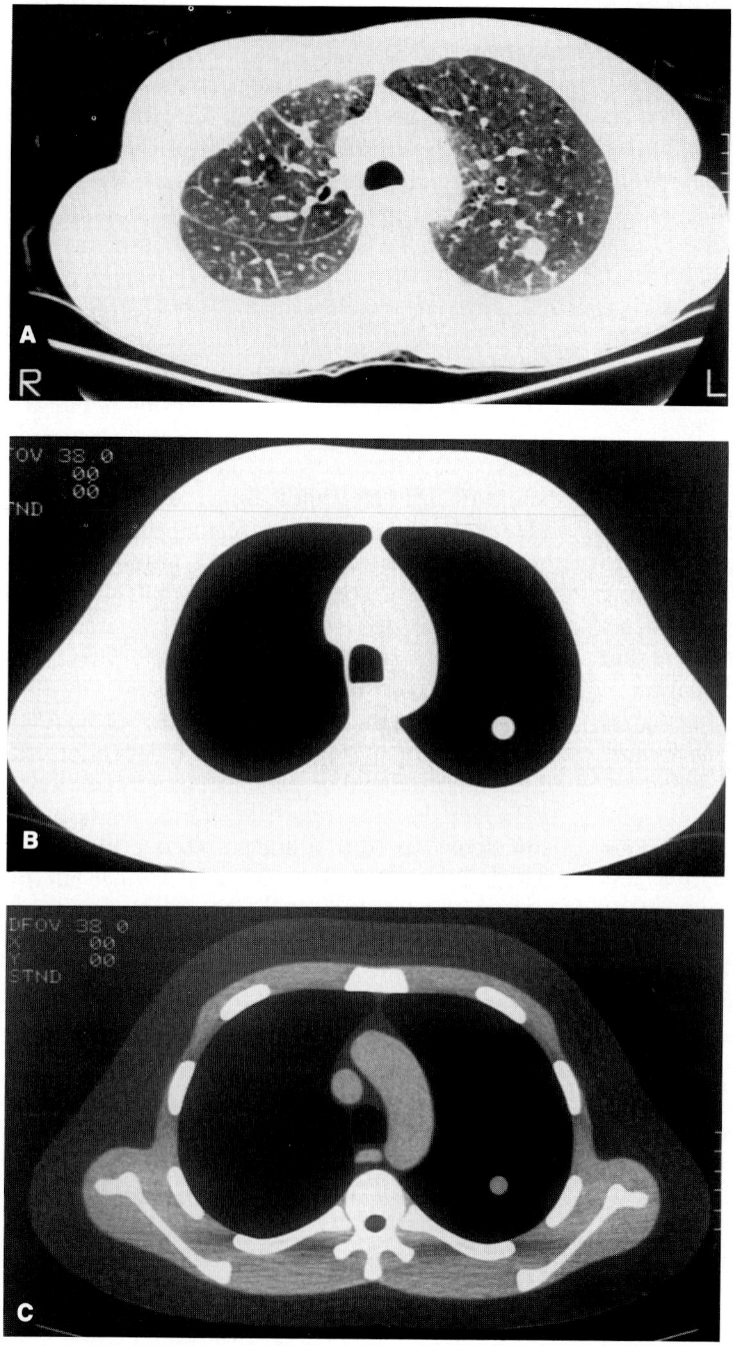


**Figure 1-5. (A)** CT scan with 1.5-mm collimation in a woman with breast carcinoma shows a solitary nodule. **(B)** CT scan of anthropomorphic chest phantom using a technique identical to that used in scanning the patient. The phantom was assembled to simulate the same CT level, chest wall thickness, and nodule size and location. **(C)** Same scan as in *B,* but photographed using a mediastinal window setting, shows the variations in density of the different components of the phantom that simulate bone, muscle, and fat.
(*Continued on facing page*)

1-cm collimation. In addition, in half of the cases in which a nodule could be called benign using CT nodule densitometry with the chest phantom, calcium was clearly visible within the lesion on thin-section scans, and there was no need for the phantom.

### Dual-Energy Techniques

Dual-energy CT scanning has been suggested as a technique for quantifying the amount of calcium in a lung nodule. Elements with high atomic numbers (*e.g.,* calcium) exhibit different

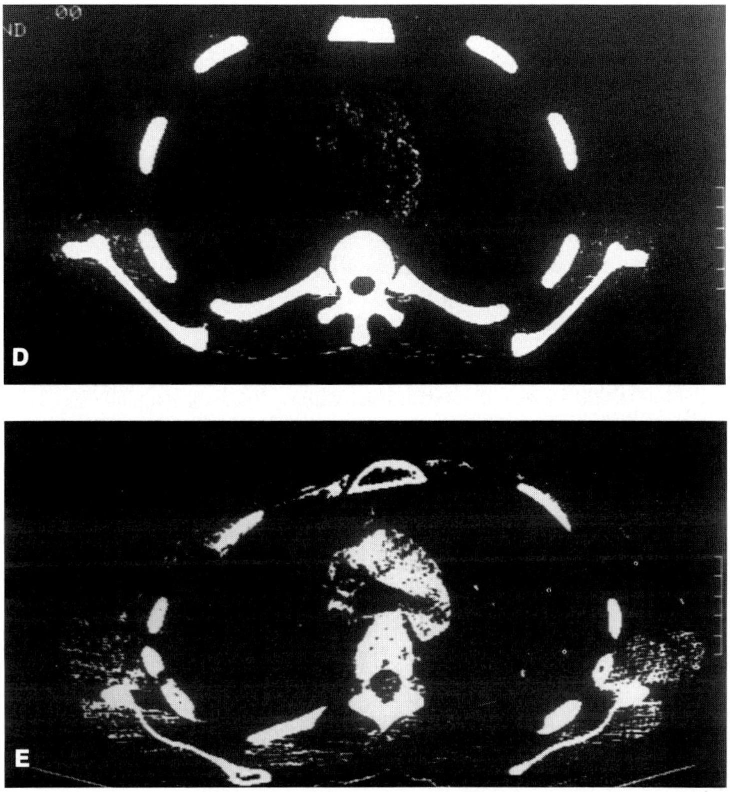


**(D)** Very narrow window (4 HU) view of the scan in *B* at the window level where the last pixel in the nodule was visible. **(E)** Scan of the patient's nodule using the same window width (4 HU) and level as in *D* shows that more pixels are visible and thus are denser than the phantom nodule. However, these pixels are too few to indicate that significant calcification is present. A metastasis was diagnosed at needle aspiration.

degrees of x-ray absorption at different energies. By noting the attenuation of the x-ray beam at different energies, the amount of calcium in an area of interest can be accurately quantified. However, this method has not yet been used clinically in a large series because of technical problems, especially the difficulty of replicating the exact level on the two different scans performed with different energies.

Preliminary experiments have been reported using dual-energy digital radiography with simultaneous energy measurements. Because there is exact registration of the dual-energy images, the problems of misregistration occurring with CT have been avoided. This technique has provided quite accurate calcium measurements of nodules in a phantom. However, as with dual-energy CT, digital radiography techniques remain experimental.

### Other Uses of CT

Computed tomography can occasionally identify other thoracic abnormalities that are useful in the diagnosis of a solitary pulmonary nodule. The CT detection of an endobronchial lesion, or bronchial narrowing at the site of a hilar mass, can direct bronchoscopy to the appropriate diagnostic level. The demonstration of multiple lung nodules suggests metastases from an extrathoracic primary tumor rather than from bronchogenic carcinoma. Scanning following the intravenous injection of contrast material can confirm that a nodule represents an arteriovenous fistula.

Computed tomography of extrathoracic regions can demonstrate metastases to other organs (*e.g.*, adrenal glands) that may lend themselves to biopsy. In the patient with a solitary pulmonary nodule suspected of being a lung cancer, any adrenal mass should be biopsied before a thoracotomy is attempted.

## Bronchography

Bronchography is of extremely limited value in the assessment of the solitary pulmonary nodule suspected of representing bronchogenic carcinoma. Occasionally, a slowly resolving pneumonia can mimic a mass on plain chest radiographs. In such cases, the bronchographic demonstration of normal bronchi within the lesion makes neoplasm a less likely possibility and permits continued radiographic observation. Bronchographic features that suggest a carcinoma are a "rat-tailed" bronchus within the lesion, an abrupt termination of a bronchus at the edge of the mass, and an annular constriction of the bronchial lumen (Fig. 1-6).

Complications of bronchography include toxic reaction to an overdose of local anesthetic, allergic reaction to contrast material, compromise of respiratory function because of bronchial or airway filling by contrast material, atelectasis, and pneumonia. Rare deaths have been reported. In recent years, bronchoscopy has all but replaced bronchography as a technique for differentiating malignant from inflammatory lesions. Although biopsy under direct vision or brush biopsy with fluoroscopic assistance may be performed during bronchoscopy, these procedures are of limited value in the diagnosis of peripheral solitary pulmonary nodules. Occasionally, bronchography is performed in conjunction with bronchoscopy.

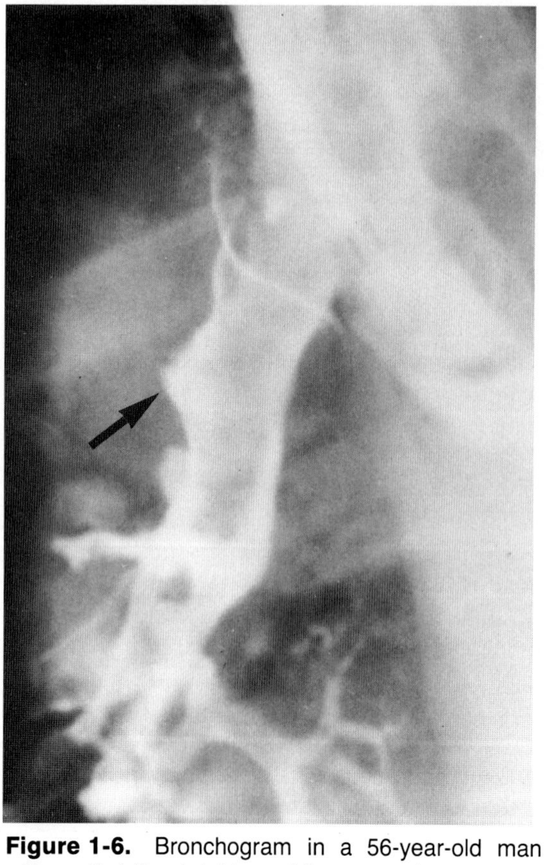

**Figure 1-6.** Bronchogram in a 56-year-old man with an ill-defined right parahilar mass shows abrupt termination (*arrow*) of the right-upper-lobe bronchus at its origin. This was proven to be a squamous cell carcinoma at thoracotomy.

## Angiography

In current radiologic practice, angiographic procedures (pulmonary arteriography, bronchial arteriography, superior venacavography) play no role in the evaluation of lung nodules or known bronchogenic carcinoma.

## Radionuclide Tumor Localization

A high proportion of bronchogenic carcinomas take up intravenously injected $^{67}$Ga citrate. However, because inflammatory lesions also demonstrate isotope uptake, the precise role of gallium scanning in characterizing and staging solitary pulmonary nodules is controversial. Some authors have concluded that the concentration of gallium in both the primary nodular lesion and the mediastinum is sufficient evidence of nonresectability, and mediastinoscopy should not be undertaken. On the other hand, if the primary tumor concentrates gallium but the mediastinum does not, these authors suggest that the patient should have thoracotomy without need for mediastinoscopy. Other authors have reported a significant percentage (22%) of false-negative mediastinal gallium scans and have recommended that mediastinoscopy still be performed in patients with no evidence of mediastinal uptake of the isotope.

Computed tomography has been shown to be superior to gallium scintigraphy in the diagnosis of mediastinal disease, and thus gallium scanning is uncommonly used in clinical practice.

## Aspiration Lung Biopsy

Aspiration lung biopsy has become firmly established in the investigation of the peripheral solitary pulmonary nodule suspected of being neoplastic. Lesions as small as 1 cm can be biopsied, although the minimum size varies with the skill of the operator. Confirmation of placement of the tip of the needle within the lesion must be obtained in two projections. Biplane fluoroscopy is the most convenient method, but single-plane fluoroscopy and CT also may be used.

Needle biopsy of the lung is a safe procedure. Although pneumothorax occurs in approximately 20% of patients, intercostal tube evacuation is required only in a small percentage. Hemorrhage and death are uncommon; in patients with carcinoma, dissemination of malignant cells from an aspiration biopsy may rarely occur. Needle aspiration yields malignant cells in more than 90% of neoplastic nodules. This percentage can be optimized by having a cytologist on hand at the time of the biopsy and by repeating the biopsy if the specimens are negative. Cytologic determination of cell type is good for squamous cell carcinomas and adenocarcinomas but poor for undifferentiated tumors. A bacterial diagnosis can be made in almost 70% of infectious nodules. The diagnosis of a benign nodule (*e.g.*, hamartoma) also can be made, although this usually requires a larger aspirate than for the diagnosis of malignancy.

In general, needle biopsy should be reserved only for those patients with solitary pulmonary nodules who are not candidates for thoracotomy because of age or complicating illnesses, or because the lesion is suspected to be a metastatic deposit (Fig. 1-7). Because of the relatively high false-negative rate (up to 10%) in patients with carcinoma, a negative biopsy should not be taken to mean that no tumor is present. If a patient can tolerate surgery, a solitary pulmonary nodule that could represent a malignancy is usually resected without needle biopsy being performed. If a nodule is suspected to be benign because of its appearance, growth rate, or the patient's age, a needle biopsy can be used to specifically diagnose benignancy or to increase the likelihood of a benign process prior to radio-

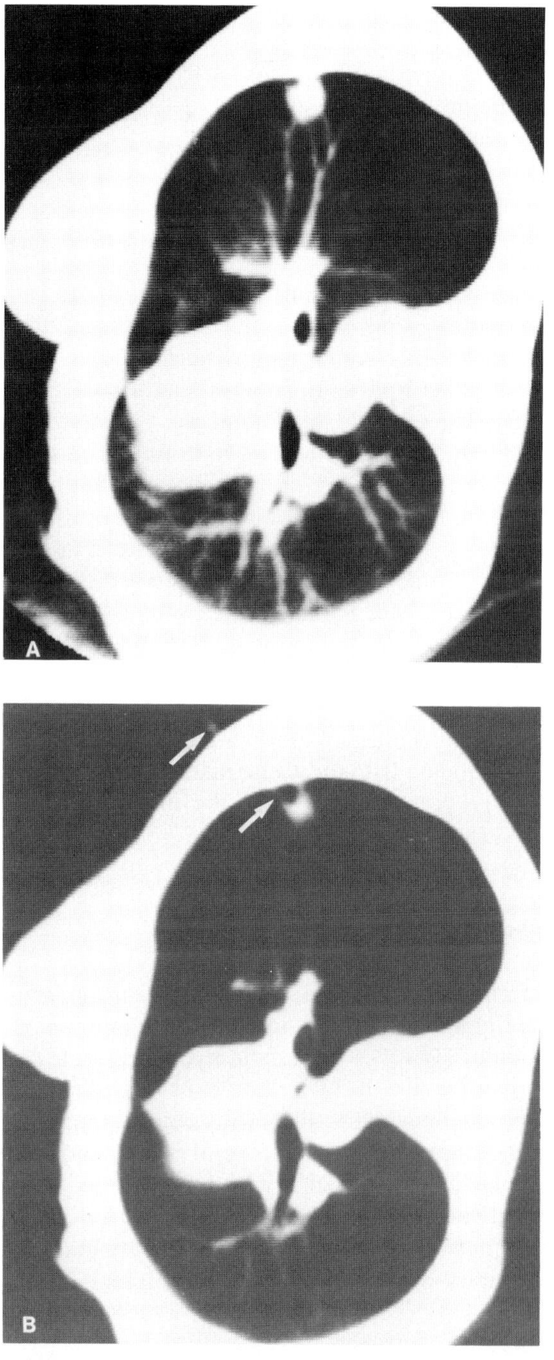

**Figure 1-7.** **(A)** CT scan of a woman with breast carcinoma shows a solitary nodule. **(B)** Needle aspiration biopsy was performed using CT because the nodule was not visible at fluoroscopy. Metastatic carcinoma was found at biopsy, and the patient was treated with chemotherapeutic agents. The needle is faintly visible (*arrows*).

graphic follow-up. It is important to note that the role of needle biopsy in the patient with a solitary pulmonary nodule varies considerably among different institutions.

## IS THE PATIENT AN OPERATIVE CANDIDATE?

In addition to the results of the clinical and radiographic examinations, the evaluation of the patient with a solitary pulmonary nodule depends at least partially on whether the patient is an operative candidate. Thoracotomy can be exceedingly risky in patients who are older, are in poor general health, or have poor pulmonary function. Practically speaking, a consideration of whether a patient with a solitary pulmonary nodule is an operative candidate often enters into the decision tree earlier in the patient's evaluation than is indicated in the algorithm at the end of this chapter. For example, if a patient is not being considered for surgery, an uncalcified nodule may be biopsied following plain radiographs. If the nodule is found to be malignant, CT may then be performed to stage the tumor prior to radiation therapy.

### Thoracotomy

Surgical exploration is, of course, the most accurate method of diagnosing a solitary pulmonary nodule. However, thoracotomy, even for a peripheral lesion, bears a significant mortality rate (approaching 1%). Primary complications include empyema, bronchopleural fistula, and persistent chest wall pain. Although thoracotomy should be avoided if possible in making a diagnosis, approximately 25% to 30% of patients with a solitary pulmonary nodule who undergo this surgical procedure do not have a definite preoperative diagnosis.

## Bibliography


Alazraki NP, Ramsdell JW, Taylor A et al: Reliability of Gallium scan chest radiography compared to mediastinoscopy for evaluating mediastinal spread in lung cancer. Am Rev Respir Dis 117:415–420, 1978

Bachynski JE: Selective bronchography of solitary mass lesions in the lung. J Can Assoc Radiol 22:65–70, 1971

Bateson EM: An analysis of 155 solitary lung lesions illustrating the differential diagnosis of mixed tumors of the lung. Clin Radiol 16:51–65, 1965

Breyer RH, Karstaedt N, Mills SA et al: Computed tomography for evaluation of mediastinal lymph nodes in lung cancer. Correlation with surgical staging. Ann Thorac Surg 38:215, 1984

Brown LR, DeRemee RA: 55° oblique hilar tomography. Mayo Clin Proc 51:89–95, 1976

Cann CE, Gamsu G, Birnberg FA et al: Quantification of calcium in solitary pulmonary nodules using single- and dual-energy CT. Radiology 145:493, 1982

Daly BDT, Jr, Faling LJ, Pugatch RD et al: Computed tomography: An effective technique for mediastinal staging in lung cancer. J Thorac Cardiovasc Surg 88:486, 1984

Edwards WM, Cox RS, Jr, Garland LH: The solitary nodule (coin lesion) of the lung: An analysis of 52 consecutive cases treated by thoracotomy and a study of preoperative diagnostic accuracy. AJR 88:1020–1042, 1962

Friedman PJ, Feigin DS, Liston SE et al: Sensitivity of chest radiography, computed tomography, and gallium scanning to metastasis of lung carcinoma. Cancer 54:1300, 1984

Godwin JD: The solitary pulmonary nodule. Radiol Clin North Am 21:709–720, 1983

Godwin JD, Speckman JM, Fram EK et al: Distinguishing benign from malignant pulmonary nodules by computed tomography. Radiology 144: 349, 1982

Hajek M, Homan van der Heide JN: Early detection of mediastinal spread of pulmonary carcinoma by mediastinoscopy. Thorax 25:720–724, 1970

Herman PG, Hessel SJ: The diagnostic accuracy and complications of closed lung biopsies. Radiology 125:11–14, 1977

Higgins GA, Shields TW, Keehn RJ: The solitary pulmonary nodule: Ten-year follow-up of Veterans Administration–Armed Forces cooperative study. Arch Surg 110:570–575, 1975

James EC, Ellwood RA: Mediastinoscopy and mediastinal roentgenology: A clinical correlation. Ann Thorac Surg 18:531–538, 1974

Khouri NF, Stitik FP, Erozan YS et al: Transthoracic needle aspiration biopsy of benign and malignant lung lesions. AJR 144:281, 1985

Libshitz HI, McKenna RJ, Jr: Mediastinal lymph node size in lung cancer. AJR 143:715, 1984

Libshitz HI, McKenna JR, Jr, Haynie TP et al: Mediastinal evaluation in lung cancer. Radiology 151:295, 1984

Martini N, Flehinger BJ, Zaman MB et al: Results of resection in non-oat cell carcinoma of the lung with mediastinal lymph node metastases. Ann Surg 198:386, 1983

Mittman C, Bruderman I: Lung cancer: To operate or not. Am Rev Respir Dis 116:477–496, 1977

Nathan MH: Management of solitary pulmonary nodules: An organized approach based on growth rate and statistics. JAMA 227:1141–1144, 1974

O'Keefe ME, Jr, Good CA, McDonald JR: Calcification in solitary nodules of the lung. AJR 77:1023–1033, 1957

Osborne DR, Korobkin M, Ravin CE et al: Comparison of plain radiography, conventional tomography, and computed tomography in detecting intrathoracic lymph node metastases from lung carcinoma. Radiology 142:157, 1982

Ray JF, Lawton BR, Magnin CE et al: The coin lesion story: Update 1976. Twenty years experience with early thoracotomy for 179 suspected malignant coin lesions. Chest 70:332–336, 1976

Rotte KH, Meiske W: Results of computer-aided diagnosis of peripheral bronchial carcinoma. Radiology 125:583–586, 1977

Siegelman SS, Zerhouni EA, Leo FP et al: CT of the solitary pulmonary nodule. AJR 135:1, 1980

Trunk G, Gracey DR, Byrd RB: The management and evaluation of the solitary pulmonary nodule. Chest 66:236–239, 1974

Zerhouni EA, Boukadoum M, Siddiky MA et al: A standard phantom for quantitative analysis of pulmonary nodules by computed tomography. Radiology 149:767, 1983

Zerhouni Ea, Spivey JF, Morgan RH et al: Factors influencing quantitative CT measurements of solitary pulmonary nodules. J Comput Assist Tomogr 6:1075, 1982

Zerhouni EA, Stitik FP: Controversies in computed tomography of the thorax. The pulmonary nodule–lung cancer staging. Radiol Clin North Am 23:407–426, 1985

## SOLITARY NODULE ON PLAIN CHEST RADIOGRAPH

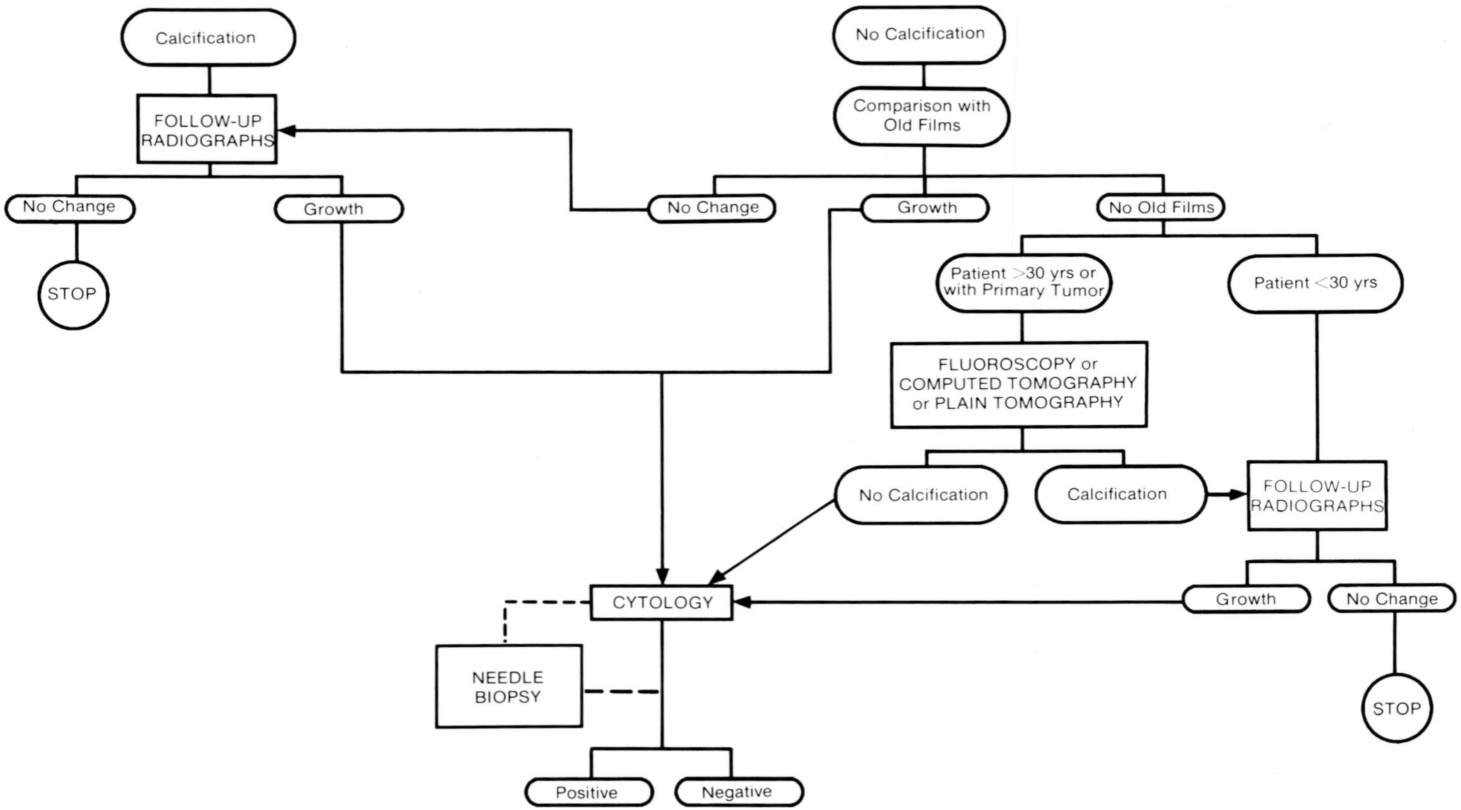

## SOLITARY NODULE ON PLAIN CHEST RADIOGRAPH

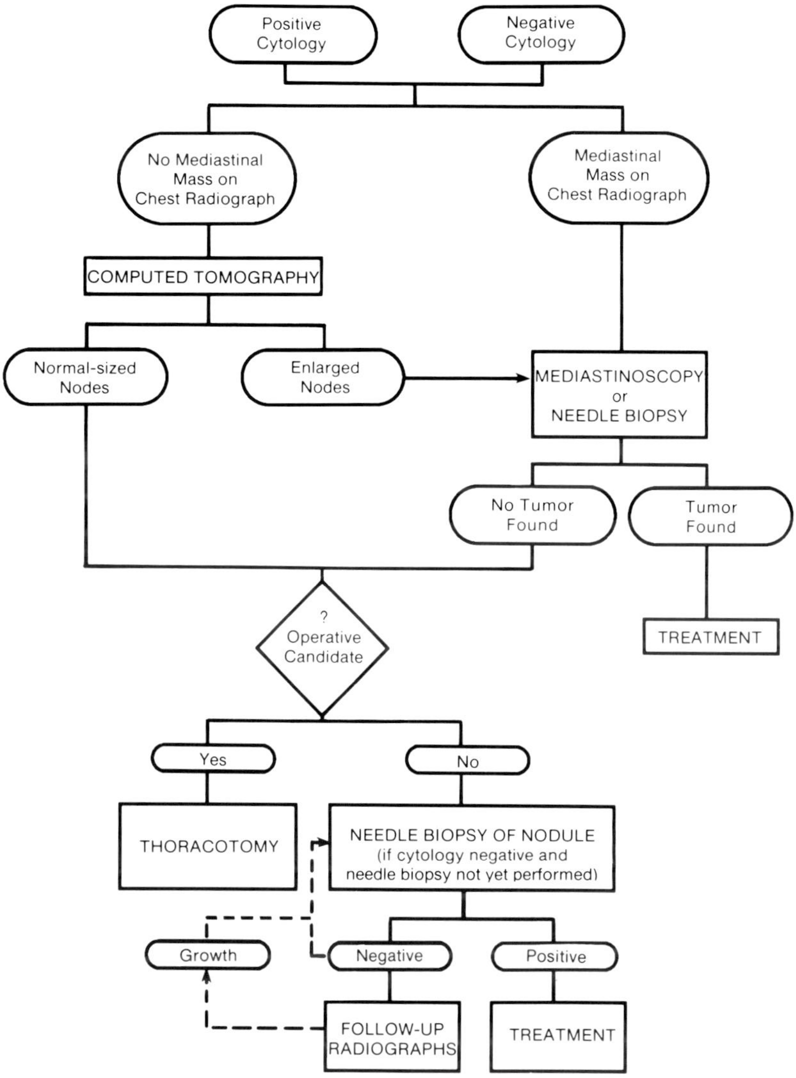

# Chapter 2

# Chest Pain

*Charles B. Higgins*
*Martin J. Lipton*

Chest pain is a symptom of a vast number of serious as well as inconsequential abnormalities (Table 2-1).

The initial step in the diagnostic approach is to define the location, radiation, severity, duration and, most important, precipitating, aggravating, and mollifying factors of the pain. This will usually allow the patient to be placed into one of four major categories of pain syndromes:

1. Transient, episodic, precordial or substernal pain (anginal pain)
2. Severe, unremitting, precordial or substernal pain
3. Sharp pain aggravated by respiration (pleuritic pain)
4. Nonspecific chest pain

## TRANSIENT, EPISODIC, PRECORDIAL OR SUBSTERNAL PAIN

Transient anginal pain generally has precipitating, aggravating, and mollifying factors. The most frequent precipitating factor is exertion (exercise). It is convenient clinically to separate this type of pain into two distinct categories: exertion pain and rest pain (frequently referred to as Prinzmetal's angina).

## DIAGNOSTIC EVALUATION

### *DIAGNOSTIC MODALITIES*

1. Plain chest radiography
2. Cardiac fluoroscopy
3. Standard electrocardiography
4. Exercise electrocardiography (exercise stress testing)
5. Radionuclide thallium scanning
6. Radionuclide exercise ventriculography (ejection fraction)
7. Coronary arteriography
8. Provocative pharmacoangiography

#### **Plain Chest Radiography**

Although the plain chest radiograph is inexpensive and without risk or patient discomfort, it is usually normal or nonspecific in a majority of

**Table 2-1** Diseases That May Be Manifested by Chest Pain

1. *Heart*
    - Myocardial disease
        - Ischemic heart disease
        - Myocarditis
        - Cardiomyopathy
    - Valvular disease
        - Aortic stenosis
        - Mitral valve prolapse
    - Pericardial disease
        - Pericarditis
2. *Aorta*
    - Dissecting aneurysm
    - Leaking or expanding atherosclerotic aneurysm
3. *Pleura*
    - Pleuritis, pneumothorax
4. *Lungs*
    - Pneumonia
    - Pulmonary embolism and/or infarction
5. *Mediastinum*
    - Emphysema
    - Mediastinitis
6. *Esophagus*
    - Rupture
    - Esophagitis
    - Esophageal tumor
    - Esophageal spasm
7. *Chest wall*
    - Arthritis
    - Tumor
    - Pleurodynia
8. *Abdominal disorders*
    - Peptic ulcer
    - Pancreatitis
    - Cholecystitis
    - Splenic flexure syndrome

patients with diseases causing chest pain. Moreover, the interpretation of the chest radiograph is highly subjective and permits considerable variability depending on the experience, proficiency, and psychological attitude of the examiner. However, even though the chest radiograph infrequently establishes a definitive diagnosis, it may be helpful in following the course, assessing the severity, providing insight into the prognosis, and detecting complications of disease processes (especially in patients with acute myocardial infarctions).

In the investigation of patients with angina, the chest radiograph is insensitive for detecting calcification of the coronary arteries, the harbinger of ischemic heart disease. In one study, coronary artery calcification was evident on the chest radiograph in only 3% of patients with ischemic heart disease. However, if the calcification is sufficiently dense and extensive to be detected on the chest radiograph, it is highly likely that the patient has hemodynamically significant coronary artery disease (Fig. 2-1).

## Cardiac Fluoroscopy

Cardiac fluoroscopy is a reliable and relatively sensitive (yet inexpensive) modality for the detection of valvular and coronary artery calcification. With disease of the aortic valve, the extent and density of calcification is roughly related to the transvalvular gradient and orifice area. Therefore, it is likely that fluoroscopy will reveal a calcified valve in the patient with angina due solely to severe or critical aortic valvular steno-

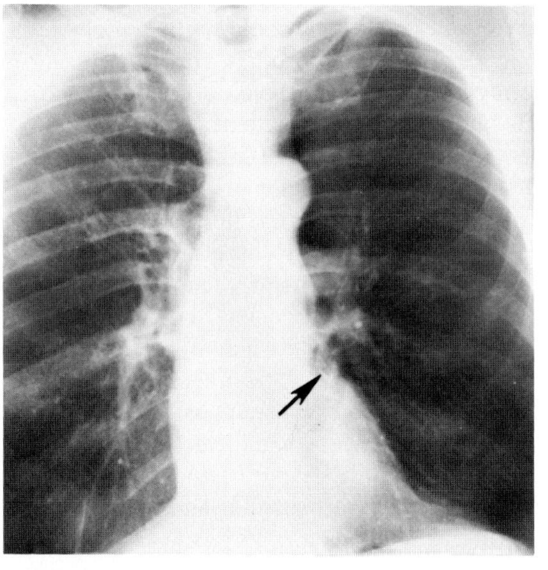

**Figure 2-1.** Chest radiograph reveals parallel lines of calcification in the proximal portion of the left coronary arterial system (*arrow*). Distinct calcification of this density has a high probability of being associated with significant obstructive disease.

sis. On the other hand, fluoroscopy cannot exclude the possibility of associated obstructive coronary artery disease as the sole or contributing factor in causing angina in the patient with aortic stenosis.

Coronary artery calcification, a manifestation of atherosclerosis, is amenable to detection by cardiac fluoroscopy. Postmortem studies suggest that most patients with coronary artery disease have dystrophic calcification of these arteries. The extent and density of this calcification found on pathologic examination is sometimes below the resolution detectable by fluoroscopy. This is the most likely explanation for 24% to 44% of patients with significant coronary artery disease having no evidence of calcification on cardiac fluoroscopy. The value of fluoroscopically detectable arterial calcification as a predictor of coronary artery disease depends on the age and sex of the patient. Coronary artery calcification in men under the age of 50 years is a moderate predictor of significant stenosis; in women under the age of 50 years, it is a strong predictor of major narrowing. Identification of calcification in older patients is not as useful, because calcification is observed in many elderly patients who do not manifest significant coronary obstructive disease. It must always be remembered that the presence of coronary artery calcification is not entirely specific for obstructive disease; this finding is detected in a small number of patients with no evidence of hemodynamically significant coronary lesions.

Until recently, cardiac fluoroscopy has been neglected by clinicians in evaluating patients with chest pain. This neglect may have been due to the high predictive value initially reported for exercise stress electrocardiography. As further experience has exposed the inherent insensitivity and inaccuracy of exercise stress electrocardiography, especially in women, cardiac fluoroscopy has been increasingly performed as an equally accurate, less time-consuming and less expensive alternative for detecting coronary artery calcification and for predicting the risk of coronary artery disease.

As the initial test in evaluating most patients with angina, cardiac fluoroscopy for coronary artery calcification has a slightly higher predictive value and sensitivity than exercise electrocardiography in detecting any degree of obstructive disease. In patients with symptomatic disease and hemodynamically significant narrowing at arteriography, the two tests have equivalent sensitivity and predictive accuracy. Only in elderly men does the predictive accuracy and specificity for exercise electrocardiography exceed that of cardiac fluoroscopy.

The inability to detect coronary artery calcification does not definitely exclude significant obstructive disease. However, in men over the age of 50 years, the lack of calcification at fluoroscopy does considerably diminish the likelihood of hemodynamically significant coronary artery disease.

## Standard Electrocardiography

The standard electrocardiogram (ECG) is probably the most frequently employed test in patients with chest pain. Although inexpensive and without risk, it is insensitive for detecting nonocclusive ischemic heart disease and therefore has very limited diagnostic utility in assessing the patient with angina. A normal resting ECG is obtained in 25% to 50% of patients with chronic coronary artery disease. In patients without a history of myocardial infarction, the ECG is normal in more than half of those with anginal pain. Even when the ECG is abnormal, the findings are frequently nonspecific. Only the presence of Q waves, indicative of a prior myocardial infarction, is a specific finding.

## Exercise Electrocardiography (Exercise Stress Testing)

Exercise electrocardiography is a physiologic test used to detect the presence of coronary artery disease by assessing the capacity of the coronary circulation to meet increased myocardial oxygen demands. One form of exercise stress testing (Master test), although simple and relatively inexpensive to perform, is so insensitive for detecting myocardial ischemia that it has been virtually abandoned. At present, patients with suspected coronary artery disease who are referred for exercise testing are usually subjected to multistage, or graded, submaximal studies. Although more difficult to perform and potentially more costly, these procedures have a far greater sensitivity.

The risk of exercise stress testing is low. A survey of 170,000 exercise tests performed in 73 medical centers revealed a mortality of approximately 0.01% and a morbidity of slightly over 0.2%. However, since there is a small potential for complications, a physician should be present at all times during a stress test.

The exercise stress test is positive when ST segments are depressed below the isoelectric line by a specified magnitude. Depression of 3 mm or more has been associated with a high frequency of severe obstructive disease (Fig. 2-2). As with most tests, the specificity and sensitivity tend to be reciprocally related and dependent on the strictness of criteria for positivity. As more patients with hemodynamically significant coronary artery disease are detected, the percentage of false positives rises dramatically. The quality of ST-segment depression is of diagnostic importance (down sloping is the most specific sign of myocardial ischemia). The occurrence of systolic hypotension accompanying the onset of angina and ST-segment depression during exercise testing is a sign of severe stenosis in the left main coronary artery or in the proximal segment of a major coronary artery.

Although initial studies reported high sensitivity, specificity, and predictive value of exercise stress testing in patients with significant obstructive coronary artery disease, more recent studies have seriously questioned the diagnostic utility of this modality. In one series of symptomatic patients, 67% with hemodynamically significant obstructive disease documented by coronary arteriography had negative exercise tests. In an asymptomatic population, exercise testing

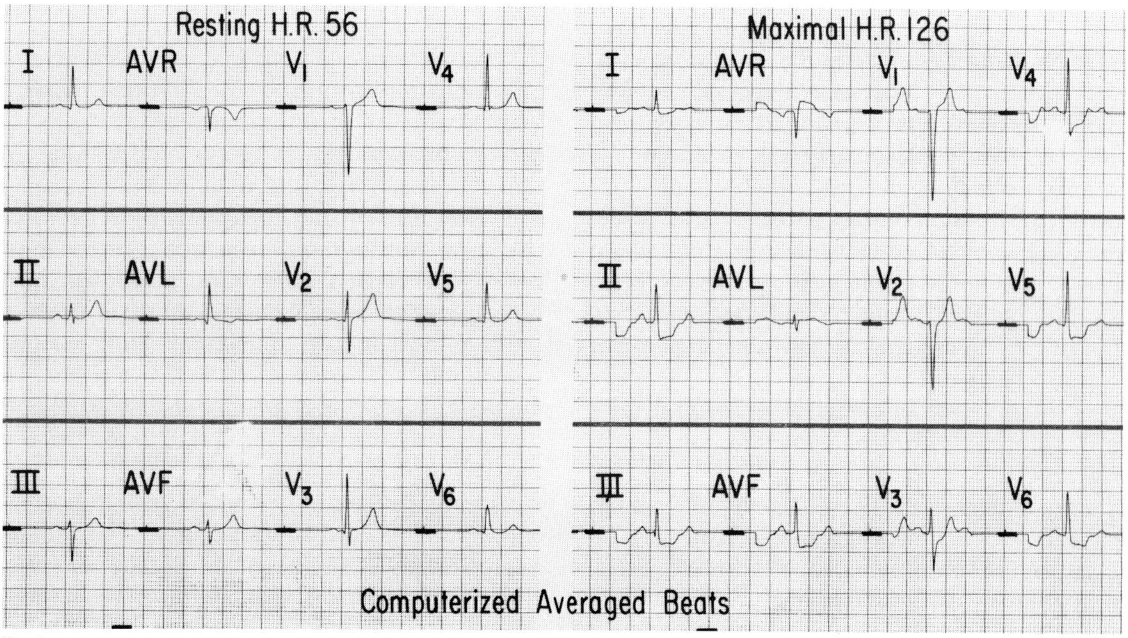


**A** **B**

**Figure 2-2.** Markedly positive exercise ECG. **(A)** Resting and **(B)** exercise electrocardiograms in a 60-year-old man with a history of inferior myocardial infarction show 3-mm depression of the ST segments. This type of exercise response is not only diagnostic of ischemic heart disease, but suggests severe obstruction of the left main coronary artery or three-vessel coronary artery disease. (Courtesy of Victor F. Froelicher, M.D.)

has been shown to be less sensitive than cardiac fluoroscopy for detecting occult disease. Exercise stress testing is particularly unreliable in women. The incidence of false-positive responses in normal women has been high. Abnormal exercise stress tests were found in 10% of healthy women aged 20 to 29 years, and in 25% of women aged 40 to 70 years. False-positive stress tests may also by caused by a multitude of other factors, including valvular heart disease, hypertension, myocardial and pericardial diseases, intraventricular conduction defects, left ventricular hypertrophy, and electrolyte abnormalities. Drugs (digitalis compounds, diuretics, sedatives, antihypertensive medications) may invalidate or complicate the interpretation of the exercise ECG.

## Radionuclide Thallium Scanning

Exercise myocardial perfusion imaging, like exercise electrocardiography, is a physiologic study that primarily assesses regional blood flow. Imaging is performed after the intravenous administration of $^{201}$Tl during maximal or near maximal exercise on a treadmill or bicycle ergometer. Rest myocardial perfusion images for comparison may be obtained several hours later after redistribution of the isotope or after a second dose of $^{201}$Tl administered at rest several days later (Fig. 2-3). Thallium myocardial imaging has a greater sensitivity and specificity than exercise electrocardiography for the detection of ischemic heart disease. In one study, $^{201}$Tl scans demonstrated rest or exercise perfusion defects in 78% of patients with hemodynamically significant coronary artery stenoses (> 50% reduction in luminal diameter). The sensitivity of thallium exercise scanning increases as more coronary arteries are significantly narrowed. In one study, the thallium scan was abnormal in 66% of patients with single-vessel disease, in 81% with two-vessel disease, and in 85% with three-vessel disease.

Thallium exercise scanning is of particular value under conditions in which exercise electrocardiography is difficult to interpret. This situation may arise in the presence of left ventricular hypertrophy, bundle-branch block, electrolyte imbalance, or medications such as digitalis.

Since the specificity of the thallium scan is considerably better than that of the exercise stress test, it has been used to detect false-positive exercise electrocardiographic responses. The finding of a negative exercise thallium scan in patients with a positive exercise ECG has sometimes obviated unnecessary coronary arteriography.

If both the exercise ECG and thallium exercise exercise scan are negative, myocardial ischemia is unlikely. However, approximately 10% of patients with significant obstructive disease of the coronary arteries are not detected by either test. In some instances, this is due to the presence of sufficient collateral vessels to avert regional ischemia in the presence of even critical obstructive lesions. Other reasons for these false negatives include the presence of areas of hypoperfusion below the limits of resolution of the technique and general myocardial ischemia resulting from severe proximal three-vessel coronary artery disease.

In practice, many thallium scans are read as "questionably positive." In addition, there is wide variability in interpretation and high observer disagreement. A recent report indicated that the sensitivity of thallium exercise scanning was not sufficient for determining the need for coronary arteriography in patients with typical or atypical anginal pain. The procedure was, however, diagnostically useful for screening patients with chest pain of uncertain etiology. The reason for these conclusions is that a history of angina indicates such a high prescan likelihood of significant coronary artery disease that the thallium scan adds little further diagnostic predictability. In the group with pain not characteristic of angina, on the other hand, the pretest likelihood of ischemic heart disease is sufficiently low that this test has diagnostic effectiveness in detecting patients with obstructive coronary artery disease.

Thallium exercise scanning may have a practical value in assessing the physiologic significance and need for coronary artery bypass grafts for coronary artery stenosis considered of borderline significance on coronary arteriography.

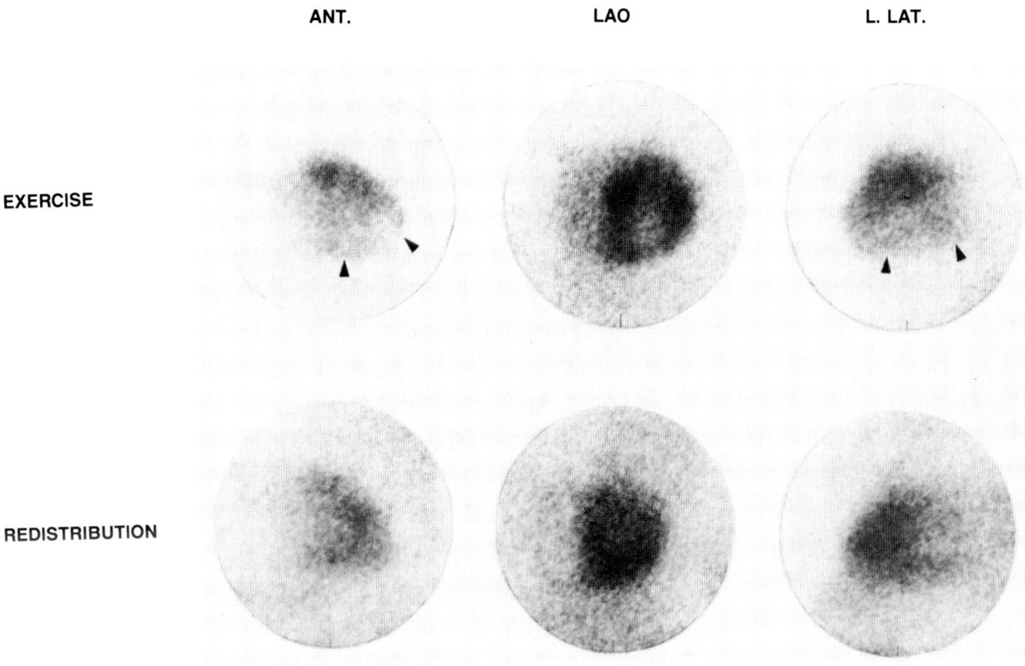


**Figure 2-3.** Exercise and redistribution $^{201}Tl$ perfusion scans show focal diminished uptake of radionuclide (*arrows*) in the inferior wall of the left ventricle. Scan after 4 hours reveals redistribution of radionuclide into the inferior wall. These findings are diagnostic for stress-induced ischemia and indicate a very high probability of hemodynamically significant stenosis of one or more coronary arteries. (Courtesy of William Ashburn, M.D.)

During exercise, if a defect in radionuclide uptake appears within the distribution of an artery with stenosis of disputed severity, this is strong evidence of the functional significance of the lesion. However, a negative test does not unequivocally indicate that a lesion is not a significant cause of ischemia.

In summary, although the thallium exercise scan has relatively high sensitivity and specificity, it is relatively expensive and has limited diagnostic usefulness in patients with anginal pain.

### Radionuclide Exercise Ventriculography (Ejection Fraction)

Radionuclide exercise ventriculography for detection of ischemic heart disease consists of multiple-gated blood-pool images of the left ventricle obtained during the cardiac cycle after *in vitro* or *in vivo* labeling of red blood cells with $^{99m}Tc$ pertechnetate. Ejection fraction and regional wall motion are determined and compared at rest and after attaining 85% of predicted maximal exercise. Normal patients increase the ejection fraction by more than 5% during exercise (*e.g.*, from 75% at rest to 80% during exercise). Patients with symptomatic and asymptomatic ischemic heart disease show no increase and often even a decrease in ejection fraction during exercise.

Abnormalities of ejection fraction are reported to be significantly more sensitive than defects on thallium exercise scanning (93% versus 71%) for the detection of ischemic heart disease. However, there are a large number of false-positive results with the ejection fraction technique. In one study, the combination of exercise thallium imaging and ejection fraction detected 100% of patients with significant coronary artery disease.

As with other forms of exercise testing, measurement of ejection fraction requires close monitoring of the study by the physician.

## Coronary Arteriography

Coronary arteriography is the "definitive test" in determining the presence and assessing the severity of coronary artery disease. This procedure is performed for the following major purposes: to establish or exclude unequivocally ischemic heart disease as the cause of chest pain, to determine the status of the coronary arteries in patients undergoing surgery for valvular heart disease, to define the location and extent of disease in patients in whom myocardial revascularization is contemplated for medically intractable angina, and to exclude ischemic heart disease in patients involved in critical occupations related to public safety.

Utilizing optimal cineangiographic techniques (particularly the axial oblique views), essentially all hemodynamically significant stenoses of the coronary arteries should be detected by this procedure. However, this ideal potential has not yet been achieved, and false-negative rates of 10% to 32% have been reported in patients with pathologically demonstrated severe stenoses. On the other hand, coronary arteriography infrequently overestimates the severity of disease; normal or mild stenosis is mistakenly considered severe in only approximately 5% of cases. The arterial segments in which errors occur most frequently are the main left coronary artery, proximal and distal segments of the circumflex artery, and the distal portion of the left anterior descending artery.

The highly subjective nature of interpretation of coronary arteriography makes the procedure liable to errors and variations of opinion. Both interobserver and intraobserver disagreements with regard to location and severity of stenoses occur approximately half the time. Diagnostically important differences are found in 25% to 35% of cases. Two different approaches should reduce these high levels of disagreement. The increased use of axial views should afford considerably greater precision of imaging of the coronary circulation, thus reducing these variabilities and inaccuracies. The use of more than one observer increases the likelihood that a stenotic lesion will be detected. When a consensus panel of three observers interprets the degree of stenosis and determines the hemodynamic significance of a lesion, the possibility of diagnostically important misinterpretation is significantly reduced (to 3%).

Despite the frequency of use and great therapeutic and prognostic implications of coronary arteriography, precise values for the diagnostic effectiveness of this procedure are not available. This lack of data arises because the results of coronary arteriography can only be fully judged by direct pathologic examination of the coronary artery circulation. Nevertheless, one measure (although questionable) of the accuracy of this procedure comes indirectly from the results of myocardial revascularization based on the anatomy demonstrated at coronary arteriography. Symptoms of angina are relieved in more than 90% of patients in whom "complete revascularization" is possible and in whom the bypass grafts remain patent.

Coronary arteriography is relatively expensive; since the procedure is usually performed on hospitalized patients, this further increases the cost.

The risk of coronary arteriography is relatively low in institutions with considerable experience. At the Cleveland Clinic, where more than 52,000 coronary arteriograms have been performed, the mortality rate is 0.07% and the incidence of major complications is less than 1%. A nationwide survey of 176 hospitals (1973–1974) found a mortality rate of 0.14% and a major complication rate (primarily ventricular fibrillation) of less than 1.5%.

## Provocative Pharmacoangiography

In some patients, spasm is a major pathogenetic mechanism contributing to or entirely responsible for coronary artery narrowing and myocardial ischemia. These patients incur chest pain unrelated to the usual inciting factors; angina occurs either exclusively at rest or both at rest and with exercise. Some display a characteristic clinical (rest angina) and electrocardiographic (transient ST-segment elevation) syndrome termed *Prinzmetal's angina.*

Many of these patients with spasm have

normal or near-normal coronary arteriograms. Others, fortuitously, may spontaneously develop spasm of one or more coronary vessels during the performance of coronary arteriography. If spasm is suspected as the underlying factor in the patient with angina who has a normal coronary arteriogram, various maneuvers have been utilized during coronary arteriography in an attempt to elicit spasm (Fig. 2-4). Provocative pharmacoangiography has been most frequently performed by intravenous administration of low doses of ergonovine maleate. Another approach has been to hospitalize the patient with episodic rest angina and to perform coronary arteriography during the spontaneously occurring periods of pain.

The ergonovine provocative test is positive in more than 90% of patients with Prinzmetal's angina and negative in 100% of patients with normal coronary arteries and without a history

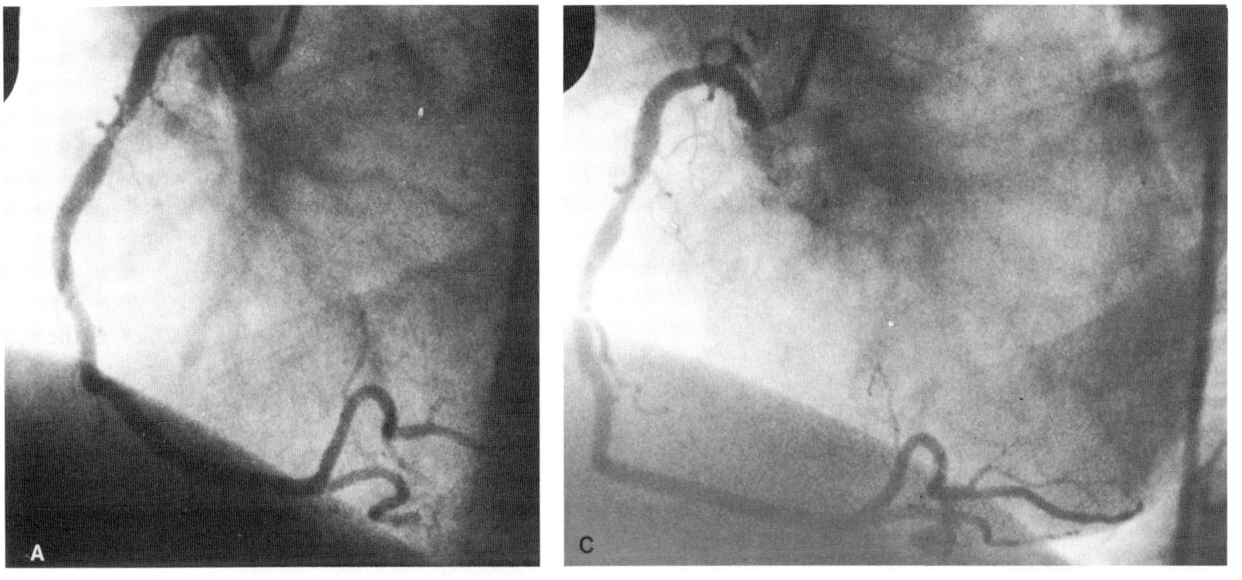


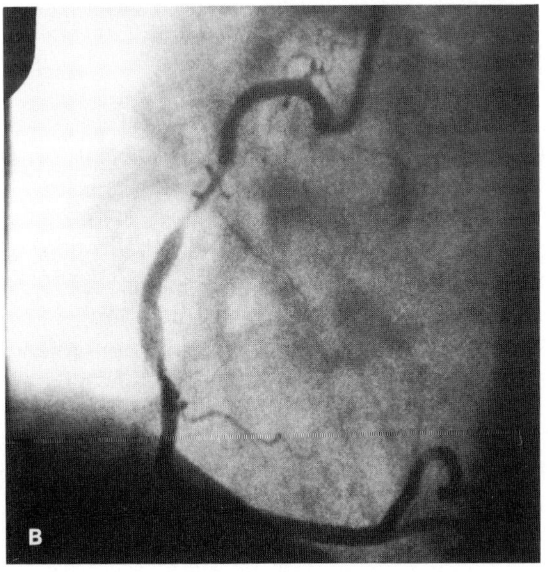


**Figure 2-4.** Coronary arteriogram with provocative pharmacoangiography (ergonovine) in a patient with Prinzmetal's angina. **(A)** Initial right coronary arteriogram reveals low-grade narrowing in the right coronary artery. **(B)** Arteriogram after ergonovine shows almost complete occlusion of the vessel due to spasm. **(C)** After nitroglycerin is administered, the spasm is reversed.

of this clinical and electrocardiographic syndrome. Although a positive test documents spasm as a predominant factor in producing myocardial ischemia, a negative study does not definitely exclude this mechanism, because patients have been reported who have had a negative response on one occasion and a positive response on subsequent challenge. It should be emphasized that this test adds definite hazard to coronary arteriography. Serious arrhythmias, myocardial infarction, and, in rare cases, deaths have resulted from this provocative test. In addition, once spasm is provoked, it may not always be readily reversed.

### Additional Procedures

New techniques such as very rapid computed tomography (CT) and digital fluoroscopy (both procedures performed after intravenous administration of contrast medium) may eventually be refined to the extent of providing direct, noninvasive visualization of coronary artery anatomy. At present, however, these procedures have no effective clinical use in assessing the patient with suspected anginal pain.

In the patient with typical angina, there is no justification for the routine use of any noninvasive diagnostic test; none of these procedures has a sensitivity and specificity greater than a clearly documented history of angina. Therefore, if the history of angina is unequivocal, medical therapy can be instituted without need for additional diagnostic procedures. If medical therapy is unsuccessful and surgical intervention is considered, coronary arteriography may be performed.

## SEVERE, UNREMITTING, PRECORDIAL OR SUBSTERNAL PAIN

Several life-threatening illnesses must be considered in the presence of severe, unremitting, precordial or substernal pain. Acute myocardial infarction is the major diagnosis to be established or excluded in patients with this type of chest pain. If the pain is cataclysmic in onset, tearing in nature, and associated with neurologic symptoms, pulse defect, or severe hypertension, acute aortic dissection must be ruled out as a diagnostic possibility. Precordial chest pain intensified by positional changes and accompanied by low-grade fever suggests the diagnosis of acute pericarditis. Chronic severe, unremitting, intractable pain in the chest is typical of an invasive and often inoperable cancer, although expanding aneurysms of the aorta (notably those involving the descending thoracic aorta) may produce this type of chronic pain by causing pressure erosion of vertebrae.

### DIAGNOSTIC EVALUATION

*DIAGNOSTIC MODALITIES*

1. Electrocardiography
2. Serum enzymes
3. Plain chest radiography
4. Radionuclide scanning ($^{99m}$Tc pyrophosphate)
5. Radionuclide scanning ($^{201}$Tl)
6. Echocardiography
7. Arteriography
8. Computed tomography
9. Position emission tomography
10. Magnetic resonance imaging

### Electrocardiography

The standard ECG is the traditional test for establishing the diagnosis of acute myocardial infarction. The positive ECG is extremely specific and clearly establishes and diagnosis of acute myocardial infarction better than does any other diagnostic modality. However, a negative ECG does not exclude this diagnosis. Almost 25% of patients with an acute myocardial infarction will have a negative ECG. The sensitivity (and predictive value) of a negative ECG is less than that for a variety of serum enzyme determinations. Performing serial ECGs over 2 to 3 days does slightly increase the sensitivity of this procedure. However, this generally entails hospitalization over the entire period and, in patients without acute myocardial infarction, adds considerable unnecessary expense.

Electrocardiographic changes (decreased amplitude of QRS complex, ST-segment elevation or depression, and arrhythmias) occur in approximately 80% of patients with acute pericarditis. However, these changes are nonspecific and frequently are not diagnostic in themselves; they are primarily used to support other findings in establishing the diagnosis of pericarditis.

### Serum Enzyme Determinations

Tests designed to identify a rise in the serum level of enzymes released by myocardial necrosis have been a standard procedure for establishing the diagnosis of acute myocardial infarction. The serum level of cardiac enzymes is usually measured initially and then serially for approximately 3 days in order to corroborate the diagnosis. In recent years, multiple frequent measurements of one of these enzymes, creatine phosphokinase (CPK), have been used to provide an indirect estimate of the volume of infarcted myocardium.

The myocardial-specific isoenzyme of creatine phosphokinase (CPK-MB) provides the greatest specificity of all enzyme tests in determining the presence of myocardial necrosis. A single measurement of this isoenzyme within 24 hours after the onset of pain is better for establishing the diagnosis of acute myocardial infarction than single or serial measurements of other cardiac enzymes and the ECG (or combinations of enzyme tests and ECGs). In one study, a positive measurement of this myocardial-specific isoenzyme obtained within 24 hours after the onset on chest pain permitted the detection of every patient with acute myocardial infarction; false-positive results were extremely low.

### Plain Chest Radiography

The plain chest radiograph is of little diagnostic value in establishing the diagnosis of acute myocardial infarction. However, assessment of pulmonary venous hypertension on the chest radiograph within the first 24 hours after onset of pain in patients with acute myocardial infarction gives considerable insight into the eventual prognosis of this disease (Fig. 2-5). Chest radiography may be of diagnostic value in some conditions producing severe, unremitting, precordial or substernal pain, such as pneumothorax, pneumomediastinum, and pericarditis accompanied by a large pericardial effusion.

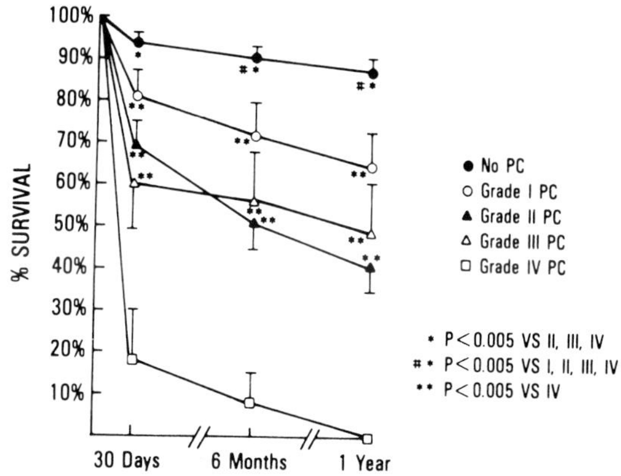


**Figure 2-5.** This graph shows the survival rate at 30 days, 6 months, and 1 year in groups of patients with various grades of pulmonary venous hypertension evident on a chest radiograph within the first 24 hours after onset of acute myocardial infarction. (Battler A, Karliner JS, Higgins CB et al: The initial chest X-ray in acute myocardial infarction. Circulation 61:1004–1009, 1980. By permission of the American Heart Association, Inc)

### Radionuclide Scanning ($^{99m}$Tc Pyrophosphate Scan)

Of the many $^{99m}$Tc-labeled compounds that concentrate in areas of acute myocardial necrosis, the pyrophosphate derivative is the one used in most clinical studies. This procedure will identify almost 90% of acute myocardial infarctions (Fig. 2-6), with a 14% false-positive rate. The diagnostic effectiveness of $^{99m}$Tc pyrophosphate scanning is thus slightly greater than electrocardiography, although significantly less than myocardial-specific isoenzyme determination, for the diagnosis of acute myocardial infarction.

The sensitivity of $^{99m}$Tc pyrophosphate scans

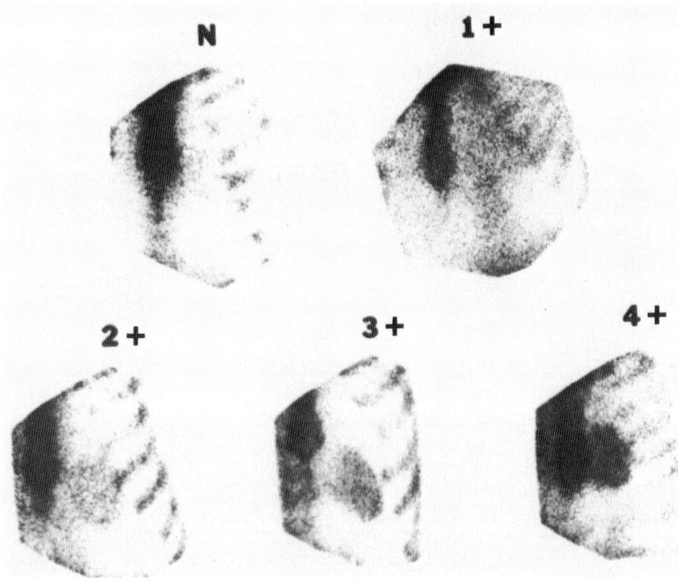


**Figure 2-6.** Anterior view of five $^{99m}$Tc pyrophosphate scans. A normal scan (*N*) is contrasted with an equivocally positive (*1* +) and three positive scans showing increasing intensity of focal uptake of the radionuclide (*2* + *to 4* +). Focal uptake of radionuclide at an intensity of *2* + or greater is highly suggestive of acute myocardial infarction in a patient with a history of recent persistent precordial or substernal pain. (Courtesy of William Ashburn, M.D.)

for detecting acute myocardial infarction depends on such factors as the elapsed time after infarction at which the scan is obtained, the location of the infarct, and the criteria used for interpreting the images. Scanning should be performed at least 12 hours after the estimated time of acute infarction, because the study is usually negative within the first few hours after the event. If the initial scan is negative, a repeat test at 48 to 72 hours following infarction will be positive in some patients. The positive image of the infarct tends to fade after 5 days, frequently disappearing after 10 to 14 days. However, follow-up studies at 6 weeks to 9 months after infarction reveal persistently positive scans in more than 50% of patients. Thus, in the patient with a prior myocardial infarction, a positive $^{99m}$Tc pyrophosphate scan may not always be diagnostic of an acute myocardial infarction.

Experimental studies have suggested that 5% or more of the myocardium must be infarcted to be routinely detectable by $^{99m}$Tc pyrophosphate scanning. Images of myocardial infarction involving the anterior and lateral segments of the left ventricle can be more precisely and reliably resolved than those located in the posterior or inferior segments. If localized cardiac uptake of isotope is considered the only positive criterion for a $^{99m}$Tc pyrophosphate scan, the accuracy of this test is good for detecting transmural acute myocardial infarctions. The diffuse pattern of cardiac uptake, however, has a considerably lower specificity and predictive value. Almost 15% of patients without acute myocardial infarction demonstrate the diffuse pattern; this pattern is frequently the only abnormality displayed on scans in patients with subendocardial myocardial infarction.

It is often difficult for $^{99m}$Tc pyrophosphate scanning to discriminate the patients with unstable angina from those with acute myocardial infarction. Forty-one percent of patients with unstable angina without definite acute infarction will have positive scans. It is unclear whether these are truly false-positive scans or are really positive examinations in which the amount of myocardial necrosis cannot be detected by any other test. False-positive $^{99m}$Tc pyrophosphate scans have also been reported in patients with valvular calcifications, high-energy cardioversion or defibrillation, ventricular aneurysms, myocardial contusions, cardiomyopathy, myocarditis, and metastases to the heart.

The $^{99m}$Tc pyrophosphate scan can provide information in addition to the mere detection of acute infarction. The scan can localize the site of infarction, provide a direct estimate of the size of the infarcted myocardium, and by the pattern and size of the area of isotope uptake, give insight into prognosis.

The major value of $^{99m}$Tc pyrophosphate scanning is in patients with suspected acute myocardial infarction in which other clinical and laboratory evidence is nondiagnostic. Scanning can be diagnostically useful in patients who present more than 48 hours after the onset of symptoms, a time at which the very sensitive myocardial-specific serum enzyme levels have usually returned to normal. Technetium-99m pyrophosphate scanning is the only method routinely available for identifying infarction of the right ventricle; scanning may also be helpful when the ECG contains preexisting abnormalities such as left bundle-branch block.

## Radionuclide Scanning ($^{201}$Tl)

Myocardial infarction appears on the $^{201}$Tl scan as an area of diminished radionuclide activity within the outline of the left ventricle, because of a regional decrease in coronary blood flow. This technique will be positive in almost all (90%–100%) patients with acute myocardial infarctions who are scanned within 6 hours after the onset of symptoms. Thus, thallium scanning has been used effectively in selecting those patients with persistent precordial pain for admission to the coronary care unit (CCU). In one study, all patients selected on this basis for treatment in the CCU were subsequently shown to have incurred a myocardial infarction. None of the patients who were rejected for admission to the CCU because of a negative scan was subsequently shown to have sustained a myocardial infarction. Since the thallium scan shows it highest sensitivity in the first 6 hours after onset of infarction, this study is frequently positive before the onset of diagnostic electrocardiographic and enzymatic abnormalities, and it is always positive before the $^{99m}$Tc pyrophosphate scan. Although thallium scanning is highly sensitive early in the course of acute myocardial infarction, the sensitivity is markedly decreased if the examination is performed 12 to 24 hours after the onset of symptoms.

As expected for any imaging test, the sensitivity of thallium scanning is closely related to the size of the infarction and its location. Within the first 6 hours, almost all small transmural or subendocardial myocardial infarctions are detected by thallium scanning. However, transmural infarctions frequently produce a questionably positive scan (*i.e.*, a diffuse and ill-defined defect).

A major limitation of thallium scanning is its inability to distinguish between acute and previous infarction. When a perfusion defect that corresponds to the site of pathologic Q waves is observed, it cannot be assumed that the defect is due to prior rather than acute myocardial infarction. It is not uncommon for an acute infarction to occur in the area immediately surrounding but not involved by an earlier infarction. Thallium scanning is also unable to distinguish infarction from acute severe ischemia without infarction (as might occur with coronary artery spasm). This dilemma can usually be solved by a delayed thallium scan after treatment with vasodilators or after spontaneous resolution of chest pain.

In summary, a normal thallium scan (uniform uptake of isotope in all views) obtained within the early hours following the suspected acute event can provide reasonable assurance that an acute myocardial infarction is unlikely. However, this does not exclude coronary artery disease or the possibility that transient ischemia may have occurred sometime prior to the imaging procedure with subsequent re-establishment of normal perfusion. An abnormal study should alert the clinician to the high probability of myocardial ischemia, which has or may lead to infarction. However, thallium scanning may be unable to differentiate acute infarction, unstable angina with transient (reversible) ischemia, or scar formation secondary to a previous acute infarction (whether apparent by history or not).

## Echocardiography

Echocardiography is of no value in the diagnostic approach to the patient with suspected acute myocardial infarction. Although M-mode and real-time sector echocardiography may demonstrate regional abnormalities of motion of the left ventricle that suggest myocardial infarction, the diagnostic efficacy of this modality is inferior to that of electrocardiography, enzyme studies, or nuclear scans. As with thallium scanning, echocardiography is unable to distinguish acute from previous myocardial infarction, or ischemic from infarcted myocardial tissue.

Echocardiography is, however, the most sensitive test available for demonstrating pericardial effusions. Therefore, echocardiography may be employed to support a clinical suspicion of acute pericarditis. The echocardiographic demonstration of pericardial effusion is a nonspecific finding, but in a patient with fever and precordial pain intensified by respiration, coughing, swallowing, or positional changes, it is almost diagnostic of acute pericarditis. The M-mode echocardiogram can detect pericardial effusions as small as 20 ml and can grossly estimate the volume of effusion, can serially monitor the accumulation and resolution of fluid, and sometimes can detect characteristic signs of pericardial tamponade. Echocardiography entails no risk or patient discomfort, is relatively inexpensive, and does not require hospitalization.

## Arteriography

Coronary arteriography and left ventriculography play no role in the diagnosis of acute myocardial infarction. The diagnosis of this condition can almost always be obtained with noninvasive studies, and the risk of coronary arteriography is increased in this condition. In a few centers, coronary arteriography has been performed in patients with evolving acute myocardial infarctions. Initial results have demonstrated that blood flow in some patients could be re-established in the occluded coronary artery by direct intracoronary injection of nitroglycerin. If it can be shown that potentially reversible spasm is an important factor in completing the occlusion of vessels narrowed by atherosclerosis, the indication for coronary arteriography in patients with persistent precordial pain may change.

Aortography does play a role in the diagnostic approach to the patient with sudden onset of persistent substernal or precordial pain suggestive of aortic dissection. This is discussed in depth in Chapter 4.

## Computed Tomography

Computed tomography can provide direct images of areas of myocardial ischemia. The area of ischemic damage has a decreased attenuation value due to the increased water content caused by intramyocardial cellular edema. The injection of intravenous contrast material has a biphasic effect on the infarcted area. During the first 1 to 2 minutes after injection (perfusion phase), the attenuation value of normal myocardium increases, while the nonperfused infarct is minimally or nonenhanced. On the other hand, CT scans obtained 5 to 10 minutes after contrast injection demonstrate relatively increased accumulation of contrast in the infarcted are (hot spot).

The greater spatial resolution of CT, compared with $^{99m}$Tc pyrophosphate scanning, suggests that this modality may be more precise in defining the site, transmural extent, and size of acute myocardial infarctions. The three-dimensional imaging capability of CT enables direct measurement of the volume of myocardial infarctions. Experimental studies have demonstrated a close relationship between the volume of the infarct determined by CT and gated magnetic resonance imaging (MRI) with that calculated by direct measurement at postmortem examination (Fig. 2-7). Computed tomography appears to have considerable accuracy in detecting infarcts of varying ages, including those as early as 2 hours after onset of symptoms. This technique may not only directly image the infarct itself, but also may identify associated left ventricular aneurysms and mural thrombi.

At present, no definite information is available regarding the diagnostic efficacy of CT; its precise role in the evaluation of the patient with suspected acute myocardial infarction has not yet been determined.

The role of CT in the patient with suspected aortic dissection is discussed in Chapter 4.

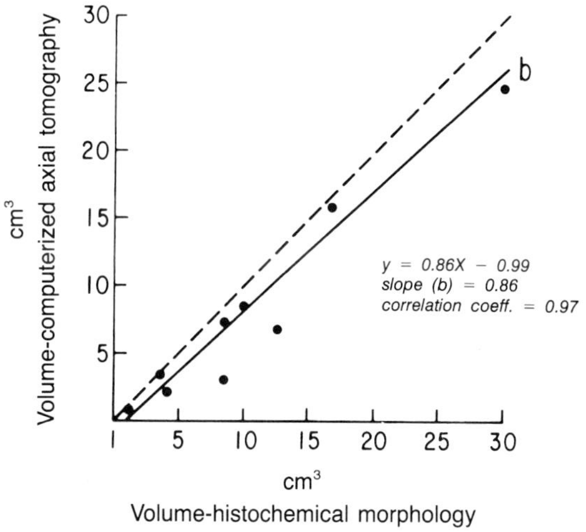


**Figure 2-7.** This graph displays the linear relationship and close correlation between the volume of myocardial infarction determined from the CT scan and histochemical morphometry. The CT scans were performed on the *ex situ* hearts of dogs with 48-hour-old myocardial infarctions. (Siemers PT, Higgins CB, Schmidt W et al: CT: Detection, quantitation and contrast enhancement of myocardial infarction utilizing computerized axial tomography: Comparison with histochemical staining and $^{99m}$Tc-pyrophosphate scanning. Invest Radiol 13:103–109, 1978)

### Magnetic Resonance Imaging

Gated MRI has demonstrated regions of acute myocardial infarction in humans. The acutely infarcted area has a high signal intensity (Fig. 2-8) and prolongation of the T2 relaxation time. However, the sensitivity and specificity of MRI for detecting acute infarction have not yet been determined.

## PLEURITIC PAIN AND NONSPECIFIC CHRONIC CHEST PAIN

Pleuritic pain, a sharp intermittent pain aggravated by respiration, will be discussed in Chapter 3 on pulmonary embolism, the most common serious disease that causes this clinical symptom.

The assessment of nonspecific chronic chest pain is critically dependent on the elicitation of associated symptoms that direct attention to a specific organ or organ system. For example, regurgitation, gaseous eructation, or dysphagia direct the diagnostic search to the esophagus. If there are no historical clues to limit the scope of

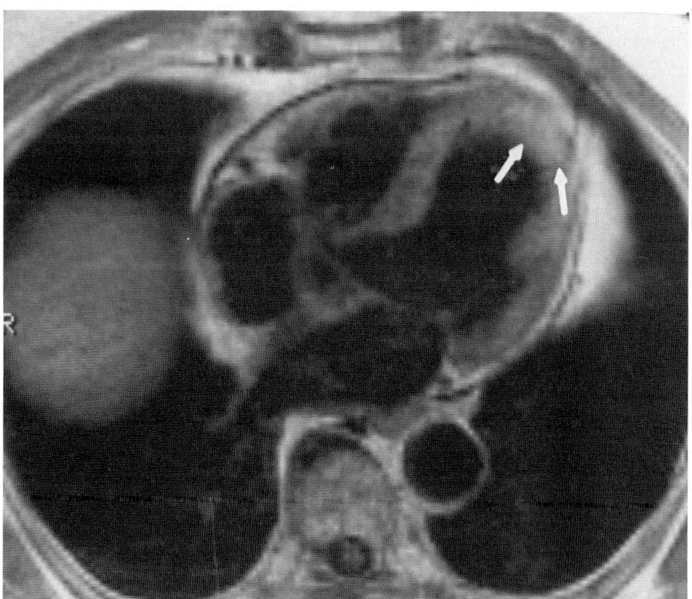

**Figure 2-8.** Gated MRI (transaxial plane) of acute myocardial infarction. The region of acute infarction in the anterior wall has increased signal intensity (*arrows*) compared with the adjacent normal myocardium.

the investigation, the radiographic evaluation becomes a low-yield "fishing expedition."

Most of the non-neuritic causes of nonspecific chronic chest pain can be excluded by performing the following three examinations: chest radiograph, upper gastrointestinal series, and computed tomography with intravenous contrast material.

In nonspecific chronic chest pain, the pretest likelihood of ischemic heart disease is low enough that the exercise $^{201}$Tl scan has been shown to have diagnostic efficacy. In this clinical situation, coronary arteriography should be performed only in those patients with positive exercise thallium scans.

## Bibliography


Adams DF, Abrams HL: Complications of coronary arteriography: A followup report. Cardiovasc Radiol 2:89, 1979

Aldrich RF, Brensike JF, Battaglini JW et al: Coronary calcifications in the detection of coronary artery disease and comparison with electrocardiographic exercise testing. Circulation 59: 1113–1124, 1979

Ascoop CA, Simoons ML, Egmond WG et al: Exercise test, history, and serum lipid levels in patients with chest pain and normal electrocardiogram at risk: Comparison to findings at coronary arteriography. Am Heart J 82:609–617, 1971

Ashburn WL, Tubau J: Myocardial perfusion imaging in ischemic heart disease. Radiol Clin North Am 18:467–486, 1980

Bartel AG, Behar VS, Peter RH et al: Graded exercise stress tests in angiographically documented coronary artery disease. Circulation 49:348–356, 1974

Bartel AG, Chen JT, Peter RH et al: The significance of coronary calcification detected by fluoroscopy. A report of 360 patients. Circulation 49: 1247–1253, 1974

Borer JS, Brensike JF, Redwood DR et al: Limitations of the electrocardiographic response to exercise in predicting coronary-artery disease. N Engl J Med 293:367–371, 1975

Botvinick EH, Taradash MR, Shames DM et al: Thallium-201 myocardial perfusion scintigraphy for the clinical clarification of normal, abnormal, and equivocal electrocardiographic stress tests. Am J Cardiol 41:43–51, 1978

Caldwell JH, Hamilton GW, Sorenson SG et al: The detection of coronary artery disease with radionuclide techniques: A comparison of rest–exercise thallium imaging and ejection fraction response. Circulation 61:610–619, 1980

Dash H, Massie BM, Botvinick EH et al: The noninvasive identification of left main and three-vessel coronary artery disease by myocardial stress perfusion scintigraphy and treadmill exercise electrocardiography. Circulation 60: 276–284, 1979

DeRouen TA, Murray JA, Owen W: Variability in the analysis of coronary arteriograms. Circulation 55:324–328, 1977

Fortuin NJ, Weiss JL: Exercise stress testing. Circulation 56:699–712, 1977

Froelicher VF, Thompson AJ, Lonzo MR, Jr et al: Value of exercise testing for screening asymptomatic men for latent coronary artery disease. Prog Cardiovasc Dis 18:265–276, 1976

Goldstein JA, Schiller NB, Lipton MJ et al: Evaluation of left ventricular thrombi by contrast-enhanced computed tomography and two-dimensional echocardiography. Am J Cardiol 57:757–760, 1986

Grande P, Christiansen C, Pedersen A et al: Optimal diagnosis in acute myocardial infarction. A cost effectiveness study. Circulation 61:723–728, 1980

Heger JJ, Weyman AE, Wann LS et al: Cross-sectional echocardiography in acute myocardial infarction: Detection and localization of regional left ventricular asynergy. Circulation 60:531–538, 1979

Higgins CB, Wexler L, Silverman JF et al: Spontaneously and pharmacologically provoked coronary arterial spasm in Prinzmetal variant angina. Radiology 119:521–527, 1976

Holman BL, Wynne J: Infarct avid (hot spot) myocardial scintigraphy. Radiol Clin North Am 18:487–500, 1980

Kelemen MH, Gillilan RE, Bouchard RJ et al: Diagnosis of obstructive coronary disease by maximal exercise and atrial pacing. Circulation 48: 1227–1233, 1973

Kramer P, Goldstein J, Herfkens R et al: Imaging of acute myocardial infarction in man with contrast-enhanced computed transmission tomography. Am Heart J 108:1514–1523, 1984

Martin CM, McConahay DR: Maximal treadmill exercise electrocardiography. Circulation 46: 956–962, 1972

Mason RE, Likar I, Biern RO et al: Multiple-lead exercise electrocardiography. Circulation 36: 517–525, 1967

McNamara MT, Higgins CB, Schechtmann N et al: Detection and characterization of acute myocardial infarction in man with use of gated magnetic resonance. Circulation 71:717–724, 1985

Pujadas G: Coronary Angiography. New York, McGraw-Hill, 1980

Rifkin RD, Parisi AF, Folland E: Coronary calcification in the diagnosis of coronary artery disease. Am J Cardiol 44:141–147, 1979

Ritchie JL, Hamilton GW, Wacker FJTH (eds): Thallium 201 Myocardial Imaging. New York, Raven Press, 1978

Ritchie JL, Zaret BL, Strauss HW et al: Myocardial imaging with thallium 201: A multicenter study in patients with angina pectoris or acute myocardial infarction. Am J Cardiol 42:345–350, 1978

Roitman D, Jones WB, Sheffield LT: Comparison of submaximal exercise ECG test with coronary cineangiocardiogram. Ann Intern Med 72: 641–647, 1970

Turner DA, Battle WE, Deshmukh H et al: The predictive value of myocardial perfusion scintigraphy after stress in patients without previous myocardial infarction. J Nucl Med 19:249–255, 1978

Zir LM, Miller SW, Dinsmore RE et al: Interobserver variability in coronary angiography. Circulation 53:627–632, 1976

**ANGINA PECTORIS**
**(TRANSIENT, EPISODIC PRECORDIAL OR SUBSTERNAL PAIN)**

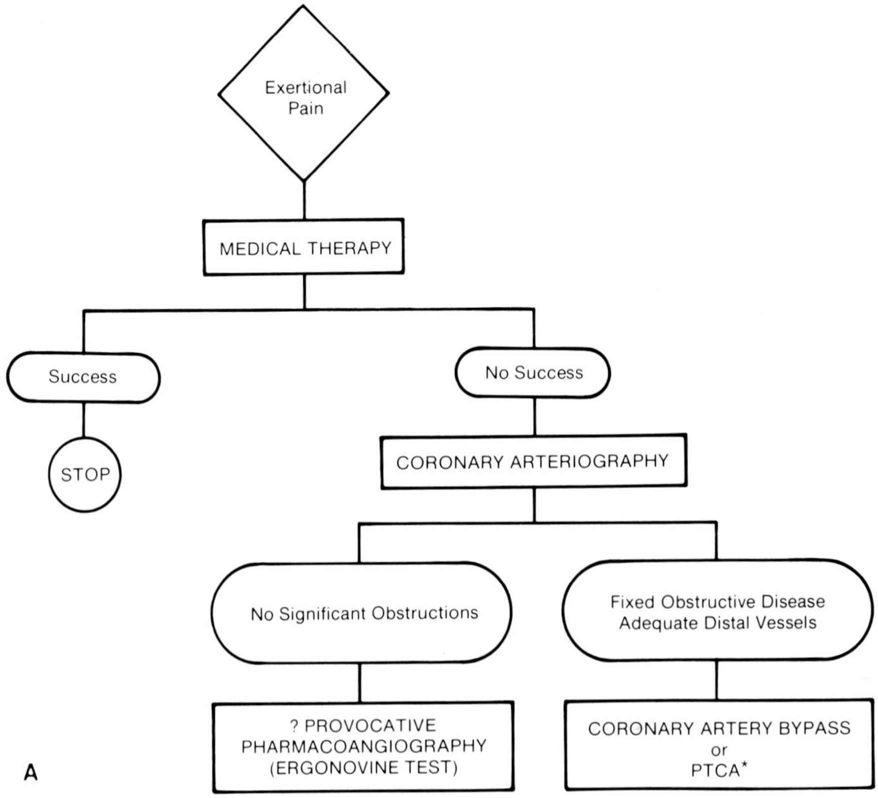


A

*PERCUTANEOUS TRANSCATHETER CORONARY ANGIOPLASTY

**ANGINA PECTORIS**
**(TRANSIENT, EPISODIC PRECORDIAL OR SUBSTERNAL PAIN)**

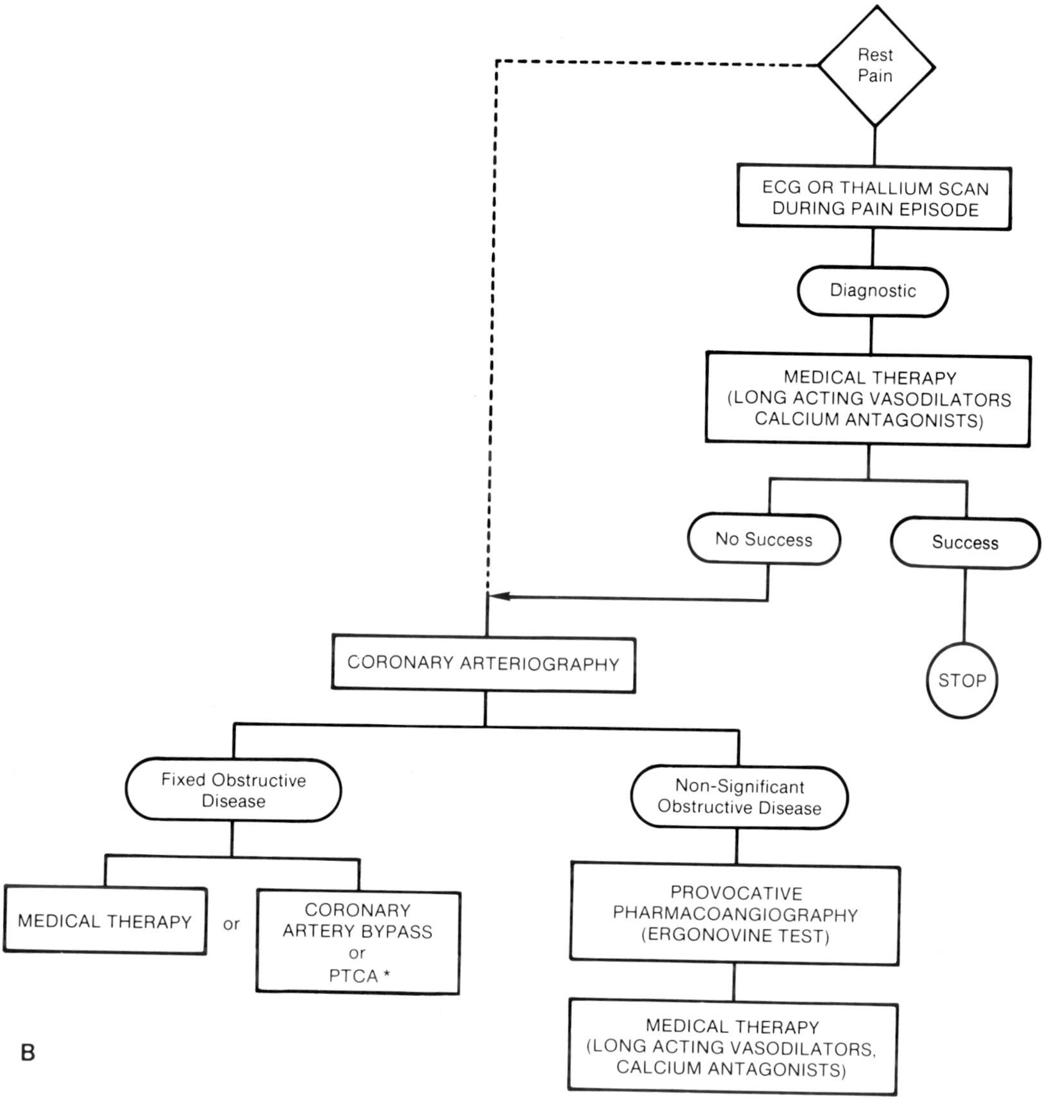


B

* PERCUTANEOUS TRANSCATHETER CORONARY ANGIOPLASTY

SEVERE UNREMITTING PRECORDIAL OR SUBSTERNAL PAIN

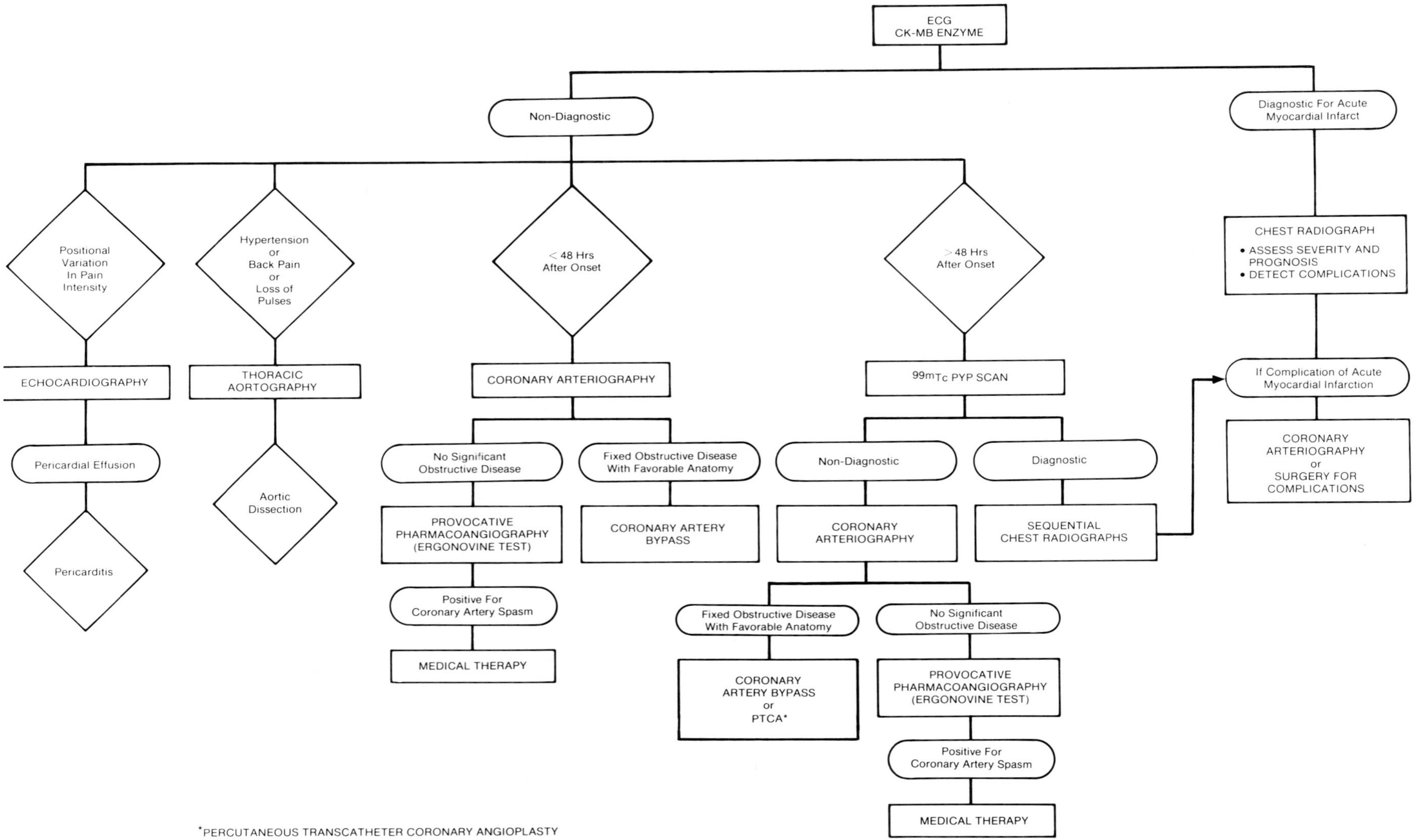


*PERCUTANEOUS TRANSCATHETER CORONARY ANGIOPLASTY

# Chapter 3

# Pulmonary Embolism

*Peter Julien*

Although pulmonary embolism is the most common acute pulmonary problem encountered in hospitalized patients, only 10% of those dying from this disorder (after having survived for at least 1 hour) are accurately diagnosed during life. In addition, half of those dying of massive pulmonary embolism have pathologic evidence of prior embolism that had gone undiagnosed. The mortality rate of patients with pulmonary embolism who are correctly diagnosed and treated (anticoagulation) is one fourth (8% compared with 30%) that of untreated patients with pulmonary embolism who survived at least 1 hour. The main problem in the diagnosis of pulmonary embolism is the nonspecific nature of the signs and symptoms and the consequent low index of suspicion. If attention is drawn to the symptom of dyspnea and the finding of tachypnea in the hospitalized patient without other clear explanation for this finding, then it is estimated that the diagnosis of pulmonary embolism will be considered in 85% of the otherwise undiagnosed patients.

The need to institute anticoagulation therapy as soon as possible in patients with pulmonary emboli and the unnecessary danger of giving these high-complication medications to those without this condition necessitate the prompt and accurate diagnosis of pulmonary embolism.

## CLINICAL AND LABORATORY FINDINGS

The Urokinase–Pulmonary Embolism Trial of patients with extensive embolic obstruction (Tables 3-1 and 3-2) indicates that certain signs and symptoms are helpful in deciding whether to study a patient for pulmonary emboli. Dyspnea and tachypnea, at least transiently, are reasonably constant in the initial presentation and represent adequate justification for proceeding with diagnostic studies. Although pleuritic chest pain is often considered to be characteristic of pulmonary embolism, this symptom is only seen when congestive atelectasis or infarction of the lung occurs. In patients with pulmonary emboli found by arteriography or autopsy, only 10% have a history of pleuritic chest pain. The finding of hypoxemia is totally nonspecific. Approximately 10% to 15% of patients with arteriographically documented pulmonary emboli will have normal $PO_2$ values. It is apparent that these clinical and

**Table 3-1** Symptoms in Patients with Pulmonary Embolism

| Symptom | Percent (%) of Patients |
|---|---|
| Dyspnea | 81 |
| Pleuritic chest pain | 72 |
| Apprehension | 59 |
| Cough | 54 |
| Hemoptysis | 35 |
| Syncope | 5 |
| Substernal chest pain | 5 |

laboratory findings are not sufficient to determine whether anticoagulation or surgical therapy should be instituted.

## DIAGNOSTIC EVALUATION

### *DIAGNOSTIC MODALITIES*

1. Chest radiography
2. Ventilation and perfusion radionuclide studies (V–Q scans)
3. Standard pulmonary arteriography
4. Digital subtraction angiography
5. Low or nonionic contrast pulmonary arteriography
6. Computed tomography
7. Magnetic resonance imaging

**Table 3-2** Physical Findings in Patients with Pulmonary Embolism

| Physical Finding | Percent (%) of Patients |
|---|---|
| Tachypnea | 88 |
| Rales | 54 |
| Wheezing | — |
| Pleural rub | — |
| Elevated $S_2P$ | 54 |
| Pulse > 100 | 43 |
| $S_3$ or $S_4$ | 34 |
| Arrhythmias | 15 |
| Blood pressure (systolic) < 100 torr | 3 |
| Diaphoresis | 33 |
| Temperature > 37.8°C | 42 |
| Thrombophlebitis | 34 |

### Chest Radiography

Although the chest radiograph in patients with pulmonary embolism is classically described as "normal," almost 90% will demonstrate some abnormality. Most of these abnormalities (Table 3-3), however, are so nonspecific that they are of little diagnostic value. The findings of focal oligemia (Westermark's sign, Fig. 3-1) or enlargement of the ipsilateral pulmonary artery (Fleischner's sign, Fig. 3-2) are unusual, although strongly suggestive when present. The pleural-based, wedge-shaped density with a rounded apex (Hampton's hump) is also uncommon but is highly characteristic of pulmonary embolism with infarction. A focal pulmonary infiltrate in the patient with a pulmonary embolism is much more likely to represent focal edema, congestive atelectasis, or hemorrhage than infarction. Infarction occurs in no more than 10% of patients with pulmonary emboli.

The lack of specificity of the chest film makes it of little value in the precise diagnosis of pulmonary embolism. A normal chest radiograph does not exclude pulmonary embolism. There are two major reasons for obtaining a chest film. The first is to exclude other causes for the patient's dyspnea, tachypnea, or pleuritic

**Table 3-3** Chest Radiograph Findings in Acute Pulmonary Embolism

| Findings | Percent (%) of Patients |
|---|---|
| Infiltrate | 54 |
| Pleural effusion | 51 |
| Atelectasis | 27 |
| Elevated hemidiaphragm | 17 |
| Two or more of the above | 44 |
| Focal oligemia only | 2 |
| Cardiomegaly or congestive failure | 17 |
| Pulmonary arterial hypertension | 5 |
| Normal | 7 |

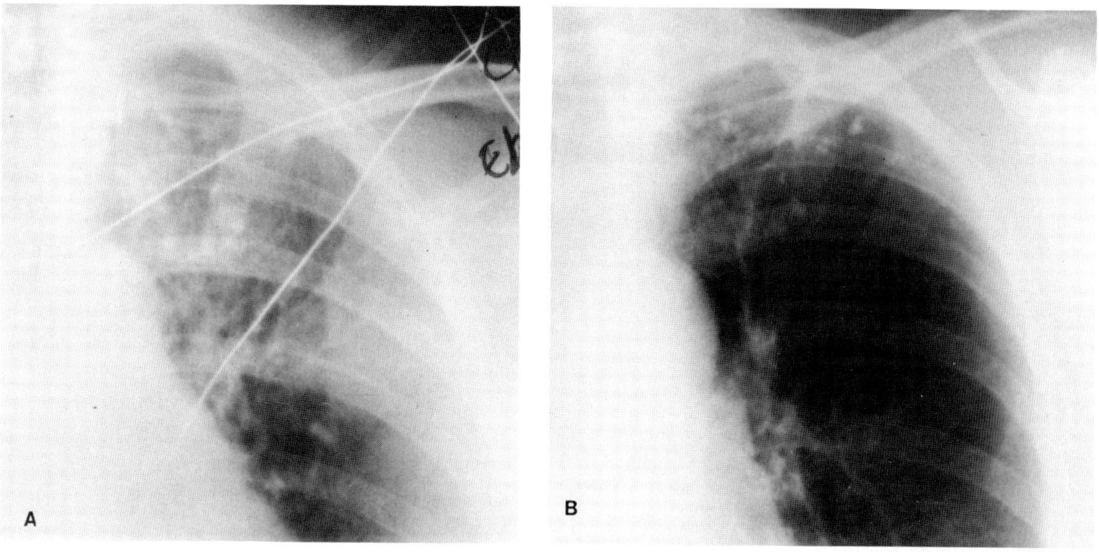

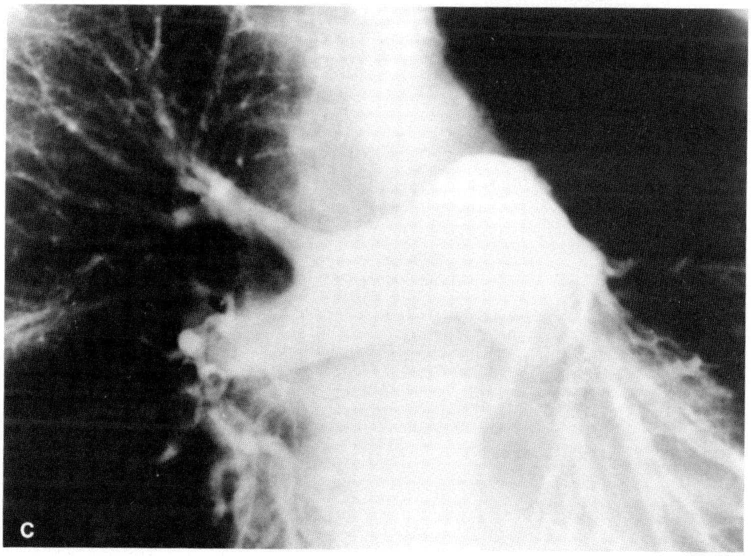

**Figure 3-1.** Westermark's sign. **(A)** Baseline chest radiograph. **(B)** Hyperlucency of left upper lobe coinciding with onset of patient's symptoms. **(C)** Arteriogram performed the same day as *B*, demonstrating an occluding clot in the left upper lobe and multiple emboli in the right lung.

chest pain (*e.g.*, a pneumothorax). The second is that the chest radiograph is indispensable for the accurate interpretation of the radionuclide lung scan (*e.g.*, do the abnormalities on the V–Q scan match abnormalities on the chest radiograph?).

### Ventilation and Perfusion Radionuclide Studies

The most controversial area in the diagnosis of pulmonary embolism is the precise value and role of the radionuclide lung scan. The perfusion lung scan, with or without a ventilation scan, is currently considered the most effective screening test for significant pulmonary thromboembolic disease. The sensitivity of the perfusion lung scan in detecting thromboembolic disease is very high; indeed, in the Urokinase–Pulmonary Embolism Trial, there were no instances in which the lung scan was completely normal when the arteriogram showed pulmonary emboli. For optimum accuracy, the perfusion study requires six views after injection of the radionuclide (most commonly $^{99m}$Tc macroaggregated particles of approximately 10μ to 50μ in diameter). The ventilation scan is performed with $^{133}$Xe and includes the washin, equilibrium, and washout phases in a single posterior projection, or additional projections after the perfusion scan to optimize the match or mismatch. These three phases of the xenon examination are necessary because air-trapping (be it on the basis of chronic obstructive pulmonary disease or tumor) is a dynamic event requiring physiologic nonstatic images for the greatest degree of diagnostic accuracy. The washout phase has clearly been shown to be the most sensitive part of the xenon examination, far exceeding the accuracy of a single equilibrium static image (Fig. 3-3). Both the ventilation and perfusion scans must be interpreted with full knowledge of the findings on chest radiography.

A newer ventilation technique involves the use of an aerosol of $^{99m}$Tc diethylenetriamine-penta-acetic acid ($^{99m}$Tc-DTPA) or $^{99m}$Tc sulfur colloid. This has the advantage of allowing ventilation imaging to be performed in the same six views as the perfusion examination because of the retention of the aerosol particles within the lung over the entire time of the examination (Fig. 3-4). Because of the shorter biologic half-life of $^{133}$Xe and the lack of retention within the lung (xenon is a gas), additional views can be obtained only with multiple separate ventilation

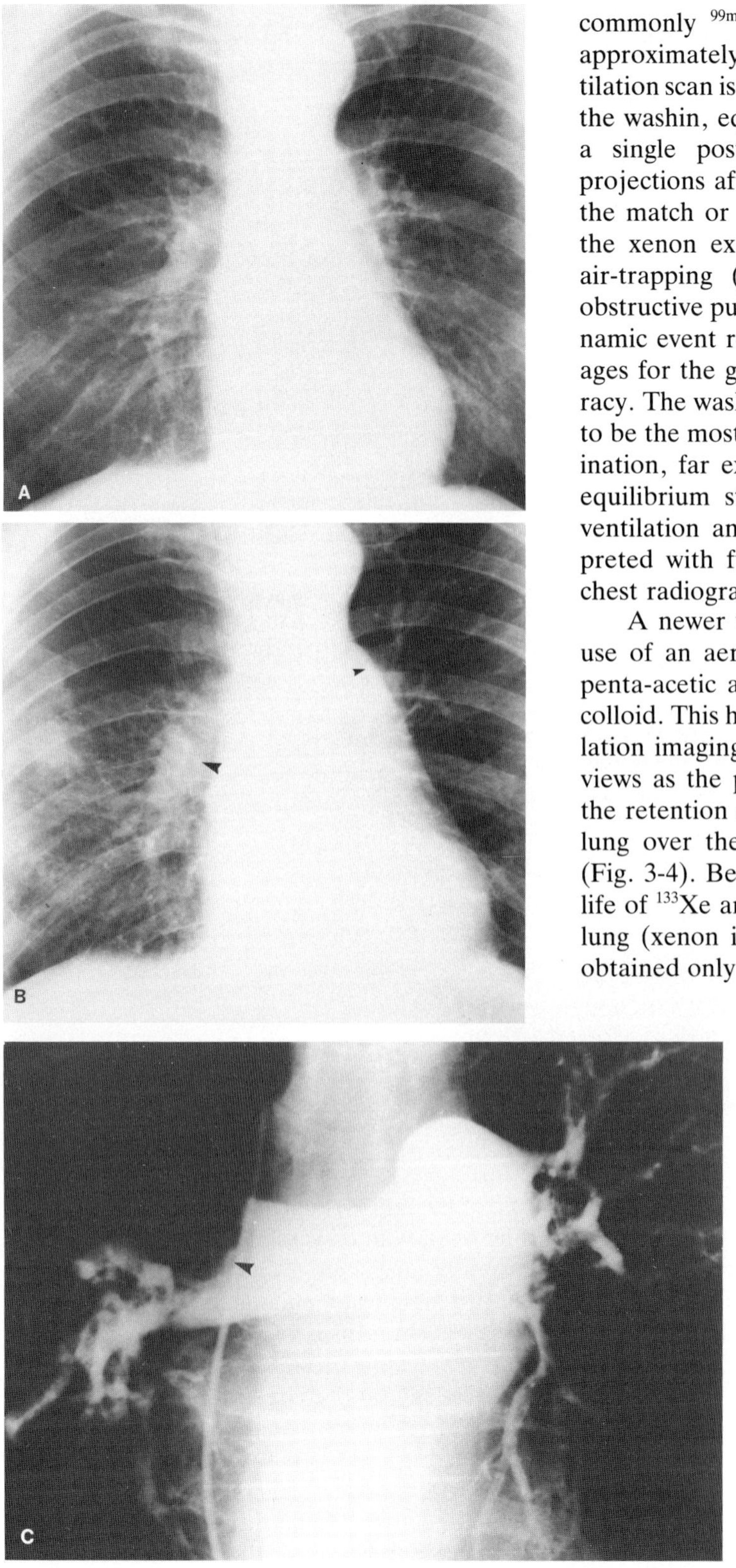


**Figure 3-2.** Fleischner's sign. **(A)** Baseline chest radiograph. **(B)** Enlargement of main pulmonary artery (*small arrow*) and right pulmonary artery (*large arrow*). **(C)** Arteriogram demonstrating multiple bilateral pulmonary emboli with large right saddle embolus (*arrow*).

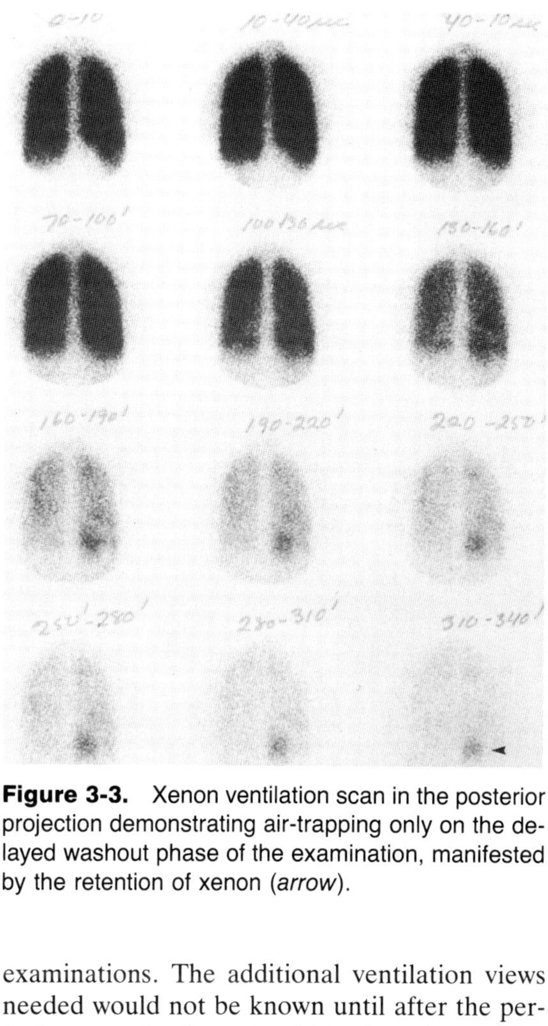

**Figure 3-3.** Xenon ventilation scan in the posterior projection demonstrating air-trapping only on the delayed washout phase of the examination, manifested by the retention of xenon (*arrow*).

examinations. The additional ventilation views needed would not be known until after the perfusion examination, at which time the quality of repeated washout images with $^{133}Xe$ (81 KeV) is limited by background activity secondary to scatter from the higher energy (164 KeV) technetium. However, by using subtraction of background technetium and a 10% window for xenon detection, postperfusion xenon ventilation views can be significantly improved. The ideal half-life and optimal energy of technetium gives it a higher inherent resolution than the xenon studies. The use of the same radionuclide for both perfusion and ventilation studies requires that the dose of aerosol be far higher (three times) than the amount given for the perfusion, or that a computer subtraction program be used. Overall, radioaerosol and xenon ventilation images appear to be diagnostically equivalent as an adjunct to perfusion scans in evaluation of patients with suspected pulmonary emboli.

The specificity of an abnormal perfusion and ventilation lung scan is not nearly as high as its sensitivity. Perfusion defects can be caused by almost any pulmonary parenchymal abnormality as well as by a number of extraparenchymal processes, such as pleural effusion (Fig. 3-5).

There are four broad interpretations of radionuclide ventilation–perfusion examinations:

1. Normal
2. Low probability for pulmonary embolism
3. Indeterminate for pulmonary embolism
4. High probability for pulmonary embolism

This classification is based on an analysis of the size and number of perfusion defects compared with the ventilation study and the chest radiograph.

1. A normal perfusion examination is considered excellent evidence for the absence of pulmonary emboli.
2. The low-probability V–Q scan is defined as small V–Q mismatches with no corresponding radiographic abnormalities or areas of V–Q match or mismatch in which the perfusion scan is substantially smaller than corresponding radiographic abnormalities (Fig. 3-6).
3. The indeterminate V–Q scan is defined as diffuse, severe airway obstruction; matched perfusion defects (regardless of ventilation); and radiographic abnormalities or a single larger subsegmental V–Q mismatch without corresponding radiographic abnormality (Fig. 3-7).
4. The high probability V–Q scan is defined as perfusion defects substantially larger than chest film abnormalities or one or more segmental or lobar, or two or more large subsegmental V–Q mismatches with no corresponding radiographic abnormalities (Fig. 3–8).

One major cause of controversy in these definitions is the comparison of the size of the perfusion defect relative to that of the radiographic abnormality. Although perfusion defects larger than the corresponding radiographic abnormality are said to have a high probability for pulmo-

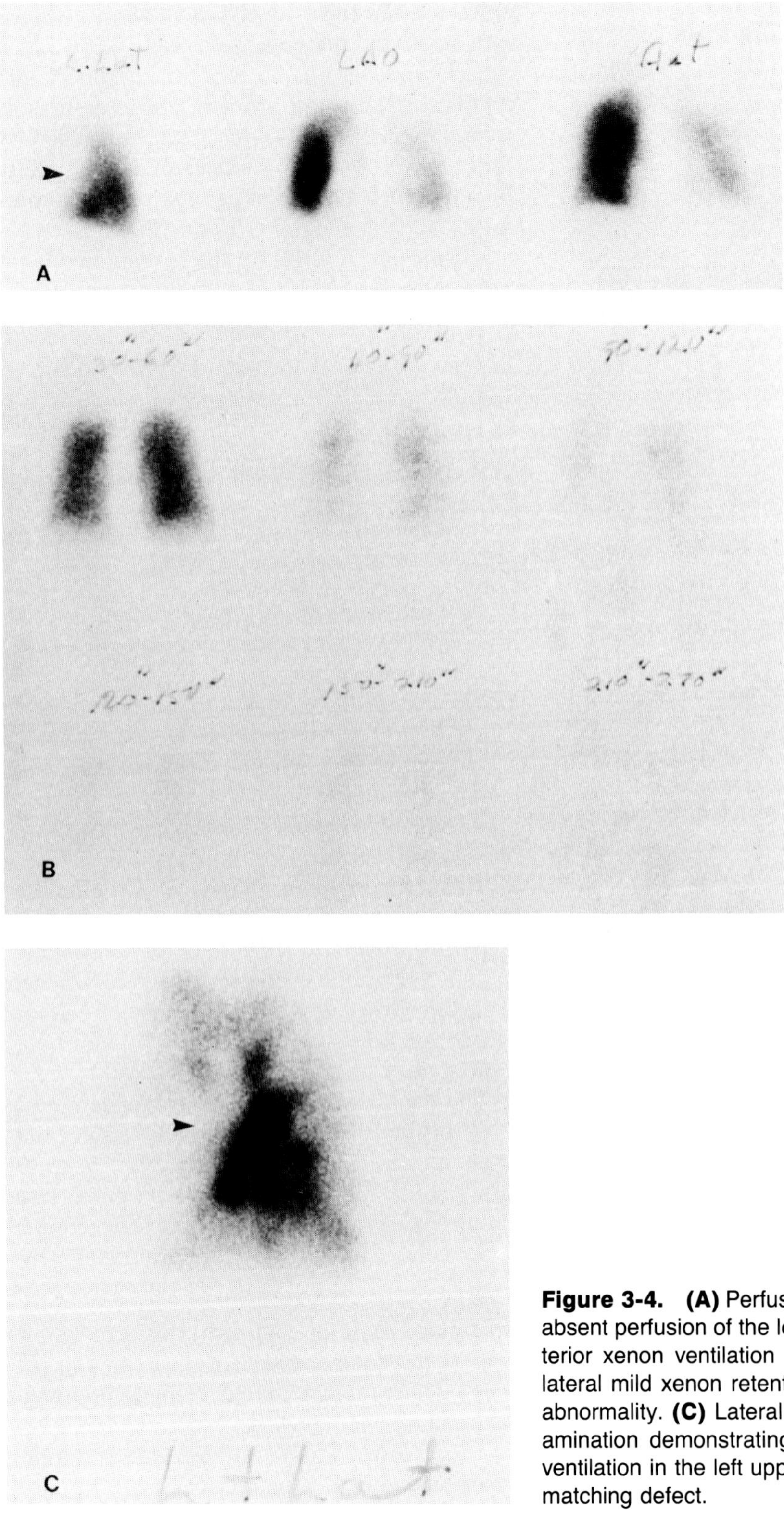


**Figure 3-4.** **(A)** Perfusion examination demonstrating absent perfusion of the left upper lobe (*arrow*). **(B)** Posterior xenon ventilation examination demonstrating bilateral mild xenon retention far less than the perfusion abnormality. **(C)** Lateral view of aerosol ventilation examination demonstrating almost complete absence of ventilation in the left upper lobe (*arrow*), representing a matching defect.

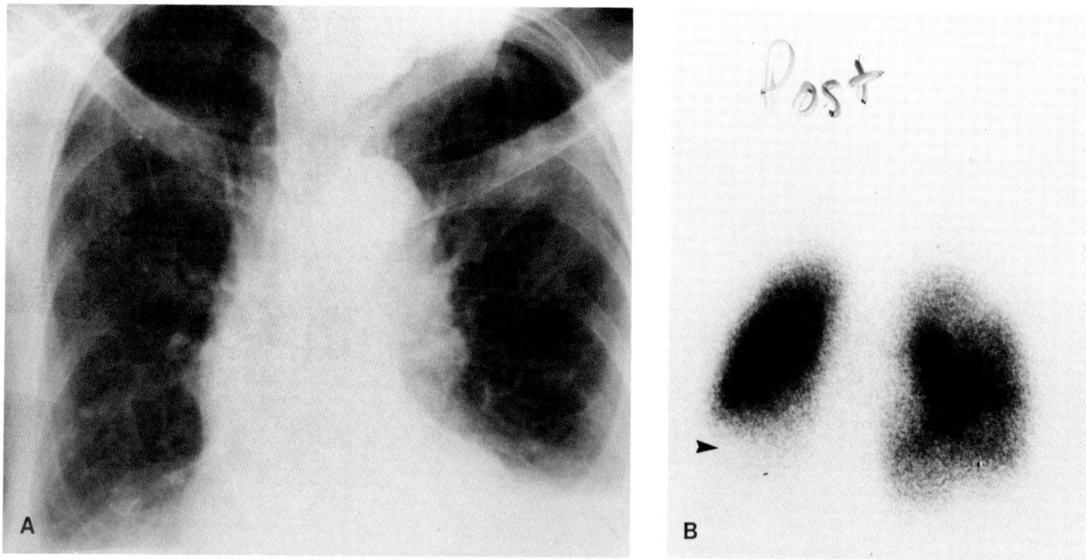

**Figure 3-5.** **(A)** Chest radiograph demonstrating a large left and small right pleural effusion. **(B)** Posterior view of perfusion examination demonstrating marked decrease in perfusion at the left base (*arrow*).

nary embolism (particularly if associated with a ventilation scan that is normal or has only minor abnormalities), I have found this pattern with well-documented pneumonia and continue to place patients with these radionuclide findings in the indeterminate category (Fig. 3-9). One other sign that I feel should probably enable the physician to put the patient in the high-probability category is a generalized decrease in perfusion to one lung with relatively normal ventilation and a normal chest film. This has usually been secondary to a large, partially occluding central embolism in the absence of evidence for a perihilar tumor (Figs. 3-10 and 3-11).

The sensitivity and specificity of the radionuclide examination using these classifications have been compared to the arteriographic data in several medical centers; the data are combined in Table 3-4. It should be remembered that patients with infarction, congestive atelectasis, or bronchospasm secondary to pulmonary embolism can have matching V–Q defects. Mismatch defects can occur in patients without pulmonary emboli who have chronic left heart failure, vasculitis, focal hypoxia, hyper- or hypocarbia, or any cause of an increased density on the chest radiograph (including pleural effusion). It is impossible to predict from the chest film whether the visible abnormalities are more likely to affect ventilation more than perfusion, or perfusion more than ventilation, or the two equally (Fig. 3-12). Therefore, these patients are placed in the indeterminate category. An apparent mismatch can also occur because of the inherent lower resolution of the xenon ventilation examination (related to the lower energy level of the isotope) or to the fact that the examination is performed in the posterior position without the advantage of the oblique views that are used in the perfusion study (see Fig. 3-4).

In summary, the overall sensitivity of the perfusion radionuclide examination is near 100%. The specificity of the high-probability perfusion examination (*i.e.*, percentage of arteriographically proven pulmonary emboli) is 75% to 80%. If the ventilation study is normal, the accuracy then climbs to 90% to 95%. The low-probability perfusion examination (less than 25% chance of pulmonary emboli) can be reduced to less than a 10% chance if a matching ventilation abnormality is demonstrated. However, only the normal perfusion scan is 100% in its diagnostic accuracy and neither the high-

*(Text continues on p. 58.)*

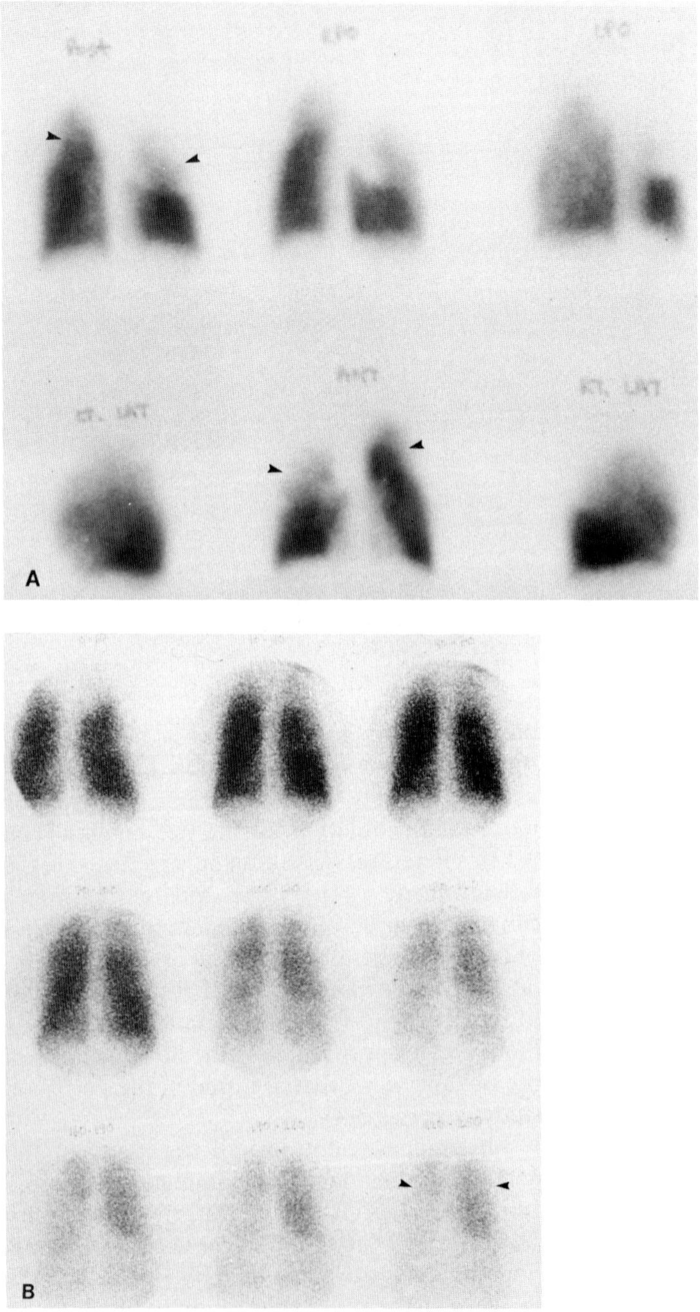

**Figure 3-6.** Low-probability examination. **(A)** Perfusion examination demonstrating decreased perfusion to both upper lobes (*arrows*). **(B)** Posterior view of xenon ventilation examination with matching retention of xenon on the washout phase (*arrows*).

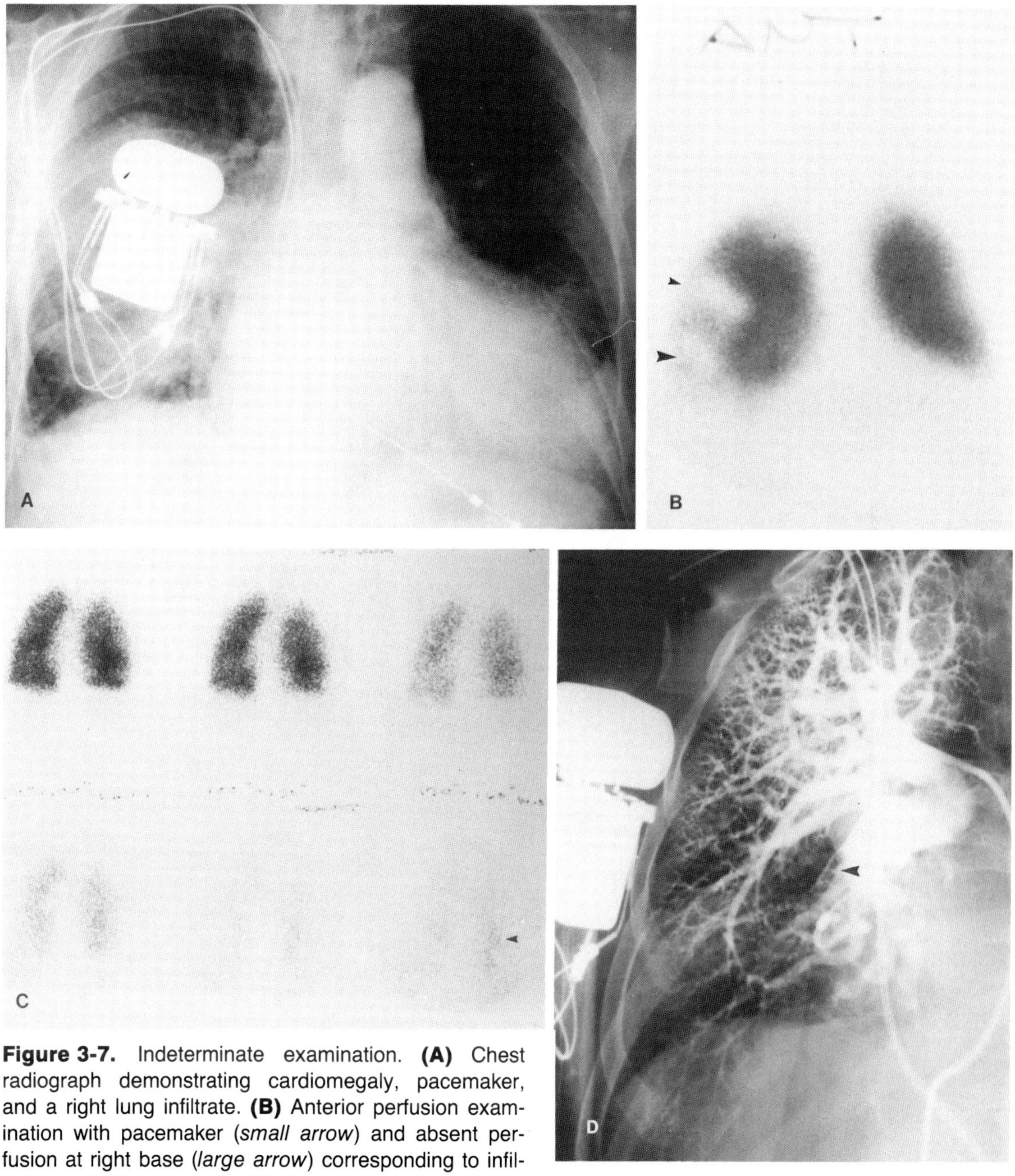

**Figure 3-7.** Indeterminate examination. **(A)** Chest radiograph demonstrating cardiomegaly, pacemaker, and a right lung infiltrate. **(B)** Anterior perfusion examination with pacemaker (*small arrow*) and absent perfusion at right base (*large arrow*) corresponding to infiltrate on chest radiograph. **(C)** Posterior xenon ventilation examination demonstrating air-trapping predominantly at the right base (*arrow*). **(D)** Arteriogram demonstrating an embolus in the branch to the right lower lobe (*arrow*).

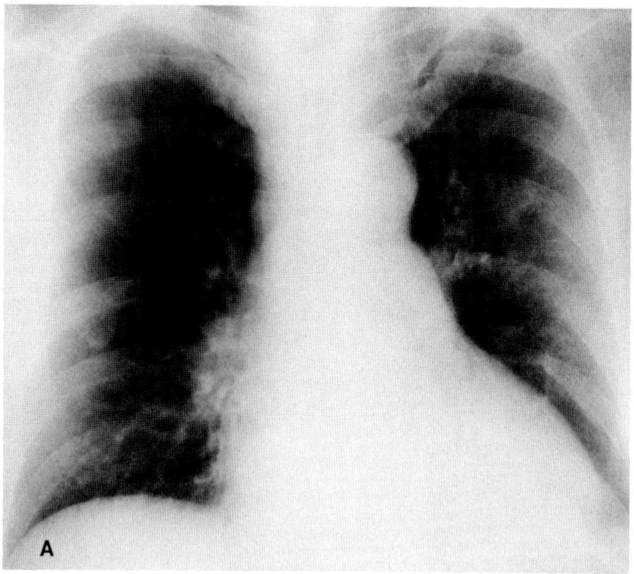

**Figure 3-8.** High-probability examination. **(A)** Chest radiograph showing small left effusion. **(B)** Perfusion lung scan demonstrating segmental perfusion defects and lobar defect in right lung (*arrow*). **(C)** Normal xenon ventilation scan on the right. **(D)** Arteriogram demonstrating multiple bilateral emboli and a large saddle embolus at the bifurcation of the right pulmonary artery (*arrow*). (*Continued on facing page*)

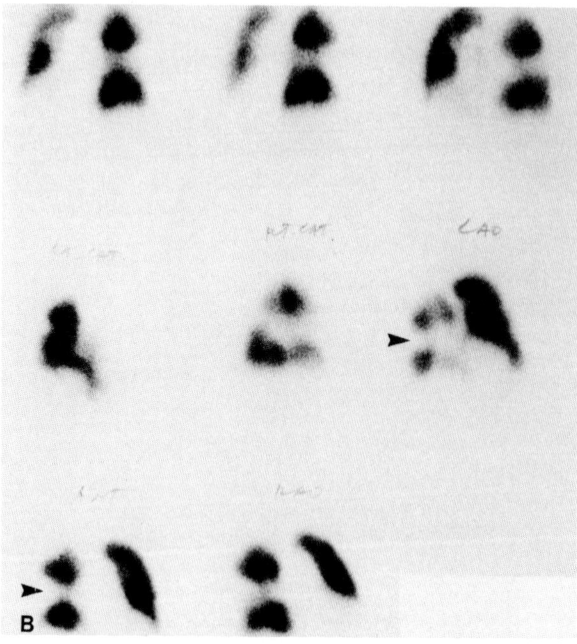

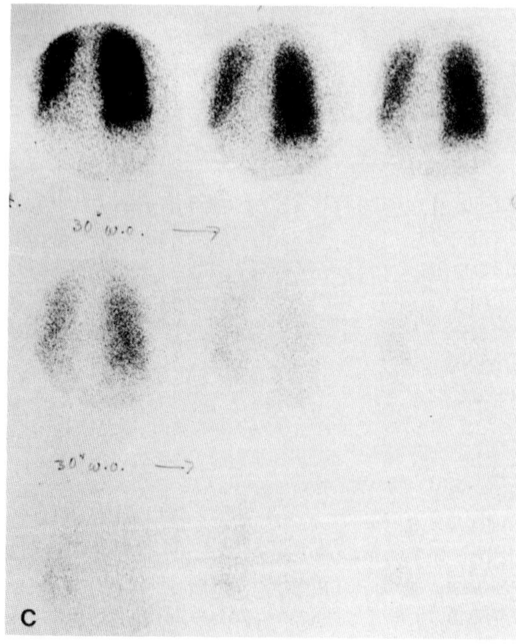

probability nor low-probability scan can be used with that degree of accuracy to prove or disprove pulmonary emboli. In an attempt to improve the accuracy of V–Q scanning for detecting pulmonary emboli, the use of Bayes theorem has become popular in some medical centers. This analysis is based on the following concept: the probability that a patient with a given V–Q finding truly has pulmonary emboli is dependent on both the pretest probability that the patient has the disease and the sensitivity and specificity of the test. The major problem with Bayesian analysis is that there is no accurate method available to assign pretest probabilities (prevalence) of pulmonary emboli based upon patients' histories, clinical findings, and laboratory tests.

Although it is generally assumed that there is no contraindication to the radionuclide exam-

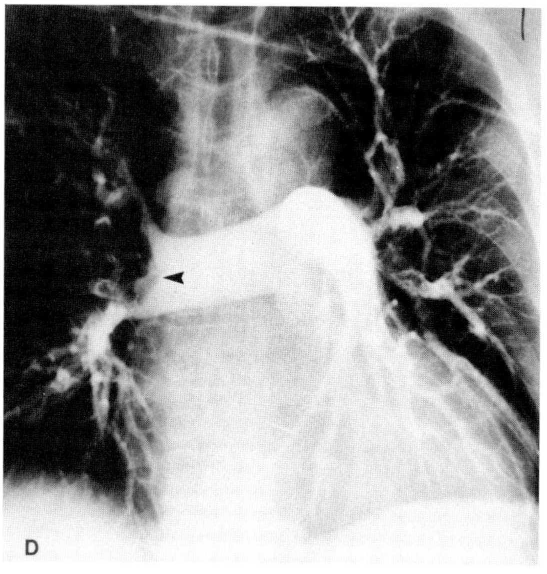

ination, four patients have been reported who died shortly after the intravenous injection of $^{99m}Tc$ macroaggregated albumin. These patients all had severe pulmonary hypertension, half on the basis of chronic pulmonary emboli and the others due to scleroderma. In the normal lung, the injection of 10-μ to 50-μ particles of $^{99m}Tc$ macroaggregated albumin will occlude approximately 0.1% of the cross-sectional area of the pulmonary vasculature at the precapillary level. The lungs of the four patients who died had severe obliterative vascular disease, and it is believed that the injected particles occluded much of the already limited vascular bed at the precapillary level, leading to marked further elevation of pulmonary artery pressure with subsequent production of severe respiratory distress, cyanosis, and shock. The current approach to patients with known severe pulmonary hypertension and possible pulmonary emboli is to give either a slow intravenous injection of uniformly small (less than 50-μ particles with high specific activity, or to use $^{99m}Tc$ human serum albumin microspheres, which have a higher specific activity, greater uniformity, and smaller size (10μ–30μ) than the macroaggregated particles. This technique should increase the margin of safety of the radionuclide lung scan in the patient with severe pulmonary hypertension.

## Pulmonary Arteriography

The pulmonary arteriogram remains the most definitive and specific test for the diagnosis of pulmonary embolism. The arteriographic criteria needed for the unequivocal diagnosis of pulmonary embolism are an intraluminal filling defect or a vascular cutoff (Fig. 3-13). The interpretation of the pulmonary arteriogram is known to have some inherent observer variability. In a large cooperative study, the use of these criteria resulted in an observer disagreement in the range of 6% compared with 67% disagreement in the interpretation of radionuclide lung scans. The findings of areas of oligemia, slow flow, or absent or delayed venous filling are secondary signs that are not sufficient to make a definitive diagnosis of pulmonary embolism. They can also be found in the previously described nonembolic conditions that produce oligemia on the radionuclide perfusion scan. Using the highly specific criteria of an intravascular filling defect or vascular cutoff, the sensitivity of a single anteroposterior injection into the main pulmonary artery (without magnification) is 80% to 85%. With the addition of oblique selective injections, magnification, and superselective injections, virtually 100% of clots 2 mm or larger can be detected and excellent correlation of the arteriogram with the perfusion radionuclide scan can be achieved. Most of the data correlating the arteriogram with the presence and size of the pulmonary emboli come from experimental evidence in dogs. In several small series of autopsies in humans, the accuracy of true-positive and true-negative arteriograms was shown to be 100%. Another clinically important method used to assess the accuracy of the negative pulmonary arteriogram is to follow those patients with negative arteriograms who are not treated with anticoagulation. In patients who have been followed for up to 6 months, no emboli have been detected clinically. Therefore, from the clinical standpoint, it does appear that the arteriogram can be considered as a "gold standard" on which the accuracy of the radionuclide studies studies can be assessed and the clinical diagnosis of pulmonary embolism confirmed.

Once the accuracy of pulmonary arteriography is established, there are three major prob-

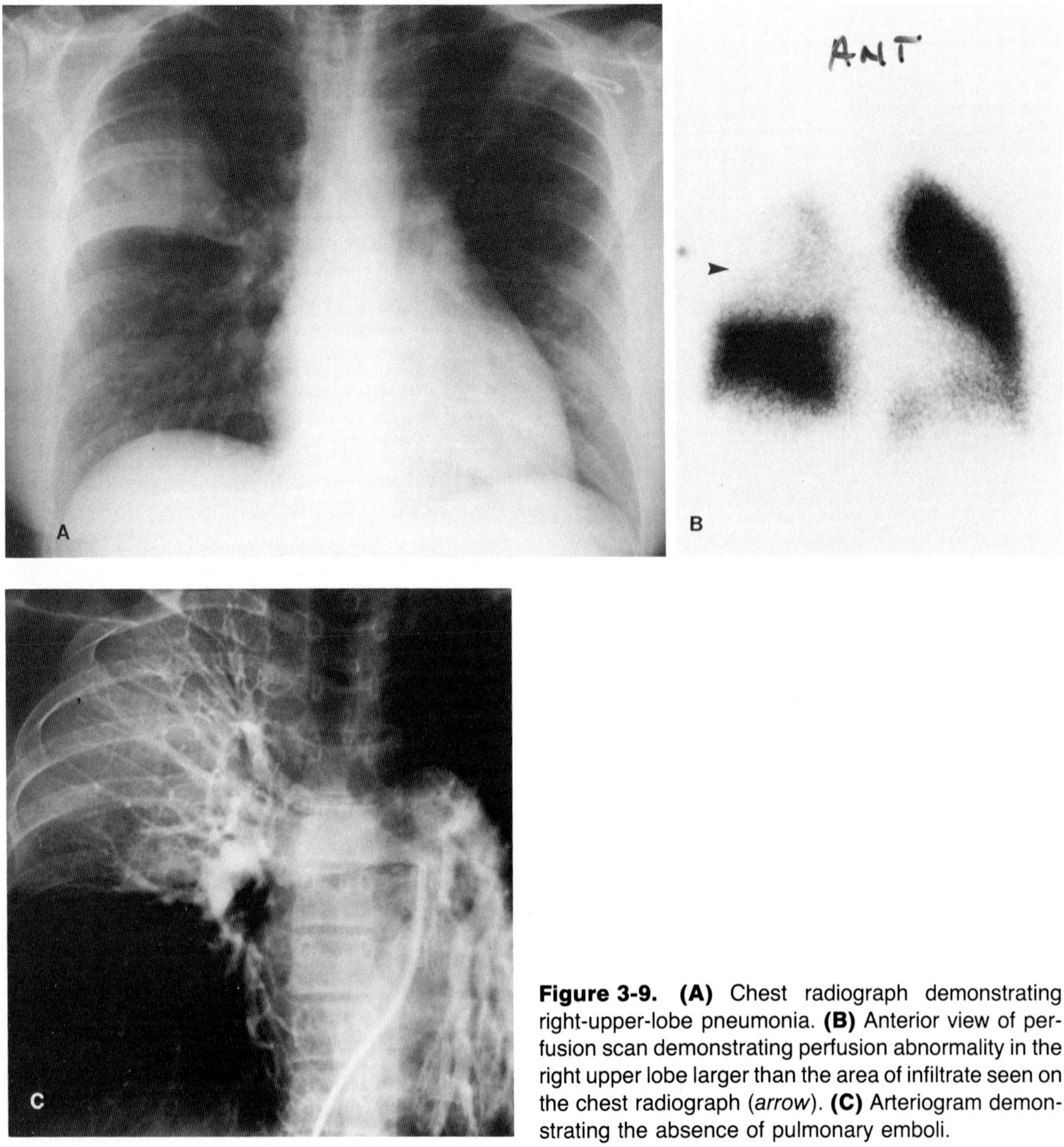


**Figure 3-9.** **(A)** Chest radiograph demonstrating right-upper-lobe pneumonia. **(B)** Anterior view of perfusion scan demonstrating perfusion abnormality in the right upper lobe larger than the area of infiltrate seen on the chest radiograph (*arrow*). **(C)** Arteriogram demonstrating the absence of pulmonary emboli.

lems that must be addressed in the evaluation of this procedure: patient selection, the problem of delay in performing the arteriogram, and complications of the procedure.

The decision to subject the patient to pulmonary arteriography is based on clinical circumstances, findings on chest radiography, and the ventilation and perfusion radionuclide scans (Table 3-4). It must be remembered that heparin administration is the leading cause of adverse drug reactions in hospitalized patients and that Coumadin (crystalline warfarin sodium) therapy also is associated with significant bleeding complications. In addition, the mere act of labeling a patient unnecessarily with the diagnosis of pulmonary embolism can have serious long-term effects, because other causes for future chest pain, dyspnea, and other symptoms may be overlooked because of the previous "documented" diagnosis. Therefore, patients for whom there is

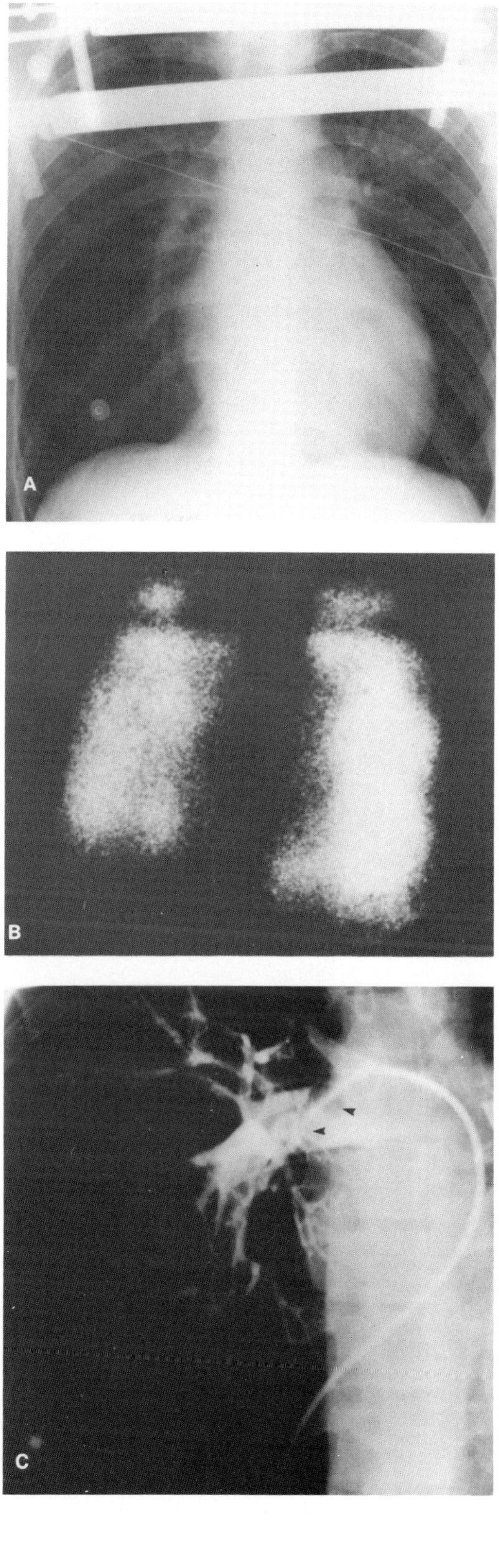

**Figure 3-10. (A)** Normal chest radiograph. **(B)** Anterior perfusion examination with decreased perfusion of entire right lung. **(C)** Arteriogram demonstrating central embolus (*arrows*) partially occluding right pulmonary artery.

a high degree of clinical suspicion of pulmonary embolism but who have low-probability or indeterminate radionuclide scans and who are candidates for treatment with anticoagulation should undergo pulmonary arteriography. Patients who are candidates for venous interruption (either surgically or through interventional radiology) or embolectomy, or who have other medical problems for which anticoagulation is extremely hazardous, also require pulmonary arteriography. Even in patients for whom the need for arteriography is quite apparent, the radionuclide examination should be performed first. If the radionuclide scan is unequivocally normal, there is no need for arteriography. If abnormalities are detected on the radionuclide study, they guide the arteriographer to specific areas requiring selective study. In patients examined by arteriography without the benefit of the radionuclide examination, less than 15% will be positive for pulmonary emboli. With chest radiographic evidence of severe lung disease (*e.g.*, diffuse pneumonia, severe bullous emphysema, severe congestive heart failure), the specificity of the radionuclide examination decreases, and in these severely ill patients one can make an argument to go directly to arteriography.

Clot lysis and an associated normal arteriogram have been reported as early as 24 hours following an acute pulmonary embolism. The natural history of pulmonary emboli indicates that most patients will have arteriographically identifiable clots for 7 to 10 days. However, because of the spontaneous dissolution of the clots, I strongly advise against performing arteriography more than 5 days after the suspected embolic episode unless the patient exhibits recurring or continuing symptoms (Fig. 3-14).

Although arteriography is the most specific of the diagnostic tests for pulmonary emboli, it also carries the greatest risk. The 1% to 2% morbidity of the procedure includes patients who develop cardiac arrhythmias, cardiac arrest,

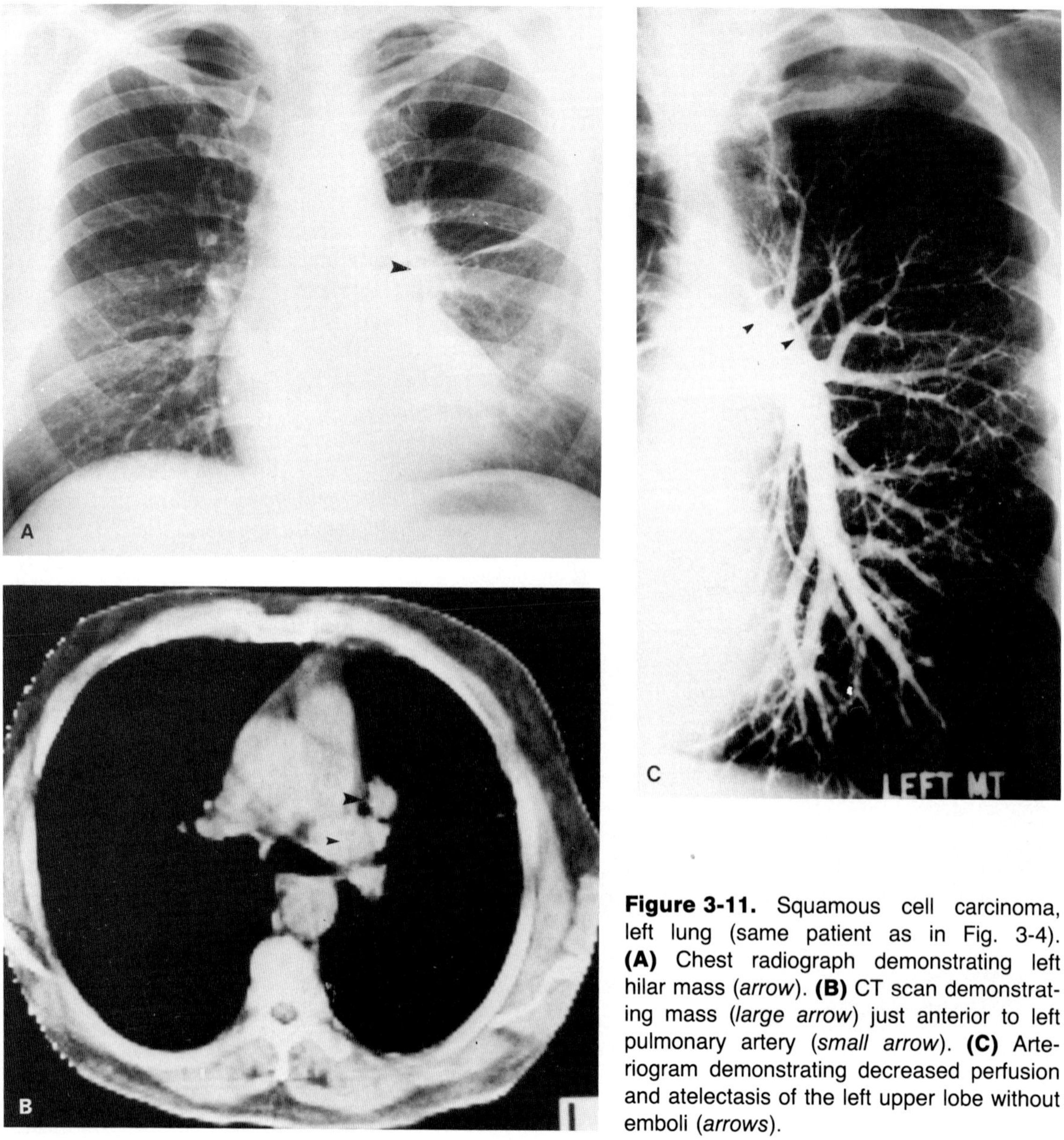


**Figure 3-11.** Squamous cell carcinoma, left lung (same patient as in Fig. 3-4). **(A)** Chest radiograph demonstrating left hilar mass (*arrow*). **(B)** CT scan demonstrating mass (*large arrow*) just anterior to left pulmonary artery (*small arrow*). **(C)** Arteriogram demonstrating decreased perfusion and atelectasis of the left upper lobe without emboli (*arrows*).

or a reaction to contrast material. Complications relating to perforation or direct injury can be avoided with the use of an end- and sidehole pigtail catheter (Grollman). Fatalities (0.1%–0.5%) usually occur in patients with severe pulmonary hypertension secondary to pulmonary emboli, congenital heart disease, or primary pulmonary hypertension. In these patients, there is the immediate development of systemic hypotension, apnea, cardiac arrest, and death despite attempts at resuscitation. Although the exact mechanism of these fatal complications is not clear, it appears to be related to the volume and tonicity of the solution injected. If the pulmonary artery mean pressure is more than 40 torr, selective rather than main pulmonary artery injections are recommended (a maximum of 40 ml/injection of contrast in each

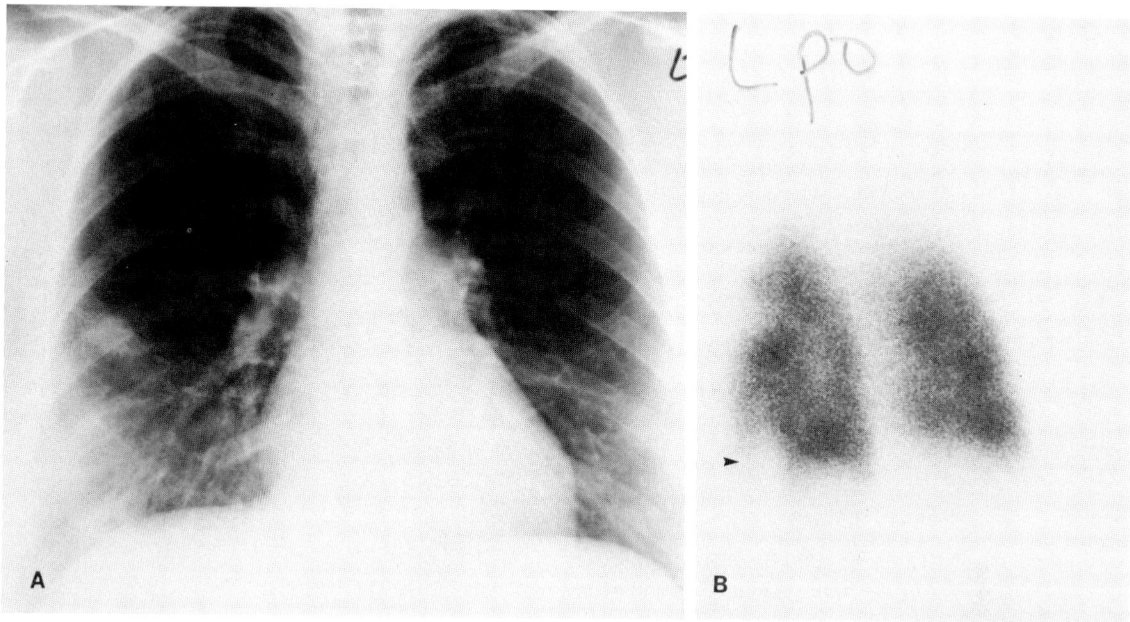


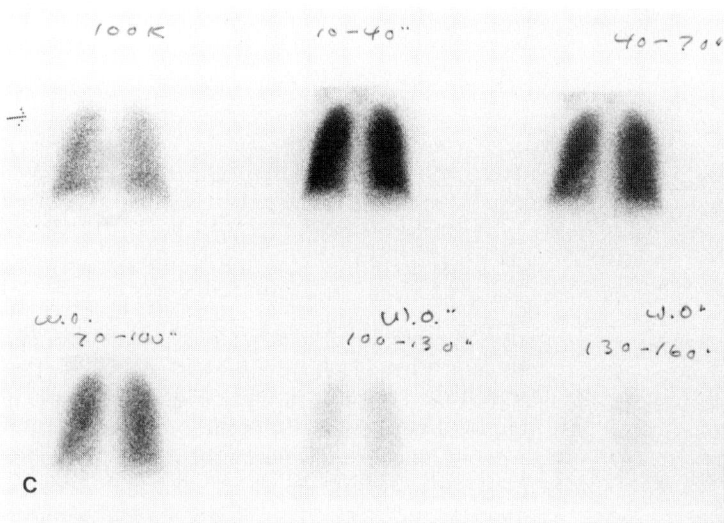


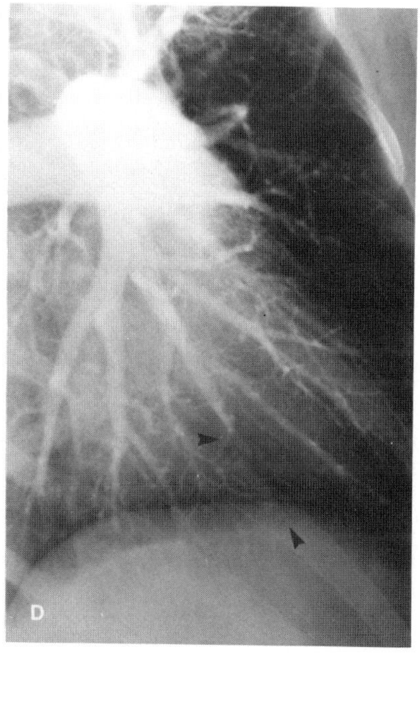


**Figure 3-12.** Wegener's granulomatosis. **(A)** Chest radiograph demonstrating bilateral infiltrates. **(B)** Left posterior oblique perfusion scan with segmental defect at left base (*arrow*). **(C)** Normal xenon ventilation scan. **(D)** Left posterior oblique pulmonary arteriogram demonstrating focal area of decreased perfusion (*arrows*), corresponding to the defect seen in *B* but secondary to vasculitis rather than emboli.

**Table 3-4** Comparison of V–Q Examinations and Pulmonary Arteriography

| Scan Interpretation | Pattern | Percent (%) of Arteriographically Proven Emboli |
|---|---|---|
| Normal | Normal perfusion | 0 |
| Low probability | Small V–Q mismatches | 0 |
| | Small V–Q mismatches with no corresponding radiograpic abnormalities | 5 |
| | Perfusion defects substantially smaller than radiographic abnormalities regardless of ventilation | 8 |
| Indeterminate | Diffuse, severe obstructive pulmonary disease | 20 |
| | Matched perfusion defects and radiographic abnormalities (regardless of ventilation) | 30 |
| | Single moderate subsegmental V–Q mismatch without radiographic abnormality | 33 |
| High probability | Perfusion defects substantially larger than radiographic abnormalities | 87 |
| | 1 or more segmental or lobar or 2 or more large subsegmental V–Q mismatches with no corresponding radiographic abnormalities | 92 |

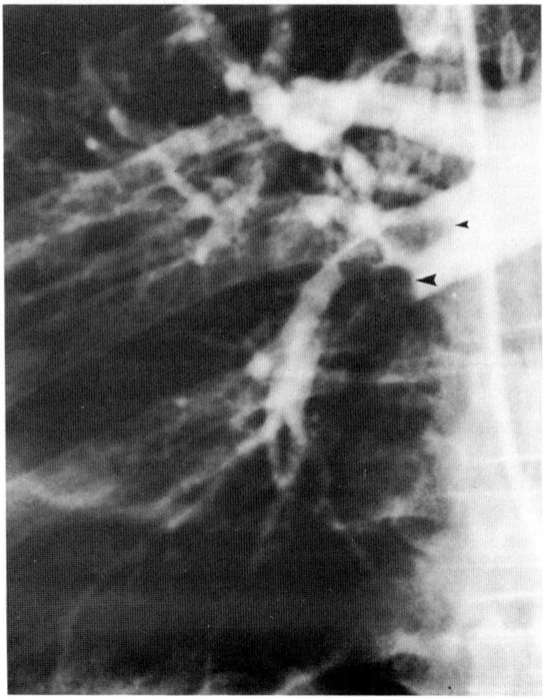

**Figure 3-13.** Pulmonary arteriogram demonstrating intraluminal filling defect (*small arrow*) and vascular cutoff (*large arrow*).

pulmonary artery). If the right ventricular end-diastolic pressure is more than 20 torr, indicating a severely compromised right heart, I recommend using either low- or nonionic contrast agents (see following section on low or nonionic contrast pulmonary arteriography). Absolute contraindications to pulmonary arteriography are a history of severe anaphylactic reaction to iodinated contrast material and the presence of an acute myocardial infarction. Relative contraindications include marked ventricular irritability, left bundle-branch block, and severe pulmonary hypertension.

Although morbidity and mortality are associated with pulmonary arteriography, they are clearly outweighed by the danger of falsely labeling a patient with the diagnosis of "pulmonary embolism" and instituting unnecessary and hazardous anticoagulation therapy.

## Digital Subtraction Pulmonary Angiography

In an attempt to decrease the complications of standard pulmonary arteriography that are re-

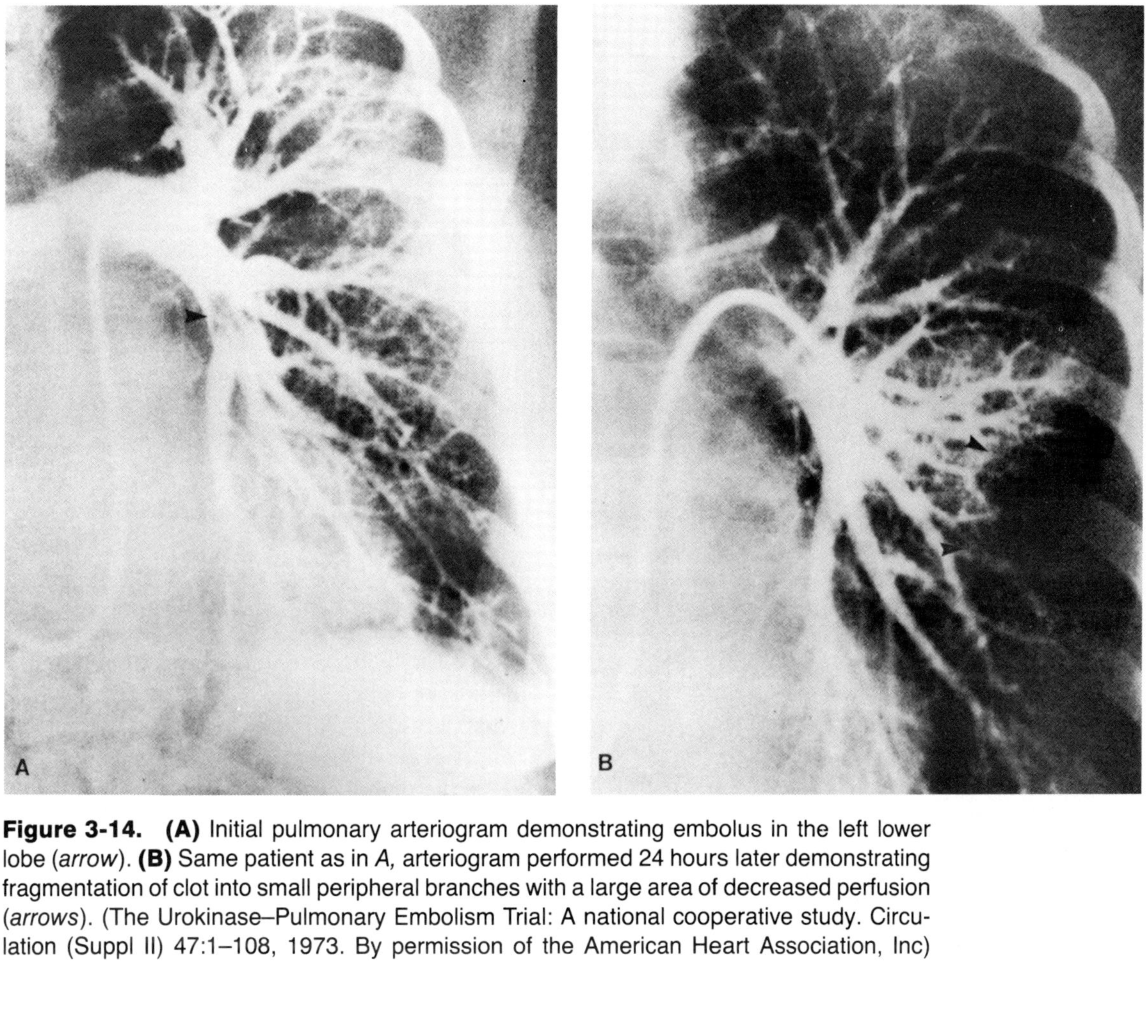


**Figure 3-14. (A)** Initial pulmonary arteriogram demonstrating embolus in the left lower lobe (*arrow*). **(B)** Same patient as in *A,* arteriogram performed 24 hours later demonstrating fragmentation of clot into small peripheral branches with a large area of decreased perfusion (*arrows*). (The Urokinase–Pulmonary Embolism Trial: A national cooperative study. Circulation (Suppl II) 47:1–108, 1973. By permission of the American Heart Association, Inc)

lated to catheter manipulation and volume of contrast, there has been a great deal of interest in replacing standard pulmonary arteriography with digital subtraction angiography. Several medical centers have shown an excellent correlation between standard arteriography and digital angiography performed with contrast injected into the superior vena cava, right atrium, or pulmonary artery. No false negatives have been reported. However, of our 17 patients who were evaluated by both digital subtraction angiography (injections of contrast into the right atrium) and standard pulmonary arteriography, emboli could be detected in only 3 using the digital technique, whereas emboli were detected in 6 patients by standard pulmonary arteriography (Fig. 3-15). Some experimental data also support this high false-negative rate using venous injections. Since it is imperative to retain the angiogram as the "gold standard" in the detection of emboli, a negative venous digital angiogram cannot be accepted as proof that no emboli are present. However, catheterization of the pulmonary artery and subsequent selective digital technique can be an acceptable alternative to conventional arteriography in cooperative patients.

### Low or Nonionic Contrast Pulmonary Arteriography

The major hemodynamic complications of pulmonary arteriography, including death, appear to be predominantly related to the hypertonicity

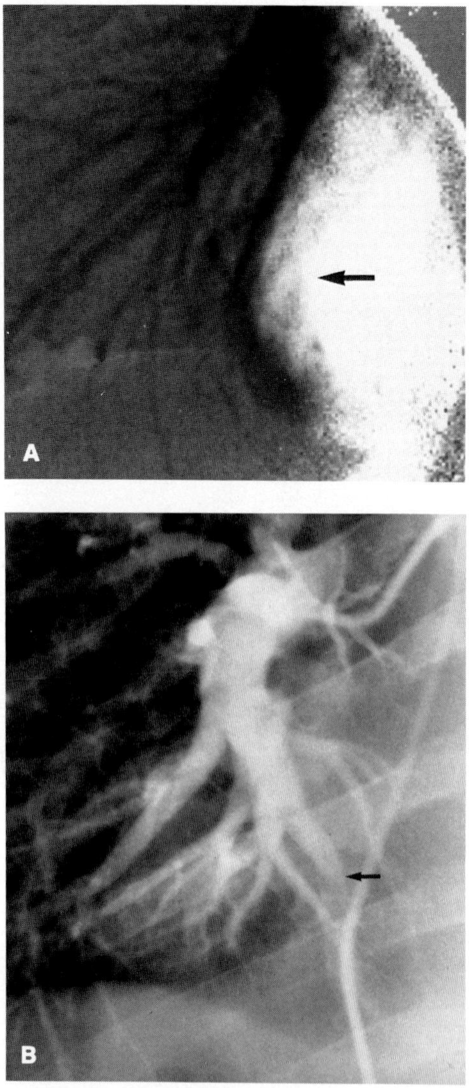


**Figure 3-15.** **(A)** Digital angiogram (RPO projection) with contrast injected into the right atrium. The medial and posterior basal segments of the right lower lobe are hidden because of subtraction artifact (*arrow*). **(B)** Selective pulmonary arteriogram (RPO projection) demonstrates clot (*arrow*) in the posterior basal segment of the right lower lobe that was hidden in *A*.

of contrast material. The use of low or nonionic contrast agents, while not detracting from image quality, produces only a minor increase in pulmonary artery pressure during injection compared with as much as a 50% increase in mean pulmonary artery pressure with standard contrast agents.

I am now using these low ionic or nonionic agents routinely in patients with elevated pulmonary artery or right ventricular end-diastolic pressure during standard pulmonary arteriography, rather than employing digital angiography using dilute hypertonic contrast. The only disadvantage of these newer agents is the tenfold increase in cost.

## Computed Tomography

Computed tomography (CT) with intravenous contrast can be used to detect central pulmonary artery clot (Fig. 3-16). However, because of cardiac-motion blurring and the transaxial plane, this technique does not play a significant role in the diagnosis of pulmonary emboli. Further experience with high-resolution cine-CT will be required to determine whether this modality has any diagnostic role in this condition.

## Magnetic Resonance Imaging

In many magnetic resonance imaging (MRI) pulse sequences, thrombus as well as turbulent and stagnant blood flow generates an excellent signal compared with normal flowing blood without the need for intravenous contrast. Using tantalum-tagged autologous clots in dogs, we were able to detect all 12 emboli larger than 3 mm (Fig. 3-17), and we have been able to detect large central clots in 2 patients (Fig. 3-18). The generation of the signal is from the clot itself and proximal slow flow. Unfortunately, MRI may produce false-positive results derived from focal areas of increased lung water, mucous plugs, and flow-related artifacts. Further clinical trials are needed to clearly determine the role of MRI in evaluating patients with suspected pulmonary embolus.

*(Text continues on p. 70.)*

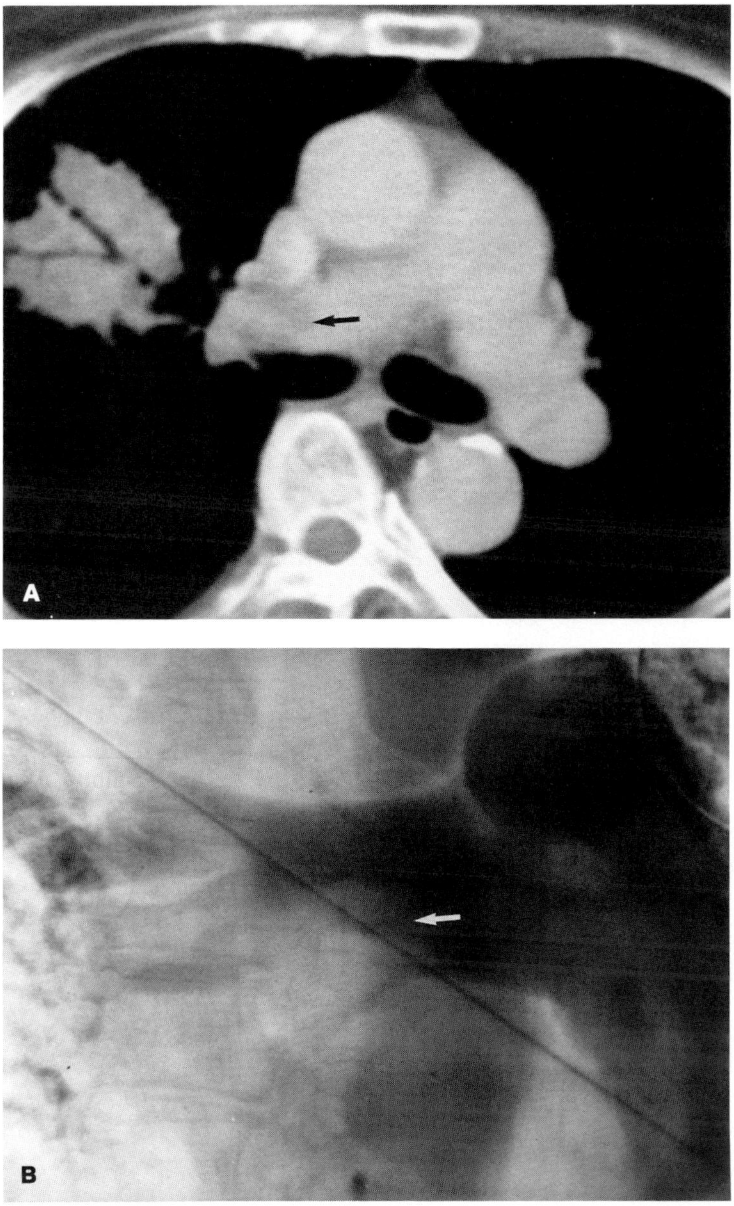

**Figure 3-16. (A)** CT demonstrates clot (*arrow*) in the right main pulmonary artery. **(B)** Pulmonary arteriogram in the same patient shows the clot (*arrow*).

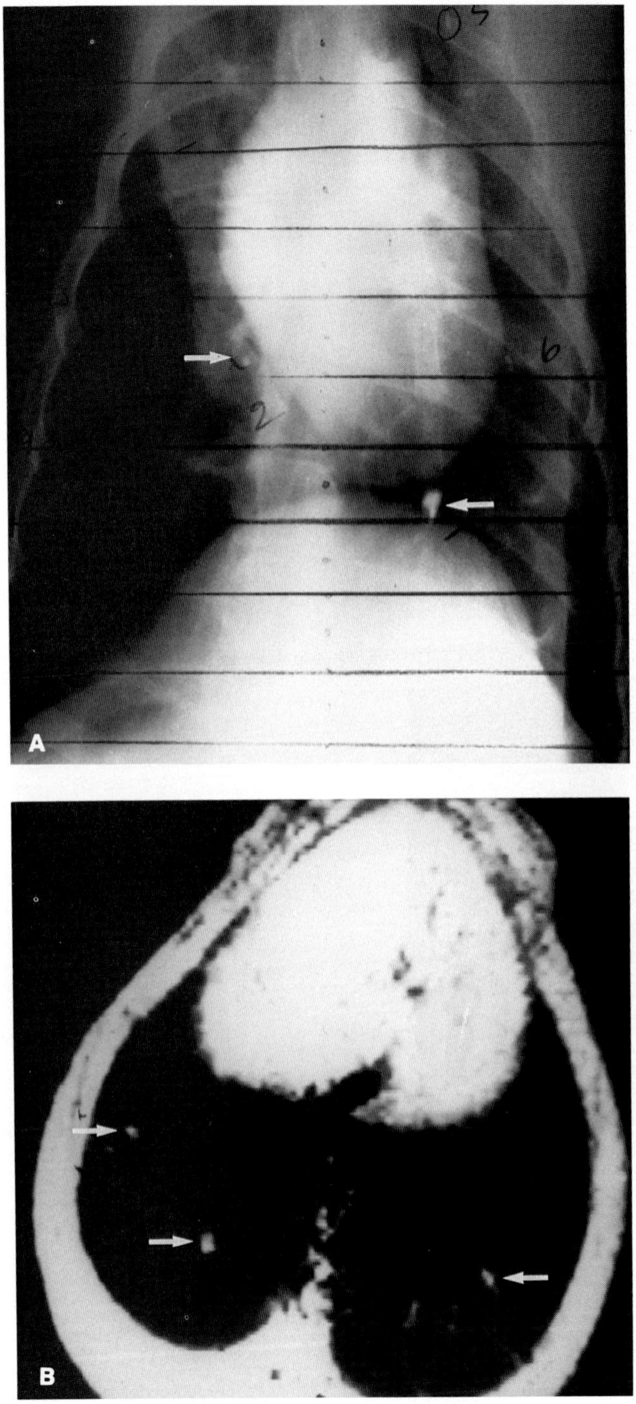


**Figure 3-17. (A)** Chest radiograph in a dog demonstrates tantalum-tagged autologous clots (*arrows*). **(B)** MRI in the same dog shows signal from these clots (*arrows*).

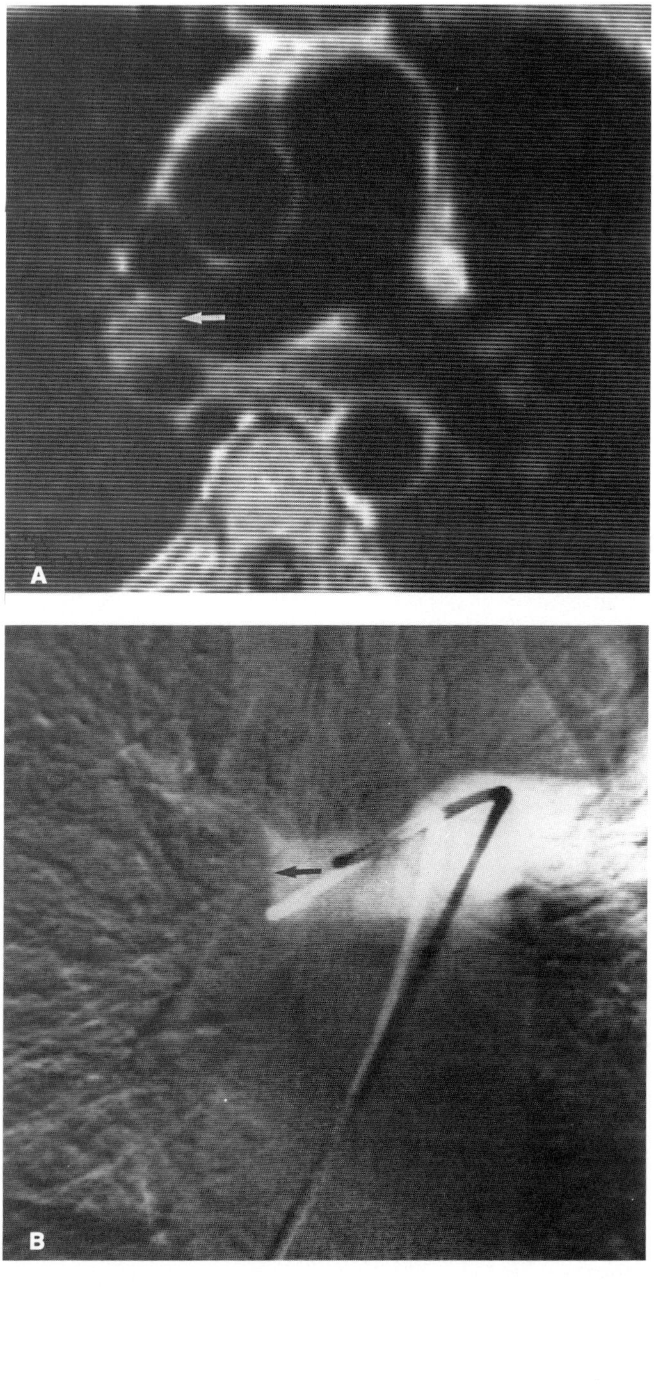

**Figure 3-18. (A)** MRI in a patient demonstrates clot (*arrow*) in the right main pulmonary artery. **(B)** Digital angiogram confirms the presence of clot (*arrow*).

## Bibliography


Alderson PO, Biello DR, Gottschalk A et al: Tc-99m DTPA aerosol and radioactive gases compared as adjuncts to perfusion scintigraphy in patients with suspected pulmonary embolism. Radiology 153: 515, 1984

Alderson PO, Gottschalk A: Letter to the Editors. Ventilation–perfusion studies for pulmonary embolism: A rebuttal to Dr. Eugene Robin. Semin Nucl Med 9:145–146, 1979

Biello DR, Mattar AG, McKnight RC et al: Ventilation–perfusion studies in suspected pulmonary embolism. AJR 133:1033–1037, 1979

Biello Dr, Mattar AG, Osel–Wusu A et al: Interpretation of indeterminate lung scintigrams. Radiology 133:189–194, 1979

Bookstein JJ, Feigen DS, Kwan WS et al: Diagnosis of pulmonary embolism: Experimental evaluation of the accuracy of scintigraphically guided pulmonary arteriography. Radiology 136:15–23, 1980

Carter WD, Brady TM, Keyes JW, Jr et al: Relative accuracy of two diagnostic schemes for detection of pulmonary embolism by ventilation–perfusion scintigraphy. Radiology 145:447, 1982

Chiles C, Guthaner DF, Djang WT: Detection of pulmonary emboli in dogs using digital subtraction angiography. Invest Radiol 18:507, 1983

Dalen JE, Alpert JS: Natural history of pulmonary embolism. Prog Cardiovasc Dis 17:259–270, 1975

Dalen JE, Babas JS, Brooks HL et al: Resolution rate of acute pulmonary embolism in man. N Engl J Med 280:1194–1199, 1969

Dalen JE, Brooks HL, Johnson LW et al: Pulmonary angiography in acute pulmonary embolism: Indications, techniques and results in 367 patients. Am Heart J 81:175–185, 1971

Fleischner FG: Pulmonary embolism. Clin Radiol 13: 169–182, 1962

Godwin JD, Webb WR, Gamsu G et al: Computed tomography of pulmonary embolism. AJR 135: 691, 1980

Goodman PC, Brant–Zawadski M: Digital subtraction pulmonary angiography. AJR 139:305, 1982

Greenspan RH, Ravin CE, Polansky SM et al: Accuracy of the chest radiograph in diagnosis of pulmonary embolism. Invest Radiol 17:539, 1982

James WS, Menn SJ, Moser KM: Rapid resolution of a pulmonary embolism in man. West J Med 128: 60–67, 1978

Komazaki T: Ioxaglate versus diatrizoate in selective pulmonary angiography. Invest Radiol 18:507, 1983

McNeil BJ: A diagnostic strategy using ventilation–perfusion studies in patients suspect for pulmonary embolism. J Nucl Med 17:613–616, 1976

Mills SR, Jackson DC, Older RA et al: The incidence, etiologies, and avoidance of complications of pulmonary angiography in a large series. Radiology 136:295, 1980

Moser KM: Pulmonary embolism. Am Rev Respir Dis 115:829–852, 1977

Moses DC, Silver TM, Bookstein JJ: The complementary roles of chest radiology, lung scanning, and selective pulmonary angiography in the diagnosis of pulmonary embolism. Radiology 49:179, 1974

Novelline RA, Baltarowich OH, Athanasoulis CA et al: The clinical course of patients with suspected pulmonary embolism and a negative pulmonary arteriogram. Radiology 126:561–567, 1978

Peck WW, Slutsky RA, Hackney DB et al: Effects of contrast media on pulmonary hemodynamics: Comparison of ionic and nonionic agents. Radiology 149:371, 1983

Pend GD, Ovitt TW, Capp MP: Comparison of conventional pulmonary angiography with intravenous digital subtraction angiography for pulmonary embolic disease. Radiology 147:345, 1983

Perlmutt LM, Braun SD, Newman GE et al: Pulmonary arteriography in the high-risk patient. Radiology 162:187, 1987

Robin ED: Overdiagnosis and overtreatment of pulmonary embolism: The emperor may have no clothes. Ann Intern Med 87:775–781, 1977

Stein MG, Crues JV, Bradley WG et al: MR imaging of pulmonary emboli: An experimental study in dogs. AJR 146:1133, 1986

Stein MG, Waxman AD, Ramanna L et al: Post-perfusion xenon-133 ventilation scintigraphy with a narrow window. AJR 145:511, 1985

Sullivan DC, Coleman RE, Mills SR et al: Lung scan interpretation: Effect of different observers and different criteria. Radiology 149:803, 1983

Taplin GV, Chopra SK: Lung perfusion–inhalation scintigraphy in obstructive airway disease and pulmonary embolism. Radiol Clin North Am 16: 491–513, 1978

The Urokinase–Pulmonary Embolism Trial: A national cooperative study. Circulation (Suppl II) 47:1–108, 1973

Vea HW, Sirotta PS, Nelp WB: Ventilation–perfusion scanning for pulmonary embolism: Refinement of predictive value through Bayesian analysis. AJR 145:967, 1985

## SUSPECTED PULMONARY EMBOLUS

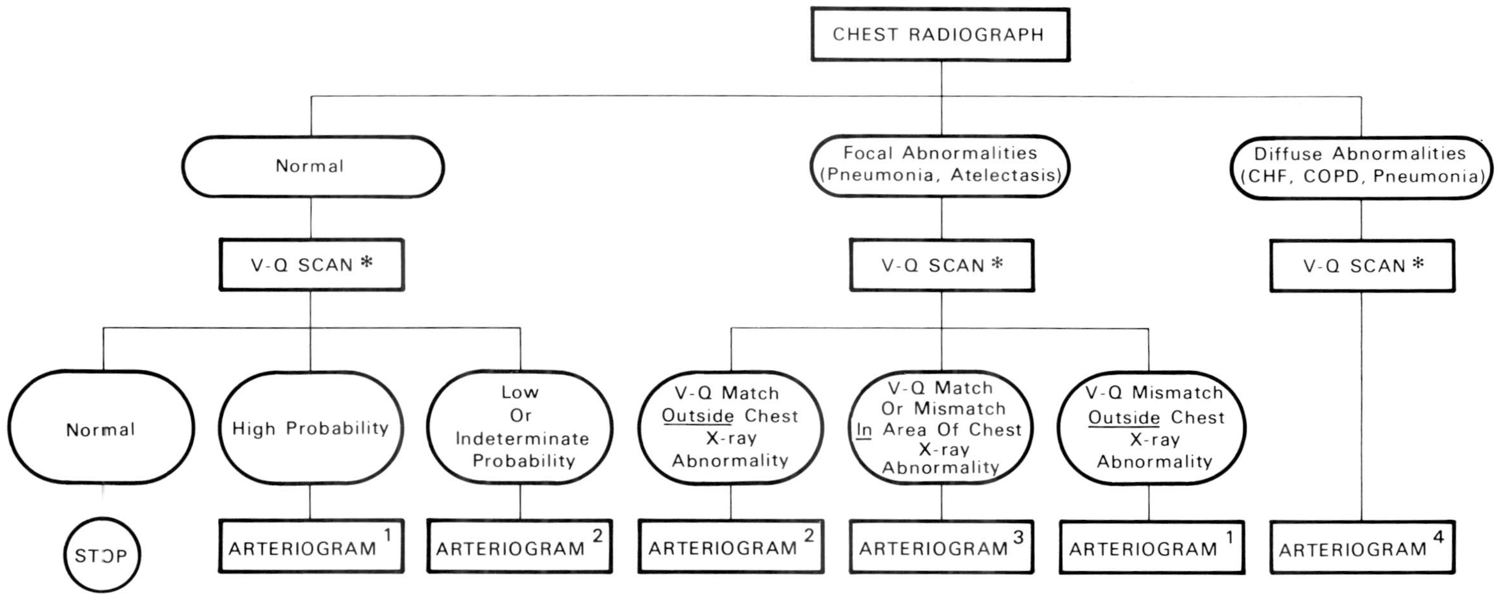


* V-Q = VENTILATION-PERFUSION SCAN

1. Only For Patients Who Are Candidates For Venous Occlusion, Embolectomy, Or Extremely High Risk For Anticoagulation.
2. If Patient Is Still Being Considered For Anticoagulation.
3. In All Patients.
4. Regardless Of Scan Findings, But Scan Is Necessary To Localize Areas For Selective Arteriography.

# Chapter 4

# Aortic Aneurysms and Dissections

*Carl-Olof Ovenfors*
*J. David Godwin*

Aneurysms and dissections of the thoracic aorta are potentially life-threatening conditions. Rupture of a thoracic aneurysm will occur in at least a third of patients; the 5-year survival rate is only approximately 50%. In aortic dissection, the mortality rate is high; 85% of patients die within 6 weeks and less than 1% survive 5 years.

Most thoracic aortic dissections occur in patients with arterial hypertension. Some are secondary to trauma, while others are due to a congenital defect, such as Marfan's syndrome. Indeed, in view of its close association, the physician should carefully search for Marfan's syndrome whenever a dissection is suspected.

A dissection most commonly begins immediately above the aortic valve and continues into the descending aorta (type I, 46%). It may extend as far as the level of the iliac bifurcation. In other cases, the dissection may stop at the origin of the brachiocephalic vessels (type II, 20%). Another frequent location for dissection is the descending aorta, just distal to the origin of the left subclavian artery (type III, 24%). The least common dissection is one limited to the aortic arch (type IV, 10%).

The differential diagnosis of thoracic aortic aneurysms and dissections includes diffuse widening and tortuosity (buckling) of the aorta, as well as such nonaortic lesions as the following:

- Mediastinal mass (tumor, lymphoma, cyst)
- Mediastinal hematoma
- Collapse of right upper lobe
- Pericardial mass or cyst
- Diaphragmatic hernia
- Cardiac aneurysm or tumor

For the radiologist, there are three basic problems to be solved in diagnosing the patient with a clinically suspected thoracic aortic aneurysm or dissection:

1. Is there a lesion?
2. What is the lesion?
3. If the lesion is an aneurysm or dissection, what must the referring physician know to properly institute medical or surgical therapy?

In most cases, the suspected aneurysm or dissection is detected on a plain chest radiograph. However, some patients have negative chest films, and the diagnosis of aneurysm or dissection can be made only on clinical grounds. The definitive diagnosis of aneurysm or dissection requires more sophisticated radiographic techniques (computed tomography, magnetic resonance imaging, or aortography).

The distinction between aneurysm and dissection is critical, because the indications for surgery are very different in the two conditions. If the patient has an aneurysm, the surgeon must know the precise location and extent of the lesion, as well as its relation to adjacent anatomic structures. In the case of a dissection, the site of entry and the point of re-entry (if one exists) must be known before a rational operative approach can be formulated.

## CLINICAL AND LABORATORY FINDINGS

Most patients with thoracic aortic aneurysms are asymptomatic, and the condition is first detected on routine chest radiographs. Aneurysms of the aortic arch may cause symptoms because of pressure on or displacement of the trachea or esophagus. Aneurysms of the ascending aorta often cause aortic valve insufficiency, which may precipitate heart failure. Descending aortic aneurysms, on the other hand, may become large before producing pain or pressure effects on adjacent organs.

Aneurysms may compress the bronchi and cause atelectasis or obstruction with secondary infection. Death may be caused by rupture of an aortic aneurysm into the pericardial or pleural spaces, or into a bronchus or the trachea, esophagus, or pulmonary artery.

In aortic dissection, severe, sharp, tearing chest pain radiating to the back is typical. Bruits, absence of peripheral pulses, and neurologic deficits in the presence of arterial hypertension are common. At times, there may be no symptoms, and the suspicion of aortic dissection may arise only from the appearance on a routine chest film.

## DIAGNOSTIC EVALUATION

### *DIAGNOSTIC MODALITIES*

1. Chest radiography
2. Computed tomography
3. Magnetic resonance imaging
4. Echocardiography
5. Aortography
6. Surgery

### Chest Radiography

Plain chest radiography (including oblique views with barium) is the initial step in the investigation of the patient with thoracic aortic aneurysm or dissection. A thoracic aneurysm usually appears as a homogeneous, circumscribed soft-tissue density protruding from the mediastinum in relation to the course of the aorta. Although usually sharply demarcated with smooth, curved borders, the margin may appear undulating or scalloped when the aneurysm is not uniform or when multiple aneurysms are present. A hazy border of an aneurysm suggests that blood is seeping out through a small perforation. Silhouetting of the border of a thoracic aneurysm occurs if there is atelectasis of the adjacent lung.

Calcifications in the wall of a thoracic aortic aneurysm are common (Fig. 4-1). Calcification in an aneurysm of the ascending aorta may sometimes be confused with the calcification seen in other mediastinal lesions (*e.g.*, thymoma or dermoid cyst). In thymomas, the calcifications are central and diffuse. The calcifications in a dermoid cyst are similar to those seen in a thoracic aneurysm, but they tend to be continuous and regular and are not seen as individual plaques.

The radiographic appearance and differential diagnosis of thoracic aneurysms depend on the portion of the aorta that is involved. Sinus of Valsalva aneurysms most often involve the noncoronary (posterior) sinus and are frequently too small to be identified on chest films. If the mass is large, however, it may project from the right side of the mediastinum at the level of the inferior pulmonary veins and simulate a pericardial cyst or thymoma in the frontal projection. The radiographic differentiation of these lesions is based on the appearance of the posterior border, which is not seen in a sinus of Valsalva aneurysm, but is usually sharply demarcated in pericardial cysts or thymomas. Aneurysms of the left sinus are contained within the mediastinum and may produce a local increase in density,

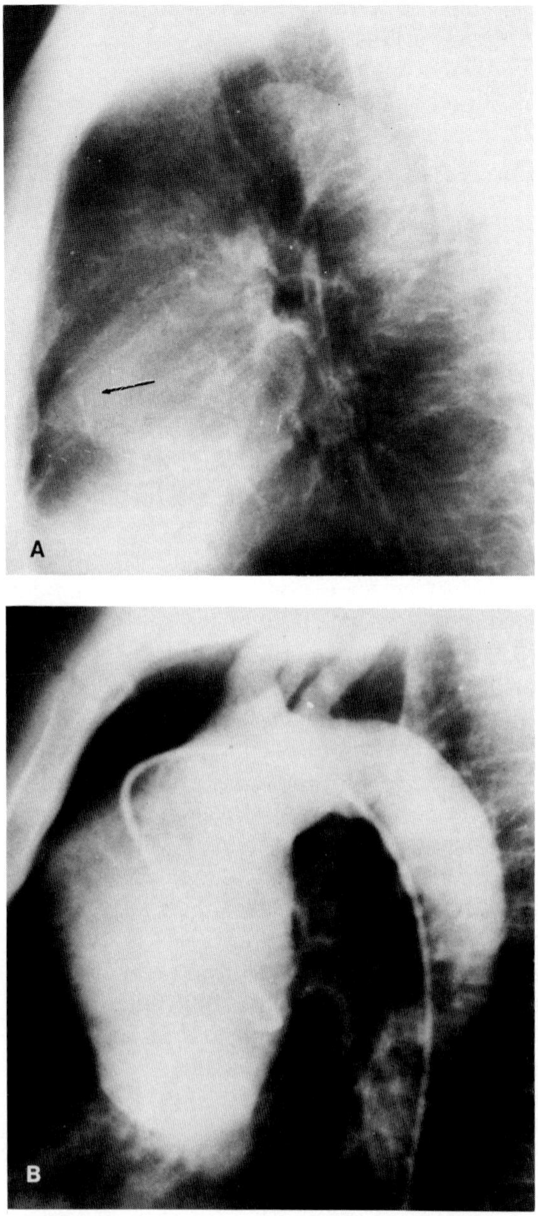

**Figure 4-1.** **(A)** Lateral chest radiograph and **(B)** aortogram demonstrate a large sacular aneurysm of the ascending aorta with calcification in the wall (*arrow*).

mimicking a brochogenic cyst in the subcarinal area or an enlarged left atrium. Aneurysms of the sinus of Valsalva are often associated with aortic valvular insufficiency and left ventricular enlargement. Perforation of an aneurysm into the right atrium or right ventricle creates an acute left-to-right shunt, which appears radiographically as increased pulmonary vascularity.

Aneurysms of the ascending aorta usually extend from the sinuses of Valsalva to the proximal aortic arch and are often associated with aortic valvular insufficiency. On the lateral view, the widened aorta fills the lower portion of the retrosternal space. On the frontal view, ascending aortic aneurysms almost always project outward from the right border of the mediastinum. Rarely, an aneurysm may arise from the medial wall of the ascending aorta and may be entirely hidden within the mediastinal shadow. If the aneurysm is large, it may even project outward from the left border of the mediastinum. It is important to remember that the medial and posterior borders of the ascending aorta are lost within the mediastinal shadow in lateral, oblique, and frontal projections. Therefore, it is extremely difficult to differentiate a fusiform aneurysm from mere tortuosity of the ascending aorta using plain chest films; in such cases, aortography, magnetic resonance imaging (MRI), or computed tomography (CT) is almost always required.

Ascending aortic aneurysms may erode the sternum or anterior ribs. Rupture of an aneurysm into the superior vena cava causes widening of the mediastinum and an increase in pulmonary vascularity caused by a large left-to-right shunt. Medially located aneurysms can rupture into the adjacent pulmonary artery; if the aneurysm is small, the only manifestations on chest films may be a wide pulmonary artery and increased pulmonary vascularity.

Aneurysms of the aortic arch may bulge in either direction, but more often they bulge to the left (Fig. 4-2). When an aneurysm is suspected in this area, the esophagus should be closely evaluated. Normally, the esophagus is closely attached to the aorta, so that mediastinal masses tend to displace both in the same direction. In cases or aortic aneurysm, however, the mass causes the esophagus to deviate toward the opposite side.

A special diagnostic problem is traumatic rupture of the aorta secondary to blunt trauma to the thorax. In approximately 95% of cases, this involves the aorta just distal to the left subclavian artery. The intima and media are torn; only the

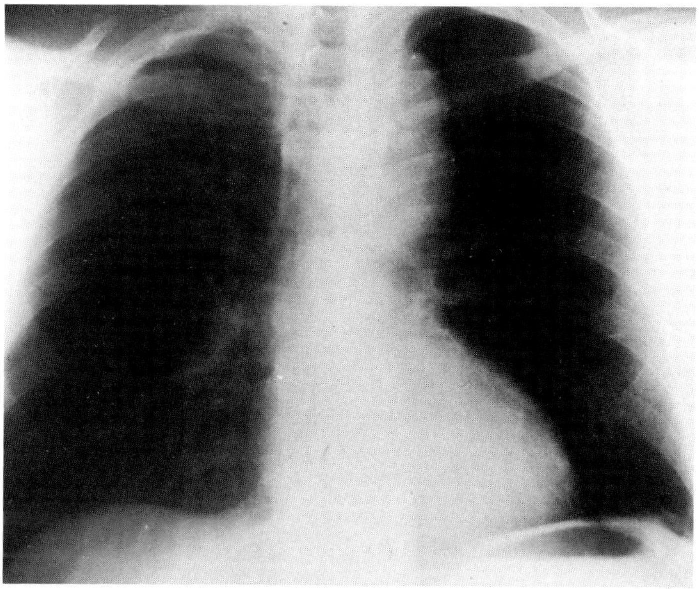

**Figure 4-2.** Arch aneurysm also involving the proximal left subclavian artery. Note the widening of the upper mediastinum with a rounded contour of the left border. The trachea is displaced to the right.

intact adventitia holds the vessel together. At times, the adventitia is also partially torn, resulting in a false aneurysm. If the adventitia is intact, a localized aneurysmal widening of the aorta is usually seen on the chest radiograph. If there is also mediastinal hemorrhage, widening of the mediastinum and shifting of the trachea to the right are seen (Fig. 4-3). The hemorrhage may extend into the extrapleural tissues over the left lung and produce an "apical cap." A large, left-sided hemothorax may also occur.

The differential diagnosis of arch aneurysms and aortic rupture includes mediastinal tumors, kinking, and coarctation of the aorta.

Aneurysms of the descending thoracic aorta are situated behind the heart. On the frontal view, they may be projected entirely within the cardiac silhouette, although they usually bulge into the left lung. In patients with arteriosclerotic or syphilitic aneurysms, changes can usually be detected in other portions of the aorta. If the remainder of the aorta appears normal, the possibility of a congenital, traumatic, or mycotic aneurysm must be considered.

The differential diagnosis of descending thoracic aortic aneurysms includes tumor, abscess, posterior diaphragmatic hernia (Bochdalek), and aneurysm of the posterior wall of the left ventricle, which is in contact with the aorta. If the aortic wall is not calcified, it may be impossible to differentiate a tortuous descending aorta from a fusiform aneurysm on the frontal projection unless the esophagus is outlined with barium.

The critical differentiation between a thoracic aortic aneurysm and dissection is often impossible to make on plain chest radiography and requires aortography, MRI, or CT. At times, the widened aortic shadow caused by a dissection has an irregular or wavy outer border (Fig. 4-4). When the dissection begins just beyond the left subclavian artery, a localized hump may be seen on the superior aspect of the distal portion of the arch, especially on lateral or left oblique projections. In most cases, however, the appearance of the aorta is normal or shows only nonspecific widening.

If it is not clear whether a soft-tissue mass on a chest film represents an aortic aneurysm or dissection, the presence and appearance of calcification within the lesion often provides the major clue to the proper diagnosis. Because calcifications are located within the intima, the thickness of the aortic wall can be estimated by observing the distance between the calcification and the outer border of the aortic shadow. With aneurysms, the intima closely follows the contour of the aneurysmal sac, and the distance between the calcification and the outer border of the aorta is only a few millimeters. In dissec-

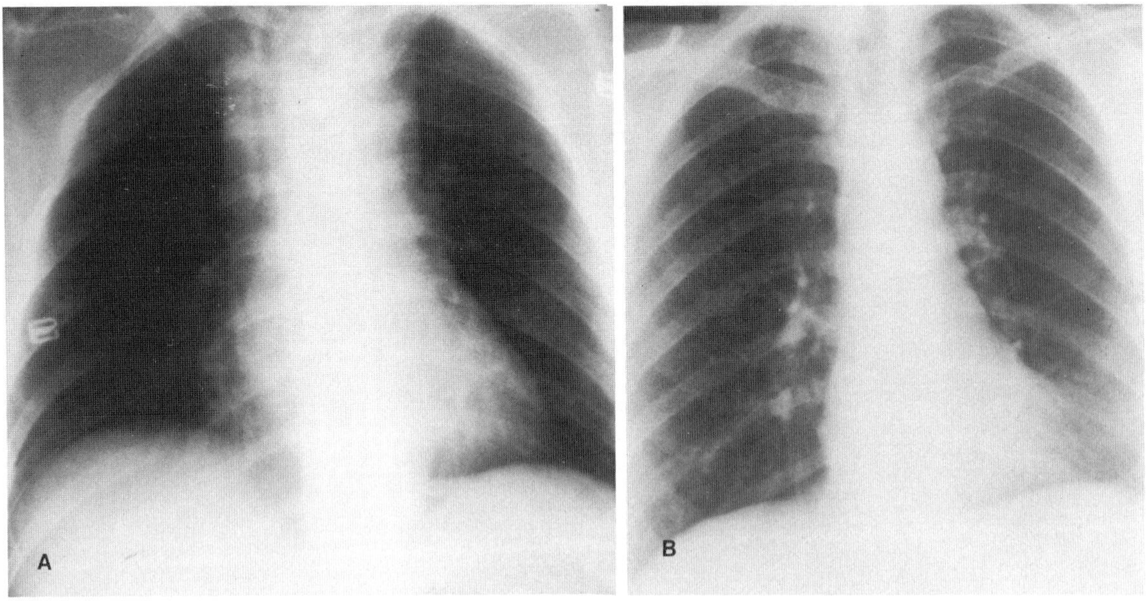


**Figure 4-3.** Aortic rupture after deceleration trauma (traffic accident). The aorta was ruptured just distal to the origin of the left subclavian artery. Note the widening of the upper mediastinum on the frontal chest radiograph taken immediately following trauma **(A)** as compared with that taken 3 months later **(B).** There was also displacement of the trachea to the right.

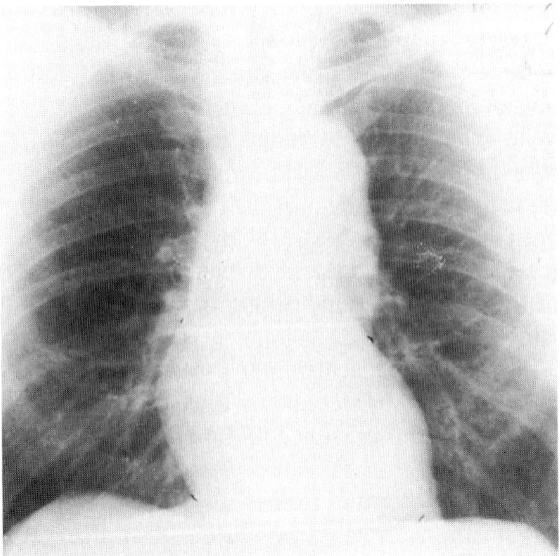

**Figure 4-4.** Aortic dissection involving the thoracic and abdominal aorta. The chest radiograph shows only diffuse widening of the descending aorta with an irregular, wavy left border.

tions, however, the accumulation of blood within the media displaces the intima inward, thus separating the calcium deposits from the aortic contour. This sign of aortic dissection is easiest to interpret in the descending portion. In the arch region, the sign must be used with caution. Because the aorta is foreshortened on the frontal projection, calcifications may lie in a portion of the aorta different from that which forms the apparent radiographic border.

An abrupt change in the configuration of the aorta suggests the presence of a dissection. If the ascending aorta is involved, the aortic valve is frequently distorted, resulting in valvular insufficiency and left ventricular dilatation.

Dissections often rupture outward through the adventitia and may result in massive hemothorax (usually on the left side) or rupture into the pericardium with subsequent acute tamponade and sudden death. At times, this process may produce a mediastinal hematoma that obscures the underlying aortic rupture.

Although the chest film may frequently suggest the presence of a dissection of the thoracic aorta, the appearance is rarely pathognomonic. A definite diagnosis of dissection must be made on the basis of CT, MRI, or aortography.

## Computed Tomography

In the nonemergency patient whose chest radiograph is suggestive of thoracic aortic aneurysm, CT offers a rapid, noninvasive, and accurate assessment and should be the next diagnostic procedure of choice after chest radiography. Unlike aortography, CT does not require catheterization and thus may be performed on an outpatient basis. Computed tomography provides more morphologic detail by better demonstrating mural calcification. It can directly identify an intraluminal thrombus, which can only be inferred from the results of aortography. If an extrapulmonary chest mass simulates a thoracic aortic aneurysm, CT can be used to make this distinction and will likely provide some information about the origin and structure of the lesion. Repeated CT is also of value in assessing growth of an aneurysm. If part of the aneurysm is filled with thrombus, aortography will not reliably assess expansion of the sac. Serial follow-up with plain chest films is also frequently unreliable, because apparent changes in the size of the aneurysm may be due to slight degrees of patient rotation.

Computed tomography for suspected thoracic aortic aneurysms employs intravenous contrast; scans are obtained at 1-cm intervals over the course of the lesion. Characteristic findings on CT are aortic dilatation (Fig. 4-5); mural calcification; intraluminal thrombus, seen as a soft-tissue density separating the contrast-filled portion of the lumen from the aortic wall (Fig. 4-6); and effects on adjacent structures, such as displacement of the mediastinum or bone erosion. Computed tomography generally supplies all the information needed by the surgeon to plan the operative approach.

In the patient in whom nonacute aortic dissection is considered in the differential diagnosis of chest pain, CT offers a low-risk, alternative diagnostic method to aortography. This technique can determine the location and extent of a suspected aortic abnormality; by demonstrating whether the dissection involves the ascending aorta or if there is rupture into the pericardial or pleural spaces, CT can aid in determining whether immediate operation is required. The major limitation of CT with respect to aortography in the patient with suspected acute dissection is that only a single level can be evaluated on a given slice, contrary to the rapid series of images covering a wide field that can be achieved with aortography.

In the patient with a nonemergent aortic aneurysm or dissection, CT is usually the definitive study and aortography is not required. The major exception to this rule is the patient with a dissection in whom it is impossible to determine by CT which major vessel branches from the aorta are blocked and which are patent. Many surgeons do not care about this information; for others, however, this knowledge is essential and an aortogram must therefore be performed prior to surgery.

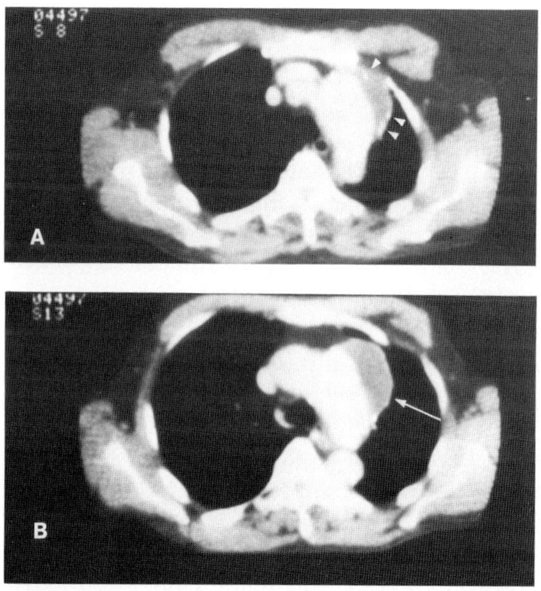


**Figure 4-5.** CT scans through the aortic arch **(A)** and slightly below **(B)** after intravenous contrast injection show calcifications in the wall of the aneurysm (*arrowheads* in *A*) and a large filling defect consisting of thrombus (*arrow* in *B*).

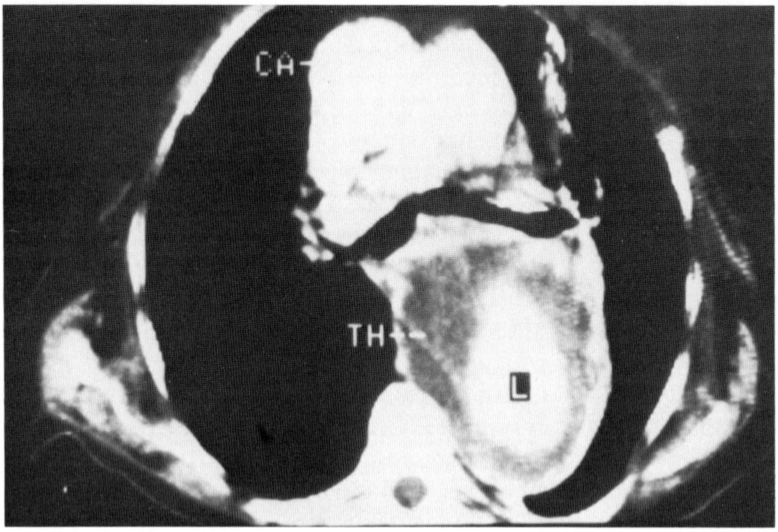


**Figure 4-6.** Descending aortic aneurysm. Contrast-enhanced CT scan at a level just below the carina shows the mildly dilated ascending aorta with calcification (*CA*) and markedly dilated descending (*L*) aorta. There is a large mural thrombus (*TH*) surrounding the lumen (*L*) of the descending aortic aneurysm.

The evaluation of suspected aortic dissection by CT utilizes intravenous contrast injection and a series of scans at 1- to 2-cm intervals from above the arch through the level of the diaphragm. Computed tomography may demonstrate a double channel with an intimal flap (Fig. 4-7). With dynamic scanning and bolus injection of contrast material, differential filling of the true and false channels can be observed, as with aortography. If partial filling of the aorta with a thrombus- or hematoma-filled channel is demonstrated, inward displacement of intimal calcification can differentiate a dissection from a simple aortic aneurysm. Other findings consistent with dissection include irregular caliber of the aorta, compression of the true lumen, and possibly pleural fluid. If an aortic abnormality extends below the level of the diaphragm, CT scanning is continued into the abdomen to the level of the iliac bifurcation. It is easier to follow the course of a dissection into the abdomen with CT scans than to attempt to combine ultrasound images with those generated by CT.

Computed tomography is also of value in the follow-up of thoracic aortic dissection after medical or surgical treatment. Complications of dissection (redissection, extension of dissection, or aneurysm formation) are more accurately detected by CT than by plain chest radiography; CT also obviates the risk of repeated aortography.

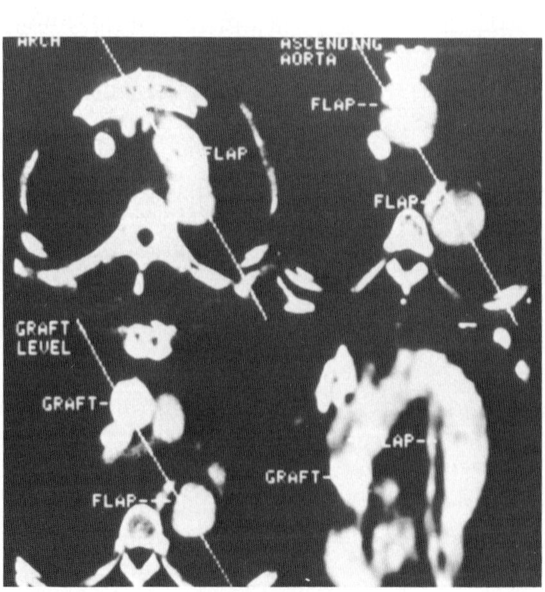


**Figure 4-7.** Persistent aortic dissection in a patient previously treated by graft replacement in the ascending aorta. CT scans through the arch (*upper left*), ascending and descending aorta (*upper right*), and at the level of the graft (*lower left*). The picture at lower right is a reformatted image of the aorta in the oblique plane indicated by the dotted lines on the previous scans. The intimal flap is well demonstrated, indicating a dissection.

## Magnetic Resonance Imaging

Electrocardiographically gated MRI in transverse, sagittal, and coronal planes provides a noninvasive method for obtaining high-quality examinations of the thoracic aorta in patients with suspected dissection, aneurysm, or traumatic rupture. Spin-echo pulse sequences are generally used, and the repetition time (TR) is determined by the heart rate and is equal to the RR interval. Dual-echo sequences with an echo time (TE) of 30 msec and 60 msec are often used.

The high contrast between rapidly flowing blood, vessel wall, and adjacent soft-tissue structures permits identification of vessels by MRI without the need for intravenous injection of contrast material. Abnormalities that either increase (*e.g.*, aneurysm) or decrease (*e.g.*, coarctation) the size of the aortic lumen can be easily demonstrated by MRI. Because sections can be obtained in multiple planes without the image degradation that occurs with CT, MRI can show the relation of an abnormality to the vessels arising from the aortic arch (Fig. 4-8). However, tortuosity of vessels and image degradation from patient motion may compromise the ability of MRI to delineate small vascular abnormalities or the relation of branch vessels to an aneurysm.

Magnetic resonance imaging, like CT and aortography, can demonstrate aortic dissections and show their extent (Fig. 4-9). Indeed, the use of respiratory gating or short TR times should

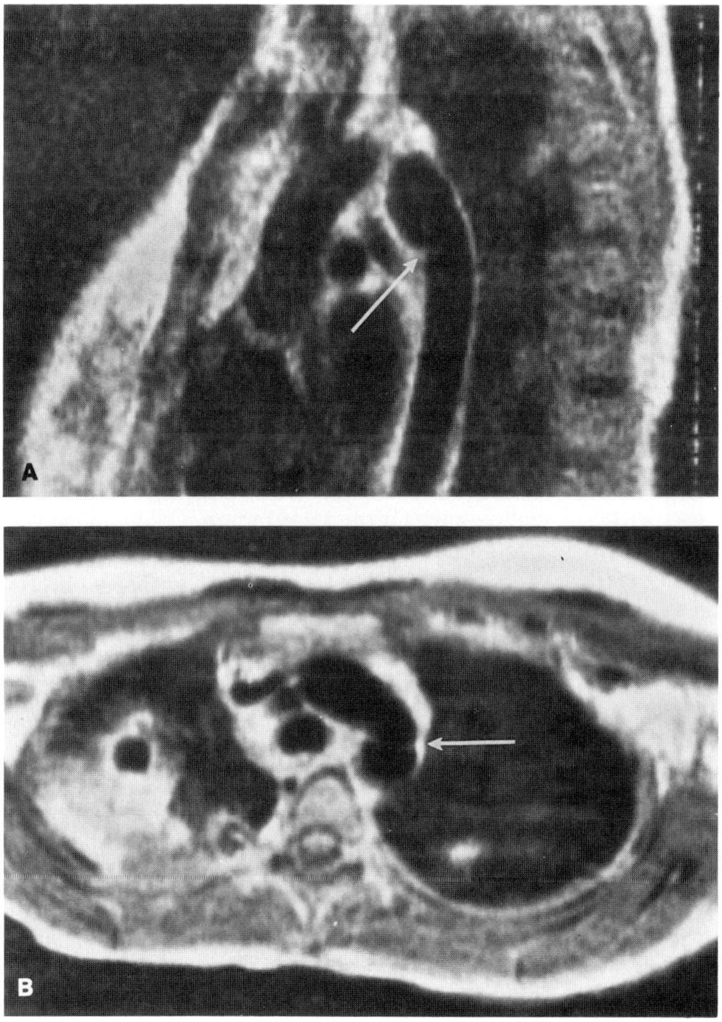


**Figure 4-8.** MRI of traumatic aortic rupture with false aneurysm. **(A)** Sagittal view shows the site of rupture just distal to the left subclavian artery (*arrow*). **(B)** Transaxial view shows the intimal flap of a local dissection (*arrow*). (Courtesy of Kathleen Brown, M.D.)

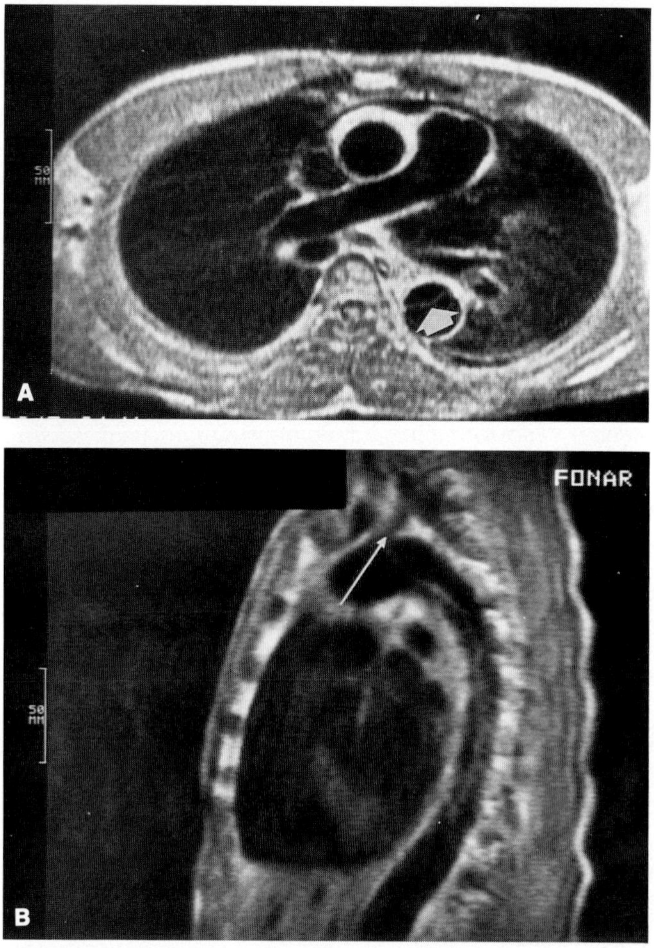


**Figure 4-9.** MRI of aortic dissection. **(A)** Transaxial image with spin-echo technique (TR, 28 msec) at the level of the main and right pulmonary arteries clearly shows the intimal flap (*arrow*) in the descending aorta. **(B)** Sagittal image shows the intimal flap extending from the left subclavian artery (*arrow*) to the level of the diaphragm.

permit a more precise display of aortic abnormalities, comparable to that now available with aortography. Because it does not use intravenous contrast material, MRI is especially valuable in diagnosing the patient with a suspected aortic dissection who is hypersensitive to iodinated contrast material or whose renal function does not permit contrast administration.

Calcification produces little or no signal on MRI, as opposed to the bright signal it produces on CT. Thus, MRI cannot distinguish an aneurysm from a dissection with a thrombosed false lumen by assessing possible displacement of intimal calcification. In the patient with an aortic dissection, an intimal flap is usually detected as a linear, medium-intensity structure separating the true and false lumens. Rapidly flowing blood in these lumens appears as either a signal void on both first- and second-echo images or as a relative increase in signal intensity on the second-echo image. If the false lumen is thrombosed, or even if it is open but the flow is slow, the intimal flap may not be visualized. In this situation, aortic dissection is difficult to differentiate from an aortic aneurysm with mural thrombosis. Aortography may be required to make this distinction. Other limitations of MRI include the inability to ensure that the entire region of interest is imaged in one section and the difficulty in examining critically ill patients who require monitoring equipment.

If there is a clinical suspicion of aortic dissection of the ascending aorta and echocardiography is difficult to perform for technical reasons, MRI offers a reliable and noninvasive alternative procedure.

Despite the ability of MRI (and CT) to demonstrate various aortic abnormalities, in selected patients aortography may be necessary to provide additional information. Neither MRI nor CT can assess the severity of aortic insufficiency, the status of the coronary arteries, or the precise location of tears in the aorta in patients with aortic dissections.

## Echocardiography

Thoracic aortic aneurysms or dissections located in the sinus of Valsalva, aortic root, or most proximal portions of the ascending aorta may be successfully diagnosed by echocardiography. Because ultrasound cannot penetrate the air-filled lung, aneurysms or dissections in other portions of the aorta cannot be diagnosed with this modality unless the lesion is so large that it is in direct contact with the chest wall.

Dilatation of the aortic root more than 4 cm implies an aneurysm or dissection. A double lumen is characteristic of dissection. Indirect signs of aneurysm or dissection include aortic valve insufficiency (demonstrated by left ventricular dilatation and fibrillation of the mitral valve and interventricular septum) and left-to-right shunts caused by rupture of an aneurysm into the superior vena cava or pulmonary artery.

## Aortography

One of the most acute situations in which an immediate diagnosis is required is laceration or rupture of the aorta. The history of a traffic accident with deceleration trauma followed by chest pain and widening of the mediastinum on the chest radiograph is strongly suggestive of this diagnosis (Fig. 4-10). An immediate aortogram is indicated not only to demonstrate the lesion prior to operation, but also to exclude laceration or rupture of the aorta in the patient in whom the mediastinum is widened due to other causes.

In the patient with a suspected acute dissection of the thoracic aorta, aortography is also the procedure of choice. In both emergency situations (acute rupture or acute dissection of the thoracic aorta), there is usually no time to perform CT or MRI.

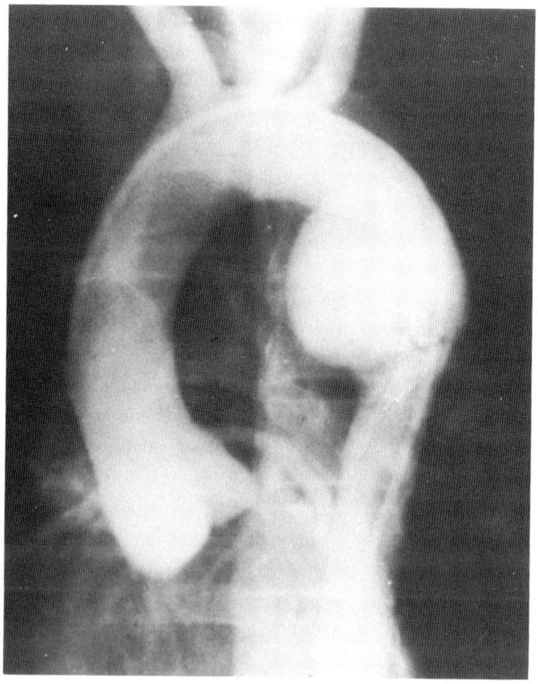

**Figure 4-10.** Aortic rupture after deceleration trauma (traffic accident). As in this case, the rupture usually occurs distal to the origin of the left subclavian artery.

In both acute rupture and acute dissection of the thoracic aorta, the tip of the catheter should be placed in the ascending aorta, 4 cm to 5 cm above the plane of the aortic valve. There is some controversy in the literature about the best approach. Some authors favor the right axillary route in order to avoid passing the injured area, which most often is located distal to the innominate artery. In our experience, catheterization using a soft pigtail catheter can be performed safely from the femoral artery if it is done with care. Because the circulation is usually decreased, a relatively slow injection rate with a large dose is required.

If CT or MRI is not available, aortography can be the definitive procedure for distinguishing between a thoracic aortic aneurysm and a para-aortic mass or generalized unexplained mediastinal widening (Fig. 4-11). If a thoracic aortic aneurysm is demonstrated, abdominal aortography should also be performed, because com-

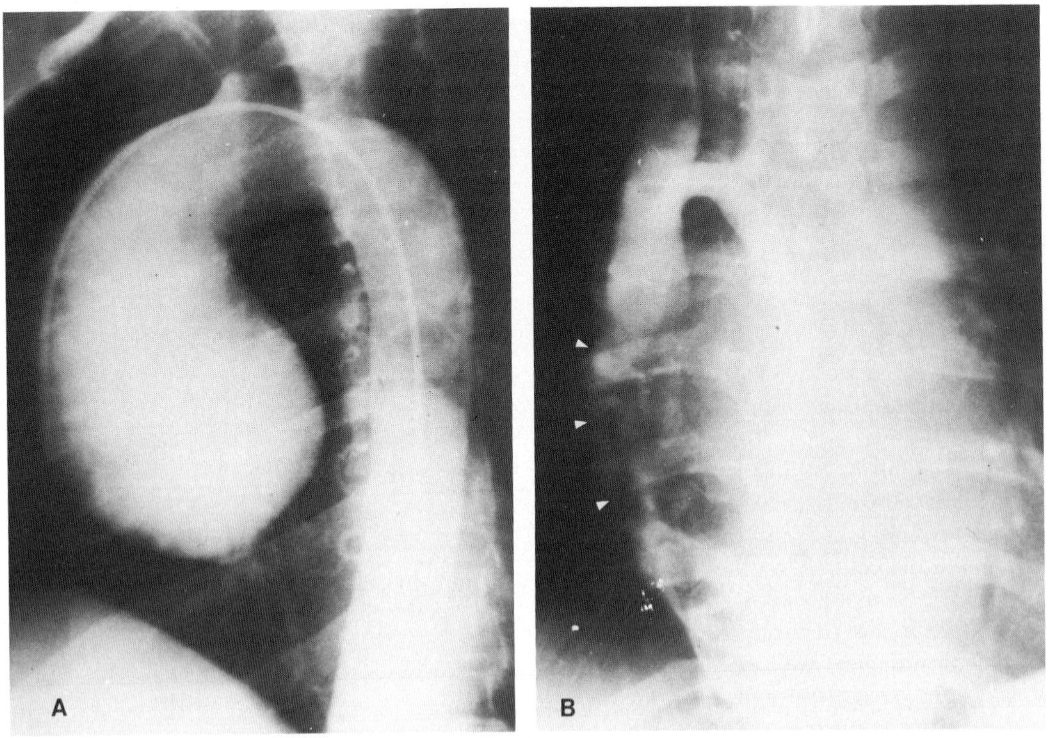


**Figure 4-11.** Aneurysm of ascending aorta in Marfan's syndrome. There is enormous dilatation of the ascending aorta **(A)**, which compresses the right atrium and superior vena cava (*arrowheads* in **B**), resulting in retrograde venous flow from the superior to the inferior vena cava via the azygos vein.

bined thoraco-abdominal aneurysms are common.

The definitive arteriographic diagnosis of an aortic dissection depends on the demonstration of two channels separated by an intimal flap (Fig. 4-12). The false channel may be filled with clot and thus impossible to opacify with contrast material. In this situation, the diagnosis can be made by demonstration of a compressed true channel (Fig. 4-13). In addition, the aortic wall will be thickened (>5 mm), although this is a nonspecific finding that may also be due to mural thrombus, aortitis, neoplasm, or abundant periaortic fat.

Flow in the false lumen indicates either runoff or re-entry. In the latter condition (associated with a much higher mortality), an effort should be made to demonstrate the points of entry and re-entry. When both lumens are filled with contrast material, the true lumen is usually located on the inner curvature of the ascending and descending aorta, and the false lumen spirals around it. The best radiographic projection for demonstrating the two lumens is usually the right posterior oblique.

At times, the false channel is inadvertently entered at aortography. The clue to this situation is the absence of filling of the coronary, brachiocephalic, or intercostal arteries, as well as the indirect sign of a lack of catheter recoil during contrast injection. Injection into the false channel of the dissection may produce aortic rupture of extended dissection and should be avoided if possible; a slow hand injection may be performed. Once it is determined that the false channel has been entered from the transfemoral approach, it is usually better to use the axillary or brachial route.

The use of digital subtraction angiography after the intra-arterial injection of contrast mate-

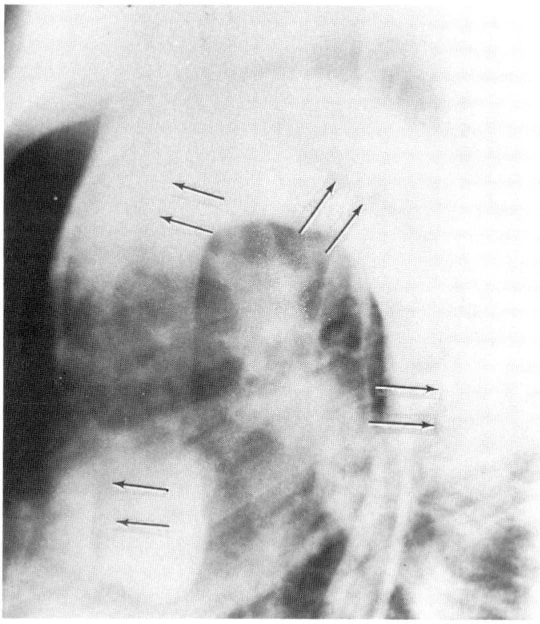

**Figure 4-12.** Type I aortic dissection. Aortogram shows the intimal flap (*arrows*) and the two channels. There was re-entry below the diaphragm.

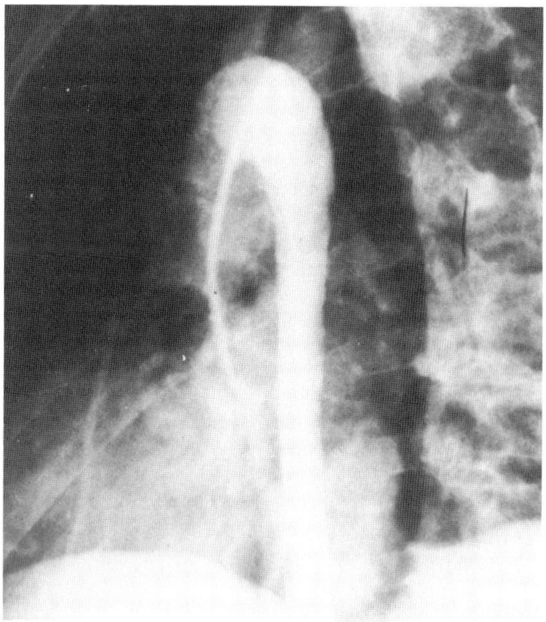

**Figure 4-13.** Type II aortic dissection. Note the narrowing of the true lumen and nonfilling of the false lumen (verified at operation).

rial for imaging of the thoracic aorta is somewhat controversial. This technique is widely employed for diagnosing aortic aneurysms, for which only gross pathologic changes need to be demonstrated. For more detailed study of anatomic structures, as in demonstrating subtle dissections, conventional aortography is usually required. Digital angiography is of value in patients with impaired renal function, because a lower dose of contrast material and nonionic contrast agents can be used.

The overall mortality rate from all types of percutaneous aortography is 0.06%. Major complications occur in approximately 0.7% of patients; minor complications are seen in less than 3% of patients.

Imaging of the thoracic aorta after intravenous contrast injection is usually not sufficient to demonstrate the anatomy of a suspected aortic aneurysm. In the patient in whom arterial catheterization is impossible because of severe arteriosclerosis, contrast injection via direct puncture of the left ventricle has been preferable to venous angiography.

## Surgery

Although the final confirmation of an aortic aneurysm or dissection is usually made at operation, surgery is rarely performed as a diagnostic procedure. Indeed, a precise diagnosis is essential before surgical treatment. Computed tomography, MRI, or aortography is required to provide the maximum preoperative information regarding the size, structure, and location of the aneurysm or dissection and its relation to the surrounding structures.

## Bibliography

Amparo EG, Higgins CB, Hricak H et al: Aortic dissection: Magnetic resonance imaging. Radiology 155:399–406, 1985

Brown OR, Popp RL, Kloster FE: Echocardiographic criteria for aortic root dissection. Am J Cardiol 36:17–20, 1975

Debakey ME, Noon GP: Aneurysms of the thoracic aorta. Mod Concepts Cardiovasc Dis 44:53, 1975

Egan TJ, Neiman HL, Herman RJ et al: Computed tomography in the diagnosis of aortic aneurysm dissection of traumatic injury. Radiology 136: 141–146, 1980

Geisinger MA, Risius B, O'Donnell JA et al: Thoracic aortic dissections: Magnetic resonance imaging. Radiology 155:407–412, 1985

Godwin JD, Breiman RS, Speckman JM: Problems and pitfalls in the evaluation of thoracic aortic dissection by computed tomography. J Comput Assist Tomogr 6:750–756, 1982

Gramiak R, Shah PM: Echocardiography of the aortic root. Invest Radiol 3:356–366, 1968

Gross SC, Barr L, Eyler WR et al: Computed tomography in dissection of the thoracic aorta. Radiology 136:135–139, 1980

Harris EJ: Aneurysms of the sinus of Valsalva. AJR 76:767–772, 1956

Hayashi K, Meaney TF, Zelch JV et al: Aortographic analysis of aortic dissection. AJR 122:769–782, 1974

Heiberg E, Wolverson MK, Sundaram M et al: CT characteristics of aortic atherosclerotic aneurysm versus aortic dissection. J Comput Assist Tomogr 9:78–83, 1985

Higgins CB, Silverman NR, Harris RD et al: Localized aneurysms of the descending thoracic aorta. Clin Radiol 26:475–482, 1975

Kanik V, Hemley SD, Kittredge RD et al: Some problems in the angiographic diagnosis of dissecting aneurysms of the thoracic aorta. AJR 91: 1283–1287, 1964

Lang EK: A survey of the complications of percutaneous retrograde arteriography. Seldinger technique. Radiology 81:257–263, 1963

Lardé D, Belloir C, Vasile N et al: Computed tomography of aortic dissection. Radiology 136: 147–151, 1980

McKusick VA: The cardiovascular aspects of Marfan's syndrome: A heritable disorder of connective tissue. Circulation 11:321–342, 1955

Mills CM, Brant–Zawadzki M, Crooks LE et al: Nuclear magnetic resonance principle of blood flow imaging. AJR 142:165–170, 1984

Moore EH, Webb WR, Verrier ED et al: MRI of chronic posttraumatic false aneurysms of the thoracic aorta. AJR 143:1195–1196, 1984

Morgan JR, Rogers AK, Fosbus RG: Ruptured aneurysms of sinus of Valsalva. Chest 61:640–643, 1972

Nishimura K, Hibi N, Kato T et al: Real-time observation of ruptured right sinus of Valsalva aneurysm by high-speed ultrasonocardiotomography. Circulation 53:732–735, 1976

Oudkerk M, Overbosch E, Dee P: CT recognition of acute aortic dissection. AJR 141:671–676, 1983

Pattison JN, Grainger RG: Congenital kinking of the aortic arch. Br Heart J 21:555–561, 1969

Pinet F, Michaud P, Amiel M et al: Aortography of traumatic aneurysms of the thoracic aorta: A study of 10 cases. Ann Radiol 16:11, 1973

Simeone JF, Minagi H, Putman CE: Traumatic disruption of the thoracic aorta: Significance of the left apical extra-pleural cap. Radiology 117: 265–268, 1975

Sutorious DJ, Schreiber JT, Helmsworth JA: Traumatic disruption of the thoracic aorta. J Trauma 13:583–590, 1973

Symbas PN, Baldwin BJ, Silverman ME et al: Marfan's syndrome with aneurysm of the ascending aorta and aortic regurgitation. Am J Cardiol 25: 483–489, 1970

Vasile N, Mathieu D, Keita K et al: Computed tomography of thoracic aortic dissection: Accuracy and pitfalls. J Comput Assist Tomogr 10:211–215, 1986

Webb WR, Gamsu G, Crooks LE: Multisection sagittal and coronal magnetic resonance imaging of the mediastinum and hila. Radiology 150: 475–478, 1984

Wyman SM: Dissecting aneurysm of the thoracic aorta: Its roentgen recognition. AJR 78:247–255, 1957

**SUSPECTED THORACIC ANEURYSM/DISSECTION**

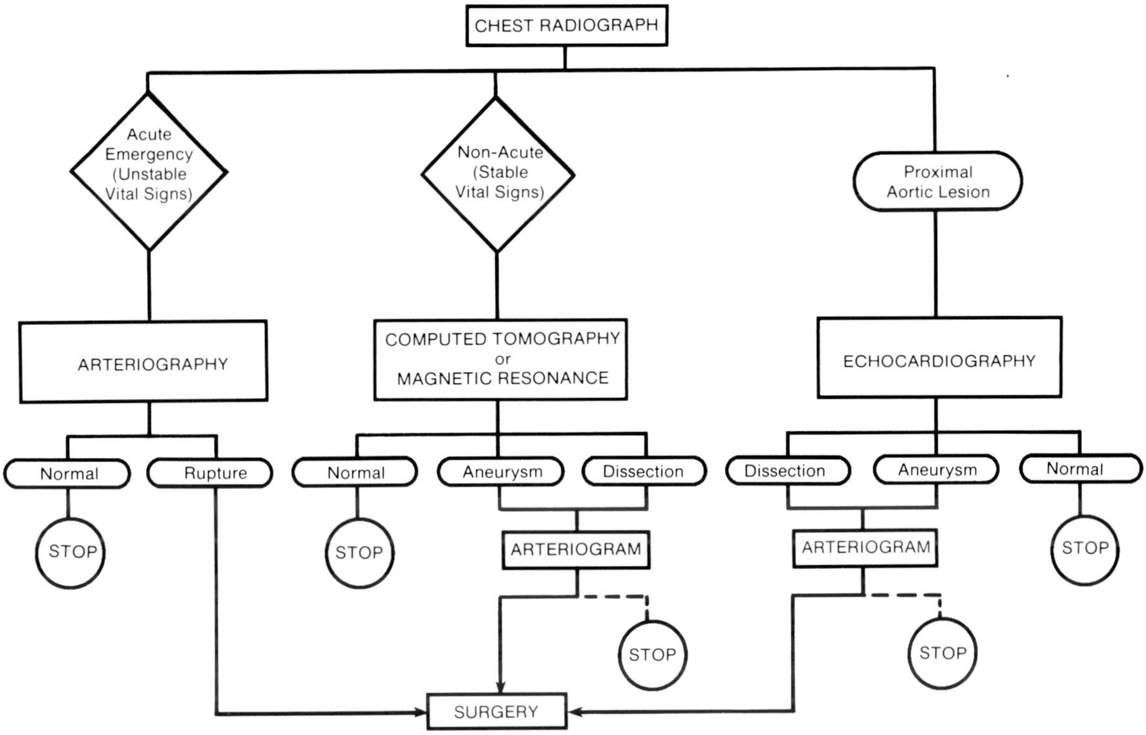

# Chapter 5

# Mediastinal Masses

*David S. Feigin*

Because virtually all normal and abnormal structures in the mediastinum have the same radiographic density, abnormal masses can be visualized only if they displace a pleural stripe to such a degree that the mass, or the structures displaced by the mass, become partially surrounded by air. Since mediastinal structures are generally movable and elastic, masses may displace them to a considerable degree before any clinical symptoms arise. For these reasons, mediastinal masses may become quite large before becoming clinically or radiographically obvious.

Of the many types of masses found in the mediastinum, the most important are

1. Neoplasms—usually benign but occasionally malignant, often without difference in radiographic appearance
2. Lymph node masses—four principal subcategories
   a. Malignant lymphoid diseases, such as Hodgkin's disease
   b. Metastatic disease
   c. Granulomatous disease—infectious and noninfectious
   d. Benign and reactive masses
3. Benign cysts—usually congenital
4. Vascular lesions, especially aneurysms
5. Diffuse fatty or fibrous infiltration

The approach to mediastinal masses has been radically altered by the increasing use of computed tomography (CT) of the chest. Unlike plain film and digital chest radiography, CT can reliably distinguish the fat, fluid, and soft-tissue densities comprising the normal and abnormal mediastinal structures, and it often plays a vital role in the subsequent evaluation and treatment of patients with mediastinal masses.

Density has emerged as a more useful criterion than location for the primary analysis of mediastinal masses. Location and characteristics of imaging appearance then become secondary criteria, to be used along with clinical information in arriving at a differential diagnosis. Eventually, magnetic resonance imaging (MRI) may replace or augment CT in the evaluation of mediastinal masses.

## CLINICAL AND LABORATORY FINDINGS

Approximately half of all mediastinal masses occur in asymptomatic persons. Exceptions include esophageal masses, which nearly always cause dysphagia, and neurofibromas, which usually cause symptoms of peripheral nerve deficit. Mediastinal masses that are symptomatic tend to produce similar symptoms because of displacement of normal mediastinal organs. Such symptoms include dysphagia, stridor, cough, wheezing, localized or diffuse chest pain, or a combination of these, and are far more a function of the size of the mass than of its identity.

The most important clinical symptom complex related to a mediastinal mass is the association of myasthenia gravis with thymoma. Since approximately 15% of all patients with myasthenia gravis have thymomas, any mediastinal mass in a patient with this condition is assumed to be a thymoma unless the findings strongly suggest different diagnosis. The association between thymoma and red blood cell aplasia and hypoplasia is definite but less common. Abnormal thyroid

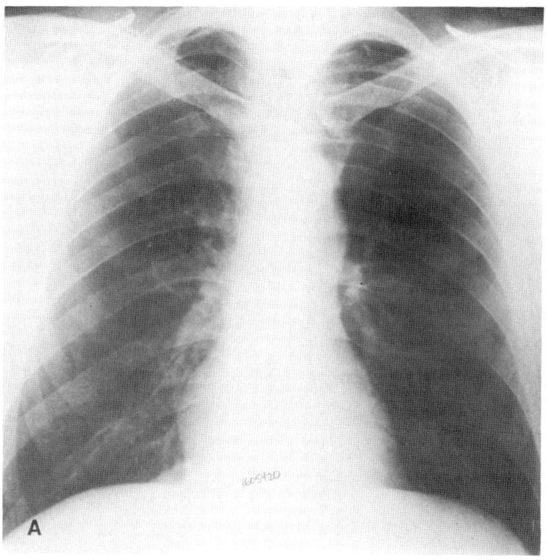


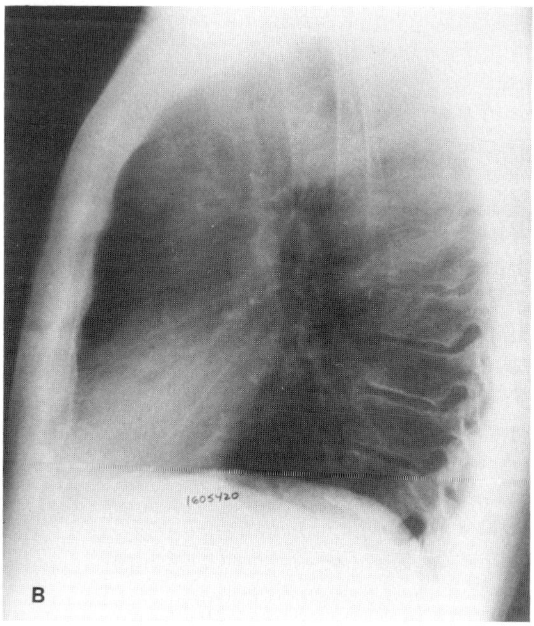


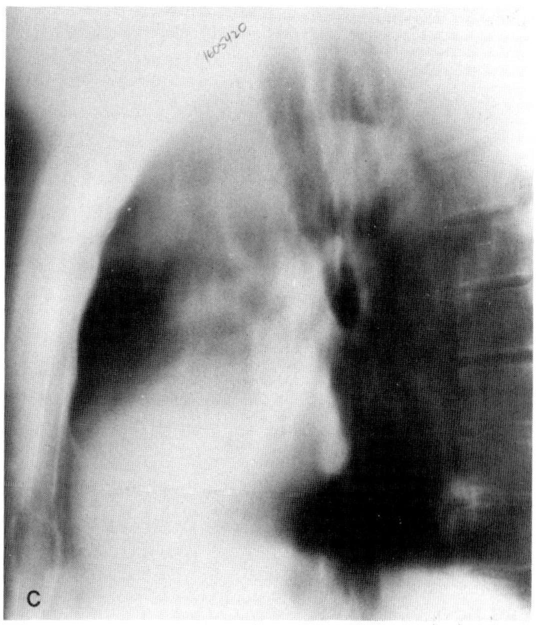


**Figure 5-1.** Anterior mediastinal mass, a thymoma, in a 55-year-old man who had myasthenia gravis. **(A)** Frontal view shows the pleural stripe anterior to the descending aorta to be displaced laterally. **(B)** Lateral view shows a mass in the upper portion of the anterior mediastinum, just anterior to the trachea and extending nearly to the sternum. **(C)** Lateral tomogram shows the anterior mediastinal mass more clearly, including its lobulated lower anterior border. (Courtesy of Armed Forces Institute of Pathology)

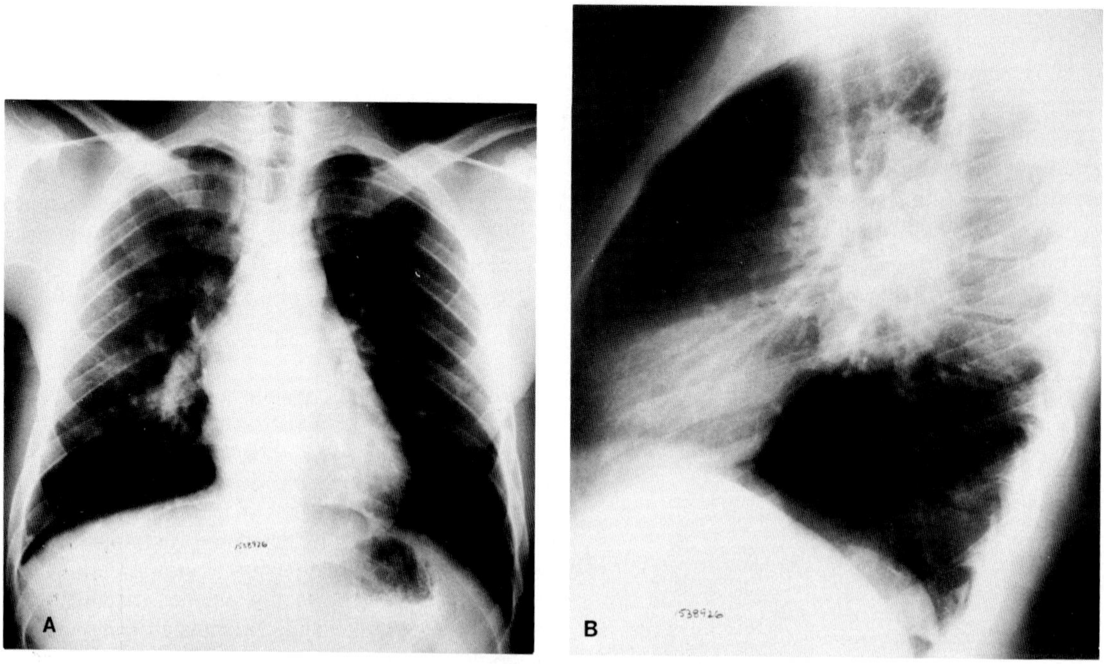

**Figure 5-2.** Middle mediastinal mass, a congenital respiratory cyst, in an asymptomatic 20-year-old man. **(A)** Frontal view demonstrates the mass by displacement of pleura overlying the right hilum. **(B)** Lateral view shows a large mass projecting posteriorly from the region of the carina in the middle mediastinum. (*Continued on facing page*)

function in a patient with a mediastinal mass, especially if the mass is in the superior mediastinum, should suggest that the mass represents abnormal thyroid tissue.

## ANATOMY OF THE MEDIASTINUM

Mediastinal masses are nearly always first discovered on chest radiographs. To arrive at a reasonable differential diagnosis among the many types of masses, it is most convenient to divide the mediastinum into four compartments: anterior, middle, posterior, and superior. It must always be remembered that the superior mediastinum is really the superior extension of the other three compartments rather than a true subdivision.

The anterior mediastinum is most usefully defined as extending from the sternum to a line drawn through the anterior wall of the trachea and posterior border of the heart (Fig 5-1). According to this definition, the anterior mediastinum includes the entire cardiopericardial silhouette, as well as the regions above and anterior to the heart. This is more useful than placing the heart and pericardium in the middle mediastinum, because masses arising from these structures project superiorly and anteriorly more often than posteriorly.

The most common anterior mediastinal masses are neoplasms and cysts. Lymph node masses occur in the anterior mediastinum, but middle mediastinal involvement is usually also visible. Hodgkin's disease, especially the nodular sclerosing form, is an exception and often arises solely in the anterior region. The most common neoplasms are thymoma and teratoma. These are often separable by the age of the patient or the clinical symptoms. The presence of myasthenia gravis favors thymoma. Teratomas are most common in patients younger than 30 years, while thymomas more fequently occur between the ages of 40 and 60 years and are usually found in men. Most anterior mediastinal cysts arise from the pericardium.

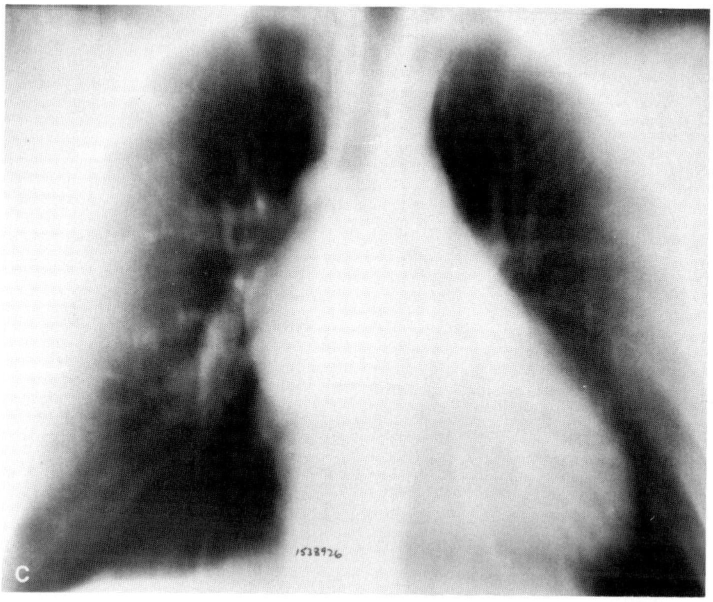

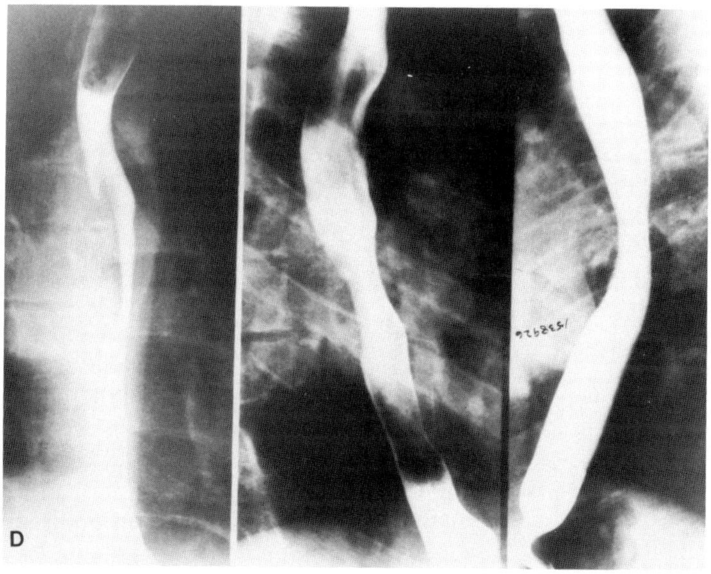

**(C)** Frontal tomogram shows the mass widening the subcarinal bronchial angle with prominent lateral displacement of the bronchus intermedius and right main stem bronchus. **(D)** Three views from an esophagogram show extrinsic compression of the esophagus by the mass. (Courtesy of Armed Forces Institute of Pathology)

The middle mediastinum extends from the anterior wall of the trachea and posterior border of the heart to the anterior border of the vertebral bodies (Fig. 5-2). Most middle mediastinal masses are lymph nodes, cysts, or aneurysms. Esophageal masses usually become symptomatic before they are radiographically apparent.

Posterior mediastinal masses are all those situated behind the anterior borders of the vertebral bodies (Fig. 5-3). Neoplasms, especially neurogenic tumors, are by far the most common posterior mediastinal masses.

Masses that appear to arise from or extend through the diaphragm may represent mediastinal projections of abdominal masses and may occur in any of the three compartments. If such masses are of soft-tissue density, they are best evaluated by liver scan, liver–lung scan, upper gastrointestinal series, or barium enema, depending on their location.

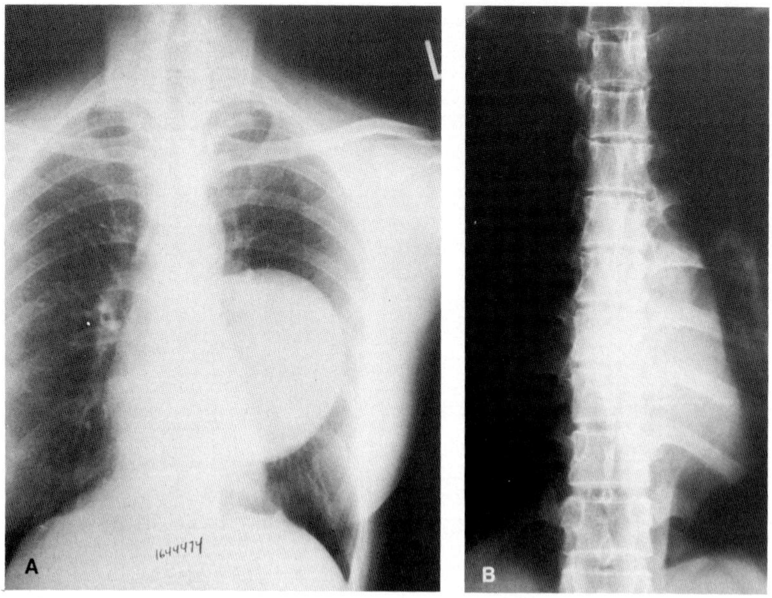


**Figure 5-3.** Posterior mediastinal mass, a neurolemmoma, in a 40-year-old woman who had vague posterior chest pain. **(A)** Frontal view shows a very large, sharply defined mass in the left chest. **(B)** Overpenetrated frontal view shows displacement of the paravertebral pleural stripe laterally, clearly indicating the posterior location of the mass and its origin from the mediastinum. (Courtesy of Armed Forces Institute of Pathology)

The superior mediastinum is defined as the portion of the other three compartments located above the top of the aortic arch. The most important mass in this region is enlargement of the most inferior part of the thyroid, often called the "substernal thyroid," which is best evaluated by radionuclide studies or by CT. All other masses in the superior mediastinum, however, should be evaluated in the same manner as those farther inferior in the same vertical compartment.

## DIAGNOSTIC EVALUATION

### *DIAGNOSTIC MODALITIES*

1. Plain film radiography, including oblique and overpenetrated views
2. Fluoroscopy
3. Digital chest radiography
4. Computed tomography
5. Conventional tomography
6. Esophagogram
7. Magnetic resonance imaging
8. Ultrasound and ultrasound-guided cyst puncture
9. Thyroid scan
10. Angiogram or venogram
11. Gallium scan
12. Myelogram
13. Percutaneous biopsy
14. Endoscopic biopsy
15. Mediastinoscopy and surgery

### Plain Film Radiography

Plain film radiography is of value not only in detecting mediastinal masses, but also in determining the location of a mass and whether there are any associated bony abnormalities. Not all mediastinal masses are sufficiently visible on the lateral view to facilitate placing the mass in its appropriate compartment. Clues from the frontal view, such as the hilum overlay sign and loss of specific pleural stripes, should be used whenever possible. Oblique views, especially shallow obliques, are often very helpful (Fig. 5-4). Overpenetrated views are essential in analysis of the posterior mediastinum and are often of value in placing other masses (see Fig. 5-3).

Bony involvement is usually visible on plain films, especially if coned-down views are obtained of areas with localized chest pain. An anterior mediastinal mass with sternal erosion is far more likely to be Hodgkin's disease than another mass in this compartment. Neurogenic tumors,

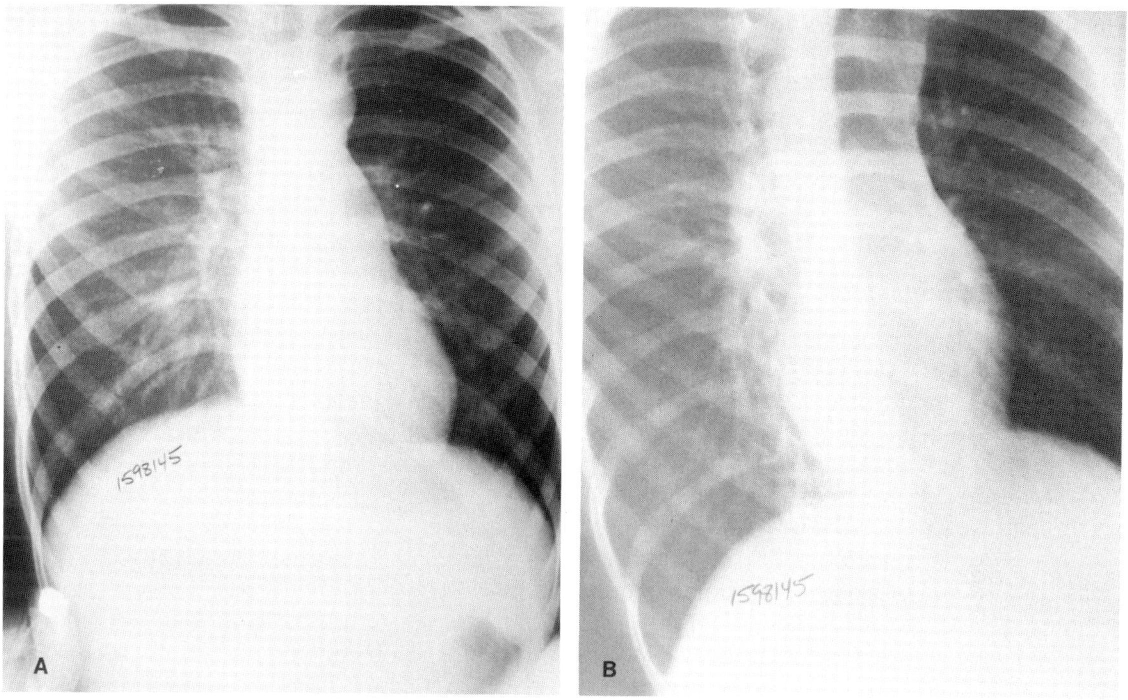

**Figure 5-4.** Middle mediastinal mass, a congenital respiratory cyst, in an asymptomatic 8-year-old girl. **(A)** Frontal view shows minimal visualization of a mass behind the heart medially. **(B)** Right anterior oblique view clearly shows a mass in the middle mediastinum with displacement of the right pleura from just below the carina to the diaphragm. (Courtesy of Armed Forces Institute of Pathology)

even when benign, often cause pressure erosion of spinal processes or ribs. Neural foraminal enlargement is seen in a sizable minority of neurolemmomas and neurofibromas because of growth of the tumor within and outside the spinal canal.

## Fluoroscopy

Fluoroscopy is occasionally of value in localizing mediastinal masses that are not clearly visualized on plain radiographs. Most advocates of fluoroscopy of mediastinal masses are those who have been pursuing this approach for many years; other radiologists favor the use of oblique views. On the average, the difference in radiation exposure is trivial. I personally favor oblique views, because their increased resolution permits careful analysis of disturbances of the pleural stripes.

## Digital Chest Radiography

Computer processing of a standard view of the chest may be performed in several ways. Digitization of density data can produce an image of exceedingly wide latitude that may be viewed with selected windows and center values similar to CT. A laser can be used to "read" an existing radiograph, again resulting in a manipulatable image of very wide latitude. Digitization of chest images results in improved demonstration of both normal and abnormal mediastinal structures. The effect is similar to having several films of varying penetration simultaneously available for interpretation.

The value of digital chest imaging is thus no greater than that of a perfect plain film of the chest in any single projection. Unlike CT, density differentiation is not improved. The radiation dose can be minimized, especially because repeat examinations necessitated by technical inadequacy are virtually eliminated. Continued improvement in digital techniques, coupled with the increasing need to find alternatives to the expense and storage of films, may increase the future usefulness of this modality.

## Computed Tomography

Two vital characteristics of CT have markedly increased the value of this modality in imaging mediastinal masses. Computed tomography can readily distinguish among the densities of fat, fluid (as in a cyst), soft tissue, and moving blood (when contrast enhanced). The cross-sectional anatomy provided by CT images allows more precise localization of masses than is possible in any conventional projection. Thus, CT has become the imaging procedure of choice whenever a mediastinal mass is present or suspected on plain radiographs. In most cases, CT obviates the need for conventional tomography, oblique and overpenetrated views, or fluoroscopy. The risks of CT are limited to those related to the administration of contrast material, which is often not needed if advanced CT equipment is available.

Masses consisting exclusively or principally of fat may be diagnosed by CT without need for further evaluation or intervention. Such masses are virtually always benign and include diffuse lipomatosis of the mediastinum, localized lipomas, thymolipomas, and similar lesions. Although most cystic masses are benign, some malignant lesions may be cystic. If the position of a cystic mass permits, cyst puncture is often performed. If the cyst is not accessible to puncture, thoracotomy still may be necessary; however, many clinicians prefer to observe the lesion if they are sure it is cystic, and especially if the patient is a significant operative risk (Fig. 5-5). The accuracy of CT diagnosis in other soft-tissue masses is variable (Figs. 5-6 and 5-7). Both highly vascular lesions and blood vessel masses themselves (such as aneurysms) usually require CT before and after the infusion of contrast material. Differences in CT number with and without contrast should be compared with the CT numbers of obvious blood vessels, such as the aorta or pulmonary artery (Fig. 5-8). Bolus injection may be necessary to provide sufficient density difference between blood vessels and dense or highly vascular masses. The difference in density between cystic and solid soft-tissue masses is variable. Nonseptated cysts with clear fluid often exhibit lower CT numbers than soft-tissue structures, but complex cysts are usually indistinguishable from soft-tissue masses.

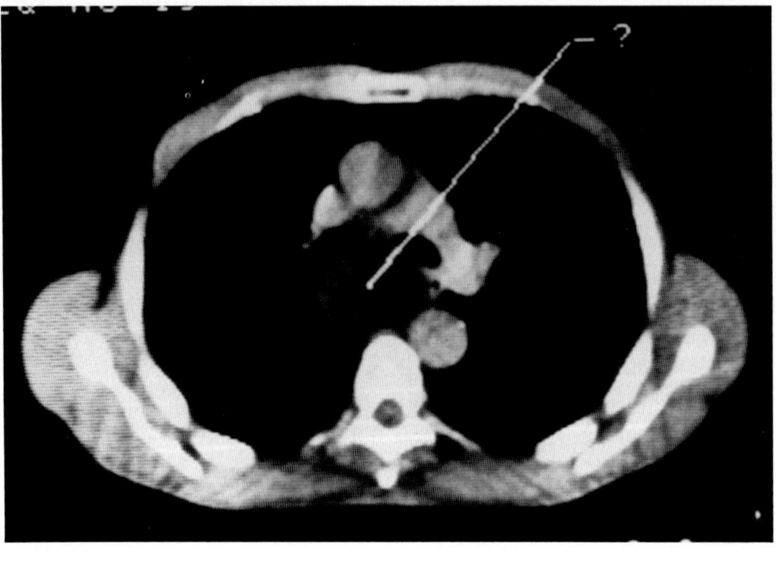


**Figure 5-5.** Congenital respiratory cyst in an elderly man. Contrast-enhanced CT at the carinal level shows a water density mass (?) located just posterior to the carina. This is the most common position for congenital respiratory cysts. (Reprinted by permission of the publisher from Mediastinal masses: A system for diagnosis based on computed tomography, by Feigin DS and Padua EM, J Comput Tomogr 10: 11–21. Copyright 1986 by Elsevier Science Publishing Co, Inc)

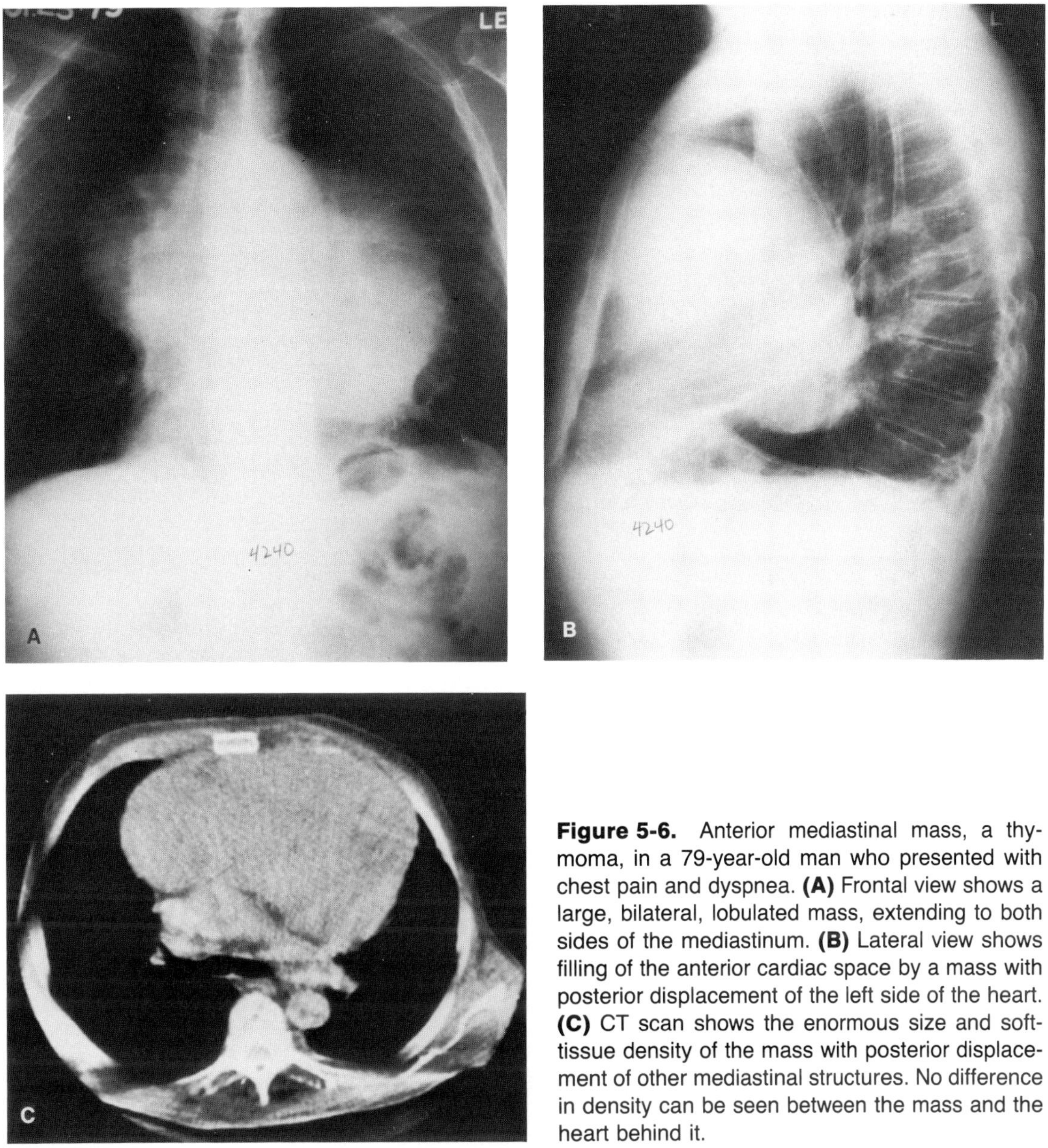

**Figure 5-6.** Anterior mediastinal mass, a thymoma, in a 79-year-old man who presented with chest pain and dyspnea. **(A)** Frontal view shows a large, bilateral, lobulated mass, extending to both sides of the mediastinum. **(B)** Lateral view shows filling of the anterior cardiac space by a mass with posterior displacement of the left side of the heart. **(C)** CT scan shows the enormous size and soft-tissue density of the mass with posterior displacement of other mediastinal structures. No difference in density can be seen between the mass and the heart behind it.

## Conventional Tomography

Conventional tomography is usually necessary only if CT is not available. The frustration that many radiologists experience with conventional tomography of the mediastinum is often caused by attempting to use the frontal view when an oblique or lateral projection is far more appropriate (see Fig. 5-1). Conventional tomograms should always be obtained in the position in which the mass is best visualized on plain films. The meanderings of the mediastinal pleura on both sides usually make the frontal view the least useful projection. Lateral tomography is often the best projection for anterior or superior mediastinal masses. Steep obliques are usually the best projections for posterior masses, because spinous process and rib involvement may be assessed at the same time as the mass.

The risks of conventional tomography are

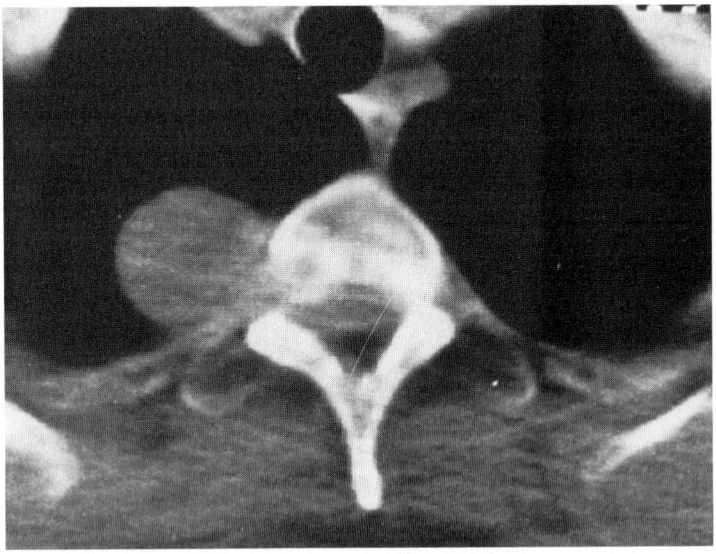

**Figure 5-7.** Posterior mediastinal mass, a neurolemmoma, in a young man. Detail of a CT scan demonstrates widening of a neural foramen with a soft-tissue density both inside and outside the spinal canal. (Reprinted by permission of the publisher from Mediastinal masses: A system for diagnosis based on computed tomography, by Feigin DS and Padua EM, J Comput Tomogr 10:11–21. Copyright 1986 by Elsevier Science Publishing Co, Inc)

limited to expense and radiation, the latter of which is similar to that from multiple plain films of the chest. Resolution can be maximized and the dose minimized by limiting the field of view to as small an area as possible.

## Esophagogram

A barium swallow is essential in the analysis of middle mediastinal masses (see Fig. 5-2). It is usually possible to differentiate primary esophageal masses from those secondarily deviating the esophagus. The esophagogram can also demonstrate the relationship between the esophagus and the heart or aorta without need for more costly studies, such as CT. The typical deviations of the esophagus by enlarged blood vessels in the upper mediastinum and by bronchogenic cysts at the level of the carina are so characteristic that they sometimes obviate the need for further investigation or lead directly to angiography or surgery. Substernal thyroids usually produce some deviation of the esophagus, and so the

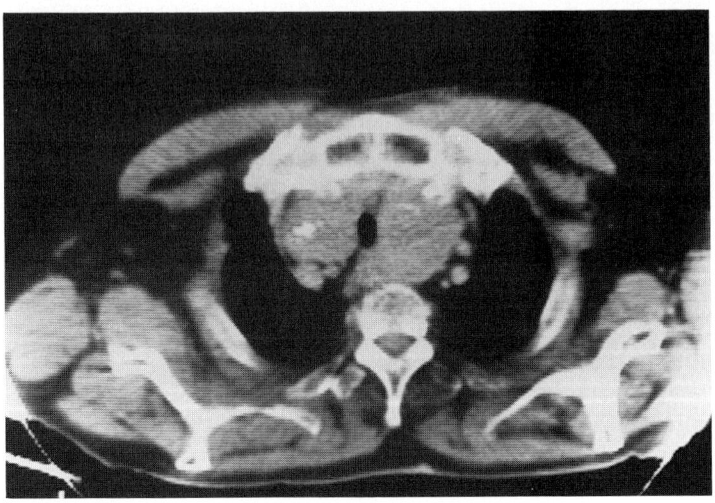

**Figure 5-8.** Multinodular goiter with diffuse thyroid enlargement. CT at the level of the sternoclavicular junction shows a large thyroid mass surrounding and narrowing the trachea with displacement of other mediastinal structures laterally and posteriorly. There is calcification in the right lobe of the thyroid, and the overall thyroid density slightly exceeds that of the average muscle. (Reprinted by permission of the publisher from Mediastinal masses: A system for diagnosis based on computed tomography, by Feigin DS and Padua EM, J Comput Tomogr 10:11–21. Copyright 1986 by Elsevier Science Publishing Co, Inc)

esophagogram is of little use in evaluating these patients. Primary esophageal masses are best approached by endoscopic biopsy rather than by further imaging of the mediastinum.

## Magnetic Resonance Imaging

Magnetic resonance imaging has not yet proven superior to CT in the evaluation of mediastinal masses. The major advantage of MRI is that it can be performed in any projection, including sagittal and parasagittal. Sagittal projections are most useful for imaging the great vessels, especially the aorta (Fig. 5-9). Because moving blood produces no signal on MRI, this modality has the potential for increasing the specificity of imaging of vascular abnormalities, such as thromboembolism, aneurysm, and dissection.

Investigations are under way to evaluate the possible use of MRI to distinguish among masses of soft-tissue density (such as inflammatory versus malignant enlarged lymph nodes) by identifying differences in signal intensity using varieties of pulse sequencing. Such differentiation would be of great value in obviating the need for biopsy or surgery in many cases (*e.g.*, preoperative evaluation of patients with bronchogenic carcinoma).

The principal disadvantages of MRI are its enormous expense and limited availability. Patient criteria for suitability also are more limited than for other imaging modalities, because pacemakers and other implanted metallic devices are contraindications and a patient cannot be examined if his girth exceeds that of the imager. Cardiac gating is essential for all mediastinal masses except those in the superior region. This requirement for gating necessitates longer acquisition times, which require significant patient cooperation and lead to less efficient utilization of the imager.

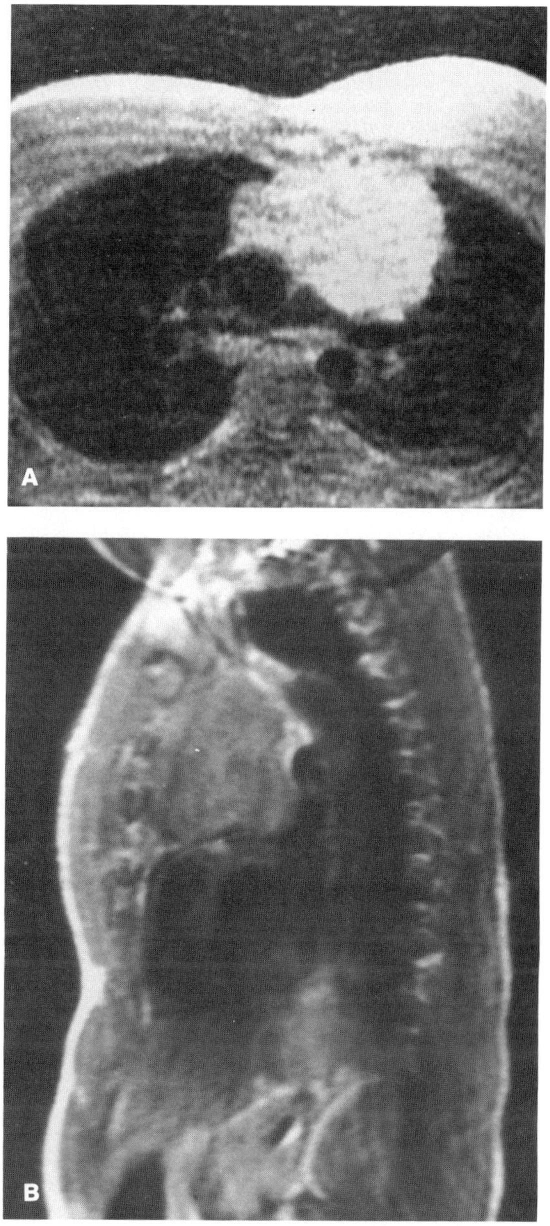


**Figure 5-9.** Anterior mediastinal mass, Hodgkin's disease, in a young man. **(A)** Transverse MRI shows a large, lobulated, anterior mass with high signal intensity on a T2-weighted image. **(B)** Sagittal view with T1 weighting shows displacement of adjacent structures inferior and posterior to the mass.

## Ultrasound and Cyst Puncture

The use of ultrasound to evaluate the mediastinum is severely inhibited by the presence of air in the lungs, which surrounds the mediastinum in most projections. An obvious exception exists in

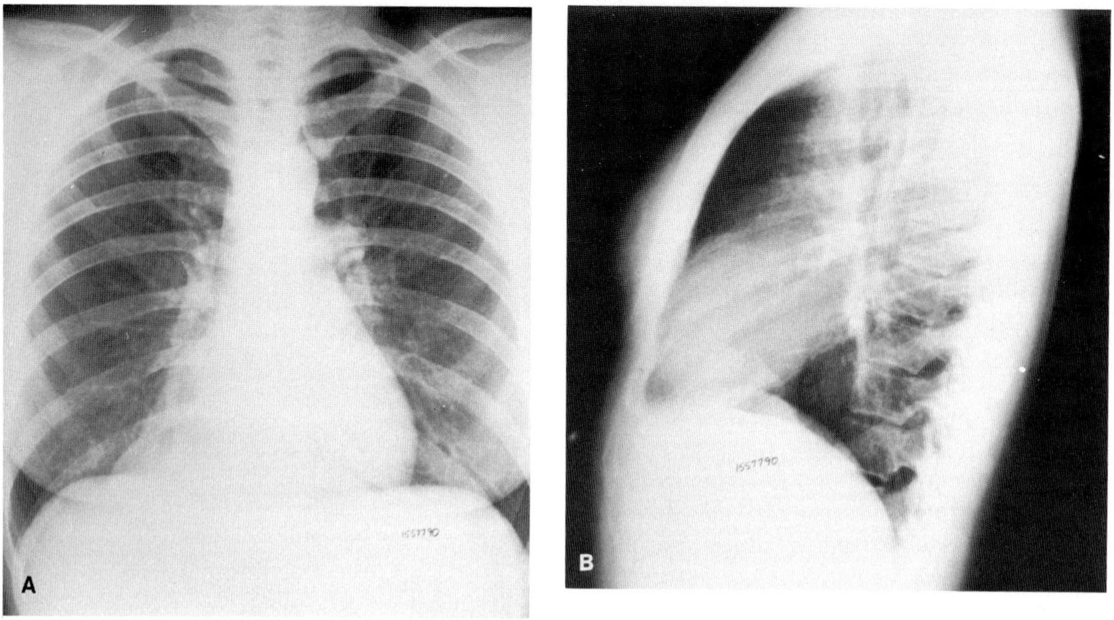

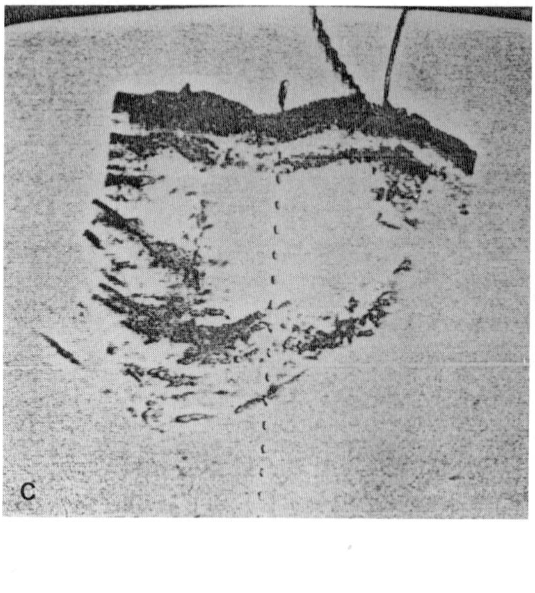

**Figure 5-10.** Anterior mediastinal mass, a pericardial cyst, in a 27-year-old woman who complained only of a cough. **(A)** Frontal view shows a mass in the right cardiophrenic angle. **(B)** Lateral view shows the mass to overlie the heart and to touch the anterior portion of the diaphragm. **(C)** B-mode ultrasound shows the cystic nature of the mass with excellent through transmission and no internal echoes. (Courtesy of Armed Forces Institute of Pathology)

the lower anterior mediastinum, where the lack of intervening air permits cysts, especially pericardial cysts, to be visualized by ultrasound (Fig. 5-10). Some radiologists recommend puncture of pericardial cysts both to confirm the presence of the cyst and to deflate it. This procedure is virtually free of complications and obviates the need for surgery or other diagnostic studies.

The use of ultrasound and cyst puncture in other areas of the mediastinum is not yet generally accepted. Middle mediastinal cysts occasionally can be evaluated by ultrasound, but it is difficult to confirm their cystic nature with sufficient confidence to eliminate the need for further diagnostic investigation. Cyst puncture in the middle mediastinum is both more difficult and more hazardous; however, its safety is increasing as more radiologists and other physicians are becoming experienced in its techniques.

### Thyroid Scan

Whenever a superior mediastinal mass deviates the trachea and displaces the upper mediastinal pleural stripe to either side, enlargement of a substernal thyroid is the most likely cause of the radiographic abnormality (Fig. 5-11). Such masses may first be evaluated by $^{99m}Tc$ thyroid scanning, followed, if necessary, by $^{131}I$ thyroid scanning or CT. Computed tomography may also be used as the initial study as an alternative to radionuclide thyroid scanning.

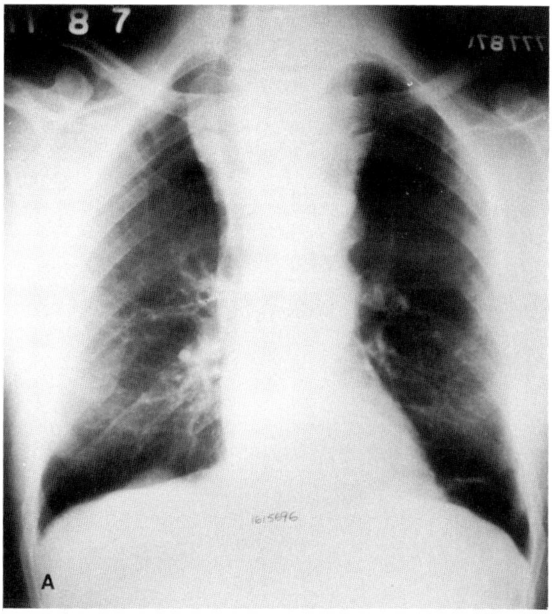

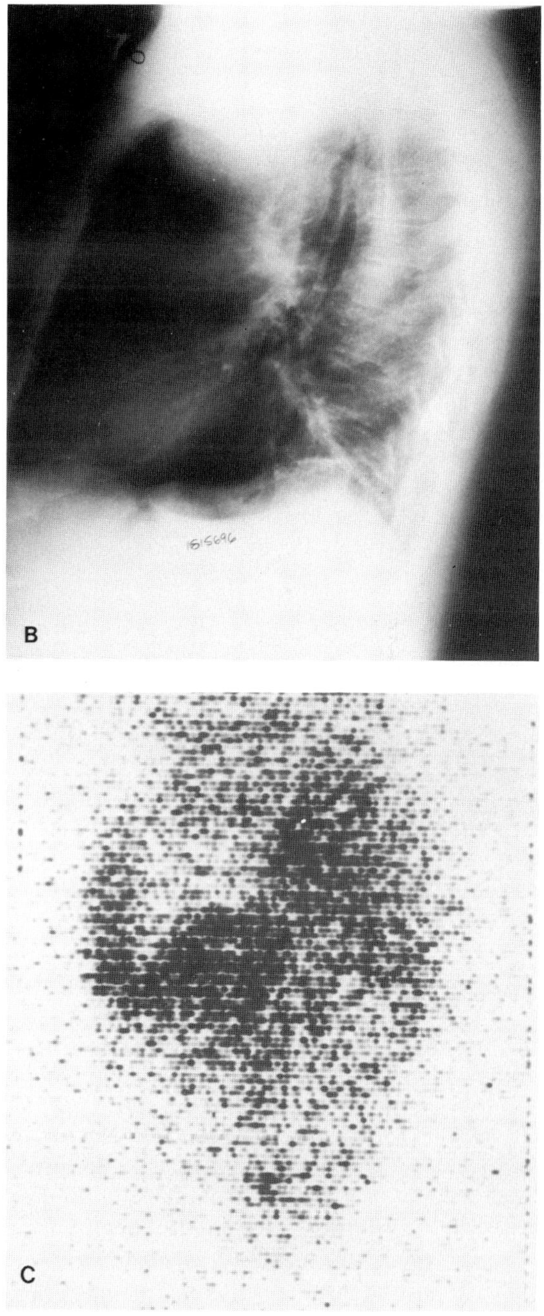

**Figure 5-11.** Superior mediastinal mass, a multinodular substernal thyroid, in a 60-year-old man who presented with dyspnea. **(A)** Frontal view shows marked widening of the superior mediastinum to both sides and severe deviation of the trachea to the right. **(B)** Lateral view shows posterior displacement of the trachea by the large superior mediastinal mass. **(C)** $^{131}I$ scan shows marked increased uptake of the radionuclide in the area of the mass seen on the radiographs. (Courtesy of Armed Forces Institute of Pathology)

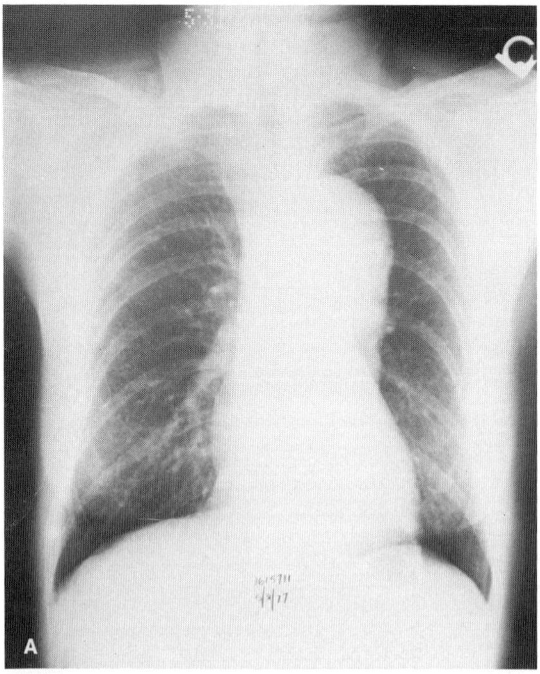

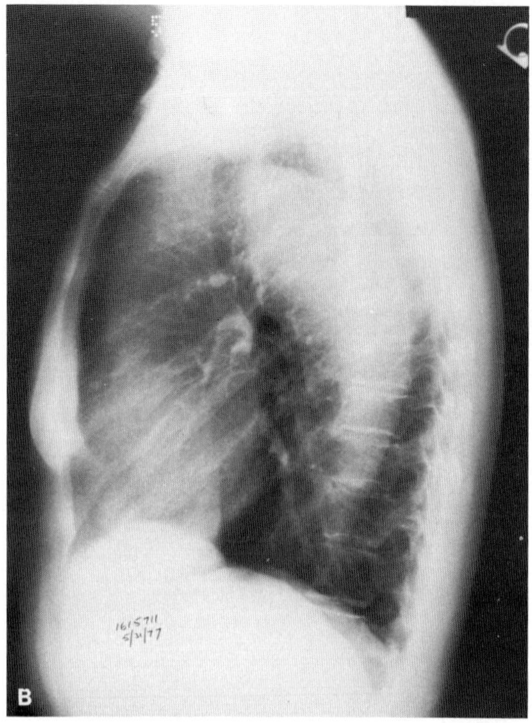

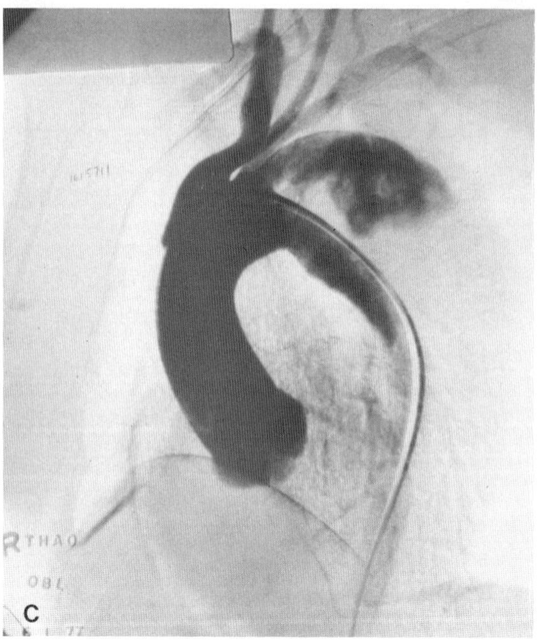

**Figure 5-12.** Middle mediastinal mass, a dissecting aortic aneurysm, in a 54-year-old woman who had experienced sharp, sudden chest pain. **(A)** Frontal view shows massive dilatation of the aortic knob and posterior thoracic aorta. **(B)** Lateral view confirms the aortic enlargement and shows some tracheal displacement anteriorly. **(C)** Oblique view of an aortogram shows contrast entering a large dissection that originates near the origin of the left subclavian artery. (Courtesy of Armed Forces Institute of Pathology)

Thyroid scanning is the most accurate method for diagnosing the presence of abnormal thyroid tissue in the neck or mediastinum. The so-called "substernal" thyroid is generally an extension of the normal thyroid gland into the anterior portion of the superior mediastinum and does not represent an independent mass. Although technetium scanning is often diagnostic, the energy of this isotope may be insufficient to penetrate the sternum. Normal structures in this region may also take up the radiopharmaceutical. For these reasons, iodine scanning is often necessary despite the significantly higher dose to the gland (50 rem or more) when $^{131}I$ is used. Iodine-123, if available, is preferred, because the dose to the gland with this isotope is less than 2% of that from a $^{131}$I scan.

If no thyroid scan demonstrates increased uptake in or around a mass deviating the trachea, the lesion should be investigated in the same manner as a mass situated lower in the mediastinum in that compartment.

## Arteriography or Venography

Arteriography is required and is extremely accurate in the investigation of masses in the middle mediastinum that are suspected of being lesions of blood vessels (especially aneurysms and dissections) (Fig. 5-12). Venography is indicated in middle mediastinal masses associated with symptoms of venous obstruction (Fig. 5-13). However, arteriography is much less useful and is not indicated in the evaluation of mediastinal lesions that are not suspected to be of blood vessel origin. The specificity of arteriography in investigating soft-tissue masses in the mediastinum is not high, although scattered reports suggest that this procedure may be of value in evaluating anterior mediastinal masses. Complications occur in 1% to 3% of patients who undergo thoracic aortography. Fatalities are very uncommon, far less than 1%, and most have been reported to involve infants. Most complications of thoracic aortography are related to the site of entry of the catheter. Significant complications in the chest include neurotoxicity secondary to inadvertent injection of contrast into an artery supplying the spinal cord, thromboembolic disease including stroke, and puncture of thoracic vessels.

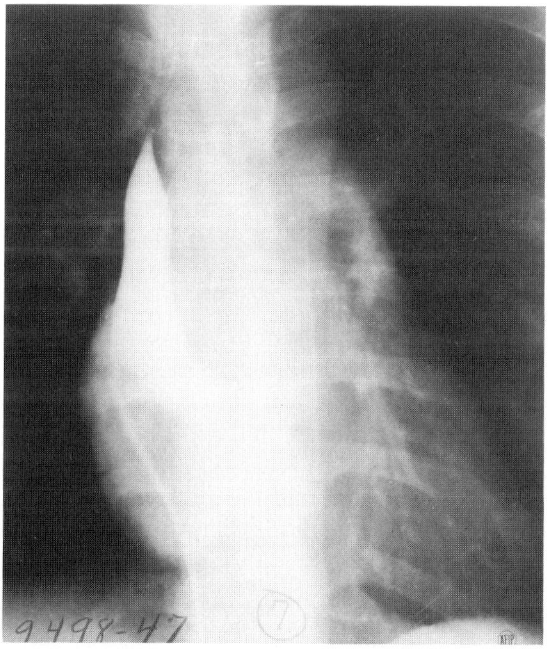

**Figure 5-13.** Sclerosing mediastinitis in a 38-year-old woman who had varicosities over her upper abdomen and lower chest. Venogram shows smooth tapering of the inferior portion of the superior vena cava. (Feigin DS, Eggleston JC, Siegelman SS: The multiple roentgen manifestations of sclerosing mediastinitis. Johns Hopkins Med J 144:1–8, 1979; reprinted with permission)

## Gallium Scan

The role of $^{67}$Ga scanning in evaluating mediastinal masses is not well established. Uptake of gallium occurs in most inflammatory and many neoplastic lesions of the mediastinum. Malignant neoplasms take up $^{67}$Ga more readily than benign ones. The overall accuracy rates of this modality are approximately 60% to 79% for malignant lesions (many false negatives) and 80% to 90% for inflammatory diseases (fewer false negatives). Gallium scanning is much less sensitive for benign tumors, although no definite accuracy rate is available.

At present, the results of gallium scanning do not significantly alter the need for thoracotomy. However, as imaging techniques improve with tomographic scanning of the mediastinum, gallium scanning may become of value when it is unclear whether a mediastinal soft-tissue mass demonstrated on tomography is a cyst or represents inflammation or neoplasm.

## Myelography

If neither conventional nor computed tomography demonstrates bony involvement associated with a posterior mediastinal mass, myelography is required to assess the possibility that a neurogenic mass may be growing into the spinal canal (Fig. 5-14). The presence of such spinal canal growth usually indicates that a neurosurgeon should be involved in the surgical removal of the mass.

Myelography is exceedingly accurate for the diagnosis of spinal cord involvement with mediastinal masses. The discomfort, expense, and possible neurologic complications associated with myelography make this procedure less desirable for the investigation of posterior masses if other methods prove or exclude spinal canal involvement.

### Percutaneous Biopsy

Percutaneous biopsy of mediastinal masses may be performed using fluoroscopic or CT guidance. The techniques are similar to those used for cyst puncture, with CT providing far better precision in placing the needle. Several systems have been developed using skin markers to precisely determine the angle and depth of needle placement.

Percutaneous biopsy often obviates the need for surgery or mediastinoscopy, especially when it results in confirmation of malignancy that is not amenable to definitive surgery.

Complications resulting from percutaneous mediastinal biopsy include hemorrhage and pneumothorax. When performed with care, the pneumothorax rate may be reduced to 10% to 15% and hemorrhage requiring specific therapy has been reported only very rarely.

### Endoscopic Biopsy

Endoscopic biopsy is the procedure of choice for histologic diagnosis of mucosal lesions of the esophagus that are demonstrated by barium swallow. The overall accuracy of this procedure is high, although it has a greater specificity than sensitivity.

Esophagoscopy with endoscopic biopsy is contraindicated when there is clinical evidence of acute esophagitis, such as from ingestion of caustic substances. In other patients, however, the procedure is quite safe, especially when a flexible endoscope is used. The major complication is perforation of the esophageal wall, which often occurs at the level of the cricopharyngeal sphincter and frequently requires surgical drainage of the mediastinum. Other complications include pneumothorax, mediastinitis, and, rarely, esophageal obstruction.

### Mediastinoscopy and Surgery

Mediastinoscopy is a procedure in which an incision in the suprasternal notch on the right is used to provide access for direct visualization of the mediastinum. The area visualized through the mediastinoscope is limited to the paratracheal region and the upper portion of the tracheal bifurcation. The accuracy rate of mediastinoscopy is more than 90% for lesions located around the trachea and above the main stem bronchi; the specificity exceeds the sensitivity. Middle mediastinal nodes are the most reliably visualized and biopsied structures.

Complications of mediastinoscopy are relatively uncommon. Mortality is less than 0.1%, and morbidity is 1% to 2%. Complications include mediastinal bleeding, vocal cord paralysis, pneumothorax, hemothorax, infection (including mediastinitis), and esophageal perforation.

Mediastinotomy, the use of a small incision that is usually made in the left parasternal region, may also be used to assess mediastinal masses that are not adjacent to the trachea. The left parasternal approach permits direct visualization of the areas surrounding the bronchus and pulmonary artery, including the aorticopulmonary window. Although the accuracy rates are similar, mediastinotomy is slightly more difficult to perform and has a slightly higher complication rate than mediastinoscopy.

Because imaging methods are frequently incapable of differentiating among various soft-tissue masses of the mediastinum, thoracotomy is required to make the definite diagnosis of most mediastinal masses. Mediastinal exploratory surgery has a very low mortality, and most of the fatalities have occurred in patients with myasthenia gravis. Complications of mediastinal surgery

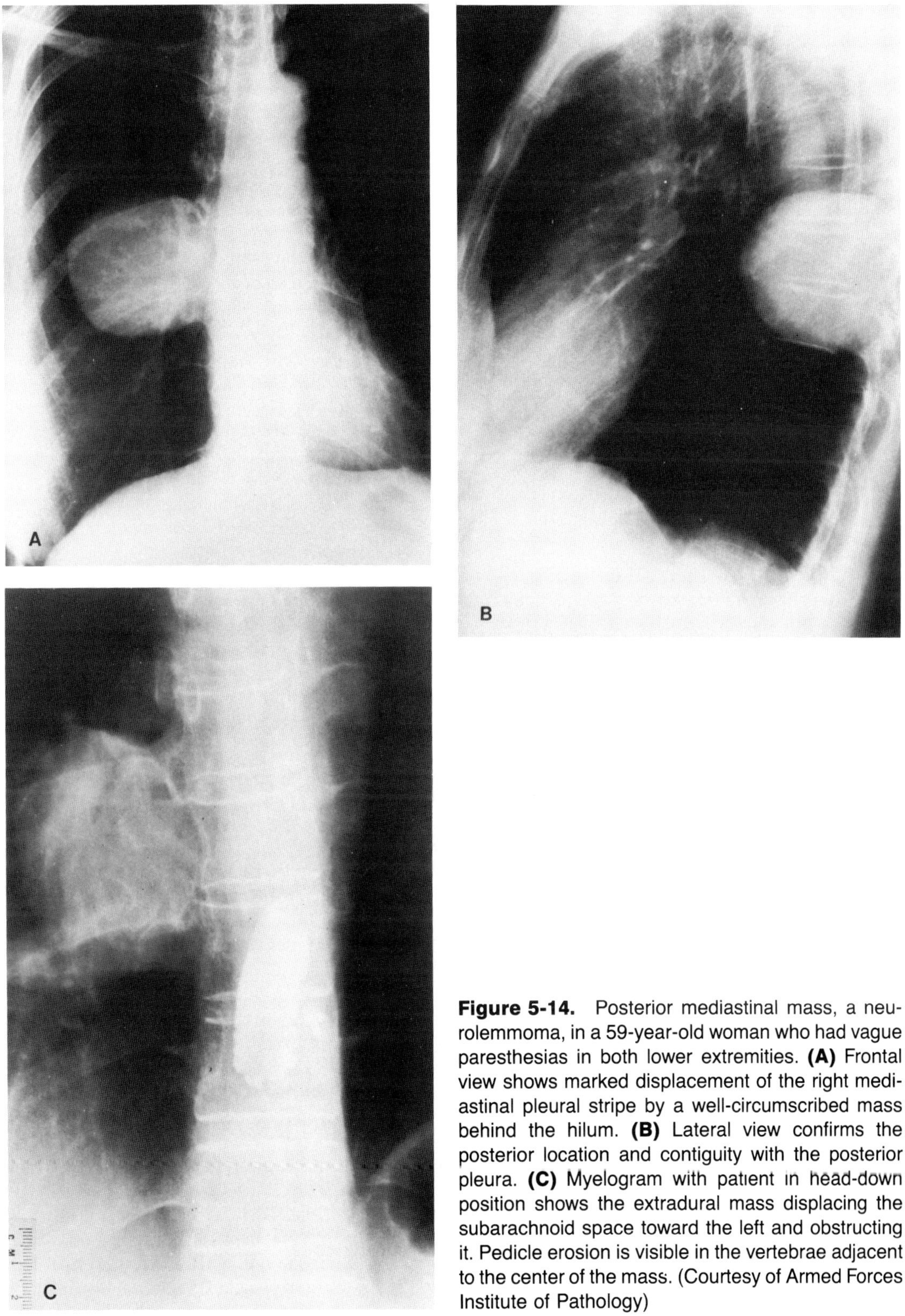

**Figure 5-14.** Posterior mediastinal mass, a neurolemmoma, in a 59-year-old woman who had vague paresthesias in both lower extremities. **(A)** Frontal view shows marked displacement of the right mediastinal pleural stripe by a well-circumscribed mass behind the hilum. **(B)** Lateral view confirms the posterior location and contiguity with the posterior pleura. **(C)** Myelogram with patient in head-down position shows the extradural mass displacing the subarachnoid space toward the left and obstructing it. Pedicle erosion is visible in the vertebrae adjacent to the center of the mass. (Courtesy of Armed Forces Institute of Pathology)

include those described for mediastinoscopy, as well as diaphragmatic paralysis and complications related to other surgical procedures involving the heart and pericardium.

## Bibliography


Aronberg DJ, Glazer HS, Sagel FS: MRI and CT of the mediastinum: Comparisons, controversies, and pitfalls. Radiol Clin North Am 23:439–448, 1985

Beeckman P, Dewilde A, Osteaux M et al: Critical evaluation of different x-ray methods in exploration of mediastinal lymphadenopathy. Belge Radiol 595:459–465, 1976

Bein ME, Mancuso AA, Mink JH et al: Computed tomography in the evaluation of mediastinal lipomatosis. J Comput Assist Tomogr 2:339–383, 1978

Benjamin SP, McCormack LJ, Effler DB et al: Primary tumors of the mediastinum. Chest 62:297–303, 1972

Brown ML, O'Donnell JB, Thrall JH et al: Gallium-67 scintigraphy in untreated and treated non-Hodgkin lymphomas. J Nucl Med 19:875–879, 1978

Brundage BH, Rich F, Spigos D: Computed tomography of the heart and great vessels: Present and future. Ann Intern Med 101:801–809, 1984

Cohen AM: Magnetic resonance imaging of the thorax. Radiol Clin North Am 22:829–846, 1984

Crowe JK, Brown LR, Muhm JR: Computed tomography of the mediastinum. Radiology 128:75–87, 1978

Day DK, Gedgaudas E: The thymus. Radiol Clin North Am 22:519–538, 1984

Feigin DS, Eggleston JC, Siegelman SS: The multiple roentgen manifestations of sclerosing mediastinitis. Johns Hopkins Med J 144:1–8, 1979

Feigin DS, Fenoglio JJ, McAllister HA et al: Pericardial cysts: A radiologic–pathologic correlation and review. Diag Radiol 125:15–20, 1977

Feigin DS, Padua EM: Mediastinal masses: A system for diagnosis based on computed tomography. J Comput Assist Tomogr 10:11–21, 1986

Francis IR, Glazer GM, Bookstein FL et al: The thymus: Reexamination of age-related changes in size and shape. AJR 145:249–254, 1985

Glazer GM, Gross BH, Quint LE et al: Normal mediastinal lymph nodes: Number and size according to American Thoracic Society mapping. AJR 144:251–265, 1985

Glazer HS, Aronberg DJ, Sagel SS: Pitfalls in CT recognition of mediastinal lymphadenopathy. AJR 144:267–274, 1985

Glazer HS, Gutierrez FR, Levitt RG et al: The thoracic aorta studied by MR imaging. Radiology 157:149–155, 1985

Godwin JD, Korobkin M: Acute disease of the aorta, diagnosed by computed tomography and ultrasonography. Radiol Clin North Am 21:551–574, 1983

Gothlin J, Jonsson K, Lunderquist A et al: The angiographic appearance of thymic tumors. Diagn Radiol 124:47–52, 1977

Haller JA, Mazur DO, Morgan WW: Diagnosis and management of mediastinal masses in children. J Thorac Cardiovasc Surg 58:385–393, 1969

Heitzman ER: Royal College Lecture. Radiologic diagnosis of mediastinal lymph node enlargement. J Can Assoc Radiol 29:151–157, 1978

Higgins CB, Stark D, McNamara M et al: Multiplane magnetic resonance imaging of the heart and major vessels: Studies in normal volunteers. AJR 142:661–667, 1984

Hyson EA, Ravin CE: Radiographic features of mediastinal anatomy. Chest 75:609–613, 1979

Irwin RS, Braman FS, Arvanitidis AN et al: $^{131}$I thyroid scanning in preoperative diagnosis of mediastinal goiter. Ann Intern Med 89:73–74, 1978

James ED, Ellwood RA: Mediastinoscopy and mediastinal roentgenology. Ann Thorac Surg 18: 531–538, 1974

Kelley MJ, Mannes EJ, Ravin CE: Mediastinal masses of vascular origin. J Thorac Cardiovasc Surg 76:559–572, 1978

Klatte EC, Yune HY: Diagnosis and treatment of pericardial cysts. Radiology 104:541–545, 1972

Levitt RG, Glazer HS, Roper CL et al: Magnetic resonance imaging of mediastinal and hilar masses: Comparison with CT. AJR 145:9–14, 1985

Livesay JJ, Mink JH, Fee HJ et al: The use of computed tomography to evaluate suspected mediastinal tumors. Ann Thorac Surg 27:305–311, 1979

Mink JH, Bein ME, Sukov R et al: Computed tomography of the anterior mediastinum in patients with gravis and suspected thymoma. AFR 130: 239–246, 1978

Oldham HN, Jr: Mediastinal tumors and cysts. Ann Thorac Surg 11:246–275, 1971

Pilepich MV, Rene JB, Munzenrider JE et al: Contribution of computed tomography to the treatment of lymphomas. AJR 131:69–73, 1978

Reed JC, Hallet KK, Feigin DS: Neural tumors of the

thorax: Subject review from the AFIP. Radiology 126:9–17, 1978

Salyer WR, Eggleston JC: Thymoma: A clinical and pathological study of 65 cases. Cancer 37: 229–249, 1976

Smathers RL, Brody WR: Digital radiography: Current and future trends. Br J Radiol 58:285–307, 1985

Sprayregen S, Jacobson HG: Angiographic differentiation of thoracic aneurysms and neoplasms. Vasc Surg 10:200–213, 1976

von Schulthess GK, McMurdo K, Tscholakoff D et al: Mediastinal masses: MR imaging. Radiology 158: 289–296, 1986

Webb WR, Jensen BG, Gamsu G et al: Sagittal MR imaging of the chest: Normal and abnormal. J Comput Assist Tomogr 9:471–479, 1985

Wieder S, Rabinowitz JG: Fibrous mediastinitis: A late manifestation of mediastinal histoplasmosis. Radiology 125:305–312, 1977

## ANTERIOR MEDIASTINAL MASS

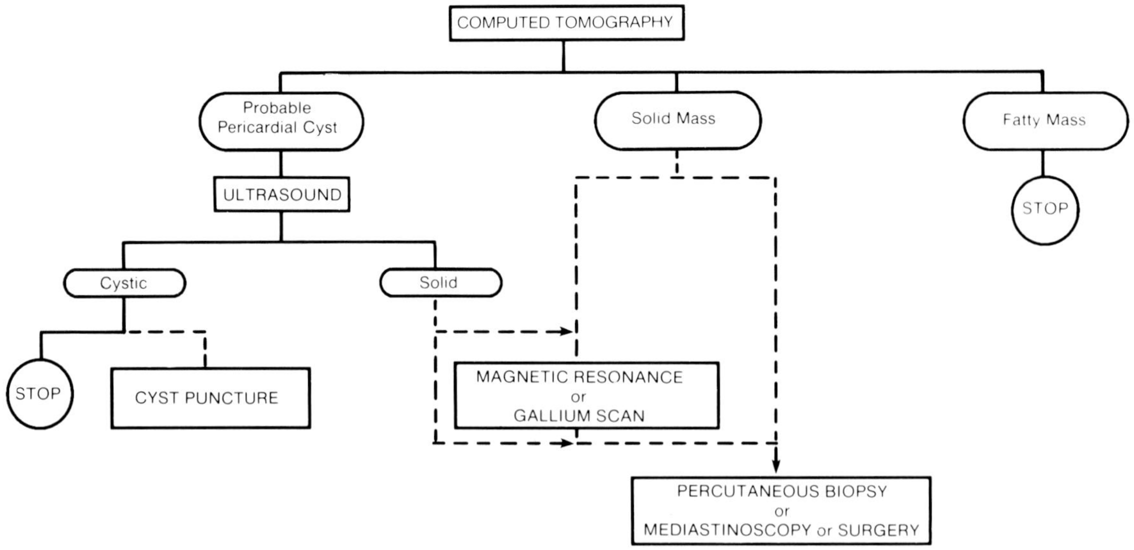


## MIDDLE MEDIASTINAL MASS

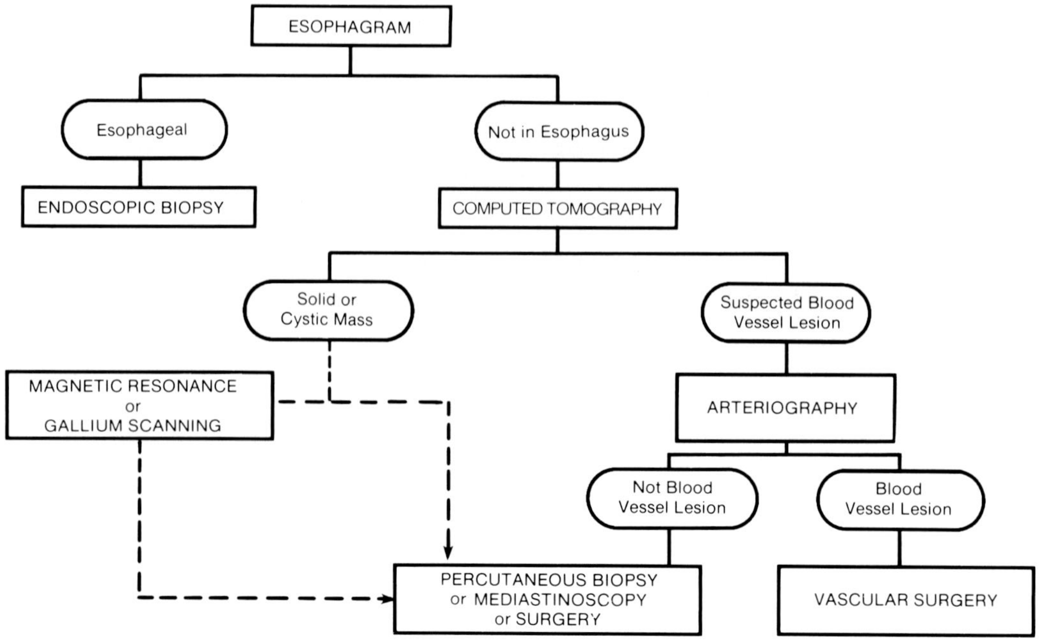

## POSTERIOR MEDIASTINAL MASS

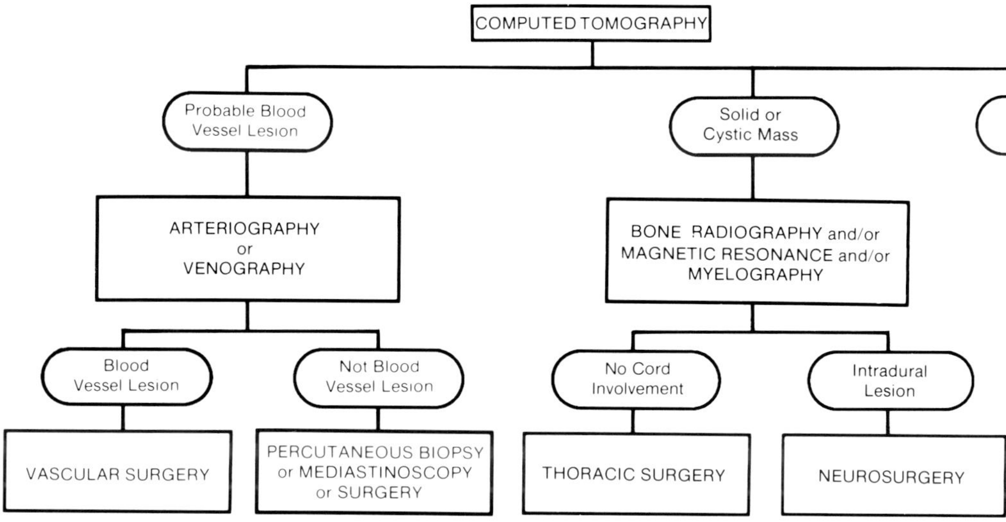


## SUPERIOR MEDIASTINAL MASS

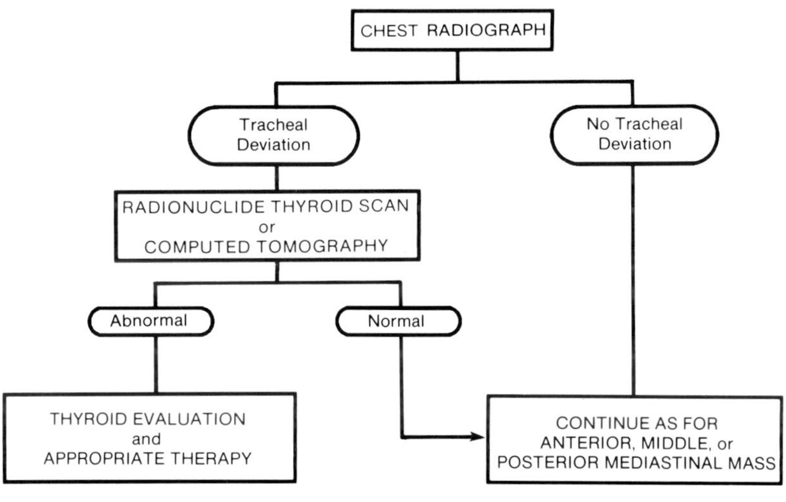

# Chapter 6

# Pleural Masses

*Marcus W. Hedgcock*

Most pleural masses are discovered fortuitously on plain chest radiographs obtained for other reasons. At times, pleural masses may produce symptoms directly referable to the lungs or chest wall, such as large mesotheliomas that cause dyspnea or chest pain. In other instances, pleural masses may produce extrathoracic symptoms, such as finger clubbing or hypertrophic osteoarthropathy.

The differential diagnosis of pleural masses includes the following:

1. Pleural fluid collections
   a. Pleural effusion
   b. Chylothorax
   c. Hemothorax
2. Solid pleural masses
   a. Pleural plaques
   b. Fibrin bodies
   c. Benign neoplasms
   d. Malignant neoplasms

## CLINICAL AND LABORATORY FINDINGS

Clinical findings, associated radiographic abnormalities, and laboratory studies can help to narrow the differential diagnosis of the pleural-based lesion. Pertinent information that should be sought is shown in Tables 6-1 and 6-2.

## DIAGNOSTIC EVALUATION

### *DIAGNOSTIC MODALITIES*

1. Plain chest radiography
2. Fluoroscopy
3. Conventional tomography
4. Ultrasound
5. Arteriography
6. Computed tomography
7. Gallium scanning
8. Needle aspiration
9. Needle biopsy
10. Diagnostic pneumothorax
11. Surgery
12. Contrast instillation

### Plain Chest Radiography

Most pleural-based masses are discovered on plain chest radiographs. A mass with a meniscus on the erect film suggests pleural fluid, usually a

**Table 6-1** Signs That Suggest the Etiology of Pleural Fluid Collections

| Clinical | Radiographic | Pleural Fluid Analysis | Suggested Etiology |
|---|---|---|---|
| Fever<br>Pain<br>Weight loss<br>Malaise<br>Positive tuberculin test | Fibronodular changes<br>Consolidation | Protein > 3 g/100 ml<br>Polymorphonuclear cells < 50%<br>Gluocse < 25 mg/100 ml<br>*p*H < 7.3<br>Positive tuberculosis smear or culture | Tuberculosis |
| Fever<br>Pain | Consolidation | Polymorphonuclear cells > 50%<br>Positive Gram stain or culture | Bacterial (nontuberculous) infection |
| Fever<br>Pain | Periosteal elevation next to empyema | Hyphae on smear<br>Positive fungal cultures | Fungal infection |
| Fever | Bilateral consolidation | Positive viral cultures | Viral mycoplasmal infection |
| Fever<br>Pain<br>Jaundice | Cavitating lesion<br>Elevation of right hemidiaphragm | Blood<br>Cytolized liver tissue<br>Bits of liver tissue | Amebiasis with hepatopleural fistula |
|  | Bilteral pleural effusion<br>Cardiomegaly with normal vasculature | Antinuclear antibodies | Systemic lupus erythematosus |
| Arthritis | Nodules or interstitial changes in lungs<br>Rheumatoid skeletal changes<br>Long-standing effusion | Nonpurulent sterile effusion without malignant cells<br>Positive rheumatoid factor<br>Glucose < 25 mg/100 ml | Rheumatoid disease |
| Weight loss<br>Hemoptysis<br>Heavy smoking | Parenchymal mass<br>Hilar adenopathy<br>Bronchial obstruction<br>Bone lesions | Malignant cells<br>Protein > 3 g/100 ml | Neoplasm |
| Sudden chest pain<br>Hemoptysis<br>Shortness of breath<br>Low arterial $pO_2$ | Defect on nuclear perfusion scan<br>Basal lung opacity<br>Elevation of ipsilateral hemidiaphragm | Serosanguinous fluid | Thromboembolism |
| Shortness of breath<br>Pedal edema | Cardiomegaly<br>Increaed pulmonary vascularity<br>Interstitial edema | Transudate | Congestive heart failure |
| History of trauma<br>Palpable rib fracture | Acute rib fracture<br>Pneumothorax | Blood<br>Serosanguinous fluid<br>Chyle | Trauma |
| Pancreatitis<br>Renal failure<br>Subphrenic abscess |  |  | Extrathoracic cause |

**Table 6-2** Signs That Suggest the Etiology of Solid Pleural Masses

| Clinical | Radiographic | Biopsy Specimen | Suggested Etiology |
|---|---|---|---|
| Asymptomatic | Unchanged for years<br>Mass calcified | Fibrous tissue | Fibrous plaque |
| Asymptomatic | Unchanging or slowly changing over years | Fatty tissue | Lipoma |
| Finger clubbing<br>Bone pain<br>Asbestos exposure | Enlarging pleural mass<br>Hypertrophic osteoarthropathy<br>Rib erosion | Mesothelioma or other neoplasm | Mesothelioma or other neoplasm |
| Asymptomatic | Pleural mass that moves | Fibrous tissue | Fibrin body |

pleural effusion (Fig. 6-1*A*). On a decubitus film, the effusion layers out (Fig. 6-1*B*). Exceptions to this rule are infrapulmonic effusions, pseudotumor (fluid collection in the pleural divisions between the lobes of a lung), and loculated pleural effusions. Even though these types of pleural fluid collections may not flow evenly, the shape of the fluid collection may change sufficiently to suggest that the density represents fluid and not a solid mass (Fig. 6-1*B*). With an infrapulmonic effusion, the apparent apex of the hemidiaphragm on the posteroanterior film may appear to be more lateral than normal, suggesting the correct diagnosis.

If a large pleural mass does not change shape or demonstrate free flow, comparison with recent radiographic examinations (within 1–2 months) may be of value. A large pleural mass that has appeared within this period is almost certainly fluid. Associated clinical or radiographic signs (Table 6-1) may also suggest a fluid, rather than solid mass. If the mechanism for fluid collection is reversed (*e.g.*, correction of congestive heart failure), subsequent films will demonstrate resolution of the pleural masses (Fig. 6-1*C*).

A small, pleural-based mass may be difficult to differentiate from a parenchymal nodule. Shallow, oblique radiographs of the chest or stereoradiography of the chest with the lesion *en face* will usually distinguish between a pleural and parenchymal location. Similarly, a radiograph of the lesion in tangent will show undercut edges if the lesion is parenchymal, rather than the smooth edges that blend with the pleural surface that are seen with pleural-based lesions. This positional radiography is most efficiently performed under fluoroscopic control.

The appearance of extrapulmonary structures on the plain film may also be of value in assessing the pleural-based mass. Rib erosion is most commonly seen with squamous cell carcinoma that has metastasized to the pleura and, less frequently, with malignant mesothelioma. Rib erosions are uncommonly seen with other benign or malignant pleural neoplasms. Calcification of the diaphragmatic pleura is practically diagnostic of asbestosis. It should be remembered, however, that the most frequent manifestation of asbestosis is an uncalcified pleural plaque. Calcification implies a long-standing process, because it usually requires at least 20 years for an asbestosis plaque to calcify. Calcification of a pleural mass does not necessarily confirm a benign process, because calcified mesotheliomas have been reported. In the patient with a known primary tumor elsewhere and metastases to other organs, a developing pleural mass may safely be assumed to represent a metastasis, because a more definitive evaluation of the lesion will not significantly change the patient's therapy. However, in the patient with no known primary neoplasm, or with a remote primary tumor with no other known metastases, further diagnostic studies are mandatory. In such patients, the identification of malignant cells in a pleural effusion or by pleural biopsy is required

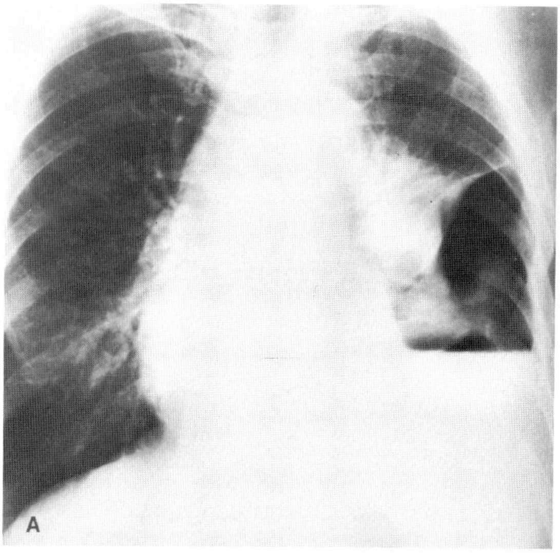

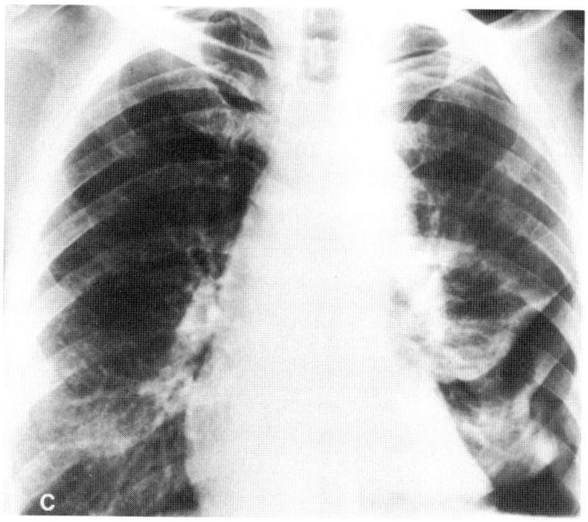

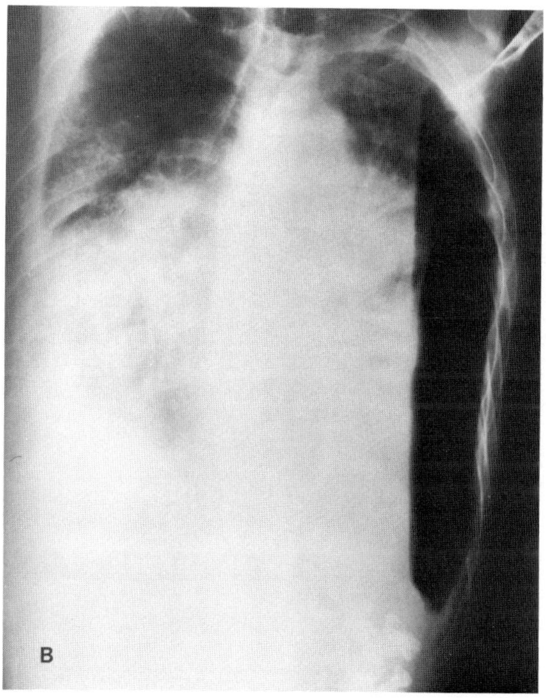

**Figure 6-1.** A 45-year-old man was evaluated for shortness of breath and chest pain. **(A)** A postero-anterior radiograph shows a large pleural lesion with a meniscus that layers out on a left lateral decubitus view **(B)** and represents a pleural effusion. The oblate left midlung lesion, which changes shape on the decubitus view and **(C)** becomes smaller after the aspiration of pleural fluid, represents a "pseudotumor" in the major fissure. There is also an area of pleural density in the upper lateral thoracic region with an erosion of the left fifth lateral rib. Open resection of the lesion found a malignant mesothelioma.

before the pleural-based mass can be unequivocally deemed to be metastatic.

## Fluoroscopy

When plain film radiography is unable to differentiate whether a mass is pleural-based or parenchymal, fluoroscopy with spot films is indicated. Under fluoroscopy, callus surrounding a healing rib fracture can be clearly distinguished from a more serious process. Fluoroscopy is also of value in localizing lesions for needle aspiration or biopsy, as well as in facilitating marking the skin over a pleural lesion for preoperative localization.

## Conventional Tomography

If a mass is clearly demonstrated to be pleural-based, conventional tomography is usually not indicated. One exception is the apical pleural mass, for which the demonstration of associated rib erosion (often not identified on plain films) is highly suggestive of a neoplastic process. Conventional tomography may be of value in determining whether a mass is pleural-based or parenchymal, although fluoroscopy is usually more efficient and less expensive in making this distinction.

Linear or polytomography of a pleural-based mass is most effective with the lesion in tangent to the x-ray beam. Tomography may identify calcification within the lesion (suggestive, but not diagnostic, of benignancy, because calcified mesotheliomas have been reported).

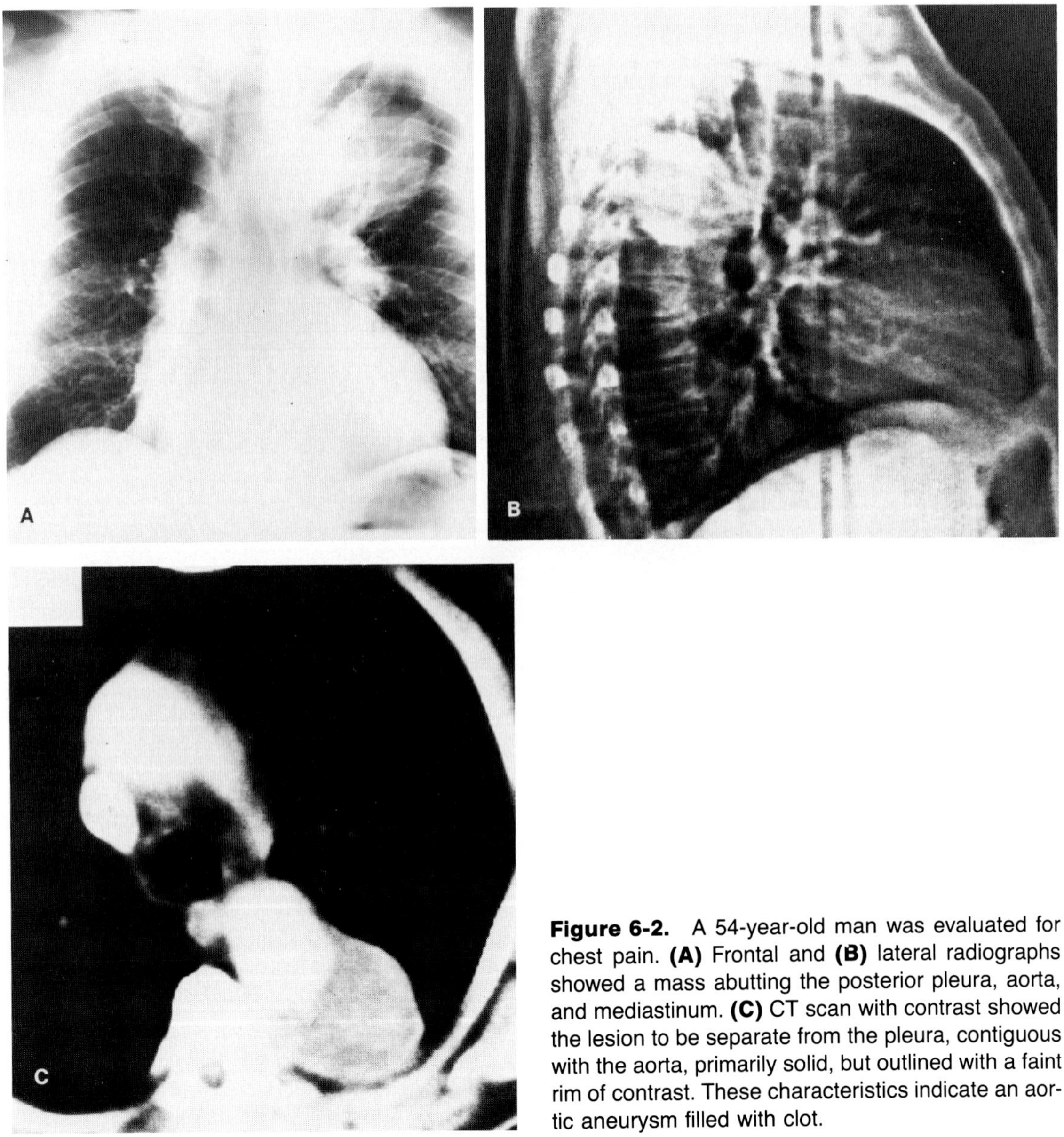


**Figure 6-2.** A 54-year-old man was evaluated for chest pain. **(A)** Frontal and **(B)** lateral radiographs showed a mass abutting the posterior pleura, aorta, and mediastinum. **(C)** CT scan with contrast showed the lesion to be separate from the pleura, contiguous with the aorta, primarily solid, but outlined with a faint rim of contrast. These characteristics indicate an aortic aneurysm filled with clot.

## Arteriography

Arteriography is of limited value in the assessment of most pleural-based lesions. The one exception is the evaluation of pleural lesions that abut the heart or great vessels in the thorax. Computed tomography, if available, is a more benign and less expensive procedure that can usually provide the same diagnostic information in these cases, and it is therefore preferable to arteriography (Fig. 6-2).

## Ultrasound

Ultrasound is extremely useful in the differentiation of pleural fluid from solid, pleural-based lesions. On ultrasound, a fluid lesion will show characteristic sonolucency, whereas a solid lesion will typically have internal echoes (Fig. 6-3). Ultrasound is also of value in localizing fluid collections for aspiration. In lesions of complex structure, such as empyema or organizing hematoma, ultrasound may be able to identify the fluid areas of a pleural-based lesion and thus define the best site for needle aspiration (Fig. 6-4).

The use of ultrasound is limited by attenuation of the sonic beam by bone and by scattering of the beam by air (Fig. 6-5). Because of these physical constraints, ultrasound cannot visualize the mediastinum (except at the sternal notch), nor can it demonstrate any parenchymal lesion surrounded by air-filled lung. In addition, certain neoplasms (such as the lymphoma group) may be so homogeneous as to mimic the sonolucent appearance of fluid on the ultrasound scan. Ultrasound is a valuable tool for defining diaphragmatic movement, especially on the right, where fluid collections below and above the diaphragm can be distinguished (see Fig. 6-3).

## Computed Tomography

Computed tomography (CT) provides imaging in the same projection as ultrasound. However, because CT is not compromised by intervening bone or air, pleural-based masses abutting the mediastinum or heart and those lying against the interlobular pleura can be assessed with this modality (see Fig. 6-2). In one study, thoracic CT provided information not otherwise available in more than one third of 75 patients with mixed pleural and parenchymal disease. In patients

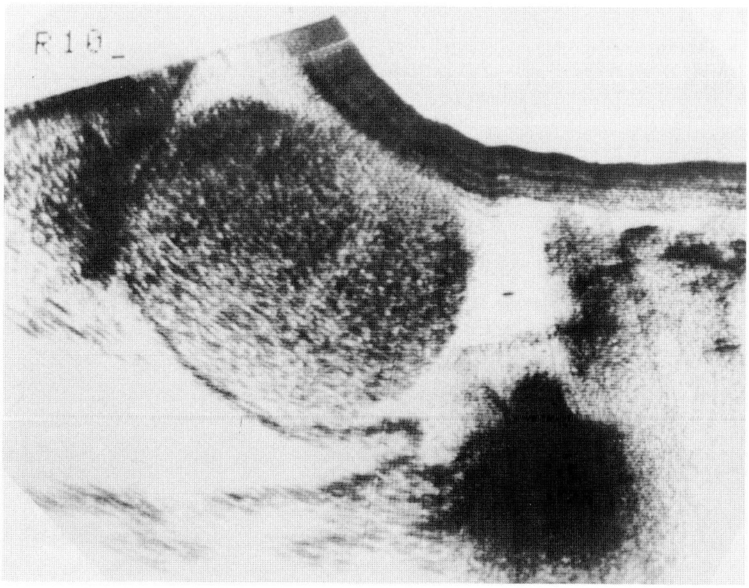

**Figure 6-3.** Ultrasound of pleural effusion. The curvilinear structure in the upper portion of the scan field is the hemidiaphragm. Above this, the pleural effusion is seen as an area of lucency with strong backwall echoes, indicating a fluid, homogeneous mass.

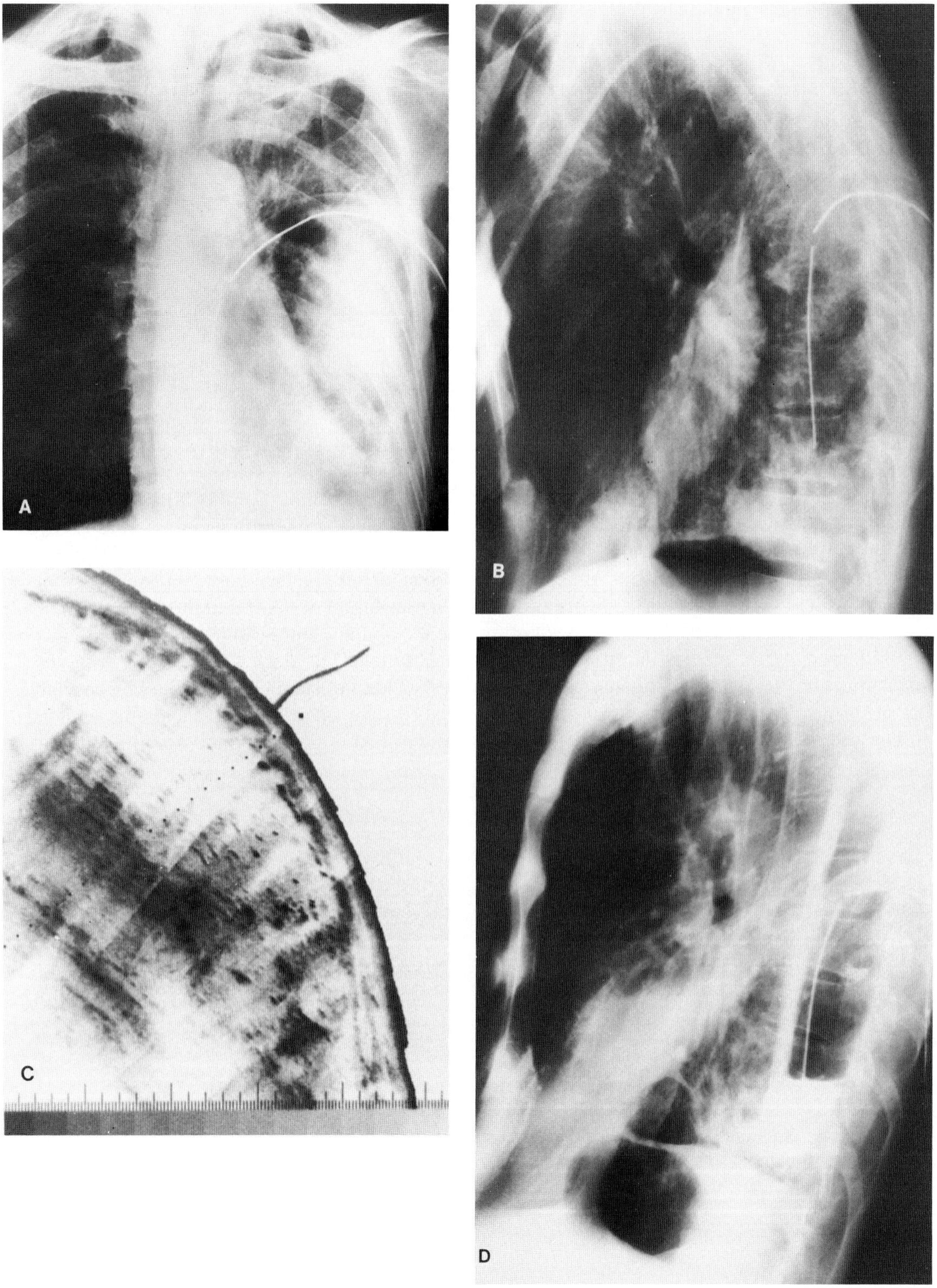

being evaluated for metastatic disease, CT can define pleural-based masses smaller than those visible on conventional tomography of the chest, although the significance of these small lesions in determining tumor resectability is not yet clear. As with plain film radiography, calcification of pleural-based masses on CT suggests benignity. In most cases, CT can differentiate solid from fluid lesions; at times this modality can even distinguish among several solid pleural lesions (*e.g.*, pleural lipomas have lower CT numbers than other pleural-based masses).

### Radionuclide Scanning

The role of radionuclide scanning in the investigation of patients with pleural masses is uncertain at this time. Although inflammatory lesions of the pleura may take up $^{67}$Ga, the use of this agent to discriminate benign from malignant processes is still not of practical clinical value.

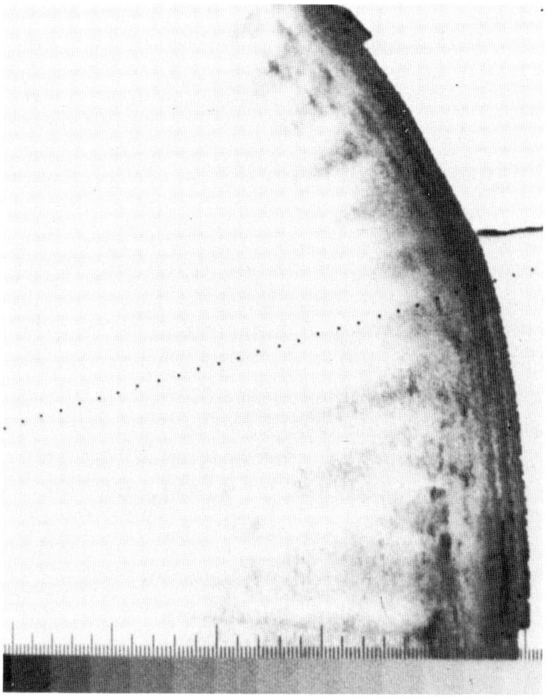

**Figure 6-5.** Ultrasound of a normal chest wall. Note that no echoes are returned through the air in the lung and that the ribs produce wedge-shaped areas of echoes ("rib artifacts").

### Needle Aspiration and Biopsy

Unless the etiology is unequivocal (*e.g.*, pleural effusion due to congestive heart failure or a pleural mass known to be unchanged for a period of at least 2 years), all pleural-based masses should be aspirated or biopsied. Needle aspiration is of value both for symptomatic relief of large pleural effusions and for chemical and cytologic analysis of pleural fluid collections (see Fig. 6-1). Needle biopsy, however, is of limited value in evaluating solid masses of the pleura. Because mesothelioma is notorious for producing false-negative results, only a needle biopsy that makes the definite diagnosis of mesothelioma is valid, and surgical resection of the lesion is still required. A needle biopsy that demonstrates only fibrous tissue does not exclude the diagnosis of mesothelioma. Therefore, if mesothelioma is suspected, open biopsy is the diagnostic procedure of choice.

If tuberculous effusion is suspected, needle biopsy of the pleura may be of great value. Positive biopsy cultures will occur in 55% to 80% of

◀ **Figure 6-4.** A 50-year-old man was treated for empyema with a chest tube. After 5 days, fluid drainage had stopped, although **(A)** a large mass in the left midlung and **(B)** a smaller mass in the left costophrenic angle posteriorly persisted. The large mass was believed to be a pseudotumor because of its oblate shape and continguity with the major fissure. **(C)** Ultrasound of the smaller posterior mass showed a mixed echo pattern consistent with an empyema or abscess. Needle aspiration utilizing ultrasound produced 200 ml of purulent fluid. **(D)** To rule out patent bronchopleural fistula, barium was instilled in the cavity with the needle left in place. Although there was no patent communication with the bronchial tree, the pseudotumor disappeared, indicating that the cavity communicated with the rest of the pleural space. The chest tube was in a cavity filled with air, which was separated from the lower cavity by a pseudomembrane, explaining why the chest tube ceased to drain fluid.

patients with tuberculous effusions, whereas culture of pleural fluid alone will reveal the diagnosis in only 25% of patients.

## Diagnostic Pneumothorax

The use of diagnostic pneumothorax for differentiating pleural from parenchymal lesions has been relegated to mere historical interest. The theory behind this technique was that a pleural-based lesion would remain fixed, whereas a parenchymal mass would move with the collapsing lung. However, because of the high morbidity of this technique and the current availability of less invasive modalities that provide identical information, diagnostic pneumothorax is no longer ever indicated.

## Surgery

Surgical biopsy is the definitive procedure for diagnosing solid lesions of the pleura. Because of the definite possibility of needle biopsy failing to demonstrate malignant cells in the face of a pleural neoplasm, open surgical biopsy is required in such patients even if needle biopsy of the lesion shows no evidence of tumor cells.

## Contrast Instillation

In cases of empyema or abscess in which a patent bronchopleural fistula is suspected, contrast material may be introduced into the cavity (see Fig. 6-4*D*). Barium is the contrast agent of choice; an oil-based agent such as Lipiodol may also be used. *Water-soluble contrast agents should never be used; they can produce sudden and massive pulmonary edema.* Bronchography may also be performed to determine whether the cavity communicates with the bronchial tree.

## Bibliography

Bern AS, Heitzman ER: The roentgenologic signs of pedunculated pleural tumors. AJR 87:892–895, 1962

Borow M, Couston A, Livornese L et al: Mesothelioma following exposure to asbestos. A review of 72 cases. Chest 64:641–646, 1973

Fraser RG, Pare JAR: Diseases of the pleura. In Fraser RG, Paré JAR (eds): Diagnosis of Diseases of the Chest, vol 3, p 1746. Philadelphia, WB Saunders, 1979

Kreel L: Computed tomography of the lung and pleura. Semin Roentgenol 13:213–225, 1978

Pugatch RD, Faling LJ, Robins AH et al: Differentiation of pleural and pulmonary lesions using computed tomography. J Comput Assist Tomogr 2:601–606, 1978

Schaner EG, Change AE, Doppman JL et al: Comparison of computed and whole lung tomography in detecting pulmonary nodules. AJR 131:51–54, 1978

Skin MS, Gray PW: Pitfalls in ultrasonic detection of pleural fluid. J Clin Ultrasound 6:421–423, 1978

Stout AP: Tumors of the soft tissues. In Atlas of Tumor Pathology, Sect II, Fasc 5. Washington, DC, National Research Council Committee on Pathology, 1953

SUSPECTED PLEURAL MASS

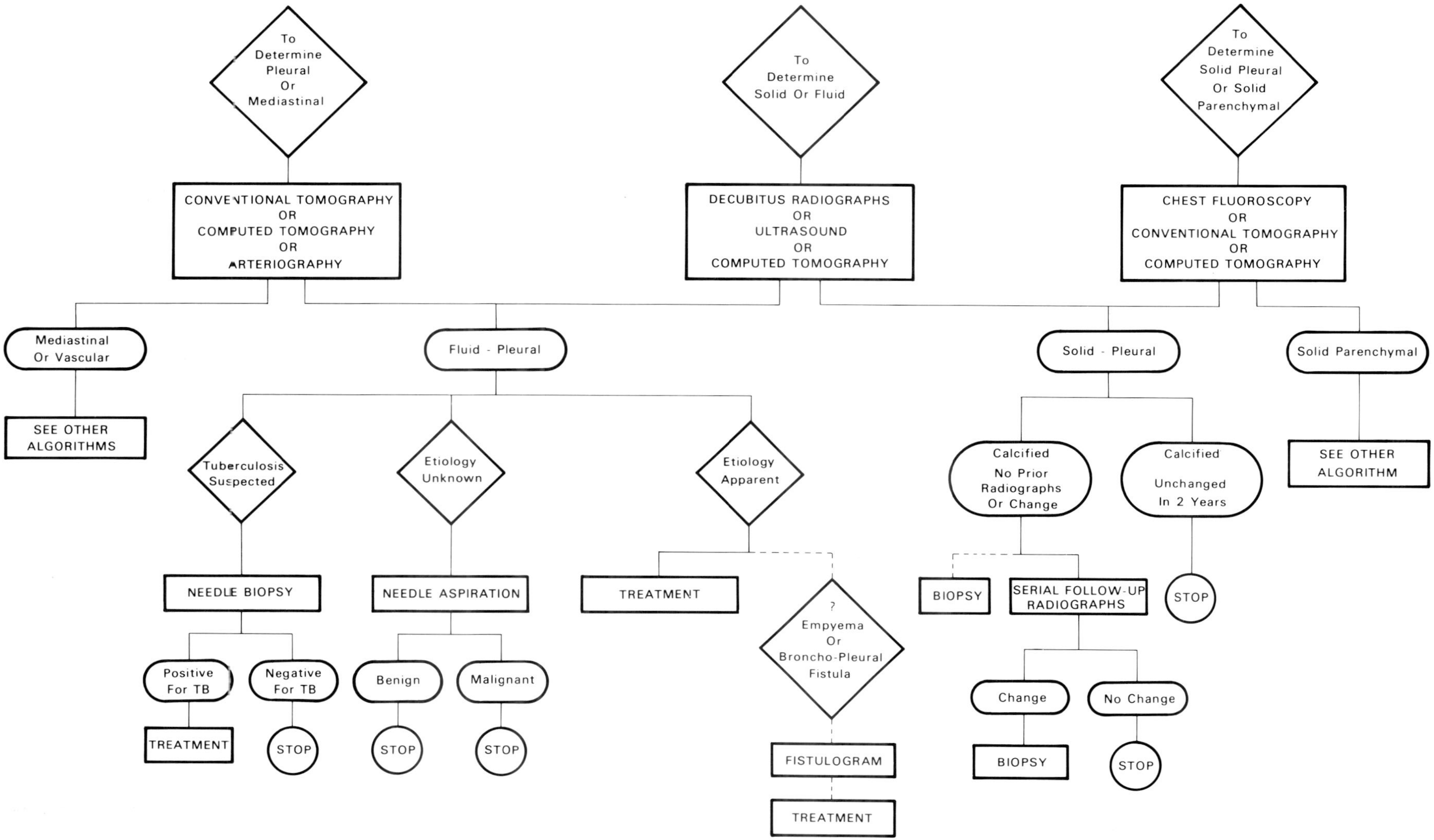

# Chapter 7

# Pericardial Disease

*Stephen W. Miller*
*Linda D. Gillam*

Pericardial diseases are often overlooked or produce diagnostic dilemmas. The advent of the new imaging modalities has revolutionized the diagnosis of the patient with clinically suspected pericardial disease and has led to an increased incidence of unsuspected pericardial disease (*e.g.*, pericardial effusions or calcifications) being detected on cardiac images obtained for unrelated reasons.

## COMMON CLINICAL PRESENTATIONS

Acute pericarditis characteristically presents with chest pain, located mainly in the sternal region. Classically, pericardial pain is described as sharp, is lessened when the patient sits up, and may radiate to the neck and back. However, because pericardial pain may be difficult to distinguish from the much more common pain arising from other organ systems (myocardial ischemia, pleuritis, aortic aneurysm and dissection, hiatal hernia, gallbladder disease), the diagnostic evaluation frequently begins with imaging of another organ system that has a higher probability of involvement.

The rapid accumulation of as little as 150 ml of fluid in the pericardial space can produce cardiac tamponade and hemodynamic compromise. If the fluid collects more gradually, the patient may be virtually asymptomatic even though there are several liters of fluid in the pericardial space. Pericardial effusion should be suspected in any patient with acute clinical signs of low cardiac output in the absence of hypovolemia if there is associated evidence of trauma to the heart or thorax, aortic dissection, or cardiac rupture after acute myocardial infarction or cardiac surgery. Chronic low-output states that may be associated with tamponade include malignancy, renal insufficiency, Dressler's syndrome, and inflammatory processes involving the heart, pericardium, or pleura.

Constrictive pericarditis also causes decreased filling of the heart and low cardiac output. Common clinical presentations include abdominal swelling (from ascites and hepatosplenomegaly) and distention of the jugular veins that increases during inspiration (Kussmaul's sign). However, clinical signs simulating pericardial constriction can also develop in patients with pericardial effusion, right or biventricular failure, tricuspid valvular disease, caval obstruction, and liver failure.

## DIAGNOSTIC EVALUATION

### *DIAGNOSTIC MODALITIES*

1. Plain chest radiography
2. Echocardiography
3. Computed tomography
4. Magnetic resonance imaging
5. Angiography

#### Plain Chest Radiography

Plain chest radiography is usually the initial imaging modality in the patient with suspected pericardial disease. Although chest radiography occasionally can provide an unequivocal diagnosis (*e.g.*, congenital absence of the pericardium), in most cases it merely identifies and localizes the abnormality prior to further imaging studies. Plain radiographic findings of importance include the size and shape of the cardiac silhouette, the presence of pleural effusions or associated pneumonia, pericardial calcification, and adjacent mediastinal masses.

#### Echocardiography

Evaluation of the pericardium was one of the earliest successful applications of M-mode echocardiography. This technique has now been largely replaced by two-dimensional echocardiography as the major modality in the initial assessment of the patient with a suspected diagnosis of pericardial disease. Under normal conditions, the space that separates the visceral and parietal layers of the pericardium contains only enough fluid (20 ml–50 ml) to act as a lubricant. On echocardiography, the two pericardial layers produce a single, highly reflective interface that can be separated from adjacent echoes by reducing either the strength of the transmitted pulse (damping) or the receiver gain. Because the pericardium surrounds the entire heart and proximal great vessels (except for a variable portion of the left atrium), portions of it are seen in virtually all standard cross-sectional image planes using the two-dimensional technique and on both the anterior and posterior surfaces of the heart by M-mode examination. Thus, almost all segments of the pericardium are evaluated during a complete echocardiographic study, and even localized pericardial pathology can be detected.

#### Computed Tomography

Computed tomography (CT) is indicated in patients with suspected pericardial disease if the echocardiographic study is limited, if there is a possibility of mediastinal extension of the pericardial process, or if there is disagreement between the clinical signs and the imaging findings. Computed tomography is of special value in demonstrating that the pericardium is normal, thus permitting the diagnostic search to shift to other organ systems. The pericardium can be identified in 95% of normal CT examinations. Its mean width is 1 mm to 2 mm and is never more than 4 mm. The pericardium is best seen anterior to the right ventricle, where it appears as a soft-tissue density bordered by mediastinal fat anteriorly and epicardial fat centrally. The pericardium along the lateral aspect of the heart frequently is not visible, either because it is quite thin in that region or because of adjacent cardiac motion. Absence of the anterior pericardial density suggests congenital absence of the pericardium, although indirect signs (interposition of the lung between the aorta and the pulmonary artery, and between the heart and the diaphragm) are probably more accurate. Cardiac motion may obscure the lateral borders of the pericardium.

#### Magnetic Resonance Imaging

Early experience with magnetic resonance imaging (MRI) indicates that this modality will be of great clinical use in the evaluation of suspected pericardial disease. The high soft-tissue contrast of this modality permits sharp delineation of the pericardium from the myocardium and pericardial fat. Unlike echocardiography, MRI is not dependent on operator technique or the patient's body habitus and provides a larger field of view. Disadvantages of MRI at this stage of its development include high cost and limited availability, lack of real-time imaging, and the requirement that the patient lie quietly up to 10 minutes during gated acquisition. In addition, patients who have pacemakers or intracranial metallic aneurysm clips are usually excluded from examination by MRI.

### Angiography

Although right atrial angiography has been used in the past to demonstrate pericardial effusion, echocardiography has effectively replaced this invasive technique. Configurational changes in the superior vena cava and right atrium can suggest cardiac tamponade and lead directly to pericardiocentesis without further imaging studies.

## APPROACH TO DIFFERENT DISEASE ENTITIES

### Pericardial Effusion

Echocardiography is well established as the gold standard for the diagnosis of pericardial effusion. It can be performed rapidly even at the bedside and, in addition to demonstrating a pericardial effusion, echocardiography can also provide information regarding the volume and distribution of the fluid and its hemodynamic significance. Echocardiography can also show associated pericardial pathology (*e.g.*, tumor, intrapericardial strands) and can provide useful guidance during pericardiocentesis.

A small pericardial effusion appears as a relatively echofree space with systolic and diastolic separation of the visceral and parietal layers of the pericardium posteriorly. Larger effusions also produce an echofree space between the anterior right ventricle and the parietal pericardium just beneath the anterior chest wall. However, the presence of an echofree space exclusively anterior to the right ventricle, or in the atrioventricular groove, more likely represents epicardial fat rather than a pathologic fluid collection. Similar separation of the pericardial layers in systole alone is considered a normal

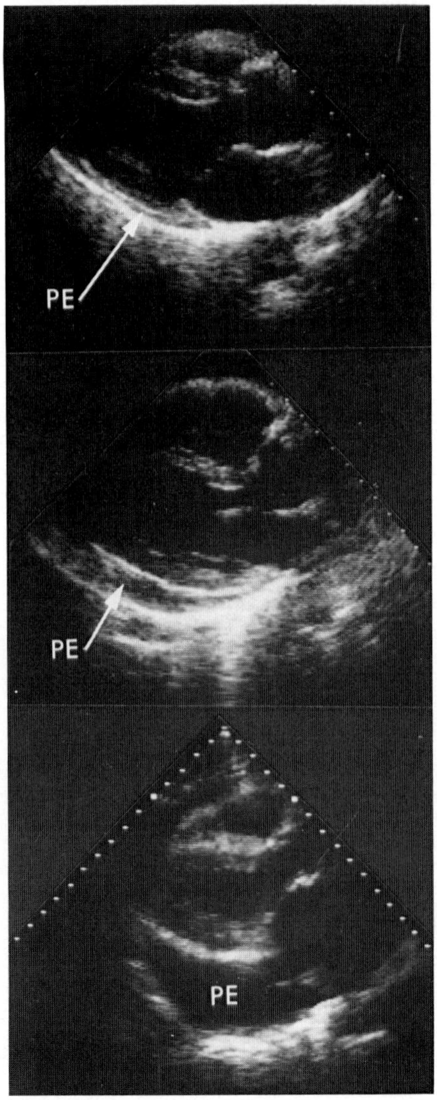


**Figure 7-1.** Parasternal long-axis echocardiograms show small (*top panel*), moderate (*middle panel*), and large (*lower panel*) pericardial effusions (*PE*). In each case, the effusion is represented by the echofree space separating the visceral and parietal layers of the pericardium.

variant. The volume of pericardial fluid demonstrated on echocardiography is generally estimated semiquantitatively, with effusions classified as small (approximately 100 ml), moderate (100 ml–500 ml), or large (more than 500 ml) (Fig. 7-1).

Two-dimensional echocardiography is generally superior to M-mode studies for evaluating a pericardial effusion, because the multiple imaging planes permit a thorough assessment of the pattern of fluid distribution. If the effusion is loculated or nonuniform, the volume of the effusion may be falsely under- or overestimated using the M-mode technique.

Although echocardiography is exquisitely sensitive to the presence of a pericardial effusion, in occasional instances the acoustic access is inadequate. The specificity of two-dimensional echocardiography for diagnosing a pericardial effusion exceeds 95%. The most common source of a false-positive diagnosis is the left pleural effusion (Fig. 7-2). Pericardial fluid generally can be differentiated from a pleural effusion, because the former classically does not extend up behind the left atrium. However, large pericardial effusions may produce retroatrial extension of fluid simulating a pleural effusion. A second method for differentiating pericardial fluid from pleural fluid is to assess the relative positions of the heart and descending aorta as seen on the parasternal long-axis view. Pericardial fluid separates the two structures, whereas the aorta remains in close proximity to the atrioventricular groove if pleural fluid is present.

Pericardial pathology coexisting with an effusion may also be demonstrated by echocardiography (Fig. 7-3). The presence of multiple nodules studding the visceral pericardium or masses within the fluid is virtually pathognomonic for a malignant effusion. Nonspecific findings such as intrapericardial strands or foamy echoes overlying the visceral pericardium can also be demonstrated.

Although the presence of pericardial fluid

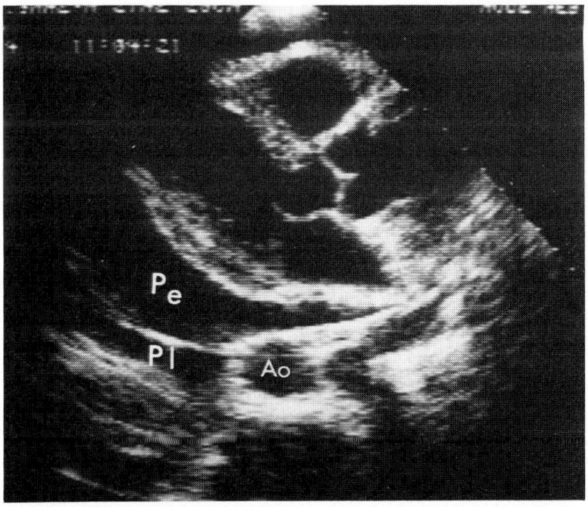


**Figure 7-2.** Parasternal long-axis echocardiogram demonstrates both pericardial (*Pe*) and pleural (*Pl*) effusions. The descending aorta (*Ao*) is separated from the heart by the pericardial effusion.

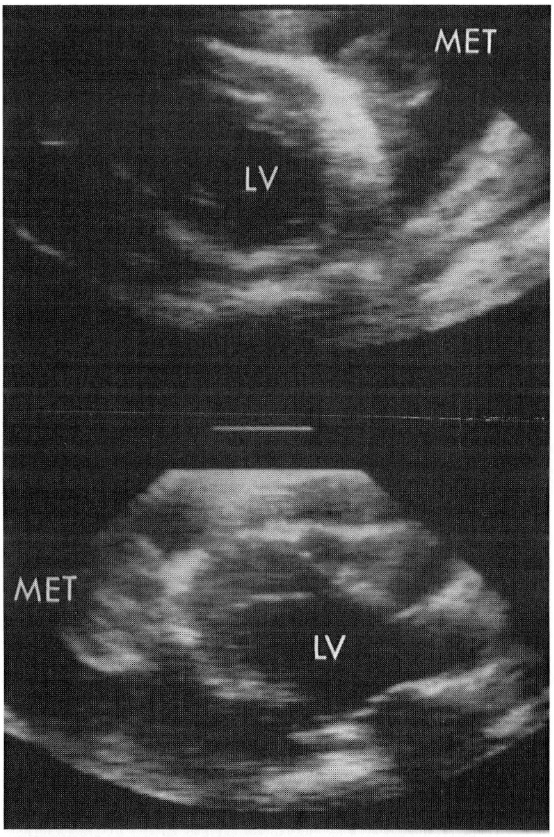


**Figure 7-3.** Parasternal long-axis (*top panel*) and short-axis (*bottom panel*) echocardiograms in a patient with a large malignant pericardial effusion demonstrate echogenic masses within the fluid that are virtually pathognomonic of metastases (*MET*). (*LV*, left ventricle)

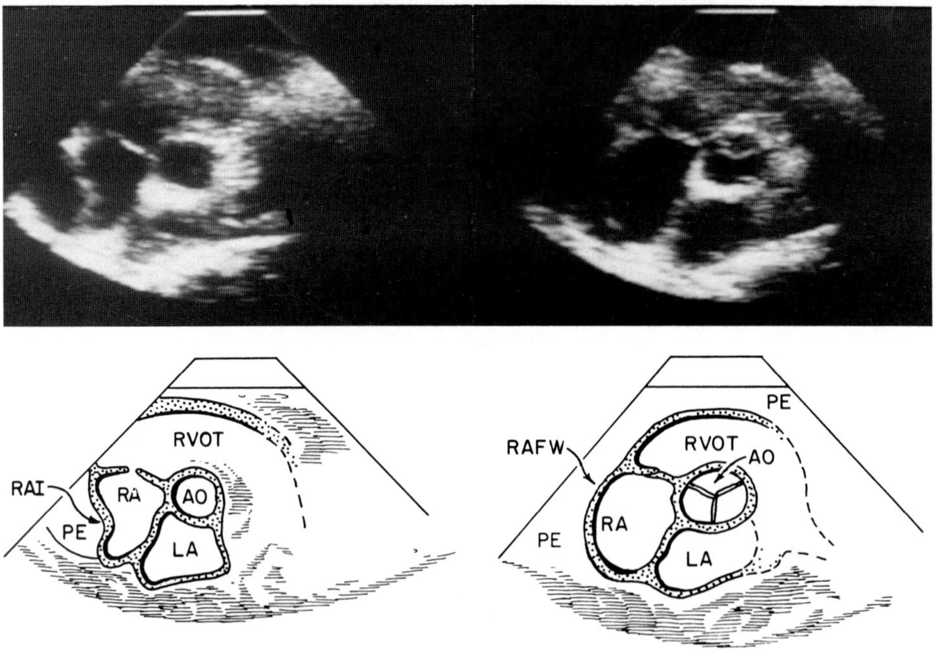


**Figure 7-4.** Parasternal short-axis echocardiogram from a patient with cardiac tamponade and right atrial inversion (*RAI*). Following atrial systole (*left panel*), the right atrial free wall (*RAFW*) buckles in and maintains this abnormal configuration throughout a variable portion of ventricular systole. By end systole (*right panel*), the right atrial wall has resumed a normal rounded shape. (*PE,* pericardial effusion; *RA,* right atrium; *LA,* left atrium; *RVOT,* right ventricular outflow tract; *AO,* aorta) (Gillam LD, Guyer DE, Gibson TC et al: Hydrodynamic compression of the right atrium: A new echocardiographic sign of cardiac tamponade. Circulation 68:294–301,1983. By permission of the American Heart Association, Inc)

can be unequivocally demonstrated by echocardiography, it is often difficult to differentiate a pericardial effusion complicated by tamponade from one without hemodynamic compromise. The echocardiographic correlates of the physical diagnostic sign of pulsus paradoxus appear to be relatively nonspecific. However, the recently improved visualization of the right heart on two-dimensional echocardiography has permitted the diagnosis of tamponade by demonstrating right atrial inversion and right ventricular collapse (Fig. 7-4). These findings are highly accurate in identifying patients with hemodynamic evidence of tamponade.

On plain chest radiographs, a pericardial effusion causes generalized enlargement of the cardiac silhouette (Fig. 7-5). On routine lateral chest radiographs, the epicardial fat pad sign is a good indication of pericardial effusion or thickening (Fig. 7-6). In many persons, the anterior mediastinal and epicardial fat can be visualized on either side of a pencil-thin line representing the normal pericardium. Separation of the epicardial fat stripe from the anterior mediastinal fat by a soft-tissue density of more than 4 mm is virtually pathognomonic of pericardial effusion or thickening. A positive demonstration of this epicardial fat pad sign is significant; the absence of the sign is of no diagnostic value.

The sudden development of enough pericardial fluid to produce tamponade may cause severe alterations in cardiac function with minimal changes in the radiographic cardiac silhouette because of either pre-existing mediastinal fibrosis or the constraining effect of the elastic pericardium. This situation can develop in patients

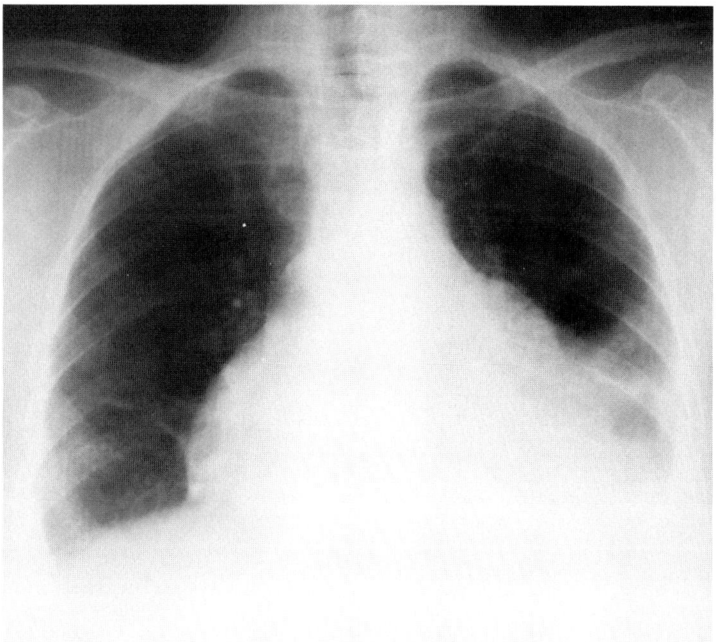

**Figure 7-5.** Dressler's syndrome. The large cardiac silhouette and bilateral pleural effusions with normal pulmonary vasculature in a patient 6 weeks following myocardial infarction suggest a pericardial effusion rather than cardiomegaly from left ventricular failure.

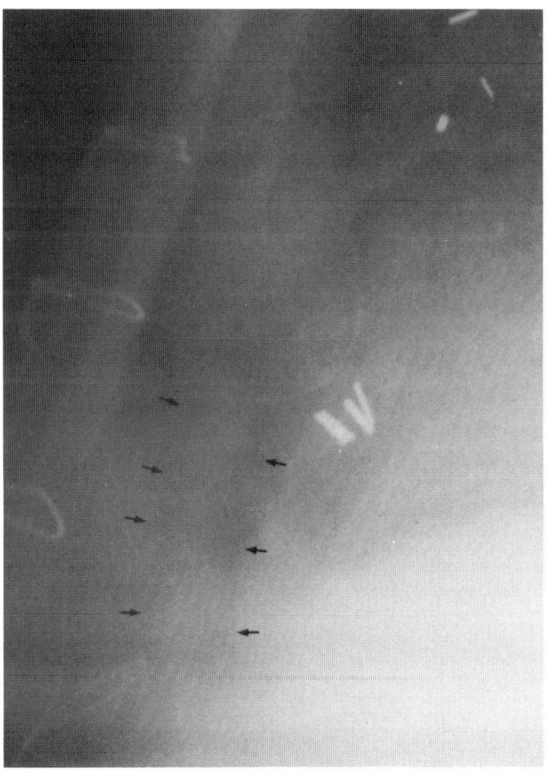

**Figure 7-6.** Epicardial fat pad sign. The distance between the epicardial fat (*right arrows*) and the pericardial fat (*left arrows*) represents the width of the pericardial effusion plus the pericardium.

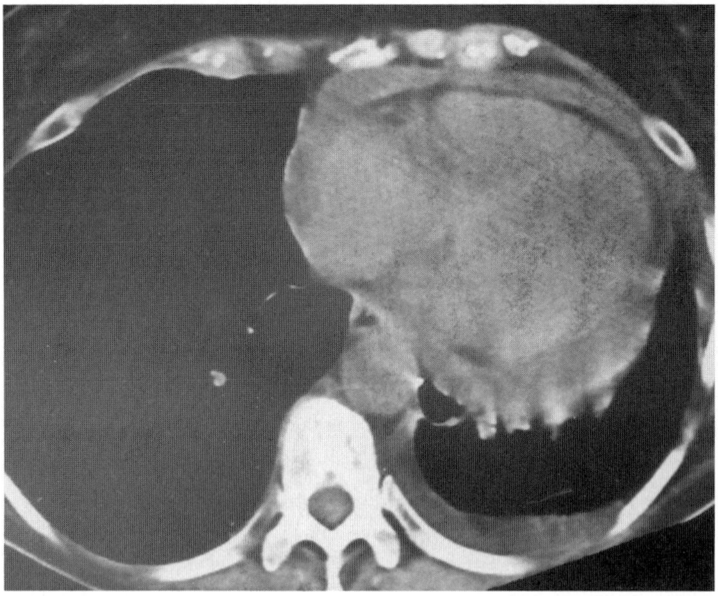

**Figure 7-7.** CT scan of pericardial effusion. The epicardial fat and the denser myocardium posteriorly outline the pericardial effusion.

with stab wounds to the heart and in those with aortic dissection and rupture into the pericardium. These patients should go directly to angiography.

Computed tomography can demonstrate pericardial effusions with a sensitivity similar to that of echocardiography. It has the advantage of not requiring an acoustic window, but it is less cost effective than echocardiography. The CT density of pericardial effusions varies depending on the protein, cellular, and fat content of the fluid. In general, the CT number tends to be high when an effusion is bloody, intermediate in hypothyroidism, and relatively low in renal failure or heart failure. In the supine patient, a small effusion tends to accumulate posteriorly. Larger effusions form a layer of fluid that surrounds the heart, separating the cardiac chambers from mediastinal fat, parietal pleura, mediastinal organs, and the lungs (Fig. 7-7).

Gated MR images show a pericardial effusion as a region of decreased signal intensity between the myocardium and the fat on the surface of the parietal pericardium (Fig. 7-8). The nor-

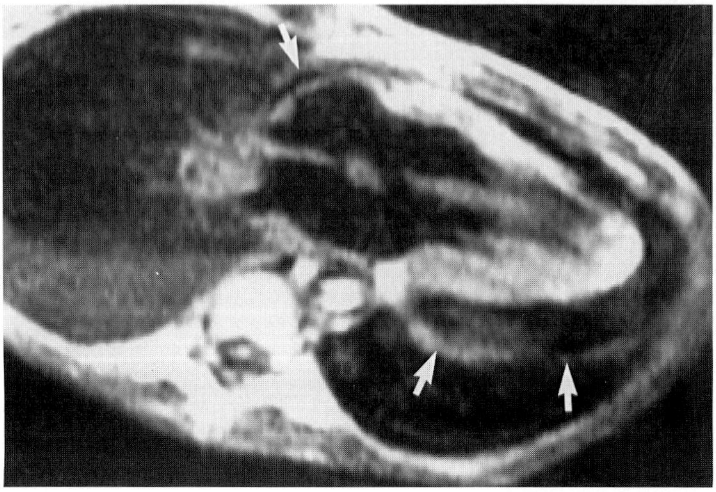

**Figure 7-8.** MR image of pericardial effusion. The pericardium (*arrows*) is displaced away from the heart by a huge pericardial effusion that has very little signal intensity. The effect of gravity is seen in the posterior location of both the pericardial and the right pleural effusions. (Miller SW, Brady TJ, Dinsmore RE et al: Cardiac magnetic resonance imaging. The Massachusetts General Hospital experience. Radiol Clin North Am 23:745–764, 1985)

mal pericardium is usually invisible when it is in direct contact with the heart. The accumulation of enough fluid to displace the pericardium (and pericardial fat) away from the heart permits identification of the intervening low signal-intensity effusion.

## Constrictive Pericarditis

In constrictive pericarditis, adherence of the visceral and parietal layers of the pericardium prevents the ventricles from filling normally, resulting in decreased stroke volume and increased venous pressure. Clinically, this condition may be difficult to distinguish from cardiac tamponade or restrictive cardiomyopathy, both of which also limit the diastolic blood volume of the heart. On plain chest radiographs, the size of the heart is often normal, although the shape of the mediastinum is abnormal and reflects adjacent pulmonary congestion and fibrosis. In approximately half the patients with constrictive pericarditis, the cardiac silhouette is enlarged because of a combination of pericardial effusion and thickening. Calcified plaques are present in the thickened pericardium of about half the patients with constrictive pericarditis. Although the heaviest deposits of calcium are located anteriorly, posterior and juxtadiaphragmatic pericardial calcification can often be seen. At times, the calcification may involve the entire pericardium so that the heart appears to be encased in a calcific shell (Fig. 7-9). It must be remembered that the pericardium may be calcified without any evidence of constriction (*e.g.,* in asbestosis); conversely, hemodynamic signs of constriction may be present without pericardial calcification. Detection of pericardial calcification is of major importance in distinguishing constrictive pericarditis from cardiac tamponade or restrictive cardiomyopathy.

Unlike pericardial effusion, in which echocardiography is an imaging modality of choice, in constrictive pericarditis the echocardiographic findings are relatively nonspecific. In addition to

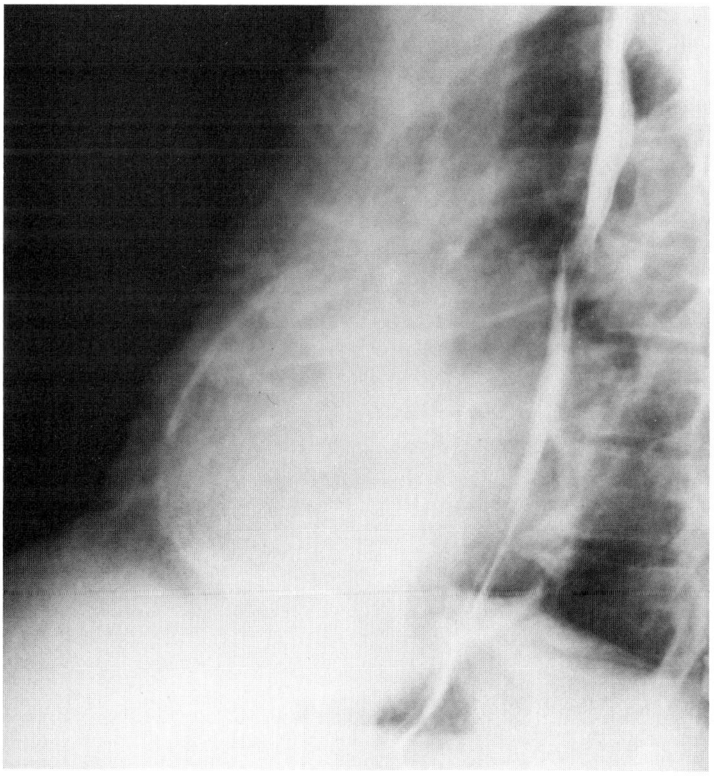

**Figure 7-9.** Pericardial calcification. There is a thin rim of calcium around the cardiac silhouette in this patient with constrictive pericarditis.

thickening and/or calcification of the pericardium, echocardiographic signs may suggest the impaired ventricular filling that is the physiologic hallmark of this condition. The signs of constrictive pericarditis include rapid early diastolic posterior movement of the left ventricular posterior wall with little or no further posterior movement as diastole continues (reflecting diminished late diastolic inflow), premature opening of the pulmonary valve (reflecting the rapid early rise in right ventricular pressure), lack of respiratory variation in the size of the inferior vena cava, and a variety of abnormalities of the interventricular septum (paradoxical motion, early and late diastolic notching, and reduced systolic thickening). Doppler echocardiographic characterization of ventricular filling also may prove to be a useful adjunct to the imaging examination.

Computed tomography is highly sensitive in detecting and measuring pericardial thickening and calcification (Fig. 7-10). By accurately differentiating a normal from a thickened pericardium, CT offers great promise in distinguishing constrictive pericarditis, in which the pericardium is thickened, from restrictive cardiomyopathy, in which the pericardium is of normal thickness. Although quantitation of ventricular function is not possible with conventional CT scanners, cine-CT techniques should soon allow measurement of systolic and diastolic volume curves.

Magnetic resonance imaging demonstrates an actively inflamed pericardium as a zone of increased signal intensity, although this finding must be interpreted with caution because of the presence of fat on both sides of the pericardium (Fig. 7-11). Unlike CT, MRI cannot demonstrate pericardial calcification, because calcium does not produce a signal. Magnetic resonance imaging can measure the thickness of the ventricular walls, which typically is normal in constrictive pericarditis and more than 12 mm in restrictive cardiomyopathy. In both of these conditions, MRI can show dilatation of the atria and venae cavae.

## Pericardial Cysts and Other Paracardiac Masses

Pericardial cysts and other paracardiac masses in the anterior mediastinum usually have a distinctive appearance on plain chest radiographs. A pericardial cyst is a fluid-filled mass that typically appears as a round or lobulated, sharply demarcated density in the right cardiophrenic angle that touches both the anterior chest wall and the anterior portion of the right hemidiaphragm. Less frequently, a pericardial cyst may arise in the left cardiophrenic angle or as a mediastinal mass anterior to the pulmonary hila or in the paratracheal region. On plain chest radiographs,

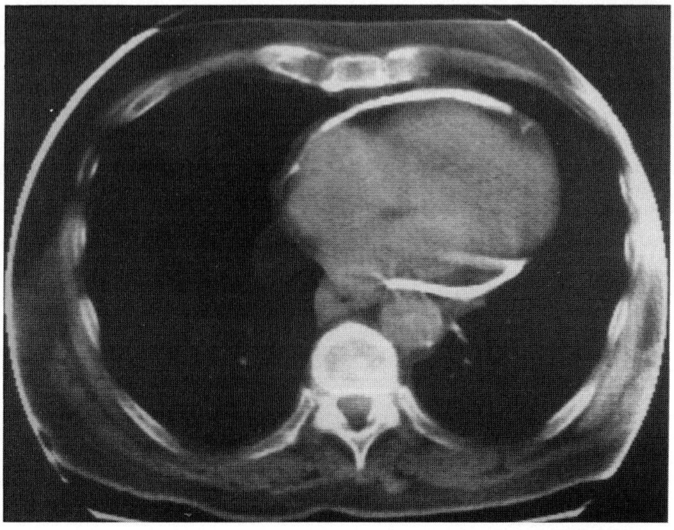

**Figure 7-10.** CT scan of pericardial calcification.

a pericardial cyst must be differentiated from a large pericardial fat pad; a diaphragmatic hernia (especially through the foramen of Morgagni); an aneurysm of the heart and great vessels; localized eventration of the diaphragm; and neoplasms of the lung, pleura, mediastinum, or pericardium (Fig. 7-12).

Additional imaging procedures are usually required to precisely diagnose a paracardiac mass. Echocardiography can demonstrate the cystic and unilocular nature of a pericardial cyst. Doppler methods can aid in distinguishing a pericardial cyst from vascular masses, which also appear sonolucent on echocardiography. Contrast-enhanced CT has become the imaging modality of choice for detecting and characterizing paracardiac masses. This technique can differentiate a fluid-filled pericardial cyst from pericardial fat pads and lipomas as well as from solid masses or aneurysms. On MRI, pericardial cysts have long T1 and T2 relaxation times and appear as uniformly low signal-intensity structures, whereas pericardial lipomas have a high signal intensity.

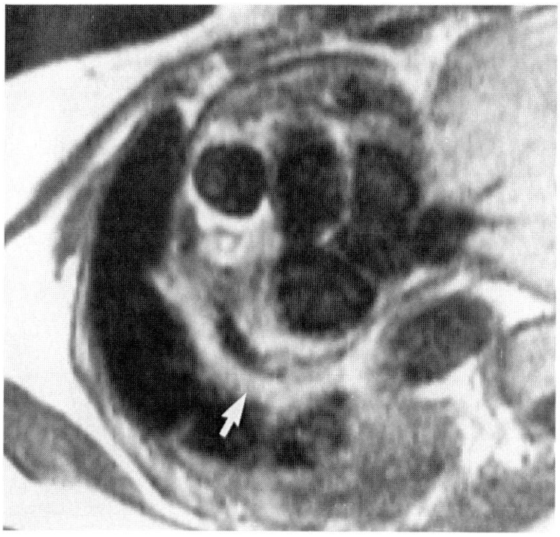

**Figure 7-11.** Pericarditis. MRI shows thickening of the pericardium (*arrow*) behind the left atrioventricular sulcus. The pericardial fluid has increased signal intensity with an irregular distribution that probably reflects fibrous stranding. (Miller SW, Brady TJ, Dinsmore RE et al: Cardiac magnetic resonance imaging. The Massachusetts General Hospital experience. Radiol Clin North Am 23:745–764, 1985)

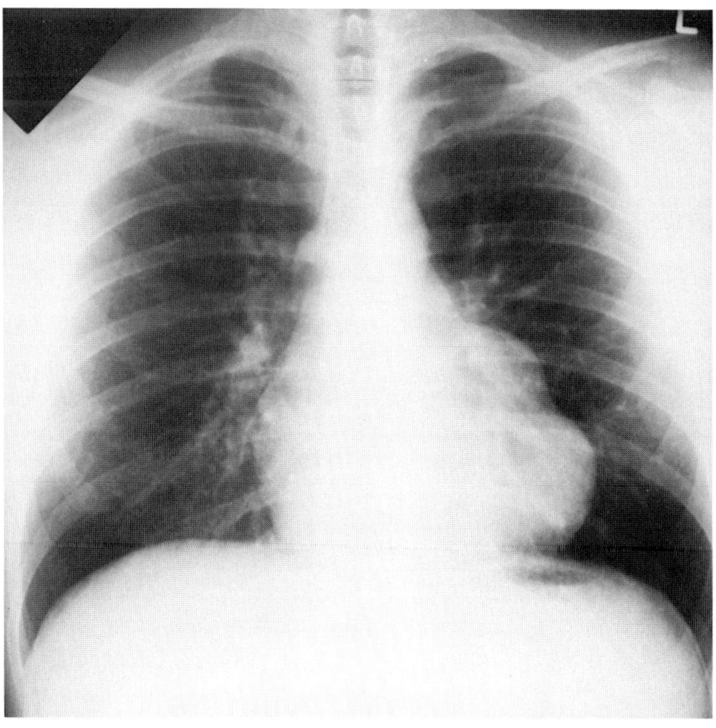

**Figure 7-12.** Pericardial dermoid tumor adjacent to the left atrial appendage.

## Bibliography


Baron MG: Pericardial effusion. Circulation 44: 294–299, 1971

Carsky EW, Mauceri RA, Azimi F: The epicardial fat pad sign. Radiology 137:303–308, 1980

Engel PJ, Fowler NO, Tei C et al: M-mode echocardiography in constrictive pericarditis. J Am Coll Cardiol 6:471–474, 1985

Feigin DS, Fenoglio JJ, McAllister HS et al: Pericardial cysts. A radiologic–pathologic correlation and review. Radiology 125:15–20, 1977

Gillam LD, Guyer DE, Gibson TC et al: Hydrodynamic compression of the right atrium: A new echocardiographic sign of cardiac tamponade. Circulation 68:294–301, 1983

Horowitz MS, Schultz CS, Stinson EB et al: Sensitivity and specificity of echocardiographic diagnosis of pericardial effusion. Circulation 50: 239–247, 1979

Isner JM, Carter BL, Bankoff MS et al: Differentiation of constrictive pericarditis from restrictive cardiomyopathy by computed tomographic imaging. Am Heart J 105:1019–1024, 1983

Miller SW: Cardiac Angiography. Boston, Little, Brown & Co, 1984

Miller SW, Brady TJ, Dinsmore RE et al: Cardiac magnetic resonance imaging: The Massachusetts General Hospital Experience. Radiol Clin North Am 23:745–764, 1985

Moncada R, Baker M, Salinas M et al: Diagnostic role of computed tomography in pericardial heart disease: Congenital defects, thickening, neoplasms, and effusions. Am Heart J 103:263–282, 1982

Schnittger I, Bowden RE, Abrams J et al: Echocardiography: Pericardial thickening and constrictive pericarditis. Am J Cardiol 42:388–395, 1978

Shiina A, Yaginuma T, Kondo K et al: Echocardiographic evaluation of impending cardiac tamponade. J Cardiogr 9:955, 1979

Singh S, Wann LS, Schuchard GH et al: Right ventricular and right atrial collapse in patients with cardiac tamponade—a combined echocardiographic and hemodynamic study. Circulation 70:966–971, 1984

Stark DD, Higgins CB, Lanzer P et al: Magnetic resonance imaging of the pericardium: Normal and pathologic findings. Radiology 150:469–474, 1984

# CARDIAC TAMPONADE

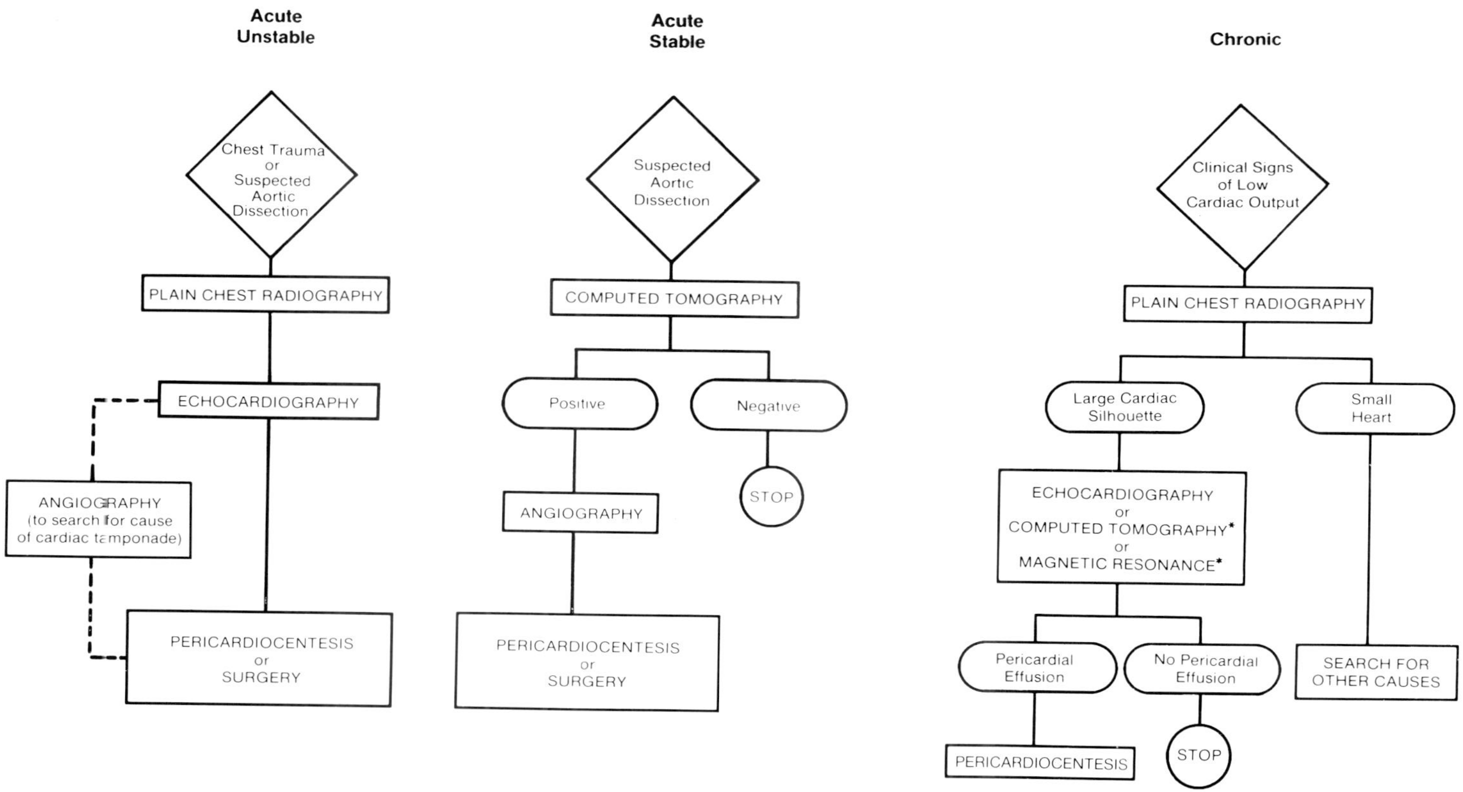


* = Less Cost Effective

**CONSTRICTIVE PERICARDITIS**

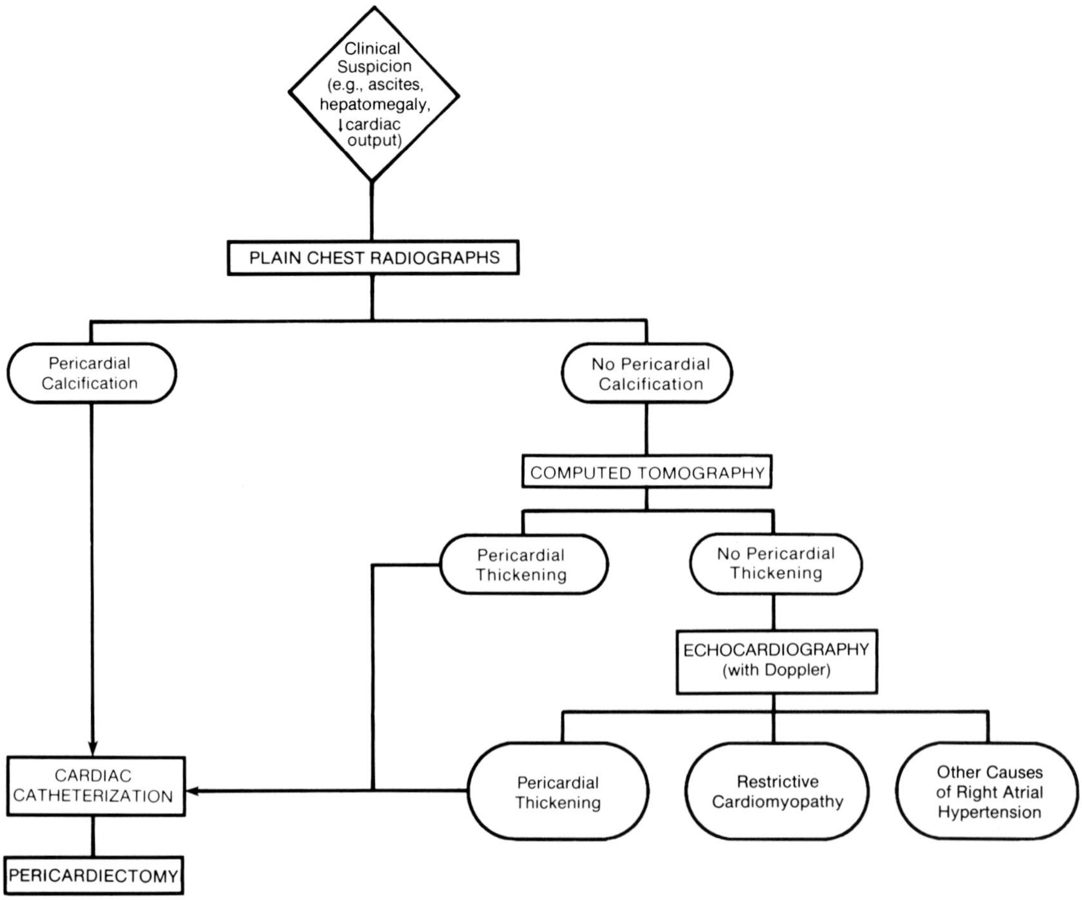

# PART TWO

# Gastrointestinal Tract

# Chapter 8

# Acute Abdominal Pain

*John R. Amberg*

Acute abdominal pain is a very common complaint, and most episodes are brief and self-correcting. The ingestion of an excessive quantity of otherwise safe products is a frequent cause of abdominal distress, and a myraid of non-prescription medications is easily available and widely used to combat the symtoms of these episodes. Medical care is infrequently sought, because the cause-and-effect relationship is so apparent. The diagnostic challenge arises only when the pain is severe, recurrent, or of unknown etiology.

The causes of abdominal pain are extensive (Table 8-1). The broad categories of intra-abdominal and extra-abdominal emphasize the importance of not confining the diagnostic search to the peritoneal cavity. The most common intra-abdominal causes of acute pain are peritoneal irritation, visceral distention, and ischemia. Although at times it may be difficult to make the precise diagnosis, it is important to remember that determining the precise etiology of acute abdominal pain may not be necessary, because the major diagnostic problem is separating those patients requiring surgery from those who only need therapy for symptomatic relief and to prevent progression of the disease.

The logical use of diagnostic imaging modalities requires more than the mere knowledge that the patient has acute abdominal pain. The initial diagnostic hypothesis must be based on the character of the pain, the history (trauma, alcoholism, inflammatory bowel disease, kidney stones), the physical findings (fever, mass, vomiting, diarrhea, hematemesis), and simple laboratory data (hematocrit, white blood count, serum amylase, serum creatinine, and urinalysis). Once a tentative diagnosis is established, an imaging procedure should be selected that will most quickly confirm or exclude that diagnosis. If the initial diagnostic suggestion is incorrect, a second diagnostic possibility should be evaluated by an appropriate imaging technique.

## DIAGNOSTIC EVALUATION

### *DIAGNOSTIC MODALITIES*

1. Plain chest radiography
2. Plain abdominal radiography
3. Ultrasound
4. Computed tomography
5. Magnetic resonance imaging

**Table 8-1** Causes of Abdominal Pain

1. Intra-abdominal
   - A. Generalized peritonitis
     1. Perforated viscus: peptic ulcer, gallbladder, colonic diverticulum
     2. Primary bacterial peritonitis: pneumococcal, streptococcal, enteric bacillus, tuberculous
     3. Nonbacterial peritonitis: ruptured ovarian cyst, ruptured follicle cyst
     4. Familial Mediterranean fever (familial periodic peritonitis)
   - B. Localized peritonitis: many types of local peritonitis may become generalized by rupture into the free peritoneal cavity
     1. Appendicitis
     2. Cholecystitis
     3. Peptic ulcer
     4. Meckel's diverticulitis
     5. Regional enteritis
     6. Acute colonic diverticulitis
     7. Colitis: ulcerative, amebic, bacterial
     8. Abdominal abscess: postoperative, hepatic, pancreatic, splenic, diverticular, tubo-ovarian
     9. Gastroenteritis
     10. Pancreatitis
     11. Hepatitis: viral, toxic
     12. Pelvic inflammatory disease, gonococcal perihepatitis (Fitz-Hugh–Curtis syndrome)
     13. Endometritis
     14. Lymphadenitis
   - C. Pain from increased tension in viscera
     1. Intestinal obstruction: adhesions, hernia, tumor, volvulus, fecal impaction, intussusception
     2. Intestinal hypermotility: irritable colon, gastroenteritis
     3. Biliary obstruction: gallstone, stricture, tumor, parasites, hemobilia
     4. Ureteral obstruction: calculi
     5. Hepatic capsule distention: acute hepatitis (toxic or viral), common duct obstruction, Budd-Chiari syndrome
     6. Renal capsule distention: pyelonephritis, ureteral obstruction
     7. Uterine obstruction: neoplasm, childbirth
     8. Aortic aneurysm
   - D. Ischemia
     1. Intestinal angina or infarction: arterial stenosis, embolism, polyarteritis
     2. Splenic infarction
     3. Torsion: gallbladder, spleen, ovarian cyst, testicle, omentum, appendix epiploica
     4. Hepatic infarction: toxemia
     5. Tumor necrosis: hepatoma, uterine fibroid
   - E. Retroperitoneal neoplasms

II. Extra-abdominal
   - A. Thoracic
     1. Pneumonitis
     2. Pulmonary embolism
     3. Empyema
     4. Myocardial ischemia
     5. Myocarditis, endocarditis
     6. Esophagitis, esophageal spasm
     7. Esophageal rupture
   - B. Neurogenic
     1. Radiculitis: spinal cord or peripheral nerve tumors, degenerative arthritis of spine, herpes zoster
     2. Tabes dorsalis
     3. Abdominal epilepsy
   - C. Metabolic
     1. Uremia
     2. Diabetes mellitus
     3. Porphyria
     4. Acute adrenal insufficiency
   - D. Toxins
     1. Hypersensitivity reactions: insect bites, reptile venoms
     2. Drugs: lead poisoning, etc.
   - E. Miscellaneous
     1. Muscular contusion, hematoma, or tumor

(Sleisenger MH, Fordtran JS: Gastrointestinal Disease. Philadelphia, WB Saunders, 1973)

6. Excretory and retrograde urography
7. Radionuclide studies
8. Gastrointestinal radiography
9. Gastrointestinal endoscopy
10. Angiography
11. Needle aspiration
12. Laparoscopy and laparotomy

### Plain Chest Radiography

The upright chest radiograph is the most sensitive method for identifying free gas in the peritoneal space. This technique also may show pulmonary infiltrates or mediastinal abnormalities that may indicate that the process responsible for the abdominal pain is actually thoracic in origin. The chest film also is of importance should general anesthesia be required during the course of diagnosis or treatment.

### Plain Abdominal Radiography

The clearest indication for obtaining plain radiographs of the abdomen is to search for gas-distended loops of bowel with gas–fluid levels in patients with a distended and tympanitic abdomen suggestive of small bowel obstruction. Plain abdominal radiography can identify calcification in the gallbladder, appendix, urinary tract, and pancreas that may (but not necessarily) reflect the underlying pain-producing process. This technique also may demonstrate gas-filled abscesses, large abdominal masses, and gas within the bowel wall associated with necrotizing enterocolitis or mesenteric ischemia.

Plain abdominal radiography has significant limitations in evaluating the patient with acute abdominal pain. It provides minimal information about the solid organs (liver, spleen, pancreas, kidneys, and genital structures). Modest amounts of fluid in the peritoneal space are difficult to detect. Many abscesses and other abdominal masses cannot be visualized, and intestinal inflammation and ulceration cannot be properly assessed (a special problem in suspected appendicitis). Plain radiographs are unable to detect ischemia in either hollow or solid organs, and the previously used signs of strangulation obstruction (*e.g.,* fixed "coffee bean" loop) have been discounted. Thus, very serious intra-abdominal pathologic processes can be present without any manifestations on plain abdominal radiographs.

It must be recognized that plain abdominal radiographs showing no abnormality are reassuring to both patient and physician. This "therapeutic" effect is probably the only justification for their current frequent use.

### Ultrasound

Ultrasound is now readily available and should replace plain abdominal radiographs as the initial imaging procedure of choice for many patients with acute abdominal pain (but not for the patient with a distended, tympanitic abdomen). Ultrasound is indicated for the evaluation of pelvic pain that is believed to originate in the ovaries, uterus, or fallopian tubes. This modality can determine the cystic versus solid nature of a palpable abdominal mass and can detect free intraperitoneal fluid, aortic aneurysm, and periaortic hemorrhage. Intussuscepted loops of bowel have characteristic sonographic features. Ultrasound is the imaging procedure of choice for patients with biliary colic, because it not only can detect stones and bile duct dilatation, but also can show abnormalities of the pancreas and liver parenchyma that may mimic cholecystitis. Some suggest that ultrasound is the only imaging procedure required in the patient with renal colic, with treatment governed by repeat assessment of the degree of hydronephrosis and the urinary sediment.

### Computed Tomography

Computed tomography (CT) is the imaging procedure of choice in patients with severe abdominal trauma, because it permits a rapid global evaluation of the abdomen in those patients who may have damage to multiple organs. Computed tomography surpasses other modalities in its depiction of the solid organs (liver, spleen, pancreas, and kidneys) as well as in its ability to identify blood in both the intra- and extraperitoneal spaces.

Computed tomography also is of great value in identifying abscesses and other fluid collections within the abdomen. Unlike ultrasound, CT is not adversely affected by a large amount of abdominal gas. In addition to abscess detection, CT permits aspiration and drainage of abdominal abscesses.

Computed tomography is superior to ultrasound for demonstrating inflammatory and ischemic insults causing bowel wall thickening, although it cannot compete with barium studies in diagnosing mucosal disease. In comparison with plain abdominal radiographs, CT can detect smaller collections of gas in the bowel wall, portal vein, and extra-alimentary tissues. Aortic aneurysms and periaortic hemorrhage also are well studied by CT.

### Magnetic Resonance Imaging

The precise role of magnetic resonance imaging (MRI) in the evaluation of patients with acute abdominal pain is still uncertain. At present, MR images of the abdomen are not as good as those obtained by CT.

### Excretory and Retrograde Urography

The clinical symptoms of acute renal colic usually are characteristic, and the associated findings of red or white blood cells in the urinary sediment often are enough to establish a reasonable diagnosis. Excretory urography can determine whether the urinary tract is obstructed and may precisely document the size and location of an obstructing stone. Following abdominal trauma, excretory urography provides functional information about the kidneys, although CT is superior in evaluating the extent of parenchymal damage. Retrograde cystourethrography is a simple method for detecting rupture of the bladder or urethra following abdominal trauma.

### Radionuclide Studies

Cholescintigraphy is an effective technique for determining cystic duct obstruction in a patient with suspected acute cholecystitis. Unlike ultrasound, cholescintigraphy provides functional data as well as anatomic information.

The selective excretion of technetium by the mucosa in a Meckel's diverticulum has made radionuclide scanning an accepted diagnostic method in patients suspected of having this condition (which more often presents with unexplained melena rather than abdominal pain).

### Gastrointestinal Radiography

Epigastric pain is very common, and thus it is unclear how much diagnostic effort to expend on patients with this symptom. Some physicians use either antacids or blockers of hydrochloric acid secretion as combined diagnostic–therapeutic agents. Upper gastrointestinal radiography is less sensitive than endoscopy in detecting erosive and ulcerative disease of the stomach, although it can identify those larger lesions that may require further evaluation.

Enteroclysis is the imaging modality of choice for evaluating patients with suspected intermittent small bowel obstruction as the cause of their pain. This technique also is of value in detecting Meckel's diverticula.

Colonic radiography can easily demonstrate obstruction caused by neoplasm, volvulus, or intussusception. It can show the luminal narrowing and sinus tracts seen in diverticulitis, with CT or ultrasound providing confirmatory evidence of bowel wall thickening or frank abscess formation. Although the demonstration of persistent changes in the ileocecal area combined with a lack of filling of the appendiceal lumen is suggestive of appendicitis, this diagnosis is often difficult to confirm or exclude on colonic radiography. Diarrhea, rather than pain, tends to be the predominant feature in most inflammatory bowel disease, which can be effectively evaluated by colonic radiography or endoscopy.

### Gastrointestinal Endoscopy

Endoscopy is the procedure of choice for directly visualizing the mucosa of the stomach or intestines. This is of major diagnostic importance in patients with upper gastrointestinal bleeding associated with abdominal pain. Not only can endoscopy localize the bleeding site, it usually can determine the underlying disease process. This information is invaluable for the surgeon faced with an emergency laparotomy to control severe bleeding.

Colonoscopy generally is not performed for patients complaining only of abdominal pain. Direct visualization of the mucosa may be indicated if there is associated bleeding or diarrhea.

### Angiography

Complete and sudden infarction in the distribution of the superior mesenteric artery is a cause of severe abdominal pain. However, the resulting bowel infarction and associated shock usually produce an abdominal catastrophe that requires emergency surgery rather than angiography. Angiography is indicated in patients with abdominal angina caused by partially occlusive disease of the mesenteric circulation. However, this is a relatively infrequent condition because of the good collateral circulation to the bowel.

### Needle Aspiration

In the past, blind four-quadrant needle aspiration was often performed in patients with suspected intra-abdominal bleeding or primary bacterial peritonitis. The presence of intraperitoneal fluid or discrete abdominal hematomas or abscesses now can be easily detected by ultrasound or CT. Needle aspiration under CT or ultrasound guidance can provide diagnostic material from intra-abdominal hematomas, abscesses, and pancreatic pseudocysts. In addition to its diagnostic value, needle aspiration can be used to drain these collections and often provides dramatic relief of symptoms.

### Laparoscopy and Laparotomy

The use of laparoscopy as a diagnostic modality has decreased with the continued improvements and increased availability of ultrasound and CT. Unlike these imaging modalities, laparoscopy has the advantage of providing direct visualization of inflammatory and neoplastic lesions.

The newer imaging modalities have substantially decreased the use of exploratory laparotomy as a diagnostic tool. Nevertheless, it must be remembered that the diagnosis of appendicitis generally is made at exploratory laparotomy and some processes, such as venous infarction of the bowel, are difficult to image.

## COMMENT

There have been relatively few studies regarding the efficacy of various imaging modalities in the diagnosis of the cause of acute abdominal pain. Consequently, the material in this chapter reflects current practice rather than the results of research. It also emphasizes the intra-abdominal causes of pain, even though extra-abdominal causes (porphyria, herniated disk, rectus muscle hemorrhage) mimicking abdominal disease also must always be considered. Unfortunately, diagnostic error is inevitable despite the many modalities currently available. Normal appendices are resected, and gallstones are removed as treatment for pain caused by functional bowel disease. Patients with acute porphyria or intestinal pseudo-obstruction may undergo unnecessary laparotomies. Nevertheless, the overall goal of relieving pain and reducing morbidity and mortality seems to have been well served by advances in diagnostic imaging procedures.

## Bibliography

Botsford TW: The Acute Abdomen: An Approach to Diagnosis and Management. Philadelphia, WB Saunders, 1977

Cope Z (Revised by Silen W): Diagnosis of the Acute Abdomen. New York, Oxford University Press, 1979

Currie DJ: Abdominal Pain. Washington, DC, Hemisphere, 1979

Eisenberg RL: Gastrointestinal Radiology: A Pattern Approach. Philadelphia, JB Lippincott, 1983

Eisenberg RL, Heineken P, Hedgcock MW et al: Evaluation of plain abdominal radiographs in the diagnosis of abdominal pain. Ann Intern Med 97:257–261, 1982

Margulis AR, Burhenne HJ: Alimentary Tract Radiology. St. Louis, CV Mosby, 1982

McCort JJ, Mindelzun RE, Filipi RG et al: Abdominal Radiology. Baltimore, Williams & Wilkins, 1981

Way LW: Abdominal pain in gastrointestinal disease. In Sleisenger MH, Fordtran JS (eds): Gastrointestinal Disease, pp 394–410. Philadelphia, WB Saunders, 1978

Weissman HS, Badia J, Sugarman LA et al: Spectrum of $^{99m}$Tc-IDA cholescintigraphic patterns in acute cholecystitis. Radiology 138:167–175, 1981

## ACUTE ABDOMINAL PAIN

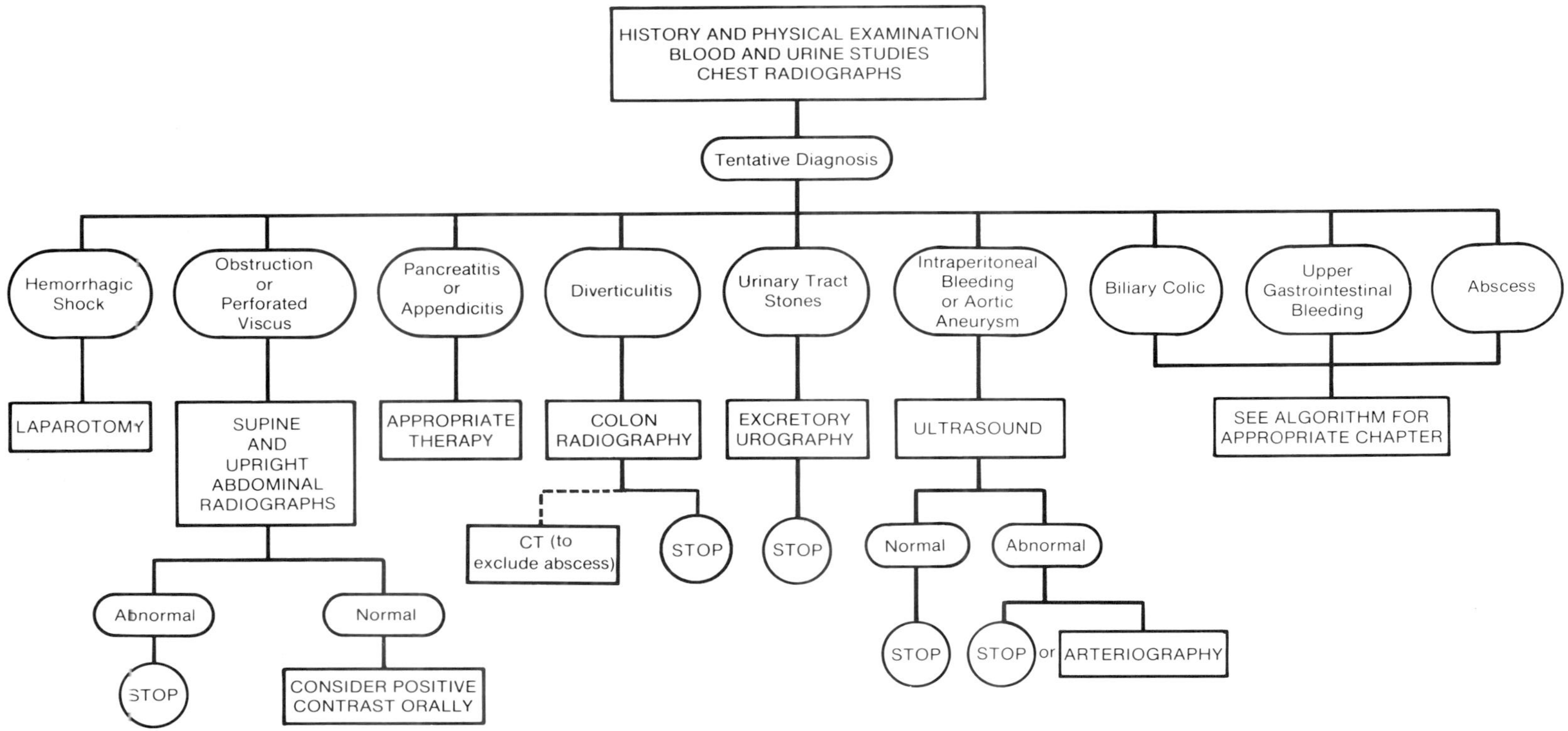

# Chapter 9

# Gastrointestinal Hemorrhage

*Peter C. Meyers*
*Mary J. Wood*

The diagnostic approach to the patient with gastrointestinal hemorrhage involves a series of decisions based on the clinically suspected origin of the bleeding, as well as on the severity of the hemorrhage and the availability of the many newer techniques for investigation. No single simple scheme can be applied to gastrointestinal hemorrhage as a whole. Patients must first be separated into those with suspected upper or lower gastrointestinal hemorrhage and then further subdivided into those with acute or chronic blood loss.

There is an extensive list of both common and uncommon causes of acute upper (Table 9-1) and lower (Table 9-2) gastrointestinal hemorrhage. Almost all of these entities can also be cited as causes for chronic gastrointestinal blood loss. Therefore, a logical approach to both diagnosis and therapy is essential, especially when one considers the 8% to 14% mortality rate for patients who present with acute gastrointestinal hemorrhage.

## CLINICAL AND LABORATORY FINDINGS

The patient with acute gastrointestinal hemorrhage usually presents with a sudden onset of hematemesis, melena, hematochezia, or a combination of these findings. The blood pressure (both upright and recumbent) and pulse rate, along with a determination of the patient's hematocrit and hemoglobin, will usually give a reasonable estimate of the magnitude of the hemorrhage. Blood in the vomitus or nasogastric aspirate indicates a bleeding site proximal to the ligament of Treitz, most often from a source in the stomach or the esophagus. The presence of melena usually implies bleeding from a site proximal to the midportion of the small bowel. Distal small bowel or ascending colon bleeding is occasionally associated with melena, but bleeding from these sites or from the distal colon usually presents as hematochezia. These simple observations play a major role in directing subsequent investigations.

**Table 9-1** Causes of Acute Upper Gastrointestinal Bleeding

| Common |
|---|
| Gastric erosions |
| Dodenal ulcer |
| Gastric ulcer |
| Varices |
| Esophagitis |
| Mallory–Weiss syndrome |
| Neoplasm |
| Esophageal ulcer |
| **Less Common** |
| Mesenteric ischemia |
| Vascular malformations |
| Anticoagulation |
| Aorta–entric fistulas |
| Hematobilia |
| Systemic and hematologic causes |
| Epistaxis |
| Hemoptysis |
| Naso- and oropharyngeal lesions |
| Factitious bleeding |

Clinical and laboratory studies are also important in identifying patients with chronic gastrointestinal blood loss who have iron-deficiency anemia or hematest-positive stools. The origin of chronic gastrointestinal hemorrhage is usually much less apparent, and the entire spectrum of available studies may have to be performed before the diagnosis is established.

## DIAGNOSTIC EVALUATION

### *DIAGNOSTIC MODALITIES*

1. Endoscopy
2. Barium upper gastrointestinal series
3. Arteriography
4. Radionuclide scan
5. Barium enema
6. Proctosigmoidoscopy
7. Colonoscopy
8. Small bowel enteroclysis
9. Retrograde small bowel enema
10. String test (seldom used)
11. Miller–Abbott tube with aspiration
12. Plain film of the abdomen
13. Surgery

**Table 9-2** Causes of Acute Lower Gastrointestinal Bleeding

| Common |
|---|
| Diverticular disease |
| Vascular malformations |
| Carcinoma |
| Polyps |
| Inflammatory bowel disease |
| Ischemia |
| Hemorrhoids |
| **Less Common** |
| Distal small bowel tumors |
| Meckel's diverticulum |
| Anal fissures |
| Rectal trauma |
| Mesenteric varices |

## ACUTE UPPER GASTROINTESTINAL HEMORRHAGE

### Endoscopy

In patients with suspected acute upper gastrointestinal hemorrhage, the prevailing medical opinion favors endoscopy as the initial diagnostic procedure of choice. The ability of the endoscopist to visualize superficial mucosal lesions, such as esophagitis, gastritis, and superficial erosions, as well as varices, Mallory–Weiss tears, and penetrating ulcers, makes endoscopy a most accurate diagnostic procedure. The endoscopist not only visualizes the abnormality but usually can say with some certainty whether or not a specific lesion is the cause of the acute bleeding episode, which cannot be done with barium studies. This is important because a significant number of patients with acute upper gastrointestinal hemorrhage are found to have more than one lesion.

The fiberoptic gastroscope was first introduced more than 20 years ago, and improvements and refinements of the original instrument have continued to date. Endoscopy is often performed in less than ideal conditions (emergencies or semi-emergencies) and in places other than the endoscopy suite. In a survey performed by the National American Society for Gastrointestinal Endoscopy, only 88.7% of all the examinations were considered to be complete, and it was estimated that endoscopy identified the lesion in 80% to 95% of patients. The procedure is contraindicated in only that small percentage of patients who have severe cardiac or pulmonary disease, or in extremely combative patients. Technical failure due to cervical spine disease is rarely encountered. The ability to visualize areas beyond strictures has been greatly enhanced by the introduction of smaller pediatric endoscopes. In the presence of large amounts of fresh blood or clots within the stomach, endoscopic diagnosis is difficult but not impossible if the endoscopist can vigorously lavage the stomach through a large-bore tube prior to endoscopy. If the blood cannot be successfully cleared by this method, the patient is usually a candidate for either arteriography or emergency surgery.

Endoscopy has been reported to have an accuracy of 80% to 95% in identifying the source of upper gastrointestinal bleeding when it lies proximal to the ligament of Treitz. However, it is unclear from the available data whether these statistics refer to the detection of the precise source of bleeding, or simply to the demonstration of any possible bleeding lesion, or if only secondary signs of hemorrhage such as a clot or a dark pigmented spot were seen. If necessary, endoscopy as a first diagnostic procedure can easily be followed by arteriography for therapeutic intervention or additional diagnostic information. If the diagnosis remains in doubt after endoscopy, barium studies can still be readily performed. The converse is certainly not true.

Despite all the obvious advantages of early endoscopy in the workup of patients with acute upper gastrointestinal hemorrhage, data showing significant patient benefit from early endoscopic diagnosis are equivocal at best. Most studies in this area have failed to demonstrate a reduction in length of hospital stay, morbidity, or mortality. However, most physicians still feel that early diagnosis via the endoscope allows them to most efficiently manage the patient.

The cost of endoscopy is greater than that of a barium study of the upper gastrointestinal tract. Complications are rare, approximately 1 per 1000 studies, and the mortality rate has been reported as 0.01% to 0.06%. The major complications relate to direct trauma, such as perforation of the esophagus, aspiration, drug reactions, and cardiopulmonary problems.

The future may hold an expanded role for endoscopy because of the many therapeutic techniques that are currently under investigation for endoscopic control of upper gastrointestinal hemorrhage (fiberoptic injection of esophageal varices; and the use of electrocautery, laser cautery, mechanical clips, or tissue adhesives via the endoscope). The exact role of these endoscopic therapeutic maneuvers remains to be determined through future studies.

## Barium Upper Gastrointestinal Series

Endoscopy, not a barium study, should be the initial diagnostic procedure in the patient presenting with acute upper gastrointestinal hemorrhage who has relatively stable vital signs. One reason for this choice is that endoscopic accuracy approaches 95%, whereas the upper gastrointestinal barium study has been variously recorded as having 30% to 80% diagnostic accuracy. The higher figure relates to studies utilizing the air-contrast examination of the stomach and duodenum. This technique increases diagnostic accuracy because of its ability to demonstrate superficial mucosal abnormalities (Fig. 9-1), but it is technically difficult to perform in the patient with acute hemorrhage, because the presence of fresh and clotted blood severely affects the quality of mucosal coating. In addition, the status of the patient and the presence of numerous intravenous lines and other resuscitative equipment limits the patient's mobility, making it difficult to achieve adequate mucosal coating.

Although the endoscopist frequently can

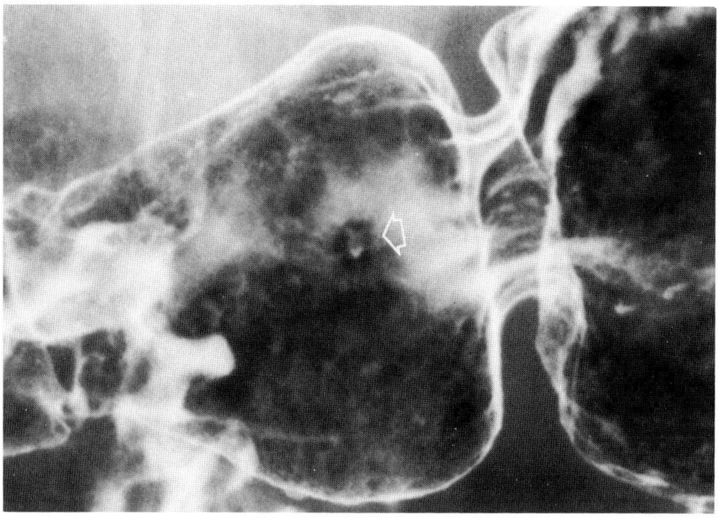

**Figure 9-1.** Superficial gastric erosion. The collection of barium represents a shallow erosion surrounded by a radiolucent halo (*arrow*). (Eisenberg RL: Gastrointestinal Radiology: A Pattern Approach. Philadelphia, JB Lippincott, 1983)

identify with certainty that a given lesion is the source of acute hemorrhage, this is usually impossible with barium studies, especially when more than one lesion is found. However, there are circumstances in the workup of patients with acute gastrointestinal hemorrhage when barium studies may be of great value. In those patients who cannot tolerate endoscopy or in whom endoscopic results have been negative, the barium study should be performed, provided that the patient is not bleeding so rapidly that arteriography or emergency surgery is required. Additionally, expert emergency endoscopy may not always be available. In this situation, an air-contrast study should be performed because of its proven diagnostic superiority over the single-contrast study. False-positive diagnoses are unusual, but false-negative examinations are all too frequent. The majority of false-negative upper gastrointestinal examinations occur in patients whose bleeding originates in superficial mucosal lesions, such as esophagitis, gastritis, and Mallory–Weiss tears.

The major advantages of the barium examination in patients with acute upper gastrointestinal bleeding are that it is readily available, has good patient acceptance, and is less expensive than other diagnostic modalities. The major disadvantages are the disappointing accuracy of the emergency barium upper gastrointestinal series and the fact that the presence of barium may preclude further diagnostic studies, such as endoscopy or arteriography or radionuclide imaging. Finally, there are no therapeutic advantages of the emergency barium upper gastrointestinal series, as there are with arteriography or endoscopy.

Complications of barium upper gastrointestinal series are virtually nonexistent and limited to aspiration of barium (usually of no clinical significance) or barium extravasation from preexisting perforations. The latter complication can be prevented by recognizing the signs of free intraperitoneal gas on a preliminary abdominal radiograph and employing water-soluble contrast material (rather than barium) to produce a limited examination.

## Arteriography

Modern arteriographic capabilities, much like endoscopy, have revolutionized the diagnostic and therapeutic approaches to acute gastrointestinal hemorrhage. Bleeding at a rate of at least 0.5 ml to 1 ml per minute will usually be detected by selective arteriography. If there is clinical evidence that acute bleeding has stopped, however, arteriography should not be considered as the first diagnostic approach.

Arteriography should be performed if endoscopy is inconclusive or if a patient who is a poor surgical candidate is so actively bleeding that therapeutic transcatheter hemostasis is required. Virtually all the causes of acute upper gastrointestinal hemorrhage, including gastritis, varices, ulcers, and Mallory–Weiss tears, can be diagnosed and treated via the arteriographic catheter. The specific etiology of the hemorrhage will generally determine whether vasoconstrictive agents or embolization will be more effective.

The accuracy of arteriography in diagnosing acute upper gastrointestinal hemorrhage is reported to be 70% to 95% when there is active bleeding. Hemorrhage usually can be stopped by transcatheter therapeutic measures in the majority of these patients. In patients in whom hemostasis fails or is only temporary, this technique will usually allow time for vascular volume replacement (to stabilize the patient's condition and to plan a more specific surgical approach).

Complications from modern arteriography are unusual. The mortality rate is less than 0.1%, and most deaths are related to contrast reactions rather than to sequelae of the catheterization itself. Serious complications such as embolization, subintimal dissection, bleeding, and hematoma formation occur in approximately 0.7% of patients. Less serious local complications at the puncture site (such as a localized hematoma) may be seen in up to 3% of patients.

### Radionuclide Scan

An *in vivo* method of labeling sucralfate with $^{99m}$Tc has been introduced for use in detecting gastric ulcers but has not yet been tested for duodenal ulcers. This radionuclide scan is less expensive and has a smaller radiation dose than the usual upper gastrointestinal series or arteriography, and therefore it may be a useful modality in the patient who is not a candidate for endoscopy or barium study.

### Surgery

Surgery is rarely utilized as a diagnostic tool in patients with acute upper gastrointestinal hemorrhage. However, for those patients whose hemorrhage is massive and whose vital signs cannot be maintained to permit arteriography, emergency surgery may be indicated for both diagnostic and therapeutic purposes. Surgery can be lifesaving in these situations, although the mortality rate is high.

The recent use of transcatheter hemostatic methods has greatly reduced the need for emergency surgery. Preoperative arteriography, if readily available and rapidly performed, will at least permit accurate locations of the bleeding site and therefore more precise surgical intervention. Even if only partially effective, transcatheter hemostasis may allow time for the patient to be stabilized before any operative procedure is undertaken. Blood-volume replacement and resuscitative methods may be carried out in the arteriography suite prior to surgical intervention.

It is difficult to establish mortality rates for patients undergoing emergency surgery for upper gastrointestinal hemorrhage. The overall mortality rate for all patients admitted with acute upper gastrointestinal bleeding ranges from 8% to 14%. Reports of the morbidity and mortality of emergency surgery vary widely depending on the patient's age and the cause of hemorrhage. The most important factor is the selection of patients for surgery and the timing of surgical intervention. Careful consultation among the radiologist, gastroenterologist, and surgeon will undoubtedly result in the most efficient use of surgery at the most appropriate time for those patients most likely to benefit from the procedure.

## ACUTE LOWER GASTROINTESTINAL BLEEDING

### Radionuclide Scanning

Radionuclide scanning is now commonly accepted as the most sensitive diagnostic study for detecting lower gastrointestinal bleeding. Technetium-99m–labeled or $^{111}$In-labeled colloid particles injected intravenously can demonstrate lesions that are actively bleeding at a rate of 0.05 ml to 0.1 ml per minute. The major limitation of this highly accurate study is that, like arteriography, the patient must be actively bleeding at the time of the injection of the isotope. In addition, the colloid particles localizing in the liver and spleen may obscure portions of the upper abdomen.

In patients with intermittent bleeding from the lower gastrointestinal tract, radionuclide scanning with $^{99m}$Tc-labeled red blood cells has a 93% sensitivity for detecting and localizing bleeding sites (Fig. 9-2). An *in vitro* or a modified *in vivo* method of labeling the red blood cells can detect bleeding at a rate of 0.1 ml to 0.3 ml per minute. Continuous imaging is performed for 90 minutes. If no bleeding is detected at this time, delayed images are obtained for up to 24 hours. If the delayed views show some isotope activity within the lumen, sequential imaging over 90 minutes is repeated with either the same dose or an additional dose of labeled

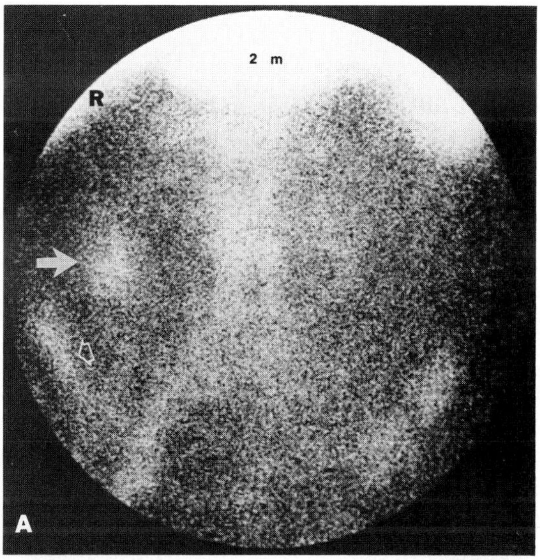


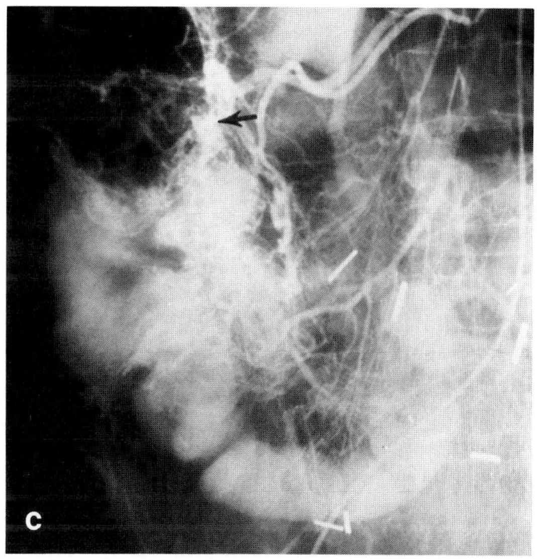


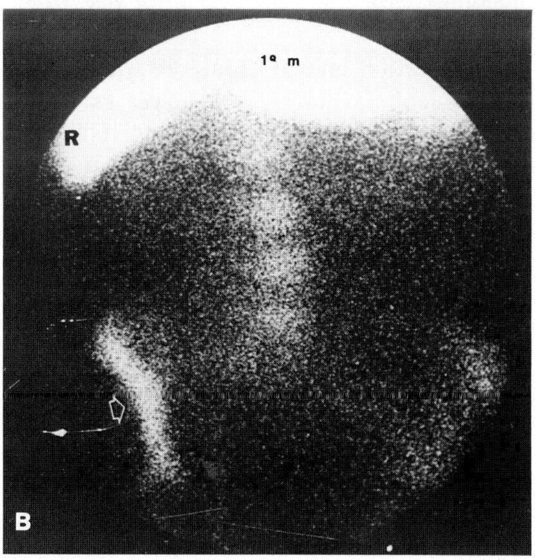


**Figure 9-2.** Angiodysplasia. **(A)** $^{99m}$Tc sulfur colloid scan 2 minutes after injection shows a large area of increased radionuclide activity (*closed arrow*) in the right lower quadrant of the abdomen. The open arrow indicates isotope activity in the right iliac crest. **(B)** Sequential nuclear image at 18 minutes after injection demonstrates complete absence of radioactivity in the gastrointestinal tract. The open arrow again denotes activity in the right iliac crest. **(C)** Arteriography shows the angiodysplasia (*arrow*) in the cecum.

red blood cells, in order to better define tne anatomic bleeding site. Movement of the radionuclide proximally or distally is the *sine qua non* of active intraluminal bleeding. Lack of movement suggests an angiodysplasia, arteriovenous malformation, or vascular tumor. Additional techniques such as pre- and postdefecation images, bedpan image, glucagon administration, or a $^{99m}$Tc diethylenetriamine pentaacetic acid ($^{99m}$Tc-DTPA) enema can be employed to enhance localization of the bleeding site.

### Arteriography

Arteriography is the imaging procedure of choice in patients with massive acute lower gastrointestinal hemorrhage, most of whom are bleeding from diverticulosis. The rate of blood loss must be more than 0.5 ml per minute to localize the bleeding site. In patients with brisk bleeding, contrast material injected into the appropriate blood vessel rapidly extravasates from the bleeding vessel into the lumen of the gut, leaving a persistent blush (Fig. 9-3). In some centers, radionuclide scanning is performed prior to arteriography in order to localize the bleeding site as closely as possible and thus permit selective catheterization of the suspected bleeding vessel. Radionuclide scanning is the procedure of choice when the patient's renal function does not permit the use of intravenous contrast material.

In addition to demonstrating hemorrhage from diverticulosis, arteriography is highly accurate in detecting bleeding from arteriovenous malformations, the second leading cause of massive acute lower gastrointestinal bleeding. Particularly in cases of diverticular hemorrhage, transcatheter hemostasis from vasopressor infusion or embolization has been highly successful, and in many patients surgery may be avoided entirely. In those patients in whom surgery is ultimately required, the diagnostic and therapeutic value of arteriography permits both stabilization of the patient and resection of the colon limited to the area of the bleeding site. An additional advantage of arteriography is its ability to identify bleeding sites in the small bowel or duodenum that may masquerade as acute colonic hemorrhage.

### Surgery

Emergency surgery in patients with massive colon hemorrhage carries a mortality of approximately 30%. Total colectomy frequently must be performed because of the inability of the surgeon to identify the specific site of bleeding. Therefore, if arteriography is available, it should be utilized prior to surgery to identify the site of bleeding. Even if transcatheter hemostasis is inadequate, surgery following arteriography will at least allow for a rational segmental colon resection.

### Barium Enema

The barium enema is indicated in the evaluation of patients with nonmassive lower gastrointestinal bleeding who present with persistent bleeding or occult blood in the stool. This procedure has no place in the diagnosis or treatment of massive bleeding. A barium enema should not be performed as an emergency examination, because it is essential that the patient be well prepared and have a colon clear of any fecal material. Ideally, an air-contrast examination should be performed to detect small lesions. A well-performed barium enema examination is an excellent screening study for colon disease, because it can detect most lesions causing rectal bleeding and can be performed as an outpatient procedure with low cost and little risk to the patient.

The barium enema should be used only to diagnose colonic lesions and *never* as a therapeutic technique to stop bleeding. For many years, there was the erroneous belief that a solid-column barium enema was helpful in controlling lower gastrointestinal hemorrhage, either because of tamponading the bleeding site or because the barium, in some unknown manner, promoted coagulation. Studies have conclusively shown that barium may in fact decrease coagulation and promote further colonic bleeding, while any tamponading effect is minimal.

Ischemia, usually nonocclusive, may appear as acute lower gastrointestinal bleeding. If the patient's history and clinical state suggest this diagnosis, the barium enema may be the procedure of choice. The demonstration of typical fea-

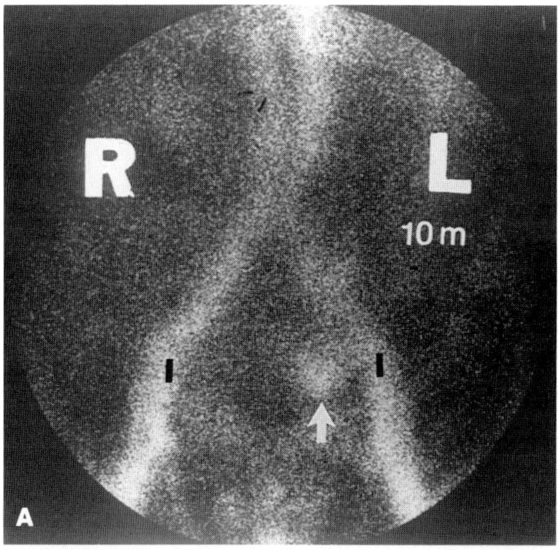


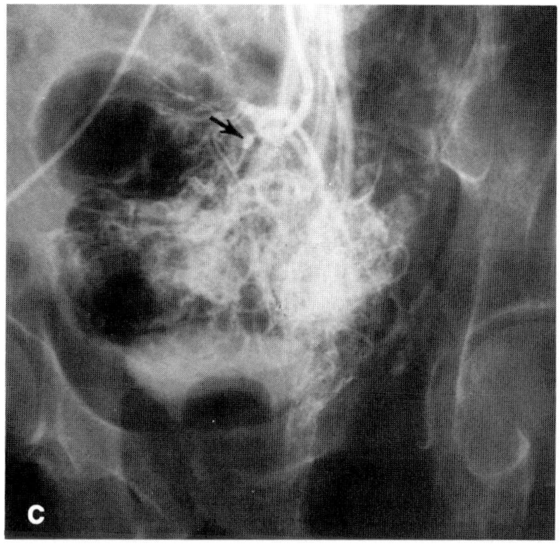


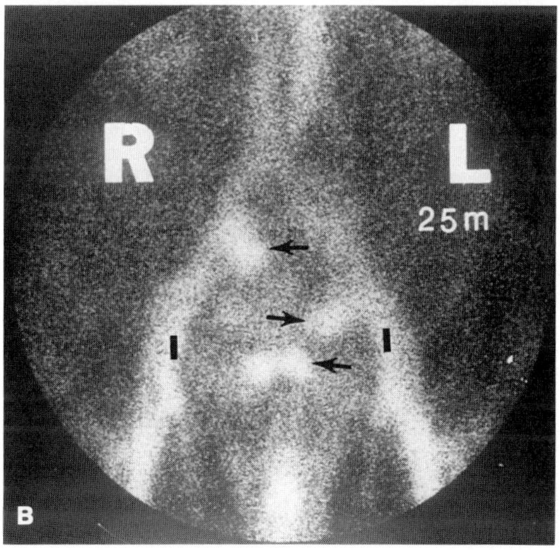


**Figure 9-3.** Active bleeding from sigmoid diverticulosis. **(A)** Radionuclide scan using $^{99m}$Tc-tagged red blood cells (modified *in vitro* method). At 10 minutes there is an area of radionuclide activity in the left pelvic region (*arrow*). **(B)** On the image taken at 25 minutes, there is intraluminal movement of the radionuclide (*arrows*) consistent with active bleeding. **(C)** Arteriography reveals "puddling" of contrast material (*arrow*) at the active bleeding site in the sigmoid colon. (*I*, iliac arteries)

tures of ischemic colitis (thumbprinting, ulceration, and stricture) will usually be diagnostic. Correction of underlying problems, such as congestive heart failure and other low cardiac output states, may permit successful conservative management without the need for acute surgical intervention. On the other hand, perforation or progression to ischemic necrosis will require immediate surgery.

Complications of barium enema studies are rare. Rectal perforation is usually related to trauma from insertion of the enema tip or use of retention balloons. Barium extravasation below the peritoneal reflection is usually well tolerated without the need for surgical intervention. Extravasation of barium into the peritoneal cavity most frequently occurs through a pre-existing colon perforation. In rare instances, the increased pressure during the barium enema examination may cause perforation in a colon predisposed to rupture because of ischemia or severe inflammatory disease. If a perforation is clinically suspected but not confirmed on plain radiographs, an adequate examination can still be obtained using water-soluble contrast material.

Cardiovascular problems and transient bacteremia have been associated with the performance of a barium enema. Ten to fifteen percent of patients over the age of 60 years have been reported to have significant electrocardiographic changes during barium enema examination, although death directly attributed to the examination is very rare. Bacteremia has been reported in patients in whom sequential blood cultures were obtained, but the risk of sepsis is negligible except in patients who are severely immunosuppressed as a result of hematologic disease or chemotherapy.

### Colonoscopy

Colonoscopy is an important technique for investigating the etiology of acute lower gastrointestinal bleeding. Even in the most tortuous colon, the endoscopist should have no problem reaching the cecum in at least 90% of patients. Colonoscopy should be preceded by a well-performed barium enema examination, because 60% to 70% of colonic lesions can be detected by contrast studies alone. Colonoscopy in patients with unexplained lower gastrointestinal bleeding will detect a polyp in approximately 15%, cancer in 10%, inflammatory disease in 7%, and an arteriovenous malformation in 5% as the cause of bleeding.

Diagnostic colonoscopy (without polypectomy or biopsy) carries a complication rate of approximately 0.1% to 0.25% (mortality is approximately 0.008%). The major complications are perforation or bleeding; cardiorespiratory problems and bacteremia are less common.

## CHRONIC GASTROINTESTINAL HEMORRHAGE

### Barium Studies

In the patient with chronic gastrointestinal bleeding who presents with hematest-positive stool or iron-deficiency anemia, barium studies take precedence as the screening procedures of choice. The entire gastrointestinal tract should be examined, including the esophagus, stomach, duodenum, small bowel, and colon. Current data, both prospective and retrospective, appear to indicate that air-contrast examinations significantly increase the yield of both upper and lower gastrointestinal barium studies. Using endoscopy and colonoscopy as the standards, air-contrast examinations have accuracy rates as high as 95% in the upper portion of the gastrointestinal tract and 75% to 90% in the colon. Although it is likely that the accuracy of air-contrast examinations will always be less than that of adequate direct visualization by upper endoscopy and colonoscopy, barium and endoscopic studies are clearly additive and complementary from a diagnostic standpoint. This is especially true for the colon, in which colonoscopy has certain "blind spots," and complete evaluation by colonoscopy is not universally accomplished.

### Enteroclysis

The peroral placement of a tube into the distal duodenum followed by rapid instillation of large volumes of barium, with or without double-contrast techniques, has become a popular method for studying the small bowel. This procedure has no place in the workup of patients with acute gastrointestinal bleeding, but it should be considered in the diagnostic workup of patients with chronic gastrointestinal bleeding when routine barium and endoscopic studies are negative. Tumors and inflammatory diseases of the small bowel that are not identified on conventional barium studies may be detected by enteroclysis. Complications are rare and can be directly related to passage of the tube. The examination generally takes 30 to 60 minutes to perform and is relatively well tolerated by the patient.

### Endoscopy

Panendoscopy of the upper gastrointestinal tract is clearly indicated in patients who have chronic gastrointestinal blood loss with negative upper and lower gastrointestinal series. The diagnostic accuracy of upper endoscopy approaches 95%. Similarly, the greatest role for colonoscopy is in the evaluation of the patient with chronic, rather than acute, lower gastrointestinal hemorrhage. Following a negative or equivocal barium enema examination, colonoscopy should be performed. Significant lesions (usually polyps) will be found in up to 25% of these patients. With the increasing use of air-contrast barium enema examinations, the false-negative rate of radiographic colon studies should be reduced, and the rate of lesions demonstrated only on colonoscopy should decrease.

Although a very high degree of accuracy is generally accorded to colonoscopic evaluation (90%–95%), most studies fail to take into account lesions not identified because of incomplete examination of the entire colon. Current data indicate that complete colonoscopy may be achieved in approximately 85% of patients.

### Arteriography

Arteriography has a definite role to play in the evaluation of patients with chronic gastrointestinal hemorrhage in whom no source has been found utilizing barium studies and endoscopy. Panabdominal arteriography can be expected to reveal a likely bleeding source in approximately 30% to 40% of these patients. The majority of the lesions will be arteriovenous malformations (also detectable by noninvasive radionuclide imaging). In this situation, however, it is usually impossible to be certain that the arteriographically demonstrated vascular malformation is in fact the cause of the patient's chronic gastrointestinal blood loss.

### Surgery

Exploratory laparotomy for patients with undiagnosed chronic gastrointestinal hemorrhage following negative barium studies, endoscopy, and arteriography will reveal a convincing source of bleeding in 15% to 30% of patients. Although the mortality rate from elective exploratory laparotomy is less than 1%, this method of diagnosis obviously should be reserved until all nonoperative diagnostic tests have been completed. Exploratory laparotomy for undiagnosed chronic gastrointestinal bleeding is controversial. The decision to perform exploratory surgery or to attempt repeated or additional diagnostic tests may depend on the severity of the anemia and the patient's age and general medical condition, as well as the overall clinical evaluation by the primary physician.

### Miscellaneous Diagnostic Tests

Approximately 55% of Meckel's diverticula contain ectopic gastric mucosa, which eventually causes bleeding in 90% of cases. Because $^{99m}Tc$ pertechnetate concentrates in gastric mucosa, a bleeding Meckel's diverticulum containing gastric mucosa typically produces a blush in the lower abdomen on the radionuclide scan within the first 30 minutes of serial imaging. This procedure has a sensitivity of 85% and a specificity of 95%. The sensitivity of technetium scanning may be enhanced by the administration of pentagastrin, cimetidine, or glucagon. If a Meckel's diverticulum is actively bleeding, a $^{99m}Tc$ sulfur colloid scan should be the initial imaging procedure.

The string test, with or without fluorescein, is used to diagnose suspected small bowel bleeding. A weighted 100-cm to 150-cm string is introduced by mouth and allowed to pass into the small bowel. After approximately 8 hours, the string is retrieved and, if there is blood staining, the proximal margin can be measured. Similarly, a Miller–Abbott tube can be passed into the small bowel with repeated aspiration until blood is noted in the aspirate. These techniques, however, give only a gross estimate of the site of gastrointestinal bleeding.

Mention must be made of the use of the abdominal radiograph in patients with gastrointestinal bleeding. Although the literature contains at least one reference to a "bubbly" radiolucency of an admixture of blood clots and air in the bowel lumen, the value of this sign is questionable. However, the appearance of toxic megacolon in inflammatory bowel disease and thumbprinting in ischemic disease may at times be very useful in the differential diagnosis of acute gastrointestinal hemorrhage when the clinical setting suggests either of these conditions.

## GENERAL CLINICAL GUIDELINES FOR EVALUATING LOWER GASTROINTESTINAL BLEEDING

### Massive Bleeding

Although there are numerous causes for massive colonic bleeding, the most common are diverticulosis, arteriovenous malformation, or brisk bleeding from the upper gastrointestinal tract.

Diverticulosis can be easily demonstrated by a barium enema examination, but this procedure cannot determine whether the diverticula are actually bleeding. Radionuclide scanning is the imaging procedure of choice to determine whether the bleeding arises from the colon and to document the precise site of hemorrhage to facilitate the next diagnostic procedure, arteriography. The presence of blood in the bowel makes colonoscopy difficult; thus, this procedure is a less valuable imaging study. A bleeding site detected by arteriography often can be controlled by embolization or drug therapy.

Bleeding from an arteriovenous malformation may be sudden and massive and may present with no symptoms. These malformations usually occur on the right side of the colon and are best diagnosed by arteriography. As with bleeding from diverticulosis, a radionuclide scan is often performed prior to arteriography to precisely localize the site of the lesion. Colonoscopy can also be employed, although the presence of blood in the colon limits the usefulness of this procedure.

### Nonmassive Acute Rectal Bleeding

If the patient notices blood dripping into the toilet bowl after defecation, the lesion is usually near the anal canal, and the initial procedure should be either anoscopy or sigmoidoscopy. A barium enema examination should be obtained, because this type of bleeding should not automatically be attributed to the anal lesion.

Bright red blood staining the underwear without defecation usually signifies a lesion that is external to the anal canal and can be diagnosed with the anoscope.

In patients with rectal bleeding and abdominal pain, the most likely cause is ischemic bowel disease, especially if there is the sudden onset of pain in a previously asymptomatic patient. The initial imaging procedure should probably be proctoscopy; if negative, an arteriogram should follow. A barium enema examination can demonstrate the typical thickening of the colonic wall due to intramural hemorrhage.

Rectal bleeding with diarrhea is a common manifestation of colitis, which often can be diagnosed by sigmoidoscopy. If the patient is not acutely ill or toxic, a barium enema examination should then be performed.

### Chronic Colonic Bleeding

Streaks of blood on the stool surface are usually due to a rectosigmoid lesion such as a polyp or cancer, although hemorrhoids or fissures can also present in this manner. The imaging modality of choice in such patients is probably the double-contrast barium enema, although some physicians prefer to begin with sigmoidoscopy and, if negative, to proceed to the barium enema to detect a lesion in the transverse or descending portions of the colon.

### Occult Blood

The demonstration of hematest-positive stools usually indicates a lesion in the right colon, because blood arising in this location has a chance to become mixed with the stool and not be visible to the eye. Initially, the patient should be evaluated with a barium enema examination; if negative, this can be followed by colonoscopy. Although other examinations are not indicated for evaluating the colon, if a colonic abnormality is not detected, it is necessary to thoroughly search for a source of bleeding above the colon.

## Bibliography

Alavi A, Dann RW, Baum S et al: Scintigraphic detection of acute gastrointestinal bleeding. Radiology 124:753–756, 1977

Amberg JR, Berk RN, Burhenne HJ et al: Colonic polyp detection: Role of roentgenography and colonoscopy. Radiology 125:255–257, 1977

Atkins HL, Srivastave SC, Meinken GE et al: Biological behavior of erythrocytes labeled in vivo and in vitro with technetium-99m. J Nucl Med Technol 13:136–139, 1985

Balint J, Sarfeh I, Fried M: Diagnostic methods: Endoscopy and Angiography. In Gastrointestinal Bleeding Diagnosis and Management. New York, John Wiley & Sons, 1977

Balint J, Sarfeh I, Fried M: Gastrointestinal hemorrhage of unknown origin. In Gastrointestinal Bleeding Diagnosis and Management. New York, John Wiley & Sons, 1977

Bunker SR, Lull RJ, Tanasescu DE et al: Scintigraphy of gastrointestinal hemorrhage: Superiority of 99m Tc red blood cells over 99m Tc sulfur colloid. AJR 143:543–548, 1984

Callahan RJ, Froelich J, McKusick KA et al: A modified method for the in vivo labeling of red blood cells with Tc 99m: Concise communication. J Nucl Med 23:315–318, 1982

Clearfield H, Dinoso V: Diagnosis and management of upper gastrointestinal hemorrhage. In Clearfield H, Dinoso V (eds): Gastrointestinal Emergencies. New York, Grune & Stratton, 1976

Eastwood GL: Does early endoscopy benefit the patient with acute upper gastrointestinal bleeding? Gastroenterology 72:737–739, 1977

Fraser GM: The double contrast barium meal in patients with acute upper gastrointestinal bleeding. Clin Radiol 29:625–634, 1978

Gelfand DW, Wu WC, Oh DJ: The extent of successful colonoscopy: Its implication for the radiologist. Gastrointest Radiol 4:75–78, 1979

Goldberger LE, Bookstein JJ: Transcatheter embolization for treatment of diverticular hemorrhage. Radiology 122:613–617, 1977

Haskin M, Pais MJ, Haskin P: Complications of routine gastrointestinal x-ray examination. In Clearfield H, Dinoso V (eds): Gastrointestinal Emergencies. New York, Grune & Stratton, 1976

Johnsrude, IS, Jackson DC: The role of the radiologist in acute gastrointestinal bleeding. Gastrointest Radiol 3:357–368, 1978

Laufer I, Smith NC, Mullen JE: The radiological demonstration of colorectal polyps undetected by endoscopy. Gastroenterology 70:167–170, 1976

Linscheer WG, Fazio TL: Control of upper gastrointestinal hemorrhage by endoscopic spraying of clotting factors. Gastroenterology 77:642–646, 1979

Lull RJ, Morris GL: Scintigraphic detection of gastrointestinal hemorrhage: Current status. J Nucl Med Technol 14:79–86, 1986

McKusick KA, Froelich J, Callahan RJ et al: 99m Tc red blood cells for detection of gastrointestinal bleeding: Experience with 80 patients. AJR 137:1113–1118, 1981

Meyers MA, Ghahremani GG: Complications of gastrointestinal fiberoptic endoscopy. Gastrointest Radiol 2:273–280, 1977

Miller KD, Tutton RH, Bell KA et al: Angiodysplasia of the colon. Radiology 132:309–313, 1979

Miller RE, Sellink JL: Enteroclysis: The small bowel enema. How to succeed and how to fail. Gastrointest Radiol 4:269–283, 1979

Morris DW, Levine GM, Soloway RD et al: Prospective, randomized study of diagnosis and outcome in acute upper-gastrointestinal bleeding: Endoscopy versus conventional radiography. Am J Dig Dis 20:1103–1109, 1975

Oddson TA, Johnsrude IS, Jackson DC et al: Acute gastrointestinal hemorrhage—the changing role of barium examinations. Radiol Clin North Am 16:123–133, 1978

Orecchia PM, Hensley EK, McDonald PT et al: Localization of lower gastrointestinal hemorrhage: Experience with red blood cells labeled in vitro with 99m Tc. Arch Surg 120:621–624, 1985

Pera A, Seevers R, Meyers K et al: Gastric ulcer localization by direct in vivo labeling of sucralfate. Radiology 156:783–786, 1985

Reuter SR, Redman HC: Gastrointestinal bleeding. In Gastrointestinal Angiography. Philadelphia, WB Saunders, 1977

Sandlow LJ, Becker GH, Spelberg MA et al: A prospective randomized study of the management of upper gastrointestinal hemorrhage. Am J Gastroenterol 61:282–289, 1974

Sfakianakis GN, Conway JJ: Detection of ectopic gastric mucosa in Meckel's diverticulum and in other aberrations by scintigraphy: I. Pathophysiology and 10-year clinical experience. J Nucl Med 22:647–654, 1981

Sfakianakis GN, Conway JJ: Detection of ectopic gastric mucosa in Meckel's diverticulum and in other aberrations by scintigraphy: II. Indications and methods—a 10-year experience. J Nucl Med 22:732–738, 1981

Sheedy PF, Fulton RE, Atwell DT: Angiographic evaluation of patients with chronic gastrointestinal bleeding. AJR 123:338–347, 1975

Sigstedt B, Launderquist A: Complications of angiographic examinations. AJR 130:445–460, 1978

Smith TK, Richards OA: A simple kit for the preparation of 99mTc-labeled red blood cells. J Nucl Med 17:126–132, 1976

Stevenson GW, Cox RR, Roberts CJC: Prospective comparison of double-contrast barium meal examination and fibreoptic endoscopy in acute upper gastrointestinal hemorrhage. Br Med J 2:723–724, 1976

Tedesco FJ, Waye JD, Raskin JB et al: Colonoscopic evaluation of rectal bleeding: A study of 304 patients. Ann Intern Med 89:907–909, 1978

Waye J: A diagnostic approach to colon bleeding. Mt Sinai J Med 51:491–501, 1984

Williams KDG, Dawson JL: Fibreoptic injection of oesophageal varices. Br Med J 2:766–767, 1979

Winzelberg GG, McKusick KA, Froelich J et al: Detection of gastrointestinal bleeding with 99m Tc labeled red blood cells. Semin Nucl Med 12:139–146, 1982

## ACUTE UPPER GASTROINTESTINAL BLEEDING
## (Hematemesis, Melena, Positive Nasogastric Aspirate)

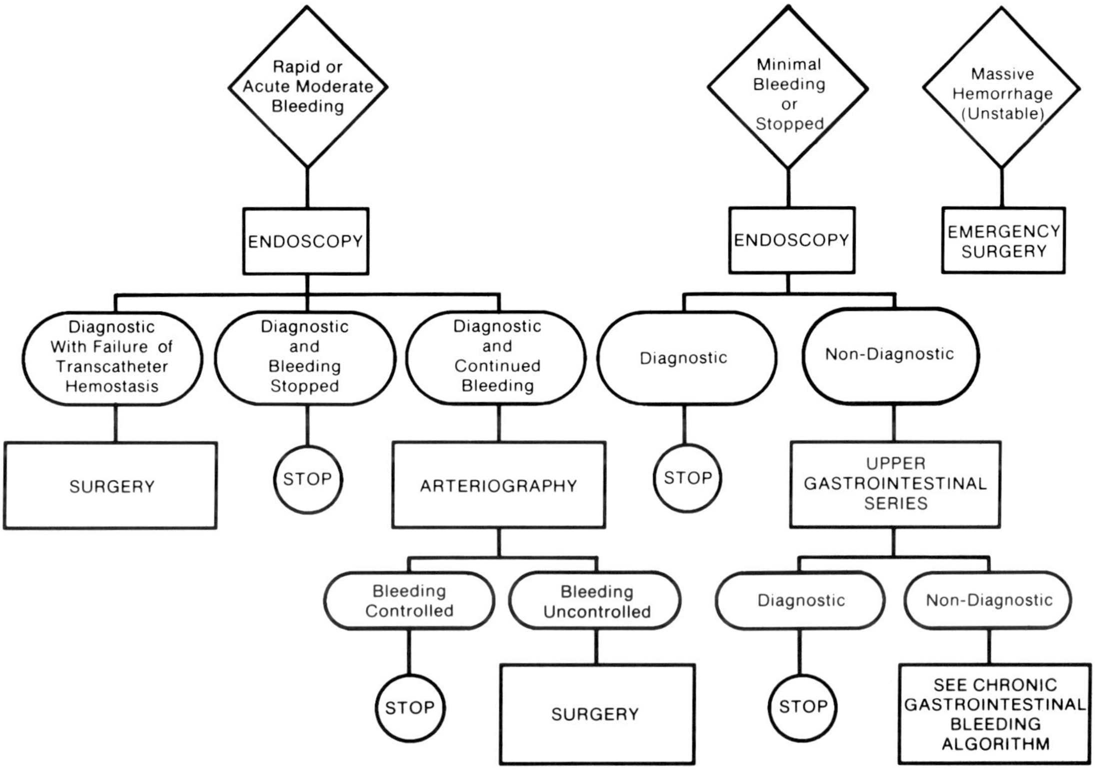

## ACUTE LOWER GASTROINTESTINAL BLEEDING

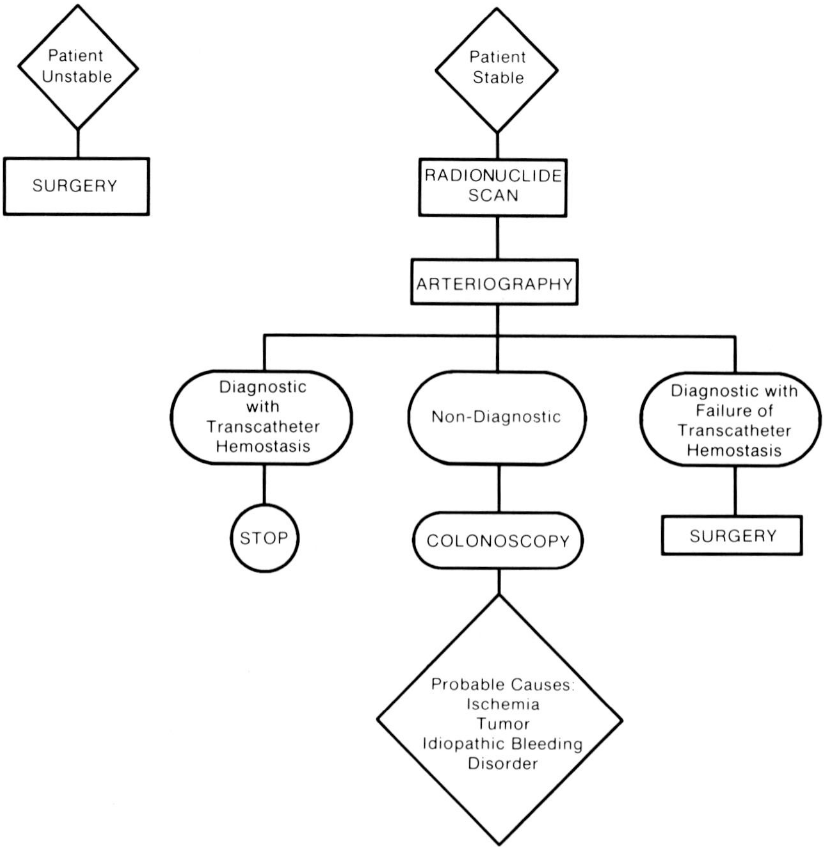

**CHRONIC GASTROINTESTINAL BLEEDING**

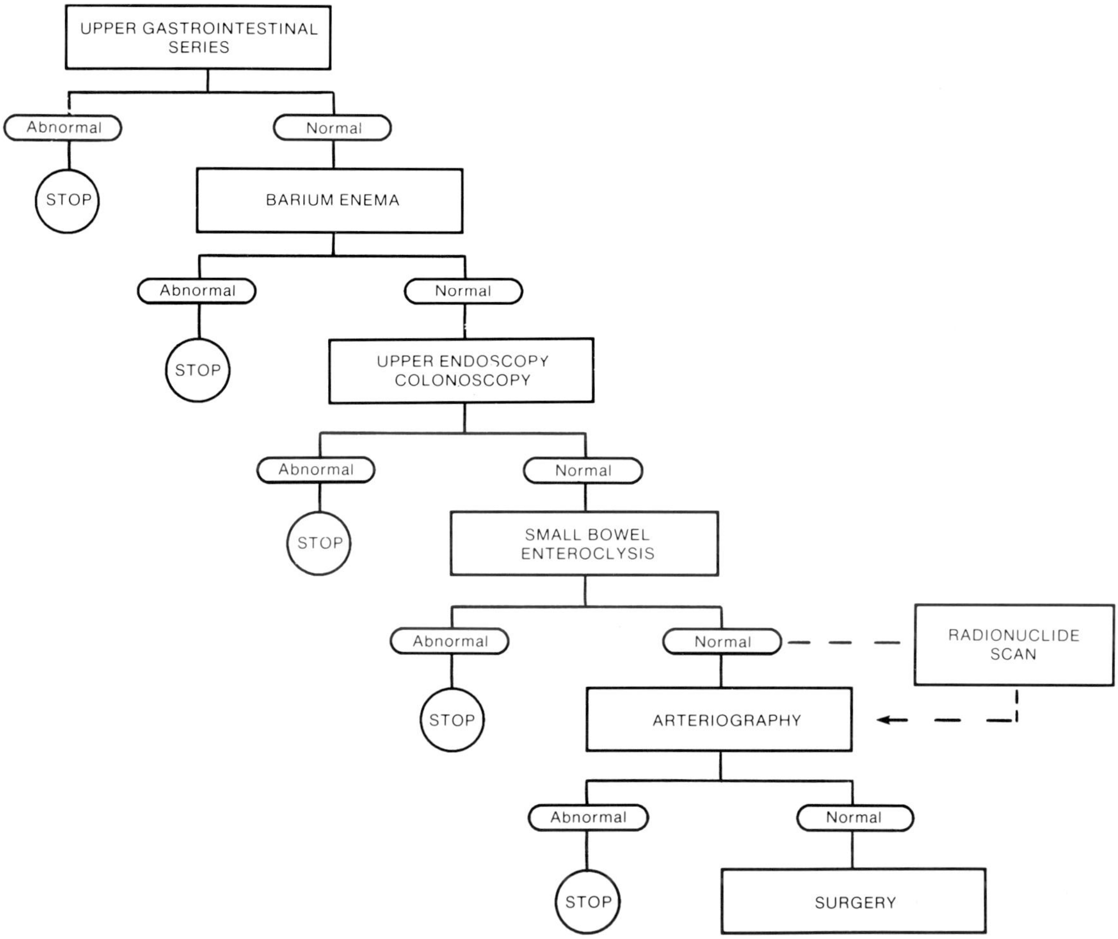

# Chapter 10

# Gallbladder Disease

*Roger K. Harned*
*Susan M. Williams*
*Joseph C. Anderson*

Cholelithiasis and its complications continue to be a common medical problem in the United States. Ten to twenty percent of the population is estimated to have gallstones, and approximately 500,000 persons per year require hospitalization for this condition and related problems. The annual cost of cholelithiasis resulting in cholecystectomy has been estimated to represent 2.5% of all health expenditures.

New imaging technologies have changed the traditional approach to gallbladder disease. Ultrasound has replaced oral cholecystography as the diagnostic procedure of choice for the detection of gallstones. Cholescintigraphy, endoscopic retrograde cholangiography, fine-needle percutaneous transhepatic cholangiography, and computed tomography (CT) have revolutionized the diagnostic approach to biliary disease.

## CHOLELITHIASIS

### CLINICAL FINDINGS

Symptomatic cholelithiasis is more common in females and is most often encountered in the 50- to 60-year-old age group. Obesity is associated with an increased incidence of gallstones in both sexes. The majority of patients with cholelithiasis consult their physicians because of episodic pain in the epigastrium or right upper abdominal quadrant (biliary colic), often accompanied by vomiting. Other symptoms such as fatty food intolerance or excessive belching may also be associated with gallbladder diseases, but these are not specific and do not always indicate the need for an imaging study.

The incidence of gallstones is higher in American Indians and Mexican-Americans, and in patients with diabetes mellitus, hemolytic anemia, cirrhosis, or any extensive small bowel disease or resection. Physicians should have a heightened awareness of the possibility of gallbladder disease in these patient groups, and the indications for diagnostic evaluation may be more liberally applied than for the general population.

There is approximately an 11% incidence of asymptomatic cholelithiasis in the general population. Although controversy exists, most physicians favor a conservative approach in dealing with this problem. However, patients with asymptomatic gallstones who are American Indians or Mexican-Americans, or who have diabetes mellitus or concomitant gallbladder wall calcification, should be considered at increased risk for complications. Cholecystectomy may be considered in this high-risk group.

## DIAGNOSTIC EVALUATION

### *DIAGNOSTIC MODALITIES*

1. Plain abdominal radiography
2. Oral cholecystography
3. Ultrasound
4. Endoscopic retrograde cholangiography
5. Cholescintigraphy
6. Computed tomography
7. Cholecystokinin cholecystography
8. Percutaneous transhepatic cholangiography

#### Plain Abdominal Radiography

Cholesterol stones and pigment stones (primarily composed of calcium bilirubinate) are the two major types of calculi that form in the gallbladder and biliary ducts. In the United States, approximately 80% of gallstones are of the cholesterol type and cannot be identified on plain abdominal radiographs. This percentage varies with different ethnic groups. About 20% of gallstones contain sufficient amounts of calcium to be detectable on plain films. They classically appear as multiple laminated, circular or rhomboid opacifications in the right upper abdominal quadrant (Fig. 10-1). However, it may be difficult to differentiate small, single calcified gallstones from other opacifications that have a similar appearance (*e.g.*, renal calculi). Ultrasound or oral cholecystography is often necessary for precise diagnosis. Nonopaque cholesterol stones occasionally can be identified on plain abdominal radiographs by a radiolucent, triradiate pattern in the center of the calculus. This lucent stellate appearance ("Mercedes-Benz" sign; Fig. 10-2) is produced by diffusion of nitrogen gas into dendritic cracks formed by shrinkage of cholesterol crystals in the stone. In most cases, however, the detection of cholelithiasis on plain abdominal radiographs is only an incidental finding in the evaluation of a patient with nonspecific abdominal pain.

#### Oral Cholecystography

Oral cholecystography, previously the unchallenged method for diagnosing cholelithiasis, has been replaced by ultrasound in most institutions. The accuracy of oral cholecystography in detecting gallstones, once believed to be almost 98%,

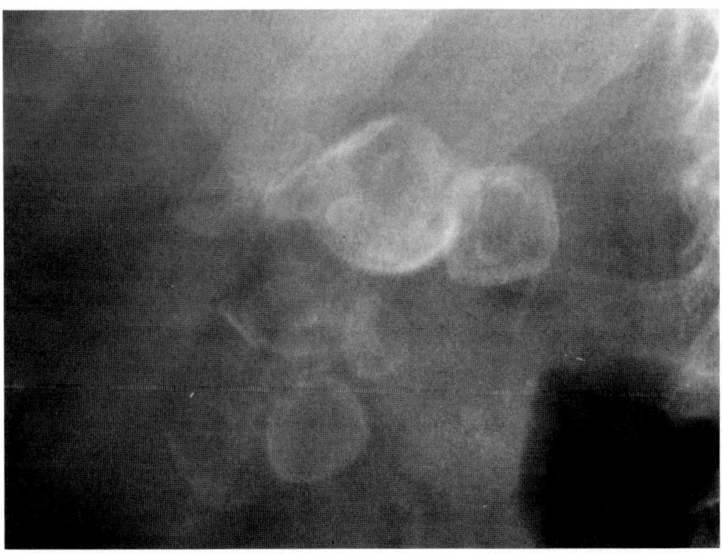

**Figure 10-1.** Multiple calcified gallstones.

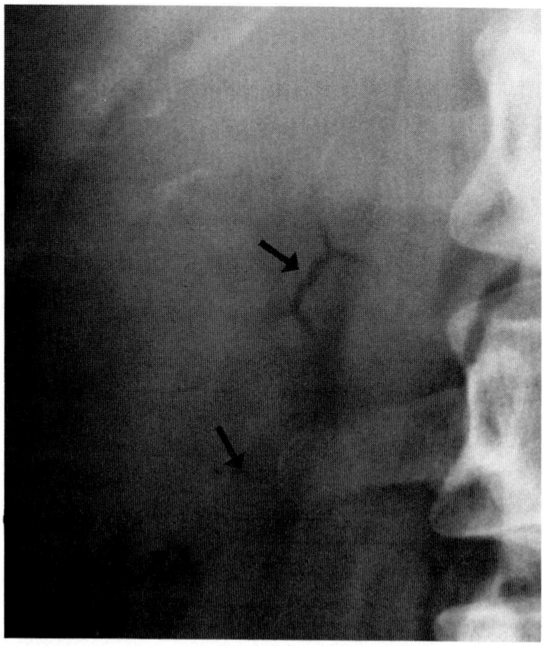

**Figure 10-2.** Radiolucent stellate patten ("Mercedes-Benz" sign, *arrows*) in cholesterol gallstones.

is now considered to be closer to 90%. Even a meticulously performed oral cholecystogram with an adequately opacified gallbladder may have a significant false-negative rate of 6% to 8%. Limitations of the technique or oral cholecystography that also make it a less desirable imaging study than ultrasound include (1) the use of a contrast agent with the potential for adverse reactions, (2) inconsistent intestinal absorption of contrast and dependence on adequate liver function, (3) the use of ionizing radiation, and (4) the uncertain significance of a nonvisualized gallbladder.

For all practical purposes, oral cholecystography is now a secondary examination that is only indicated if ultrasound is not available or equivocal, or if persistent clinical symptoms suggest gallbladder disease even if the ultrasound is normal.

### Dissolution of Gallstones

Oral cholecystography continues to play a role in the selection of patients for the medical dissolution of gallstones. Pretreatment visualization of the gallbladder by oral cholecystography is important, because gallstone dissolution is unsuccessful in the patient with a nonfunctioning gallbladder. Chenodeoxycholic acid is currently the most commonly used, orally administered drug for dissolution therapy, but it is only effective against stones containing at least 50% cholesterol. The gallstones that are most likely to be successfully dissolved are single, radiolucent, and 6 mm to 10 mm in size. An analysis of these characteristics combined with a complicated mosaic of clinical variables can predict the composition of gallstones in 80% to 90% of patients, thus aiding in the selection potential candidates for medical dissolution therapy.

## Ultrasound

### Technique

Ultrasound is now the procedure of choice for the diagnosis of cholelithiasis. However, careful technique is mandatory to provide accurate evaluation of the gallbladder. Real-time B-mode sonography is preferred over articulated-arm B-scanners because real-time equipment provides rapidly formed, high-resolution images that allow a gallbladder study to be completed within 5 to 15 minutes. Real-time scanners also can be moved to the patient's bedside and allow the examination to be performed with greater technical ease without sacrificing resolution. Real-time sonography can adequately study approximately 97% of patients, whereas articulated-arm scanning results in approximately an 11% incidence of inadequate examinations. Transducers with 3.5 mHz to 5 mHz frequency and medium-to-short focal length are most useful in adults. Patients should fast for 8 to 12 hours prior to the ultrasound examination, because there is a significant reduction in accuracy in approximately half of nonfasting patients because of gallbladder contraction and increased bowel gas. The gallbladder should be imaged in the supine, left posterior oblique, and sitting positions. The oblique and sitting positions allow the liver edge and gallbladder to descend below the costal margin and facilitate the movement of stones to the dependent gallbladder fundus.

## Diagnostic Signs

The ultrasound diagnosis of cholelithiasis is primarily based on the ability to detect gallstones in the lumen of the gallbladder. The most accurate sonographic appearance of cholelithiasis is a high-amplitude intraluminal reflection from the surface of a stone that is associated with a posterior acoustic shadow (Fig. 10-3). This finding can be demonstrated in two thirds of patients with gallstones and is virtually 100% specific for the diagnosis of cholelithiasis. Most stones gravitate to the dependent portion of the gallbladder. However, stones containing gas may float (Fig. 10-4), and calculi impacted in the gallbladder neck do not move (Fig. 10-5). The demonstration of a posterior acoustic shadow caused by a gallstone may be difficult and requires high-frequency transducers, optimal focusing, and fine adjustment of the time-gain compensation. The chemical composition of gallstones does not affect their shadowing characteristics. However, the size of a gallstone is important, because small stones (less than 5 mm) usually do not cast an acoustic shadow.

The sonolucent lumen of the gallbladder cannot be identified in approximately 20% of patients with cholelithiasis, because it is completely filled with calculi. In such cases, the diagnosis of cholelithiasis is made by demonstrating a high-amplitude echo in the gallbladder fossa associated with a posterior acoustic shadow (Fig.

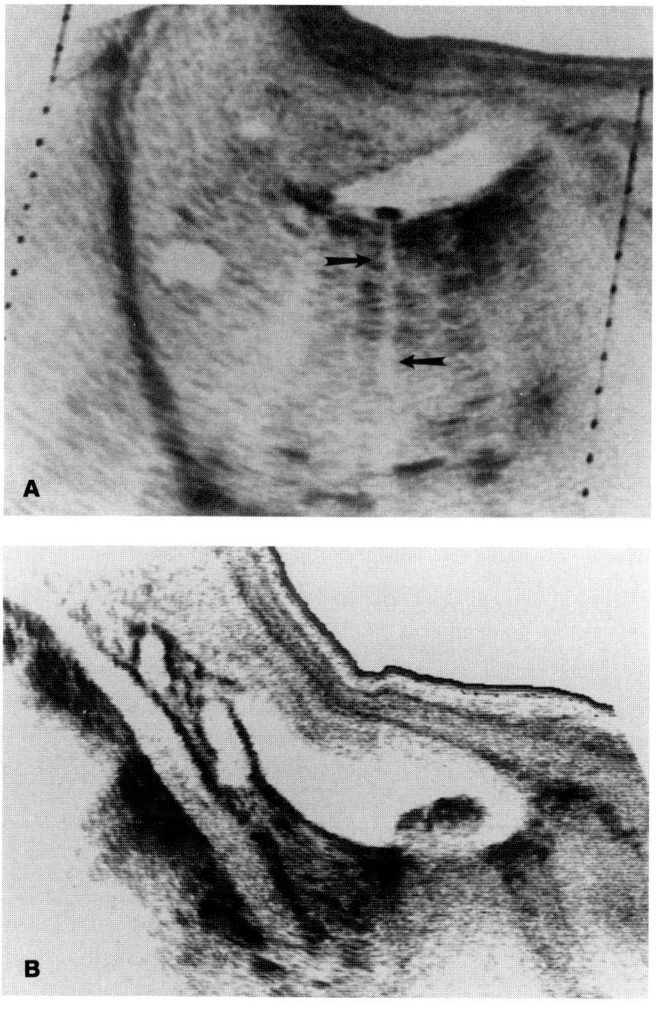


**Figure 10-3.** Ultrasound of cholelithiasis. **(A)** High-intensity intraluminal echoes with posterior acoustic shadow (*arrows*). **(B)** With the patient in a sitting position, gallstones roll to the dependent portion of the gallbladder fundus.

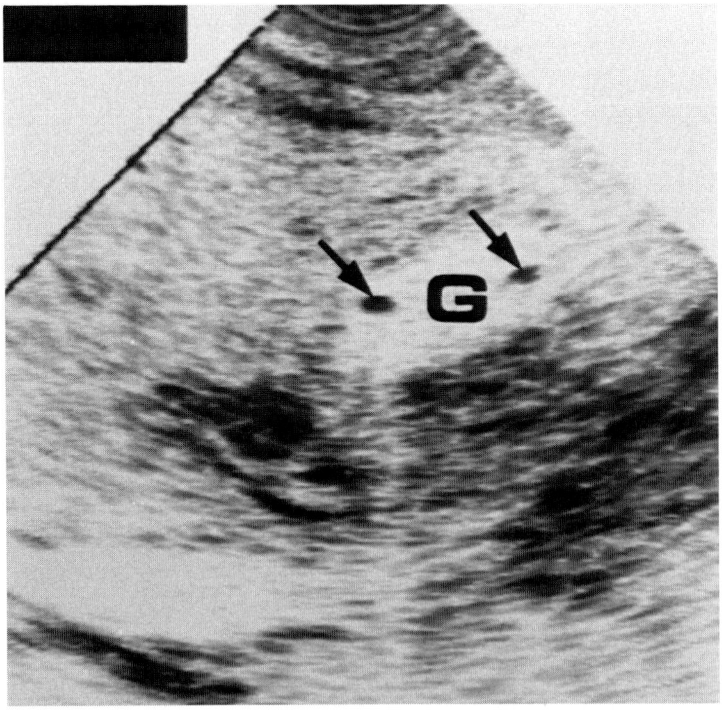


**Figure 10-4.** Floating calculi (*arrows*) in gallbladder (*G*). Gallstones may float if they contain gas, or if the bile is highly viscous or has a high specific gravity.

10-6). It is often difficult to differentiate the calculus-filled gallbladder from surrounding gas-containing bowel. Demonstration of the double-arcuate echo sign with posterior shadowing can aid in identifying the stone-filled gallbladder (Fig. 10-7). In addition, the characteristics of the shadow are important, because shadows caused by gallstones are usually free of reverberations whereas shadows caused by bowel gas are cluttered with reverberation artifacts. The differential diagnosis of the gallbladder without a sonolucent lumen includes previous cholecystectomy, gas in the gallbladder from biliary surgery or fistula, emphysematous cholecystitis, gallbladder wall calcification, nonfasting status, and extreme obesity.

Ultrasound has a specificity, true sensitivity, and overall accuracy of approximately 95% for

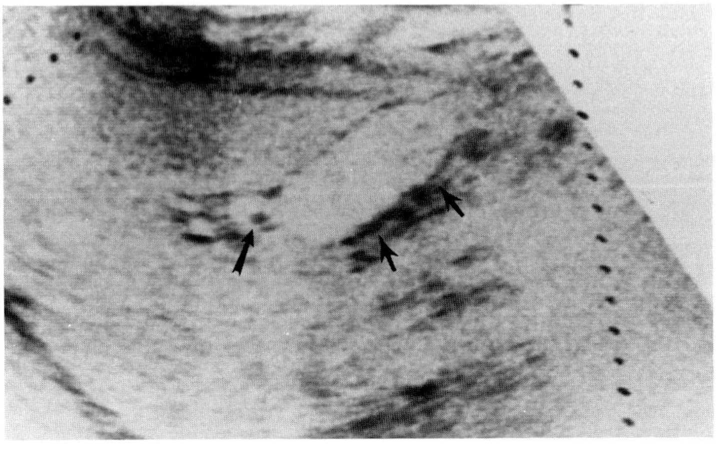

**Figure 10-5.** Impacted stone (*arrow*) in neck of gallbladder. Note also the thin layer of nonshadowing tiny gallstones (*arrowheads*) along the posterior wall of the gallbladder.

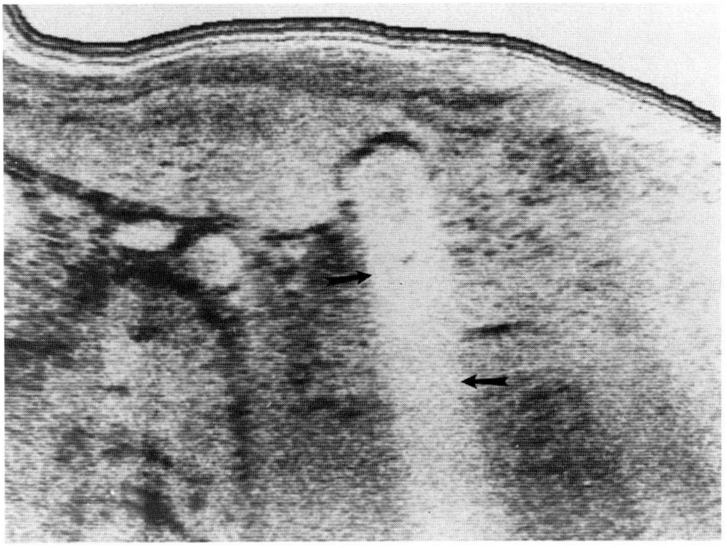

**Figure 10-6.** Nonvisualization of gallbladder lumen. The echogenic contour with posterior shadowing (*arrows*) from the gallbladder fossa is diagnostic of cholelithiasis.

diagnosing cholelithiasis. comparative studies have shown that ultrasound can occasionally detect calculi that were not seen on oral cholecystography; the reverse situation rarely occurs.

### Echogenic Bile

Echogenic bile, or biliary sludge, is caused by filterable particulate matter, usually cholesterol crystals and calcium bilirubinate granules. On Ultrasound biliary sludge appears as low-level echoes in the gallbladder lumen with no associated acoustic shadowing (Fig. 10-8). The echogenic material tends to incompletely fill the gallbladder and usually layers out in the dependent portion of the gallbladder as the patient changes position; infrequently, it may completely fill the gallbladder. Echogenic bile can be evanescent, presenting after a prolonged fast or hyperalimentation and disappearing following the resumption of food intake. Biliary sludge may form in patients with obstruction of the cystic or common bile duct. Other causes include pus, blood, and cellular debris. Because it is not known whether echogenic bile is a cause for stone formation, cholecystectomy is not indicated for this finding alone.

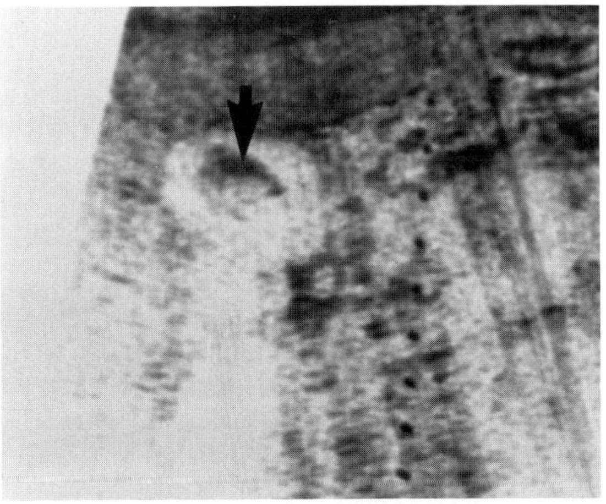

**Figure 10-7.** Double-arcuate echo sign in nonvisualization of gallbladder lumen. The outer arcuate contour is from the gallbladder wall, and the inner echogenic arc with acoustic shadowing is from gallstones (*arrow*).

## Endoscopic Retrograde Cholangiopancreatography

Although primarily used to evaluate the biliary and pancreatic ducts, there may be a role for endoscopic retrograde cholangiopancreatography (ERCP) in the diagnosis of cholelithiasis in the rare patient who has persistent symptoms suggesting cholelithiasis and who has abnormal liver function tests and negative sonography and

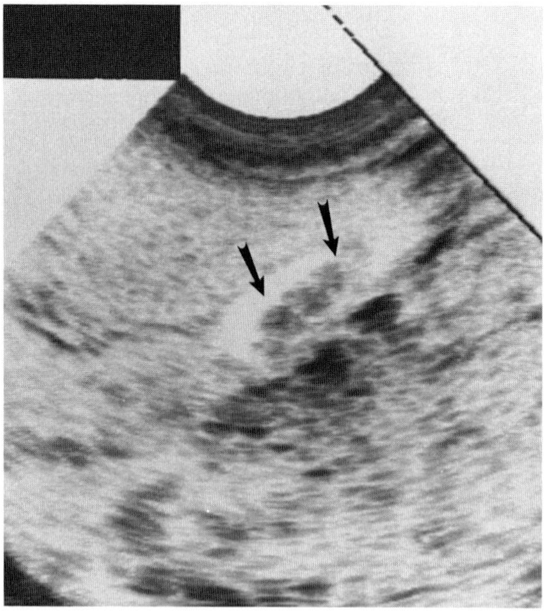

**Figure 10-8.** Tumefactive biliary sludge. Four rounded, echogenic, nonshadowing gallbladder opacifications (*arrows*) are demonstrated.

oral cholecystography. Opacification of the gallbladder by ERCP may occasionally demonstrate small gallstones (Fig. 10-9). However, because of the slightly increased risk and relatively high cost, ERCP should be used infrequently in the diagnosis of cholelithiasis.

### Computed Tomography

Computed tomography is neither as accurate nor as cost effective as ultrasound for the diagnosis of cholelithiasis. This imaging modality fails to detect many gallstones because of their small size and isodensity with bile.

## CHOLECYSTITIS

### ACUTE CHOLECYSTITIS

Approximately 95% of cases of acute cholecystitis are caused by a calculus obstructing the cystic duct. This complication is estimated to develop in 3% to 10% of patients with cholelithiasis. Cholesterol-saturated bile, altered lymphatic and venous drainage, and bacterial infection have all been implicated in the inflammatory process. The patient with acute cholecystitis presents with colicky right-upper-quadrant abdominal pain, tenderness, fever, nausea, and vomiting. The disease may progress to gangrene of the gallbladder wall and perforation.

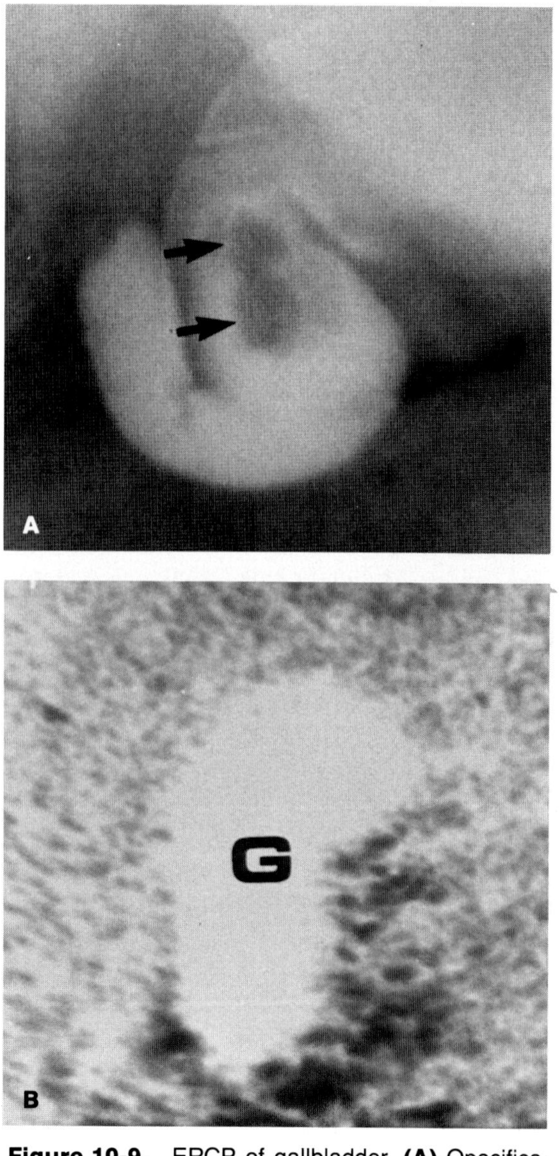


**Figure 10-9.** ERCP of gallbladder. **(A)** Opacification of the gallbladder by ERCP shows small stones (*arrows*) in the tortuous gallbladder neck. **(B)** Ultrasound of the gallbladder (*G*) was normal.

## Cholescintigraphy

Radionuclide scanning with iminodiacetic derivatives (*e.g.*, $^{99m}$Tc-IDA) is of particular value in the assessment of cystic duct patency in patients with suspected acute cholecystitis. The radionuclide is administered intravenously and is excreted by the hepatocytes into the biliary ducts. Radionuclide accumulation in the gallbladder indicates patency of the cystic duct and thus is strong evidence against acute cholecystitis, which almost always is associated with cystic duct obstruction. For all practical purposes, visualization of the gallbladder within 1 hour following radionuclide injection excludes the diagnosis of acute cholecystitis. Conversely, nonvisualization of the gallbladder in the clinical setting of right-upper-quadrant pain is strongly suggestive of acute cholecystitis (Fig. 10-10). If the gallbladder is not visualized initially, delayed scans up to 4 hours are required, because some patients with chronic cholecystitis may have delayed gallbladder visualization. Cholescintigraphy has a sensitivity of approximately 98% and a specificity of approximately 92% in patients with cystic duct obstruction. The uncommon false-positive results occur in patients with chronic cholecystitis, prolonged hyperalimentation, local invasive cancer or inflammation around the cystic duct, and previous cholecystectomy. False-negative results (less than 5%) usually occur in patients with acalculous cholecystitis.

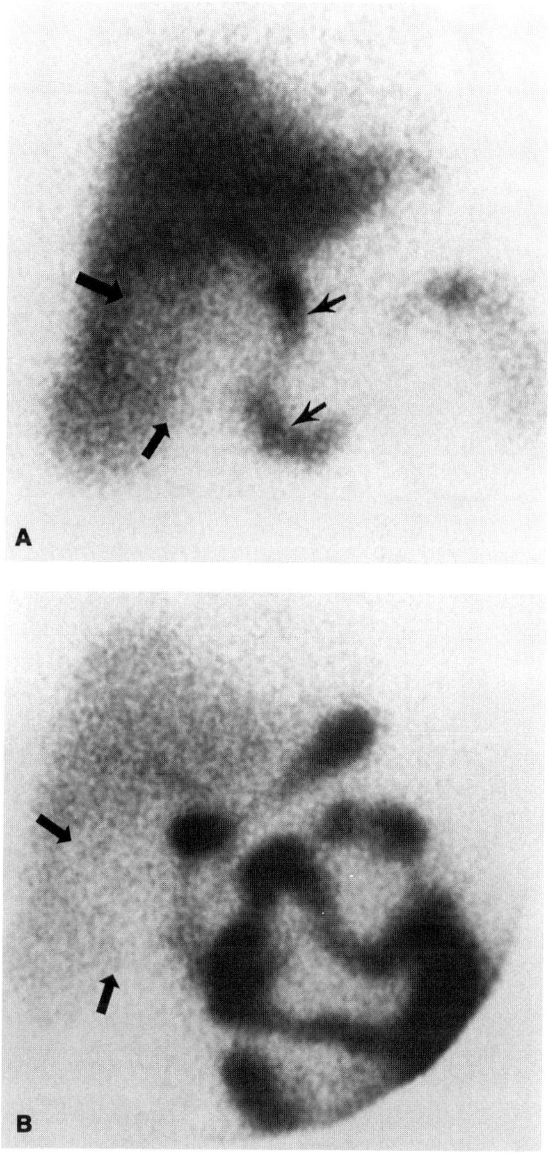


**Figure 10-10.** Acute cholecystitis. **(A)** Cholescintigram obtained 1 minute after injection of $^{99m}$Tc DISIDA shows visualization of the common bile duct and duodenum (*arrowheads*) but photopenia in the gallbladder fossa (*arrows*). **(B)** One-hour study confirms nonvisualization of the gallbladder (*arrows*), indicating cystic duct obstruction.

## Ultrasound

Ultrasound also is an excellent imaging modality for evaluating patients with suspected acute cholecystitis. As with cholelithiasis, the diagnosis of acute cholecystitis is primarily dependent on the detection of gallstones. This finding is not necessarily pathognomonic, however, because patients with "silent" gallstones may have abdominal pain unrelated to cholecystitis. Therefore, major secondary signs are important in the sonographic diagnosis of acute cholecystitis. These signs include point tenderness directly over the gallbladder (Murphy's sign) and thickening of the gallbladder wall (Fig. 10-11). Other

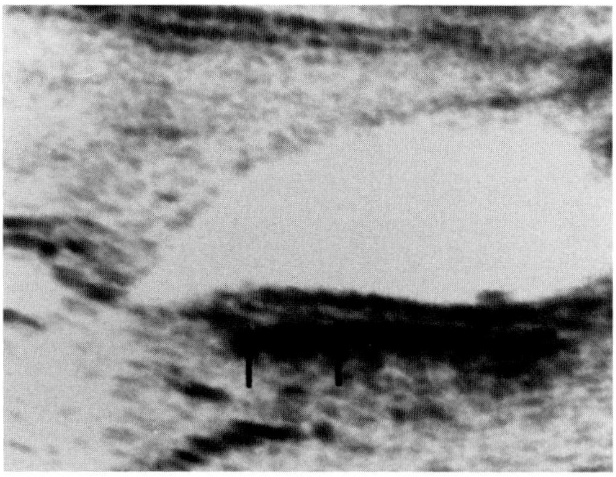

**Figure 10-11.** Acute cholecystitis. Thickening of the gallbladder wall (*arrows*) and a small, non-shadowing gallstone are demonstrated.

sonographic findings suggesting the diagnosis of acute cholecystitis include biliary sludge, pericholecystic fluid collections, enlargement and rounded shape of the gallbladder, and gas in the gallbladder lumen or wall (Fig. 10-12). Occasionally, an impacted stone in the neck of the gallbladder may be detected as the cause of acute

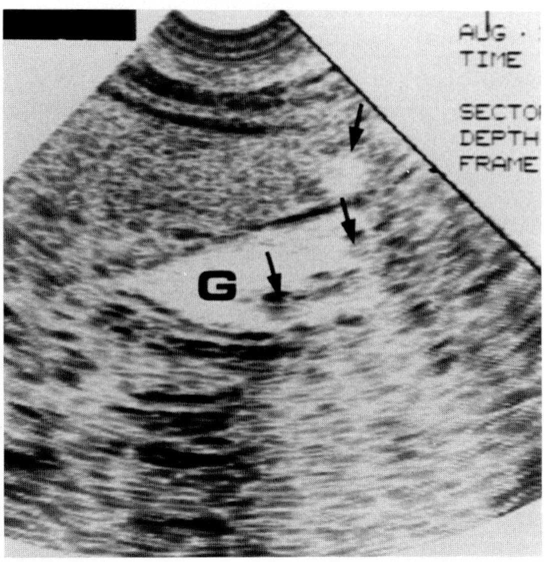


**Figure 10-12.** Acute cholecystitis. Classic gallstones (*intraluminal arrows*), thickening posterior gallbladder wall, and pericholecystic fluid collection (*extraluminal arrow*) are demonstrated.

cholecystitis. Because one third of patients presenting with right-upper-quadrant pain have symptoms originating from nonbiliary sources, ultrasound is of value in detecting other abdominal lesions causing pain, such as liver abscess. pancreatitis, periaortic adenopathy, pelvic inflammatory disease (Fitzhugh–Curtis syndrome), and primary or metastatic liver neoplasms.

The issue of whether ultrasound or cholescintigraphy should be the primary diagnostic modality in evaluating patients with suspected acute cholecystitis is controversial. Currently, ultrasound is the more popular modality at many institutions, because it is relatively inexpensive, rapid (5–15 minutes compared with 1–4 hours for cholescintigraphy), highly accurate (88%–95%) and can detect nonbiliary causes of right-upper-quadrant pain (cholescintigraphy almost exclusively evaluates the liver and biliary ducts).

## Ultrasonic Evaluation of Gallbladder Wall Thickening

The echogenic contour produced by the gallbladder wall normally has a thickness of 3 mm or less. Although diffuse thickening of the gallbladder wall was once considered pathognomonic of acute cholecystitis, an identical appearance can be produced by localized and systemic conditions, such as chronic and acute cholecystitis, hypoalbuminemia, portal hypertension, ascites, pancreatitis, heart failure, hepatitis, obesity, renal failure, and multiple myeloma. A thickened wall can also be seen in the contracted gallbladder of a nonfasting patient. Focal areas of gallbladder wall thickening or polypoid lesions can be seen with primary adenocarcinomas, metastatic neoplasms, adenomyomatosis, cholesterosis, adenomatous polyps, and gallbladder varices.

The sonographic character of the gallbladder wall may help to differentiate benign from malignant causes of ascites. Ascites due to portal hypertension and hypoproteinemia is usually associated with a hypoechoic wall, whereas ascites caused by a malignant peritoneal neoplasm is generally accompanied by a thin hyperechoic wall.

### Computed Tomography

Although CT can demonstrate signs of acute cholecystitis such as a thickened gallbladder wall, gas within the gallbladder wall, and pericholecystic fluid collections, it is not recommended as the initial procedure in patients with suspected acute cholecystitis.

## EMPHYSEMATOUS CHOLECYSTITIS

In contrast to cholelithiasis and acute cholecystitis, emphysematous cholecystitis is more common in males, and 20% to 30% of cases occur in patients with diabetes mellitus. Infection with gas-forming bacteria such as clostridia, *Escherichia coli, Klebsiella, Aerobacter aerogens,* and nonhemolytic streptococci results in the accumulation of varying amounts of gas in the lumen and wall of the gallbladder as well as in the pericholecystic soft tissues. The abnormal gas can often be identified on plain abdominal radiographs (Fig. 10-13). The cystic duct is almost always obstructed by edema and inflammation, even though gallstones are not always present. Distention of the gallbladder, causing vascular compromise and ischemia, is important in the pathogenesis of this condition, and there is an increased risk of gangrene and perforation as compared with nonemphysematous cholecystitis.

Gangrene of the gallbladder wall can sometimes be recognized, before perforation occurs, by the sonographic demonstration of an intraluminal membrane and an irregular wall contour (Fig. 10-14). Perforation of the gallbladder may present acutely with free intraperitoneal bile that has the sonographic characteristics of ascites. In subacute cases in which the perforation has been walled off, ultrasound may identify loculated fluid collections in the pericholecystic region. Gas within the lumen or wall of the gallbladder produces high-intensity echoes with posterior shadowing containing reverberations.

## ACALCULOUS CHOLECYSTITIS

The term *acalculous cholecystitis* refers to the 5% to 10% of cases of acute cholecystitis that occur in the absence of gallstones. Acalculous cholecystitis is more common in older, male patients with multisystem disease. In many cases, the cystic duct is obstructed by inflammation and edema. Suggested etiologic factors include infected bile and the development of gallbladder

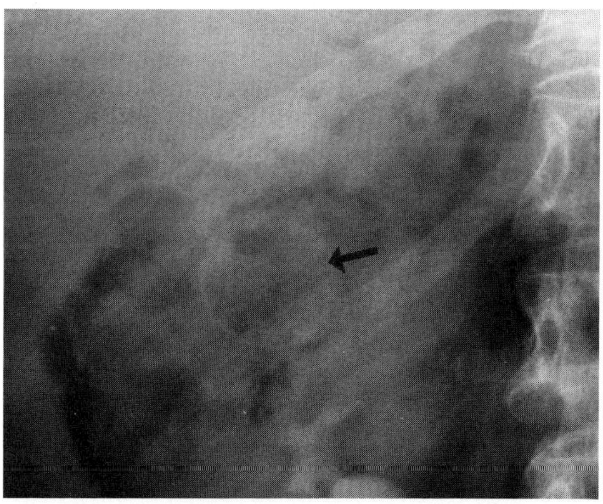

**Figure 10-13.** Emphysematous cholecystitis. Plain abdominal radiograph shows gas in the gallbladder wall and pericholecystic soft tissues. Note the calcified gallstone (*arrow*).

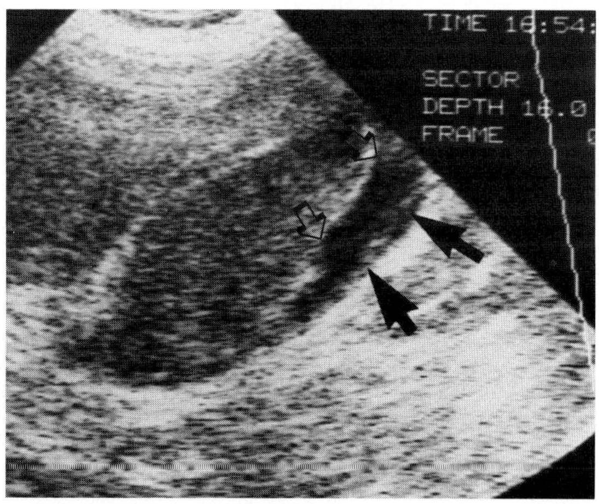


**Figure 10-14.** Gangrenous cholecystitis. There is biliary sludge, an irregular posterior wall (*closed arrows*), and an intraluminal membrane (*open arrows*) paralleling the posterior gallbladder wall.

ischemia and stasis due to spasm of the sphincter of Oddi that causes reflux of pancreatic enzymes into the cystic duct.

Cholescintigraphy can be diagnostic of acalculous cholecystitis, although false-negative rates of 25% to 30% have been reported. Ultrasound may show pericholecystic fluid collections and/or a thickened gallbladder wall. The use of cholecystokinin or a fatty meal to show alterations in the size or shape of the gallbladder during an ultrasound examination has produced inconsistent results.

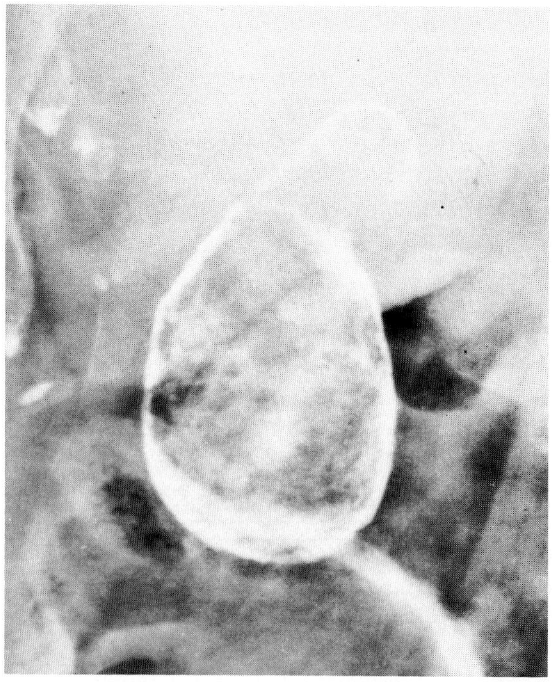

**Figure 10-15.** Porcelain gallbladder. Curvilinear intramural calcification in a patient with adenocarcinoma of the gallbladder. (Eisenberg RL: Gastrointestinal Radiology, p 821. Philadelphia, JB Lippincott, 1983)

## CHRONIC CHOLECYSTITIS

The preoperative diagnosis of chronic cholecystitis is made by the demonstration of gallstones in a patient with symptoms that suggest gallbladder disease. Exact histologic criteria for this diagnosis are not clearly defined. Almost all patients undergoing cholecystectomy for biliary symptoms and cholelithiasis have some histologic changes of cholecystitis; autopsy and operative series of incidentally removed gallbladders have shown that some degree of inflammatory change is often present. In addition, cholelithiasis may occasionally be present without cholecystitis; conversely, chronic acalculous cholecystitis may occur.

### Porcelain Gallbladder

The inflammatory changes of chronic cholecystitis may result in calcification of the gallbladder wall ("porcelain gallbladder"). Gallstones are usually present, and the cystic duct is often obstructed. Calcification of the gallbladder wall has a characteristic appearance on plain abdominal radiographs (Fig. 10-15). Although the true incidence is not known, extensive calcification of the gallbladder wall is found in less than 1% of cholecystectomy specimens. Patients with gallbladder wall calcification are often asymptomatic and the condition is usually an incidental finding. Because several series have reported the development of adenocarcinoma in up to 60% of gallbladders with calcified walls, prophylactic cholecystectomy should be considered whenever a porcelain gallbladder is encountered.

### Milk of Calcium Bile

Opacification of intraluminal bile (limey bile syndrome; milk of calcium bile) may develop in patients with chronic cystic duct obstruction if there is a high enough concentration of calcium salts. The opacified bile often contains floating stones and can be clearly identified on plain abdominal radiographs (Fig. 10-16). Patients with milk of calcium bile have histologic changes of chronic cholecystitis but no increased incidence of carcinoma.

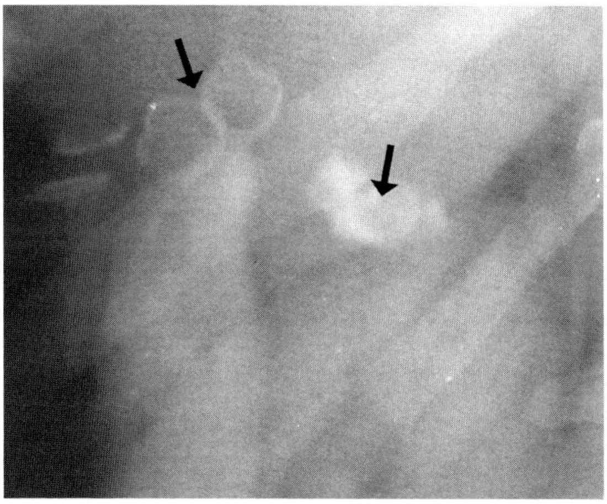

**Figure 10-16.** Milk of calcium bile. Plain abdominal radiograph (no oral contrast) shows opacification of the gallbladder with calculi in the gallbladder neck and cystic duct (*arrows*).

### Cholecystokinin Cholecystography

There is an interesting group of patients who have classic symptoms of cholelithiasis but normal-appearing gallbladders on ultrasound, oral cholecystography, and ERCP. These cases have been variously classified as "biliary dyskinesia," "cystic duct syndrome," or "chronic acalculous cholecystitis." Although some of these patients will improve or be relieved of their symptoms following cholecystectomy, it is difficult to recommend surgery without objective evidence of gallbladder disease. One suggested diagnostic approach is cholecystokinin cholecystography, in which opacification of the gallbladder using oral contrast material is followed by the administration of cholecystokinin or one of its analogs. Serial films are obtained to measure gallbladder contractility, and the patient is simultaneously evaluated for reproduction of symptoms. The use of cholecystokinin has also been combined with ultrasound and cholescintigraphy. However, no consistent diagnostic criteria have resulted from any of these studies. Thus, there are currently no reliable, objective imaging procedures to confirm the diagnosis of biliary dyskinesia.

## DIAGNOSTIC EVALUATION OF GALLBLADDER PATHOLOGY OTHER THAN CHOLELITHIASIS AND CHOLECYSTITIS

### CHOLESTEROSIS

Cholesterosis is a benign condition (present in 10%–20% of gallbladders in surgical and autopsy series) in which triglycerides and cholesterol esters accumulate in the macrophages within the lamina propria of the gallbladder wall. The lipid deposits may be diffuse and less than 1 mm in size (strawberry gallbladder) or appear as single or multiple polypoid masses as large as 1 cm. There is usually no evidence of associated inflammation. On oral cholecystography, the larger cholesterol deposits appear as fixed filling defects that do not move with compression or positional changes and thus can be distinguished from gallstones. Ultrasound shows the cholesterol deposits as nonmobile, nonshadowing intraluminal echoes (Fig. 10-17). Cholecystectomy usually is not indicated unless gallstones and/or biliary colic are present.

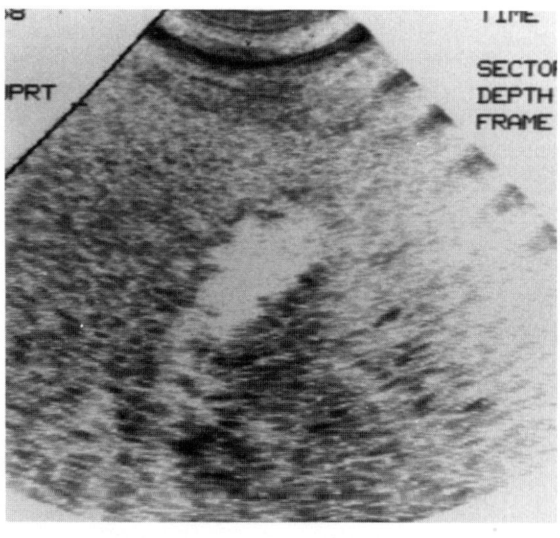


**Figure 10-17.** Polypoid cholesterosis. Ultrasound shows multiple nonshadowing polyps protruding into the gallbladder lumen.

## ADENOMYOMATOSIS

Adenomyomatosis of the gallbladder is characterized by hyperplasia of the mucosa and hypertrophy of the muscularis. Proliferation of the mucosa often extends into the muscularis, forming diverticula termed Rokitansky–Aschoff sinuses. Adenomyomatosis is best diagnosed by oral cholecystography and may involve the gallbladder in one of three ways. The diffuse type presents with a thickened wall and opacification of intramural diverticula paralleling the gallbladder lumen. The segmental variety consists of circumferential, localized wall thickening and contrast-filled diverticula. The localized form presents as a soft, pliable mass (adenomyoma) that is located in the gallbladder fundus and is secondary to focal hyperplasia.

Ultrasound can show the Rokitansky–Aschoff sinuses as anechoic or hyperechoic foci within the thickened gallbladder wall (Fig. 10-18). Reverberation artifacts or acoustic shadows can emanate from these foci. However, because ultrasound may only suggest the presence of adenomyomatosis, oral cholecystography is often necessary to confirm the sonographic findings.

Clinical management and treatment of these patients is controversial, because the exact significance of the disease is not understood. The patients may be asymptomatic or may present with symptoms indistinguishable from uncomplicated cholelithiasis or cholecystitis. Cholecystectomy is probably not indicated unless there are calculi or prolonged symptoms of biliary colic.

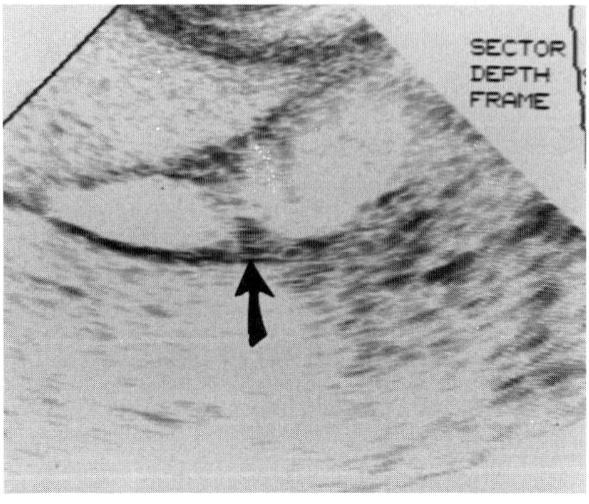


**Figure 10-18.** Segmental adenomyomatosis. Localized circumferential thickening (*arrow*) of the gallbladder wall is shown.

## BENIGN NEOPLASMS OF THE GALLBLADDER

Most true benign neoplasms of the gallbladder are papillary or nonpapillary adenomas, which are found in less than 5% of cholecystectomies. They are either sessile or pedunculated, usually solitary, and smaller than 1 cm. On ultrasound or oral cholecystography, these tumors appear as fixed, intraluminal masses. Because there is no evidence to indicate that these tumors have malignant potential, cholecystectomy is not indicated unless growth is demonstrated or a large polypoid mass raises the possibility of carcinoma. The differential diagnosis of these benign tumors includes other fixed masses such as solitary cholesterol polyp, adherent gallstone, localized adenomyomatosis, inflammatory polyp, and, rarely, heterotopic pancreatic or gastric tissue or a mesenchymal neoplasm.

## CARCINOMA OF THE GALLBLADDER

Carcinoma of the gallbladder accounts for less than 2% of all malignant tumors in the United States, but it is the fifth most common cause of death from gastrointestinal malignancy. Most cases occur after the age of 50 years. The incidence is three times greater in females than in males, and 70% to 95% of cases are associated with cholelithiasis. Carcinoma is reported to develop in up to 60% of patients with calcification of the gallbladder wall (porcelain gallbladder). Because the patient is often relatively asymptomatic during the early stages of the disease, the tumor is usually advanced by the time of diagnosis, and death commonly ensues within 1 to 5 years. The majority of lesions are well-differentiated adenocarcinomas, of which more than 50% are scirrhous. Contiguous tumor invasion, often directly into the liver, is the most frequent mode of extension. Carcinoma of the gallbladder commonly spreads into the pericholedochal, pancreaticoduodenal, celiac, and periaortic nodes; biliary obstruction frequently develops.

Although ultrasound and CT have improved the preoperative diagnosis of carcinoma of the gallbladder, detection of a resectable tumor remains unusual. The most common manifestation of carcinoma of the gallbladder on ultrasound or CT is a mass in the gallbladder fossa with extension into the liver (Fig. 10-19). Frequently associated findings include thickening of the gall-

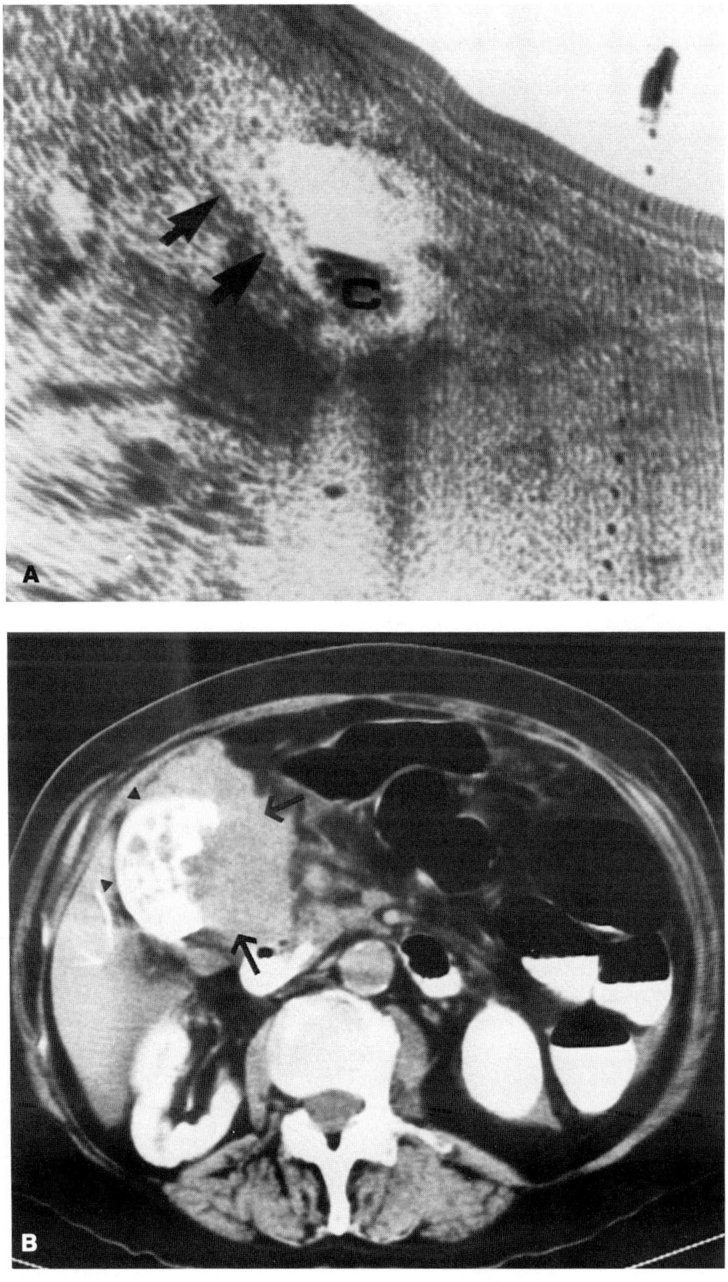


**Figure 10-19.** Carcinoma of the gallbladder. **(A)** Ultrasound shows cholelithiasis (*C*) and asymmetric thickening of the posterior gallbladder wall (*arrows*). **(B)** CT demonstrates an irregular mass (*arrows*) arising from the wall of the contrast-filled gallbladder (*arrowheads*).

bladder wall, an intraluminal polypoid mass, cholelithiasis, biliary obstruction, nodal involvement, and hematogenous metastases. Although chronic cholecystitis may produce a thickened gallbladder wall simulating carcinoma, visualization of a thin halo of fluid around the wall favors an inflammatory etiology. Percutaneous transhepatic cholangiography can permit biliary decompression, as well as aiding and localizing the point of bile duct obstruction secondary to direct tumor extension or nodal involvement (if neither CT nor ultrasound can provide this information).

## Bibliography

Berk RN, Ferrucci JT, Fordtran JS et al: The radiological diagnosis of gallbladder disease. Radiology 141:49–56, 1981

Berk RN, Ferrucci JT, Leopold GR: Radiology of the Gallbladder and Bile Ducts. Philadelphia, WB Saunders, 1983

Berk RN, van der Vegt JH, Lichtenstein JE: The hyperplastic cholecystoses: Cholesterolosis and adenomyomatosis. Radiology 146:593–601, 1983

Cohen S, Soloway RD: Gallstones. New York, Churchill Livingstone, 1985

Cooperberg PL, Burhenne HJ: Real-time ultrasonography—diagnostic technique of choice in calculous gallbladder disease. N Engl J Med 302:1272–1279, 1980

Davis GB, Berk RN, Scheible FW et al: Cholecystokinin cholecystography, sonography and scintigraphy: Detection of chronic acalculous cholecystitis. AJR 139:1117–1121, 1982

Gale ME, Robbins AH: Computed tomography of the gallbladder: Unusual diseases. J Comput Assist Tomogr 9(3):439–443, 1985

Jeffrey RB, Laing FC, Wong W et al: Gangrenous cholecystitis: Diagnosis by ultrasound. Radiology 148:219–221, 1983

Laing FC, Federle MP, Jeffrey RP et al: Ultrasonic evaluation of patients with acute right upper quadrant pain. Radiology 140:449–455, 1981

Madrazo BL, Francis I, Hricak H et al: Sonographic findings in perforation of the gallbladder. AJR 139:491–496, 1982

Parulekar SG: Sonographic findings in acute emphysematous cholecystitis. Radiology 145: 117–119, 1982

Raghavendra BN, Subramanyam BR, Balthazar EJ et al: Sonography of adenomyomatosis of the gallbladder: Radiologic–pathologic correlation. Radiology 146:747–752, 1983

Ralls PW, Colletti PM, Halls JM et al: Prospective evaluation of $^{99m}$Tc-IDA cholescintigraphy and gray-scale ultrasound in the diagnosis of acute cholecystitis. Radiology 144:369–371, 1982

Ralls PW, Colletti PM, Lapin SA et al: Real-time sonography in suspected acute cholecystitis—prospective evaluation and secondary signs. Radiology 155:767–771, 1985

Raptopoulous VD, D'Orsi CJ, Smith EH et al: Dynamic cholecystosonography of the contracted gallbladder. AJR 138:275–278, 1982

Shuman WP, Rogers JV, Rudd TG et al: Low sensitivity of sonography and cholescintigraphy in acalculous cholecystitis. AJR 142:531–534, 1984

Simeone JF, Mueller PR, Ferrucci JJ et al: Significance of non-shadowing focal opacities at cholecystosonography. Radiology 137:181–185, 1980

Venu RP, Greenen JE, Toouli J et al: Endoscopic retrograde cholangiopancreatography diagnosis of cholelithiasis in patients with normal gallbladder x-ray and ultrasound studies. JAMA 249:758–761, 1983

Weiner SN, Koenigsberg M, Morehouse H et al: Sonography and computed tomography in the diagnosis of carcinoma of the gallbladder. AJR 142:735–739, 1984

Weissman HS, Rosenblatt R, Sugarman LA, Freeman LM: An update in radionuclide imaging in the diagnosis of cholecystitis. JAMA 246:1354–1357, 1981

Yoo J, Beal W, Ware R et al: Hepatobiliary imaging reveals high percentage of abnormalities. Radiology Today, pp 15, 31, May–June, 1985

## ACUTE RIGHT UPPER QUADRANT PAIN

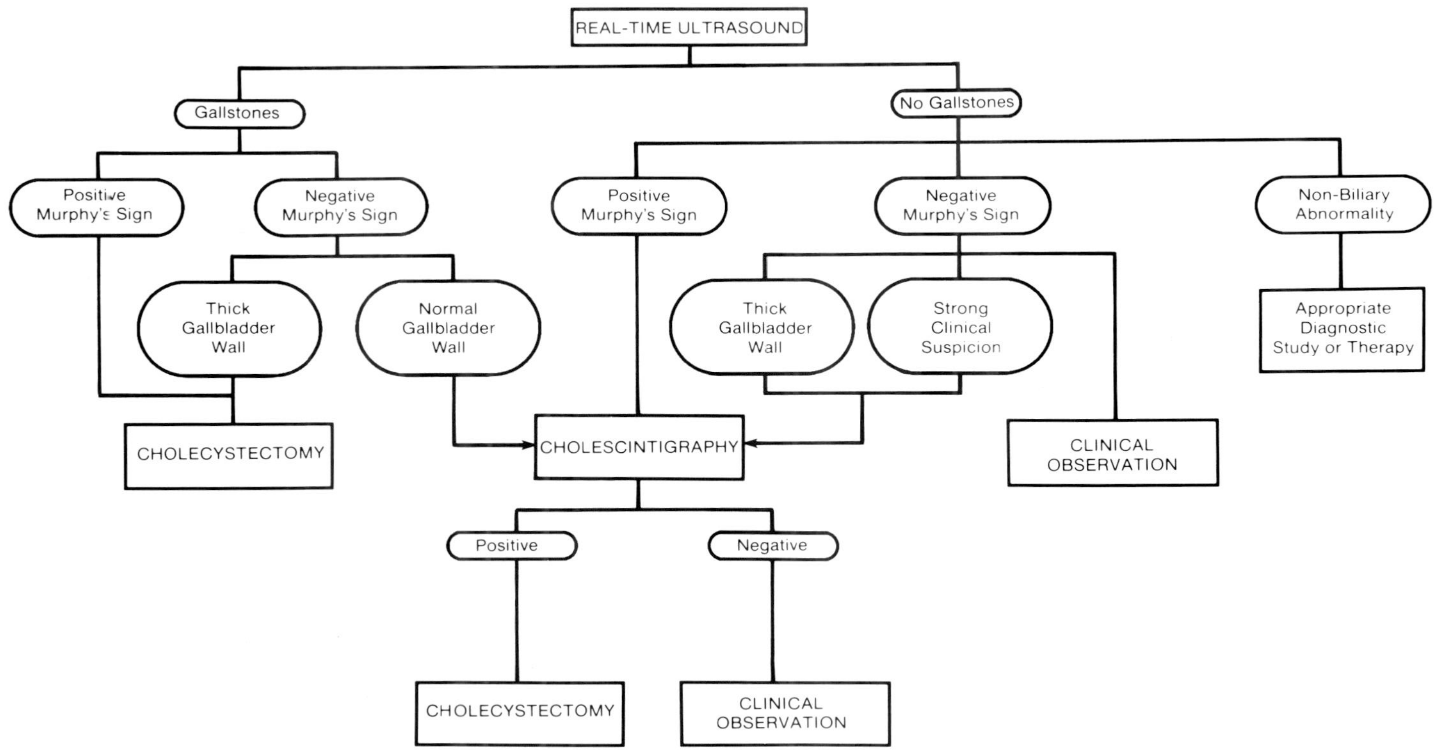


Adapated from: Ralls PW, Colletti PM, Lapin SA, et al: Real-time sonography suspected acute cholecystitis — Prospective evaluation and secondary signs. Radiology 155:767-771, 1985.

## CHRONIC RIGHT UPPER QUADRANT PAIN

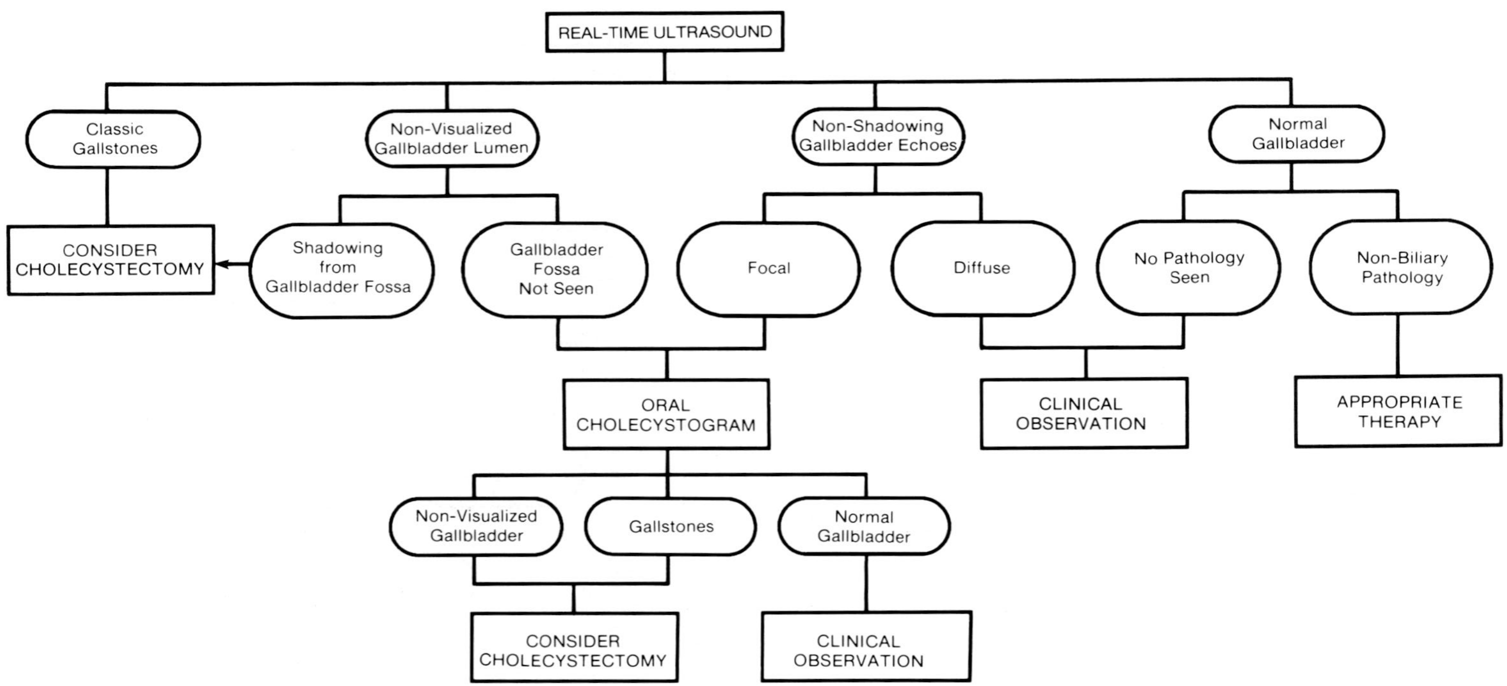


Adapted from: Ralls PW, Colletti PM, Lapin SA, et al: Real-time sonography suspected acute cholecystitis — Prospective evaluation and secondary signs. Radiology 155:767-771, 1985.

# Chapter 11

# Jaundice

*Jefferson O. Janes*
*James A. Nelson*

The observation of jaundice by the patient's friends or physician often sets in motion an extensive diagnostic workup. Anxiety is particularly high in the patient of middle age or older, since cancer may be the causative agent. Clinical jaundice is only a sign of underlying disease for which there are many diagnostic possibilities. Sometimes features suggesting hepatocellular disease are so typical that treatment and prolonged observation follow naturally without any need for imaging procedures. At other times, the history and physical examination, combined with serum liver function studies, are either consistent with biliary obstruction or are equivocal. It is in this setting that radiologic evaluation is indicated.

There are many etiologies of obstructive jaundice. Biliary stone disease is the most common cause in the United States. Fortunately, trauma to the bile ducts at the time of surgery with subsequent stricture formation is diminishing in frequency. Ascaris can infest the common bile duct and cause jaundice. Chronic pancreatitis may produce an inflammatory mass or pseudocyst large enough to obstruct the duct. An increasingly frequent cause of obstructive jaundice is malignancy of the bile ducts, the pancreas, or adjacent nodes. The etiology of obstructive jaundice in children is most often congenital (*e.g.,* biliary atresia, intrahepatic cystic disease, choledochal cyst).

The early recognition of obstructive jaundice has important therapeutic and prognostic implications. Prolonged obstruction leads to progressive biliary cirrhosis with ultimate deterioration of liver function. It also predisposes the patient to bouts of ascending cholangitis, hepatic abscess formation, or life-threatening sepsis. The relief of benign obstruction (*e.g.,* stones, strictures, pseudocysts of the pancreas) usually allows the patient to return to a normal life. Radiological interventional biliary procedures, which are becoming increasingly used, require precise localization and characterization of lesions. In addition, identification of the site of obstruction permits more rational surgical planning or may obviate the need for surgery.

## CLINICAL FINDINGS

Patients with unexplained jaundice are frequently subjected to delay in diagnosis because of futile attempts to delineate obstructive from nonobstructive jaundice by means of liver function tests. Ideally, the patient with obstructive jaundice should have a high percentage (>30%) of direct-reacting bilirubin, a high or moderately elevated serum glutamic oxaloacetic transaminase (SGOT), and a markedly increased level of alkaline phosphatase. Unfortunately, this is not always the case, and laboratory studies often are insufficient to discriminate between obstructive and nonobstructive jaundice.

## DIAGNOSTIC EVALUATION

### *DIAGNOSTIC MODALITIES*

#### *Noninvasive*

1. Conventional radiographic studies
   a. Plain abdominal radiography
   b. Intravenous cholangiography
   c. Barium studies
   d. Infusion hepatomography
   e. Oral cholecystography
2. Ultrasound examination
3. Computed tomography
4. Radionuclide imaging
5. Magnetic resonance imaging

#### *Invasive*

1. Percutaneous transhepatic cholangiography
2. Endoscopic retrograde cholangiopancreatography
3. Arteriography
4. Biopsy
5. Surgery

### Conventional Radiographic Studies

#### Plain Abdominal Radiography

The plain abdominal radiograph should be obtained after initial history, physical examination, and laboratory studies. Its use is cost effective to search for obvious causes of jaundice, such as calcified stones in the region of the biliary tract, calcified cysts, or large mass lesions (Fig. 11-1).

#### Intravenous Cholangiography

Intravenous cholangiography (IVC) was formerly the mainstay of diagnosis in mild obstructive jaundice, especially in the postcholecystectomy syndrome patient. However, the advent of ultrasound, computed tomography (CT) and thin-needle percutaneous transhepatic cholangiography (PTHC) has greatly reduced the clinical

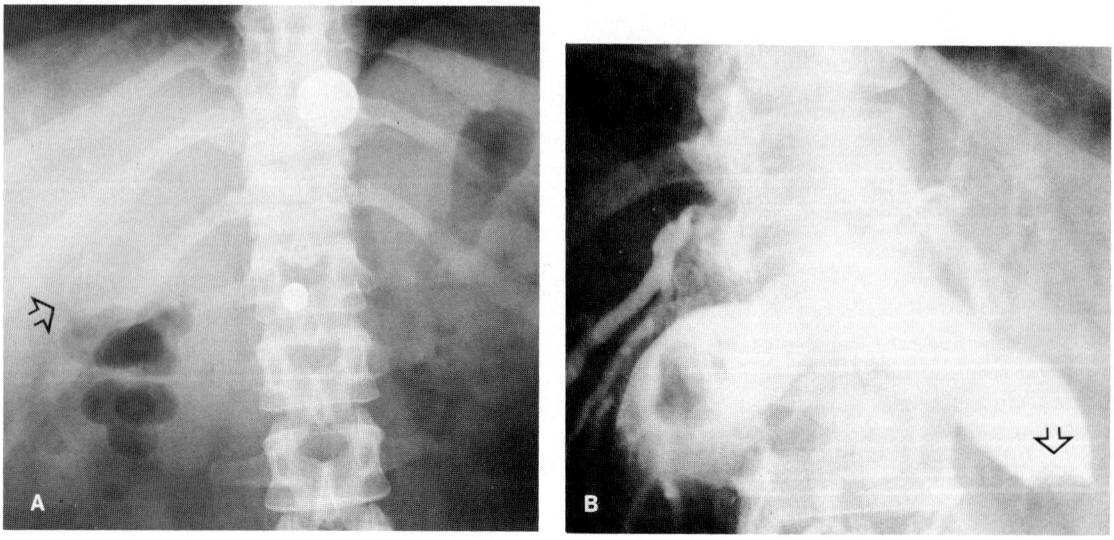


**Figure 11-1. (A)** Plain abdominal radiograph obtained prior to PTHC demonstrates a calcified gallstone (*arrow*). Metallic artifacts are seen overlying the spine. **(B)** PTHC demonstrates two gallstones. Arrow indicates the obstructing stone in the common bile duct.

application of IVC, because these techniques provide the same information without the morbidity (approximately 25%) and occasional death associated with the contrast material used for cholangiography. The IVC visualizes 80% to 100% of ducts with bilirubin less than 2 mg per 100 ml, but only 40% to 60% with bilirubin higher than 3 mg per 100 ml, and even fewer if serial values are rising. The most valuable role of IVC has been the detection of retained common bile duct stones in the postoperative patient. Frequently, such patients have minimal or fluctuating jaundice caused by a ball-valve stone and may not have dilated ducts. Patients with choledochal cysts without jaundice are also candidates for IVC evaluation (Fig. 11-2*A*).

### Barium Studies

Barium studies of the duodenum may be helpful in the occasional patient who has a tumor of the papilla causing jaundice. This method, or endoscopy or CT, can find these lesions. Because tumors at the papilla have the most favorable prognosis of any obstructing biliary tract cancer, their detection greatly alters the therapeutic approach.

Barium studies may also demonstrate secondary invasion or displacement of the gut due to adjacent pancreatic, gallbladder, or common bile duct lesions. However, this information can be obtained in a more direct fashion using ultrasound or CT.

### Infusion Hepatomography

Infusion hepatomography based on the concept of total body opacification has been advocated for diagnosis of intrahepatic duct dilatation. It is of no clinial usefulness.

### Oral Cholecystography

Oral cholecystography should not be performed in the patient with jaundice. The failure rate of

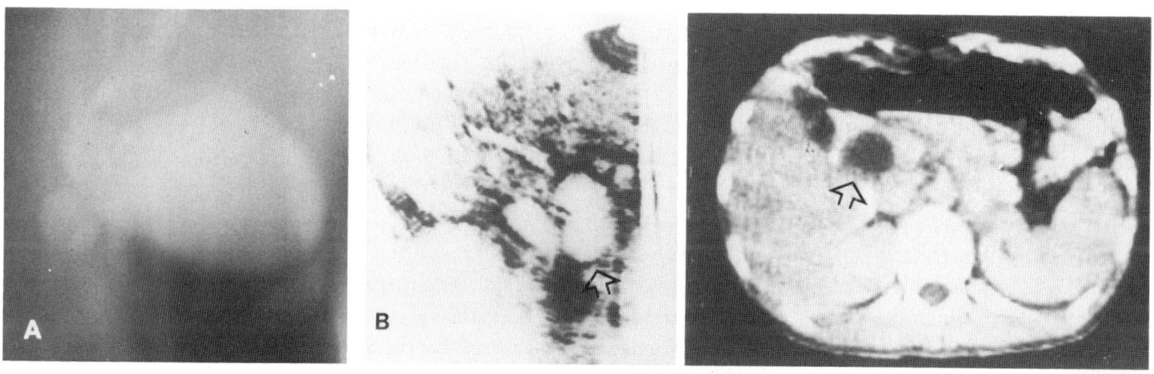


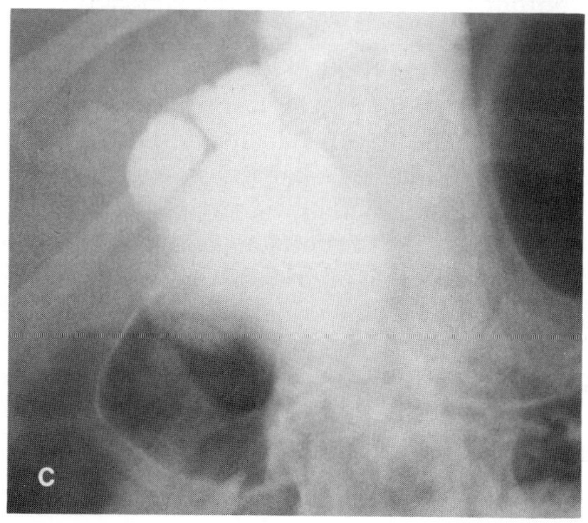


**Figure 11-2.** **(A)** IVC demonstrates filling of a choledochal cyst with contrast. **(B)** Oblique sonogram (*left*) demonstrates dilated intrahepatic bile ducts and fluid-filled structures near the porta hepatis. CT scan in the region of the porta hepatis (*right*) shows two fluid-filled structures. Arrows point to the choledochal cyst. Laterally placed fluid-filled structure is the gallbladder. **(C)** Radiograph following ERCP demonstrates filling of the choledochal cyst.

this procedure is very high, and increased renal toxicity has been observed after the use of oral cholecystographic agents in the jaundiced patient.

## Ultrasound Examination

After a supine abdominal radiograph is obtained, ultrasound should be the next imaging procedure used whenever the initial history, physical examination, and laboratory studies suggest that obstructive jaundice may be present. Ultrasound will be positive in approximately 95% of patients with dilated bile ducts; it can be performed with no morbidity, excellent patient acceptance, and reasonable cost (Fig. 11-2*B*). False-negative results may occur when the ducts are filled with thick bile that makes the dilated ducts indistinguishable from liver parenchyma. In some patients with obstructive jaundice, the ducts do not dilate (*e.g.,* sclerosing cholangitis); occasionally, clinical jaundice will precede ductal dilatation (the reverse occurs as well). In these situations ultrasound is not helpful.

To recognize intrahepatic biliary duct dilatation by ultrasound, it is essential to differentiate portal venous structures from ducts, especially in the mild or moderately jaundiced patient. This appears to be more easily determined with real-time techniques than with static imaging methods. Distal duct enlargement requires sagittal scanning with identification of the inferior vena cava, which is closely associated with the vertical portion of the common bile duct. Dilation of the gallbladder is of little significance, because it is frequently unrelated to distal common bile duct obstruction. The precise location of an obstructing lesion can be found in approximately 50% of patients. In the remainder, it is usually possible to determine whether the site of obstruction is above or below the porta hepatis. It is important to remember that ultrasound frequently does not demonstrate the cause of biliary obstruction. Although a large tumor or nodal masses may be identified, strictures or stones will rarely be detected.

There is little difference in overall diagnostic accuracy between ultrasound and CT. Indeed, if the results of ultrasound are inconclusive, CT is seldom more dependable in delineating the problem. The advantages of ultrasound include shorter scanning time, allowing for decreased motion artifact; longitudinal, oblique and transverse scanning; lower cost; and no ionizing radiation exposure. Disadvantages of ultrasound are related to the dependence on operator experience, limitations due to an irregular abdominal wall (*e.g.,* bandages, wounds, ostomies), rib cage interference, decreased spatial resolution with image degradation in the obese patient, interference related to intestinal gas, and fluctuating jaundice seen with ball-valve common bile duct stones with intermittent obstruction.

## Computed Tomography

Computed tomography is highly accurate (90%–95%) in demonstrating a dilated biliary system in patients with obstructive jaundice. Potential sources of error include motion artifacts, especially respiratory motion caused by prolonged scan times; a dilated common bile duct that goes unrecognized in the absence of intrahepatic ductal dilatation; dilatation of portal venous branches that mimics dilated biliary radicals; metastases with low CT numbers that simulate dilated intrahepatic ducts; and fluctuating jaundice seen with ball-valve common bile duct stones with intermittent obstruction.

Some of these sources of error have been obviated by the use of intravenous renal contrast agents to enhance surrounding liver parenchymal tissue, thus highlighting the low-density, bile-filled dilated ducts. It should be remembered that contrast will also enhance a dilated portal structure. This is an important consideration in the occasional patient with severe anemia in whom lowered CT numbers of portal venous structures may suggest dilated ducts. Observations of lack of branching, irregular shape, and higher CT numbers (40–50 CT units for metastases compared to 10–20 CT units for bile) have aided in differentiating metastases from dilated bile ducts. Computed tomography will demonstrate the lesion causing biliary obstruction in approximately 75% of patients. However, as

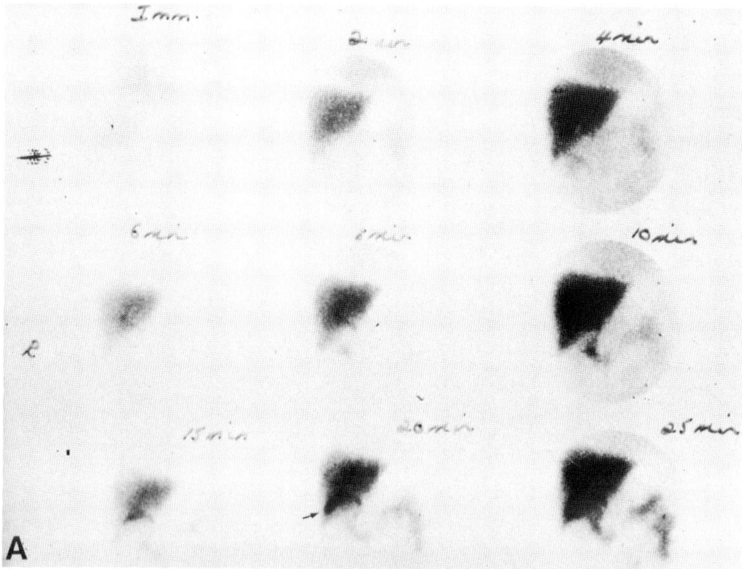

A

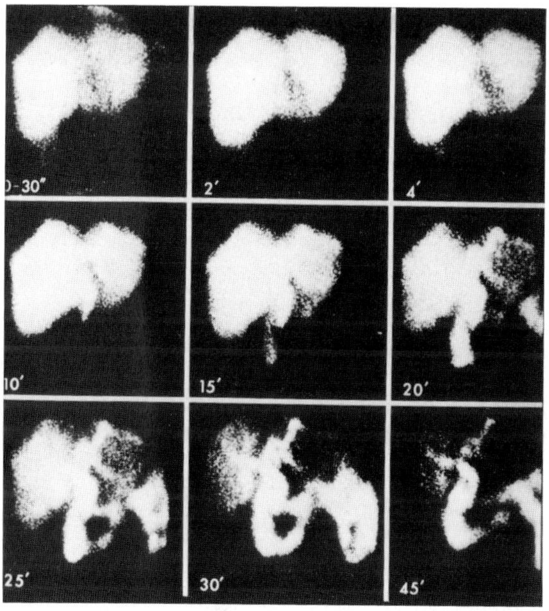


B

**Figure 11-3. (A)** Normal $^{99m}$Tc-hepatobiliary iminodiacetic acid cholescintigram shows immediate filling of bowel with radionuclide and no intrahepatic or choledochal dilatation. Arrow points to the gallbladder. **(B)** $^{99m}$Tc-HIDA cholescintigram demonstrates dilated bile ducts (secondary to postsurgical changes following common bile duct exploration) with normal emptying of radionuclide into the bowel. Ultrasound showed dilated ducts.

with ultrasound, sclerosing cholangitis or acute obstruction with normal or small intrahepatic ducts may result in failure to appreciate the fact that obstructive jaundice is present.

Computed tomography may be the technique of choice in obese or gaseous patients in whom ultrasound is unable to demonstrate intra- or extrahepatic ductal structures. On the other hand, the inability of CT to adequately visualize structures in the emaciated patient with little perivisceral fat requires ultrasonography. The advantages of CT (high patient acceptance, noninvasive) are generally similar to those of ultrasound. The disadvantages are the higher cost of CT and the exposure to ionizing radiation.

## Radionuclide Imaging (Cholescintigraphy)

The attempt to use $^{131}$I rose bengal to adequately visualize the biliary ductal system in the jaundiced patient has had limited success. Recently, biliary imaging agents have been developed that have rapid hepatic uptake from the plasma, rapid metabolism by hepatocytes, and prompt excretion into the bile at high concentration. There is little or no intestinal absorption and minimal renal excretion of these agents. The compounds are $^{99m}$Tc-labeled iminoacetic acid analogs of lidocaine and are available in instant kit form. Visualization of the ductal system with these agents has been achieved at bilirubin levels up to 10 mg to 15 mg per 100 ml. A satisfactory radionuclide study will show the size of the common duct and the dynamics of the excretion into the duodenum (Fig. 11-3). This examination, like ultrasound, is not helpful in identifying the cause of the obstruction.

Cholescintigraphy is infrequently required in the workup of the adult jaundiced patient. It is primarily a backup procedure that can be used in the rare instances in which ultrasound, CT, and percutaneous cholangiography fail to solve the diagnostic problem. It is useful in childhood jaundice and obstructed biliary–enteric anastomoses.

Liver–spleen scanning may also play some diagnostic role, particularly in the search for diffuse metastatic disease as a cause of a patient's jaundice.

### Magnetic Resonance Imaging

Use of magnetic resonance imaging, although promising in initial studies, is at present of limited value.

### Percutaneous Transhepatic Cholangiography

Although first accomplished over 45 years ago, PTHC with large, sheathed needles has been considered too risky to perform unless surgical intervention was immediately available. With the development of the thin (23 gauge), flexible needle in Japan, PTHC has become the primary modality for localizing the proximal extent and character of obstructing lesions of the biliary system (Figs. 11-4*A*, 11-5*A*, 11-6*A*). If a sufficient number of needle passes into the liver substance are made (10–15 attempts), PTHC will demonstrate almost 100% of dilated biliary systems. This technique will also demonstrate 50% to 75% of nondilated biliary systems. Some authors consider that the inability to demonstrate the biliary system after 10 to 15 unsuccessful passes implies that the patient is suffering from nonobstructive rather than obstructive jaundice. This technique is particularly useful in the patient with a Billroth II anastomosis or choledocho-enterostomy (Fig. 11-7).

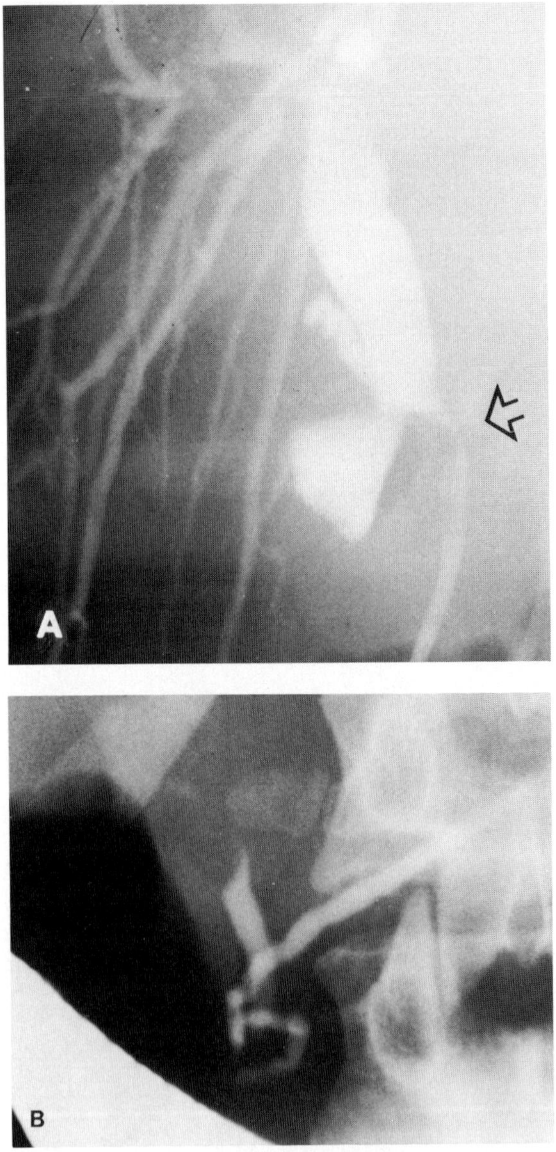


**Figure 11-4. (A)** PTHC demonstrates incomplete obstruction (*arrow*) of the proximal common bile duct. Lesion proved to be a benign tumor of the common bile duct. **(B)** ERCP shows complete retrograde obstruction of the common bile duct with a normal pancreatic duct.

Although much safer than the larger sheathed-needle approach, thin-needle PTHC has a complication rate of 5% to 8%. Fever or other signs of sepsis occur in 3.5% of patients, and the incidence of this complication appears to increase in the completely obstructed system, especially if the ductal system becomes overdistended with contrast material. The small size of the needle used often precludes evacuation of

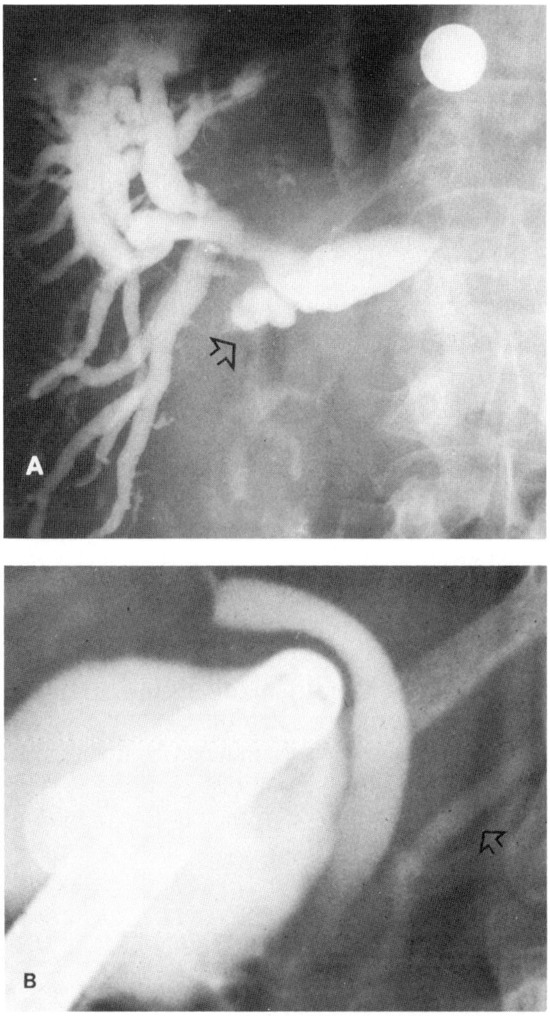


**Figure 11-5. (A)** PTHC demonstrates complete obstruction of the common bile duct due to a cholangiocarcinoma. Arrow points to the partially filled cystic duct, indicating that the gallbladder is available for palliative surgical drainage of the obstructed system. **(B)** ERCP shows complete obstruction of the common bile duct and a normal pancreatic duct (*arrow*).

bile and contrast following examination, further contributing to the problem. Other complications of PTHC are bile leakage with peritonitis, hemoperitoneum (usually not life threatening), and an occasional pneumothorax from puncture of the pleural space.

Distinct advantages of the thin-needle PTHC approach include high success rates with

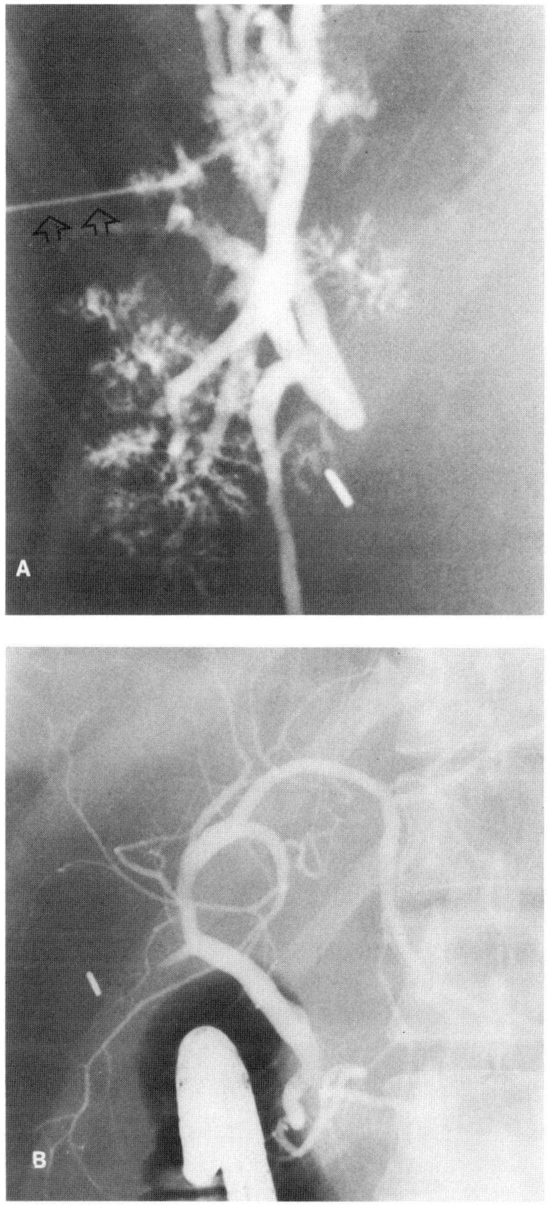


**Figure 11-6. (A)** PTHC shows a nondilated, completely obstructed right intrahepatic biliary ductal system with filling of intrahepatic abscesses following surgical ligation of the system. Arrow points to the needle tract. **(B)** ERCP in the same patient demonstrates a hypertrophied left-lobe ductal system, which is otherwise normal. Clinically, the patient was having episodes of sepsis secondary to the abscesses in the atrophic right lobe.

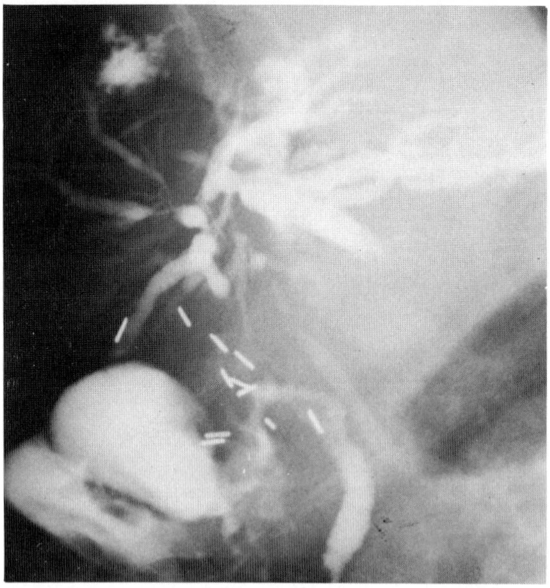

**Figure 11-7.** PTHC in a patient with choledochoenterostomy who developed jaundice secondary to sclerosing cholangitis. PTHC shows normal-sized ducts (also seen on ultrasound).

minimal time expenditure, modest operator skill requirements, use of routine fluoroscopic equipment, minimal and controllable complications, modest cost, and wide availability. This technique has rapidly become the procedure of choice in demonstrating the precise site of obstruction in patients with a dilated biliary system. It is an excellent examination for making the diagnosis in patients with sclerosing cholangitis, a condition that is poorly evaluated by ultrasound and CT. Percutaneous transhepatic cholangiography is also of value in unequivocally demonstrating a nonobstructed ductal system in patients whose preliminary liver enzyme studies suggest an obstructive rather than a hepatocellular origin of their jaundice.

### Endoscopic Retrograde Cholangiopancreatography

Endoscopic retrograde cholangiopancreatography (ERCP) is becoming increasingly available in medical centers. With experienced operators, there is a 70% to 90% success rate for cannulation of the biliary tract via duodenal intubation (Figs. 11-4*B*, 11-5*B*, 11-6*B*). This method has several unique advantages, including endoscopic observation of the intestine, visualization of the lower portion of a completely obstructed common bile duct, evaluation of a nodilated intrahepatic system (*e.g.*, sclerosing cholangitis), and delineation of the pancreatic duct. Endoscopic retrograde cholangiopancreatography is the procedure of choice for precise visualization of the biliary tract in patients with abnormal bleeding parameters. This technique can be used when PTHC cannot be successfully performed.

There are several major disadvantages of ERCP. The availability of the study is severely limited by the need for the operator to have extensive experience in biliary cannulation. The examination is time consuming and expensive (personnel time and the significant cost of the endoscope itself). Endoscopic retrograde cholangiopancreatography may be difficult to perform in patients with biliary–enteric anastomoses. The most important disadvantage is the fairly high morbidity rate (10%–15%). Pancreatitis and endoscopically induced complications are the major adverse sequelae. It is our feeling that ERCP should be reserved for those instances in which PTHC is either unsuccessful or contraindicated.

### Arteriography

The limited yield and high morbidity of arteriography make this procedure of little value in the workup of the patient with obstructive jaundice. If other diagnostic modalities reveal a solitary intrahepatic lesion, arteriography may be helpful in determining its extent, nature, and vascular anatomy. In such instances, arteriography is primarily an immediate preoperative measure.

### Biopsy

The specifics of the lesion causing jaundice can often be obtained only by a biopsy. A liver biopsy may be appropriate if biliary obstruction has been excluded. A percutaneous aspiration biopsy with a narrow-gauge needle may be useful if a liver, pancreatic, or bile duct mass has been demonstrated. This procedure is becoming increasingly popular, although the aspiration of nonmalignant cells does not provide complete confidence of benign disease.

### Surgery

The place of surgery in the differential diagnosis of jaundice has been markedly changed since the advent of newer radiological imaging procedures. However, laparotomy or laparoscopy and biopsy are more extensive steps that may ultimately be required to complete the diagnostic investigation.

## Bibliography

Bree RL, Reuter SR: Angiographic findings in patients with cholelithiasis and obstructive jaundice. Radiology 112:291–295, 1974

Conrad MR, Landay MJ, Janes JO: Sonographic "parallel channel" sign of biliary tree enlargement in mild to moderate obstructive jaundice. AJR 130:279–286, 1978

Cooperberg PL, Ayre–Smith G, Garrow DG: Gray-scale ultrasound of biliary tract disease: A correlative study with percutaneous transhepatic cholangiography. J Can Assoc Radiol 28:237, 1977

Cooperberg PL, Li D, Wong P et al: Accuracy of common hepatic duct size in the evaluation of extra-hepatic biliary obstruction. Radiology 135: 141–144, 1980

Elias E, Hamlyn AN, Jain S et al: A randomized trial of percutaneous transhepatic cholangiography versus endoscopic retrograde cholangiography for bile duct visualization in obstructive jaundice. Gastroentrology 71:439–443, 1976

Ferrucci JT, Jr: Medical progress: Body ultrasonography (second of two parts). N Engl J Med 300: 590–602, 1979

Ferrucci JT, Jr, Wittenberg J: Refinements in Chiba needle transhepatic cholangiography. AJR 129: 11–16, 1977

Gold RP, Casarella WJ, Stern G et al: Transhepatic cholangiography: The radiological method of choice in suspected obstructive jaundice. Radiology 133:39–44, 1979

Goldberg HI, Filly RA, Korobkin M et al: Capability of CT body scanning and ultrasonography to demonstrate the status of the biliary ductal system in patients with jaundice. Radiology 129: 731–737, 1978

Goldstein LI, Sample WF, Kadell BM et al: Gray-scale ultrasonography and thin-needle cholangiography: Evaluation in the jaundiced patient. JAMA 238:1041–1044, 1978

Harbin WP, Mueller PR, Ferrucci JT: Transhepatic cholangiography: Complications and use patterns of the fine-needle technique (a multi-institutional survey). Radiology 135:15–22, 1980

Havrilla TR, Haaga JR, Alfidi RJ et al: Computed tomography and obstructive biliary disease. AJR 128:765–768, 1977

Kessler RE, Falkenstein DB, Clemett AR et al: Indications, clinical value and complications of endoscopic retrograde cholangiopancreatography. Surg Gynercol Obstet 142:865–870, 1976

Lee T, Henderson S, Ehrlich R: Ultrasound diagnosis of common bile duct dilatation. Radiology 124: 793–797, 1977

Leopold GR: Ultrasonography of jaundice. Radiol Clin North Am 17:127–136, 1979

Levitt RG, Sagel SS, Stanley RJ et al: Accuracy of computed tomography of the liver and biliary tract. Radiology 124:123–128, 1977

Rosenthall L: Clinical experience with the newer hepatobiliary radiopharmaceuticals. Can J Surg 21:297–300, 1978

Rosenthall L, Fonseca C, Arzoumanlan KA et al: $^{99m}$Tc-IDA hepatobiliary imaging following upper abdominal surgery. Radiology 130:735–739, 1979

Rosenthall L, Shaffer EA, Lisbona R et al: Diagnosis of hepatobiliary disease by $^{99m}$Tc-HIDA cholescintigraphy. Radiology 126:467–474, 1978

Sample WF, Sarti DA, Goldstein LI et al: Gray-scale ultrasonography of the jaundice patient. Radiology 128: 719–725, 1978

Shanser JD, Korobkin M, Goldberg HI et al: Computed tomographic diagnosis of obstructive jaundice in the absence of intrahepatic ductal dilatation. AJR 131:389–392, 1978

Taylor KJW: Diagnostic Ultrasound in Gastrointestinal Disease. New York, Churchill Livingstone, 1979

Weissmann HS, Frank M, Rosenblatt R et al: Cholescintigraphy, ultrasonography and computerized tomography in the evaluation of biliary tract disorders. Semin Nucl Med 9:22–35, 1979

Whalen JP: Radiology of the abdomen: impact of new imaging methods. Caldwell lecture. AJR 130:61, 1978

Zimmon DS, Falkenstein DB, Riccobono C et al: Complications of endoscopic retrograde cholangiopancreatography. Analysis of 300 consecutive cases. Gastroenterology 69:303–309, 1975

## CLINICAL OBSTRUCTIVE JAUNDICE

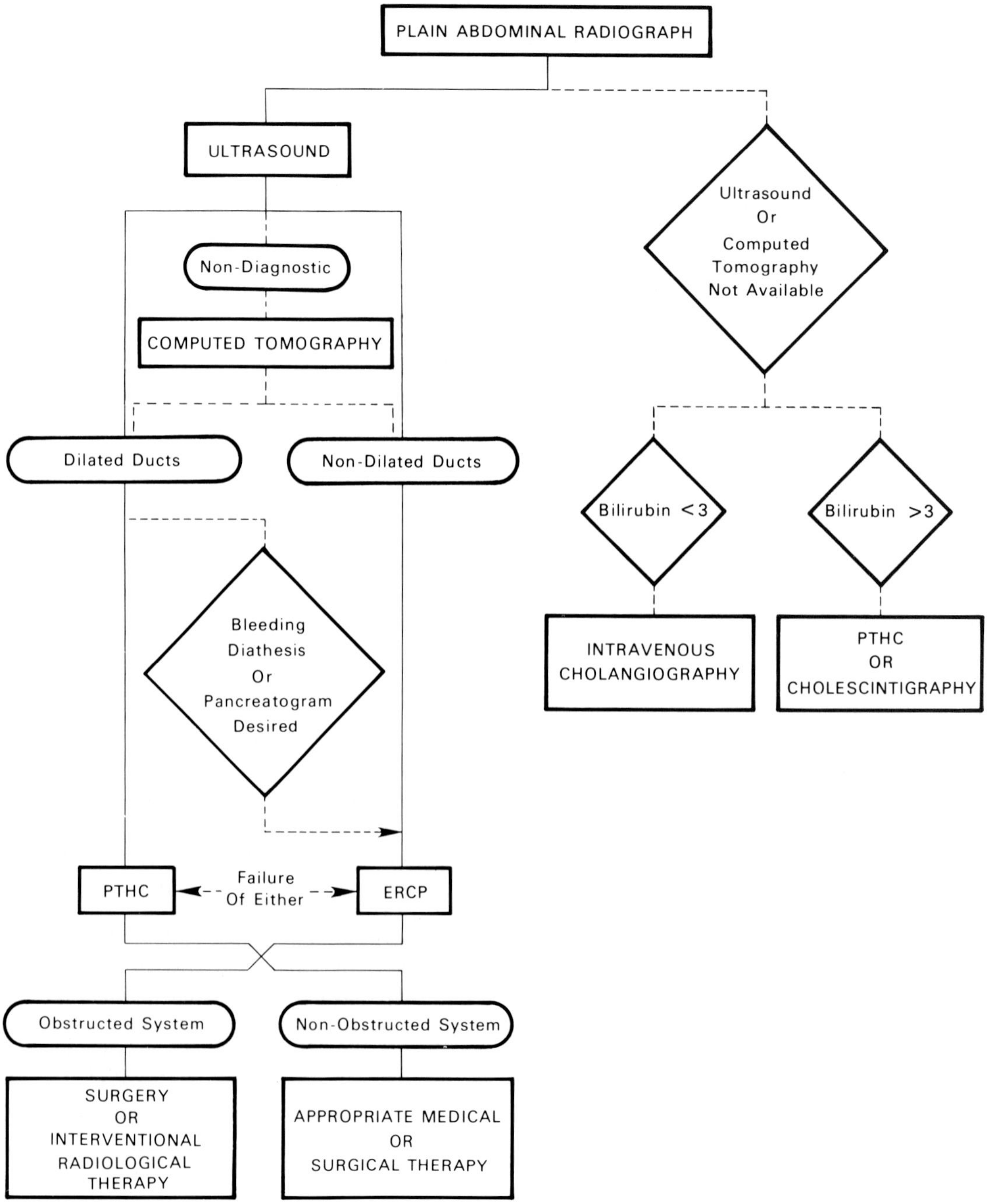

# Chapter 12

# Hepatic Masses

*William M. Marks*
*Patrick C. Freeny*

Hepatic masses may be suspected on the basis of clinical signs and symptoms, or they may be discovered incidentally during a broader diagnostic evaluation, such as staging of a primary malignancy. Once a liver mass is identified, however, knowledge of both clinical findings and hepatic imaging techniques must be integrated to permit an efficient workup, leading to a specific diagnosis.

## DIAGNOSTIC EVALUATION

The radiologic diagnosis of hepatic masses is based on careful evaluation of the gross morphologic features demonstrated on a variety of imaging modalities. If the diagnostic accuracy is to be high, it is essential that each examination be performed with precise techniques and up-to-date equipment.

### *DIAGNOSTIC MODALITIES*

1. Computed tomography
2. Hepatic arteriography
3. Hepatic scintigraphy
4. Ultrasound
5. Magnetic resonance imaging
6. Percutaneous interventional procedures

#### Computed Tomography

The essence of hepatic lesion detection by computed tomography (CT) is the demonstration of a difference in attenuation between the mass and the surrounding normal hepatic parenchyma (relative contrast attenuation). Masses with relative contrast attenuation values less than 10 Hounsfield units (HU) are difficult to detect by CT. With the exception of trauma studies and localization scans for single-level bolus dynamic studies, most investigators now agree that there is no need to obtain a noncontrast CT scan of the liver prior to bolus dynamic contrast-enhanced scans.

Various CT techniques are available to increase the relative contrast attenuation of a hepatic mass. The most sensitive technique for detecting hepatic lesions is incremental bolus dynamic scanning, which involves the use of contiguous 10-mm collimated slices and automatic table incrementation. Using state-of-the-art scanners with scan speeds of 2 seconds per scan, an image repetition rate of 9 scans per minute can be achieved. Scanning is performed during a rapid intravenous bolus injection of 150 ml of 60% iodinated contrast material (injected over 1.5 to 2 minutes), and the CT scanning sequence is initiated after the first 50 ml of contrast has been injected. This method results in a 70- to 80-HU increase in the contrast attenuation of normal hepatic parenchyma and a relative contrast attenuation of 30 HU to 40 HU between the normal liver and most solid hepatic lesions.

The single-level bolus dynamic scanning technique is used to assess the vascularity of known hepatic lesions. Using 10-mm collimated scans, a 2-second scan speed, and a 2.5-second interscan delay, 10 scans per minute can be obtained at the same slice level. The single-level bolus dynamic scan is most effective for evaluating hepatic hemangiomas and has also been used for investigating other vascular lesions, such as hepatocellular carcinoma.

Computed tomography can also be performed during the selective arterial infusion of contrast material via a catheter placed in the hepatic artery (computed tomographic arteriography, CTA). Computed tomographic arteriography is performed using a cluster (group) of three 2-second scans, a 3.5-second interscan delay, and a 10-second intergroup delay. Using automatic table incrementation, 10-mm collimated contiguous scans are obtained while 10 ml to 15 ml of a 30% iodinated contrast material is injected during each cluster. It is important to avoid reflux of contrast into the splenic artery, which results in return of contrast into the liver via the splenic vein–portal venous system and thus may obscure hepatic lesions. Computed tomographic arteriography improves the relative contrast attenuation of hepatic masses by significantly increasing the degree of contrast enhancement of these lesions. Tumors that are only minimally vascular on angiography usually show intense peripheral contrast enhancement on CTA. In one series, CTA identified additional tumor nodules in 40% of patients with known or suspected primary hepatic malignancies or hepatic metastases. Thus, CTA is primarily of value in patients who are candidates for partial hepatectomy in whom unifocal or unilobar lesions have been identified using conventional CT techniques.

A potential source of error using CTA is the production of unusual patterns of enhancement of liver parenchyma (perfusion abnormalities) following the arterial injection of contrast material. These perfusion abnormalities may be related to catheter position, variations of vascular anatomy, and altered hepatic hemodynamics due to tumor or cirrhosis. Perfusion abnormalities usually can be distinguished from tumor nodules by obtaining delayed scans, on which perfusion abnormalities generally become isodense while most tumor nodules become hypodense.

### Hepatic Arteriography

Although hepatic arteriography is now infrequently used for the evaluation of hepatic masses, it may occasionally indicate the definitive diagnosis because of specific arterial or venous changes. Currently the most important use of arteriography is in the evaluation of tumor resectability and in defining hepatic arterial and venous anatomy prior to hepatic resection. Infusion hepatic arteriography is the most efficacious technique and is performed by the injection of 45 ml of 76% iodinated contrast material (3 ml per second for 15 seconds) via a catheter placed selectively into the hepatic artery. A slow infusion rate is necessary to prevent reflux of contrast material into the splenic artery, which would eventually enter the portal venous system and obscure the lesion relative to the surrounding hepatic parenchyma. Filming is performed every 3 seconds for a 30-second period to include both the initial arterial phase ad the hepatogram phase, in which there is maximum contrast difference between primary or secondary hepatic tumors and the normal hepatic parenchyma.

### Hepatic Scintigraphy

Hepatic scintigraphy remains a very useful technique for evaluating both focal and diffuse hepatic parenchymal disease. It is widely available, highly reproducible, and much less expensive than CT or magnetic resonance imaging (MRI). The $^{99m}$Tc sulfur colloid liver–spleen scan can be completed within 30 minutes, gives a relatively low dose of radiation (1.7 R to the liver; 0.1 R whole body), and has an accuracy rate of 80% to 85% for detecting hepatic masses. False-negative errors usually involve lesions less than 2 cm to 3 cm in diameter or masses deep within the liver. Single-photon-emission computed tomography (SPECT imaging) has even higher accuracy and can consistently detect masses as small as 1 cm in diameter. Thus, SPECT imaging is particularly useful for detecting and evaluating "hot" lesions (which accumulate more radionuclide than the surrounding liver parenchyma), such as hemangiomas studied with $^{99m}$Tc-red blood cell scanning. Gallium-67 scintigraphy may be of value in diagnosing the patient with suspected hepatocellular carcinoma.

### Ultrasound

Ultrasound is an important adjunct to other imaging modalities for the evaluation of known or suspected hepatic parenchymal disease. This technique uses no ionizing radiation, requires no intravenous contrast material or radionuclides, is generally available at relatively low cost, and has achieved great patient acceptance. The major disadvantage of ultrasound is its marked operator dependency. Most ultrasound examinations of the liver are currently performed with real-time equipment using focused, high-frequency transducers. Continued technological advances, such as computed sonography, have improved the accuracy of this technique. Nevertheless, ultrasound remains more useful for directed or focal studies of hepatic disease rather than as a screening procedure.

### Magnetic Resonance Imaging

Experience with MRI of hepatic diseases is quite limited. It is still unclear which type of magnet or field strength is best for hepatic imaging. The major limitation of MRI in the upper abdomen is relatively poor resolution due to respiratory motion and prolonged scanning times. However, the technology is evolving rapidly, and MRI should soon play an important role in specific clinical situations.

## EVALUATION OF SPECIFIC TYPES OF HEPATIC MASSES

A variety of imaging techniques can be employed to aid in detecting and characterizing neoplastic and non-neoplastic masses in the liver. The choice of a specific imaging modality depends on factors such as the patient's clinical symptomatology and laboratory studies as well as the presence of an associated systemic disease or underlying hepatic abnormality. Patients with liver parenchymal disease have an increased incidence of developing hepatic tumors. Patients with alcoholic or postnecrotic cirrhosis, hemochromatosis, and alpha$_1$-antitrypsin deficiency have an increased incidence of hepatocellular carcinoma. Occupational exposure may cause hepatic tumors (*e.g.*, angiosarcomas in vinyl chloride workers), whereas patients with glycogen storage disease may develop liver cell adenomas.

### Hepatocellular Carcinoma

In most patients, the suspicion of hepatocellular carcinoma is based on the presence of underlying liver disease and abnormal laboratory studies (routine liver function tests and alpha-fetoprotein). Confirmatory imaging modalities include hepatic scintigraphy, ultrasound, and CT. Hepatocellular carcinoma appears as a photon-deficient ("cold") region on $^{99m}$Tc sulfur colloid scans and as a corresponding "hot" region on $^{67}$Ga scanning. Although other tumors may also take up $^{67}$Ga, the intensity is usually much less than with the typical hepatocellular carcinoma. Fine-needle percutaneous aspiration biopsy under ultrasound or CT guidance may be performed to confirm the histologic diagnosis.

Incremental bolus dynamic CT is probably

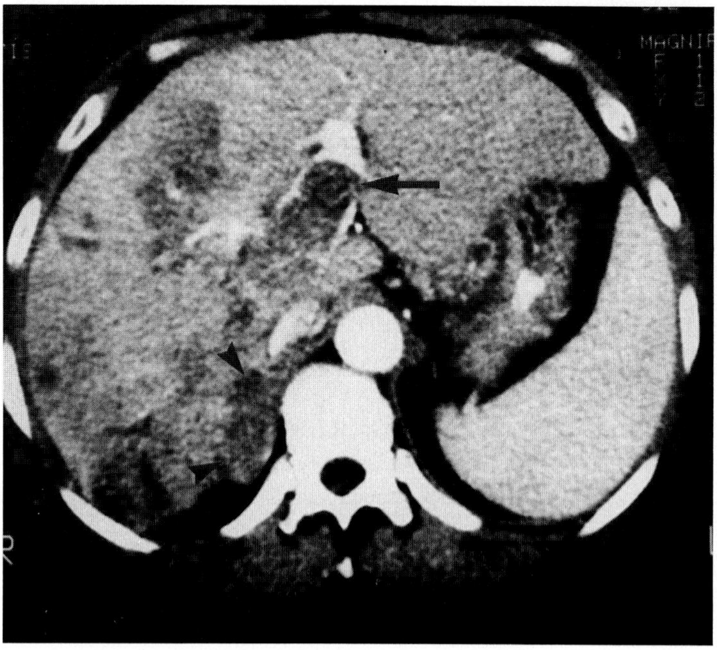

**Figure 12-1.** Hepatocellular carcinoma. Dynamic bolus CT scan shows multiple low-attenuation lesions in the right lobe of the liver. There is tumor invasion of the main portal vein (*arrow*) and a right adrenal metastasis (*arrowheads*).

the single most accurate modality for the detection of hepatocelluar carcinoma, as well as for determination of tumor resectability. The tumor usually appears as a unifocal or multifocal mass of diminished attenuation, often with peripheral or inhomogeneous contrast enhancement (Fig. 12-1). Signs of tumor unresectability on CT include multifocal or multilobar distribution, invasion of portal or hepatic veins, and extrahepatic metastases. In most patient, hepatocellular carcinomas are unresectable at the time of initial presentation. If there is no CT evidence of unresectability, and if the patient is a candidate for surgery, additional imaging studies should be performed for more precise assessment of resectability and for the preoperative definition of hepatic vascular anatomy. Infusion hepatic arteriography can detect additional lesions and can serve as a vascular road map for the surgeon, and CTA scans can identify additional tumor nodules that were not detected by infusion arteriography or incremental bolus dynamic CT (Fig. 12-2).

A variant of hepatocellular carcinoma is fibrolamellar carcinoma. This tumor occurs with equal frequency in males and females, although it generally develops in young patients (5–35 years) who have otherwise normal livers, unlike hepatocellular carcinoma, which typically arises in patients with cirrhosis or other underlying parenchymal disease. The imaging features are often nonspecific. The presence of a central scar or bizarre neovascularity suggests the diagnosis of focal nodular hyperplasia, liver cell adenoma, or hepatocellular carcinoma. Hepatic scintigraphy may be of value in excluding focal nodular hyperplasia. In most cases, however, percutaneous or open surgical biopsy is necessary to provide a specific diagnosis.

## Metastatic Disease

Metastatic disease is the most common hepatic malignancy, and its detection is one of the most important roles of diagnostic hepatic imaging. Computed tomographic arteriography is the most sensitive modality (≥95%) for detecting hepatic metastases. Computed tomography and angiography have sensitivity rates of 85% to 90% for detecting liver metastases, while the sensitivity rates of hepatic scintigraphy and nondirected ultrasound are 80% to 85% and 60% to 80%, respectively. Although experience is

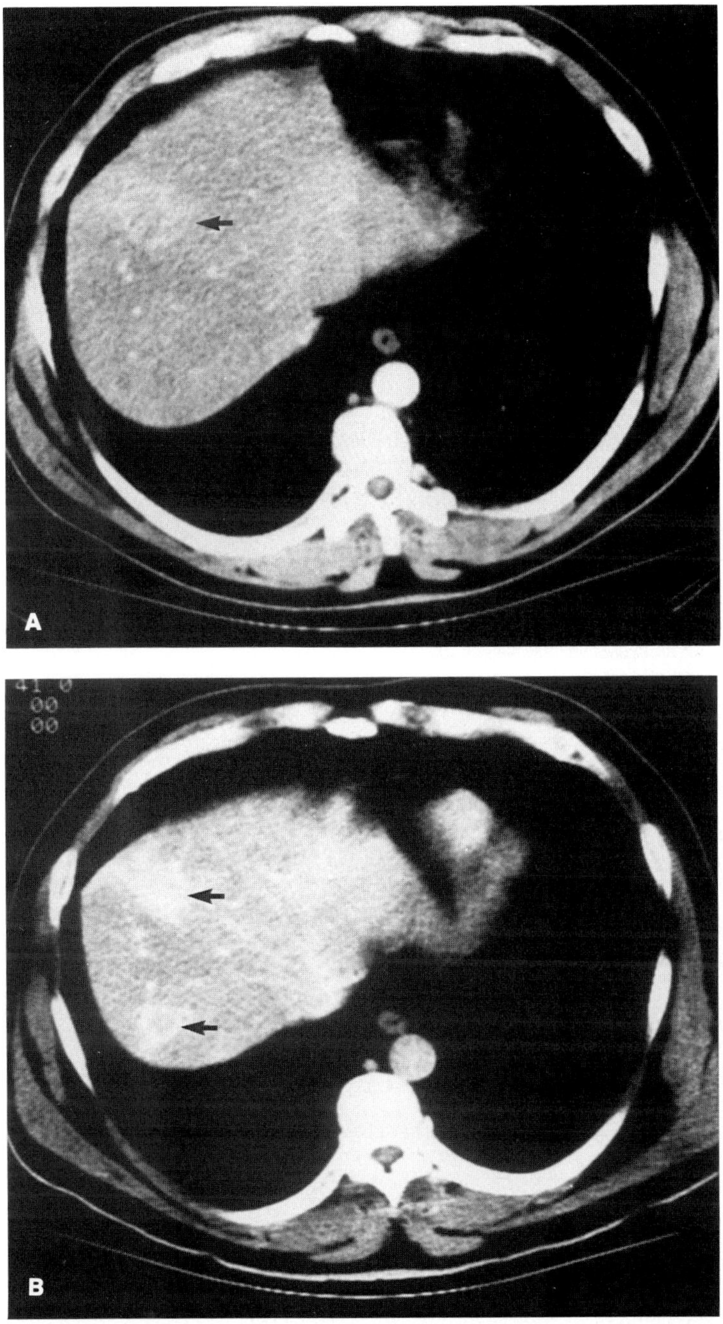

**Figure 12-2.** Hepatocellular carcinoma. **(A)** Dynamic bolus CT scan through the upper portion of the right lobe of the liver shows a suspicious area of contrast enhancement (*arrow*). **(B)** CTA scan shows two definite hypervascular tumor nodules (*arrows*) high in the right lobe of the liver.

limited, MRI using T1-weighted sequences with very short echo times (TE) and short repetition times (TR) may be even more sensitive than conventional CT for detecting hepatic metastases.

It is helpful to divide oncology patients into two groups for determining the optimal sequencing of imaging procedures. The first group is composed of patients with a known primary tumor who have a high suspicion of metastatic disease based on clinical and laboratory findings. The second group is composed of patients with a known or suspected primary tumor, but in whom

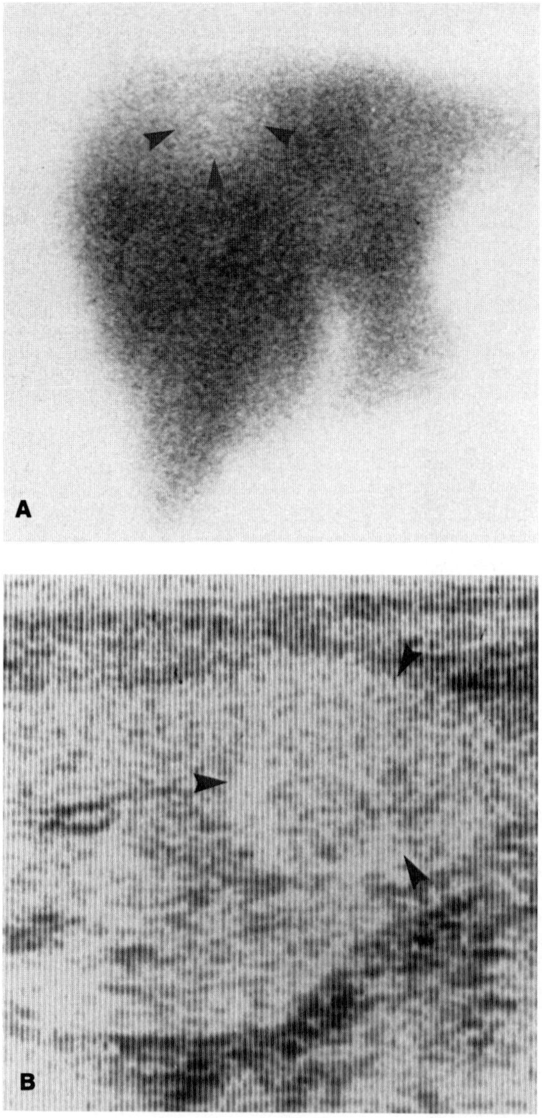

**Figure 12-3.** Liver metastasis from colon carcinoma. **(A)** Radionuclide sulfur colloid liver scan shows a photopenic ("cold") defect (*arrowheads*) in the left lobe of the liver. **(B)** Linear-array real-time ultrasound shows a solid tumor nodule (*arrowheads*) corresponding to the photopenic area on the radionuclide scan. Ultrasound-guided biopsy confirmed the diagnosis of metastatic disease.

there is no clinical or laboratory suspicion of metastases. In the first group, rapid confirmation of the clinical diagnosis can be obtained by real-time ultrasound combined with fine-needle aspiration biopsy under ultrasound guidance. If a reproducible imaging modality is required to follow the response of a lesion to chemotherapy or radiation therapy, $^{99m}$Tc sulfur colloid liver scanning is usually satisfactory (Fig. 12-3).

Incremental bolus dynamic CT scanning is the most accurate imaging modality for the initial evaluation of group-two patients with no clinical suspicion of metastatic disease. This technique can detect hepatic metastases, identify the primary tumor, and define the presence and extent of extrahepatic disease (Fig. 12-4). Fine-needle aspiration biopsy may be performed under either ultrasound or CT guidance. The aspirated material may be examined with routine staining, although more sophisticated techniques with electron microscopy and immunoperoxidase staining may provide a more specific diagnosis.

Patients with unifocal or unilobar hepatic metastases who are candidates for surgical resection should undergo careful preoperative imaging. An incremental bolus dynamic CT scan should be the initial study. In most cases, this

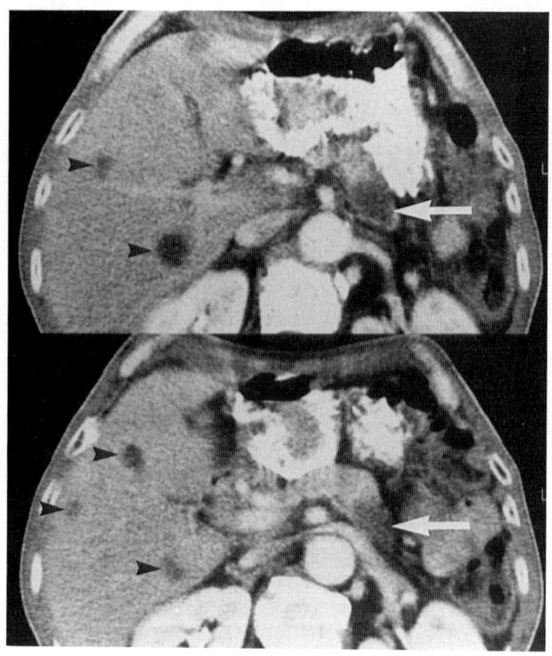

**Figure 12-4.** Liver metastases from pancreatic carcinoma. Dynamic bolus CT scans show multiple low-attenuation liver metastases (*black arrowheads*). Note the low-attenuation mass in the tail of the pancreas (*white arrows*) representing the primary pancreatic carcinoma.

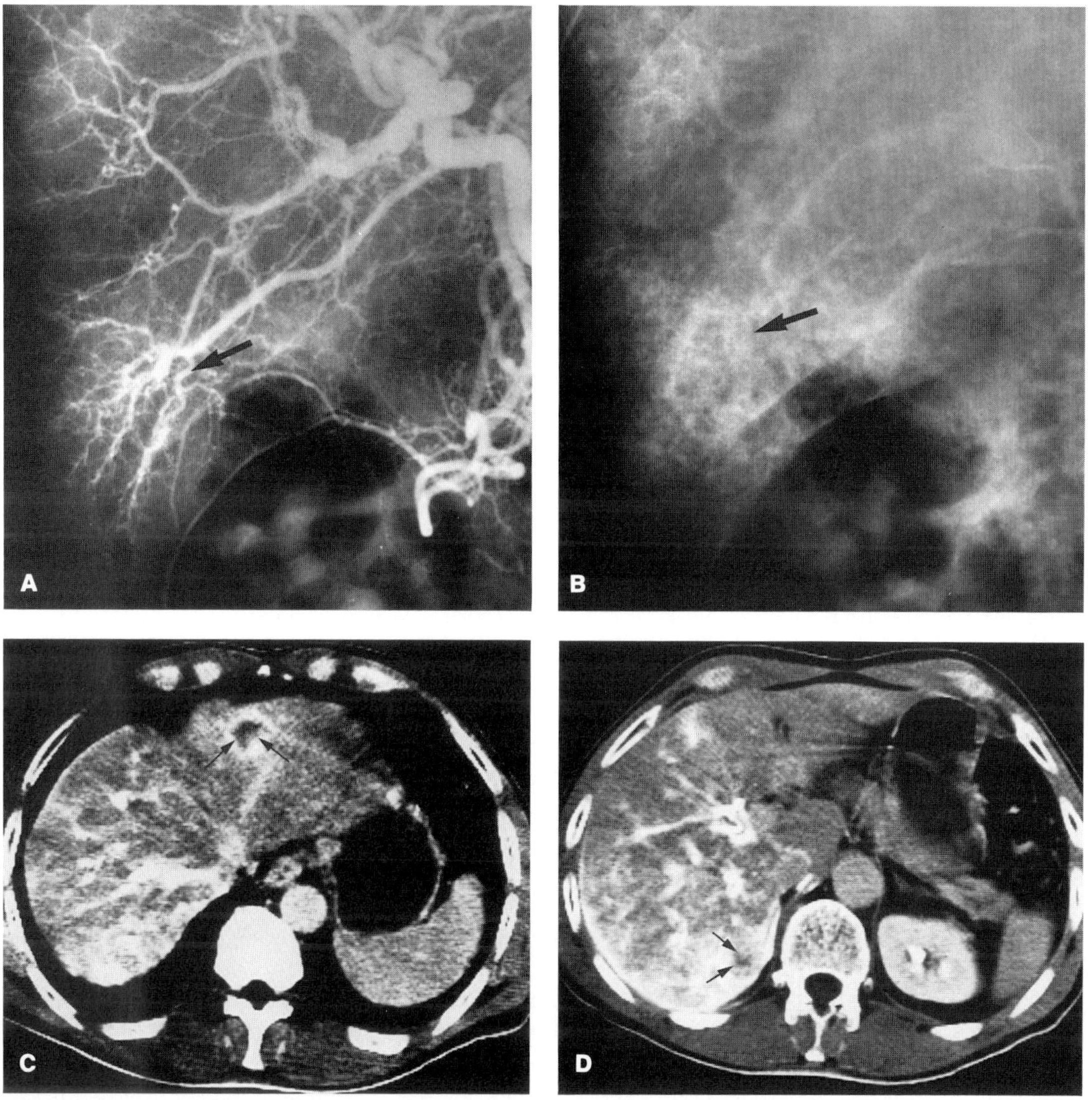


**Figure 12-5.** Liver metastases from colon carcinoma. An initial CT scan showed only a single metastasis in the posteroinferior segment of the right lobe of the liver. **(A)** Arterial and **(B)** capillary phase films from a right hepatic arteriogram show a single, hypervascular lesion in the inferior portion of the right lobe (*arrows*), corresponding to the initial lesion seen on CT. No additional tumor nodules were identified on this examination or on a selective left hepatic arteriogram. (**C** and **D**) CTA scan shows two additional tumor nodules (*arrows*), one in the anterolateral portion of the left lobe **(C)** and one in the inferomedial portion of the right lobe **(D)**.

examination will detect any multifocal or multilobar hepatic metastases or evidence of extrahepatic metastatic disease, all of which indicate unresectability of the tumor. If tumor unresectability is questionable on the bolus dynamic CT scan, CTA and/or infusion hepatic arteriography may be indicated to confirm this therapeutically critical diagnosis. The small group of patients believed to have resectable tumor should have hepatic arteriography and CTA prior to surgery to ensure resectability (Fig. 12-5).

## Benign Hepatic Tumors

Focal nodular hyperplasia and liver cell adenoma are two benign hepatic tumors that are believed to be associated with the use or oral contraceptives. Focal nodular hyperplasia is a relatively common tumor that rarely causes symptoms and is often detected incidentally during imaging procedures performed for other reasons. Liver cell adenoma is a rare benign tumor that is more likely to be symptomatic and typically causes pain and an abdominal mass. Rupture of the tumor with spontaneous bleeding into the peritoneal cavity may result in the acute onset of pain and hypotension.

The most efficacious imaging modality for the initial detection of these tumors is real-time ultrasound of the liver. If a lesion is detected, additional imaging studies must be performed to provide a specific diagnosis.

The ultrasound appearance of focal nodular hyperplasia is nonspecific, with lesions appearing hyperechoic, hypoechoic, or of mixed echogenicity. On incremental bolus dynamic CT, focal nodular hyperplasia may be hyperdense, but it is often isodense with the liver and therefore undetectable (Fig. 12-6*A*). The demonstration of a central hypodense scar is highly suggestive of this diagnosis.

Hepatic scintigraphy is the major imaging modality in the diagnosis of focal nodular hyperplasia. In adults, focal nodular hyperplasia is the only primary hepatic tumor that contains a sufficient number of Kupffer cells to take up the sulfur colloid. More than half of patients with focal nodular hyperplasia will therefore have normal scintigrams, with the tumor isodense with normal liver (Fig. 12-6*B*). In some patients, the tumor may take up more isotope than the normal parenchyma and thus appear as a "hot" nodule. Thus, if ultrasound or CT detects a hepatic mass larger than 3 cm (*i.e.*, large enough to be detected by conventional hepatic scintigraphy), a normal sulfur colloid study confirms the diagnosis of focal nodular hyperplasia. If the scintigram reveals a focal photopenic defect, or if the lesion is smaller than 3 cm in diameter (*i.e.*, too small to be accurately detected by hepatic scintigraphy), hepatic arteriography should be performed. In about 80% of cases, arteriography shows the typical appearance of focal nodular hyperplasia as a well-marginated, hypervascular lesion with a dense parenchymal stain containing a central cleft and/or radial septations. If the arteriographic findings are atypical, percutaneous or surgical biopsy is required.

Liver cell adenomas have a broad spectrum of findings and usually cannot be diagnosed specifically. They generally appear on ultrasound as discrete hepatic masses with inhomogeneous echo patterns. Rarely, the tumors may be homogeneous and hypoechoic. On CT, liver cell adenoma appears as a discrete hepatic mass with inhomogeneous contrast enhancement (Fig. 12-7). If the tumor has undergone recent hemorrhage, a nonenhanced scan may show areas of increased attenuation due to intratumoral blood. The arteriographic features of liver cell adenoma, which may simulate hepatocellular carcinoma, include a dilated feeding hepatic artery, peripheral arterial supply, mixed areas of hypo- and hypervascularity, and, often, neovascularity.

## Incidentally Detected Hepatic Lesions

Several benign hepatic masses may be detected incidentally in asymptomatic patients during radiologic imaging procedures performed for other (nonhepatic) reasons. In addition to focal nodular hyperplasia (discussed previously), other benign, incidentally detected hepatic lesions include hemangioma and non-neoplastic processes, such as hepatic cyst and focal fatty infiltration.

### Hemangiomas

Hemangiomas are the most common benign tumors of the liver. They occur in all age groups, have a strong female predominance, and are found in about 4% of autopsies. Because hepatic hemangiomas are benign and usually require no therapy, they must be distinguished from malignant tumors. The majority of hepatic hemangiomas are detected incidentally during ultra-

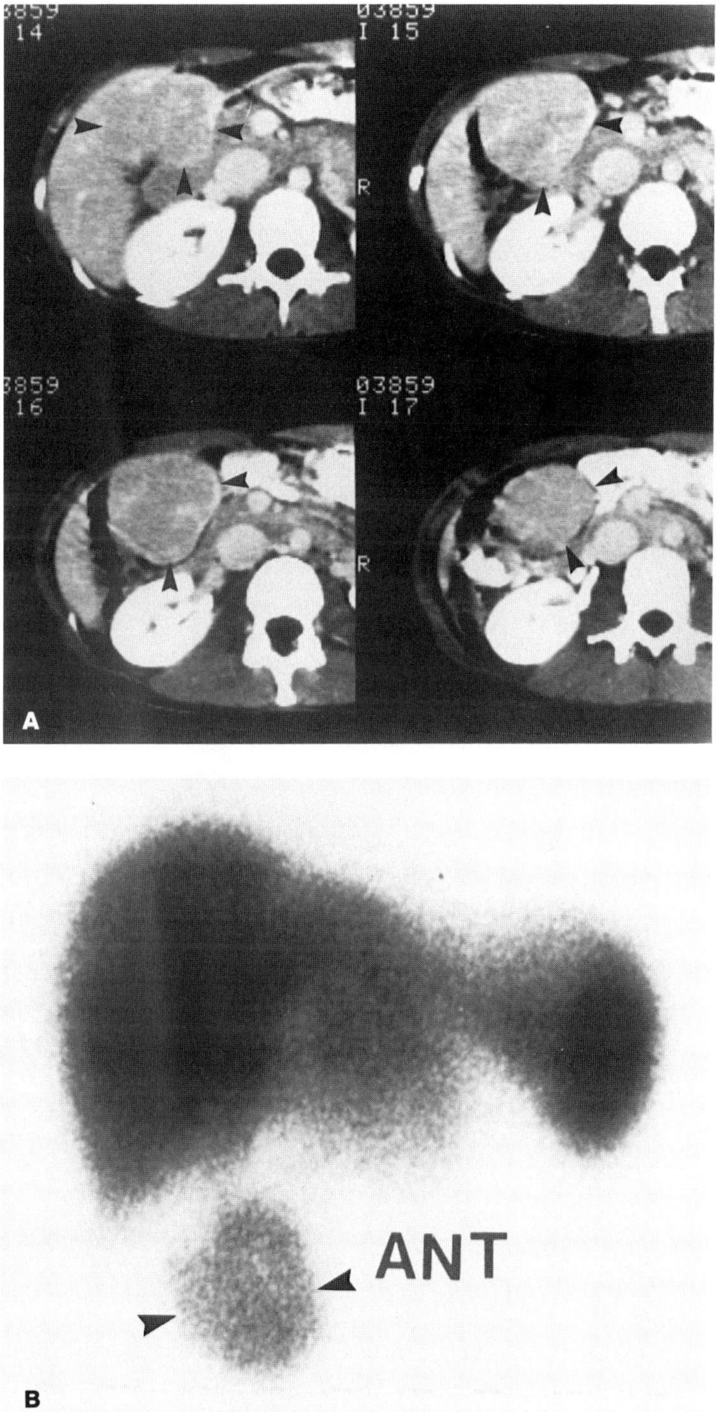


**Figure 12-6.** Focal nodular hyperplasia. **(A)** Dynamic bolus CT scan shows an isodense mass (*arrowheads*) arising from the inferior portion of the medial lobe of the liver. **(B)** Radionuclide sulfur colloid liver–spleen scan shows isotope uptake (*arrowheads*) in the mass.

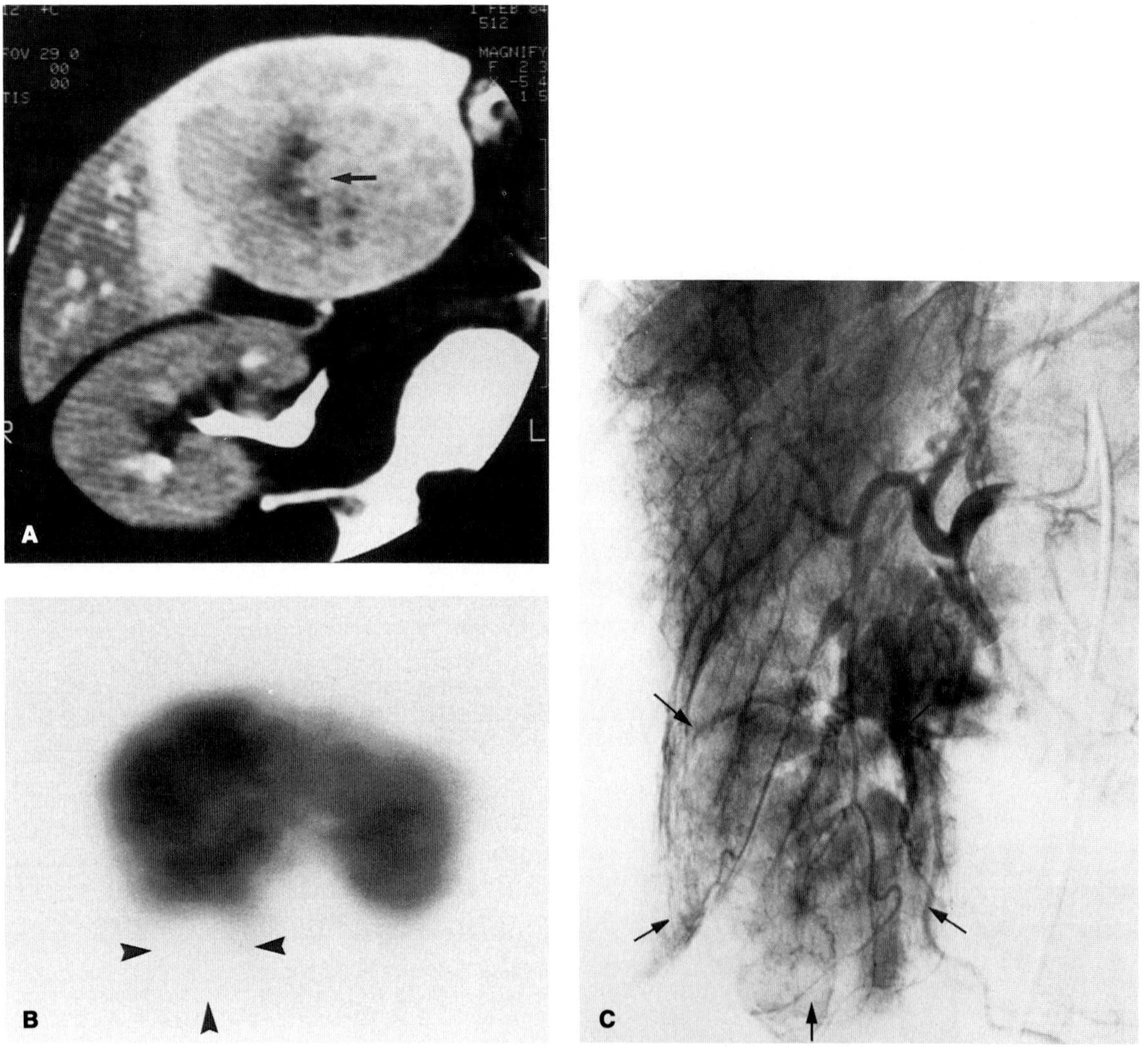


**Figure 12-7.** Liver cell adenoma. **(A)** Dynamic-bolus CT scan shows an isodense mass arising from the right lobe of the liver. Note the inhomogeneous center (*arrow*). **(B)** Sagittal view from a radionuclide sulfur colloid liver scan with SPECT imaging shows a photopenic ("cold") mass (*arrowheads*). **(C)** Selective hepatic arteriogram shows a moderately vascular mass (*arrows*) with subtle neovascularity arising from the right lobe of the liver.

sound of the gallbladder. Most appear as focal hyperechoic masses with posterior acoustic enhancement; occasionally, they may be hypoechoic or have a mixed echogenic pattern (Fig. 12-8*A*). Until recently, arteriography has been the major modality for diagnosing hepatic hemangiomas. The classic arteriographic appearance of this tumor is an early circular or C-shaped collection of contrast material that persists long into the venous phase and is supplied by normal feeding vessels (Fig. 12-8*B*).

The typical CT appearance of hepatic hemangioma consists of a low-attenuation lesion on noncontrast scans, peripheral contrast enhancement during the bolus phase, and an isodense appearance in comparison with the normal surrounding hepatic parenchyma on delayed scans (Fig. 12-8*C*). A recent study has shown that this

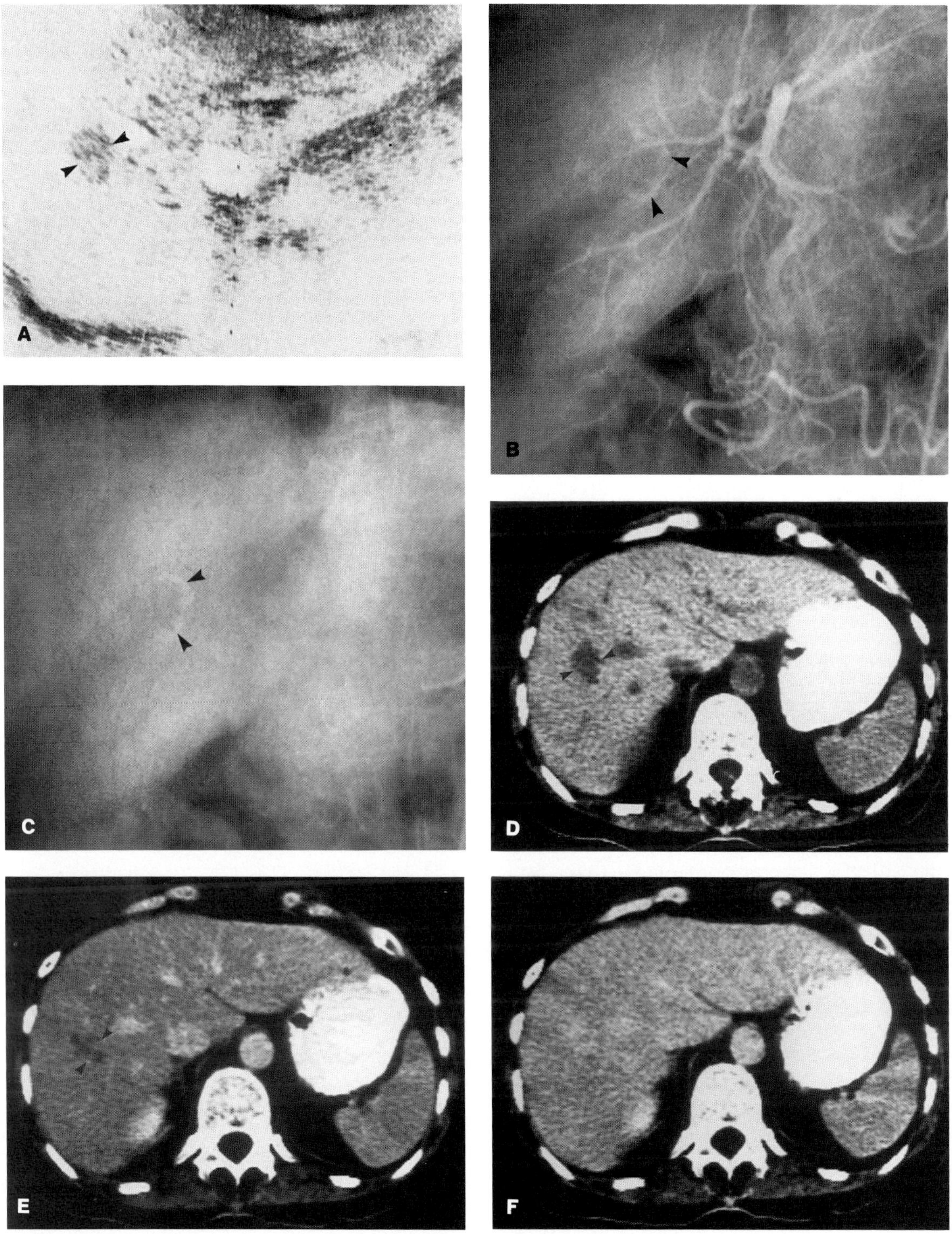


**Figure 12-8.** Hepatic hemangioma. **(A)** Ultrasound shows a focal hyperechoic lesion (*arrowheads*) in the right lobe of the liver. **(B)** Arterial and **(C)** capillary phase films from a selective hepatic arteriogram show the characteristic ring-shaped configuration of contrast accumulation (*arrowheads*). **(D)** Initial CT scan without intravenous contrast shows the low-attenuation mass. **(E)** Scan obtained during intravenous contrast injection shows faint peripheral contrast enhancment of the lesion (*arrowheads*). **(F)** Delayed scan following contrast injection shows the lesion to be isodense with the surrounding liver parenchyma.

characteristic CT pattern is seen in only approximately half of hepatic hemangiomas. Nevertheless, the demonstration of this typical pattern makes malignant neoplasm a highly unlikely possibility.

Hepatic scintigraphy, using SPECT imaging and $^{99m}$Tc-labeled red blood cells, is a highly sensitive and specific imaging modality for diagnosing hepatic hemangiomas. It is rapidly becoming the primary diagnostic modality, replacing arteriography and CT. The tumor characteristically appears normal on initial scans but shows increased isotope activity ("hot" lesion) in comparison to normal surrounding liver on delayed scans (1 to 24 hours following injection) (Fig. 12-9). Although increased activity on delayed scans has also been seen in patients with hepatocellular carcinoma, in this group there is also increased activity on the initial or flow-study scans. Metastatic tumors show no increased activity on either initial or delayed scans.

In our opinion, when an echogenic hepatic lesion is discovered incidentally on ultrasound in a patient who is asymptomatic, has normal liver function tests, and has no known primary tumor, the patient can simply be followed with a repeat sonogram in 6 months without the need for additional imaging procedures. However, additional diagnostic evaluation is required if the hepatic lesion is hypoechoic or of mixed echogenicity, or if the patient is symptomatic (relative to the liver lesion), has abnormal liver function tests, or has a known primary tumor. In such cases, our experience has indicated that the $^{99m}$Tc-red blood cell scan is the most efficacious imaging technique. If the red blood cell scan is equivocal, arteriography is the next procedure of choice for making a specific diagnosis.

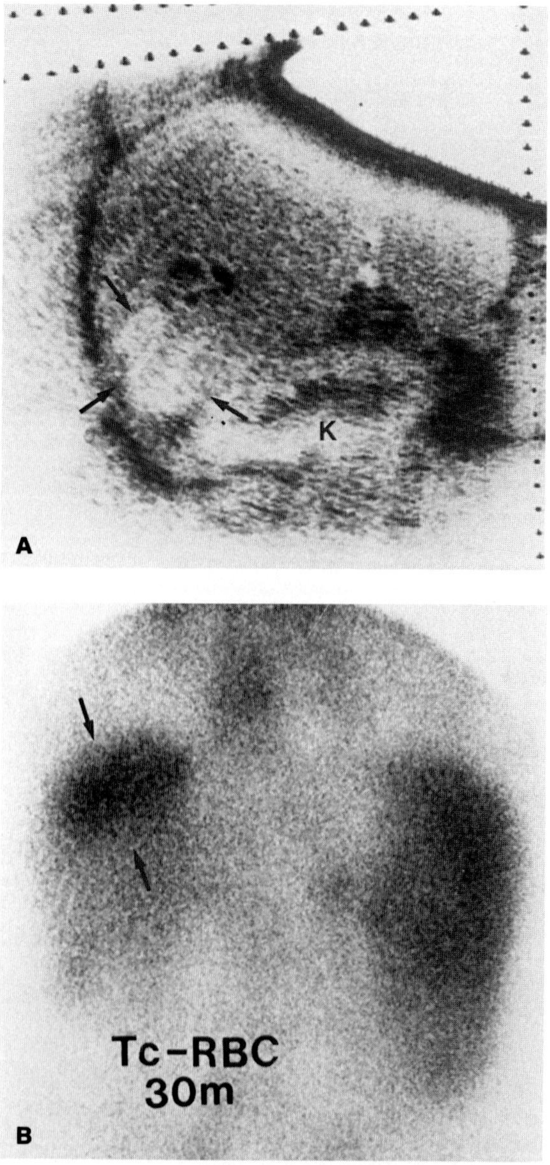


**Figure 12-9.** Hepatic hemangioma. **(A)** Sagittal ultrasound shows a focal hypoechoic mass (*arrows*) in the posterior right lobe of the liver (*K*, kidney). **(B)** Technetium-99m red blood cell scan at 30 minutes shows a focal area of increased radionuclide uptake ("hot") corresponding to the abnormality seen on ultrasound.

## Hepatic Cysts

Hepatic cysts are common lesions that are usually detected incidentally but may cause symptoms due to mass effect and pressure. They may be unifocal, multifocal, or part of the polycystic disease syndrome (associated with polycystic renal disease in approximately 80% of cases). On scintigraphy, hepatic cysts appear as non-

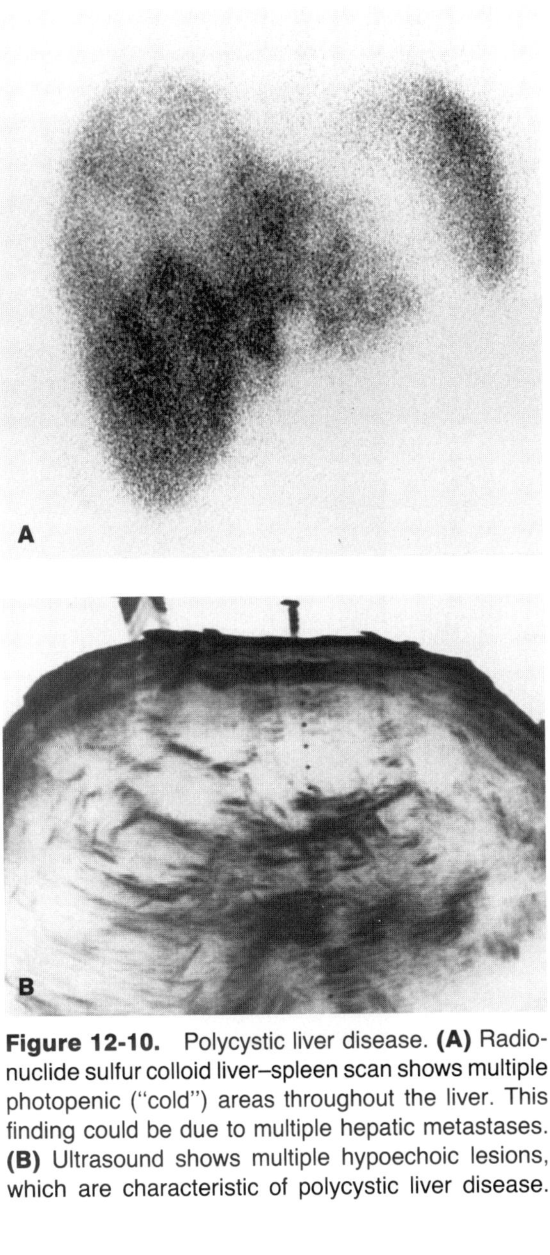

**Figure 12-10.** Polycystic liver disease. **(A)** Radionuclide sulfur colloid liver–spleen scan shows multiple photopenic ("cold") areas throughout the liver. This finding could be due to multiple hepatic metastases. **(B)** Ultrasound shows multiple hypoechoic lesions, which are characteristic of polycystic liver disease.

specific photopenic ("cold") areas that may be indistinguishable from other lesions, such as metastases. Ultrasound is highly accurate in diagnosing simple hepatic cysts. The classic findings consist of a sonolucent lesion with thin, well-defined walls and posterior acoustic enhancement (Fig. 12-10). If these precise ultrasound criteria are not demonstrated, the mass should be biopsied or the patient should have further imaging studies (CT and guided fine-needle aspiration biopsy) to exclude the possibility of a cystic tumor (cystadenoma, cystadenocarcinoma), a cystic or necrotic primary tumor or metastasis, or an abscess.

## Focal Fatty Infiltration

Focal or diffuse fatty infiltration may develop in a variety of clinical settings, such as hyperalimentation, steroid therapy, chronic alcoholism, cirrhosis, and diabetes mellitus. Focal fatty infiltration, which may mimic a discrete liver mass, is usually detected incidentally on a CT scan performed for other reasons. The focal collection of fat appears as a discrete area of diminished attenuation with no evidence of contrast enhancement (Fig. 12-11). Normal contrast-enhancing vessels (hepatic or portal veins) can often be seen coursing through the areas of fat. The process is evanescent and may appear and disappear frequently. Radionuclide scanning occasionally may be of value in difficult cases. Although most $^{99m}$Tc sulfur colloid scans are normal in focal fatty infiltration, there may be increased isotope uptake by the fat on $^{133}$Xe scans.

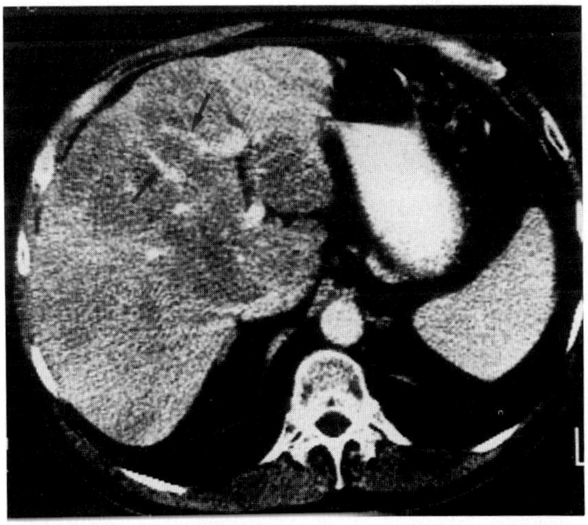

**Figure 12-11.** Focal fatty infiltration. Dynamic bolus CT scan shows multifocal areas of decreased attenuation in both lobes of the liver. Note the normal-appearing portal veins (*arrows*) coursing through the areas of decreased attenuation.

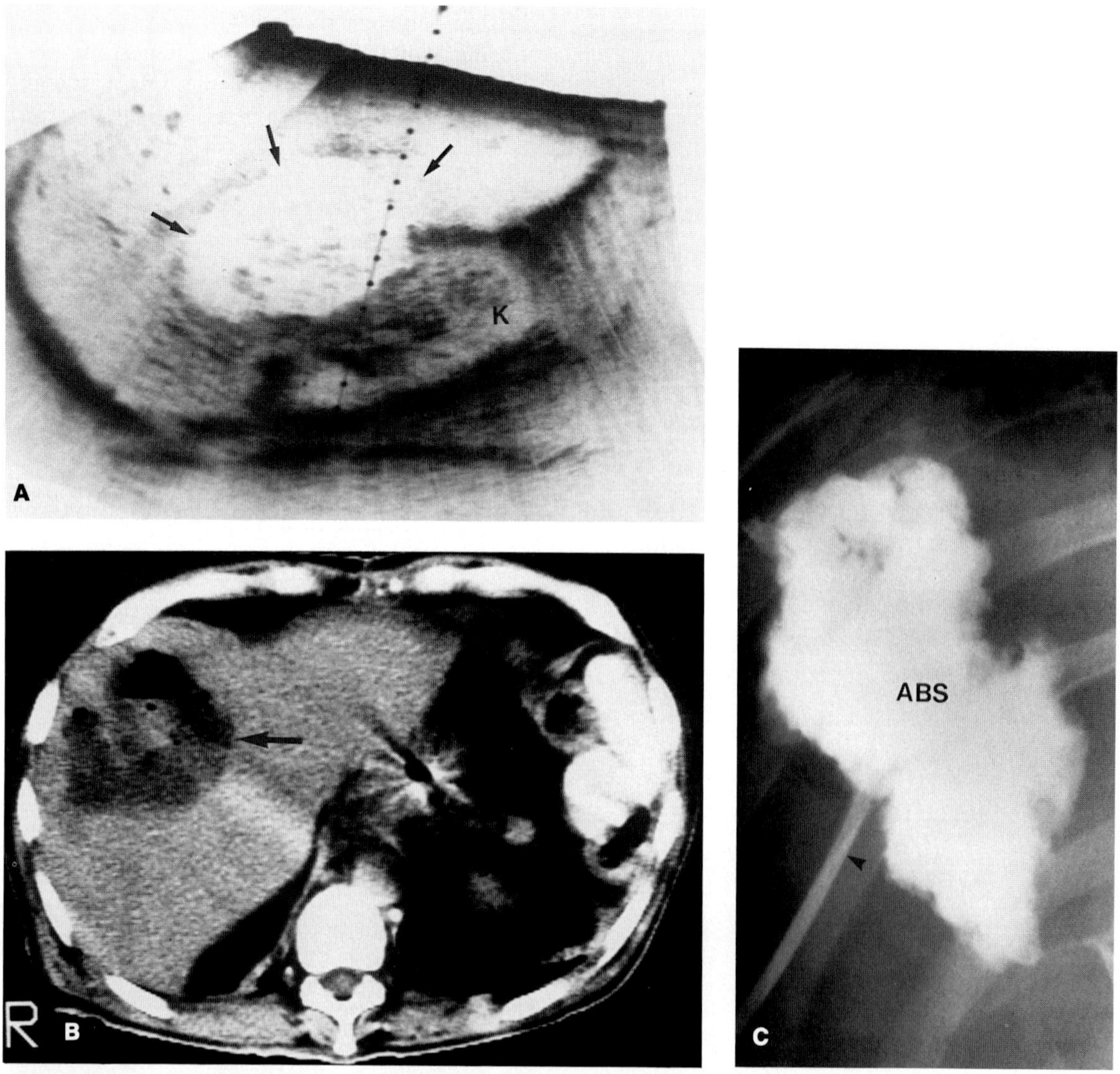


**Figure 12-12.** Hepatic abscess. **(A)** Sagittal ultrasound shows a pyogenic abscess as a hypoechoic mass with internal echoes (*arrows*) in the right lobe of the liver (*K,* kidney). **(B)** CT scan in a different patient shows a gas-containing abscess (*arrow*) in the right lobe of the liver. **(C)** Contrast injection through a percutaneous catheter (*arrowhead*) fills the abscess cavity (*ABS*).

Percutaneous biopsy may be helpful in difficult cases, but it is seldom needed to make the diagnosis.

### Hepatic Abscesses

The patient with a suspected hepatic abscess is usually first studied with CT or ultrasound. Fever of unknown origin or diffuse signs and symptoms are generally indications for CT scanning; if there is specific clinical information to suggest a hepatic abscess, ultrasound is the initial imaging procedure of choice. On ultrasound, an abscess usually appears as a fluid-filled mass that often contains some degree of internal echogenicity depending on the amount of debris or gas within it (Fig. 12-12*A*). The wall of an abscess is thicker and more irregular than that of a typical cyst. On CT, an abscess usually has low attenuation (0–30 HU) and an irregular, thickened wall; gas may be identified within the abscess in about 20% of cases (Fig. 12-12*B*).

The demonstration of a normal liver on a technically satisfactory CT or ultrasound examination virtually excludes the possibility of a hepatic abscess. If diffuse parenchymal disease, such as cirrhosis or fatty infiltration is present, $^{67}$Ga or $^{111}$In-white blood cell scanning may be of value in demonstrating focal isotope uptake within the abscess. Although an abscess usually can be distinguished from a simple cyst. differentiation from a necrotic or cystic tumor may require aspiration with analysis of the fluid. Once the diagnosis of a hepatic abscess has been definitively established, percutaneous drainage is usually the therapeutic procedure of choice (Fig. 12-12*C*).

## Bibliography


Alpern MB, Lawson TL, Foley WD et al: Focal hepatic masses and fatty infiltration detected by enhanced dynamic CT. Radiology 158:45–59, 1986

Berland, LL, Lawson TL, Foley WD et al: Comparison of pre- and postcontrast CT in hepatic masses. AJR 138:853–858, 1982

Bree RL, Schwab RE, Neiman HL: Solitary echogenic spot in the liver: Is it diagnostic of a hemangioma? AJR 140:41–45, 1983

Foley, WD, Berland LL, Lawson TL: Contrast enhancement technique for dynamic hepatic computed tomographic scanning Radiology 147: 797–803, 1983

Freeny PC: Angiography of hepatic neoplasms. Semin Roentgenol 18:114, 1983

Freeny PC, Marks WM: Computed tomographic arteriography of the liver. Radiology 148:193–197, 1983

Freeny PC, Marks WM: Hepatic perfusion abnormalities during CT angiography: Detection and interpretation. Radiology 159:685–691, 1986

Halvorsen RA, Korobkin M, Ram PC et al: CT appearance of focal fatty infiltration of the liver. AJR 139:277–281, 1982

Kunstlinger F, Federle MP, Moss AA et al: Computed tomography of hepatocellular carcinoma. AJR 134:431–437, 1980

LaBerge JM, Laing FC, Federle MP et al: Hepatocellular carcinoma: Assessment of resectability by computed tomography and ultrasound. Radiology 152:485–490, 1986

Marks WM, Jacobs RP, Goodman PC et al: Hepatocellular carcinoma: Clinical and angiographic findings and predictability for surgical resection. AJR 132:7–11, 1979

Moinuddin M, Allison JR, Montgomery JH et al: Scintigraphic diagnosis of hepatic hemangioma: Its role in the management of hepatic mass lesions. AJR 145:223–228, 1985

Rabinowitz SA, McKusick KA, Strauss HW: $^{99m}$TC red blood cell scintigraphy in evaluating focal liver lesions. AJR 143:63–68, 1984

Roemer CE, Ferrucci JT, Mueller PR: Hepatic cysts: Diagnosis and therapy by sonographic needle aspiration. AJR 136:1065–1070, 1981

Rogers JV, Mack LA, Freeny PC: Hepatic focal nodular hyperplasia: Angiography, CT, sonography, and scintigraphy. AJR 137:983–990, 1981

Scott WW, Sanders RC, Siegelman SS: Irregular fatty infiltration of the liver: Diagnostic dilemmas. AJR 135:67–71, 1980

Welch, TJ, Sheedy PF, Johnson CM: Focal nodular hyperplasia and hepatic adenoma: Comparison of angiography, CT, US, and scintigraphy. Radiology 156:593–595, 1985

## SUSPECTED HEPATOCELLULAR CARCINOMA

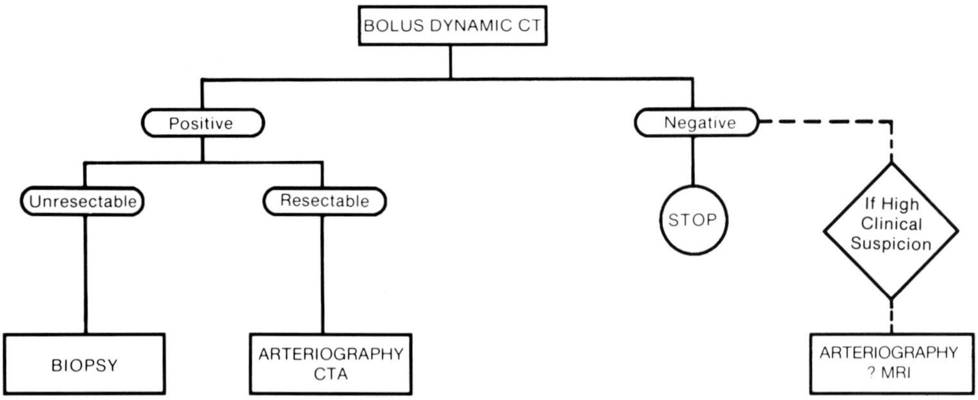


## KNOWN PRIMARY TUMOR
### Clinical Suspicion of Liver Metastases

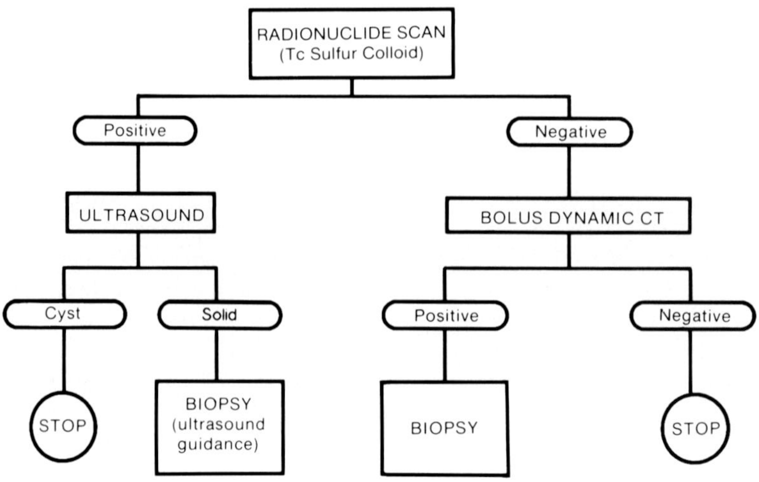

**KNOWN OR SUSPECTED PRIMARY TUMOR**
**No Clinical Suspicion of Liver Metastases**

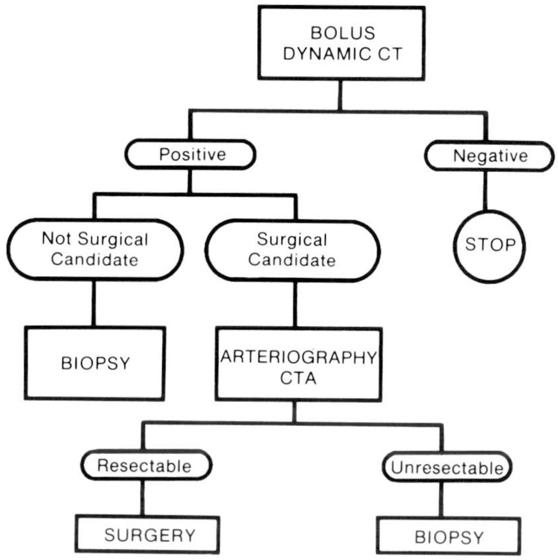


**SUSPECTED FOCAL NODULAR HYPERPLASIA**
**(Positive Ultrasound or CT)**

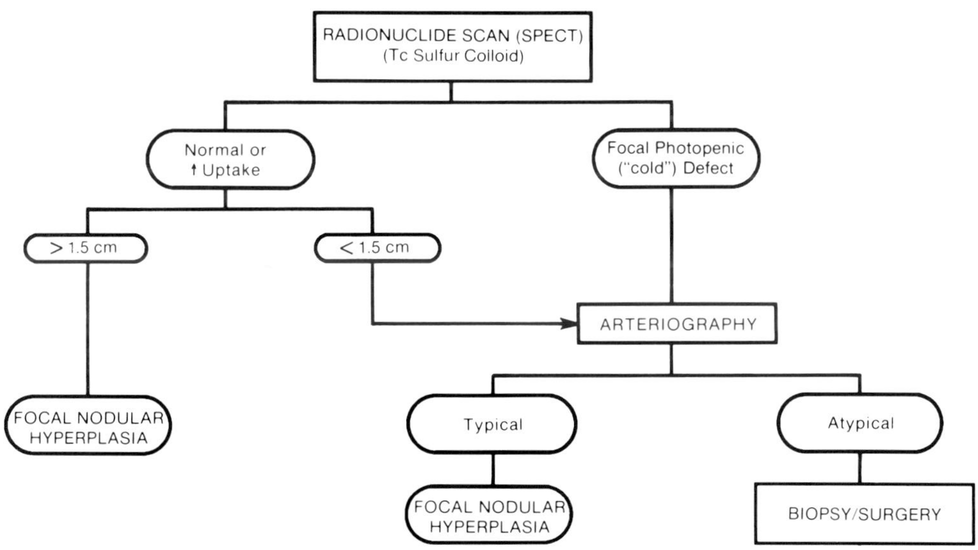

**SUSPECTED HEMANGIOMA**

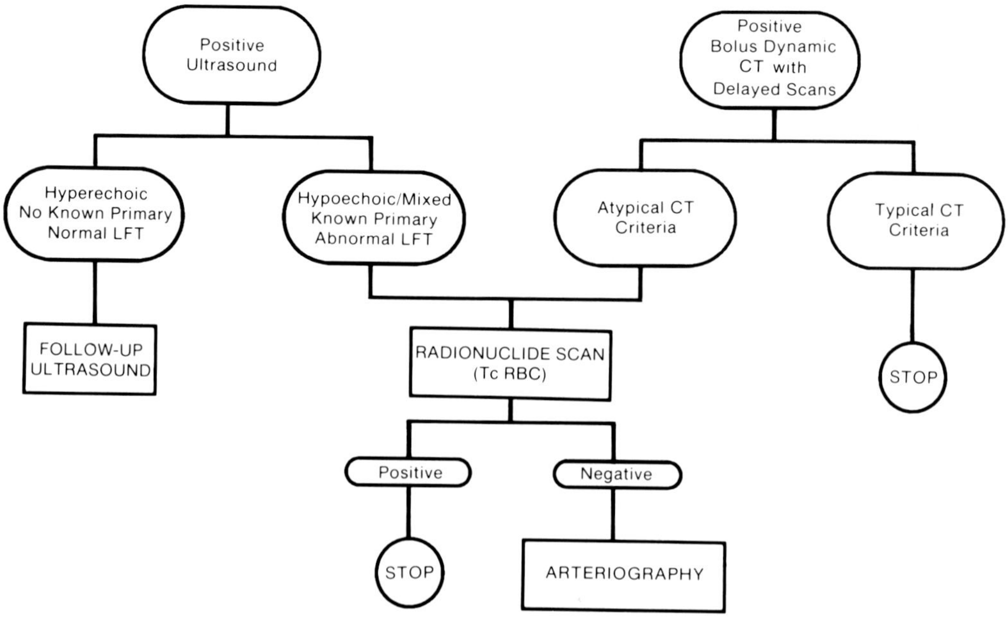

# Chapter 13

# Pancreatic Disease

*Edward T. Stewart*

Epigastric pain unexplained by studies of other abdominal organs is the usual event that triggers a search for pancreatic disease. The decision to investigate the pancreas is one that not only has an impact on medical costs but is anxiety producing for both patient and physician. Basic questions in the assessment of the patient with suspected pancreatic disease are twofold:

1. Is the pancreas abnormal?
2. If abnormal, is the cause an inflammatory or neoplastic process?

Pancreatitis is a common disorder. In the United States, it is most frequently related to alcohol. Common duct stones, trauma, and drugs such as corticosteroids may precipitate this benign disease. There are also rare cases of familial pancreatitis. The spectrum of pancreatitis is broad, ranging from a single event free of residual sequelae to recurrent attacks leading to progressive destruction of the pancreas. A major complication of pancreatitis is the formation of pseudocysts. More than half of these cysts can be shown to communicate with the pancreatic duct at a site of ductal disruption. In approximately 30% of patients, pseudocysts are multiple. Extrapancreatic pseudocysts are less likely to resolve spontaneously, and surgical intervention is frequently necessary. Pseudocysts also can become infected, resulting in pancreatic abscess.

Carcinoma of the pancreas remains an elusive tumor. Cures are few because identification rarely occurs prior to extensive local growth or metastatic spread. The majority of pancreatic cancers (60%–70%) occur in the head of the gland, commonly presenting with painless jaundice. Most of the remaining tumors arise in the body, with only a few occurring in the tail. The prognosis for most carcinomas of the pancreas remains dismal, with a mean survival of 4 months despite new diagnostic capabilities.

A small percentage of pancreatic tumors arise in the islet cells and secrete hormones (*i.e.*, insulin, gastrin, glucagon), which produce a variety of unusual syndromes. These endocrine tumors may secrete more than one hormone at a time. Islet cell tumors frequently have metastasized to adjacent lymph nodes and the liver at the time of initial laparotomy. The primary lesion is often extremely small, and despite extensive metastasis, it may never be positively identified.

Tumors arising from structures adjacent to the pancreas (bile ducts, kidney, colon, stomach adrenals) may masquerade as primary pancreatic malignancies. Lymph node involvement in metastatic carcinoma or lymphoma may also mimic primary pancreatic malignancy.

## CLINICAL AND LABORATORY EVALUATION

Although many laboratory tests, such as stool analysis, digestive tolerance test, pancreatic enzyme studies, and pancreatic secretion studies, have been used to evaluate the function of the pancreas, most are very nonspecific. Even though there is considerable overlap between benign and malignant disease, these laboratory tests are of value in identifying patients in whom suspected pancreatic disease should be further evaluated.

Duodenal intubation and aspiration of pancreatic secretions may be of value in the patient with suspected pancreatic cancer. The failure to collect adequate pancreatic juice following stimulation with cholecystokinin has resulted in a greater than 80% positive predictability. In the absence of a history of pancreatitis, this test appears to be one of the most sensitive in screening patients for malignant disease. At this time, there are no reliable tumor-specific antigens. In most patients, however, when carcinoma of the gland is to be excluded, these tests are bypassed in favor of more specific imaging procedures, such as computed tomography (CT) or endoscopic retrograde cholangiopancreatography (ERCP).

Amylase and lipase levels in the serum and urine, combined with clinical symptomatology, are important in the initial diagnosis of pancreatitis and may be sufficient to follow patients with uncomplicated inflammatory disease of the gland.

## DIAGNOSTIC EVALUATION

### *DIAGNOSTIC MODALITIES*

1. Plain radiographs and barium studies
2. Ultrasound
3. Computed tomography
4. Pancreatic arteriography
5. Endoscopic retrograde cholangiopancreatography and transhepatic cholangiography
6. Magnetic resonance imaging
7. Radionuclide imaging
8. Aspiration cytology

### Plain Radiographs and Barium Studies

In patients with pancreatitis, plain abdominal radiographs may demonstrate calcification or a mass in the region of the pancreas, as well as sentinel loops due to localized adynamic ileus. Saponification of the peritoneal fat by the pancreatic enzymes very infrequently causes a mottled appearance on plain films. The results of plain abdominal radiographs rarely influence the treatment of patients with suspected pancreatic disease.

The value of barium studies in patients with pancreatic disease has always been limited, because they detect changes only when the pathologic process displaces or infiltrates the gut. Even large pancreatic lesions may not do this. Conventional techniques may be augmented with either tube or tubeless hypotonic duodenography achieved with the aid of glucagon. High accuracy rates have been reported with hypotonic duodenography, but these rates were achieved prior to the availability of ultrasound and CT and thus are undoubtedly much too optimistic.

Barium studies are far more sensitive for detecting lesions in the head of the pancreas and in the region of the papilla of Vater than for processes involving the body or tail of the pancreas. These studies of the duodenum may not permit a distinction between benign and malignant disease. The sensitivity and specificity of barium studies are now recognized to be so low that the new imaging modalities have relegated them to a less important role, especially in the search for pancreatic malignancy.

### Ultrasound

Ultrasound is an extremely useful noninvasive screening procedure that is now available throughout the medical community. Most examinations are performed in real-time, using either linear-array or sector scanners. Medium-focus transducers of 3 mHz or 5 mHz are generally adequate for examining patients of average size. Advantages of ultrasound include its noninvasiveness, lack of ionizing radiation, wide availability, and generally low cost. Disadvantages include the technical problem of gas or obesity, wich severely limits the quality of the examination, and the strong dependence on operator expertise.

Technically satisfactory ultrasound examinations have sensitivity and specificity rates greater than 75% (but less than CT) for detecting pancreatic abnormalities. False-positive studies are infrequent. Ultrasound can show the size and echogenicity of the gland, the appearance of the pancreatic duct, and any pancreatic calcifications and stones. Complications of pancreatitis, such as pseudocysts and pancreatic ascites, can be detected and followed. Ultrasound can detect gallstones as the etiologic agent in some patients with pancreatitis. It can also show the effects of pancreatitis on the biliary tree, primarily bile duct dilatation proximal to a distal common bile duct stricture caused by fibrosis, edema, or pseudocyst compression. On ultrasound, carcinoma of the pancreas appears as a mass that may be associated with dilated pancreatic and/or biliary ductal structures due to obstruction by tumor (Fig. 13-1). Distal metastases, especially to the liver, also may be detected. However, small tumors of both the exocrine and endocrine portions of the gland are poorly detected by ultrasound.

Ultrasound cannot differentiate benign and malignant masses of the pancreas. Therefore, the clinical setting influences the diagnostic possibilities. A pancreatic mass in a nonalcoholic patient is most likely malignant. In patients with chronic pancreatitis, it is usually impossible to determine whether a pancreatic mass is benign or malignant because of the nonspecific nature of the sonographic findings.

## Computed Tomography

High-resolution CT is now widely available and is the major imaging modality for evaluation of the pancreas. Computed tomography has greater spatial resolution than ultrasound, is not operator dependent, and is not adversely affected by large amounts of intestinal gas. Thin-slice thicknesses (<10 mm), dynamic scanning, enhancement with intravenous contrast, and bowel opacification with oral contrast are required for optimal pancreatic imaging.

Computed tomographic findings consistent with pancreatitis include mass, edema, peripancreatic phlegmon, calcification (usually ductal), intra- or extrapancreatic pseudocysts (Fig. 13-2), obstruction of the pancreatic or bile ducts, pancreatic abscess, and pancreatic ascites. Extension of pancreatic pseudocysts into unusual locations (thorax, various retroperitoneal spaces) is best demonstrated on CT.

Percutaneous drainage of pancreatic abscesses and pseudocysts is now the therapeutic procedure of choice if the fluid collection is accessible and not complex. Computed tomographic guidance is usually preferable to ultrasound, because adjacent bowel loops, liver, spleen, and blood vessels are better demonstrated. Proper patient selection is essential for percutaneous procedures, and the route of entry must be planned carefully.

Carcinoma of the pancreas generally appears on CT as a mass with (or without) dilatation of the pancreatic and/or bile ducts because of obstruction. Computed tomography can demonstrate spread of tumor into the peripancreatic fat planes, direct extension into adjacent organs, and distant metastases. It can also show encasement or occlusion of peripancreatic arteries and veins and evidence of malignant ascites.

Computed tomography has a sensitivity of approximately 95% for detecting carcinoma of the pancreas. It is equally sensitive in detecting complications of pancreatitis, especially the location and extension of pseudocysts. A major shortcoming of CT is the inability to discriminate between benign and malignant pancreatic masses in patients with chronic pancreatitis (usually on the basis of alcohol abuse). Because of the overlap in CT findings (mass and evidence of ductal obstruction) in these two entities, percutaneous aspiration cytology may be of great value.

Because of the relatively high cost of CT,

ultrasound is usually the screening procedure of choice in the patient with vague, unexplained abdominal complaints that are believed to relate to the pancreas. However, CT scanning is usually the initial imaging modality if carcinoma of the pancreas is suspected.

## Pancreatic Arteriography

The inadequacies of barium studies in the 1960s and 1970s led to extensive use of arteriography to detect pancreatic disease. The use of subselective injections and magnification techniques significantly improved the diagnostic capabilities of arteriography. Claims are made that more than 90% of patients could be correctly identified as being normal or abnormal and that a correct diagnosis of carcinoma or pancreatitis could be achieved in 85% of abnormal cases (Fig. 13-3). However, ultrasound and CT have markedly diminished the role of arteriography as a primary diagnostic modality for pancreatic disease. Arteriography is of value for detecting

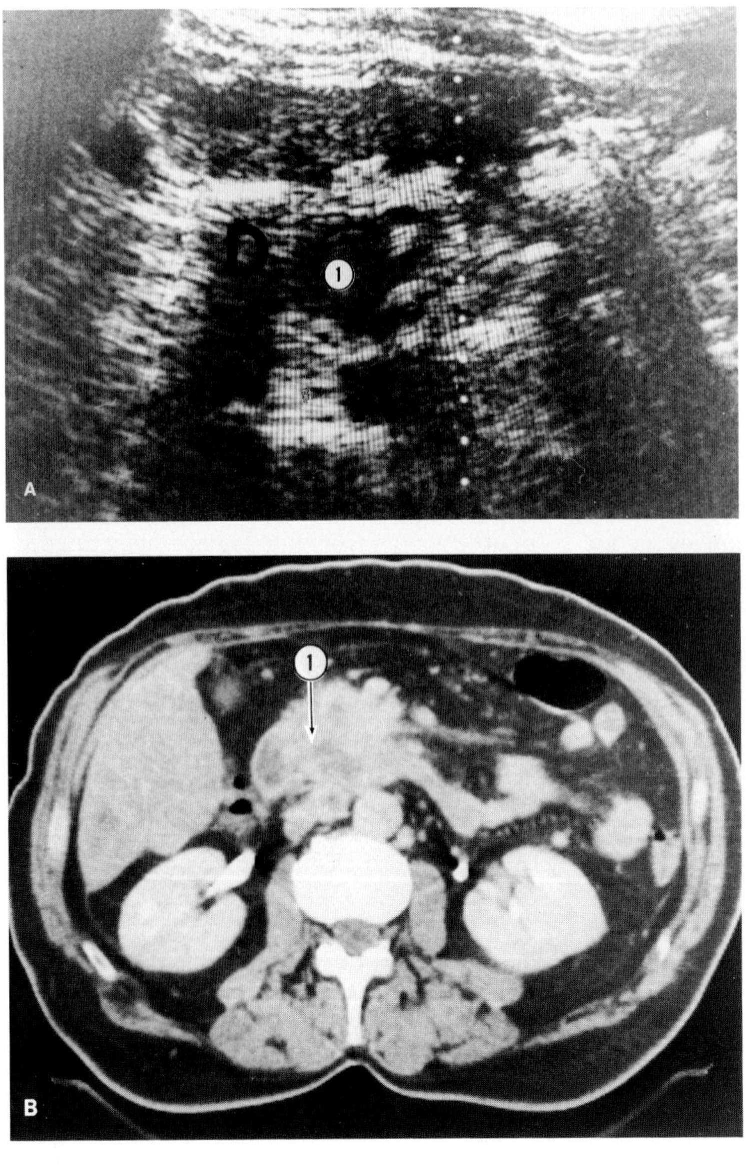


**Figure 13-1. (A)** Screening ultrasound in an elderly man who presented with symptoms consistent with pancreatic carcinoma demonstrates a mass in the head of the pancreas (*1*). The duodenum (*D*) and aorta (*A*) are seen in relation to the pancreatic mass. **(B)** CT scan demonstrates a large mass, with areas of low attenuation, that is located primarily within the head of the pancreas (*1*). This appearance is compatible with both inflammatory and malignant disease. In this patient, there was no history of previous pancreatic pathology.

(*Continued on facing page*)

complications of pancreatitis, such as arterial pseudoaneurysms and stenotic or occlusive lesions of peripancreatic arteries or veins. The demonstration of splenic vein occlusion and the presence of collateral venous channels can be important surgically. The onset of acute hemorrhage in a patient with pancreatitis is an indication for immediate arteriography. In staging patients with pancreatic malignancy, arteriography may show tumor neovascularity and encasement of arteries and veins.

Arteriography plays an important role in detecting small endocrine tumors of the pancreas. These lesions, and any hepatic metastases, are typically extremely hypervascular.

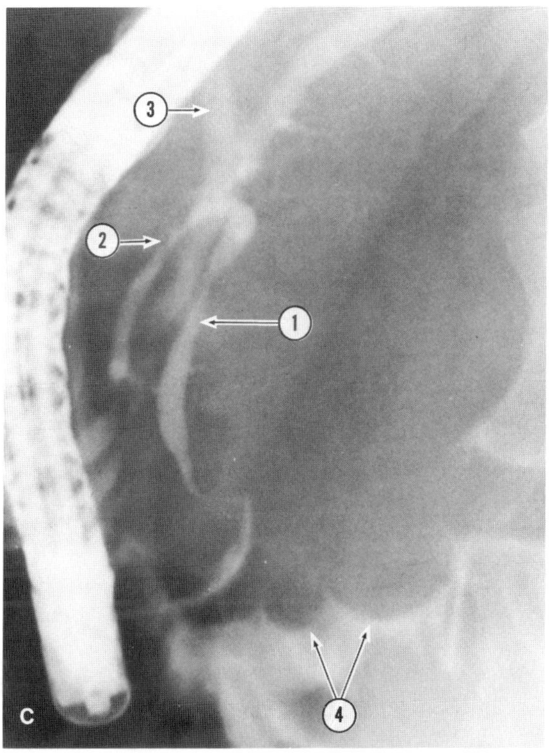


**(C)** ERCP demonstrates a stricture involving the main pancreatic duct (*1*) as well as a stricture at the origin of the duct of Santorini (*2*), with amputation of the lateral branches in these areas, consistent with carcinoma of the pancreas. The common duct (*3*) is not dilated even though it must pass through the very large tumor mass. Scalloping along the duodenal sweep (*4*) indicates invasion of the wall of the duodenum. Aspiration cytology performed at the time of ERCP confirmed the malignant nature of the mass. Cytology also could have been easily performed using CT. The patient's tumor was obviously unresectable, and he died of multiple metastases within 6 weeks. Laparotomy was never performed because the aspiration cytology confirmed the diagnosis.

## Endoscopic Retrograde Cholangiopancreatography and Transhepatic Cholangiography

Endoscopic retrograde cholangiopancreatography has been a valuable addition in the evaluation of patients with both benign and malignant pancreatic disease. Although the procedure is primarily an endoscopic technique, the radiographic detail recorded at the time of filling of ductal structures is the most important aspect of the examination. Because of the endoscopic skill required to be routinely successful, ERCP tends to be less readily available than other diagnostic procedures for evaluating the pancreas.

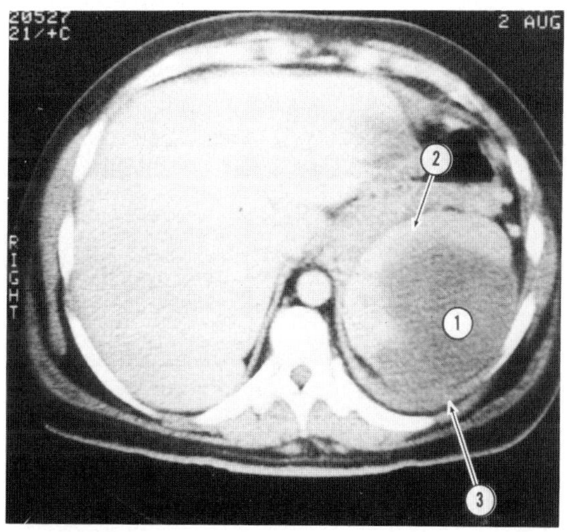


**Figure 13-2.** CT scan shows a large pancreatic pseudocyst (*1*) intimately related to the hilum of the spleen (*2*). There is edema of the soft-tissue planes posterior to the cyst (*3*). The patient had a history of chronic pancreatitis with unremitting abdominal pain and abnormal pancreatic function studies. The serum amylase level was persistently elevated. The pancreatic pseudocyst was removed in its entirety along with the spleen.

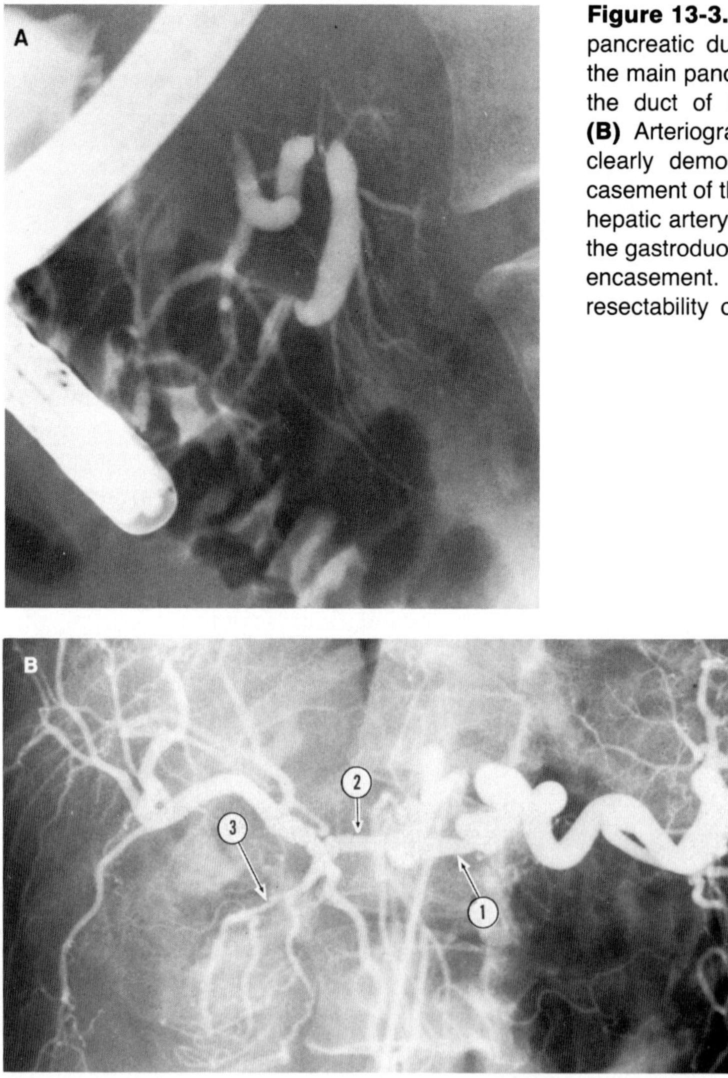


**Figure 13-3. (A)** Retrograde cannulation of the pancreatic duct demonstrates sharp amputation of the main pancreatic duct at the level of the takeoff of the duct of Santorini, consistent with carcinoma. **(B)** Arteriography performed for staging purposes clearly demonstrates malignant invasion and encasement of the splenic artery at its origin (*1*) and the hepatic artery (*2*). Other abnormal vessels related to the gastroduodenal artery (*3*) demonstrate malignant encasement. Arteriography thus verified the unresectability of this patient's pancreatic carcinoma.

Endoscopic retrograde cholangiopancreatography can establish the diagnosis of pancreatic carcinoma with great accuracy (approximately 95%). The most common finding in pancreatic malignancy is partial or complete stricture of the pancreatic duct. Carcinomas in the head of the pancreas also tend to produce strictures and varying degrees of obstruction of the common bile duct early in the course of the disease. In the absence of a history of pancreatitis, strictures of both the pancreatic and biliary ducts ("double-duct" sign) are characteristic of carcinoma. Like CT, ERCP has difficulty in separating benign from malignant strictures in patients with chronic pancreatitis. Aspiration cytology via the cannula can provide malignant cells in approximately 50% of patients with carcinoma (Fig. 13-4). Endoscopic retrograde cholangiopancreatography is of little value in staging cancer of the pancreas, because it gives little or no information about invasion of local structures or distant metastases to lymph nodes or liver. Some islet cell tumors with findings similar to carcinoma have been detected by ERCP, and ERCP also can demonstrate carcinoma of the papilla of Vater and provide an opportunity for a confirming biopsy at the same time.

Patients with acute pancreatitis usually do

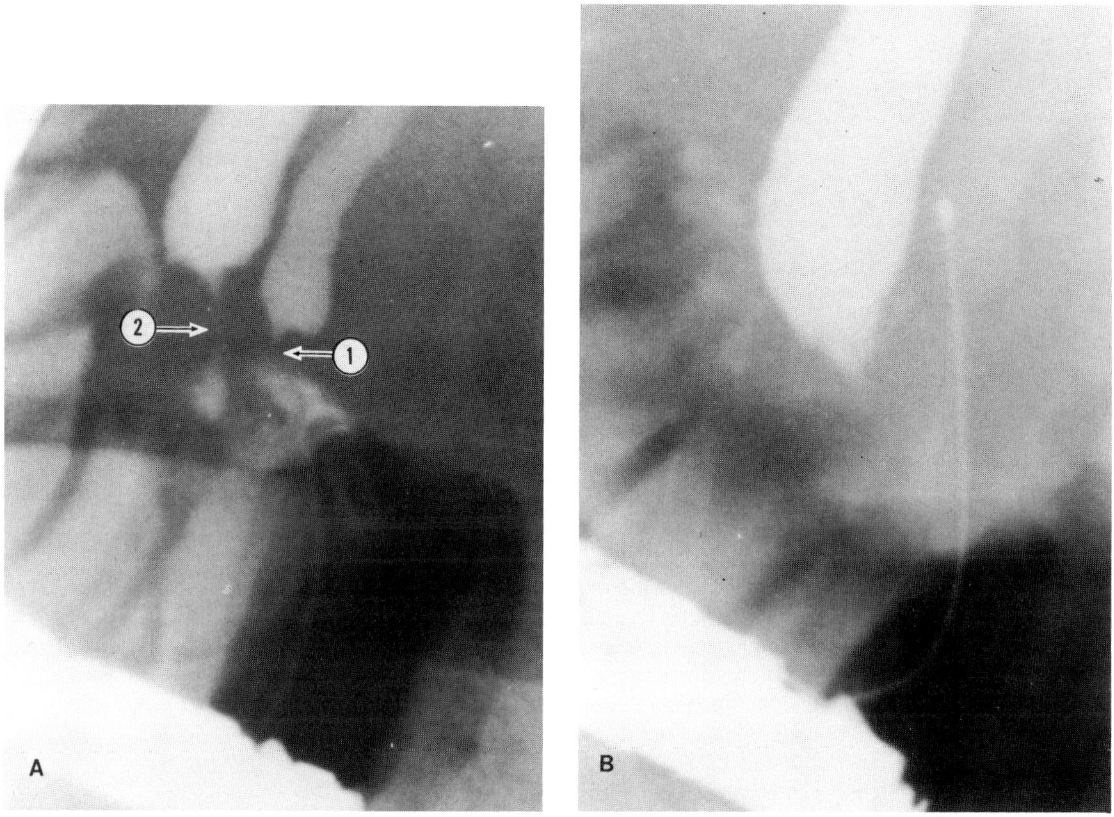


**Figure 13-4.** **(A)** ERCP demonstrates short strictures of the main pancreatic duct (*1*) and the common bile duct (*2*), findings that are characteristic of carcinoma of the pancreas involving the distal common duct. **(B)** A magnified film demonstrates the cytology brush inserted into the pancreatic duct at the time of ERCP to obtain cytologic material, which in this case was positive for malignancy.

not have any significant abnormalities on ERCP; indeed, the procedure is generally contraindicated in acute disease. In patients with chronic pancreatitis, ERCP is generally not used as a diagnostic tool but rather as a method for determining the extent and nature of the disease and for evaluating complications. It can confirm the diagnosis and detect the presence of strictures, ductal stones, and areas of ductal disruption and communication with previously known or unknown pseudocysts (Fig. 13-5). Endoscopic retrograde cholangiopancreatography is usually not indicated in patients with known pseudocysts because of the danger of introducing pancreatic sepsis. However, it can be employed as a preoperative planning procedure to evaluate the level of ductal disruption and to document strictures or stones that may need to be bypassed or removed at surgery.

In the presence of congenital nonfusion between the dorsal and ventral pancreatic anlagen (5% of normals), the majority of the pancreas may be unavailable for direct study by cannulating the major papilla. With experience, the minor papilla can now be cannulated in most of these patients so that the complete pancreas can be evaluated. Annular pancreas can be diagnosed with certainty by ERCP.

Transhepatic cholangiography (THC) has been widely used to evaluate patients with obstructive jaundice who may have severe narrowing of the common bile duct due to pancreatic disease. The use of this procedure has decreased since the advent of ERCP, although the choice of

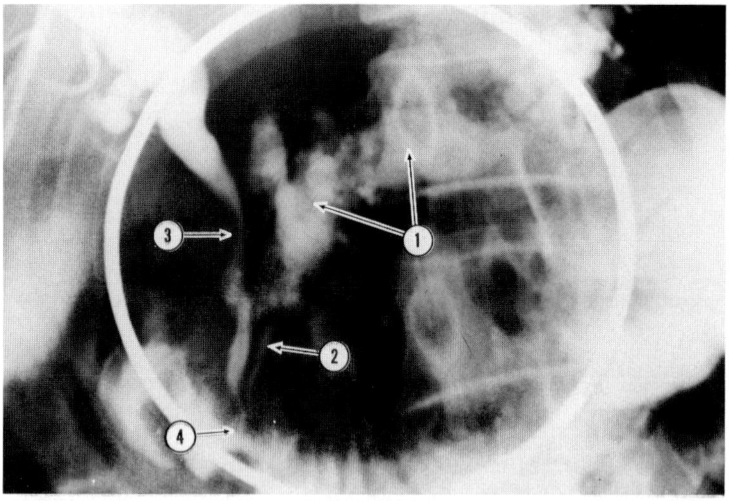


**Figure 13-5.** Compression spot film taken at the time of ERCP demonstrates the changes involving the pancreatic duct (*1*) seen in chronic pancreatitis. There is ectasia and irregularity of the main duct and lateral branches, as well as numerous calcifications that are not well demonstrated on this film. No communicating pseudocysts are shown. The main pancreatic duct in the head of the pancreas is narrowed (*2*). The common bile duct is also stenotic as it passes through the head of the pancreas (*3*). The stenosis of the common duct causes partial obstruction to the biliary tree, as evidenced by the dilated biliary structures above this stricture. Although a malignant obstruction in the head of the pancreas could be present in this patient with chronic pancreatitis, no malignancy was subsequently found. Aspiration cytology directed at the stricture of the main pancreatic duct could easily be performed at the time of this ERCP. Note that the location of the papilla of Vater (*4*) must be clearly demonstrated radiographically to evaluate the length of any strictures that might be present.

procedure is generally determined by local expertise and the questions to be answered. Endoscopic retrograde cholangiopancreatography has the advantage of being able to directly visualize the pancreatic duct. Patients with conditions such as cholodocholithiasis or papillary stenosis who are likely to benefit from therapeutic papillotomy are candidates for ERCP rather than THC. Conversely, THC is recommended for patients with high bile duct strictures at the porta hepatis. In the presence of high-grade or complete bile duct obstruction, ERCP cannot adquately delineate the upper margin of the lesion, a determination that is essential in the selection of the appropriate interventional procedure or surgery to treat the biliary obstruction. In some cases, both ERCP and THC are necessary to completely define the anatomy of an obstructing process. Both THC and ERCP can be used for interventional biliary duct procedures such as balloon dilatation of benign strictures and stenting of benign or malignant strictures. In many patients with carcinoma of the pancreas, nonoperative management of malignant biliary strictures is now the treatment of choice.

## Magnetic Resonance Imaging

Although the anatomic information provided by CT scanning may eventually be augmented by magnetic resonance imaging (MRI), the current role and usefulness of MRI in evaluating the pancreas has not been firmly established. It is hoped that MRI will assist in the detection and staging of pancreatic neoplasms as well as in following the response to therapy. In the future, the ability to generate sagittal and coronal images may prove to be of significant benefit in patients with both benign and malignant pancreatic disease.

### Radionuclide Imaging

For a time there was hope that radionuclide imaging could solve the problems associated with detecting pancreatic disease. Scans with $^{75}$Se methionine have a reported sensitivity of 75% to 80%. However, the procedure has an unacceptably high false-positive rate (30%–35%). Because nuclear scanning is so nonspecific, it is of little value in screening for pancreatic disease or in other stages of the diagnostic workup.

### Aspiration Cytology

Fine-needle aspiration cytology of the pancreas, using a 21- to 23-gauge needle, has become an acceptable and rapid method for confirming the presence of pancreatic malignancy. After the mass is localized by CT, ultrasound, THC, or ERCP, a percutaneous approach is made with transabdominal sampling (Fig. 13-6). In the presence of cancer, positive cytologic findings can be expected in 75% to 100% of patients. Because it is common to find a small primary malignancy with much surrounding inflammatory disease, tissue-sampling errors may occur. This means that negative cytologic findings do not exclude malignancy.

The ability to obtain a cytologic diagnosis without laparotomy makes fine-needle aspiration an extremely useful procedure. When cou-

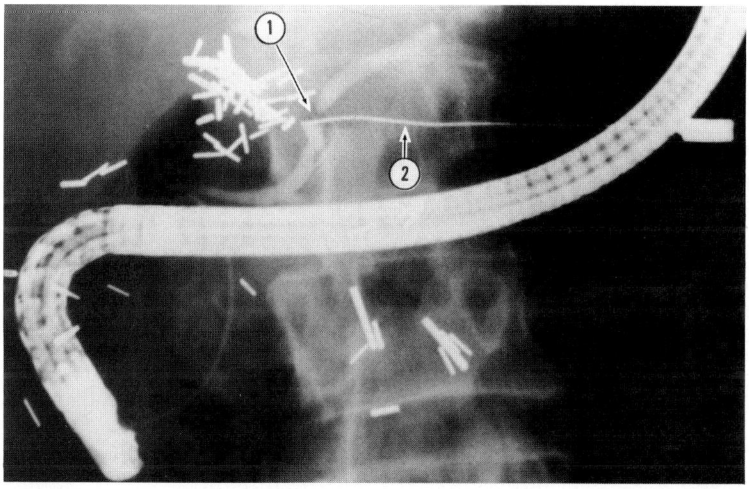


**Figure 13-6.** Repeat ERCP in a young patient with recurrent bouts of abdominal pain in whom exploratory surgery (leaving many clips) was performed 6 weeks previously because of a stricture found in the main pancreatic duct on a prior ERCP. No malignancy was found at surgery. The current study documents the stricture (*1*), which is quite short and could easily be due to malignant disease. Aspiration cytology directed to the point of stricture was very accurately performed using the percutaneous approach. The needle and its tip are well seen (*2*). Benign cells were repeatedly aspirated from this site. Although malignancy was not unequivocally excluded by this procedure, the patient maintained a benign clinical course and the lesion apparently represents a benign stricture of unknown etiology in this young, nonalcoholic man.

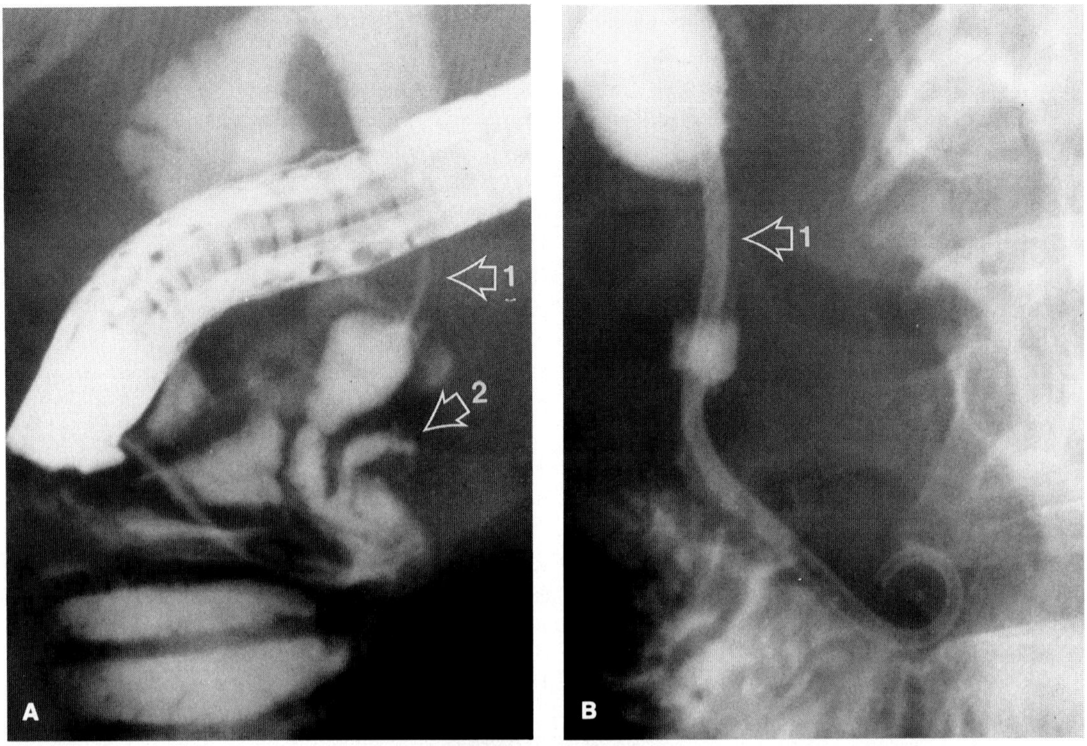


**Figure 13-7. (A)** ERCP shows a tight stricture of the common bile duct (*1*) associated with complete obstruction of the main pancreatic duct in the head of the pancreas (*2*). The location and appearance of these two strictures is virtually pathognomonic of pancreatic carcinoma in the absence of a history of pancreatitis or alcohol intake. **(B)** Percutaneous transhepatic stent (*1*) passes through the strictured segment of the common bile duct with the tip located in the duodenum providing both external and internal drainage.

pled with new transhepatic biliary drainage procedures for alleviating obstructive lesions of the pancreas, the radiologist now has an opportunity to significantly improve the quality of life remaining in patients with unresectable tumors causing biliary obstruction (Fig. 13-7).

The limiting factor of fine-needle aspiration is probably the availability of a good cytologist—a requirement for accurate diagnosis. Fine-needle aspiration cytology has few complications. Although potential tumor-seeding is a theoretical complication of needle aspiration biopsy, only rare cases have been reported, and in view of the dire prognosis of pancreatic carcinoma, this does not appear to represent a practical problem.

## COMMENT

Elegant and accurate diagnostic techniques are now available for evaluating the once elusive pancreas. It is tempting to apply these techniques liberally and often. Unfortunately, malignant disease of the pancreas carries such a grave prognosis that the only advantage to the patient in detecting a lesion may be to cease any further evaluation. It is extremely difficult to economically justify diagnostic "overkill" in this situation. By the same token, the patent with benign pancreatic disease, such as pancreatitis, should be followed by the least invasive, most inexpensive technique available. Expensive technology should not replace good judgment.

## Bibliography

Bachrach WH, Virsner JW, Izenstark JL et al: Pancreatic scanning: A review. Gastroenterology 63: 890–910, 1972

Barkin J, Vining D, Miale A, Jr et al: Computerized tomography, diagnostic ultrasound, and radionuclide scanning. JAMA 238:2040–2042, 1977

Blackstone MO, Cockerham L, Kirsner JB et al: Intraductal aspiration for cytodiagnosis in pancreatic malignancy. Gastrointest Endosc 22:221, 1976

Bookstien JJ, Reuter SR, Martel W: Angiographic evaluation of pancreatic carcinoma. Radiology 93:757–764, 1969

Cosgrove H, Legge D, O'Connell FX et al: Angiographic evaluation of gastrointestinal hemorrhage complicating pancreatic disease. Clin Radiol 29:289–293, 1978

Cubilla AL, Fitzgerald PJ: Classification of pancreatic cancer (nonendocrine). Mayo Clin Proc 54: 449–458, 1979

DiMagno EP, Malagelada JR, Taylor WF et al: A prospective comparison of current diagnostic tests for pancreatic cancer. N Engl J Med 297: 737–741, 1977

Eaton SB, Ferrucci JT, Jr, Benedict KT, Jr: A comprehensive evaluation of radiologic exploration of the pancreas. CRC Crit Rev Radiol Sci 1: 165–205, 1970

Feinberg SB, Schreiber DR, Goodale R: Comparison of ultrasound pancreatic scanning and endoscopic retrograde cholangiopancreatograms: A retrospective study. J Clin Ultrasound 5:96–100, 1977

Ferrucci JT, Jr, Mueller Pr, Harbin MN: Percutaneous transheptaic biliary drainage. Radiology 135: 1–13, 1980

Ferrucci JT, Jr, Wittenberg J: A comprehensive approach for diagnosis of pancreatic disease. Radiology 136:255–256, 1980

Ferrucci JT, Jr, Wittenberg J, Margolies MN et al: Malignant seeding of the tract after thin-needle aspiration biopsy. Radiology 130:345–346, 1979

Fitzgerald PJ, Fortner JG, Watson RC et al: The value of diagnostic aids in detecting pancreas cancer. Cancer 41:868–879, 1978

Foley, WD, Stewart ET, Lawson TL et al: Computed tomography, ultrasonography, and endoscopic retrograde cholangiopancreatography in the diagnosis of pancreatic disease: A comparative study. Gastrointest Radiol 5:29–35, 1980

Freeny PC, Ball TJ: Evaluation of endoscopic retrograde cholangiopancreatography and angiography in the diagnosis of pancreatic carcinoma. AJR 130:683–691, 1978

Freeny PC, Ball TJ: Rapid diagnosis of pancreatic carcinoma. Radiology 127:627–633, 1978

Freeny PC, Ball TJ, Ryan J: Impact of new diagnostic imaging modalities on pancreatic angiography. AJR 133:619–624, 1979

Freeny PC, Lawson TL: Radiology of the Pancreas. New York, Springer-Verlag, 1982

Goldman ML, Naib ZM, Galambos JT et al: Preoperative diagnosis of pancreatic carcinoma by percutaneous aspiration biopsy. Am J Dig Dis 22:1076–1082, 1977

Goldstein HM, Neiman HL, Bookstein JJ: Angiographic evaluation of pancreatic disease. Radiology 112:275–282, 1974

Goldstein HM, Zornoza J, Wallace S et al: Percutaneous fine needle aspiration biopsy of pancreatic and other abdominal masses. Radiology 123:319–322, 1977

Haaga JR, Alfidi RJ, Havrilla TR et al: Definitive role of CT scanning of the pancreas. Radiology 124:723–730, 1977

Hatfield ARW, Wilkins SR, Levi AJ: Assessment of endoscopic retrograde cholangiopancreatography (ERCP) and pure pancreatic juice cytology in patients with pancreatic disease. Gut 17:14–21, 1976

Ho CS, Taylor B: Percutaneous transgastric drainage for pancreatic pseudocyst. AJR 143:623–625, 1984

Husband JE, Meire HB, Kreel L: Comparison of ultrasound and computer-assisted tomography in pancreatic diagnosis. Br J Radiol 50:855–862, 1977

Karlson KB, Martin EC, Fankuchen EI et al: Percutaneous drainage of pancreatic pseudocysts and abscesses. Radiology 142:619–624, 1982

Lawson TL: Sensitivity of pancreatic ultrasonography in the detection of pancreatic disease. Radiology 128:733–736, 1978

McLoughlin MJ, Ho CS, Langer B et al: Fine needle aspiration biopsy of malignant lesions in and around the pancreas. Cancer 41:2413–2419, 1978

Mueller PR, Ferrucci JT, Jr, Simeone JF et al: Lesser sac abscesses and fluid collections: Drainage by transhepatic approach. Radiology 155:615–618, 1985

Osnes M, Hanssen AS, Myren J: Endoscopic retrograde brush cytology (ERCP) of the biliary and pancreatic ducts. Scand J Gastroenterol 10: 829–831, 1975

Reuter SR: Superselective pancreatic angiography. In

Anacker H (ed): Efficiency and Limits of Radiologic Examination of the Pancreas, pp 149–158. Acton, MA, Thieme-Edition, 1975

Ring EJ, Aleaga JA, Freiman DB et al: Therapeutic applications of catheter cholangiography. Radiology 128:333–338, 1978

Smith EH, Bartrum RJ, Jr, Chang YC: Ultrasonically guided percutaneous aspiration biopsy of the pancreas. Radiology 112:737–738, 1974

Stanley RJ, Sagel SS, Levitt RG: Computed tomographic evaluation of the pancreas. Radiology 124:715–722, 1977

Stewart ET, Geenen JE: Endoscopic retrograde cholangiography. In Berk RN, Ferrucci JT, Jr, Leopold GR (eds): Radiology of the Gallbladder and Bile Ducts: Diagnosis and Intervention, pp 367–400. Philadelphia, WB Saunders, 1983

Stewart ET, Vennes JA, Geenen JE: Atlas of Endoscopic Retrograde Cholangiopancreatography. St. Louis, CV Mosby, 1977

## ACUTE PANCREATITIS

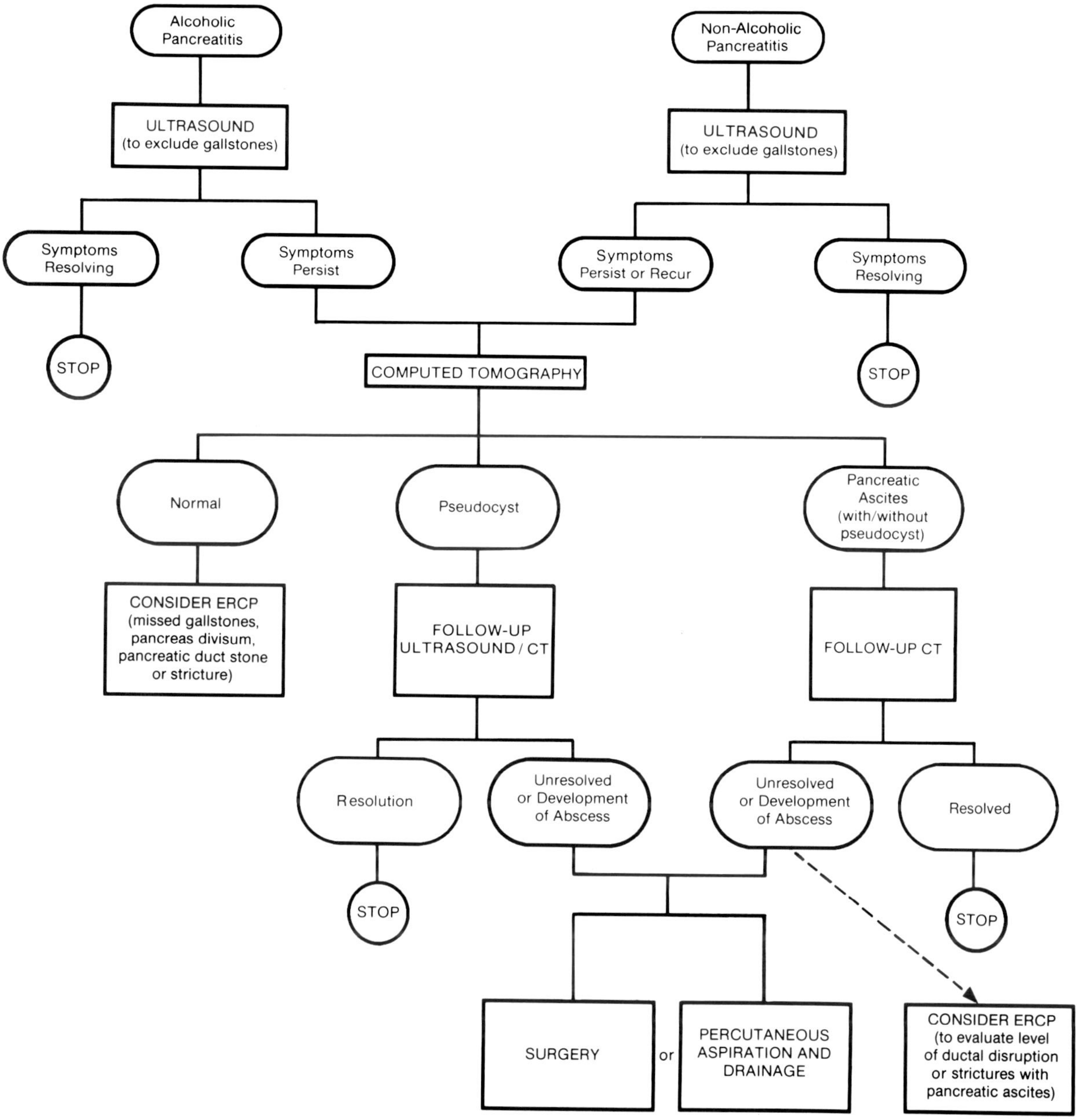

# CHRONIC PANCREATITIS

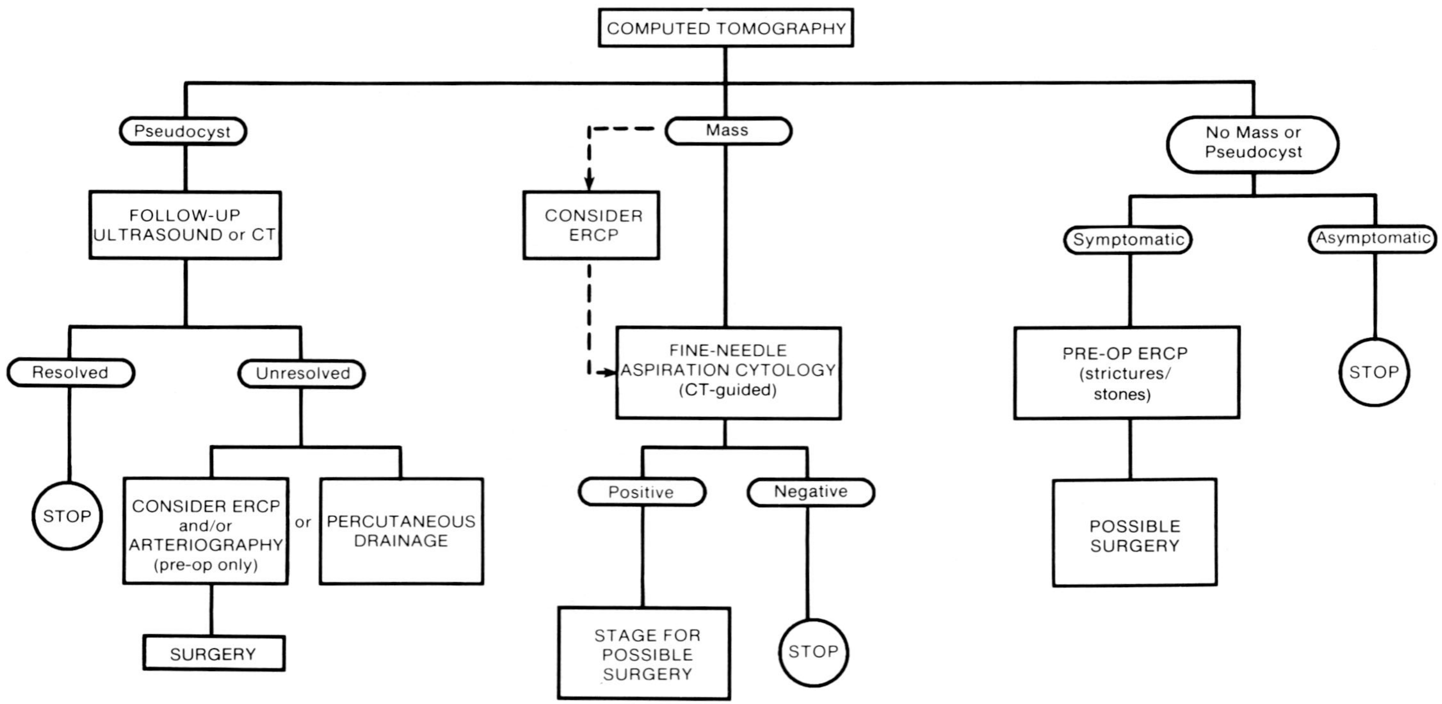

## SUSPECTED CARCINOMA OF THE PANCREAS
(No History of Pancreatitis)

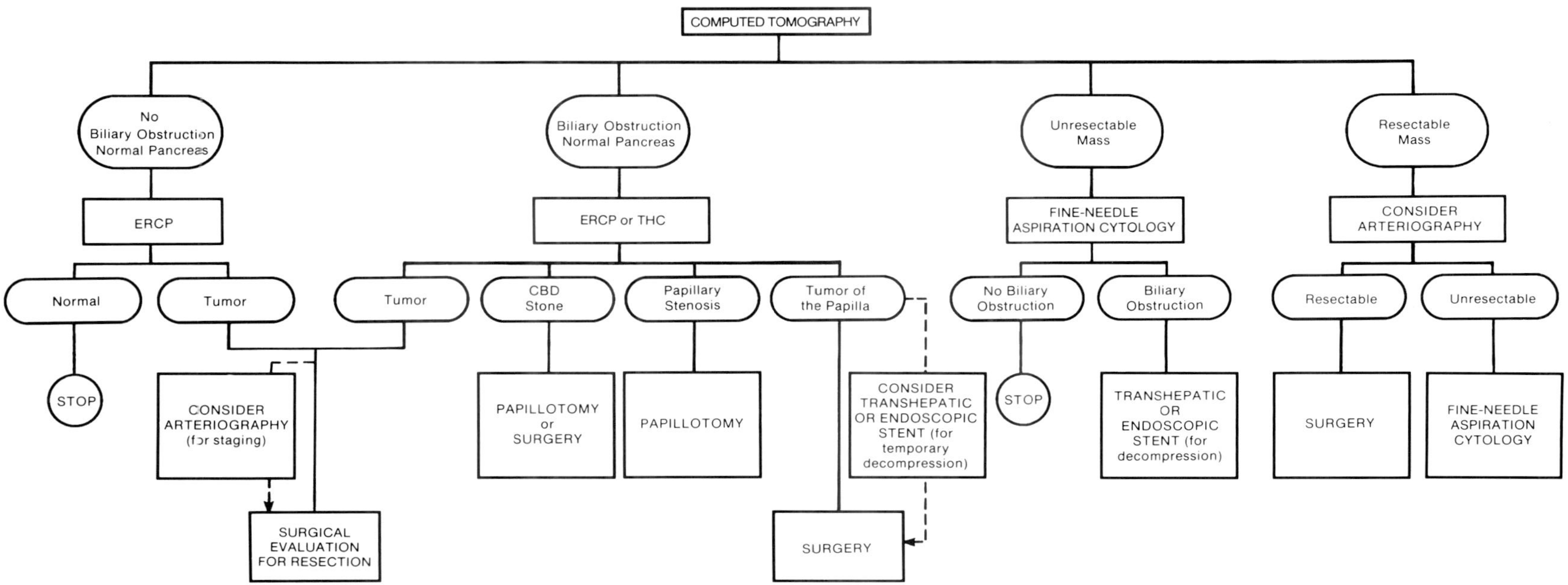

# Chapter 14

# Palpable Abdominal Masses

*Richard M. Gore*

The traditional radiographic evaluation of a palpable abdominal mass consists of plain abdominal radiographs, excretory urography, oral cholecystography, and conventional barium studies of the stomach, small bowel, and colon. Although these techniques occasionally suggest a specific diagnosis, they most often reveal only indirect evidence of an abdominal mass, such as displacement of normal structures and obliteration of normal interfaces. Consequently, exploratory laparotomy is frequently necessary to provide a definite diagnosis. During the past decade, advances in computed tomography (CT), ultrasound, and magnetic resonance imaging (MRI) have made the characterization of abdominal masses relatively simple and direct. The exquisite spatial and density resolution of these imaging modalities permits more accurate diagnosis, preoperative staging, and follow-up of disease than was ever previously possible. Indeed, when combined with percutaneous aspiration biopsy, these modalities now obviate the need for exploratory laparotomy in most instances.

## CLINICAL CONSIDERATIONS

It is essential to correlate the clinical location of a palpable abdominal mass with the history and laboratory findings in order to select the most expeditious and cost-effective imaging workup. For ease of discussion, the location of clinically palpable masses can be categorized as follows: right upper quadrant; epigastric; left upper quadrant; midline or midabdominal; right lower quadrant; hypogastric; left lower quadrant; and diffusely enlarged abdomen. Once a mass is detected, it is necessary to determine the organ or space of origin, size, relation to other structures, and whether the mass is cystic or solid, benign or malignant.

## DIAGNOSTIC EVALUATION

### *DIAGNOSTIC MODALITIES*

1. Plain abdominal radiographs
2. Conventional barium studies

3. Excretory urography
4. Arteriography and venography
5. Radionuclide scanning
6. Magnetic resonance imaging
7. Ultrasound
8. Computed tomography
9. Percutaneous aspiration biopsy

## IMAGING SEQUENCE

Although each palpable abdominal mass requires an individualized radiographic approach, there are certain fundamental principles that determine imaging sequence. If ultrasound, CT, MRI, angiography, or radionuclide studies are likely to provide a reasonably specific diagnosis, these procedures should be used prior to barium studies. Barium causes streak artifacts on CT, attenuates the photons emitted by radioisotopes, scatters the insonating ultrasound beam, degrades MR images, and obscures intravascular contrast material. Therefore, barium studies are not generally advocated in the initial imaging of palpable abdominal masses, with the exception of those located in the lower abdomen.

### Plain Abdominal Radiographs

Although the plain abdominal radiograph may seem an anachronism in this era of high-technology cross-sectional imaging, this low-yield, albeit low-cost, technique occasionally can make a specific diagnosis, such as a calcified aortic aneurysm, gastric pseudotumor, fecal impaction, or an enlarged porcelain or "milk of calcium" gallbladder. Most often, the plain abdominal radiograph only yields nonspecific and indirect evidence of a mass, such as alteration in the size or density of an organ, displacement of normal structures or bowel, and obscuration of fat planes.

### Conventional Barium Studies

Air-contrast barium studies provide unmatched radiographic visualization of mucosal abnormalities of the alimentary tract. However, in recent years, barium studies have been relegated to an adjunctive role in the evaluation of upper and midabdominal masses. Unless the mass arises from the alimentary tract, barium studies only show indirect signs of a mass, such as separation and displacement of bowel loops or traction and spiculation of the mucosa by a subserosal mass.

Barium studies do have a primary role in the adult patient with a lower abdominal mass whose history suggests gastrointestinal pathology, such as a neoplasm (anemia and weight loss) or an inflammatory mass (fever, leukocytosis). The role of barium studies in these clinical situations is discussed later in this chapter in the sections on right- and left-lower-quadrant masses.

### Excretory Urography

Excretory urography is not recommended as a primary examination in the evaluation of a patient with a palpable abdominal mass. Unless the mass originates in the kidney, the excretory urogram only demonstrates indirect signs, such as displacement or obstruction of the kidney and ureter. In addition, CT, ultrasound, and MRI can more directly image renal masses that have reached a palpable size. If it is important for the surgeon to know the status of the ureters prior to abdominal surgery, this information can be obtained on a plain abdominal radiograph taken following contrast-enhanced CT.

### Arteriography and Venography

Computed tomography, ultrasound, and MRI have relegated arteriography and venography to secondary roles in the evaluation of palpable abdominal masses. The major use of arteriography and venography is to provide a vascular road map prior to surgery. These modalities also remain as the "gold standard" for assessing vascular occlusion or tumor invasion into blood vessels (inferior vena cava, aorta, renal artery and vein, splenic vein) and for confirming the presence of an aneurysm detected by other modalities.

## Radionuclide Scanning

The cross-section imaging modalities have virtually eliminated the use of radionuclide studies in the evaluation of palpable abdominal masses. Although $^{67}$Ga can be used to detect occult infections and tumors, this technique is nonspecific and may take up to 72 hours to perform. Scanning with $^{99m}$Tc sulfur colloid can demonstrate the size of the liver and spleen but is nonspecific in terms of characterizing space-occupying lesions within these organs. Sulfur colloid scanning is still of value in determining whether a left-upper-quadrant mass represents an accessory spleen or residual splenic tissue following splenectomy.

## Magnetic Resonance Imaging

Magnetic resonance imaging can provide unique, clinically useful images of the lower abdomen and pelvis and can directly display masses in sagittal, coronal, oblique, and transverse planes. Because of its exquisite soft-tissue density discrimination, MRI can detect subtle invasion of tumors into adjacent structures. Mass effects on and invasion of vascular structures such as the inferior vena cava, renal veins, and aorta can be well demonstrated. Current limitations of the use of MRI in the upper abdomen include respiratory motion artifacts, length of data acquisition, lack of optimal oral contrast material to outline the alimentary tract, and high cost. With the exception of the last problem, most of the other limiting factors should be resolved in the near future. At the present time, MRI is too expensive to be advocated as a primary imaging modality for upper and middle abdominal masses, because its cost effectiveness in relation to CT and ultrasound has yet to be established.

## Ultrasound

The advantages of ultrasound in the evaluation of palpable abdominal masses include its general availability, speed, lack of ionizing radiation, relatively low cost, ability to be transported to the bedside, and minimum need for patient preparation and cooperation. This modality can distinguish solid from cystic structures and can be used regardless of organ function.

The major limitation of ultrasound in the abdomen is the adverse effect of acoustic barriers (gas, bone, barium) that reflect the insonating beam and do not permit the evaluation of deeper structures. Thus, internal lesions of the gas-filled alimentary tract are difficult to demonstrate. Ultrasound is most effective in regions where "acoustic windows" exist. These include the right upper quadrant, where the liver and right kidney displace bowel gas; the pelvis, where the fluid-filled bladder acts as a window; and to a lesser extent the left upper quadrant, where the window is provided by the spleen and left kidney. Another important limitation of ultrasound is the need for direct contact of the transducer to the skin using an acoustic coupling agent. Overlying dressings, retention sutures, stomas, drains, and open wounds prevent effective scanning. The spatial resolution of ultrasound also decreases with increasing penetration depth.

## Computed Tomography

Computed tomography has evolved as the most efficient imaging modality for evaluating the palpable abdominal mass. Among the many advantages of CT are its excellent spatial resolution (1 mm–2 mm), exquisite density discrimination, and fast scanning time ($\leq$2 sec) as well as its ability to provide cross-sectional images unaffected by bowel gas, bone, excessive abdominal fat, or skin wounds. Computed tomography provides good visualization of vascular structures and can assess the vascularity of an abdominal mass after the intravenous administration of contrast material. Computed tomography routinely visualizes the retroperitoneal structures and displays the peritoneal compartments well, defining tissue planes and relations between masses and organs. With adequate bowel opacification, an absolute necessity for evaluating abdominal masses, mural and serosal abnormalities of the gastrointestinal tract may be demonstrated. Indeed, CT has proven useful for staging alimentary tract neoplasms and for evaluating patients with inflammatory bowel disease. If the patient cannot or will not allow opacification of the gut, the accuracy of CT in evaluating the alimentary tract, omentum, mesentery, and pelvis is dramatically reduced. Unopacified bowel loops can simulate an abscess, mesenteric tumor, or enlarged lymph nodes.

### Percutaneous Aspiration Biopsy

Once a palpable abdominal mass is detected, localized, and partially characterized by the various imaging techniques, percutaneous aspiration biopsy is the final radiographic diagnostic step. Aspiration biopsy has achieved uniform acceptance as a safe, effective means of establishing the tissue diagnosis of an abdominal mass. Biopsies can be performed with "skinny" needles (22 gauge) that provide cytologic material or larger cutting needles (18–20 gauge) that can give histology as well. Both CT and ultrasound can be used for biopsy localization. If a mass has reached sufficient size to become palpable, biopsy localization is generally performed using ultrasound, which is less time consuming and expensive. The position of the needle can be confirmed either by using a biopsy transducer or by angling the ultrasound transducer toward the mass, away from the sterile field, and observing the echoes cast by the biopsy needle. Computed tomography–guided biopsies have a 90% to 95% accuracy and are recommended for small masses and masses adjacent to infected structures, and in those instances in which the entire path of the biopsy needle must be monitored. Computed tomographic guidance is also valuable in patients who are obese, who are difficult to position, or who have skin wounds and drains.

## SPECIFIC ANATOMIC CONSIDERATIONS

### Right-Upper-Quadrant Masses

Right-upper-quadrant masses can originate from the right lobe of the liver, gallbladder, bile ducts, hepatic flexure of the colon, right adrenal gland, right kidney, or duodenum. Because the liver and kidney provide an acoustic window, ultrasound is recommended as the initial imaging modality for palpable masses in this region.

Ultrasound has a greater than 95% accuracy in detecting significant gallbladder disease. Acute cholecystitis (Fig. 14-1), hydrops, carcinoma of the gallbladder, and a Courvoisier gallbladder are common causes of right-upper-quadrant masses that are well demonstrated by ultrasound. If there is coexistent dilatation of the bile ducts and ultrasound fails to show an obstructing mass, CT should be obtained. Ultrasound can usually detect choledochal cysts that enlarge sufficiently to present as a right supramesocolic mass unless the cyst lies behind the second portion of the duodenum and is thus obscured by overlying bowel gas.

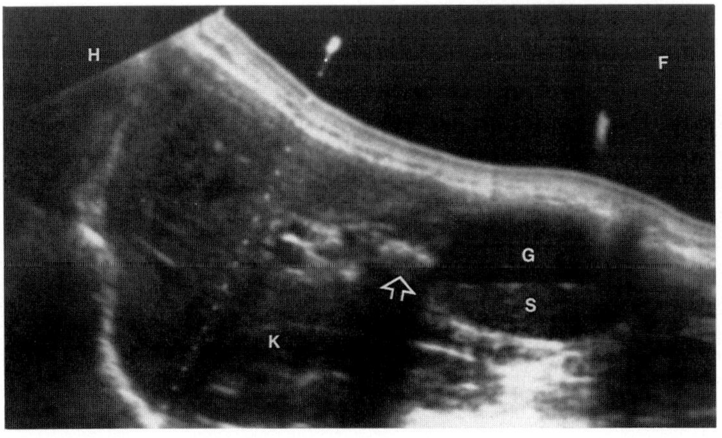


**Figure 14-1.** Acute cholecystitis. Longitudinal sonogram in a 56-year-old woman with a tender right-upper-quadrant mass demonstrates distention of the gallbladder (G) and sludge (S) within its lumen. Obstructing stones (*open arrows*) in the neck of the gallbladder cast an acoustic shadow. (*H,* cephalic; *F,* caudal; *K,* kidney)

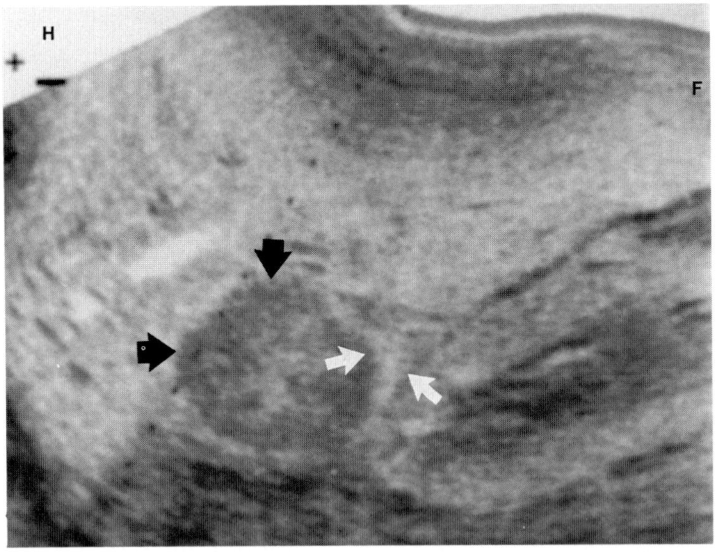


**Figure 14-2.** Adrenal metastases. Longitudinal sonogram in a 47-year-old woman with ill-defined right-upper-quadrant pain and fullness demonstrates a large adrenal mass (*black arrows*) and hepatomegaly. The mass can be localized to the adrenal gland because it causes wedging (*white arrows*) of the retroperitoneal fat between the mass and the kidney. (*H,* cephalic; *F,* caudal)

Renal lesions comprise the largest group of retroperitoneal tumors that present as abdominal masses. Ultrasound is an excellent screening modality for differentiating the common renal cysts from solid tumors or abscesses. If a renal mass is solid, a CT scan is recommended for confirmation and tumor staging.

Adrenal masses such as metastases (Fig. 14-2), nonfunctioning adenomas, and carcinomas are best diagnosed on CT; but if they are large, these lesions can be accurately shown by ultrasound. Diffuse hepatomegaly (Fig. 14-3), large primary (Fig. 14-4) or secondary neoplasms, and abscesses may present as right-upper-quadrant masses and are well demonstrated on CT, ultrasound, MRI, and radionuclides studies. Ultrasound is the most cost-effective method for evaluating hepatic size and has a 97% accuracy in detecting hepatic masses.

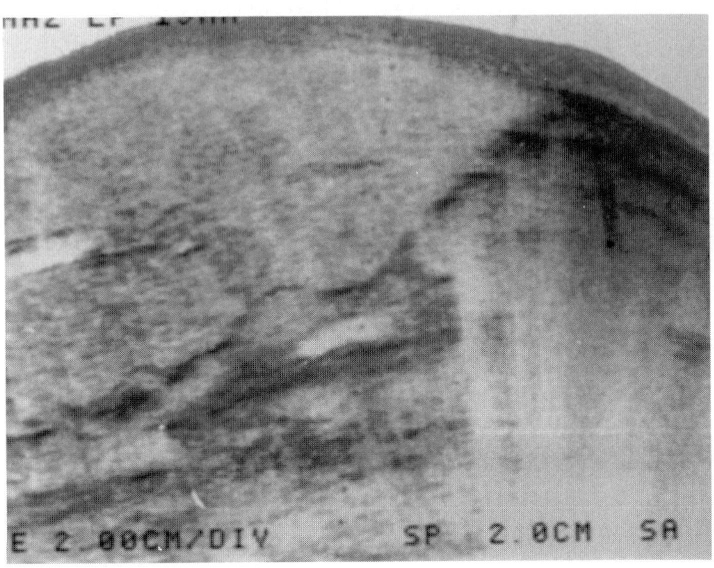


**Figure 14-3.** Diffuse hepatomegaly. Longitudinal sonogram of the right upper quadrant in a patient with non-Hodgkin's lymphoma shows generalized liver enlargement but no discrete masses.

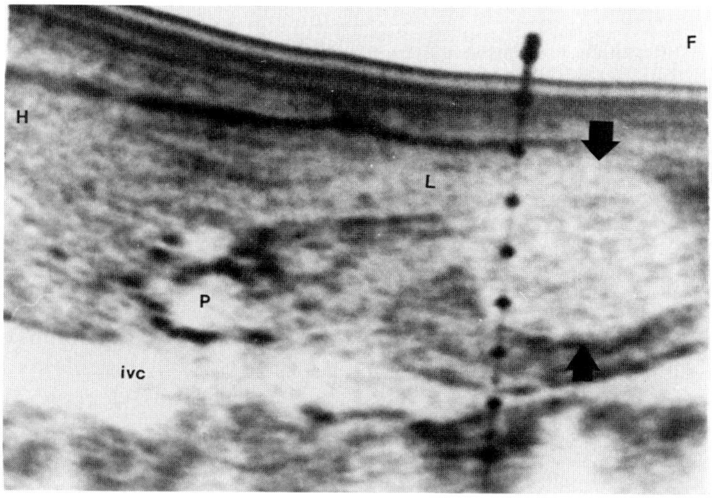


**Figure 14-4.** Hepatic adenoma. Longitudinal sonogram in a 29-year-old patient with the acute onset of right-upper-quadrant pain and an associated mass demonstrates a large hypoechoic mass (*arrows*) extending from the inferior aspect of the liver (*L*). (*H,* cephalic; *F,* caudal; *P,* portal vein; *ivc,* inferior vena cava)

Although barium studies are needed to establish the diagnosis of carcinoma of the duodenum or hepatic flexure presenting as a right-upper-quadrant mass, ultrasound and CT can show distinctive abnormalities. On ultrasound, the abnormal bowel produces a "target" or "cockade" sign consisting of an echogenic center (lumen, mucosa, gas) that may be eccentrically placed and is surrounded by the hypoechoic thickened bowel wall. This appearance is nonspecific and can be seen in Crohn's disease, ulcerative colitis, lymphoma, intussusception, leiomyosarcoma, and other benign and malignant disorders of the alimentary tract. On CT, the bowel wall is thickened, and if the tumor is advanced, spread into the surrounding fat or adjacent organs may be detected (Fig. 14-5).

If a right-upper-quadrant mass is extremely large, it may be difficult to determine the organ and peritoneal space of origin. A useful guide on ultrasound is the appearance of the retroperitoneal fat stripe located between the liver and right kidney. Hepatic masses cause inferior and posterior displacement of this echogenic fat line. Renal masses produce anterior and cephalic deviation of the fat, whereas adrenal masses

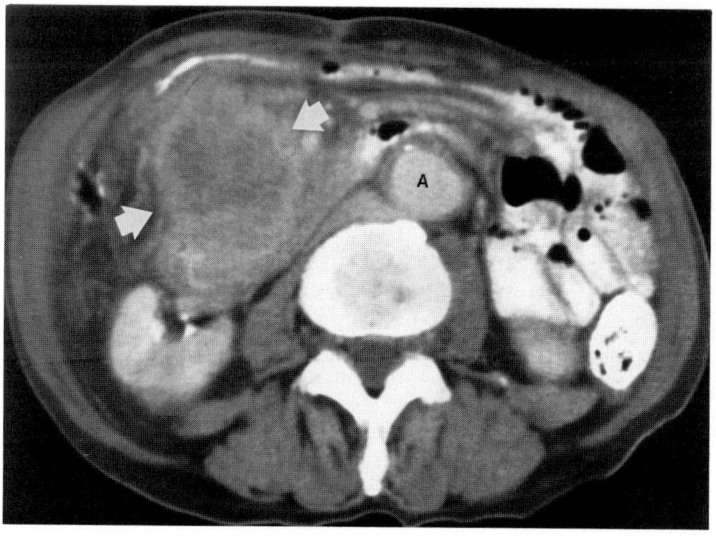


**Figure 14-5.** Adenocarcinoma of the colon. CT scan in a 63-year-old man with nonspecific constitutional complaints and a right-upper-quadrant mass demonstrates a large soft-tissue lesion of predominantly low attenuation (*arrows*). Surprisingly, the patient had no specific gastrointestinal complaints. (*A,* aneurysm of the abdominal aorta)

typically wedge the fat into a triangular configuration (see Fig. 14-2). Computed tomography can localize a right-upper-quadrant mass to the retroperitoneum by demonstrating obliteration of the perinephric fat outlining the psoas muscle, lateral displacement of fat outlining the posterior right lobe of the liver, rotation of the intrahepatic veins to the left, anterior displacement of the inferior vena cava and renal vein, or anterior displacement of the ascending colon or pancreatic head.

## Epigastric Masses

Epigastric masses most commonly arise from the liver, spleen, stomach, duodenum, or pancreas. Most pancreatic masses become symptomatic (jaundice, weight loss) before they can be palpated. Exceptions to this rule include pancreatic pseudocysts (Fig. 14-6) that may dissect anywhere in the abdominal cavity, masses of the pancreatic tail that may become huge before they are clinically apparent, phlegmonous pancreatitis, and cystadenomas and cystadenocarcinomas. Barium studies generally show lateral displacement and widening of the duodenal sweep with effacement or spiculation of the duodenal folds bordering the pancreas. The inferior margin of the gastric antrum and the posterior wall of the body or antrum may also be involved. In such cases, CT is recommended as the initial imaging modality, because ultrasound may be limited by bowel gas and body habitus. An epigastric mass can also be caused by enlargement of the left lobe of the liver due to generalized hepatomegaly, tumor (Fig. 14-7), or cirrhosis.

If the patient with an epigastric mass presents with a succussion splash or other signs and symptoms of gastric outlet obstruction, supine and erect radiographs of the abdomen should be obtained to search for a gastric pseudotumor consisting of an air-filled (Fig. 14-8) or fluid-filled stomach. A barium study can then be performed to exclude peptic ulcer disease or gastric malignancy as the cause of obstruction. If the diagnosis is still uncertain, CT is recommended as the initial modality, because it can directly image the gastric wall, pancreas, liver, and spleen and yet is not limited by bowel gas or body habitus.

## Left-Upper-Quadrant Masses

Left-upper-quadrant masses may arise from either the retroperitoneal space or the peritoneal cavity. The most common cause is splenomegaly, which may result from portal hypertension, cystic degeneration, leukemia, lymphoma, ex-

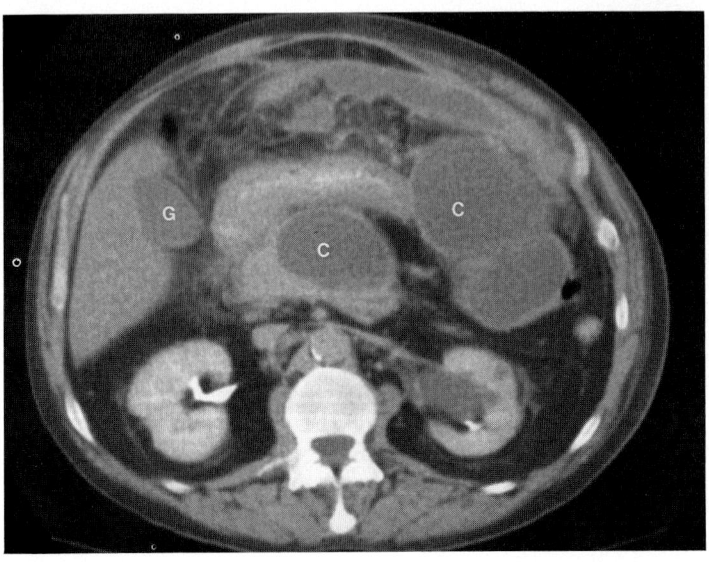


**Figure 14-6.** Pancreatic pseudocyst. CT scan obtained at the level of the left renal vein in a 42-year-old man with palpable epigastric and left-upper-quadrant masses and a history of pancreatitis shows pseudocysts (*C*) in the lesser sac, anterior pararenal space, and region of the transverse mesocolon. Note the postinflammatory changes in the peripancreatic fat. (*G,* gallbladder)

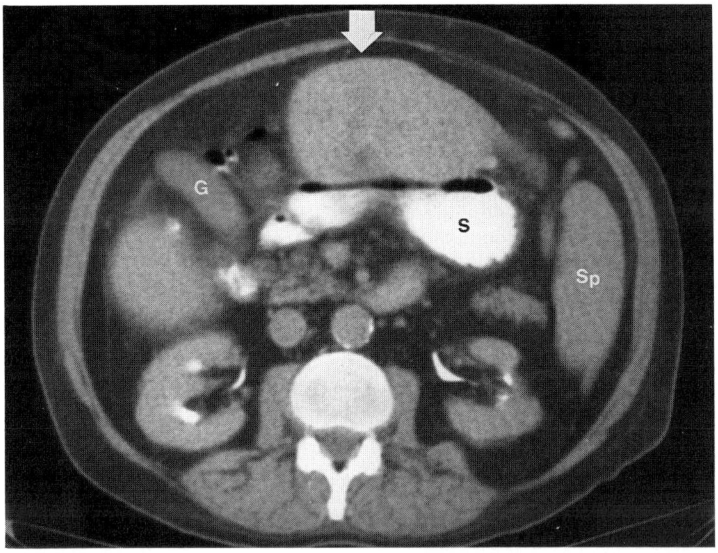


**Figure 14-7.** Hepatoma. CT scan in a 64-year-old man with weight loss and a palpable epigastric mass demonstrates marked enlargement of the left lobe of the liver (*arrow*), which contains regions of decreased attenuation. (*S,* stomach; *Sp,* spleen; *G,* gallbladder)

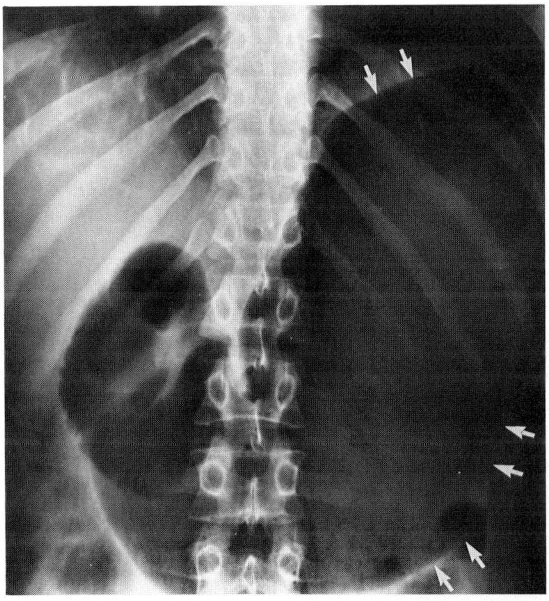

**Figure 14-8.** Gastric pseudotumor. Plain abdominal radiograph in a 38-year-old woman with nausea and epigastric pain and mass demonstrates massive dilatation of the stomach (*arrows*) and proximal duodenum. The patient was a diabetic in ketoacidosis, and the gastric distention resolved following placement of a nasogastric tube and control of her diabetes.

tramedullary hematopoiesis (Fig. 14-9), abscess, or traumatic or spontaneous hemorrhage. Other causes of palpable left-upper-quadrant masses include an enlarged left lobe of the liver, leiomyomas and other spindle cell tumors of the stomach or small bowel, primary exophytic gastric neoplasms, gastric distention due to chronic outlet obstruction, and carcinoma of the splenic flexure. Less frequent causes of left-upper-quadrant masses include mesenteric duplications or cysts, and retroperitoneal lesions such as renal, adrenal, and pancreatic masses (Fig. 14-10).

Computed tomography should be the initial imaging procedure in most patients who present with a left-upper-quadrant mass, because gas contained within the stomach, small bowel, and colon often precludes an adequate ultrasound study.

## Midabdominal Masses

Midabdominal masses are best divided into those lying in the superficial tissues or within the peritoneal or retroperitoneal compartments. Because there is such a large list of differential possibilities, it is difficult to suggest a single best imaging approach.

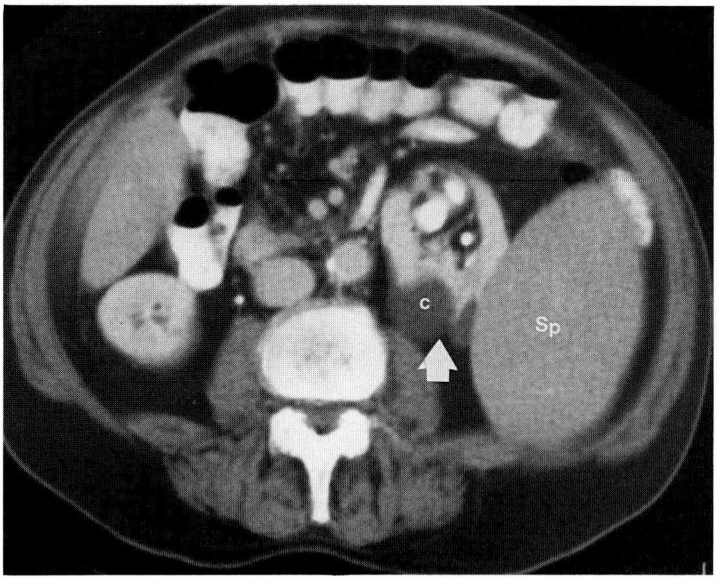


**Figure 14-9.** Splenomegaly. CT scan in a 63-year-old man with weakness, anemia, and a palpable left-upper-quadrant mass shows marked splenomegaly causing medial and anterior displacement of the left kidney (*arrow*). The patient was ultimately found to have myelofibrosis and extramedullary hematopoiesis. (*C,* left renal cyst; *Sp,* spleen)

### Superficial Masses

Rectus sheath hematomas are common sequelae of trauma, anticoagulant therapy, and bleeding diatheses. Although ultrasound can show evidence of muscle enlargement, CT and MRI can also provide better distinction between abscess and hemorrhage. If massive intra-abdominal retroperitoneal or extraperitoneal hemorrhage is suspected, CT or MRI is required for optimal evaluation of the musculature and retroperitoneum. Ventral and peristomal hernias are often detected on plain radiographs and can be confirmed by barium studies. If the hernia contains only fat, CT may be required to document this situation.

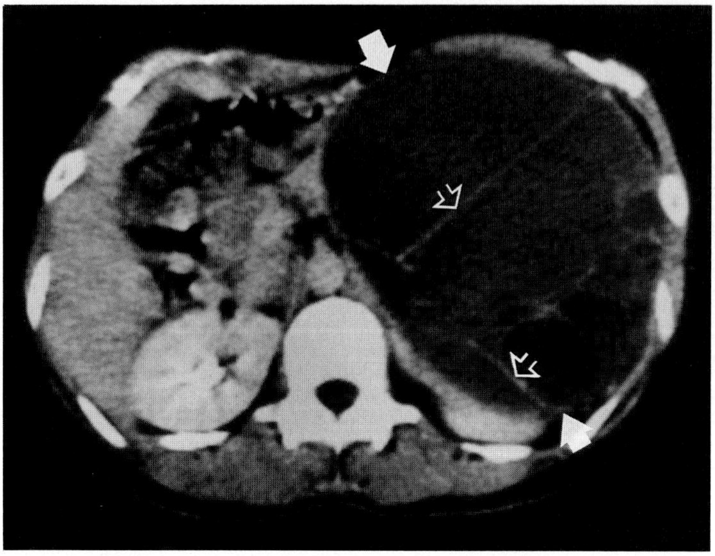

**Figure 14-10.** Cystadenocarcinoma of the pancreas. CT scan shows a huge, well-marginated, predominantly low-attenuation mass (*solid arrows*) occupying almost all of the left upper quadrant. The mass contains multiple septae (*open arrows*).

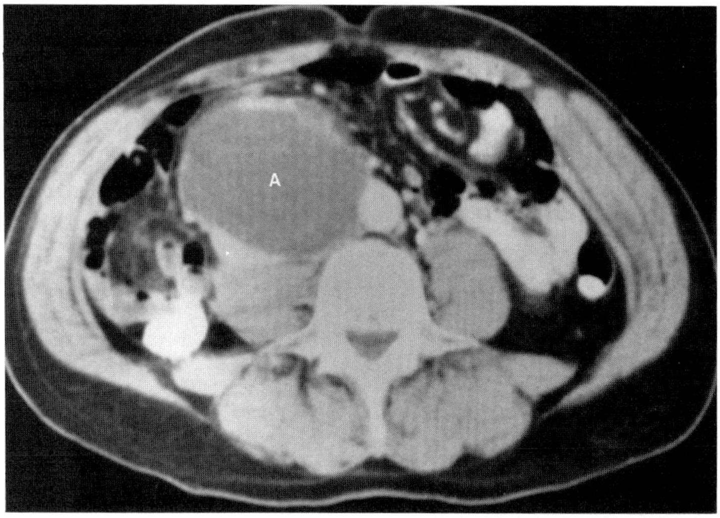


**Figure 14-11.** Abdominal abscess. CT scan in a 47-year-old man with low-grade fever, mild leukocytosis, and a palpable midabdominal mass demonstrates a low-attenuation abscess (*A*) with peripheral contrast enhancement. The abscess was aspirated and then drained percutaneously.

## Peritoneal Masses

The most common intraperitoneal midabdominal masses arise from the gastrointestinal tract and include adenocarcinoma, lympoma, leiomyoma, leiomyosarcoma, or secondary neoplasms of the small bowel and colon. Although these lesions are best evaluated by barium studies, they uncommonly present as palpable masses. When they are large enough to be felt, these neoplasms can usually be detected by CT performed after contrast opacification of the bowel.

Other intraperitoneal midabdominal masses include Meckel's diverticulum, interloop abscess (Fig. 14-11), inflammatory mesenteric masses (Crohn's disease, tuberculosis, amebiasis), duplications (jejunal, ileal), mesenteric cysts, enlarged lymph nodes (Fig. 14-12), and peritoneal implants ("omental cakes") on the

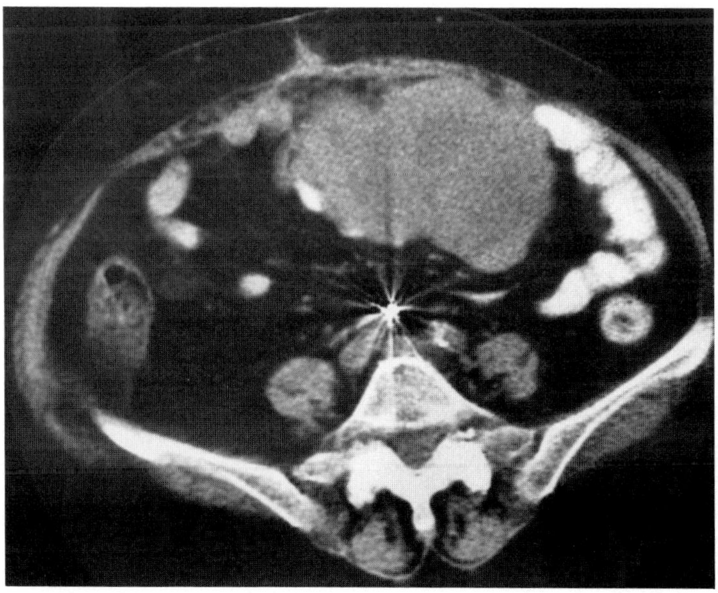

**Figure 14-12.** Non-Hodgkin's lymphoma. CT scan in a 64-year-old man with a history of lymphoma in remission for 4 years who presented with a midline abdominal mass shows a large mesenteric mass displacing bowel loops.

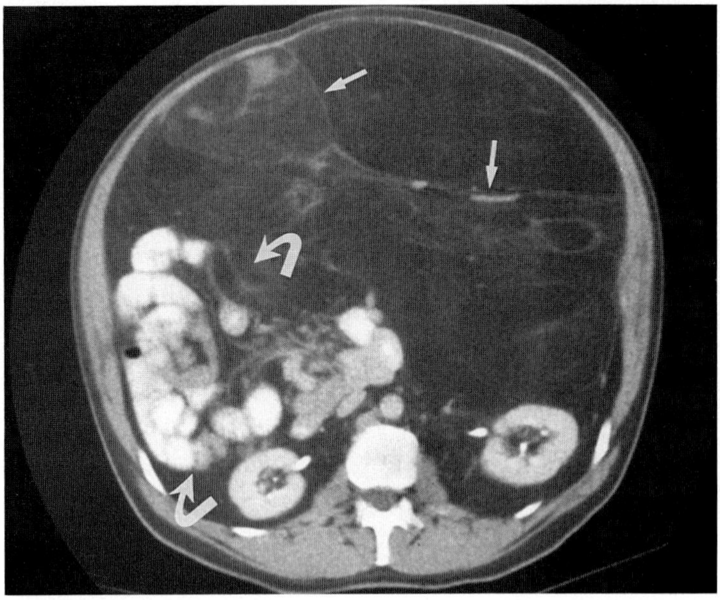

**Figure 14-13.** Liposarcoma. CT scan in a 48-year-old man who presented with slowly increasing abdominal girth demonstrates a huge mass originating in the left retroperitoneum and occupying the majority of the abdomen. The gastrointestinal tract (*curved arrows*) is compressed and displaced to the right and posterior portion of the abdomen. Multiple septations (*straight arrows*) and regions of increased attenuation are seen within this fatty mass.

greater omentum and small bowel mesentery from cancer of the colon, pancreas, stomach, or ovary.

Computed tomography is recommended as the initial imaging procedure for peritoneal mid-abdominal masses, because this modality can detect both mesenteric disease and mural abnormalities of the alimentary tract.

## Retroperitoneal Masses

Retroperitoneal masses often reach enormous proportions before the patient seeks medical attention. The most common primary retroperitoneal tumor is liposarcoma, which is best imaged by CT and classically appears as a fatty, low-attenuation mass (Fig. 14-13) with enhanc-

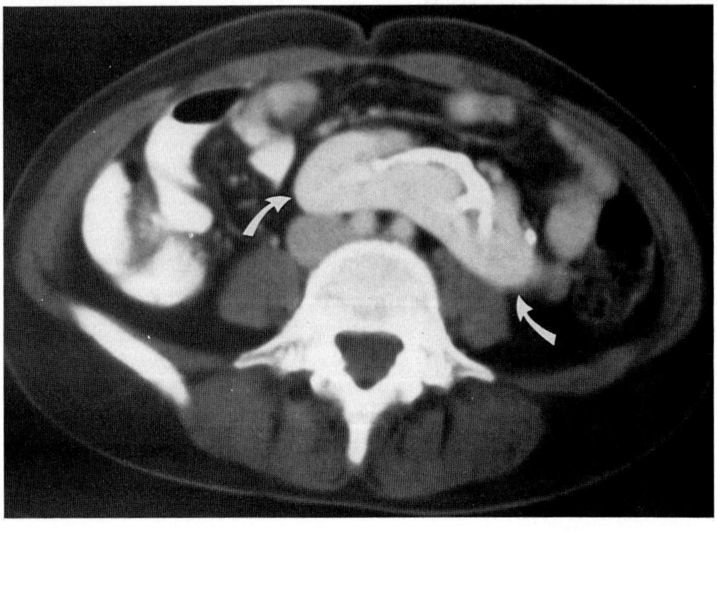

**Figure 14-14.** Horseshoe kidney. CT scan in an otherwise healthy 37-year-old woman who presented with a midline abdominal mass shows that the mass represents a horseshoe kidney (*arrows*).

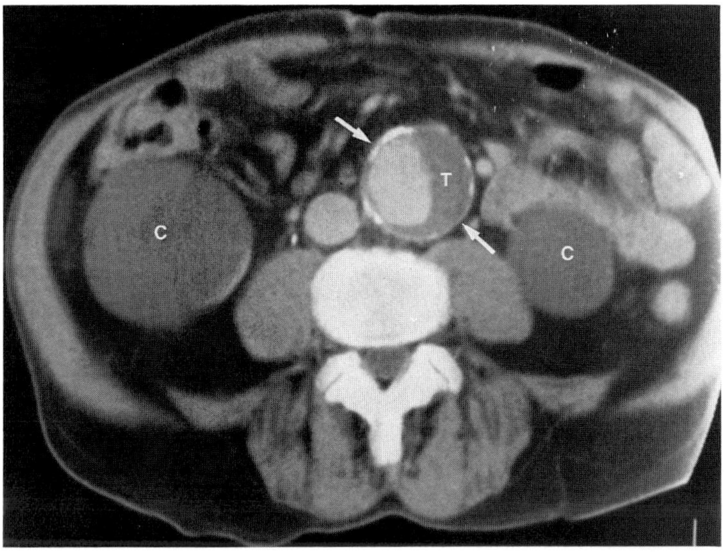


**Figure 14-15.** Aneurysm of the infrarenal abdominal aorta (*arrows*). Postcontrast CT scan in a 72-year-old man who presented with a pulsatile midline mass and a right flank mass demonstrates the aneurysm (*arrows*) and the thrombus (*T*) within it. Note also the large renal cysts (*C*) bilaterally.

ing interstices and thick, irregular fibrous strands. Computed tomography is also the best modality for evaluating less common retroperitoneal masses including rhabdomyosarcoma; teratoma; lymphangioma; and fluid collections such as abscess, hematoma, lymphocele, urinoma, and horseshoe kidney (Fig. 14-14).

A pulsatile midline mass suggests an aortic aneurysm (Fig. 14-15). In an asthenic patient ultrasound is sufficient to establish or exclude the diagnosis of aortic aneurysm. In most patients, however, CT or MRI should be employed to better demonstrate the full extent of a suspected aortic aneurysm.

## Right-Lower-Quadrant Masses

Most right-lower-quadrant masses are related to the gastrointestinal tract. A plain abdominal radiograph should first be obtained to identify any mass effect and to exclude a bowel obstruction, appendicolith, or fecal impaction (Fig. 14-16). If an obstruction is suspected, an enema with water-soluble contrast is recommended, because it will show any obstructing lesion, will not lead to impaction, and will even assist in cleansing the bowel (especially in patients with fecal impaction). Because the water-soluble contrast

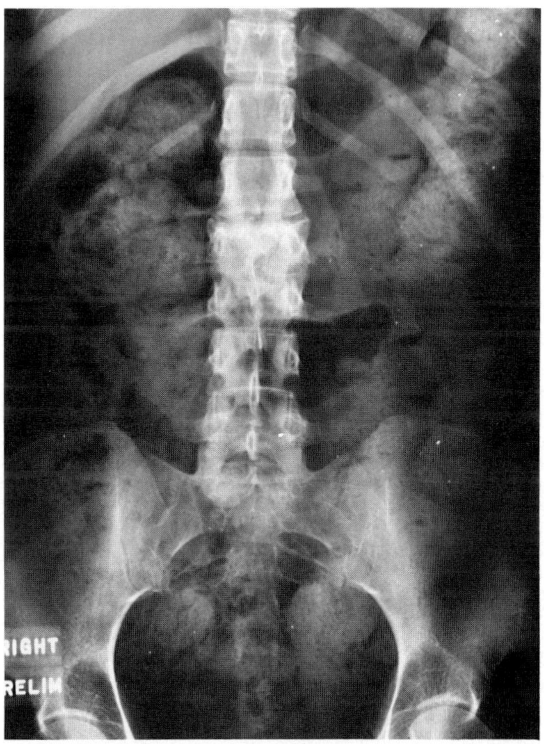

**Figure 14-16.** Focal impaction. Plain abdominal radiograph in a 27-year-old quadriplegic with a right-lower-quadrant mass demonstrates copious amounts of fecal material scattered throughout the colon and even filling the cecum.

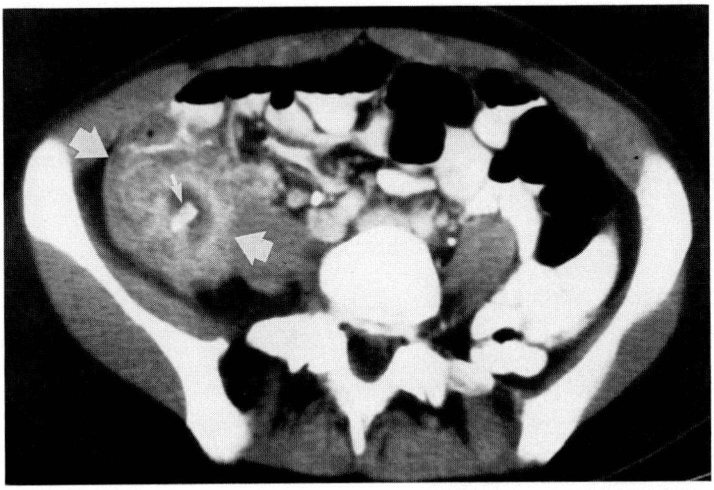

**Figure 14-17.** Appendiceal abscess. CT scan in a 27-year-old woman who presented with a right-lower-quadrant mass, vague lower abdominal pain, low-grade temperature, and mild leukocytosis shows a periappendiceal abscess (*large arrows*) surrounding an appendicolith (*small arrow*).

evacuates more readily than barium, once a colonic obstruction is excluded, a small bowel follow-through or enteroclysis can be performed on the same day to rule out a small bowel obstruction. If appendicitis is the clinical diagnosis, the patient is most often subjected to laparotomy without additional imaging studies. Confirmation of appendiceal obstruction or a periappendiceal mass can be obtained by a barium enema; CT can demonstrate an appendiceal (Fig. 14-17) or periappendiceal abscess in questionable cases. If a large cancer of the right side of the colon is suspected clinically, a barium enema should be performed to detect the lesion, and CT is the procedure of choice for staging.

Crohn's disease often presents as a palpable abdominal mass (Fig. 14-18), usually in the right lower quadrant. Computed tomography is the procedure of choice for differentiating the various causes of the mass, which include bowel wall thickening, abscess, phlegmon, enlarged lymph nodes, and creeping fat of the mesentery (enlarged, inflamed, and edematous mesenteric fat that often presents as a palpable mass). Conventional barium studies in these patients with Crohn's disease typically show only a mass effect, spiculation, or fistula in addition to mucosal abnormalities.

Lymphomas occurring in the right lower quadrant can reach enormous size (Fig. 14-19).

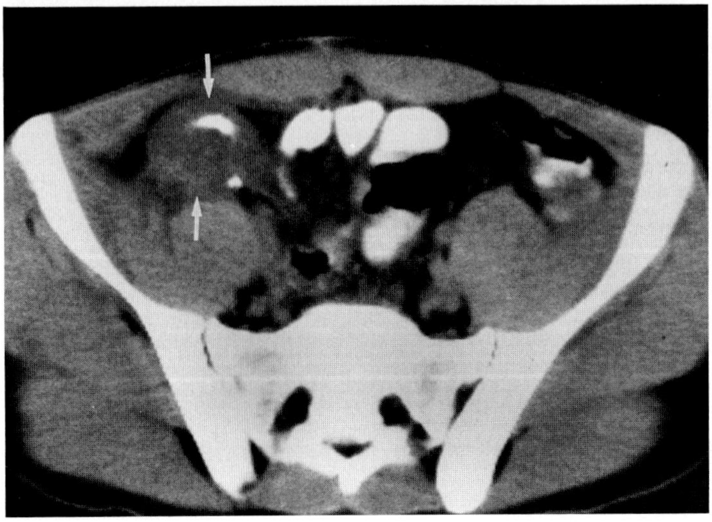

**Figure 14-18.** Crohn's disease. CT scan in an 18-year-old woman with a 5-year history of Crohn's disease and a palpable right-lower-quadrant mass shows that the mass does not represent an abscess but is merely due to marked thickening of the wall of the cecum (*arrows*).

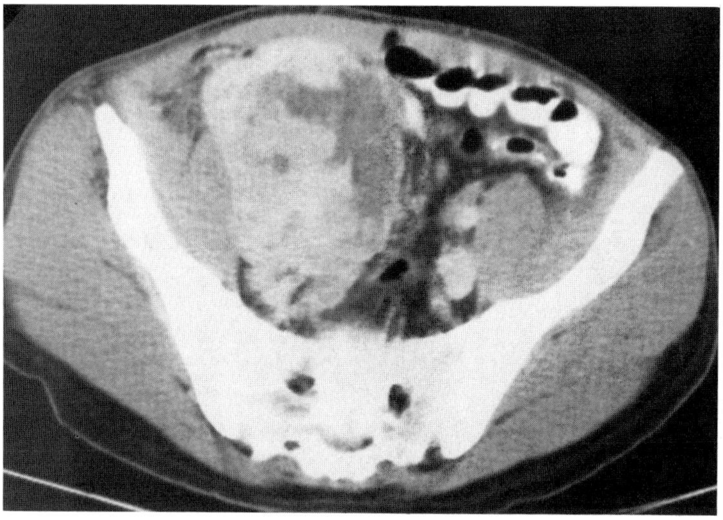

**Figure 14-19.** Hodgkin's disease. CT scan in a 43-year-old man with constitutional symptoms and a large right-lower-quadrant mass demonstrates the irregular, inhomogeneous lesion, which was seen to cause obstruction of the right kidney on more cephalic scans.

Huge dilatation of the cecum, which can occur in Ogilvie's syndrome and in patients with fecal impactions, can be demonstrated on plain abdominal radiographs.

Female patients with tubo-ovarian abscesses or ovarian cysts or tumors may present with right-lower-quadrant masses. Ultrasound is the imaging modality of choice in the true pelvis. Computed tomography is preferred if the mass extends into the right lower quadrant, because this modality provides better anatomic localization and is not adversely affected by overlying gas-filled loops of bowel.

## Hypogastric Masses

Hypogastric masses usually arise in the pelvis and are often related to the bladder, colon, uterus, or ovary. A distended urinary bladder may extend to the level of the umbilicus, usually in the midline, where it may be mistaken for a tumor because of its extreme size or because a lateral diverticulum makes it appear asymmetric. If urinary retention is suspected and direct catheterization is not revealing, ultrasound should be performed to establish the diagnosis. Ovarian cysts or neoplasms (Fig. 14-20) may occasionally

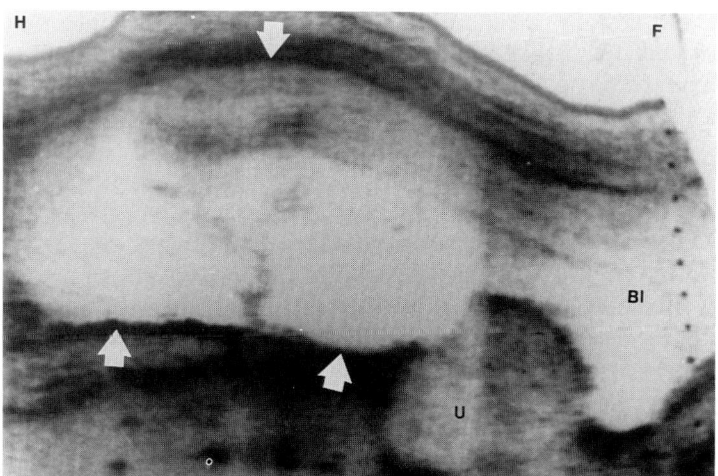


**Figure 14-20.** Ovarian cystadenocarcinoma. Longitudinal sonogram in a 64-year-old woman with a midabdominal and hypogastric mass demonstrates a huge, septated, predominantly anechoic mass arising from the pelvis and extending into the abdomen. (*H,* cephalic; *F,* caudal; *U,* uterus; *Bl,* bladder)

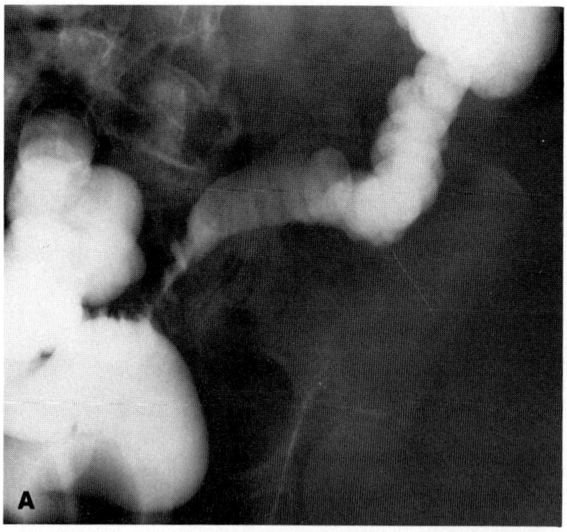


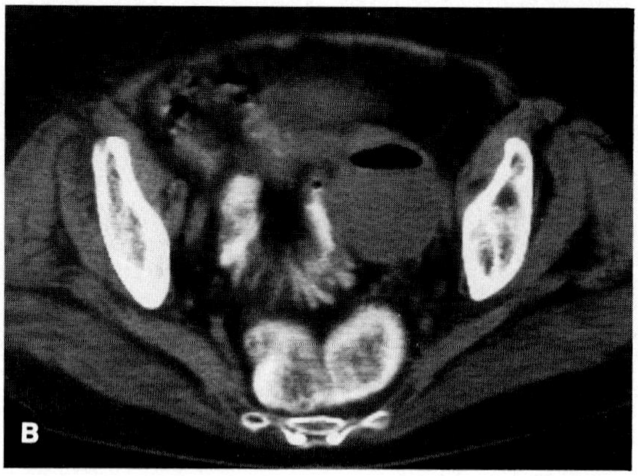


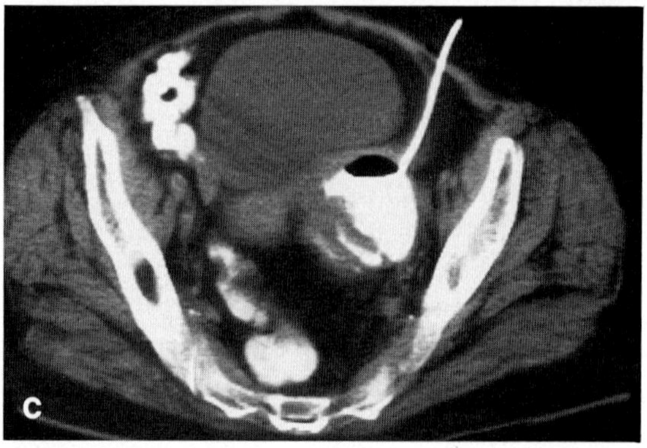


**Figure 14-21.** Diverticulitis. **(A)** Barium enema in a 72-year-old woman with fever and left-lower-quadrant pain and mass shows narrowing of the sigmoid colon with a mass effect along its inferior aspect. **(B)** Because the patient was a poor operative risk, a CT scan was performed and demonstrates a large fluid collection with an air–fluid level. **(C)** The mass was aspirated and a catheter placed percutaneously to drain the abscess. (Gore RM et al: Computed tomographic evaluation of the gastrointestinal tract in diseases other than primary adenocarcinomas. Radiol Clin North Am 20:781,1982)

become so large that they simulate ascites or a distended bladder. The lesions may not be palpable on vaginal examination because they are located too high in the uterus. In such patients, ultrasound is the imaging modality of choice for establishing the cystic nature of the mass. If the mass is solid, the extent of the lesion is best defined by CT or MRI.

## Left-Lower-Quadrant Masses

Most palpable left-lower-quadrant masses in adults arise from the colon. Approximately one third of patients with diverticulitis have a palpable abdominal mass; if this is clinically suspected, a plain abdominal radiograph should be the first imaging procedure. If the patient is acutely ill and an obstruction is suspected, a single-contrast barium enema should then be obtained (Fig. 14-21*A*), because air-contrast barium enemas are unreliable in demonstrating the fistulas and sinus tracts associated with diverticulitis. If the barium study is equivocal and the patient remains stable, a CT scan following the rectal administration of dilute contrast material may define the extent of a diverticular abscess (Fig. 14-21*B*) and act as a guide for percutaneous catheter drainage (Fig. 14-21*C*).

Carcinomas of the sigmoid colon can produce left-lower-quadrant masses. Although these neoplasms usually cause obstructive symptoms before they grow large enough to be palpated, a barium enema should be performed to exclude a sigmoid tumor if the patient has a clinical history of anemia, partial obstruction, or

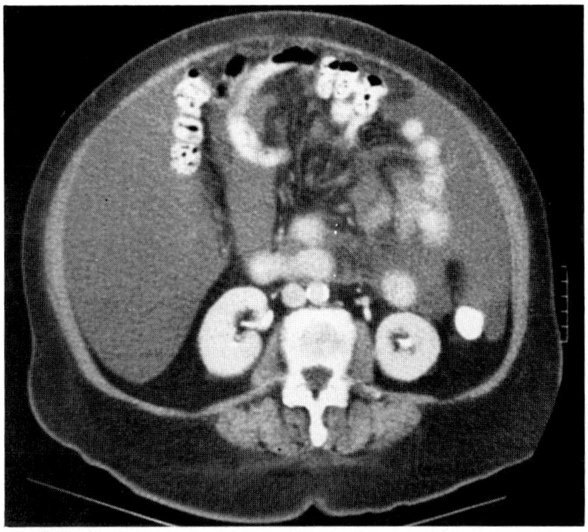

**Figure 14-22.** Massive ascites. CT scan in a 50-year-old woman who presented with increasing abdominal girth shows a large amount of intraperitoneal fluid and centralization of bowel loops.

hemoccult-positive stools. In older patients, the irregular masses of stool representing fecal impaction may be palpated in the sigmoid and diagnosed on plain abdominal radiographs. A water-soluble enema should be performed to exclude an underlying obstructing mass.

### Diffusely Enlarged Abdomen

The differential diagnosis of a diffusely enlarged abdomen is extensive and includes ascites (Fig. 14-22), lipodystrophy due to alcohol abuse or steroids, and massive peritoneal or retroperitoneal tumors. Computed tomography is the recommended initial imaging modality, because it is not inhibited by fat or bowel gas and permits visualization of the various peritoneal compartments, which is useful in defining the organ of origin of the mass. In patients with massive ascites, CT can also suggest the etiology of the peritoneal fluid by detecting masses, metastases, loculation, and the relative distribution of fluid in the lesser and greater sacs. The demonstration of a large collection of fluid in the greater and lesser sacs mandates a careful search for an abdominal malignancy.

## Bibliography

Bernardino ME, Lewis E: Imaging hepatic neoplasms. Cancer 50:2666–2671, 1982

Bree RL, Schwab RE: Contribution of mesenteric fat to unsatisfactory abdominal and pelvic ultrasonography. Radiology 140:773–776, 1981

Coscina WF, Arger PH, Levine MS et al: Gastrointestinal tract focal mass lesions: Role of CT and barium evaluations. Radiology 158:581–588, 1986

Engel IA, Auh YH, Rubenstein WA et al: Large posterior abdominal masses: Computed tomographic localization. Radiology 149:203–209, 1983

Filpi RG, Mindelzun RE, McCort JJ: Abdominal masses. In McCort JJ (ed): Abdominal Radiology, pp 301–366. Baltimore, Williams & Wilkins, 1981

Frick MP, Feinberg SB: Deceptions in localizing extrahepatic right-upper-quadrant abdominal masses by CT. AJR 139:501–504, 1982

Gore RM, Callen PW: Ultrasonography in the evaluation of malignant disorders. In Moossa AR, Robson MC, Schimpff SC (eds): Comprehensive Textbook of Oncology, pp 107–121. Baltimore, Williams & Wilkins, 1986

Gore RM, Callen PW, Filly RA: Displaced retroperitoneal fat: Sonographic guide to right upper quadrant mass localization. Radiology 142: 701–705, 1982

Gore RM, Callen PW, Filly RA: Lesser sac fluid in predicting the etiology of ascites: CT findings. AJR 139:71–74, 1982

Gore RM, Marn CS, Kirby DF et al: CT findings in ulcerative, granulomatous, and indeterminate colitis. AJR 143:279–284, 1984

Gore RM, Moss AA, Margulis AR: The assessment of abdominal and pelvic neoplasia: The impact of CT. Curr Probl Surg 19:494–552, 1982

Harter LP, Moss AA, Goldberg HI et al: CT-guided fine needle aspirations for diagnosis of benign and malignant disease. AJR 140:363–367, 1983

Holm J, Jacobsen B: Accuracy of dynamic ultrasonography in the diagnosis of malignant liver lesions. J Ultrasound Med 5:1–4, 1986

Kreel L: Masses, cysts, and abscesses. In Margulis AR, Burhenne HJ (eds): Alimentary Tract Roentgenology, vol 3, pp 504–514. St. Louis, CV Mosby, 1979

Kumari–Subaiya S, Phillips G, Weinreb J et al: Gray scale sonography in the diagnosis and differential diagnosis of the left upper quadrant masses. RadioGraphics 4:331–353, 1984

Megibow AJ, Balthazar EJ, Hulnick DH et al: CT

evaluation of gastrointestinal leiomyomas and leiomyosarcomas. AJR 144:727–731, 1985

Pelaez JC, Hill MC, Dach JL et al: Abdominal aspiration biopsy. Sonographic v. computed tomographic guidance. JAMA 250:2663–2666, 1983

Saini S, Mueller PR, Wittenberg J et al: Percutaneous drainage of diverticular abscesses: An adjunct to surgical therapy. Arch Surg 121:475–478, 1986

Simone JF, Ferrucci JT: New trends in gallbladder imaging. JAMA 246:380–383, 1981

Stark DD, Wittenberg J, Middleton MS et al: Liver metastases: Detection by phase-contrast MR imaging. Radiology 158:327–332, 1986

Sundaram M, Wolverson MK, Heiberg E et al: Utility of CT-guided abdominal aspiration procedures. AJR 139:1111–1115, 1982

Weill FS: Of humps, lumps, and swamps; pitfalls; the normal and pathological digestive tract; the acute abdomen. In Weill FS: Ultrasonography of Digestive Diseases, 2nd ed, pp 382–436. St. Louis, CV Mosby, 1982

Whitmire LF, Galambos JT, Phillips VM et al: Imaging guided percutaneous hepatic biopsy: Diagnostic accuracy and safety. J Clin Gastroenterol 7:511–515, 1985

## RIGHT UPPER QUADRANT MASS

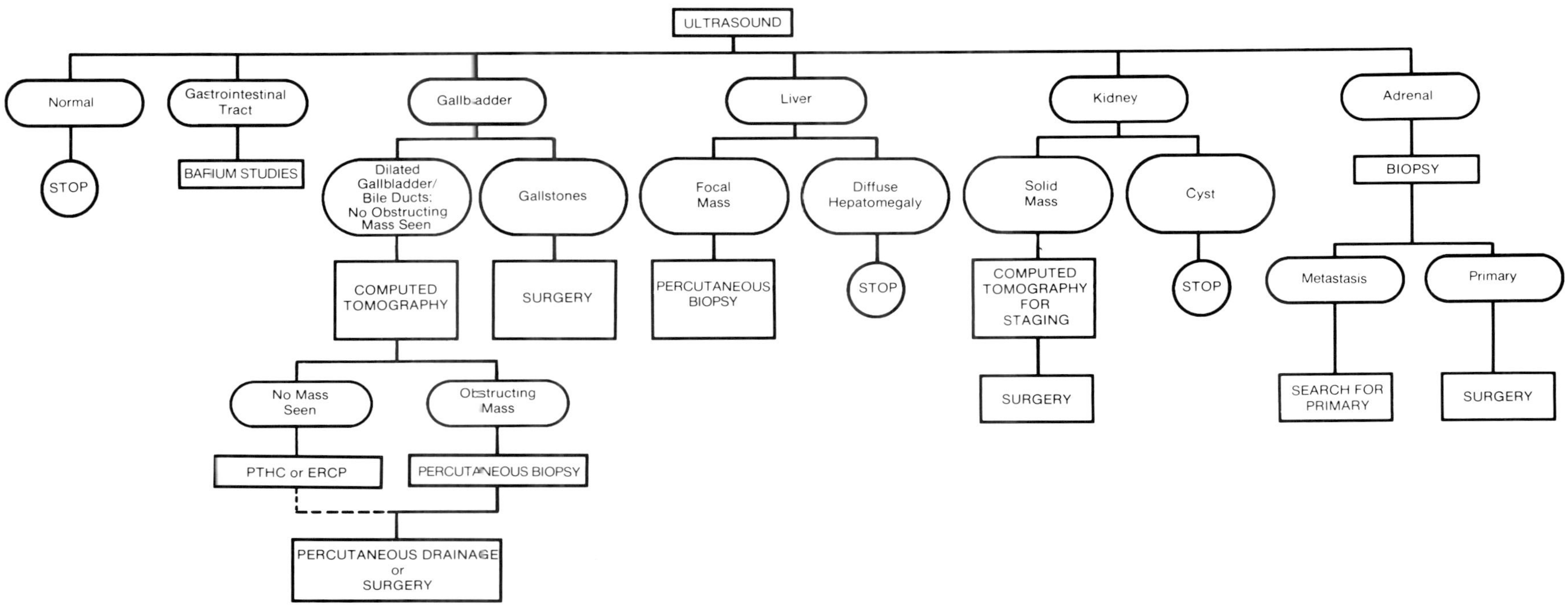

## EPIGASTRIC MASS

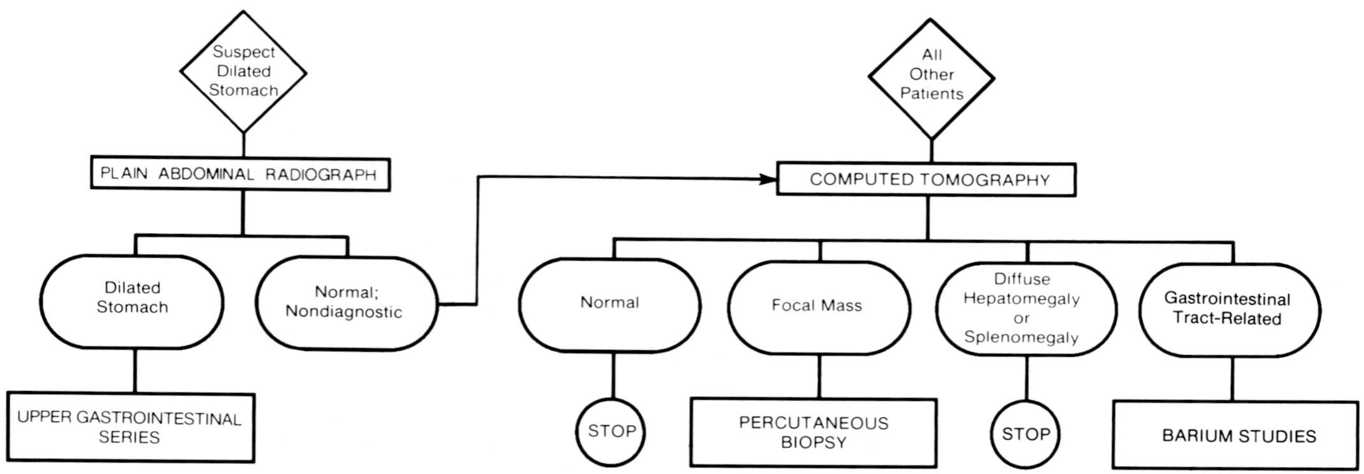

# LEFT UPPER QUADRANT MASS

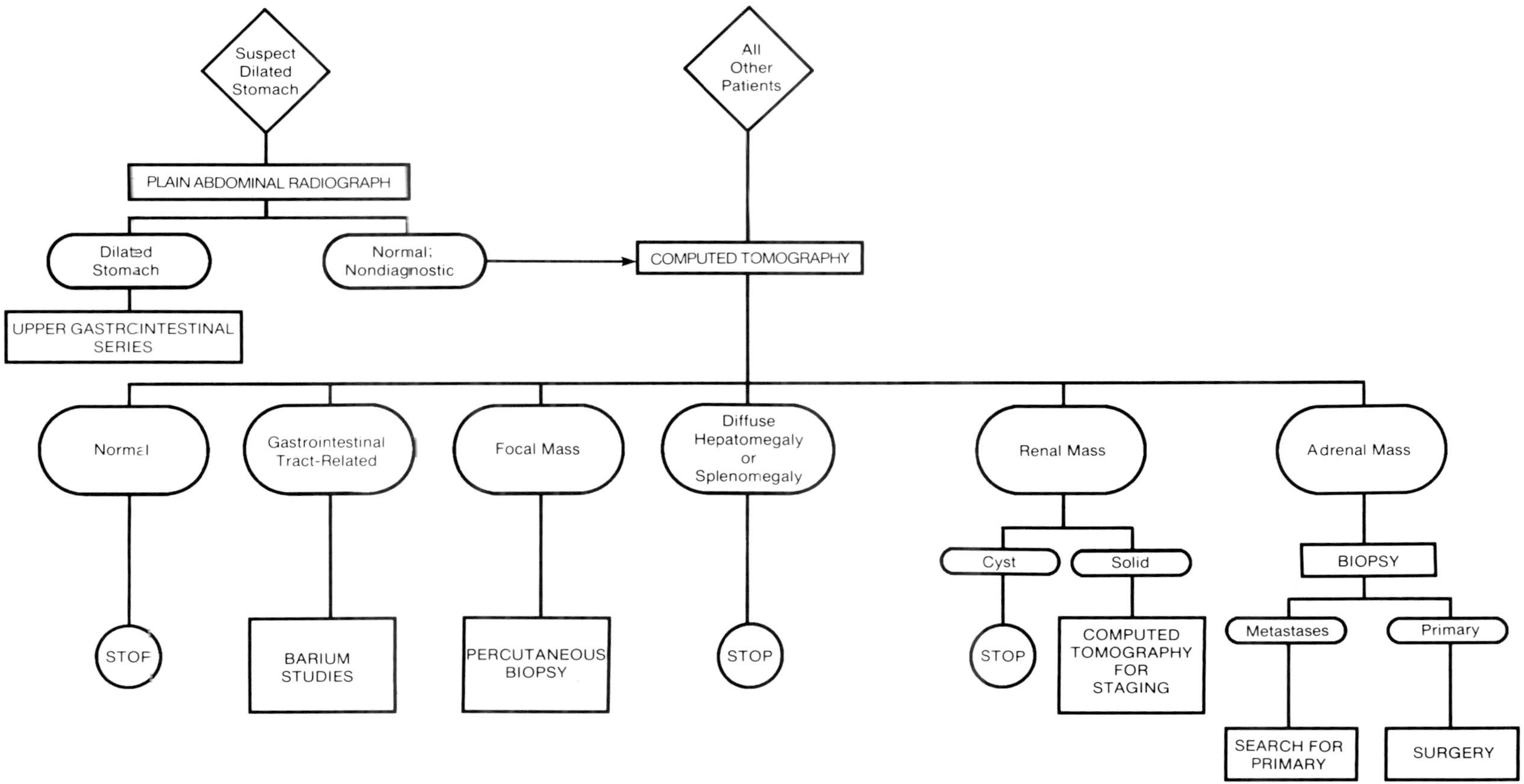

## MID ABDOMINAL MASS

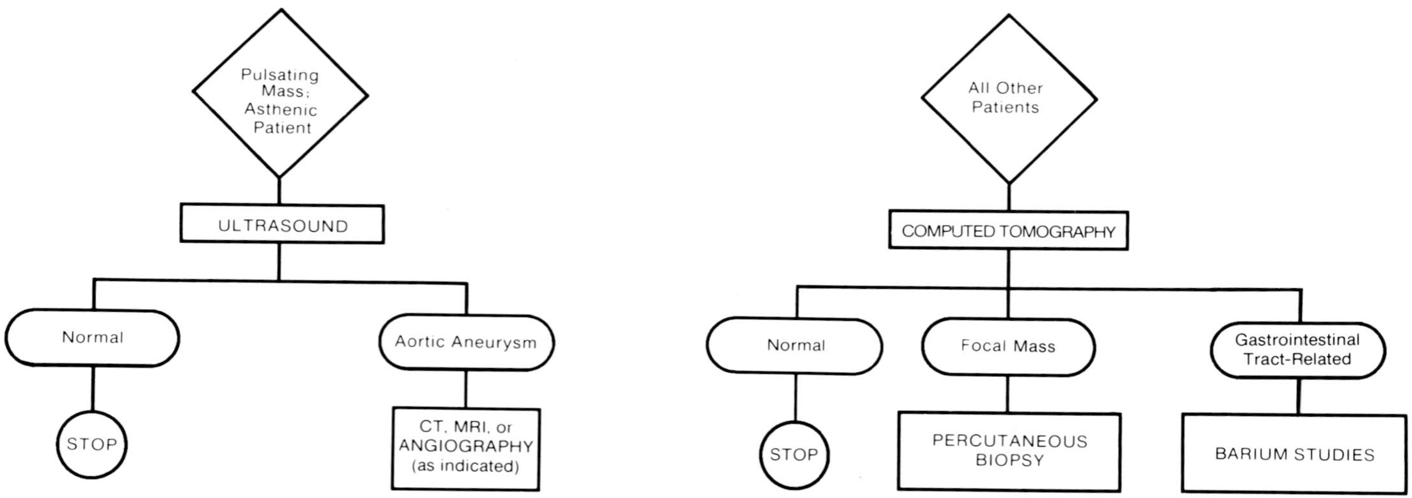

## RIGHT LOWER QUADRANT MASS

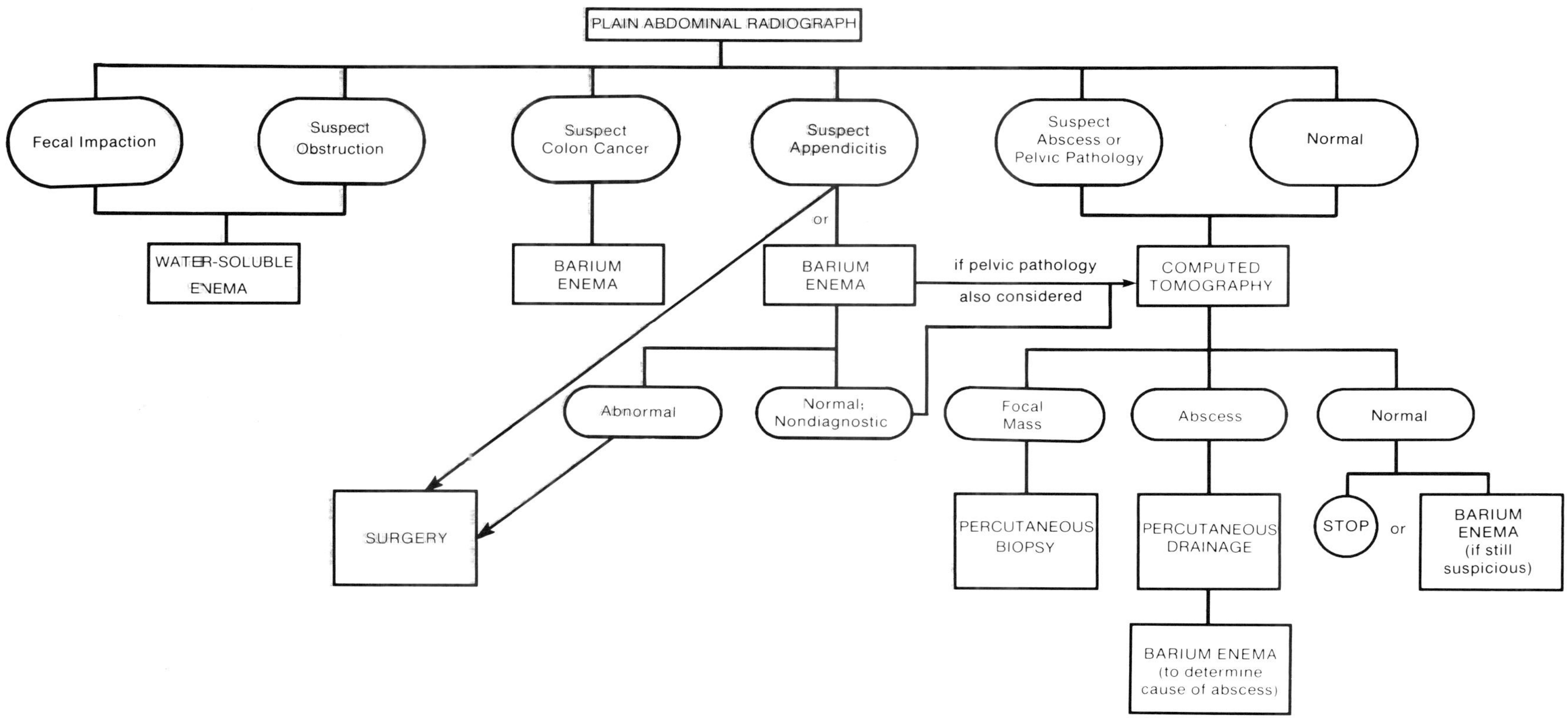

## HYPOGASTRIC MASS

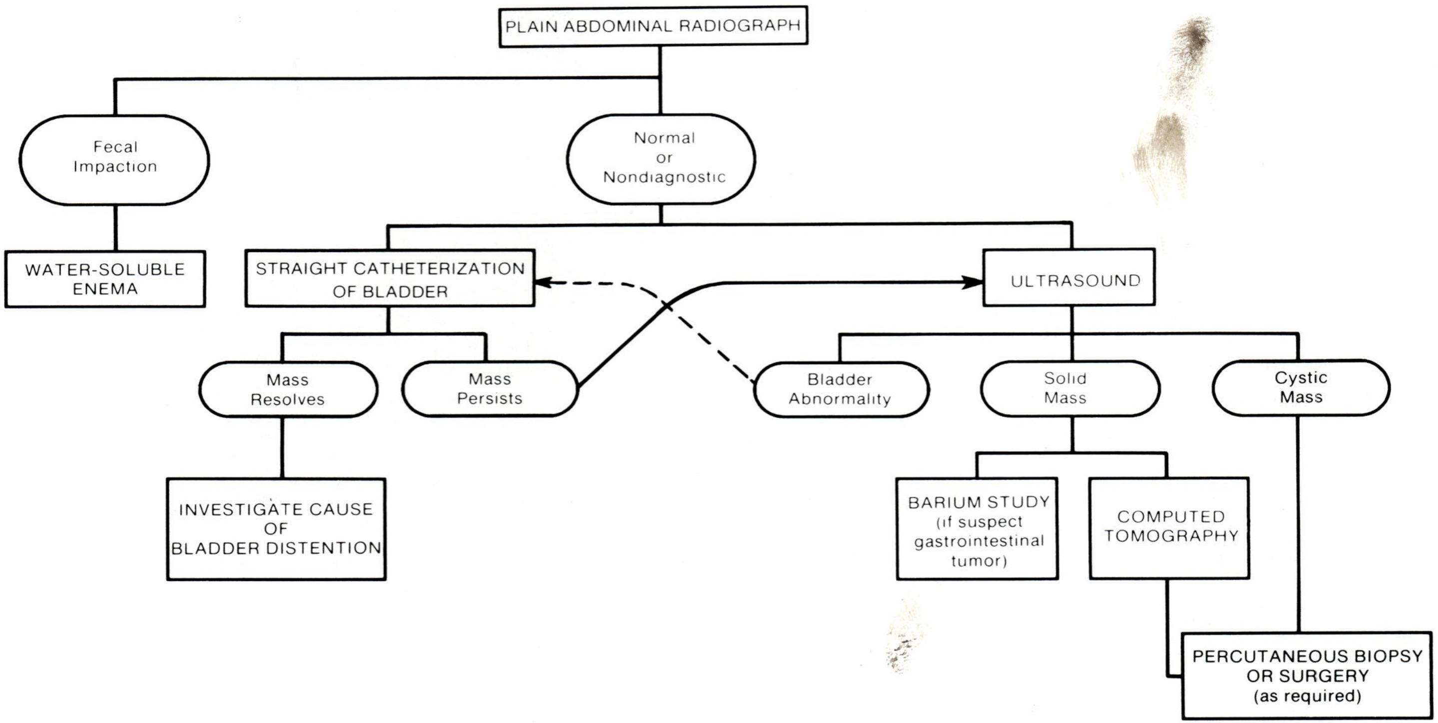

## LEFT LOWER QUADRANT MASS

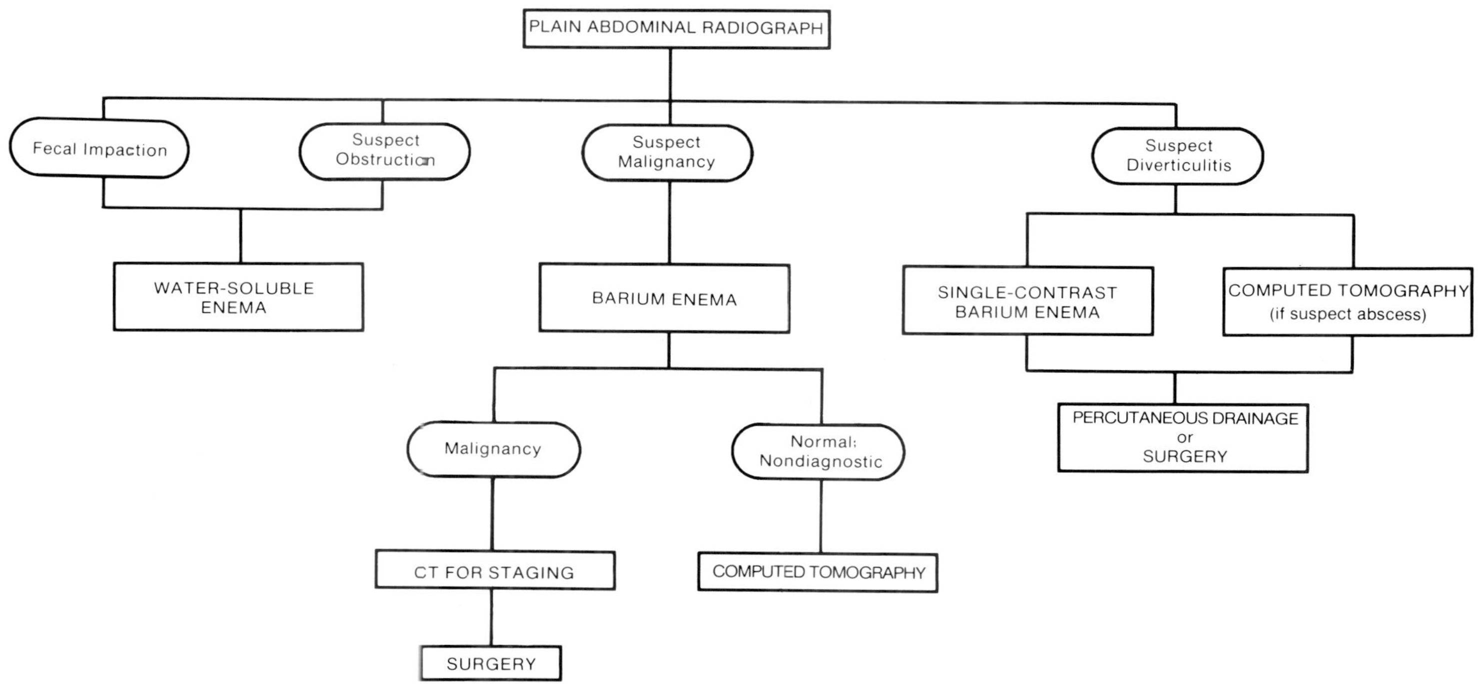

## DIFFUSELY ENLARGED ABDOMEN

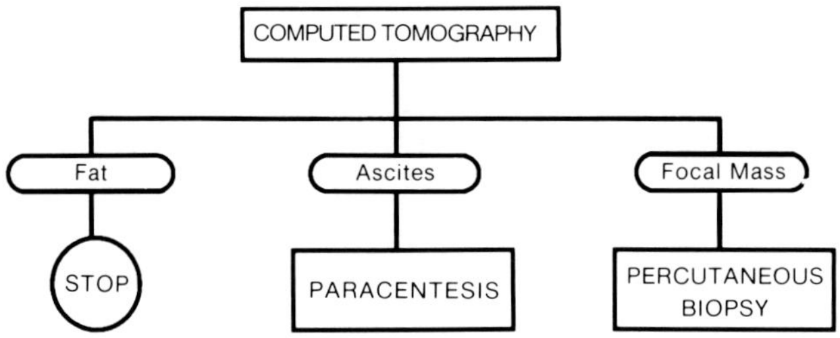

# Chapter 15

# Abdominal Masses in Children

*David F. Merten*
*Donald R. Kirks*

Abdominal masses in the pediatric age group are diverse in origin yet present an urgent and challenging problem in which diagnostic imaging plays an increasingly important role. The age of the patient is a major determinant influencing the imaging approach, because the neonate is subject to a different spectrum of conditions than is the older infant and child.

## DIAGNOSTIC EVALUATION

### *DIAGNOSTIC MODALITIES*

1. Plain abdominal radiography
2. Excretory urography
3. Voiding cystourethrography
4. Ultrasound
5. Computed tomography
6. Radionuclide studies
7. Angiography
8. Magnetic resonance imaging

#### Plain Abdominal Radiography

A plain abdominal radiograph should be obtained as the initial imaging study in all infants and children with an abdominal mass. Conventional radiographs can confirm the general location of the mass, the presence or absence of calcification, and concomitant involvement of the spine or other skeletal structures. However, in view of the intrinsically limited density range of plain radiography, more sophisticated techniques are generally required to make a definitive diagnosis.

#### Excretory Urography

Because most abdominal masses in children arise from the kidneys, the excretory urogram has traditionally been the cornerstone of radiographic evaluation. However, the use of this modality in assessing abdominal masses in children has now been largely replaced by newer imaging techniques. Although it can provide information regarding renal anatomy and function, excretory urography is surpassed by radionuclide imaging in assessing renal function, by ultrasound in characterizing the contents of the mass, and by computed tomography (CT) in depicting anatomic detail and the extent of the pathologic process. In addition, the use of excretory urography is particularly limited in the first 2 weeks of life because of the decreased glomerular filtration rate and concentrating ability of the kidneys during this time.

### Voiding Cystourethrography

Voiding cystourethrography can accurately evaluate lower urinary tract masses as well as genital masses arising in or adjacent to the bladder and urethra. It is the modality of choice in assessing disorders associated with upper-tract abnormalities (ectopic ureterocele, obstructed renal duplication) and is recommended in patients with cystic masses of the upper urinary tract, because these may be associated with or caused by vesicoureteral reflux.

### Ultrasound

Ultrasound is of particular value in imaging the pediatric patient, because it does not utilize ionizing radiation and yet can provide anatomic information (solid versus cystic, intrarenal versus extrarenal, organ of origin) that is difficult or impossible to determine by conventional radiographic techniques. The current trend in pediatric sonography is a complete reliance on computed real-time imaging (focused, phased-array) rather than on static imaging. Doppler techniques are also being increasingly employed to provide important parameters of blood flow in vascular structures.

Ultrasound is currently the screening modality of choice for abdominal masses in children. This modality is especially valuable for the anatomic delineation of neonatal abdominal masses, because many of these are cystic and benign. Because ultrasound provides less anatomic detail and smaller areas of interest, CT is the superior modality for determining the extent of malignant disease.

Limitations of ultrasound include its strong dependence on available equipment and operator expertise, the absence of functional information, and the adverse effects of bone and gas artifacts. Although ultrasound provides less precise anatomic detail than CT, in children the paucity of abdominal fat may decrease the effectiveness of CT examination.

### Computed Tomography

Computed tomography is currently the best imaging modality for providing anatomic detail of malignant abdominal masses in children. In addition to defining the anatomic and morphologic characteristics of a mass, CT can also demonstrate the extent of involvement of adjacent structures and any spread to distant foci. Enhancement with intravenous contrast material evaluates the relative blood flow to an organ or mass lesion; a bolus injection of contrast material can opacify adjacent vascular structures, such as the aorta, inferior vena cava, and renal veins. Computed tomography can provide anatomic and physiologic information in functionally compromised organs, and structures may be clearly visualized despite overlying bowel gas and bone.

It must be emphasized that, unlike ultrasound, CT is "less invasive" rather than "noninvasive," because it uses ionizing radiation, requires sedation or anesthesia in infants and small children, usually requires oral and intravenous contrast material, and alters the patient environment by requiring lower ambient temperatures. The relative paucity of fat in children may make the delineation of anatomic margins in the retroperitoneum difficult, although bolus intravenous contrast enhancement, adequate oral contrast, dynamic scanning, and careful attention to technique can usually overcome this inherent lack of tissue contrast.

### Radionuclide Studies

Radionuclide scanning is an excellent modality for demonstrating organ function and tissue vascularity. Dynamic imaging permits an evaluation of the vascularity of mass lesions and, in conjunction with static imaging, may provide a definitive diagnosis (*e.g.*, hepatic hemangioendotheliomatosis). Renal scintigraphy is superior to excretory urography for assessing and quantitating renal function, particularly in the neonate. The relatively poor anatomic detail and resolution of radionuclide scanning limits the use of this modality in evaluating malignant tumors and their extent of spread. However, if ultrasound or CT is not available, liver–spleen scanning remains a useful screening procedure for possible hepatic metastases.

### Angiography

Abdominal angiography has very limited application in the diagnostic evaluation of abdominal masses in children. It remains the only method for demonstrating detailed anatomy of parenchymal vessels and can provide information about the tissue or origin, vascularity, and anatomy of an abdominal mass. However, the dramatic advances in ultrasound, radionuclide scanning, CT, and magnetic resonance imaging (MRI) have drastically altered the indications for abdominal angiography in children. Currently, angiography is indicated only if a precise knowledge of segmental vascular anatomy is required (primary liver malignancy) or if interventional techniques (tumor embolization, arterial infusion for malignancy) are contemplated. Digital subtraction angiography has increased the contrast resolution of angiography while decreasing the risk of the procedure by permitting the use of smaller catheters and decreased volume and osmolarity of contrast material.

### Magnetic Resonance Imaging

Both magnetic resonance imaging and spectroscopy have tremendous potential in the evaluation of abdominal masses in children. Magnetic resonance imaging already is capable of producing anatomic sections of superb diagnostic quality that rival or exceed CT in demonstrating abnormalities of the brain and spinal cord.

The advantages of MRI in children include the lack of ionizing radiation, the large-field image display, and improved contrast resolution. The ability of this modality to image flowing blood is especially valuable in assessing retroperitoneal tumors, because these lesions may cause displacement, invasion, or tumor thrombus of the aorta, inferior vena cava, and other vessels. Magnetic resonance imaging is a superb technique for assessing possible extradural extension of paravertebral masses, such as neuroblastoma or sarcoma. *In vivo* spectroscopy may become a valuable technique for assessing the tissue characteristics of an abdominal mass as well as the response of a malignant tumor to therapy. Current limitations of MRI include its lack of general availability, expense, and various technical difficulties unique to the pediatric patient.

## DIFFERENTIAL DIAGNOSIS

### Neonatal Abdominal Masses

Abdominal masses in the neonate (the first month of life) are usually benign (Fig. 15-1). More than half of all neonatal abdominal masses are renal in origin, few are malignant, and the overall prognosis is good to excellent. The anatomic sites of origin of neonatal abdominal masses are renal (55%), genital (15%), gastrointestinal (15%), nonrenal retroperitoneal (10%), and hepatosplenobiliary (5%).

Real-time sonography is generally the best initial imaging study in a neonate with a suspected abdominal mass. An exception to this rule is the neonate who presents clinically with intestinal obstruction or other evidence of a gastrointestinal mass. Ultrasound can provide detailed anatomic information about the neonatal kidney and, in conjunction with renal scintig-

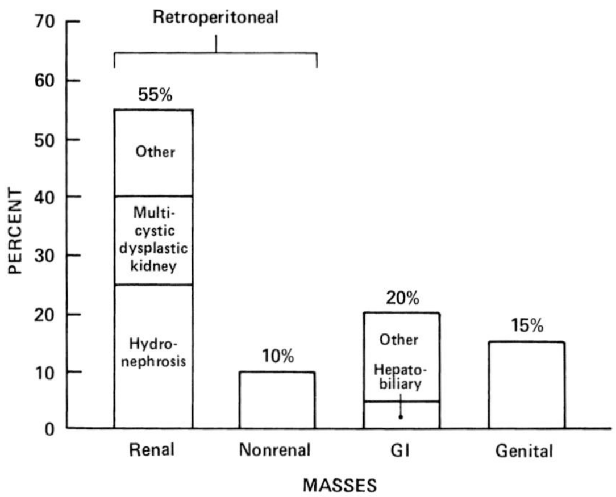


**Figure 15-1.** Neonatal abdominal masses. (Merten DF, Kirks DR: Diagnostic imaging of pediatric abdominal masses. Pediatr Clin North Am 32: 1397–1425, 1985)

raphy, provides anatomic and functional information without the limitations of excretory urography described previously.

## Hydronephrosis

Hydronephrosis is the most common abdominal mass in the neonate. The clinical diagnosis may not be suspected during the first 24 hours of life because of the normally decreased glomerular filtration rate and diminished urine production. The widespread use of ultrasound during pregnancy has dramatically increased the number of cases of hydronephrosis that are diagnosed *in utero* and confirmed in the newborn infant. The major causes of hydronephrosis in neonates include ureteropelvic junction obstruction (22%), posterior urethral valves (18%), ectopic ureterocele (14%), prune-belly syndrome (12%), and ureterovesical obstruction (8%).

Ultrasound of neonatal hydronephrosis demonstrates a large cystic mass within the kidney (Fig. 15-2*A*). There are multiple intercommunicating hypoechoic cystic spaces, with the largest located medially and representing the dilated renal pelvis. The infundibula, calyces, and surrounding renal parenchyma usually can be identified. If hydronephrosis is caused by distal ureteral obstruction or prune-belly syndrome, ultrasound also shows dilatation of one or both ureters. The combination of hydronephrosis and hydroureter suggests an obstruction of the distal ureter or bladder, such as ureterocele or posterior urethral valves. Hydronephrosis due to an obstructed duplication produces a cystic mass of the upper-pole moiety that is drained by a dilated ureter.

Dynamic renal scanning in the neonate with hydronephrosis initially shows an area of decreased activity in the kidney caused by the mass effect of the dilated renal collecting system and resultant decreased perfusion. Static scans show delayed accumulation of isotope in the renal parenchyma (Fig. 15-2*B*). In neonates with hydronephrosis due to ureteropelvic junction obstruction, delayed renal scans (4 to 6 hours after injection) show central migration of isotopic activity toward the dilated renal pelvis (Fig. 15-2*C*).

All patients with sonographic and scintigraphic evidence of hydronephrosis should have a voiding cystourethrogram to assess for possible ureterocele, posterior urethral valves, or vesicoureteral reflux. Gross vesicoureteral reflux can simulate a ureteropelvic junction obstruction, and patients with pyelocaliectasis may have associated vesicoureteral reflux or primary megaureter.

## Multicystic Dysplastic Kidney

Multicystic dysplastic kidney is the second most frequent neonatal abdominal mass and is usually discovered during the first day of life. In addition to showing the cystic anomaly, anatomic and functional imaging of both kidneys is essential, because 25% of patients with this condition have an associated abnormality of the contralateral kidney.

Ultrasound of the more common pelvoinfundibular form of multicystic dysplastic kidney demonstrates the dilated calyceal remnants as multiple hypoechoic cystic masses of variable size throughout the kidney (Fig. 15-3*A*). Unlike in hydronephrosis, in multicystic dysplastic kidney the largest of these cysts is not medial in location and the cysts do not communicate.

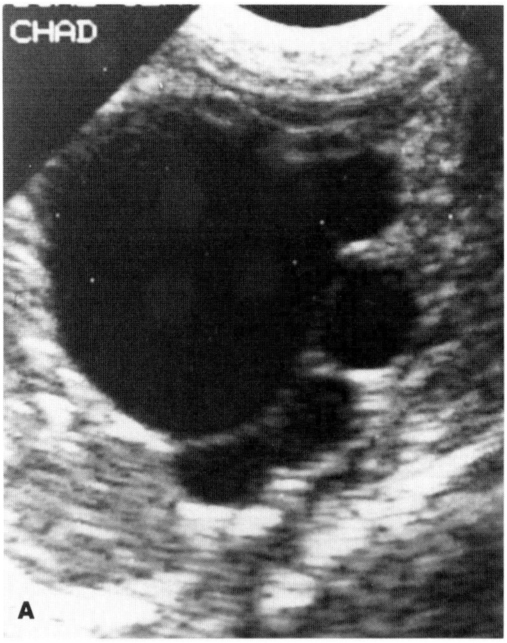


**Figure 15-2.** Congenital hydronephrosis. **(A)** Longitudinal sonogram in a newborn girl with a left flank mass shows a single, large, anechoic cystic mass (the dilated renal pelvis) surrounded by communicating smaller cysts (dilated calyces). **(B)** Immediate static renal scintigram ($^{99m}$Tc-DTPA) shows a rim of isotope activity in the thinned renal parenchyma surrounding the photon-deficient, dilated pelvocalyceal collecting system on the left. **(C)** Delayed scintigram (4 hours) demonstrates slow excretion and accumulation of tracer within the dilated left renal pelvis.

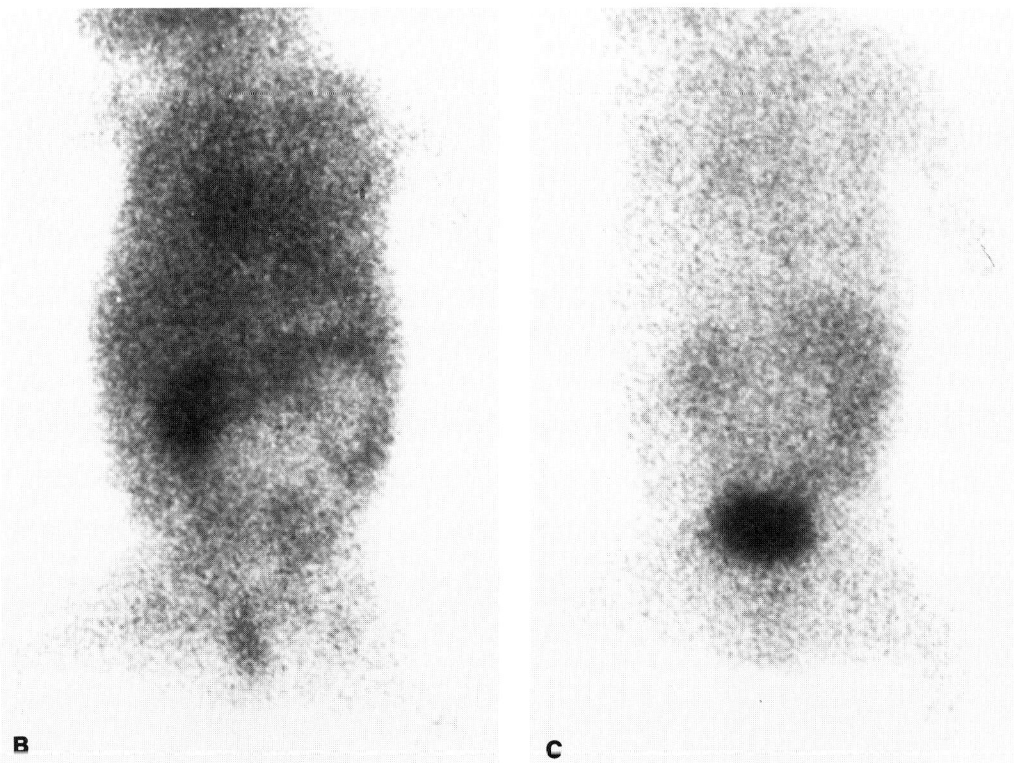

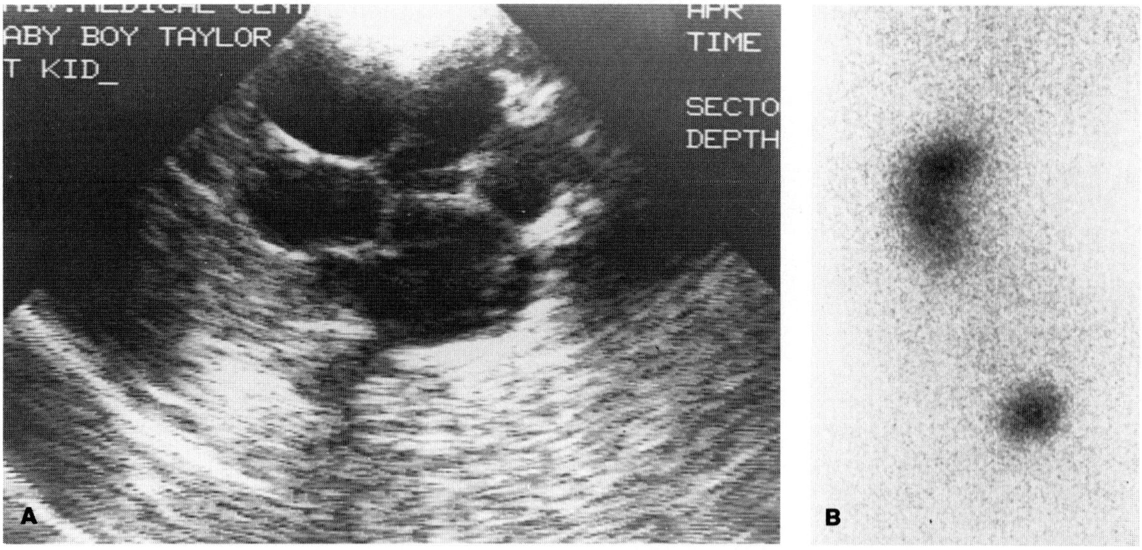


**Figure 15-3.** Multicystic dysplastic kidney. **(A)** Ultrasound of a newborn infant with a right-sided abdominal mass shows multiple anechoic cysts of variable size and haphazard arrangement replacing the right kidney. The noncommunicating cysts are separated by echogenic septa. **(B)** Posterior view of a renal scintigram obtained 1 hour following injection of $^{99m}$Tc-DTPA reveals a large photon-deficient area that represents the nonfunctioning, dysplastic right kidney.

Infundibula and peripheral renal parenchyma cannot be identified. The sonographic appearance of the hydronephrotic type of multicystic dysplastic disease, in which the cysts represent the entire pelvocalyceal system, is highly variable and may mimic congenital ureteropelvic junction obstruction or demonstrate features of hydronephrosis and pelvoinfundibular multicystic dysplastic kidney. Radionuclide studies demonstrate no isotope activity within the kidneys on early images and a lack of central isotope migration on delayed scans (Fig. 15-3*B*).

## Hepatic Hemangioendotheliomatosis

Diffuse hemangioendotheliomatosis of the liver typically presents in the neonatal period with hepatomegaly, cardiomegaly, and congestive heart failure due to massive arteriovenous shunting within the tumors. At least half the patients have cutaneous hemangiomas. The treatment of this condition is directed at stabilizing the cardiovascular system, because most hemangioendotheliomas involute spontaneously or rapidly respond to steroid therapy.

Ultrasound shows the hemangioendotheliomas as multiple mixed echogenic lesions throughout an enlarged liver (Fig. 15-4*A*). The imaging modality of choice is liver–spleen radionuclide scintigraphy, which shows increased blood flow to the liver on dynamic scans and multiple isotope-deficient areas throughout the hepatic parenchyma on static images (Fig. 15-4*B*, *C*). Although infrequently indicated for diagnosis, angiography should be performed if embolization, vascular ligation, or surgical resection is contemplated (Fig. 15-4*D*). Ultrasound is the imaging modality of choice for following the response of these benign vascular tumors to conservative therapy.

## Hydrometrocolpos

Hydrometrocolpos refers to massive dilatation of both the uterus (metro) and vagina (colpos) with an accumulation of mucinous secretions caused by vaginal atresia or, less frequently, imperforate hymen. Neonatal hydrometrocolpos is often part of a broader spectrum of congential malformations of the urogenital sinus and

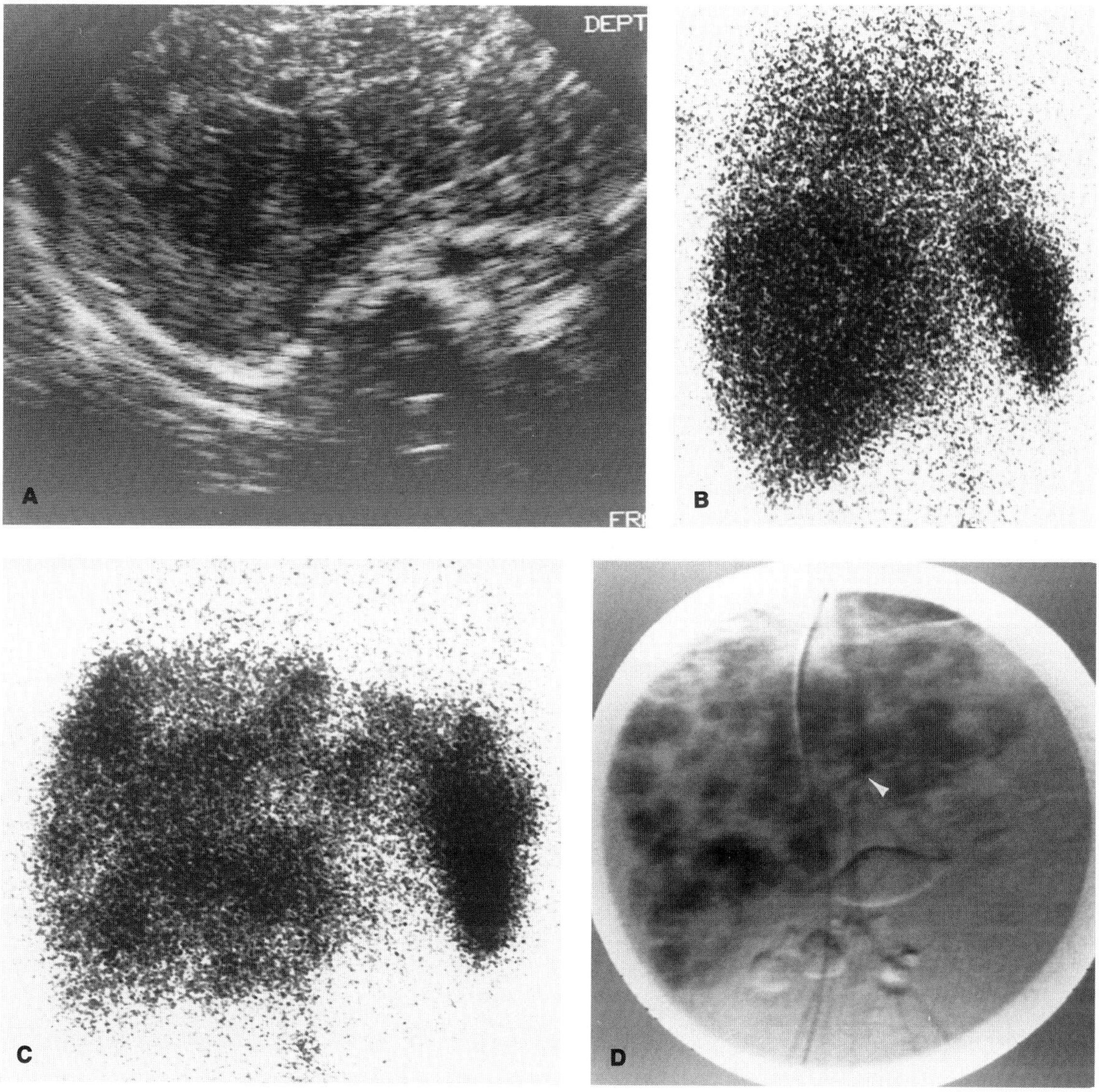


**Figure 15-4.** Hemangioendothelioma. **(A)** Transverse sonogram in a 2-week-old infant with congestive heart failure and right-upper-quadrant abdominal mass shows multiple round, sonolucent intrahepatic foci. **(B)** Dynamic liver–spleen scintigram ($^{99m}$Tc sulfur colloid) reveals preferential tracer flow into the greatly enlarged liver with rapid recirculation of radionuclide into the heart and lungs because of intrahepatic arteriovenous shunting. **(C)** Static scintigram after tracer uptake by reticuloendothelial cells shows multiple photon-deficient areas that represent intrahepatic cavernous vascular spaces. **(D)** Digital subtraction angiogram shows contrast material filling multiple cavernous intrahepatic vascular spaces. The abdominal aorta is of normal caliber above the origin of the celiac axis, but it is markedly diminished in caliber below this level (*arrowhead*).

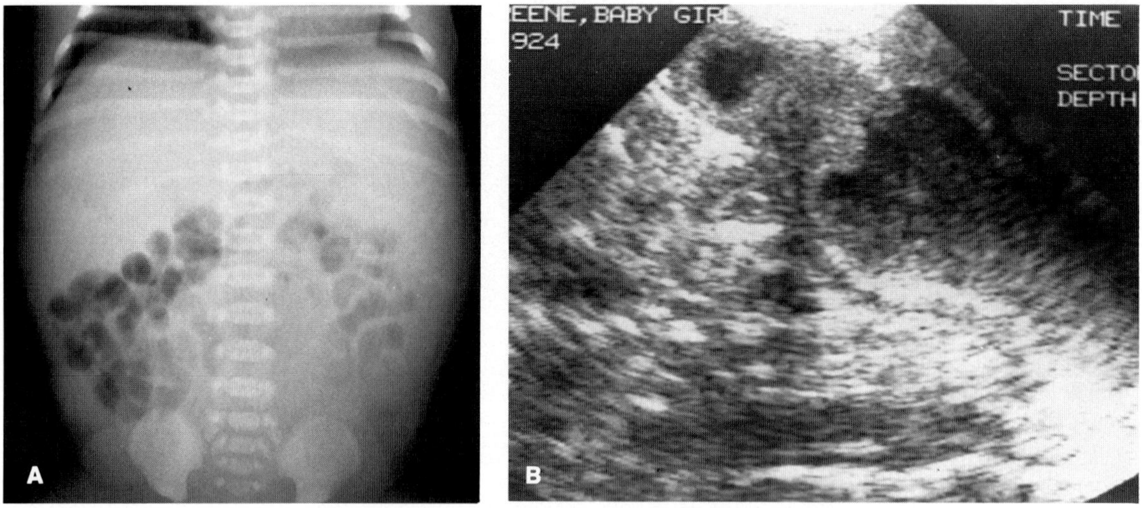


**Figure 15-5.** Hydrometrocolpos. **(A)** Plain abdominal radiograph of a newborn girl with a lower abdominal mass shows displacement of bowel loops by a midline lower abdominal mass extending from the pelvis. There is ascites and faint intraperitoneal calcification in the left upper quadrant. **(B)** Longitudinal pelvic sonogram shows the dilated vagina and the uterus, which appears as a large, "light bulb-shaped" cystic mass containing scattered echoes.

cloaca. The dilated vagina and/or uterus presents clinically and radiographically as a fixed midline abdominal mass that appears to arise from the pelvis (Fig. 15-5*A*). *In utero* obstruction of the urinary tract by the large pelvic mass may be associated with hydronephrosis or fetal anuria, oligohydramnios, and pulmonary hypoplasia. The reflux of secretions through the fallopian tubes may result in an adhesive ("plastic") peritonitis. Ultrasound shows a cystic mass, representing the fluid-filled, dilated vagina and uterus, lying between the bladder and rectum (Fig. 15-5*B*); the scattered echo pattern reflects cellular debris, mucoid material, or blood. Excretory urography or renal scintigraphy should be performed to evaluate renal function and any possible obstruction of the upper urinary tract. Cystography, genitography, and contrast enema may be required to define more complex urogenital and cloacal malformations.

## Abdominal Masses in Infants and Children

After the neonatal period, there are important differences in the frequencies of specific abdominal masses and a significant increase in the incidence of malignant tumors (Fig. 15-6). Approximately 80% of abdominal masses in this age group arise in the retroperitoneum. Although renal masses occur with approximately the same frequency as in the neonate, there is an increased incidence of Wilms' tumor with a concomitant decrease in cystic anomalies.

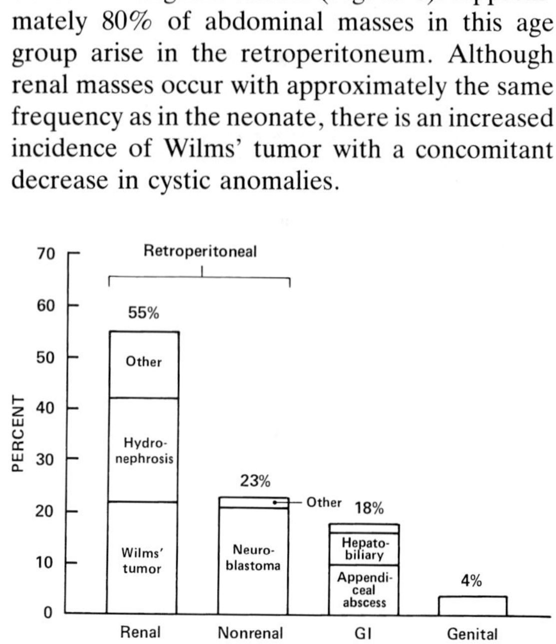


**Figure 15-6.** Abdominal masses in infants and children. (Merten DF, Kirks DR: Diagnostic imaging of pediatric abdominal mass. Pediatr Clin North Am 32:1397–1425, 1985)

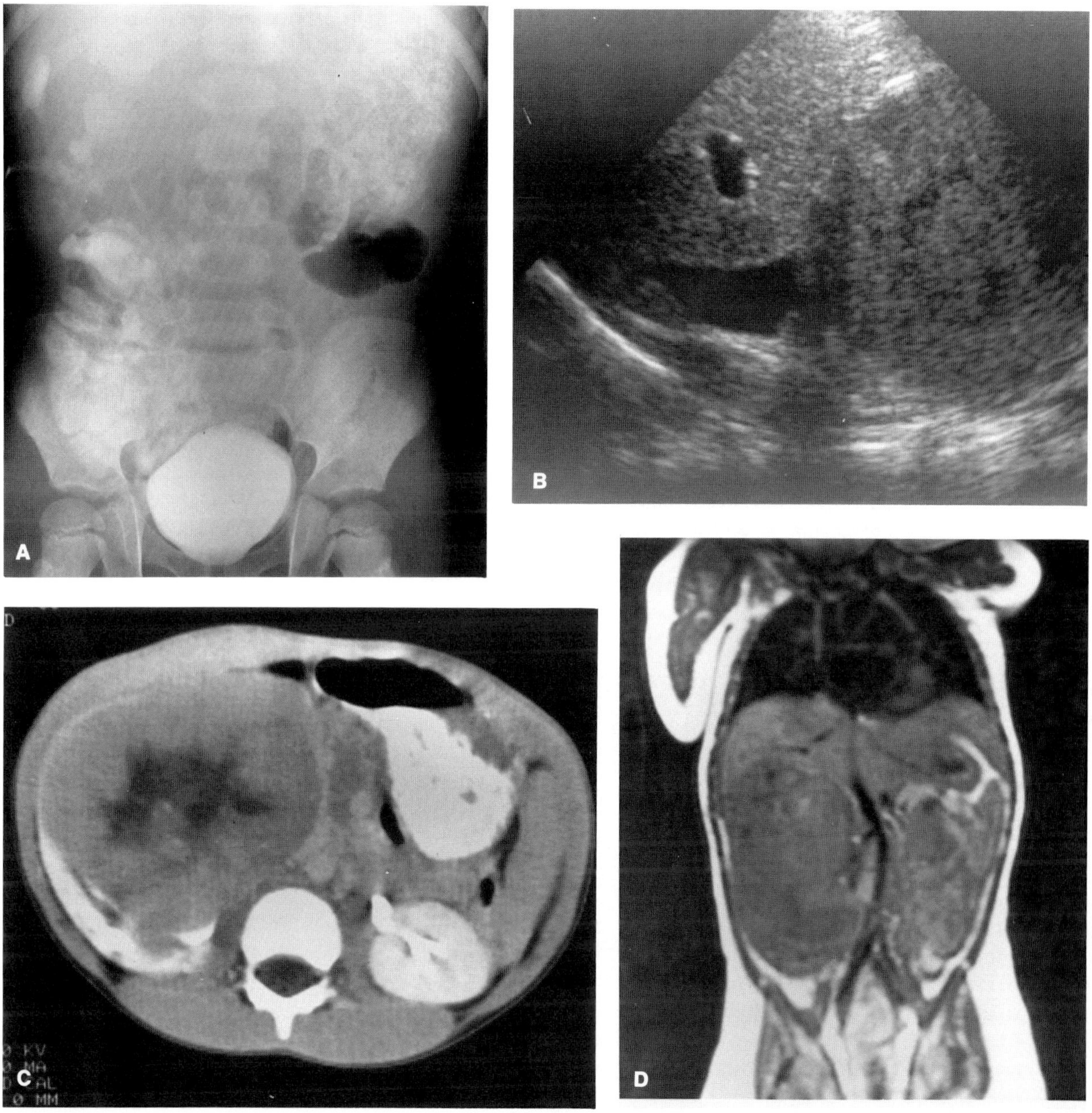

**Figure 15-7.** Wilms' tumor. **(A)** Post-CT excretory urogram of a 4-year-old boy with a right flank mass and hypertension shows displacement and effacement of the pelvocalyceal collecting structures by a large intrarenal mass. **(B)** Ultrasound shows a solid echogenic mass impinging on the inferior vena cava. **(C)** CT demonstrates a bulky mass that nearly replaces the right kidney. Scattered low-attenuation areas represent hemorrhage and necrosis. **(D)** T1-weighted MRI in coronal section shows a sharply marginated infrahepatic mass that is clearly distinct from the liver. The inferior vena cava, while displaced by the mass, shows no evidence of intracaval tumor extension.

Although ultrasound is frequently used as a screening technique to distinguish cystic from solid masses, CT plays an increasingly important role in the diagnosis and management of abdominal masses in older infants and children because of its ability to better define the anatomy as well as any local or metastatic spread of malignant tumors.

### Wilms' Tumor

Wilms' tumor (nephroblastoma) is the most common primary neoplasm of childhood, with a peak incidence at 3 years of age. The bulky renal tumor usually expands to ultimately replace most of the involved kidney and may spread by extension into the renal vein or inferior vena cava, by hematogenous and lymphatic dissemination, or, less frequently, directly to adjacent organs. The lungs are the most frequent site of distal metastases; skeletal metastases are infrequent, with the exception of the uncommon (10%) tumors with sarcomatous or clear-cell histology. The prognosis of patients with Wilms' tumors with a favorable histology is excellent (5-year survival rate of approximately 95%); sarcomatous or clear-cell lesions have a much poorer prognosis.

Excretory urography in Wilms' tumor shows stretching and distortion of the pelvocalyceal system without renal displacement (Fig. 15-7*A*). Ultrasound demonstrates an intrarenal, usually homogeneous echogenic mass (Fig. 15-7*B*); hemorrhage and necrosis may appear as scattered sonolucent areas. Computed tomogaphy further defines the location and extent of the tumor as well as spread to adjacent lymph nodes, liver, and lungs (Fig. 15-7*C*). Extension of tumor thrombus to the renal vein and superior vena cava can be demonstrated by ultrasound or by contrast-enhanced CT. Computed tomography is the modality of choice for demonstrating tumors in the contralateral kidney, which develop synchronously in up to 7% of cases and at a later time in up to 4%. Because of its ability to define vascular structures and flowing blood, MRI may eventually prove to be the imaging modality of choice for assessing tumor invasion of the inferior vena cava (Fig. 15-7*D*).

### Neuroblastoma

Neuroblastoma is the second most common primary neoplasm of childhood. Approximately 85% of these tumors develop within the first 5 years of life; half the patients are less than 2 years old at the time of diagnosis. Although the tumor may arise anywhere along the sympathetic chain, approximately 60% of neuroblastomas arise in the abdomen, and 70% of these are suprarenal in location. Neuroblastoma metastasizes early and may be widely disseminated to bone, liver, bone marrow, orbit, and skin. Clinical symptoms may be due to compression or invasion of adjacent anatomic structures, metastases, or tumoral hormonal activity.

Plain radiographs can demonstrate calcification (stippled, diffuse, or coalescent) in approximately half of abdominal neuroblastomas (Fig. 15-8*A*). Excretory urography typically shows renal displacement without distortion of pelvocalyceal structures. Ultrasound demonstrates the solid, usually inhomogeneous, nature of the mass and may be of value in assessing the relation of the tumor to the major abdominal vessels (Fig. 15-8*B*). Computed tomography is the

**Figure 15-8.** Neuroblastoma. **(A)** Plain abdominal radiograph of a 22-month-old girl ▶ shows a left paraspinous mass that contains faint stippled calcification and extends superiorly above the diaphragm. **(B)** Ultrasound demonstrates a dense, solid mass containing scattered bright echoes (psammomatous calcification). **(C)** CT scan shows a large mass anterior to the intact, functioning left kidney. The mass crosses the midline and contains extensive tumoral calcification. **(D)** Skeletal scintigram reveals uptake of tracer by the tumor (*arrow*) but no skeletal metastases. **(E)** T1- and **(F)** T2-weighted transaxial MR images reveal the left-sided paravertebral mass that involves lymph nodes and displaces the aorta and renal arteries. There is no evidence of intraspinous extension.

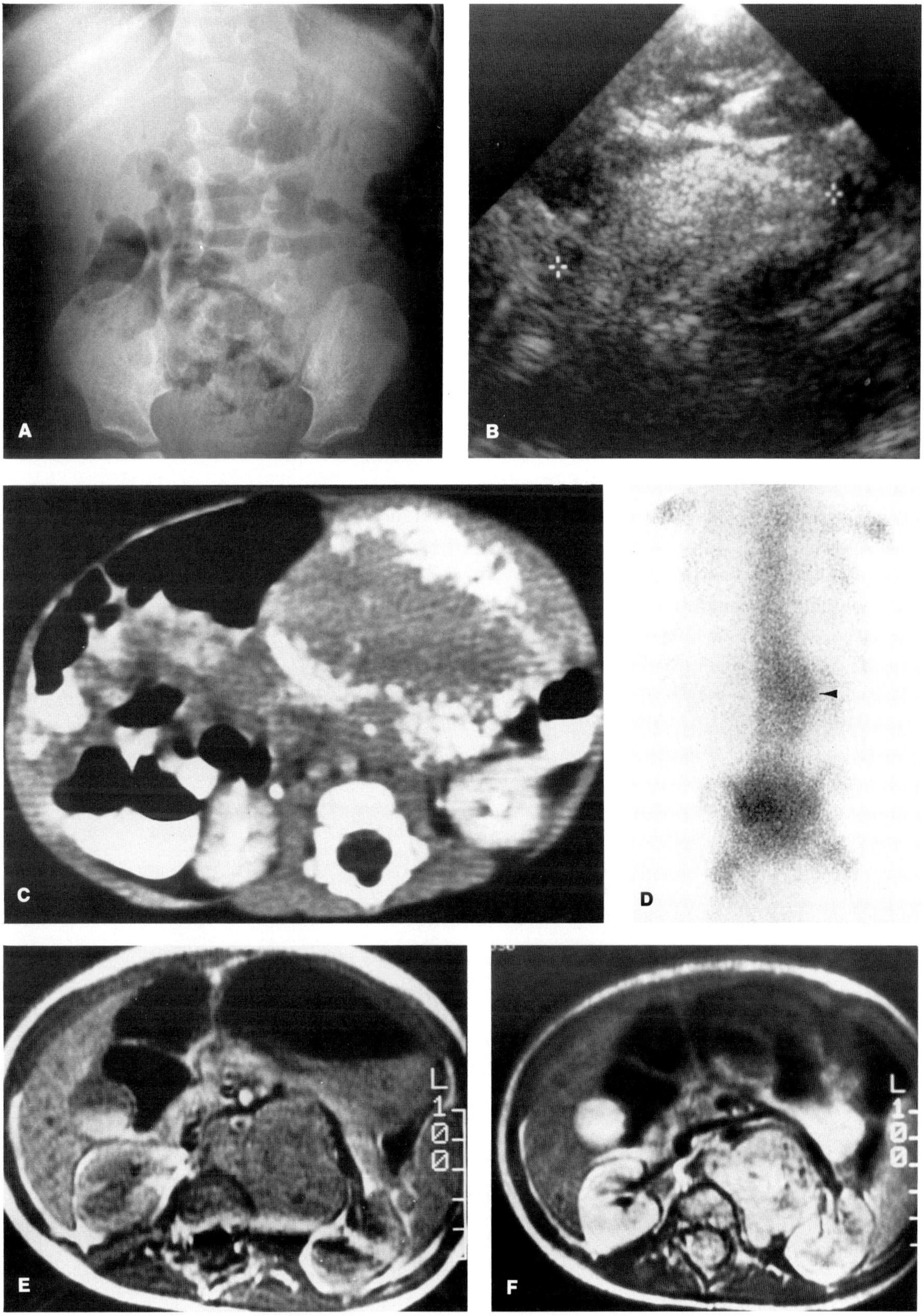
A
B
C
D
E
F

best modality for showing calcification of the mass (seen in at least 85% of cases by CT), documenting tumor extension to adjacent organs and lymph nodes, and identifying small tumors in locations other than the usual suprarenal site (Fig. 15-8*C*). The combination of CT and water-soluble contrast myelography can show intraspinal extension of tumor. Radionuclide scanning may be of value in detecting skeletal metastases, although this modality may be less sensitive than plain skeletal radiographs, especially in the metaphyseal regions. In at least 60% of patients with neuroblastoma, isotope uptake by the primary tumor is shown on radionuclide bone scans. Magnetic resonance imaging is of particular value in patients with neuroblastoma, because it defines the relation of the tumor to central vascular structures and any extradural tumor extension (Fig. 15-8*E, F*).

### Appendiceal Abscess

Appendiceal abscess is the most common gastrointestinal mass in older infants and children. Appendiceal perforation may result in generalized peritonitis (usually in the younger infant) or a localized periappendiceal abscess that often extends into the pelvis. Plain abdominal radiographs may demonstrate a mass containing gas or a calcified appendicolith (Fig. 15-9*A*). Ultrasound may show a mixed echogenic mass in the right lower quadrant or pelvis (Fig. 15-9*B*). The major value of CT is to localize an occult or atypical appendiceal abscess as well as subhepatic or subphrenic extension of the inflammatory process (Fig. 15-9*C*).

## OVERALL APPROACH TO THE IMAGING OF ABDOMINAL MASSES IN CHILDREN

In the neonate, the initial imaging study should be a plain abdominal radiograph. If there is evidence of intestinal obstruction, a gastrointestinal contrast study should be performed. Otherwise, abdominal ultrasound should be the next imaging technique employed. If the ultrasound is normal, no further imaging is required. If a mass

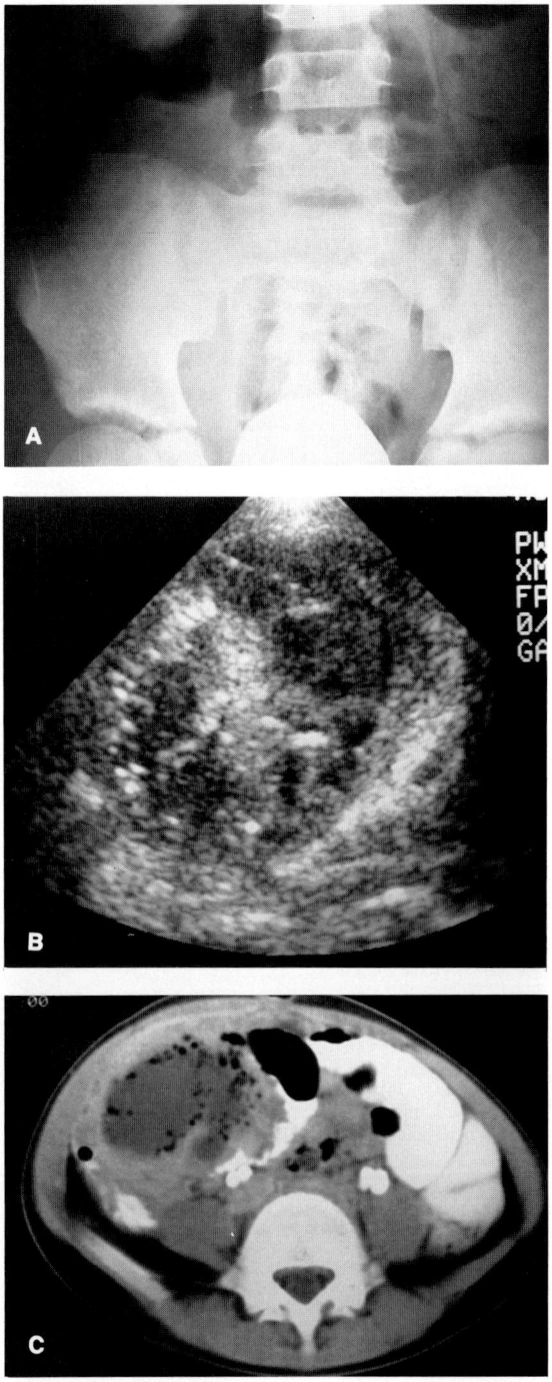


**Figure 15-9.** Appendiceal abscess. **(A)** Plain abdominal radiograph of an 8-year-old girl shows a right-lower-quadrant soft-tissue mass that appears to contain small gas bubbles. **(B)** Ultrasound demonstrates an inhomogeneous echogenic mass containing multiple bright echoes (gas bubbles). **(C)** CT scan shows that the multiple gas bubbles are contained in a large abscess.

is identified, further imaging depends on the anatomic location and sonographic characteristics of the mass.

In the older infant and child, initial plain abdominal radiography may be followed by ultrasound or excretory urography, depending on the clinical setting and the apparent location of the mass. Patients with noncalcified renal, retroperitoneal, or pelvic masses should undergo abdominal and pelvic sonography. If a renal mass is cystic, voiding cystourethrography and renal scintigraphy or excretory urography may be performed to further define the bladder anatomy, to confirm or exclude vesicoureteral reflux, and to evaluate renal function. If the plain abdominal radiography shows calcification suggestive of neuroblastoma, or if ultrasound demonstrates a solid mass, CT should be performed. Because most gastrointestinal masses that develop after the neonatal period are appendiceal abscesses or are hepatobiliary in origin, ultrasound is the screening modality of choice if one of these lesions is suspected. Radionuclide liver–spleen scanning, CT, and angiography may also be indicated. Genital masses arising in the pelvis are best evaluated by ultrasound.

## Bibliography


Baker MD, Kirks DR, Korobkin M et al: The association of neuroblastoma and myoclonic encephalopathy: An imaging approach. Pediatr Radiol 15:184–190, 1985

Bearman SB, Hine PL, Sanders RM: Multicystic kidney: A sonographic pattern. Radiology 118: 685–688, 1976

Bousvaros A, Kirks DR, Grossman H: Imaging of neuroblastoma: An overview. Pediatr Radiol 16:89–106, 1986

Felson B, Cussen LJ: The hydronephrotic type of unilateral congenital multicystic disease of the kidney. Semin Roentgenol 10:113–123, 1975

Fletcher BD, Kopiwoda SY, Strandjord S et al: Abdominal neuroblastoma: Magnetic resonance imaging and tissue characterization. Radiology 155:699–703, 1985

Griscom NT: The roentgenology of neonatal abdominal masses. AJR 93:447–463, 1965

Griscom NT, Vawter GF, Fellers FX: Pelvoinfundibular atresia: The usual form of multicystic kidney: 44 unilateral and two bilateral cases. Semin Roentgenol 10:125–131, 1975

Grossman H: Evaluating common intra-abdominal masses in children—A systematic roentgenographic approach. CA 26:219–235, 1976

Grossman H: Wilms' tumor. In Parker BR, Castellino RA (eds): Pediatric Oncologic Radiology, pp 237–263. St. Louis, CV Mosby, 1977

Grossman H, Sullivan DC, Kirks DR et al: Integrated imaging for childhood diseases. Pediatr Ann 9:15–25, 1980

Hope JW, Koop CE: Abdominal tumors in infants and children. Med Radiogr Photogr 38:2–51, 1962

Kasper TE, Osborne RW, Jr, Semerdjian HS et al: Urologic abdominal masses in infants and children. J Urol 116:629–633, 1976

Kirks DR: Computed tomography of pediatric urinary tract disease. Urol Radiol 5:199–208, 1983

Kirks DR: Pediatric imaging: Body compuerized tomography. In Lockhart JD (ed): Current Problems in Pediatrics, pp 3–63. Chicago, Year Book Medical Publishers, 1984

Kirks DR: Practical Pediatric Imaging: Diagnostic Radiology of Infants and Children, pp 593–595. Little, Brown & Co, Boston/Toronto, 1984

Kirks DR, Merten DF, Grossman H et al: Diagnostic imaging of pediatric abdominal masses: An overview. Radiol Clin North Am 19:527–545, 1981

Kirks DR, Rosenberg ER, Johnson DG et al: Integrated imaging of neonatal renal masses. Pediatr Radiol 15:147–156, 1985

Lebowitz RL, Griscom NT: Neonatal hydronephrosis: 146 cases. Radiol Clin North Am 15:49–59, 1977

Melicow MD, Usan AC: Palpable abdominal masses in infants and children: A report based on a review of 653 cases. J. Urol 81:705–710, 1959

Moore AV, Kirks DR, Mills SR et al: Pediatric abdominal angiography: Panacea or passe? AJR 138:433–438, 1982

Slovis TL, Perlmutter AD: Recent advances in pediatric urologic ultrasound. J. Urol 123:613–620, 1980

Smith FW: The value of NMR imaging in pediatric practice: A preliminary report. Pediatr Radiol 13:141–147, 1983

Smith FW, Gilday DL, Ash JM et al: Primary neuroblastoma uptake of 99m technetium methylene diphosphonate. Radiology 137:501–503, 1980

## ABDOMINAL MASS IN NEONATE

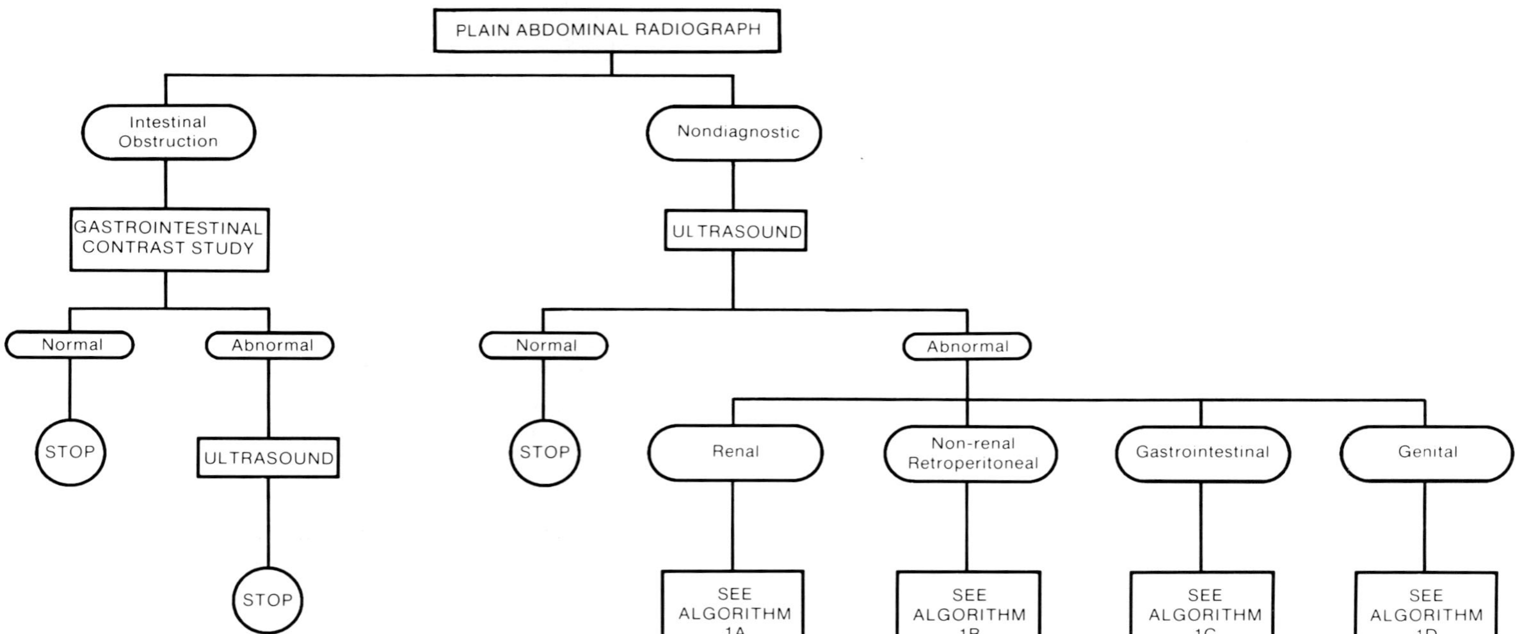

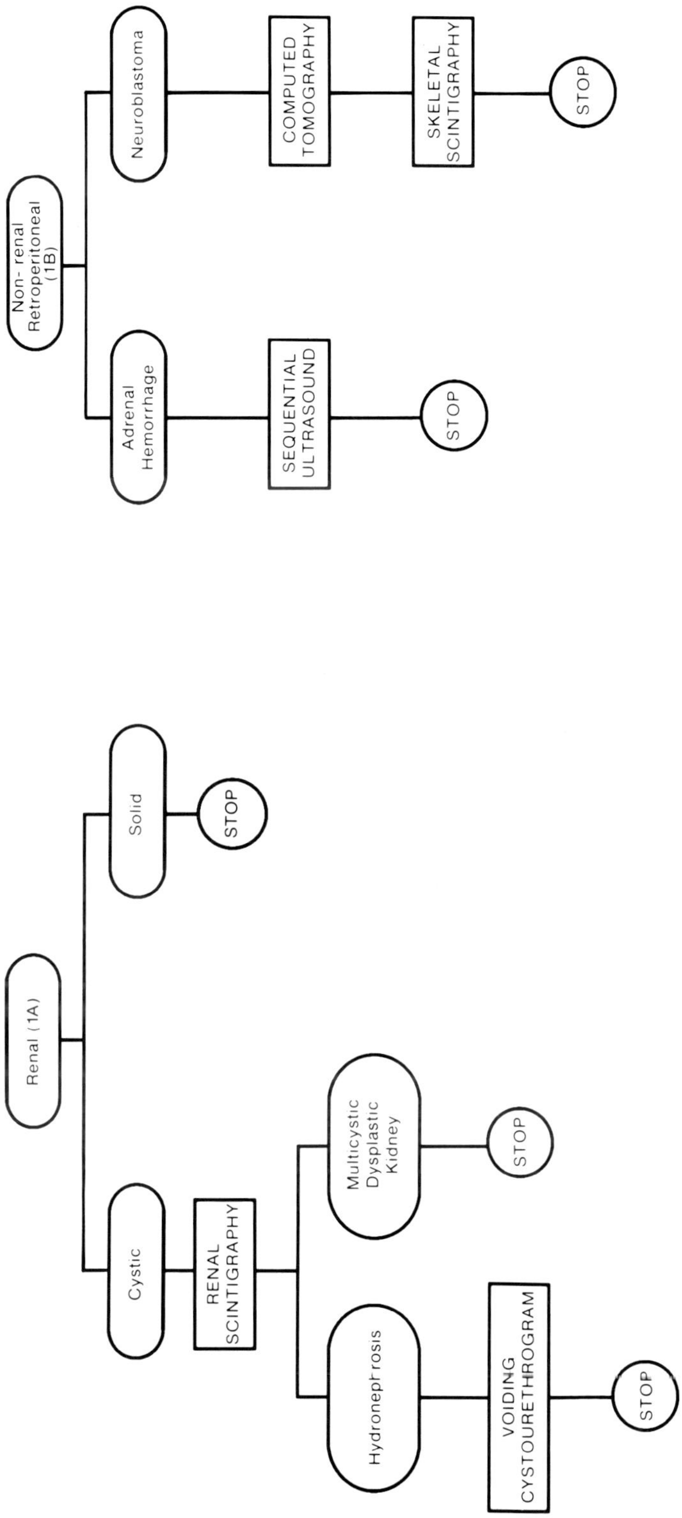

Non-renal Retroperitoneal (1B)
Adrenal Hemorrhage
SEQUENTIAL ULTRASOUND
STOP
Neuroblastoma
COMPUTED TOMOGRAPHY
SKELETAL SCINTIGRAPHY
STOP
Renal (1A)
Cystic
RENAL SCINTIGRAPHY
Hydronephrosis
VOIDING CYSTOURETHROGRAM
STOP
Multicystic Dysplastic Kidney
STOP
Solid
STOP

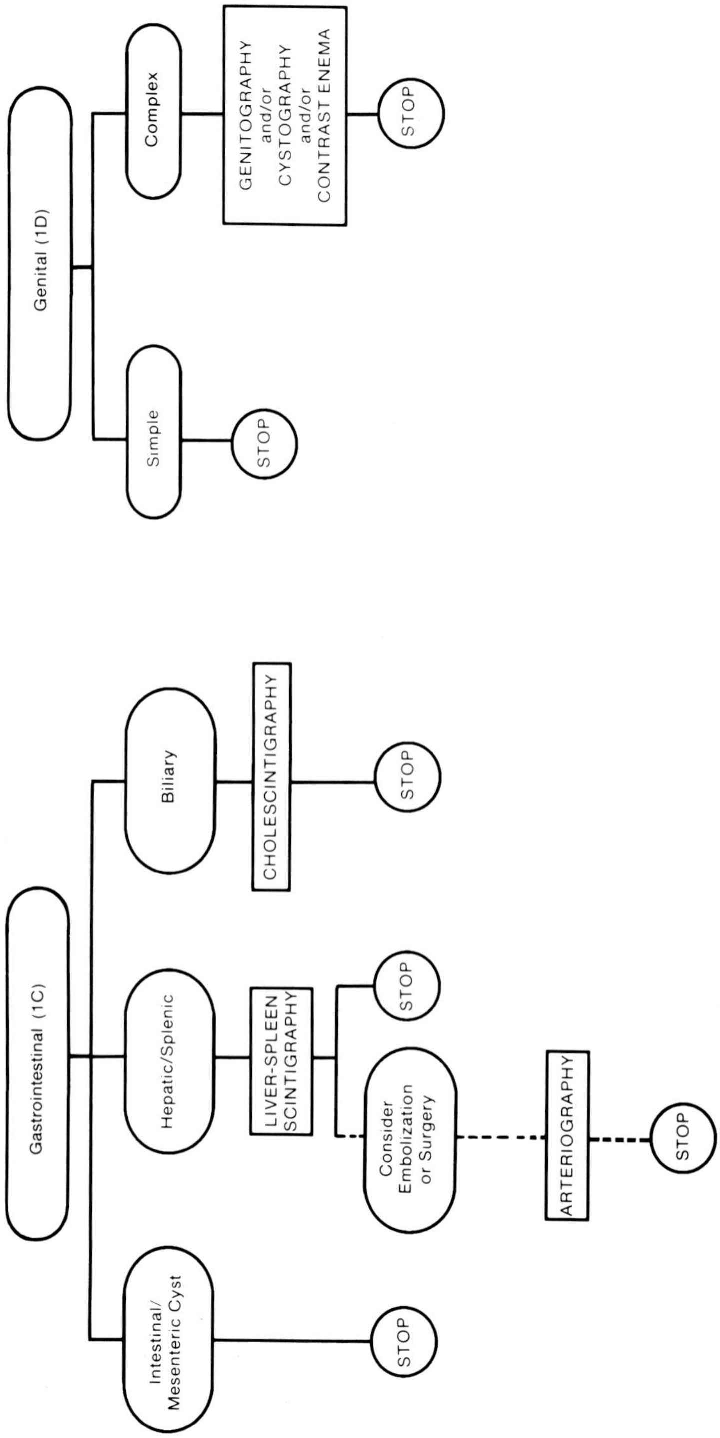

Genital (1D)
Simple
STOP
Complex
GENITOGRAPHY
and/or
CYSTOGRAPHY
and/or
CONTRAST ENEMA
STOP
Gastrointestinal (1C)
Intestinal/
Mesenteric Cyst
STOP
Hepatic/Splenic
LIVER-SPLEEN
SCINTIGRAPHY
STOP
Consider
Embolization
or Surgery
ARTERIOGRAPHY
STOP
Biliary
CHOLESCINTIGRAPHY
STOP

**ABDOMINAL MASS IN CHILD**

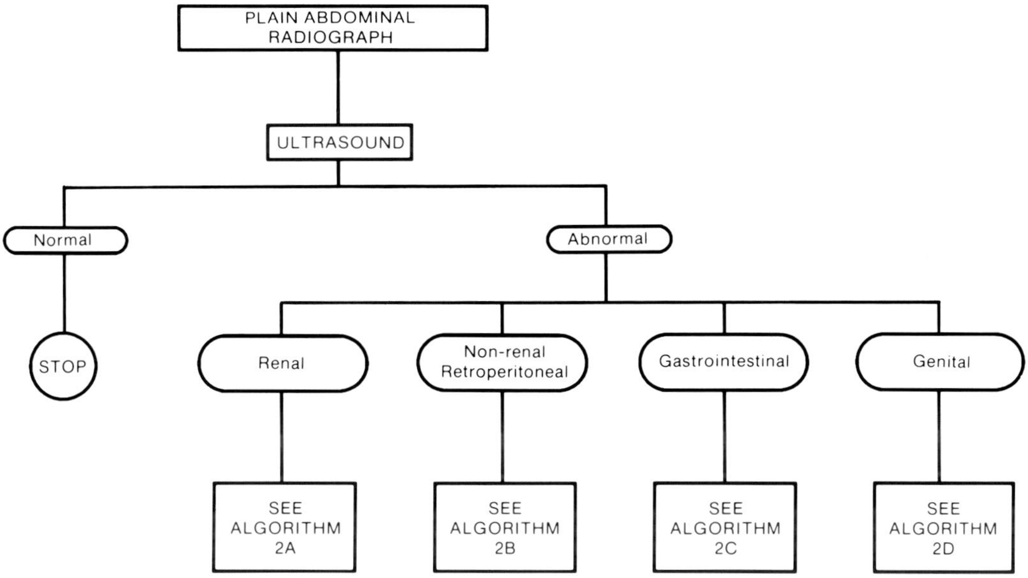

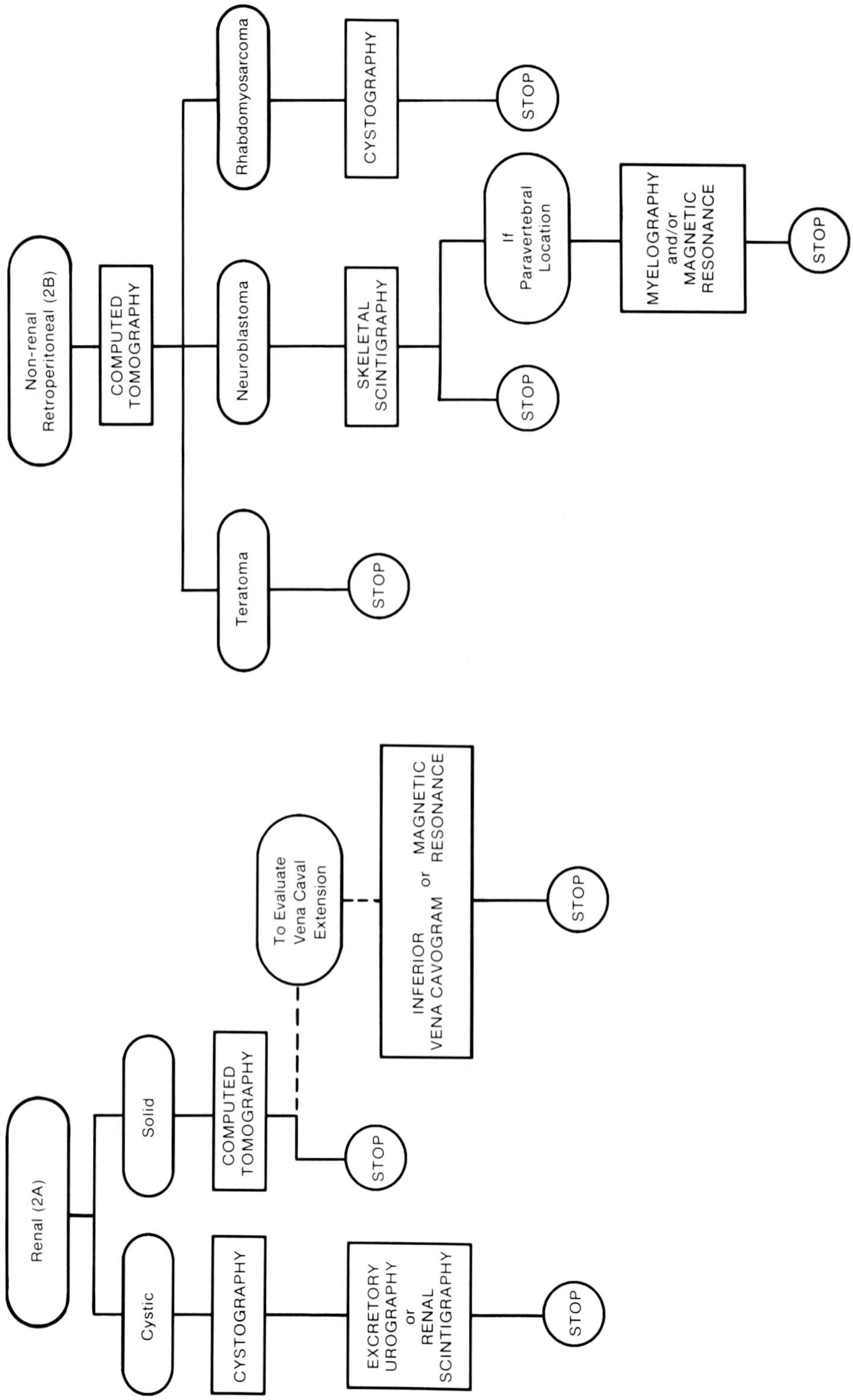

Non-renal Retroperitoneal (2B)
COMPUTED TOMOGRAPHY
Rhabdomyosarcoma
CYSTOGRAPHY
STOP
Neuroblastoma
SKELETAL SCINTIGRAPHY
STOP
If Paravertebral Location
MYELOGRAPHY and/or MAGNETIC RESONANCE
STOP
Teratoma
STOP
Renal (2A)
Cystic
CYSTOGRAPHY
EXCRETORY UROGRAPHY or RENAL SCINTIGRAPHY
STOP
Solid
COMPUTED TOMOGRAPHY
STOP
To Evaluate Vena Caval Extension
INFERIOR VENA CAVOGRAM or MAGNETIC RESONANCE
STOP

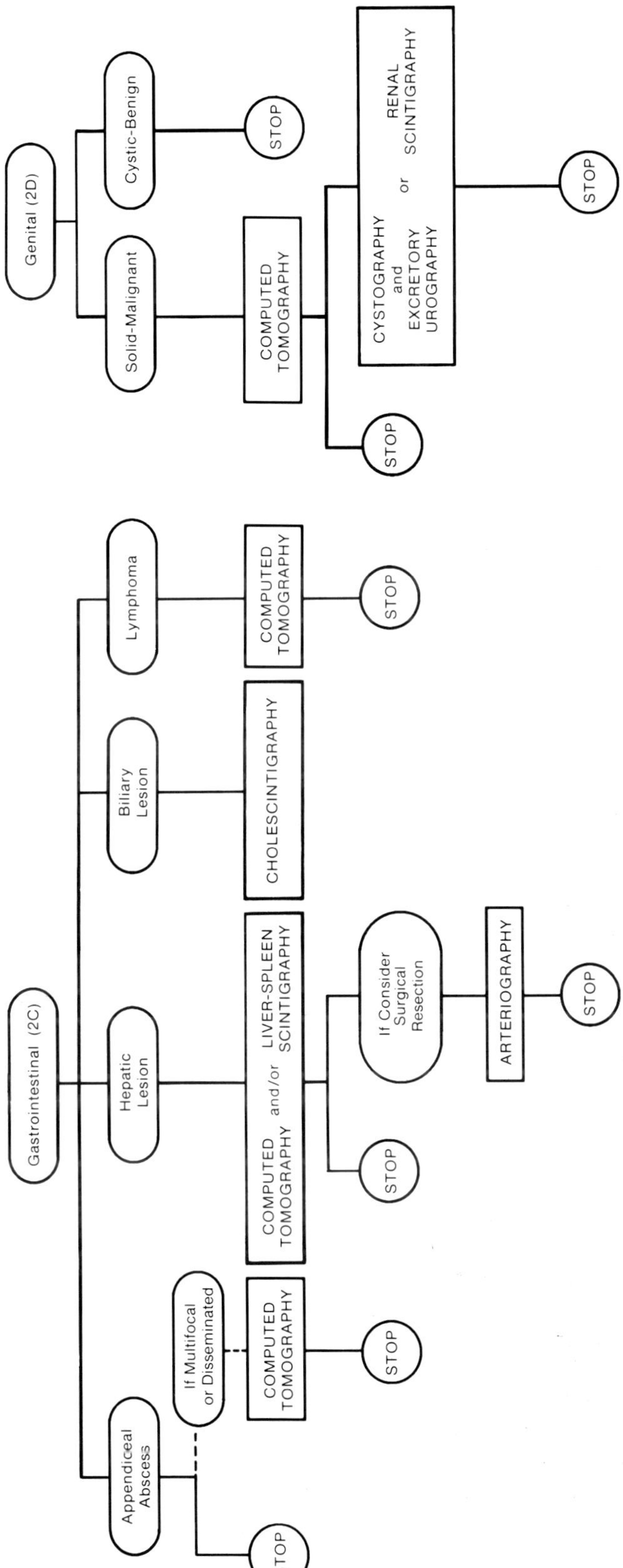
Gastrointestinal (2C)
Appendiceal Abscess
If Multifocal or Disseminated
COMPUTED TOMOGRAPHY
STOP
STOP
Hepatic Lesion
COMPUTED TOMOGRAPHY and/or LIVER-SPLEEN SCINTIGRAPHY
STOP
If Consider Surgical Resection
ARTERIOGRAPHY
STOP
Biliary Lesion
CHOLESCINTIGRAPHY
Lymphoma
COMPUTED TOMOGRAPHY
STOP
Genital (2D)
Solid-Malignant
COMPUTED TOMOGRAPHY
STOP
CYSTOGRAPHY and EXCRETORY UROGRAPHY or RENAL SCINTIGRAPHY
STOP
Cystic-Benign
STOP

# Chapter 16

# Abdominal Abscess

*William E. Fulcher*
*Gordon K. McLean*

The diagnosis of abdominal abscess has been revolutionized by the use of gray-scale ultrasound, computed tomography (CT), and abscess-avid radionuclides. When combined with clinical data, these modalities should result in almost 100% accuracy in detecting abdominal abscesses. In addition, percutaneous drainage under CT or ultrasound guidance can permit the successful treatment of abdominal abscesses without need for surgery.

## CLINICAL CONSIDERATIONS

Abdominal abscesses result from a complex and shifting spectrum of etiologies. Diseases that have predominated in the past have been supplanted by other causes. For example, appendicitis was once responsible for almost half of all intra-abdominal abscesses, but now it accounts for less than 10%. Currently, the majority of abdominal abscesses occur after surgery or trauma. Other causes include hematogenous dissemination from an infectious focus elsewhere in the body and the obstruction of drainage from an organ.

The radiologist and referring physician should be aware of those patients who are at an increased risk for developing abdominal abscesses. Patients who have sustained recent surgery or trauma; alcoholics; parenteral drug abusers; chronically ill patients; and patients receiving chemotherapy, immunosuppressive medication, or steroids all have an increased likelihood of developing abdominal infections.

The clinical manifestations of abdominal abscesses are protean. The presentation may be straightforward, with spiking fever, leukocytosis, and chills. However, other patients (particularly those who are immunosuppressed) may follow such an indolent course that an occult abscess is placed rather low on the list of diagnostic possibilities.

## ANATOMIC CONSIDERATIONS

Abdominal abscesses may occur in or adjacent to one of the solid organs or the bowel. Collections within the parenchyma of the liver, spleen, or kidneys are easily identified, because they can be directly imaged by a variety of means. Abscesses arising or extending outside the confines of a solid organ or the bowel are often limited by the surrounding fascial compartments, so that the location of the original infection may be deduced correctly.

Abscesses resulting from the free intraperitoneal spread of infection pose more imaging problems than those occurring in the solid parenchymal organs. Because of intraperitoneal contamination, approximately one third of all abdominal abscesses occur at some distance from the original site of infection. Fortunately, abscess localization within the peritoneal cavity is not a random event. The dynamics of intra-abdominal fluid movement are well defined and reliable. Sites of preferred abscess localization include the following:

1. The pelvis—below the transverse mesocolon, free fluid preferentially flows into the pouch of Douglas and paravesical spaces.
2. The right subhepatic space—from the pelvis, fluid ascends the right paracolic gutter into Morison's pouch, the most dependent portion of the right upper quadrant. Because the right paracolic gutter provides the easiest outflow from the pelvis, subphrenic and subhepatic abscesses occur two to three times more often on the right than on the left side.
3. The right subphrenic space—from Morison's pouch, fluid drains around the coronary ligament and up over the dome of the liver. Because free fluid will usually enter the subphrenic space only if Morison's pouch is filled first, the occurrence of a right subphrenic abscess generally implies previous contamination of the right subhepatic space.

Abscesses in locations not easily or preferentially reached by free intraperitoneal fluid usually result from direct spread of infection from a contiguous organ. Abscesses of the lesser sac or left subphrenic space are more likely to be the sequelae of pancreatitis or perforation of a gastric ulcer or colonic diverticulum than the result of intraperitoneal spread from a distant site.

## BACTERIOLOGY

An intra-abdominal abscess often contains multiple organisms, frequently an admixture of aerobic and anaerobic strains. Overall, *Escherichia coli* remains predominant; other frequently cultured aerobes are *Klebsiella* and *Proteus*. Anaerobic organisms are being identified with increasing frequency, possibly because of the growing awareness of their role and refinements in anaerobic culture techniques. The anaerobes most commonly identified in abdominal abscesses are, in descending order of frequency, bacteroides, enterococci, clostridia. Determination of the most appropriate antibiotic regimen requires a precise bacteriologic identification. The responsibility for obtaining bacteriologic information is falling increasingly on the radiologist, because percutaneous aspiration of abscesses under radiologic guidance often provides the first available material for culture and Gram staining.

## DIAGNOSTIC EVALUATION

### *DIAGNOSTIC MODALITIES*

1. Plain radiography of the abdomen
2. Ultrasound
3. Computed tomography
4. Radionuclide scanning
5. Excretory urography and barium studies
6. Arteriography
7. Magnetic resonance imaging

### Plain Radiography of the Abdomen

Before any of the more sophisticated modalities are employed, supine and horizontal-beam plain films of the abdomen and pelvis should be obtained. These are examined for any evidence of an abscess, such as mass effect or the presence of localized extraluminal gas. Particular scrutiny is directed to the high-yield areas (*e.g.*, pelvic, subhepatic, and subphrenic spaces). Collections of extraluminal gas may be subtle and difficult to differentiate from gas normally occurring within the bowel (Fig. 16-1). Radiographs obtained shortly after surgery may be misleading, because extraperitoneal gas collections are commonly seen postoperatively and need not indicate infection. Dilated gas-filled loops of bowel in an adynamic ileus may obscure the presence of an abnormal gas collection. If the ileus is very localized, however, its presence can aid in the identification of an area of particular concern. The obliteration of normal soft-tissue planes is a helpful but not very constant sign. For example, approximately one half of patients with a psoas abscess do not demonstrate a psoas sign. Occasionally, a very large abscess displaces the bowel or a solid organ enough to be apparent on the plain film. A unilateral pleural effusion may suggest the presence of a subphrenic infection.

Conventional radiographs are of limited use in the diagnosis of abdominal abscess. Although recent retrospective analyses of plain films claim up to 70% sensitivity for detecting abscesses, other studies suggest that only 50% of abdom-

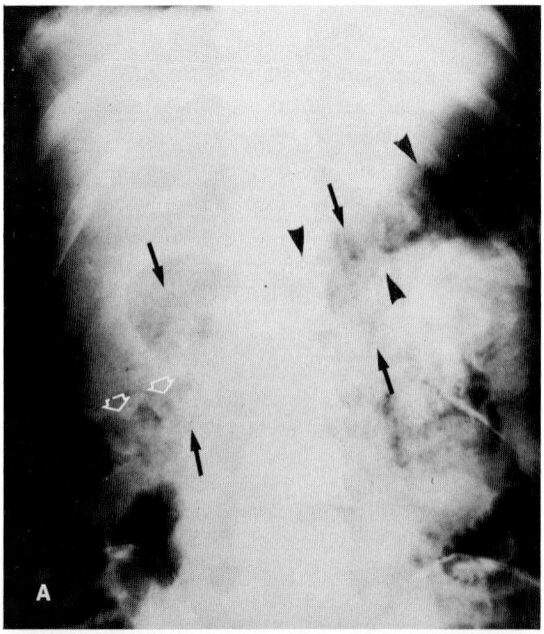


**Figure 16-1.** Pancreatic abscess. **(A)** Abdominal radiograph in a 36-year-old woman with fever and abdominal pain shows ill-defined extraluminal gas collections located centrally in the abdomen (*arrows*). Intraluminal gas in the transverse colon (*open arrows*) and stomach (*arrowheads*) makes identification of the extraluminal gas more difficult. **(B)** CT scan shows extensive gas in the pancreatic bed (*arrows*). The pancreatic abscess was drained at surgery.

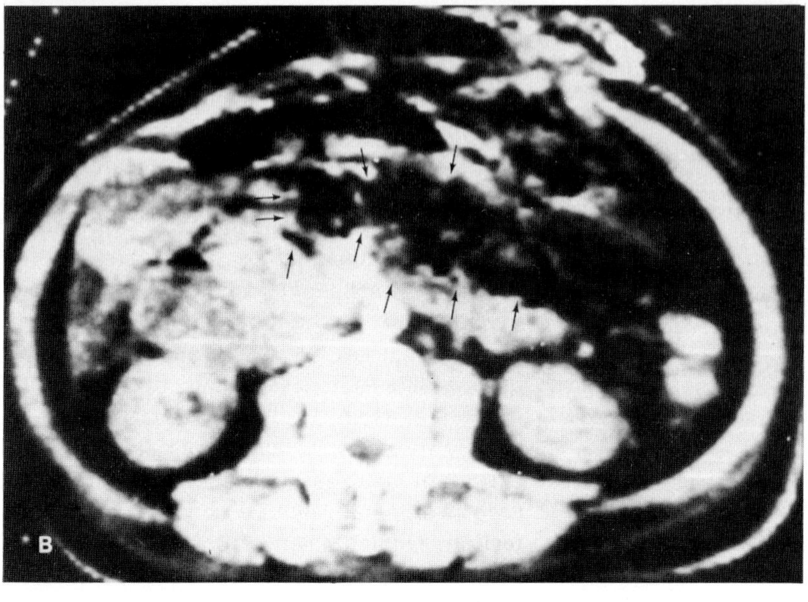

inal abscesses can be found prospectively using this technique.

## Ultrasound

Ultrasound is an extremely sensitive technique for detecting abdominal fluid collections and abscesses. With the development of real-time technology, many previous difficulties have been resolved and ultrasound has become of even greater value.

The classic ultrasound appearance of an abscess is a sonolucent collection surrounded by thick, irregular walls and clearly separable from the normal structures of the abdomen, pelvis, and retroperitoneum (Fig. 16-2*A*). In practice, many, if not most, abscesses do not present this classic pattern. A spectrum of appearances ranging from purely cystic to purely solid may occur (Fig. 16-2*B, C*). The thick, purulent contents of an abscess often produce a pattern of diffuse, weak echoes. If septations or clumps of necrotic debris are present within the central cavity, coarse, irregular echoes are seen. Internal layering of different components of the abscess may produce the bandlike pattern of a "fluid–fluid" level (Fig. 16-2*D*). Gas collections, either large or in the form of "microbubbles" reflect incident sound waves almost completely, resulting in distal "shadowing." An air–fluid level within an abscess cavity may be obscured on frontal scans and yet may be obvious on transverse or posterior oblique sonograms. Both the irregularity of abscess walls and the nature of the abscess fluid itself result in poorer definition of the wall–fluid interface than might be expected. Similarly, the through transmission of sound that is characteristic of simple cysts need not be present in abscesses (Fig. 16-2). The cross section of most abscesses is roughly elliptical; however, if the infection is confined by adhesions, fascia, or other strong barriers, the geometry is atypical. Because fluid may communicate between various intra-abdominal compartments, additional abscesses may occur in areas that are not suspected clinically. For this reason, it is important to sonographically evaluate not only the area of interest but also the entire abdomen.

Although the wide variety of sonographic appearances may seem confusing, most abscesses are readily recognized. Experienced observers can consistently detect more than 90% of abdominal abscesses, particularly those in the right upper quadrant. Like CT, ultrasound may not be able to differentiate among the various causes of abdominal fluid collections. Cysts, seromas, hematomas, necrotic tumors, abscesses, and bowel loops may have identical appearances. Occasionally, real-time sonography can identify bowel loops by showing peristalsis or changes following an enema or the drinking of fluid. Otherwise, differentiation may depend on needle aspiration of the fluid collection.

Because the liver, spleen, and bladder provide good acoustical windows, ultrasound is most useful in the detection of abscesses in the right upper quadrant, left upper quadrant, and pelvis. With the development of portable real-time units, critically ill patients can now be evaluated at the bedside. If a fluid collection is present, ultrasound can be used to guide both needle aspiration and subsequent catheter drainage.

The principal advantage of ultrasound is its sensitivity for detecting abdominal fluid collections. The examination is a flexible one; manipulation of the ultrasound transducer allows an almost infinite variety of planes to be imaged, thereby clearly identifying the anatomic relations of the lesion. Ultrasound may be performed rapidly. A single sweep of the transducer across the skin takes only a few seconds, so that good cross-sectional images can be obtained from very sick patients who can suspend respiration only briefly. Since ultrasound is a totally noninvasive procedure and delivers no ionizing radiation, it is especially suitable for the examination of children or women of childbearing age.

The principal disadvantage of ultrasound is its dependence on the technical proficiency of the operator. This has undoubtedly resulted in the wide disparity of the reported accuracy rates of this modality in abscess detection. Since the examination requires close contact between the transducer and the skin, ultrasound may be diffi-

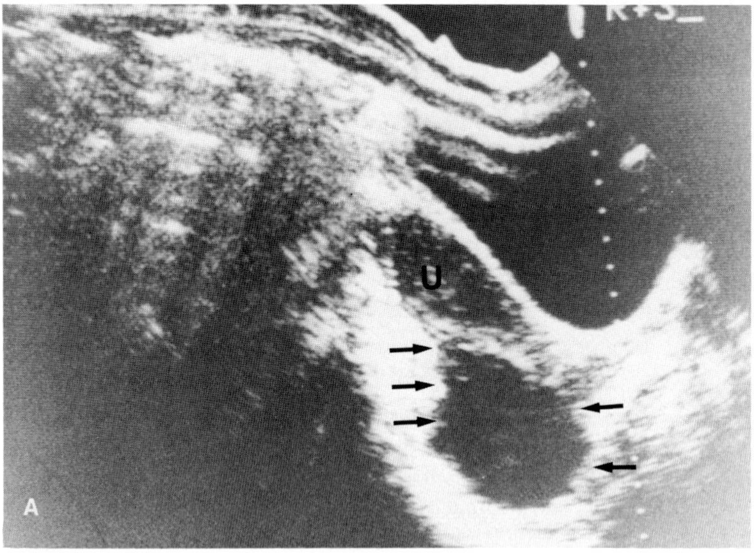


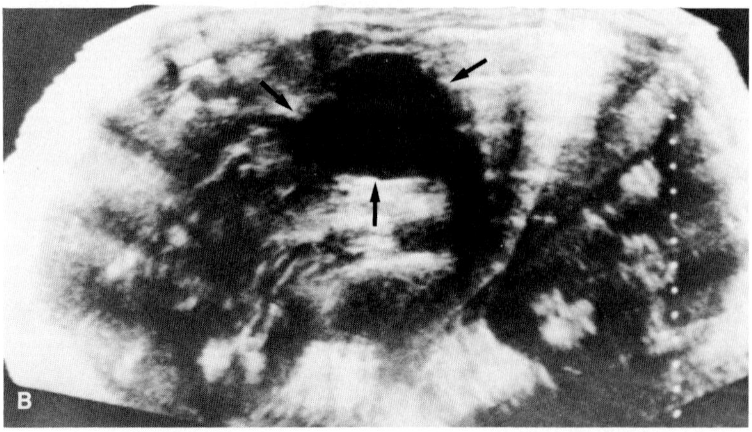


**Figure 16-2.** Sonographic features of abscess. **(A)** Sagittal sonogram through the right midpelvis in a 22-year-old woman shows a large sonolucent collection with scattered weak internal echoes (*arrows*) posterior to the uterus (*U*). Note the irregular walls of the collection and the good through sound transmission. **(B)** Cystic-appearing pancreatic abscess. Transverse sonogram through the pancreas demonstrates a large sonolucent mass (*arrow*) with good posterior acoustic enhancement. Note the smooth walls and absence of internal echoes that are characteristic of cystic lesions.

(*Continued on facing page*)

cult to employ in postsurgical patients with recent incisions, wound dressings, drains, superficial infections, or stomas. Images may also be of poor quality if the patient is particularly obese or has ascites. Since air completely reflects sound, it would seem reasonable to assume that any abscesses would be obscured by the extensive surrounding bowel gas of a reactive ileus. This problem is more theoretical than real, because most abscesses tend to localize adjacent to or adherent to the solid organs or body wall.

Although most abscesses can be imaged by ultrasound, some anatomic areas are intrinsically unsuited to this diagnostic modality. The lesser sac, for example, may be inaccessible to the ultrasound beam even in normal patients because of complete acoustic reflection by the posterior vertebrae and the anterior gastric and colonic gas. Indeed, the presence of gas may obscure a large portion of the abdominal cavity and retroperitoneum.

### Computed Tomography

The CT appearance of an abdominal abscess varies with age and maturity. Before a mature abscess cavity forms, a phlegmon may alter normal organ contours and obliterate adjacent soft-tissue planes. In the appropriate clinical setting, such changes may allow very early detection of a focal infective process. However, care must be

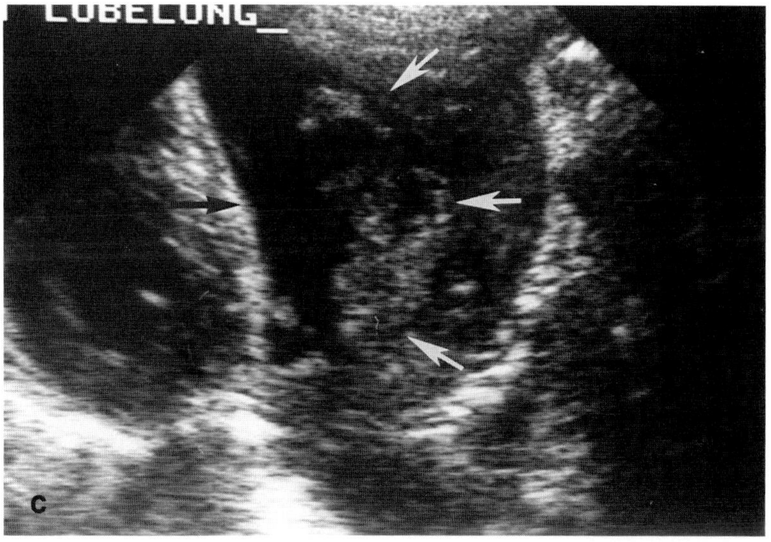


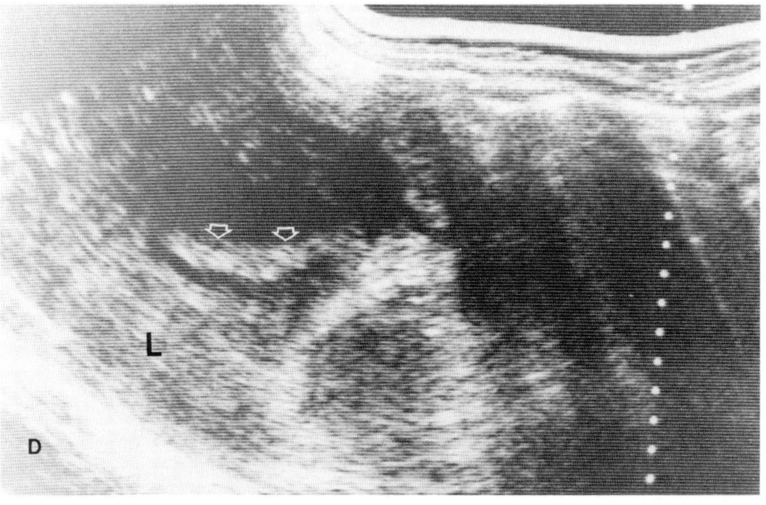


**(C)** Abscess in left lobe of the liver (*arrows*). Longitudinal sonogram shows extensive echoes within the lesion and poor posterior acoustic enhancement. **(D)** Layering of debris in an abscess. Parasagittal sonogram through the liver (*L*) in a patient with a liver abscess shows a sonolucent collection with layering of echogenic material posteriorly (*open arrows*).

exercised in interpretation because these findings are nonspecific, and infiltrating tumors or noninfectious inflammatory processes may have an identical appearance. A well-formed abscess appears as a soft-tissue or low-density mass that neither conforms to the contour of the usual parenchymal organs nor lies within the confines of the bowel (Fig. 16-3). Density values may be helpful, although they are nonspecific. The liquefied center of a mature abscess usually has a low density with attenuation values ranging from 0 to 20 Hounsfield units (HU). Abscesses with extensive necrotic debris may have attenuation numbers up to 50 HU that overlap the range usually seen with neoplasms. Abscesses commonly appear homogenous, but septations and necrotic debris may present a pattern of varying densities. The thick, irregular wall of the mature abscess can be demonstrated by CT in approximately 40% of patients. The most specific CT finding of abdominal abscess (seen in approximately 40% of cases) is the presence of gas within the central cavity (Fig. 16-3). The exquisite sensitivity of CT to minor differences in density permits the detection of minute amounts of gas. Intravenous contrast agents may be used to advantage in the detection of abscesses by CT. Following contrast administration, the hyper-

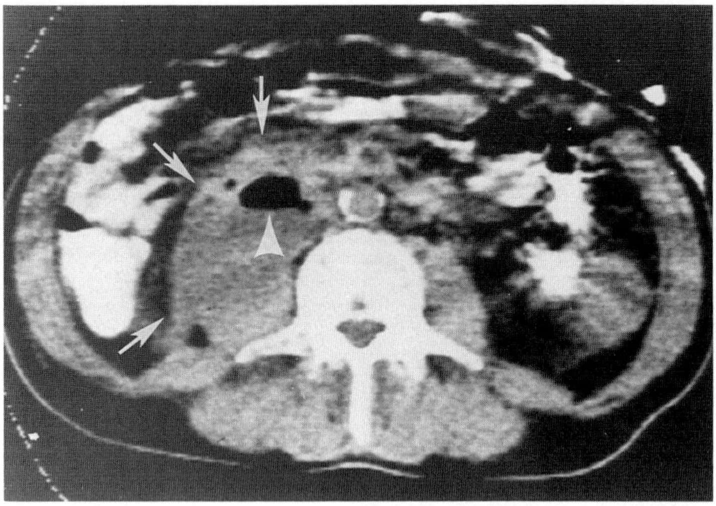

**Figure 16-3.** Psoas abscess. CT scan shows a low-density mass (*arrows*) in the region of the right psoas muscle. Note the air–fluid level (*arrowhead*) within the abscess.

vascular abscess wall may be enhanced while the central cavity remains unchanged.

Overall, CT has the highest accuracy (90%–100%) of any modality in detecting abdominal abscesses. Unlike ultrasound, false-negative CT scans are very uncommon. Nevertheless, CT is similar to ultrasound in its lack of specificity. Since even classic CT appearances can be misleading, needle aspiration is usually recommended for definitive diagnosis.

The chief advantage of CT is its unsurpassed depiction of anatomic detail. This not only facilitates abscess detection and localization, but may also be particularly valuable in directing the best surgical approach or route for percutaneous drainage. The skill of the technologist is not a major determinant of the quality of the CT image, and excellent studies are readily obtained. Since no direct machine contact with the patient is necessary, the presence of wounds, dressings, or surgical drains in no way impedes CT examination. Obese patients and those with ascites or extensive ileus can all be examined effectively. There are no anatomic regions that are not amenable to CT scanning, and it is of special value in imaging the pancreas and retroperitoneum.

Computed tomography does have several unique disadvantages. The attenuation values from which the image is constructed are not those of a true plane, but rather reflect the average density of a volume of tissue. When there is close juxtaposition of areas with widely differing densities (*e.g.,* the dome of the liver and the air-filled lung), the CT image reflects the average density of the two tissues and results in a "partial volume error." Such errors may create pseudolesions or, conversely, may obfuscate small and subtle real pathologic entities. Abrupt and extreme changes in density (*e.g.,* metallic clips or residual barium) often produce such pronounced "streaking" artifacts that the CT scan is almost uninterpretable. Since motion can degrade the image, patients must suspend respiration during each scanning cycle (a significant problem when very sick patients are examined on older CT units). Similarly, if peristaltic activity is excessive, intravenous glucagon may be necessary. Thin patients or those with poor bowel opacification may have scans that are difficult to interpret. Although CT scanners are now widely available, it is often difficult to schedule an examination quickly. In addition, the cost of CT remains several times that of ultrasound or radionuclide studies.

## Radionuclide Scanning

There are two basic approaches to the detection of abdominal abscesses by radionuclide scanning. If agents that accumulate in normal parenchyma are used, negative defects, or "cold spots," indicate displacement of the normal tissue by a pathologic process. For example, the reticuloendothelial agent $^{99m}Tc$ sulfur colloid is quite effective in locating intrahepatic or intrasplenic abscesses. However, the development of radionuclides that selectively accumulate at sites of inflammation has largely supplanted parenchymal imaging agents in abscess detection. The most widely used of these is $^{67}Ga$ citrate. This isotope selectively tags leukocytes *in vivo,* so that the migration of white blood cells to sites of infection results in an increasing local concentration of radioactivity, which usually reaches its maximum level at 24 to 72 hours after injection. More recently, $^{111}In$ oxine-tagged leukocytes ($^{111}In$-white blood cells [WBC]) has been used for localizing abscesses. A small volume of the patient's blood is removed, and the white cells are tagged *in vitro* with $^{111}In$-WBC. Since the normal characteristics of the cell are unchanged by the radionuclide tagging, as soon as the labeled leukocytes are injected into the patient they migrate to sites of infection.

Both $^{67}Ga$ and $^{111}In$-WBC allow the entire abdomen to be imaged simultaneously. Abscesses appear as a concentration of radioactivity greater than that of normal background (Fig. 16-4). The time required to develop a sufficient contrast between the site of abnormal radionuclide accumulation and the background is variable. If $^{67}Ga$ is used, large, mature abscesses that have a greater affinity for the isotope than do those in the early stages of their formation may be apparent as early as 6 hours after injection. However, most $^{67}Ga$ scans do not become positive until 24 hours have elapsed, and delays of 72 hours or more may be necessary. Scans using $^{111}In$-WBC are obtained at 18 hours after injection of the tagged cells. If the initial scans are not positive, repeat studies are obtained up to 48 hours after injection.

Gallium-67 citrate traditionally has been used as a screening test for abscesses because of its ability to examine the entire body at a low radiation dose. The sensitivity of this radionuclide is approximately 90%, although its specificity has been only approximately 65% in the face of a low pretest probability for abscess. False-positive scans may result from any inflammatory process (*e.g.*, wound healing) as well as from

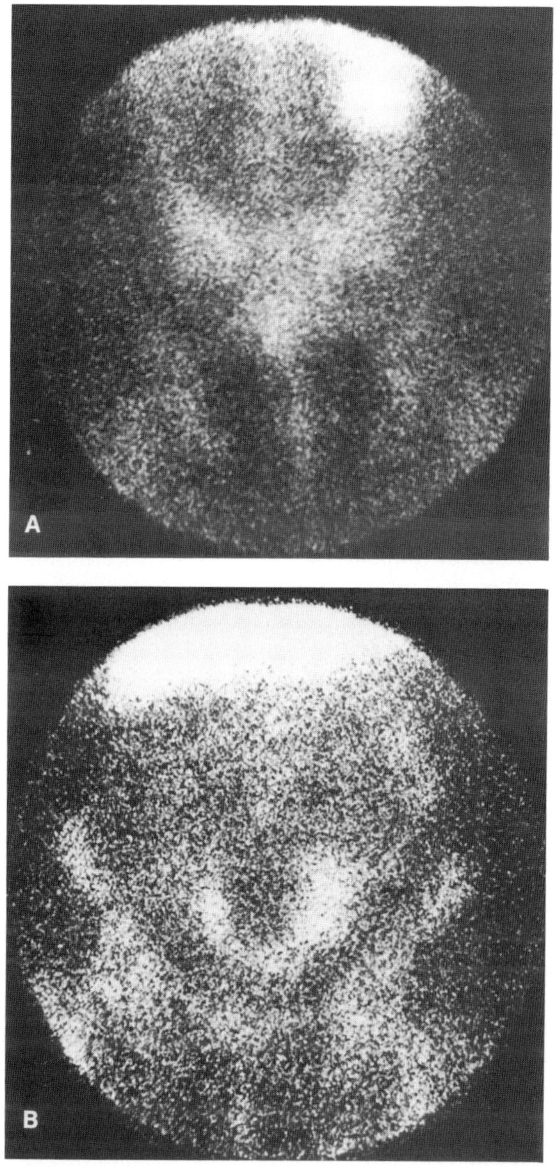


**Figure 16-4.** Radionuclide scanning of abdominal abscesses. **(A)** $^{67}Ga$ scan in a patient with a pelvic abscess. It is difficult to separate colonic activity from abscess uptake. **(B)** $^{111}In$-WBC scan in the same patient. There is no colonic uptake and the abscess is easily identified.

certain neoplasms. The major disadvantage of $^{67}$Ga is its accumulation in normal structures, such as the liver, spleen, and colon. Abscesses in these areas may be obscured, requiring imaging over a 3-day period that may represent an unacceptable diagnostic delay in critically ill patients.

Scans using $^{111}$In-WBC have higher target-to-background ratios and superior image quality than $^{67}$Ga scans. Moreover, $^{111}$In is not excreted by the bowel or kidneys, so that confusing images are minimized and scanning is generally not delayed beyond 24 hours. Indium-III scanning has a sensitivity (90%) equivalent to that of $^{67}$Ga and a much higher specificity (95% or greater). Intense focal uptake of $^{111}$In is uncommon in lesions other than abscesses or hematomas. Less prominent intensity may be seen in any inflammatory lesion as well as in some noninflammatory processes. Unlike with $^{67}$Ga, with $^{111}$In-WBC there are few, if any, false-positive results from healing wounds, alimentary or genitourinary tract activity, acute respiratory distress syndrome, or cystic fibrosis. Limitations to the use of $^{111}$In-WBC include hypokalemia, hypoglycemia, malnutrition, hemodialysis, hyperalimentation, and immunosuppressants—conditions that can alter leukocyte function and cause false-negative results.

The current radionuclide procedure of choice for detecting an abdominal abscess in the acute setting is $^{111}$In-WBC scanning because of its higher specificity and equal sensitivity to $^{67}$Ga. In the subacute or chronic setting (infections more than 2 weeks in duration), $^{67}$Ga may be the more reliable agent. Initial evidence suggests that the combination of a $^{99m}$Tc sulfur colloid scan after the $^{111}$In-WBC study may be the most accurate radionuclide approach.

Because radionuclide scans can image the entire abdomen and pelvis simultaneously, they are, theoretically, the best initial examinations for patients with suspected abdominal abscesses who present without localizing signs. Of all the diagnostic modalities, only radionuclide imaging provides physiologic information and can distinguish between inflammatory and noninflammatory lesions. If an area of increased radionuclide uptake is demonstrated, CT or ultrasound should be performed to establish the precise nature and location of the lesion. Conversely, nonspecific collections detected by ultrasound or CT may be positively identified as foci of inflammation by the use of radionuclide scanning.

### Excretory Urography and Barium Studies

Excretory urography and barium studies may help to localize an abscess by demonstrating reactive inflammatory changes or a mass effect. However, since these conventional contrast examinations are neither sensitive nor specific, their routine use is not warranted in this setting. Selected clinical situations (*e.g.,* appendicitis, diverticulitis, renal carbuncle) may provide exceptions. If barium studies are to be performed, they should follow the ultrasound, CT, or radionuclide examinations, because the quality of the latter studies may be significantly compromised by residual barium in the bowel.

### Arteriography

Arteriography has been used to localize abscesses and to narrow the differential diagnosis of mass lesions. Classically, an abscess appears as an avascular mass surrounded by a hypervascular rim. However, this pattern is not always seen, nor is it exclusive to abscesses. Avascular or necrotic tumors, metastases, cysts, and hematomas may present similar findings. Ultrasound, CT, and radionuclide scanning have largely eliminated the role of arteriography in the diagnostic workup or abdominal abscesses.

### Magnetic Resonance Imaging

Because of limited experience, the role of magnetic resonance imaging (MRI) in the detection of abdominal abscesses remains to be determined. A preliminary report suggests that the ability of MRI to directly scan in sagittal and coronal planes may make it slightly better than CT for delineating the location and extent of an abdominal abscess (Fig. 16-5). Magnetic resonance imaging also appears to demonstrate the

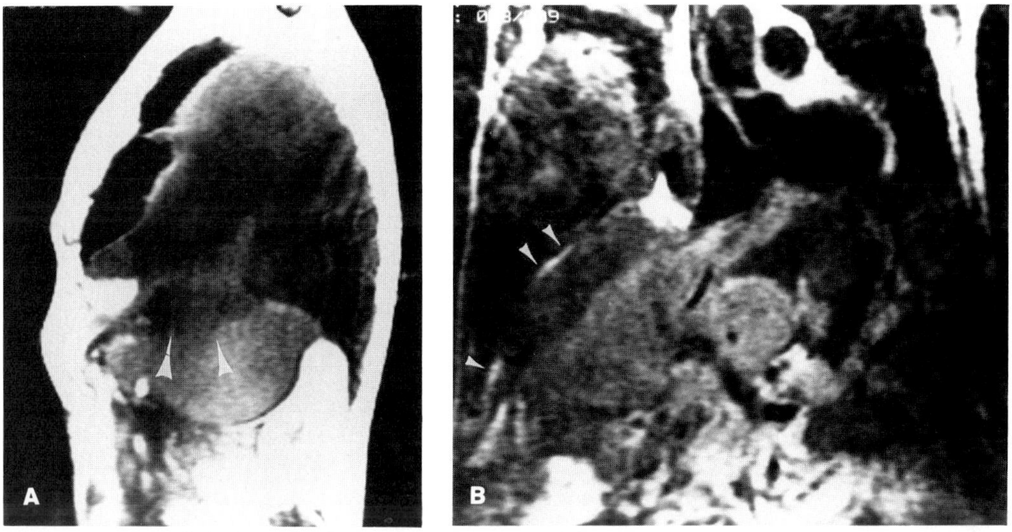


**Figure 16-5.** MRI of subdiaphragmatic abscess. **(A)** Sagittal section (SE, 300/25) shows the relatively low signal intensity of a right subphrenic abscess. Note the air–fluid level (*arrowheads*) and the right pleural effusion. **(B)** Coronal section (SE, 600/25) demonstrates the relatively high signal intensity of the diaphragm (*arrowheads*), which permits localization of the fluid.

capsule of an abscess more often than does contrast-enhanced CT. Unlike CT, MR images in postoperative patients are not degraded by artifacts from metallic surgical clips. There is also no exposure to ionizing radiation with MRI.

Disadvantages of MRI include its poor ability to evaluate areas of bone and calcification and the need for long scanning times that degrade spatial resolution in patients who are unable to suspend respiration. Magnetic resonance imaging is still not widely available and is clearly the most expensive imaging modality.

Until prospective comparisons of MRI with CT and other imaging modalities have been performed, the already proven high accuracy rate of CT makes it the imaging modality of choice for abscess localization.

## A CORRELATIVE APPROACH TO SOME REGIONAL PROBLEMS

Each imaging modality has its unique strengths and weaknesses. Integrating the information provided by an examination with that obtained in the preceding and succeeding studies will result in a high degree of diagnostic accuracy. Clearly, every available mode of investigation should not be used in each patient. The radiologic workup must be individualized so that an accurate diagnosis is reached in the shortest possible time using the least possible number of diagnostic examinations. The appropriate use of ultrasound, CT, and radionuclide scanning, in conjunction with plain radiographs and clinical data, should result in almost 100% accuracy in the detection of abdominal abscesses.

### The Perihepatic Spaces

The perihepatic spaces are the most common sites of abdominal abscesses. Approximately 85% of these infections are attributable to surgery or trauma. In the presence of an appropriate clinical history, the suspicion of a perihepatic abscess should be high even in the absence of positive physical findings. The initial plain films of the abdomen must be carefully searched for perihepatic gas collections; a right lateral decubitus view is often helpful if there is overlying

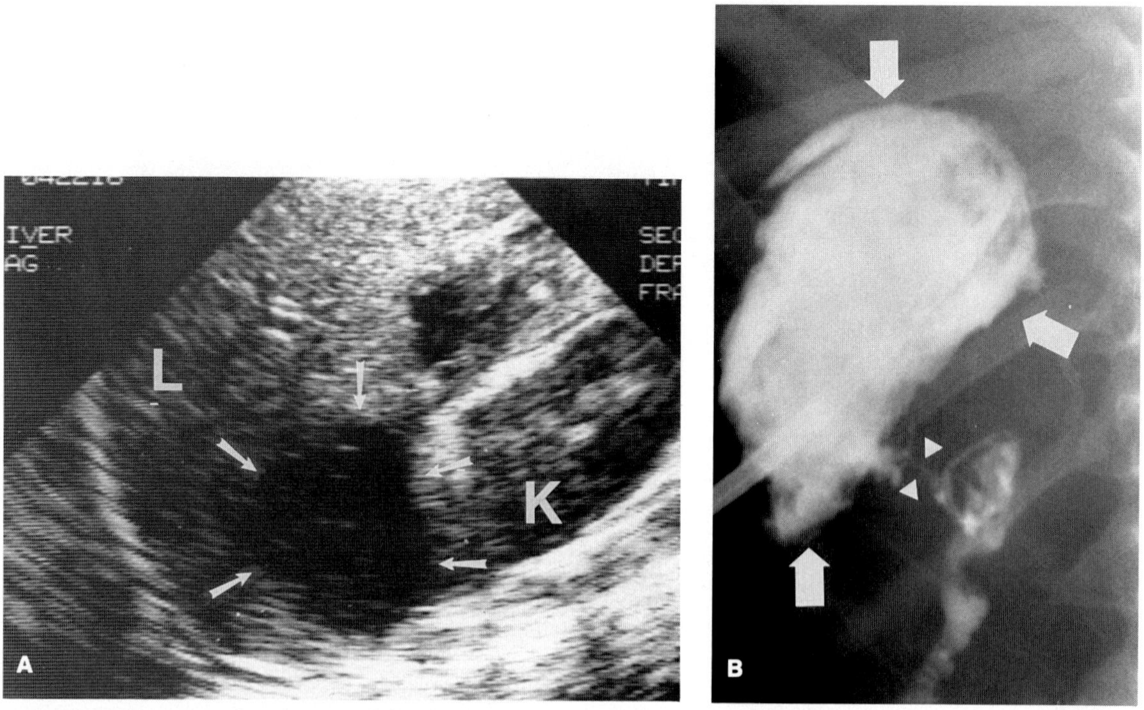


**Figure 16-6.** Postoperative abscess. **(A)** Right parasagittal sonogram demonstrates an irregular fluid collection with multiple internal echoes (*arrows*) in the subhepatic space between the liver (*L*) and kidney (*K*). **(B)** Under fluoroscopic guidance, a 12-French sump catheter has been inserted percutaneously into the subhepatic space. A contrast injection demonstrates the size of the abscess cavity (*arrows*) and a connection to the small bowel (*arrowheads*).

colonic gas. Secondary signs, such as a localized ileus of the hepatic flexure or a right pleural effusion, are suspicious but may simply reflect nonspecific postoperative changes.

Ultrasound is the procedure of choice for detecting a suspected abscess in the perihepatic spaces (Fig. 16-6). The liver parenchyma serves as an excellent acoustic window for examining these areas. If the findings are characteristic, no further diagnostic examination need be performed, and definitive therapy may be instituted. If a suspicious lesion is found, radionuclide scanning with either $^{67}$Ga or $^{111}$In-WBC may be performed or the lesion may be immediately aspirated for diagnosis if time is critical. If the radionuclide study is positive, the diagnosis of an abscess is made and the radiologic workup is complete. If the lesion does not accumulate the radionuclide, it is unlikely to represent an abscess and should be further characterized by CT.

If the ultrasound examination is negative or equivocal, CT should be the next imaging procedure. Positive CT findings should be further characterized by needle aspiration or a radionuclide study. If the CT findings or clinical data are equivocal, radionuclide scanning with either $^{67}$Ga or $^{111}$In-WBC is indicated. If the radionuclide study shows active inflammation, the diagnosis of an abscess is made and the workup is complete. A negative radionuclide scan effectively rules out an abscess. If a CT study of the perihepatic space is negative, the study should be extended to search the remainder of the abdomen and pelvis. If, despite a negative CT study, an occult abscess is still suspected clinically, the entire abdomen and pelvis should be scanned with $^{67}$Ga or $^{111}$In-WBC.

## The Left Subphrenic Space

Left subphrenic space abscesses are less common than those occurring on the right. Most follow surgery or trauma; pancreatitis or perforation of a gastric ulcer or colonic diverticulum may also produce this condition. Plain radiographs of the abdomen may demonstrate displacement of the air-filled gastric fundus, thus providing the first evidence of a left subphrenic collection. Left-sided pleural effusions may occur in association with many subphrenic processes and therefore are not specific.

Computed tomography is the preferred initial examination for a suspected abscess in the left subphrenic space. A negative CT study excludes a left subphrenic abscess. A positive CT study or an equivocal one (not uncommon if there has been recent surgery or trauma) should be followed by radionuclide scanning, because the overlapping spectrum of findings may preclude the differentiation of an infected from a sterile (*e.g.*, perisplenic hematoma) collection. Alternatively, a positive CT scan can be immediately followed by needle aspiration.

Ultrasound is occasionally an effective method for examining the left upper quadrant. More often, however, the presence of gas in the left upper quadrant anteriorly and the absence of good acoustic windows posteriorly and laterally usually preclude satisfactory ultrasound examination. A thorough ultrasound examination is possible only if the transducer can be angled up steeply under the ribs and moved freely in the intercostal spaces. Much of the perisplenic space is frequently inaccessible to the ultrasound beam.

The barium enema examination is contraindicated in patients with suspected left subphrenic space abscess. Although barium examination of the stomach may confirm the presence of a mass in the left upper quadrant, it usually gives little information about the nature or extent of the process. Of more importance, the presence of retained barium within the stomach significantly delays the performance of more sensitive and specific studies, such as CT, radionuclide scanning, and ultrasound.

## The Accessible Parenchymal Organs

### The Liver

Ultrasound is the preferred method of screening for a suspected intrahepatic abscess. A positive ultrasound study should be followed by $^{67}$Ga or $^{111}$In-WBC scanning or needle aspiration to differentiate abscesses from liquefied hematomas, necrotic tumors, or simple hepatic cysts. If ultrasound is not available, conventional liver–spleen radionuclide scanning can be performed. Computed tomogrpahy is rarely indicated unless the presence of additional abscesses in other portions of the abdomen is suspected or unless there is a high clinical suspicion of a liver abscess in the face of negative ultrasound and radionuclide studies.

### The Spleen

Either CT or $^{99m}$Tc sulfur colloid scanning can be used to screen for space-occupying lesions of the spleen. Scanning with $^{67}$Ga and $^{111}$In-WBC or direct needle aspiration is then performed to specifically identify the intrasplenic mass as an abscess. Ultrasound is of less value in this area, because the greater portion of the spleen lies beneath the ribs and is largely hidden from the ultrasound beam.

### The Kidneys

Excretory urography is still the most widely used screening examination for suspected renal abscess. Ultrasound is the preferred second examination, because it can demonstrate and characterize not only intrarenal collections (*e.g.*, renal carbuncle) but also the perirenal and pararenal abscesses commonly associated with intraparenchymal infection. If the infection is so widespread as to make precise definition of its extent impossible by ultrasound alone, CT may be helpful. Thickening of Gerota's fascia may be the first sign of a perirenal infection; this subtle change can be consistently demonstrated by CT and is also occasionally apparent on ultrasound.

### Difficult Areas

#### The Pancreas and Lesser Sac

Radiographic imaging of abscesses of the pancreas or lesser sac can be extremely difficult. The superimposition of the stomach and transverse colon often makes confident identification of abnormal gas collections on plain radiographs impossible (Fig. 16-1). If there is any significant ileus, the pancreas generally cannot be imaged adequately by ultrasound. The lesser sac is frequently inaccessible to ultrasound because of the spine posteriorly and gas in the stomach and colon anteriorly. Computed tomography is the procedure of choice, because it can most consistently image abscesses of the pancreas or lesser sac (Fig. 16-7). To determine whether fluid collections detected on CT represent abscesses, they should be further characterized by needle aspiration. If the patient has a paucity of intra-abdominal fat, precise definition of the pancreatic boundaries by CT may not be possible. In some cases, abscesses of the pancreas or lesser sac can be detected only by radionuclide scanning with $^{67}$Ga or $^{111}$In-WBC.

#### The Pelvis

Because the vagina provides a direct route of access to the pelvis, the majority of pelvic infections (*e.g.*, tubo-ovarian abscesses, infected ovarian cysts) occur in women; most patients have no history of surgery or trauma. Pelvic abscesses can be mimicked closely by a variety of pathologic processes, such as endometriomas, ovarian cysts, ectopic pregnancies, and necrotic uterine fibroids.

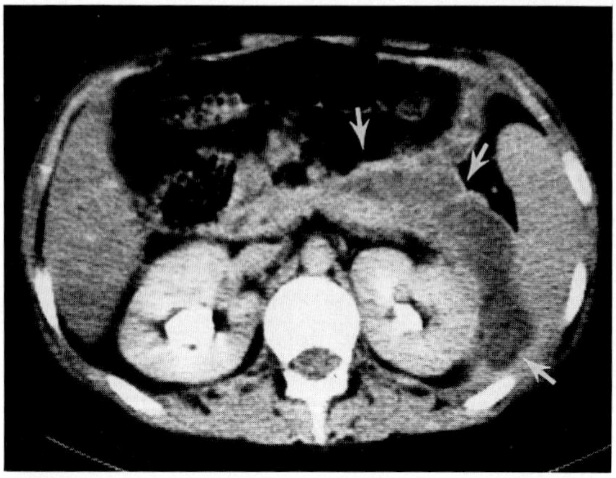

**Figure 16-7.** Pancreatic abscess. Contrast-enhanced CT scan in a 14-year-old girl with abdominal pain and fever shows a low-density fluid collection (*arrows*) in the region of the pancreatic body and tail adjacent to the spleen.

Plain radiographs of the pelvis are usually of little value in detecting pelvic abscesses. Abnormal gas collections may be masked by fecal material in the rectum and in loops of small bowel. Asymmetry of the soft-tissue contours (*e.g.*, the obturator internus muscle) is frequently present but is nonspecific.

Ultrasound is the diagnostic procedure of choice for detecting pelvic abscesses. The fluid-filled urinary bladder provides an excellent acoustic window for examining the supravesical and paravesical spaces and the pouch of Douglas. When the bladder is fully distended (occasionally requiring infusion of saline through a Foley catheter), confusing loops of small bowel are displaced out of the pelvis. If fecal material in the rectum cannot be differentiated from an abscess, an enema may be required. Additionally, filling the rectum with water permits ultrasound examination of the presacral space.

Computed tomography also may be used to examine the pelvis, but it is neither as sensitive nor as versatile as ultrasound. Since the differential diagnosis of cystic masses in the pelvis is large, radionuclide scanning may be necessary to confirm the inflammatory nature of the lesion. The normal accumulation of $^{67}$Ga in the sigmoid colon and rectum may seriously limit the use of this isotope. Therefore, $^{111}$In-WBC is the preferred agent for radionuclide scanning of the pelvis. Needle aspiration can reliably determine whether a fluid collection is infected.

## RADIOGRAPHIC APPROACH TO THERAPY OF ABDOMINAL ABSCESS

Once a fluid collection is detected and defined by ultrasound or CT, percutaneous needle aspiration should be performed to characterize the fluid. Ultrasound or CT is used to plan the easiest and safest route and to guide the needle puncture. The aspirated fluid is sent for Gram staining, culture, and, occasionally, chemical analysis.

If the aspirate is grossly purulent, or contains white blood cells or bacteria on Gram staining, drainage is indicated. In the past, surgery was the only method of drainage, although it was associated with a mortality rate of 25% and a cure rate of only 70% to 85%. With current techniques of percutaneous catheter drainage, the cure rate is approximately 90% and there is only a 10% mortality rate. In addition, the less invasive percutaneous technique permits a shorter period of hospitalization and is associated with fewer complications.

Patient selection criteria for percutaneous drainage continue to evolve. Initially, drainage was recommended for simple, solitary, well-defined, unilocular collections. More recent experience has shown that a variety of more complicated abscesses (*e.g.*, complex loculated, ill-defined, or extensively dissecting collections; multiple abscesses; abscesses associated with enteric fistulae) also respond well to catheter drainage. Although drainage is certainly more difficult with phlegmons, infected hematomas, interloop abscesses, or collections with very thick debris, even in such cases there can be a beneficial temporizing effect. The only absolute contraindication to percutaneous drainage is the lack of a safe access route. At present, in some institutions the only indication for open surgical drainage of an abdominal abscess is the lack of response to percutaneous catheter drainage.

Computed tomography is generally the preferred imaging modality for planning the access route for catheter drainage. Whenever possible, the approach should avoid unaffected parenchymal organs or spaces and allow for optimal drainage with the shortest catheter path that is safe. Commercially available catheters range from 8 French to at least 24 French in diameter. In general, nonviscous collections can be adequately drained with smaller catheters, whereas extensive or thick purulent collections need catheters of much larger diameter.

## Bibliography


Aeder MI, Wellman JL, Haaga JR, Han T: Role of surgical and percutaneous drainage in the treatment of abdominal abscesses. Arch Surg. 118: 273–280, 1983

Alexander ES, Colley DP, Clark RA: Computed tomography of retroperitoneal fluid collections. Semin Roentgenol 16:268, 1981

Brolin RE, Nosher JL, Leiman S et al: Percutaneous catheter versus open surgical drainage in the treatment of abdominal abscesses. Am Surg 50: 102–108, 1983

Callen PW: Computed tomographic evaluation of abdominal and pelvic abscesses. Radiology 131: 171–175, 1979

Casola G, van Sonnenberg E: Diagnosis and percutaneous drainage of abdominal abscesses. Clin Gastroenterol 14:469, 1985

Cronan JJ, Amis ES, Dorfman GS: Percutaneous drainage of renal abscesses. AJR 142:351–354, 1984

Datz FL, Luers P, Baker WJ et al: Improved detection of upper abdominal abscesses by combination of $^{99m}$Tc sulfur colloid and $^{111}$In leukocyte scanning. AJR 144:319, 1985

Froelich JW, Swanson D: Imaging of inflammatory processes with labeled cells. Semin Nucl Med 14:128, 1984

Gerzof SG, Johnson WC, Robbins AH et al: Expanded criteria for percutaneous abscess drainage. Arch Surg 120:227–232, 1985

Gerzof SG, Robbins AH, Johnson WC et al: Percutaneous abscess drainage. Semin Roentgenol 16:62–71, 1981

Johnson WC, Gerzof SG, Robbins AH, Nabseth DC: Treatment of abdominal abscesses. Ann Surg 194:510–520, 1981

Johnson RD, Mueller PR, Ferrucci JT, Jr: Percutaneous drainage of pyogenic liver abscesses. Radiology 144:463, 1985

Kay CJ, Pawar SU, Rosenfield A: Sonography of splenic abscesses. Semin Ultrasound 4:91, 1983

Koehler PR, Moss AA: Diagnosis of intraabdominal and pelvic abscesses by computerized tomography. Radiology 138:265, 1981

Korobkin M, Callen PW, Filly RA et al: Comparison of computed tomography, ultrasonography, and gallium-67 scanning in the evaluation of suspected abdominal abscess. Radiology 129:89–93, 1978

Kuligowska E, Newman B, White SJ, Caldarone AG:

Interventional ultrasound in the detection and treatment of renal inflammatory disease. Radiology 147:521, 1983

Lerner RM, Spataro RF: Splenic abscess: Percutaneous drainage. Radiology 153:643, 1984

McAfee JG, Samin A: In-lll labeled leukocytes: Review of problems in image interpretation. Radiology 155:221, 1985

Meyers MA: Dynamic Radiology of the Abdomen: Normal and Pathologic Anatomy. New York, Springer-Verlag, 1976

Mintz MC, Arger PH, Kressel HY: Algorithmic approach to the radiologic evaluation of a suspected abdominal abscess. Semin Ultrasound 4:80, 1983

Mueller PR, Simeone JF: Intraabdominal abscesses: Diagnosis by sonography and computed tomography. Radiol Clin North Am 21:425, 1983

Papanicolau N, Butch RJ, Mueller PR: Percutaneous abscess drainage. Semin Ultrasound 4:117, 1983

Papanicolau N, Mueller PR, Ferrucci JT, Jr et al: Abscess–fistula association: Radiologic recognition and percutaneous management. AJR 143: 811, 1984

Sfakianakis GN, Al-Sheikh W et al: Comparisons of scintigraphy with In-lll leukocytes and Ga-67 in the diagnosis of occult sepsis. J Nucl Med 23: 618–626, 1982

van Sonnenberg E, Mueller PR, Ferrucci JT, Jr: Percutaneous drainage of 250 abdominal abscesses of fluid collections. Part I—Results, failures, and complications; Part II—Current procedural concepts. Radiology 151:343, 1984

van Sonnenberg E, Wittlich GR, Casola GI et al: Complicated pancreatic inflammatory disease: Diagnostic and therapeutic role of interventional radiology. Radiology 155:335, 1985

Wall SD, Fisher MR, Amparo RF: Magnetic resonance imaging in the evaluation of abscesses. AJR 144:1217, 1985

## SUSPECTED PERIHEPATIC ABSCESS

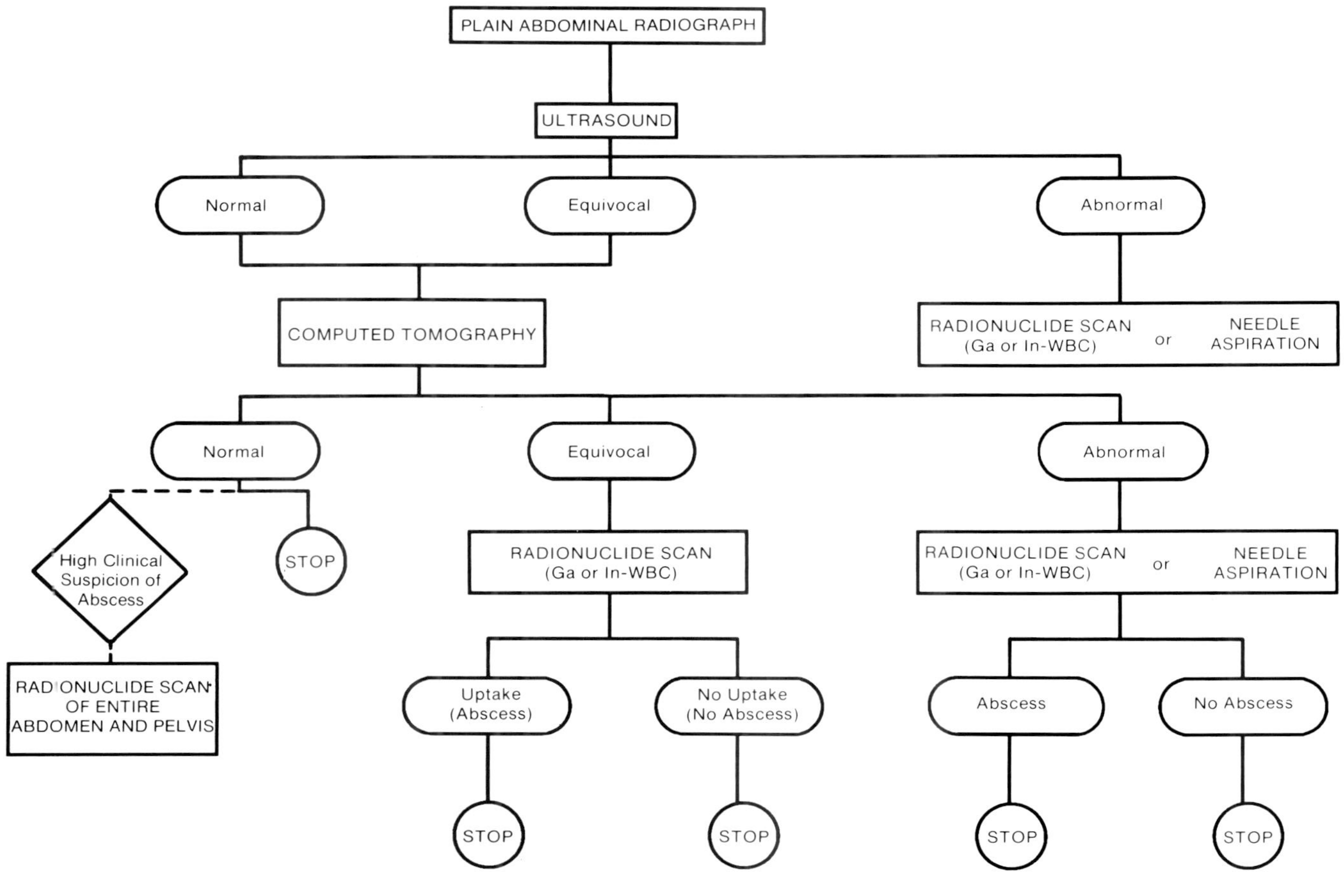

## SUSPECTED LEFT SUBPHRENIC ABSCESS

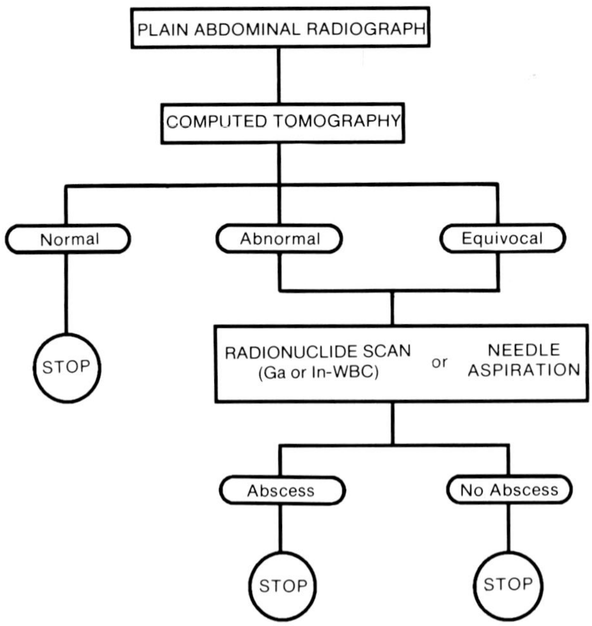

## SUSPECTED ABDOMINAL ABSCESS
## (No Localized Findings)

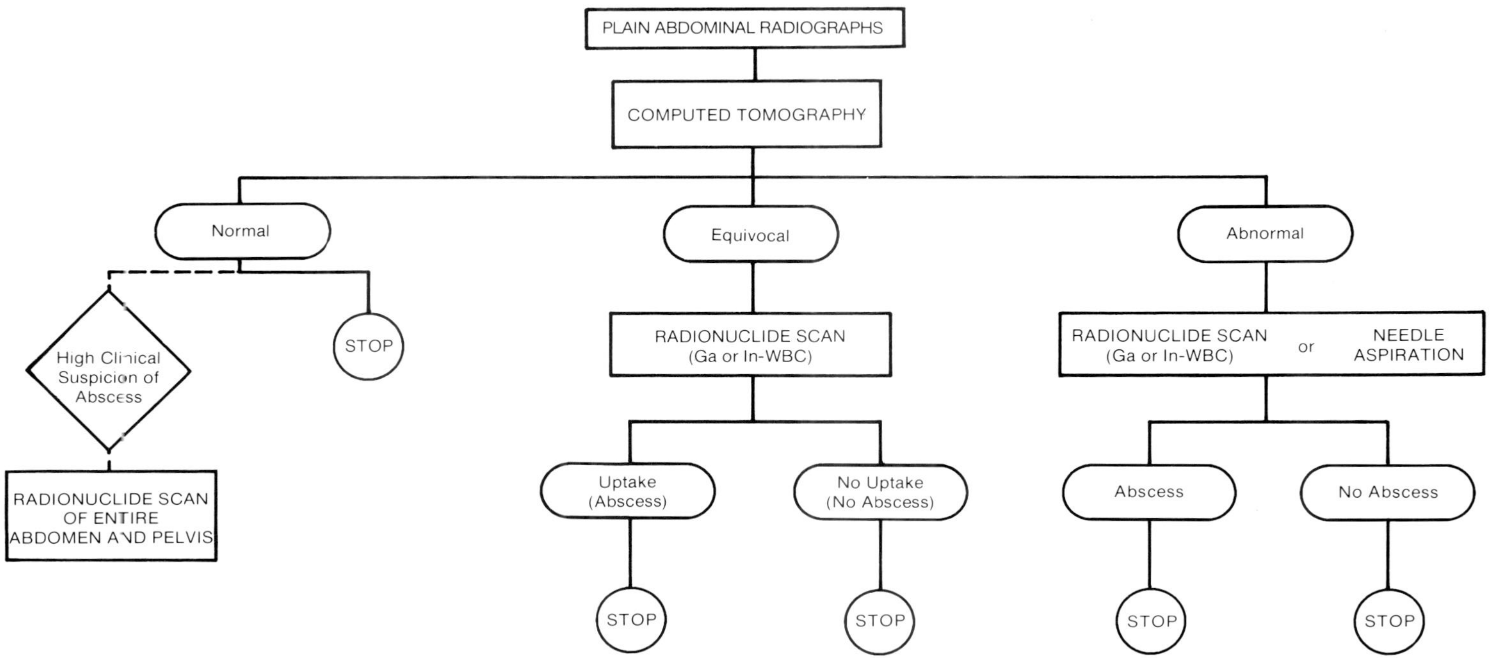

## SUSPECTED SPLENIC ABSCESS

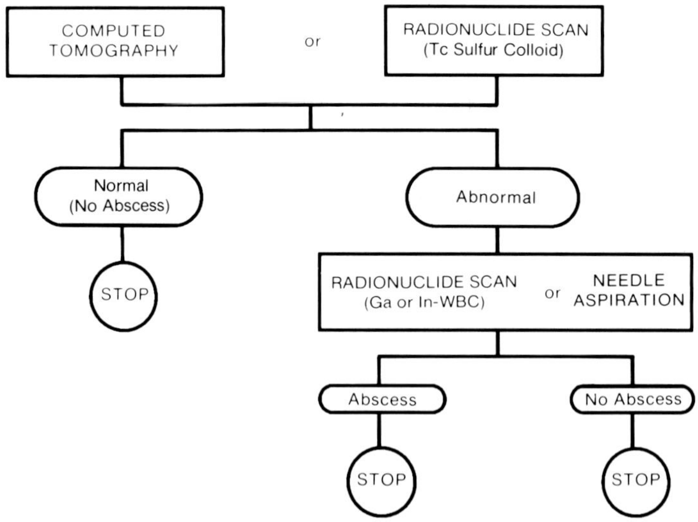


## SUSPECTED RENAL OR PERIRENAL ABSCESS

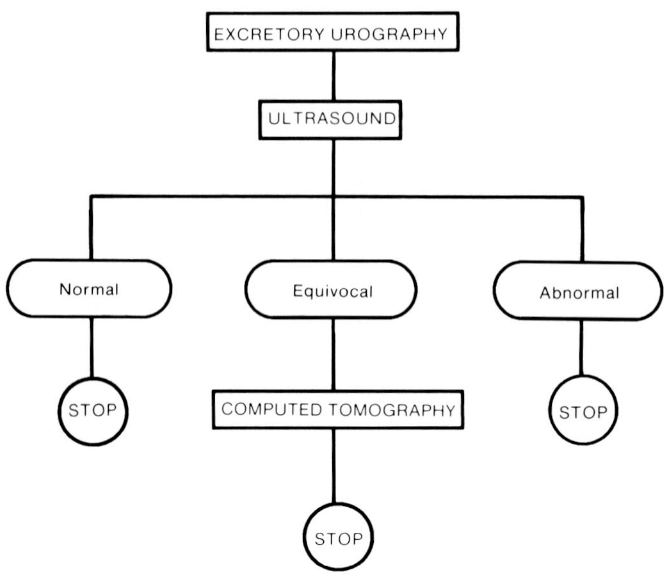

## SUSPECTED PANCREATIC OR LESSER SAC ABSCESS

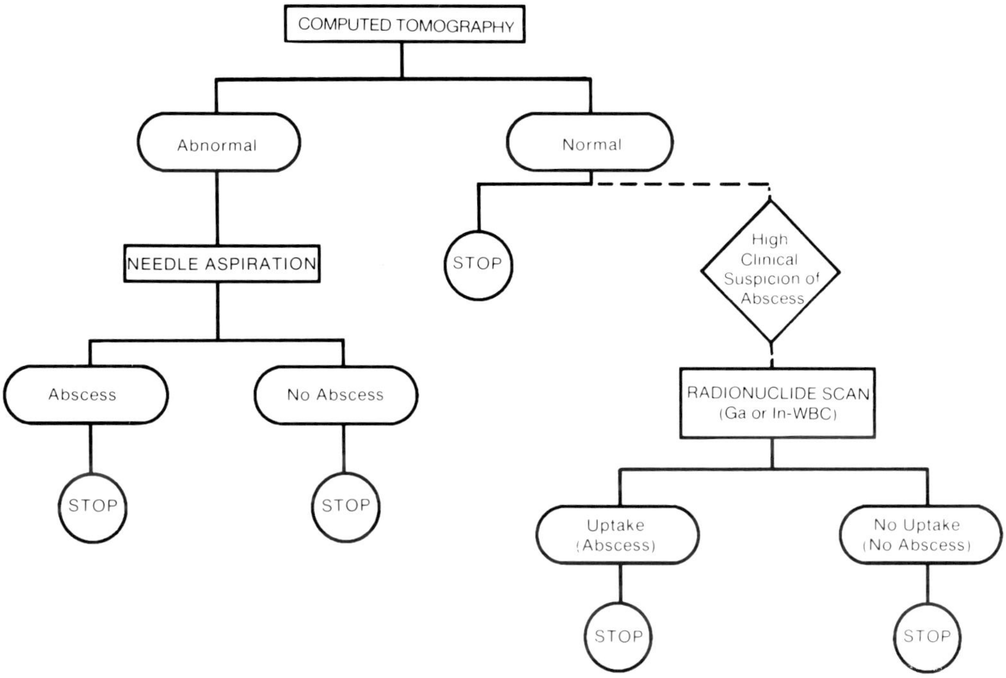


## SUSPECTED PELVIC ABSCESS

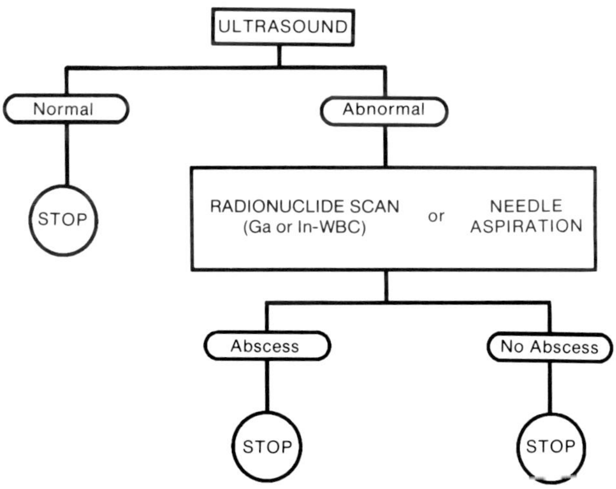

**SUSPECTED ABDOMINAL ABSCESS**
**(No Localized Findings)**

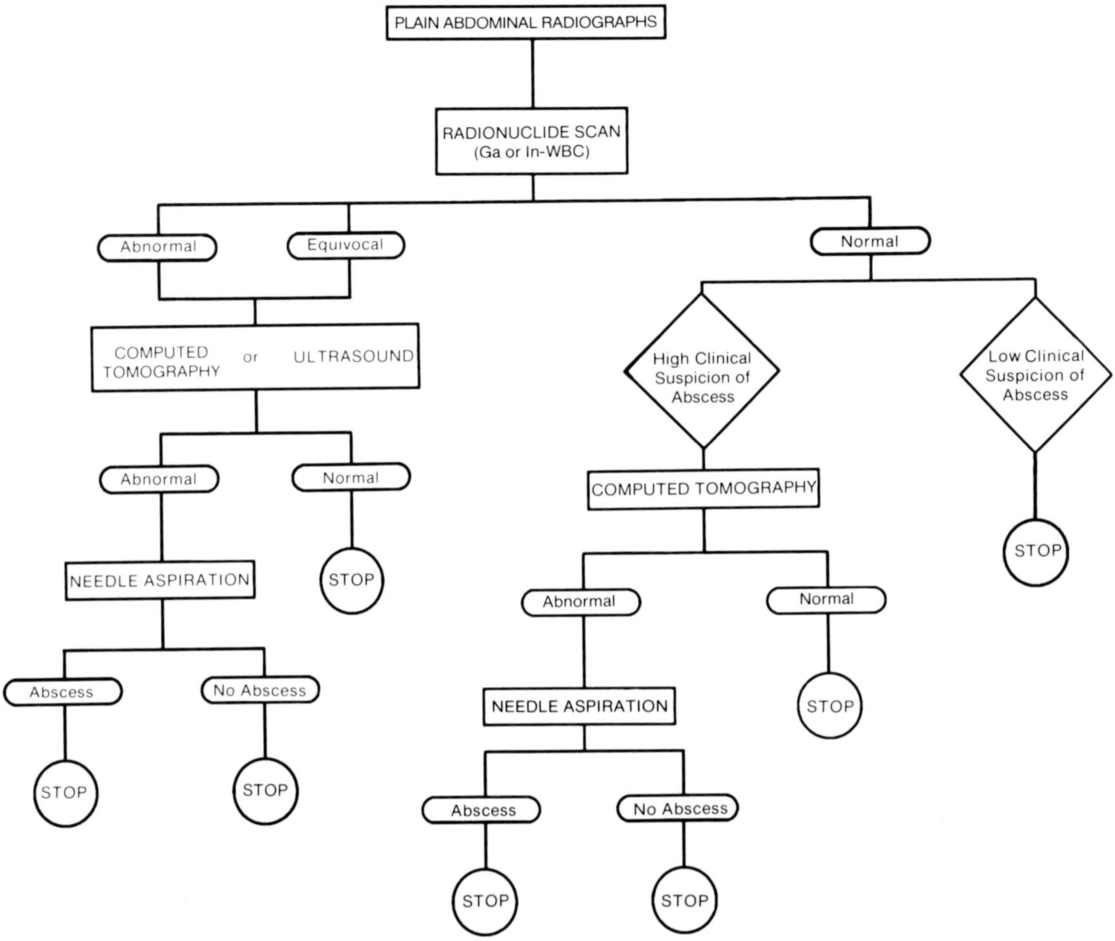

# Chapter 17

# Abdominal Aortic Aneurysm

*Madeleine R. Fisher*
*Barbara E. Demas*
*Robert L. Vogelzang*

Aneurysms of the abdominal aorta develop in approximately 1% to 2% of patients and most are of arteriosclerotic origin. Less common causes include infection, cystic medial necrosis, and trauma. Aneurysmal dilatation is defined as a diameter of the abdominal aorta greater than 3 cm. Almost all abdominal aortic aneurysms arise below the level of the renal arteries; approximately 2% to 5% are suprarenal in origin and usually represent extension of a thoracic aortic aneurysm into the abdomen. Patients with abdominal aortic aneurysms often have aneurysms in other arteries as well. Approximately 12% have thoracic aneurysms, 10% have aneurysms of the lower extremity (especially involving the popliteal artery), and almost two thirds have aneurysmal dilatation of one or both of the iliac arteries. Abdominal aortic aneurysms commonly affect men over 60 years of age; more than half of these patients have associated hypertension, and cigarette smoking is a proven contributing factor.

Most abdominal aortic aneurysms are fusiform and involve the entire circumference of the aorta. The less common saccular aneurysms affect only a portion of the circumference and consist of an outpouching with a mouth. In true aortic aneurysms, which involve all three layers of the aortic wall, the primary defect is destruction of the elastic fibers in the media that permits the remaining fibrous tissue to stretch and results in an increased diameter that raises wall tension. Laminated thrombi frequently form in areas of sluggish blood flow within the aneurysm, and this may lead to embolization of thrombotic and arteriosclerotic debris. Expanding aneurysms can compress contiguous structures and may eventually rupture. Abdominal aortic aneurysms with a diameter greater than 6 cm have about a 50% likelihood of rupture within a 10-year period, whereas only 15% to 20% of aneurysms with a diameter of less than 6 cm will rupture during this time. Almost 90% of abdominal aortic aneurysms that eventually rupture do so into the retroperitoneum, with a mean survival of 1 day between rupture and death. The remainder rupture into the peritoneal cavity and cause rapid death from exsanguination.

The differential diagnosis of a suspected abdominal aortic aneurysm is extensive and includes diffuse ectasia of the aorta, primary and metastatic tumors of the peritoneal and retroperitoneal spaces, mesenteric cysts and sarcomas, pancreatic lesions (abscess, pseudocysts, carcinoma), lymphadenopathy, horseshoe kidney, retroperitoneal hematoma, and retroperitoneal fibrosis.

## CLINICAL AND LABORATORY FINDINGS

Most abdominal aortic aneurysms are asymptomatic and are discovered incidentally on routine physical examination or a plain abdominal radiograph. A vague sense of fullness within the epigastrium may be the only subjective complaint. If pain is present, it most commonly is centered in the hypogastrium and lower back, and it tends to be steady, gnawing in nature, and persistent for hours or days at a time. Unlike musculoskeletal pain, movement does not alter the pain associated with an abdominal aortic aneurysm. The sudden onset of pain, or constant severe pain, located in the back or lower abdomen and occasionally radiating into the groin, buttocks, or legs should suggest an expanding abdominal aortic aneurysm with impending rupture. Actual rupture of the aneurysm produces extreme abdominal or back pain, hypotension, and usually shock.

On physical examination, an abdominal aortic aneurysm commonly presents as a pulsatile mass extending a variable distance from the upper to lower abdomen. However, even large aneurysms may be difficult to palpate, especially in obese individuals. The size of the aneurysm is usually overestimated on physical examination because of overlying structures. At times, a tortuous, ectatic aorta may be confused with aneurysmal dilatation. Some aneurysms are tender on palpation, especially if they are rapidly expanding or ready to rupture. Occasionally, a bruit may be heard over the site of an aneurysm.

Ruptured abdominal aortic aneurysms produce several patterns of physical findings including hemorrhagic shock with hypotension, vasoconstriction, diaphoresis, and oliguria; retroperitoneal hemorrhage with hematoma extending into the flanks and groin; peritoneal rupture with abdominal distention; and rupture into the duodenum with massive gastrointestinal hemorrhage.

## DIAGNOSTIC EVALUATION

### *DIAGNOSTIC MODALITIES*

1. Plain abdominal radiographs
2. Ultrasound
3. Computed tomography
4. Magnetic resonance imaging
5. Aortography
6. Digital subtraction aortography

### Plain Abdominal Radiographs

Traditionally, plain abdominal radiographs have been an easy and useful aid for establishing the diagnosis of an abdominal aortic aneurysm when the physical findings are inconclusive. Frontal and lateral views may show curvilinear calcification in the wall of an aneurysm; if both walls are calcified, the dimensions of the aneurysm can be estimated. In approximately 20% of cases, a previously unknown abdominal aortic aneurysm is detected on a preliminary abdominal radiograph obtained as part of a gastrointestinal or urologic evaluation. Unfortunately, more than one fourth of all abdominal aortic aneurysms do not have detectable calcification on plain radiographs and thus cannot be detected by this modality. Rarely, an abdominal aortic aneurysm may erode the anterior margin of a vertebral body, which can be seen on a lateral view. Thus, although plain abdominal radiographs may suggest the presence of an abdominal aortic aneurysm, the sensitivity of this modality is so low that it cannot be considered an adequate screening examination. In addition, the plain film affords no information regarding the extent or exact dimensions of an aneurysm, the presence of thrombus within it, or possible involvement of the renal and iliac arteries.

### Ultrasound

Ultrasound provides a noninvasive, rapid, accurate, and relatively inexpensive screening test for the patient with a suspected abdominal aortic aneurysm. It is highly sensitive and specific for delineating aneurysmal dilatation of the aorta. Disadvantages of ultrasound include the difficulty to routinely demonstrate the origins of the renal arteries and the entire extent of the aneurysm (both suprarenally and into the iliac arteries), as well as the frequent inability to demonstrate relatively fresh thrombus that is poorly organized. In addition, patient obesity, contrast material within the gastrointestinal tract, and excessive gas within the bowel may preclude satisfactory ultrasound imaging of the abdominal aorta.

The sonographic criterion of an abdominal aneurysm is dilatation of the aorta to greater than 3 cm (Fig. 17-1). Most aneurysms are fusiform in shape and appear on transverse images as round, sonolucent structures that may contain concentric or eccentric intraluminal echoes representing thrombus. Laminated thrombus within an aneurysm, particularly when well organized, appears as echoes between the sonolucent lumen and the aortic wall. The echo pattern of mural thrombus is related to its age and homogeneity. Ultrasound may fail to detect poorly organized thrombus or thrombus that is homogeneous (especially if the aorta is occluded). Mural calcification produces thick, regular, nonlinear echoes with acoustic shadowing.

The current indications for the use of ultrasound in patients with suspected aortic aneurysm depend on the institution. In some, ultrasound is the imaging modality of choice for detection and evaluation of the aneurysm. In others, computed tomography (CT) is considered to be more accurate and thus is performed as the initial imaging procedure.

### Computed Tomography

Computed tomography is a sensitive and specific modality for detecting aneurysmal dilatation of the abdominal aorta. Studies have shown CT to be more accurate than ultrasound in determining the true diameter and longitudinal extent of an aneurysm, showing intraluminal thrombus (Fig. 17-2) and assessing the effects of an aneurysm on branch vessels and surrounding structures. Computed tomography also can demonstrate the retroperitoneal hematoma associated with acute rupture of an aneurysm. Compared with ultrasound, however, CT is more costly and time consuming, uses ionizing radiation, and usually requires the intravenous injection of contrast material. Residual barium within the gastrointestinal tract may produce scanning artifacts. At times, the superior margin of an abdominal aortic aneurysm may angulate forward because of saccular buckling and may cause the incorrect CT diagnosis of renal artery involvement.

Computed tomography can differentiate an abdominal aortic aneurysm from a tortuous aorta regardless of whether there is calcification in the aortic wall. On plain radiographs, calcification limited to a portion of the wall of a tortuous, normal-sized aorta that is deviated laterally may mimic the curvilinear calcification of an abdominal aortic aneurysm. Unlike plain abdominal radiographs, on which calcification within the wall of an aortic aneurysm cannot be identified in more than 25% of cases, on CT scans aortic wall calcification can be detected in almost every patient with an aneurysm. An intravenous injection of contrast material generally is required to show intraluminal thrombus. A repeat bolus of contrast and imaging with thin sections may be needed to demonstrate the renal arteries. Displacement or obstruction of the inferior vena cava or ureters by an abdominal aortic aneurysm can be easily detected on CT.

The current indications for the use of CT in patients with suspected abdominal aortic aneurysms depend on the institution. Although CT has a higher overall accuracy than ultrasound in detecting and characterizing an abdominal aortic aneurysm, the lower cost and lack of ionizing radiation often make the latter the preferred modality for initial screening.

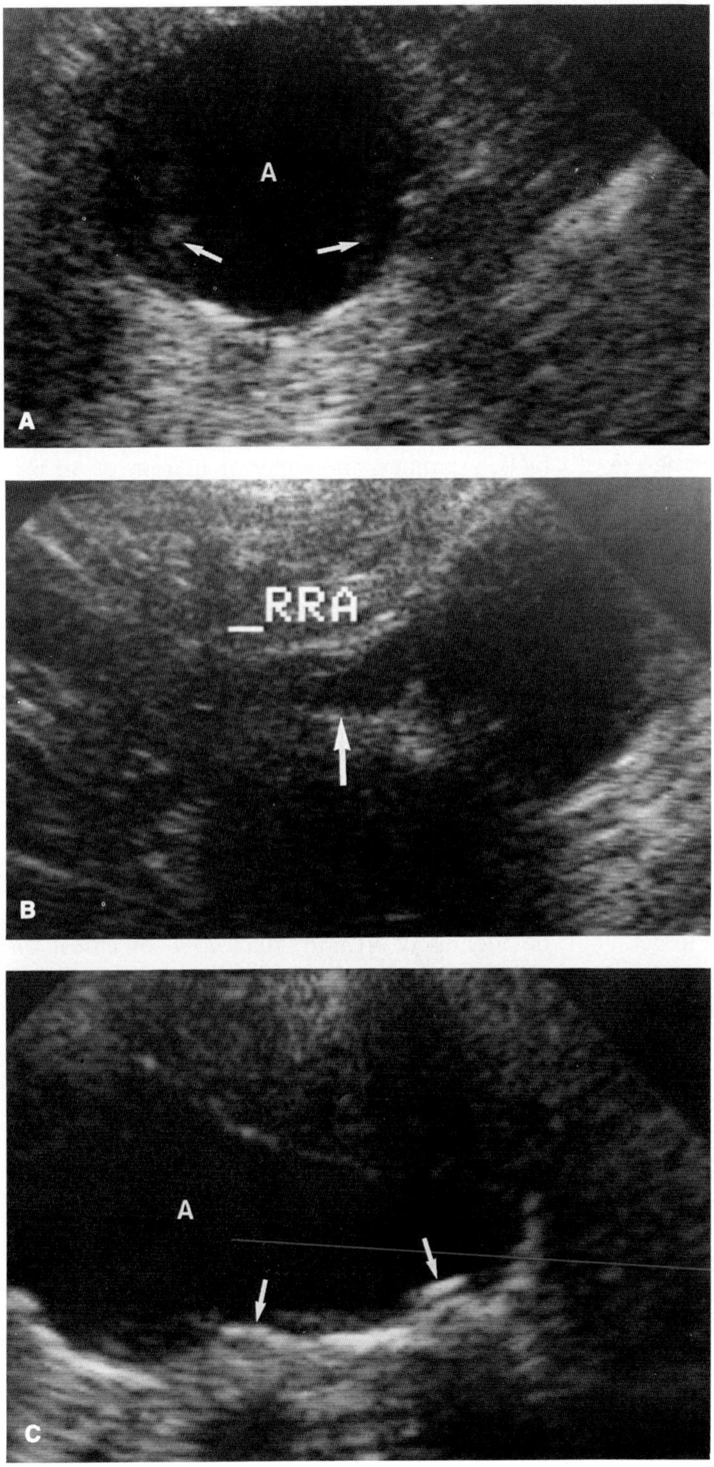


**Figure 17-1.** Abdominal aortic aneurysm arising at the renal artery level. **(A)** Transverse sonogram demonstrates the anechoic residual lumen (labeled *A*) containing low-level internal echoes (*arrows*) that represent eccentric mural thrombus. **(B)** Transverse sonogram shows the origin of the right renal artery (*arrow*) in addition to the aneurysmal dilatation of the aorta. Visualization of the renal arteries is often difficult on ultrasound. **(C)** Longitudinal sonogram through the aneurysm (*A*) demonstrates mural calcifications as thick, irregular, nonlinear echoes (*arrows*) with acoustic shadowing.

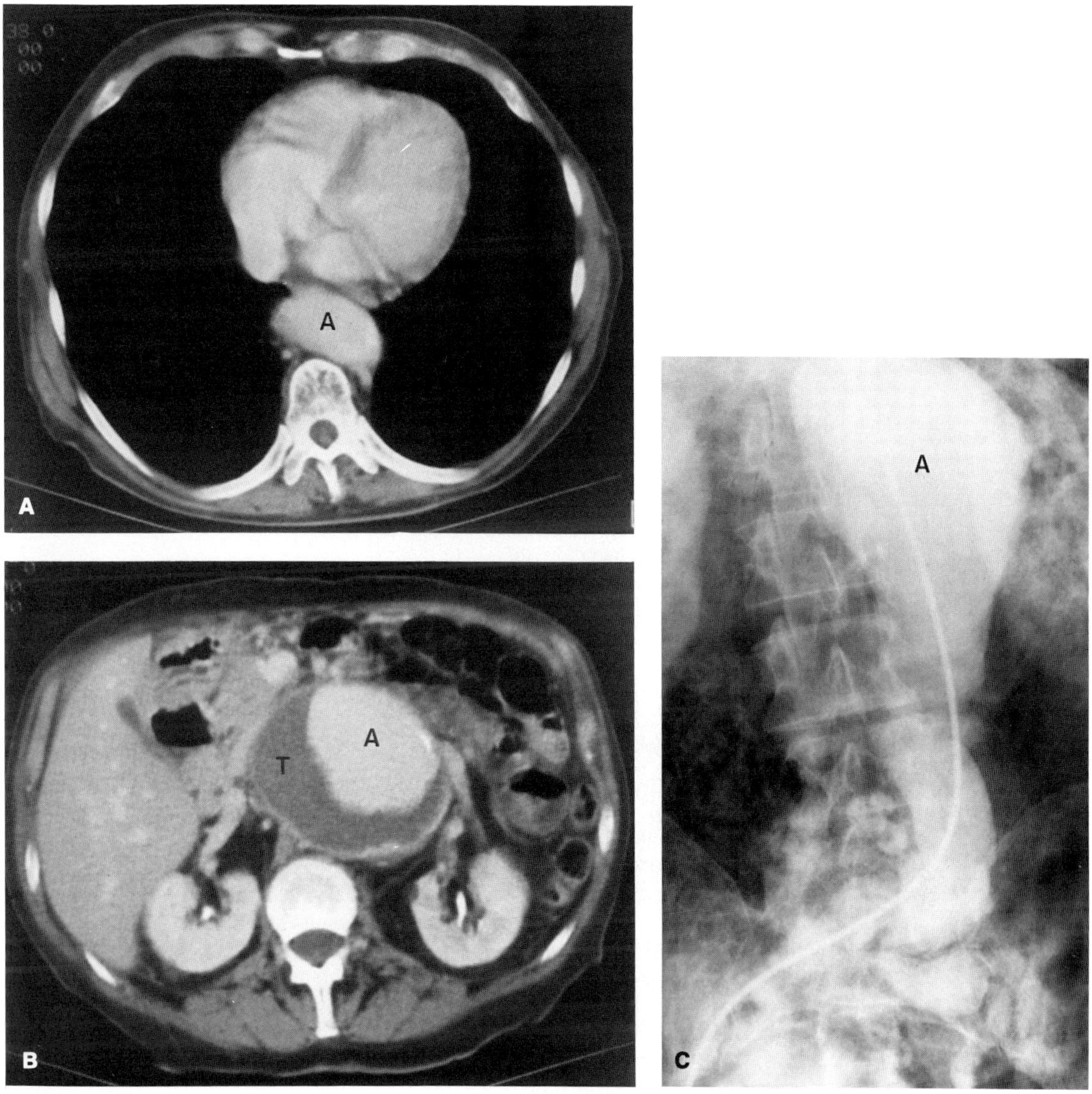


**Figure 17-2.** Thoracoabdominal aortic aneurysm. **(A)** Transverse CT scan through the thorax demonstrates an aneurysm of the descending thoracic aorta (labeled *A*). **(B)** More caudal section through the abdomen demonstrates the massively dilated abdominal aorta at the level of the renal hilum. Note the contrast-enhanced residual lumen (*A*) and the eccentric thrombus (*T*) that fills the remainder of the aneurysm. **(C)** Aortogram shows the contrast-filled lumen (A) but underestimates the size of the aneurysm, because the lack of sufficient mural calcification does not allow delineation of its true dimensions.

## Magnetic Resonance Imaging

Magnetic resonance imaging (MRI) can provide information about the dimensions and internal constituents (thrombus, atherosclerotic debris) of abdominal aortic aneurysms as well as about the extension of an aneurysm into the iliac arteries and involvement of branch vessels (Fig. 17-3). Magnetic resonance imaging is superior to ultrasound in demonstrating the renal arteries and involvement of visceral vessels. It is superior to aortography for delineating intraluminal thrombus and demonstrating the thickness of the aortic wall, but it is of less value for showing

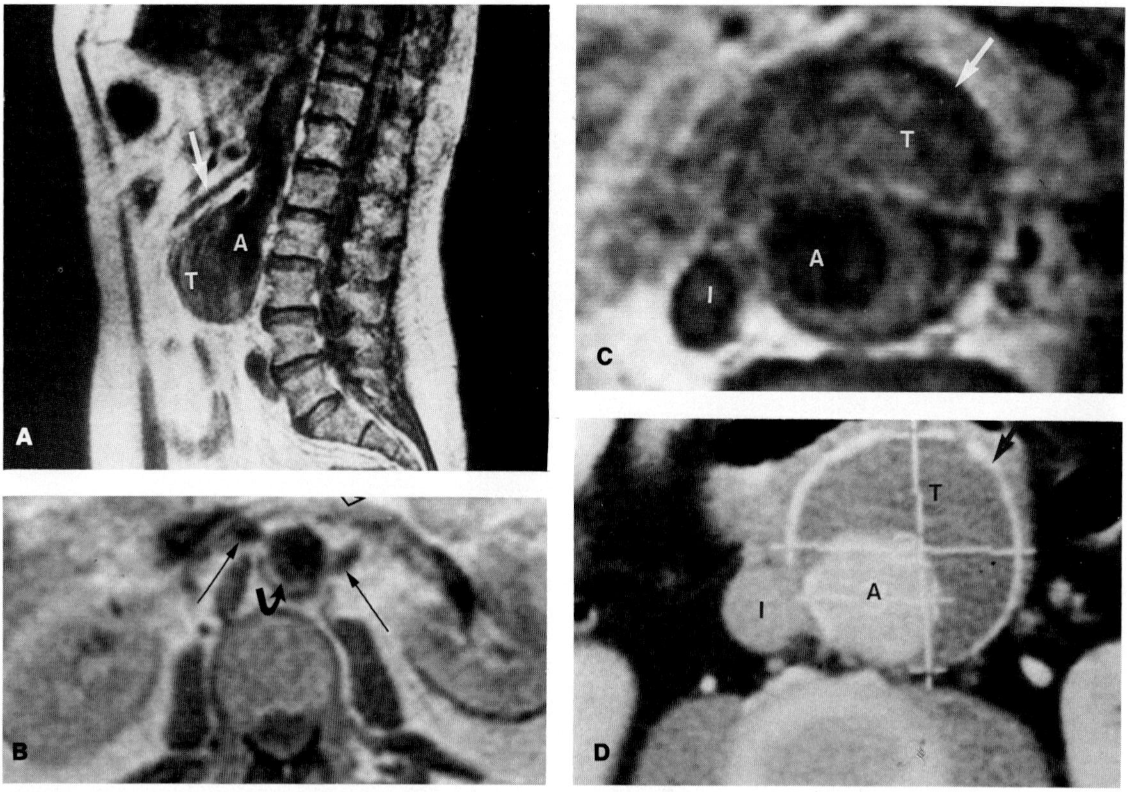


**Figure 17-3.** Infrarenal abdominal aortic aneurysm. **(A)** Sagittal MRI demonstrates dilatation of the infrarenal aorta (labeled *A*), which is almost filled with thrombus (*T*). Note that the superior mesenteric artery (*arrow*) lies above the aneurysm. **(B)** Transverse MRI shows that the aorta is of normal size at the level of the right and left renal arteries, both of which are well seen (*straight arrows*). Arteriosclerotic plaques eccentrically thicken the posterior wall of the aorta (*curved arrow*). The left renal vein (*open arrow*) crosses anteriorly. **(C)** Transverse MRI through the infrarenal aneurysm demonstrates the residual lumen (*A*) as a region of signal void representing flowing blood. The remainder of the aneurysm is filled with thrombus (*T*). The low-intensity rim in the wall of the aneurysm (*arrow*) represents calcification (*I,* inferior vena cava). **(D)** Transverse CT scan at the same level shows the contrast-filled residual lumen (*A*) surrounded eccentrically by thrombus (*T*). The calcified wall has a high attenuation (*arrow*).

renal artery stenosis or the presence of multiple renal arteries.

Magnetic resonance imaging is nonionizing, and its ability to directly acquire images in multiple planes is particularly useful for defining the full extent of an abdominal aortic aneurysm. In contrast to ultrasound, MRI provides a larger field of view and is not affected by patient obesity. Magnetic resonance imaging offers better soft-tissue contrast than CT and provides a similar degree of spatial resolution. The intravenous injection of contrast material is unnecessary with MRI, because flowing blood results in a signal void that provides natural contrast between the blood and cardiovascular structures. Disadvantages of MRI include slower scanning times, leading to image degradation as a consequence of patient motion; the possibility of claustrophobia; the contraindication to imaging patients with pacemakers and other implants with ferromagnetic properties (*e.g.*, intracranial aneurysm clips); and the inability to image hemodynamically unstable patients because of the limited patient-monitoring capabilities currently available.

Abdominal aortic aneurysms can be detected by MRI regardless of whether calcification is present within the aortic wall. Unlike with

CT, mural calcification produces a low signal intensity with MRI and thus is often not well delineated. Transverse MRI sections are obtained to differentiate an abdominal aortic aneurysm from mere tortuosity and to delineate the origin of the renal arteries. Sagittal sections complement the transverse plane in demonstrating the longitudinal extent of the aneurysm and showing the celiac and superior mesenteric arteries. The identification of organized thrombus within an aneurysm is based on differences in signal intensity between the first and second echo images. In most cases, organized thrombus decreases in relative signal intensity from the first to the second echo image, while atheromatous debris has nearly the same signal intensity on both. These internal constituents of an aneurysm often can be differentiated from slowly flowing blood, which produces an increase in relative signal intensity from the first to second echo image. In difficult cases, as in aneurysms containing less well-organized thrombus that may have a brighter signal intensity, the use of cardiac gating may aid in differentiating slow flow from thrombus. With this technique, slow flow produces changes in signal intensity between diastole and systole, whereas a thrombus shows no change in signal intensity relative to the cardiac cycle. Another technique to differentiate flow from thrombus is the use of phase images.

As with CT, the current indications for the use of MRI vary with the institution and depend on the availability of the equipment, the expertise of the operator, and the precise information required. Ultrasound or CT is generally the initial screening modality for the patient with a suspected abdominal aortic aneurysm. Magnetic resonance imaging is performed if ultrasound and CT fail to provide information about renal, visceral, and iliac artery involvement, if contrast material is contraindicated, or if the direct acquisition of images in the coronal or sagittal planes is needed with a larger view than that provided by ultrasound.

## Aortography

Before the advent of the noninvasive imaging modalities described previously, aortography was the procedure of choice for evaluating the patient with a suspected abdominal aortic aneurysm. Currently, aortography is no longer performed as a screening procedure in such patients and, indeed, is rarely required. Aortography is invasive and is associated with potential complications (although rare if performed by an experienced angiographer), such as perforation, peripheral embolization, bleeding, false aneurysm or thrombus formation at the site of catheterization, acute renal failure, cardiac decompensation, and hypersensitivity reaction to the contrast material.

A major disadvantage of aortography is that the contrast material fills only the aortic lumen and not the entire circumference of the aneurysm. If there is intraluminal thrombus, aortography may fail to detect dilatation of the aorta unless its wall is calcified (Fig. 17-2*C*). Ultrasound, CT, and MRI are equally or more accurate than aortography in detecting an aortic aneurysm and determining its actual diameter, and these relatively noninvasive modalities may also be used to demonstrate any progressive dilatation of the aneurysm.

At present, the specific indication for aortography in the patient with an abdominal aortic aneurysm is to assess involvement of the major visceral arterial branches (*e.g.*, renal and mesenteric arteries). Clinical findings that may possibly require arteriography include intestinal angina, suspicion of a horseshoe kidney, the presence of an abdominal or flank bruit (especially in young, hypertensive patients with impaired renal function), and the need to evaluate the arterial supply to the lower extremities.

## Digital Subtraction Aortography

Digital subtraction aortography (DSA) can be used if the relation of an abdominal aortic aneurysm to the renal or iliac arteries has not been shown adequately by CT or MRI. Aortography, rather than DSA, is generally employed if a more complex abnormality is suspected (*e.g.*, stenosis of the renal or visceral arteries). Although intravenous injections were used initially, DSA is now most commonly performed via a direct injection through an intra-arterial catheter (Fig. 17-4).

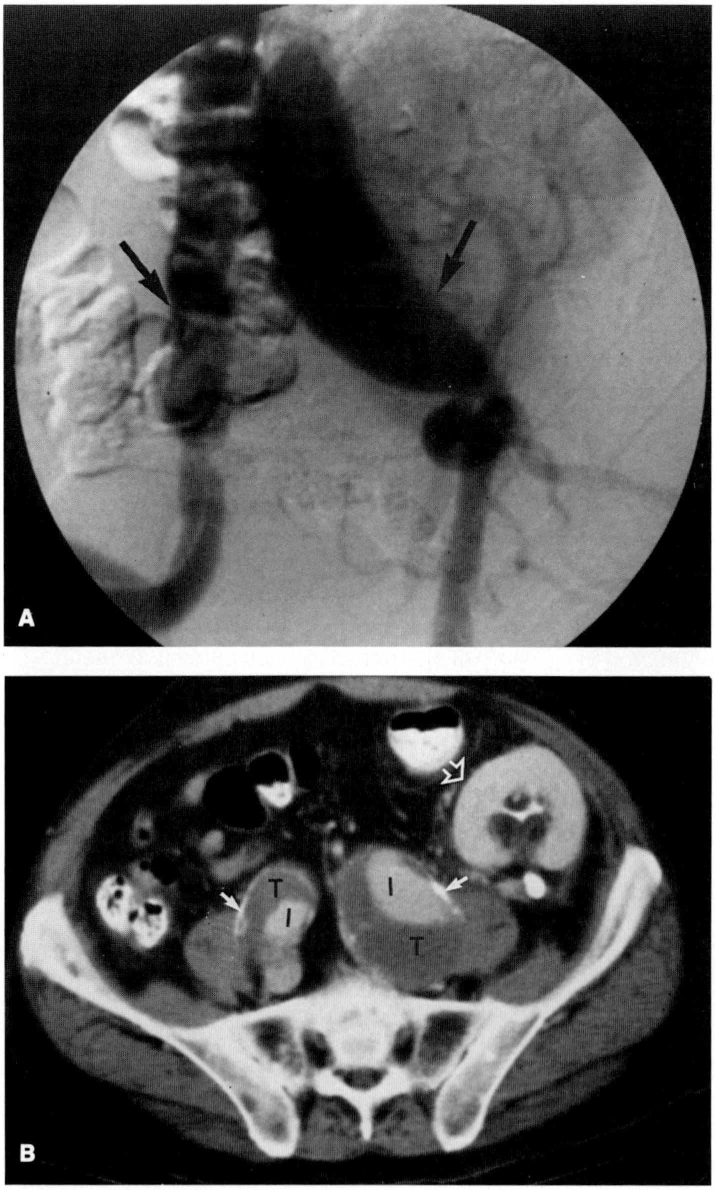


**Figure 17-4.** Infrarenal aneurysm extending into the iliac arteries. **(A)** Intra-arterial DSA shows that the aneurysm involves both iliac arteries (*arrows*) but greatly underestimates its extent. **(B)** CT scan shows the true size of the iliac aneurysms. The eccentric contrast-filled lumens (*I*) are surrounded by thrombus (*T*), and the walls of the aneurysms contain scattered calcifications (*closed arrows*). A renal transplant (*open arrow*) lies within the left iliac fossa.

## IMAGING FOR COMPLICATIONS AND POSTOPERATIVE EVALUATION OF ABDOMINAL AORTIC ANEURYSMS

### Inflammatory Fibrosis

Inflammatory fibrosis develops about an abdominal aortic aneurysm in up to 25% of cases. Inflammatory fibrosis is important clinically, because it frequently obstructs the ureters and inferior vena cava and is adherent to the duodenum. Its presence requires important modifications in the usual surgical approach. The appearance of inflammatory fibrosis on the various imaging modalities must not be confused with conditions such as lymphadenopathy and retroperitoneal hematoma from a ruptured aneurysm.

On ultrasound, the inflammatory mass appears as a hyperechoic region surrounding the

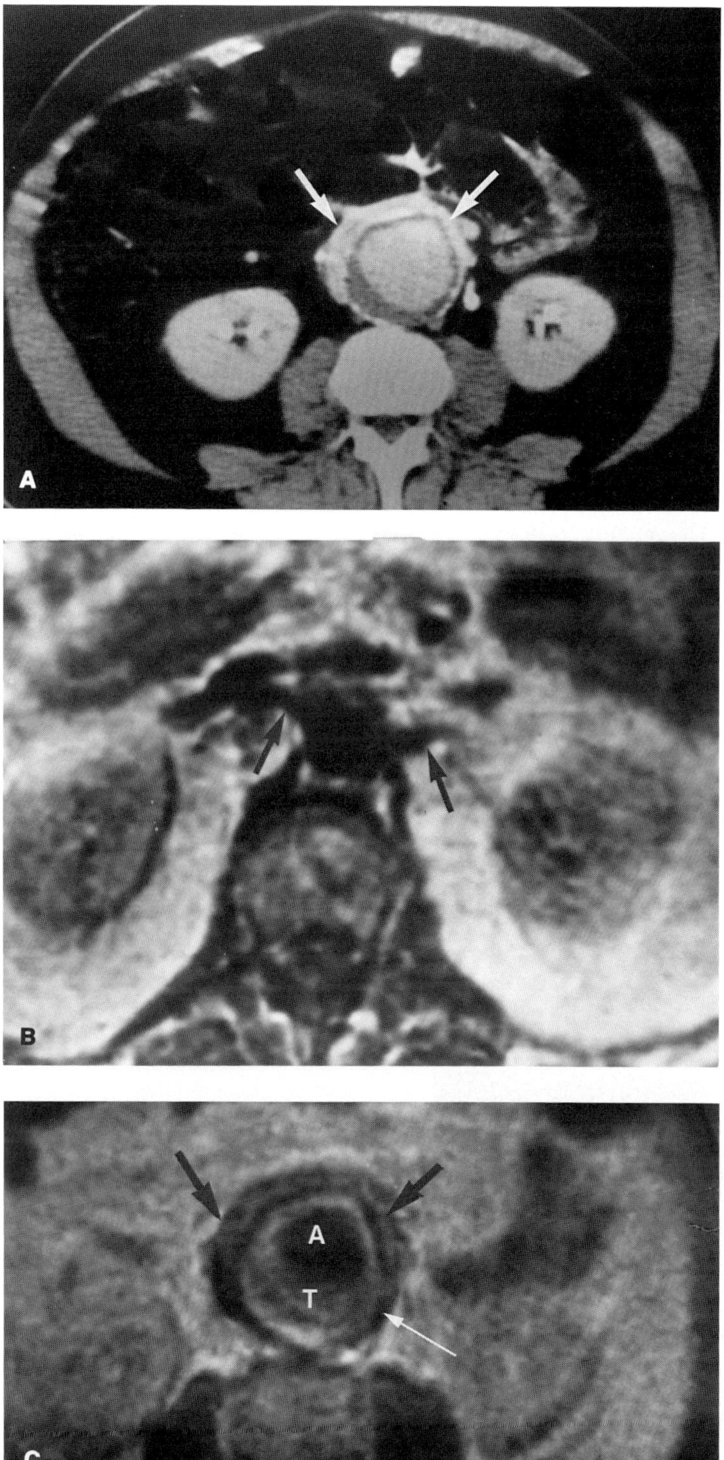


**Figure 17-5.** Inflammatory fibrosis. **(A)** Transverse CT scan demonstrates an infrarenal aneurysm with mural calcification surrounded by material that has a high attenuation (*arrows*) after the intravenous administration of contrast. Although this is compatible with inflammatory fibrosis, an aortic rupture could not be excluded because of the patient's severe pain. **(B)** Transverse MRI through the level of the renal arteries (*arrows*) shows that neither the ostia nor the proximal portions are involved by the aneurysm. **(C)** Transverse MRI through the infrarenal aneurysm demonstrates the residual lumen (*A*), thrombus (*T*), and calcified wall (*white arrow*). On this T2-weighted image, note the ring of low signal-intensity material (*black arrows*) surrounding the aneurysm. This appearance is compatible with fibrosis and is very different from the expected MRI intensity of a hematoma.

echogenic and thickened aortic wall. The fibrosis generally surrounds the anterior and lateral walls of the aorta, sparing the posterior wall. On CT, the low-attenuation inflammatory mass surrounds the thickened aortic wall, which often contains calcification (Fig. 17-5*A*). After the intravenous administration of contrast material, the inflammatory material is enhanced less than the aortic lumen. This produces four concentric layers which, proceeding outward from the center, represent enhanced lumen, unenhanced thrombus, calcified wall, and enhanced perianeurysmal inflammatory fibrosis. Computed tomography is superior to ultrasound in demonstrating complications of inflammatory fibrosis, such as ureteral encasement and involvement of the bowel and the inferior vena cava. However, it is difficult to distinguish periaortic inflammatory fibrosis from a hematoma associated with aneurysm rupture with both modalities. This dilemma can be solved with MRI, in which periaortic fibrosis has a signal intensity much less than fat and slightly more than muscle on both T1- and T2-weighted sequences (Fig. 17-5*B, C*), while recent hematoma has a signal intensity greater than muscle and less than fat on the T1-weighted image and an intensity similar to fat on the T2 image. As the hematoma becomes more chronic, the signal intensity becomes similar to fat on both the T1- and T2-weighted images.

## Aneurysm Rupture

Computed tomography is currently the imaging modality of choice for determining the age and site of rupture of an abdominal aortic aneurysm and for assessing the extent of the surrounding hematoma. A retroperitoneal collection with attenuation values of 40 to 60 Hounsfield units indicates an acute or subacute hematoma associated with rupture (Fig. 17-6). As the hematoma matures, its attenuation value decreases. Because acute rupture of an abdominal aortic aneurysm requires emergency treatment, few patients receive preoperative ultrasound examinations. An acute hematoma associated with aneurysm rupture may produce a complex echogenic mass adjacent to the aneurysm. A chronic hematoma appears as a hypoechoic collection around the aneurysm that extends into the flanks. In a stable patient, MRI should play an important role in detecting a hematoma and delineating its extent. The MRI variation in signal intensity of hematomas of different ages has been described previously.

## Infection

Mycotic aneurysms, which most frequently are due to salmonella or staphylococcus, generally involve the abdominal portion of the aorta.

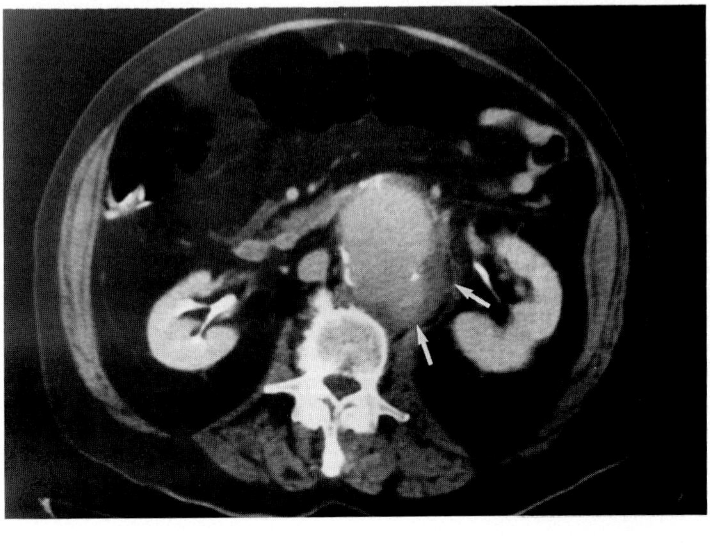

**Figure 17-6.** Aortic aneurysm rupture. CT scan shows the hematoma (*arrows*) along the left posterolateral aspect of the aneurysm.

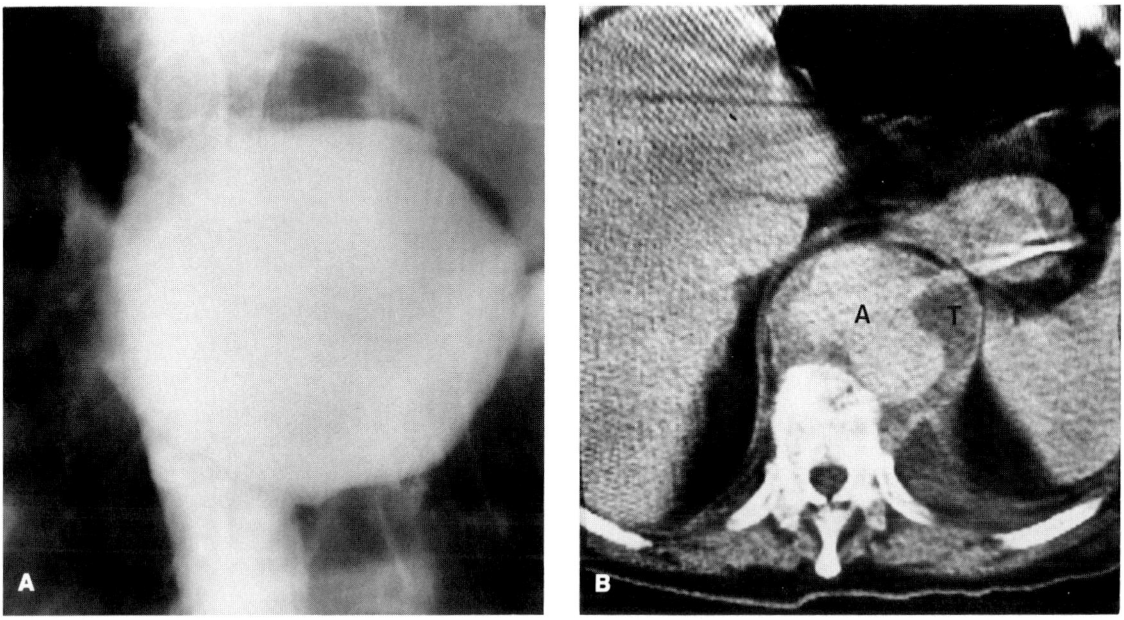


**Figure 17-7.** Mycotic aneurysm. **(A)** Aortogram shows a huge suprarenal aneurysm in a patient with *Salmonella* infection. **(B)** CT scan better demonstrates the irregular lumen (*A*) surrounded by thrombus (*T*) as well as the true dimensions of the aneurysm and its erosion of the underlying vertebral body.

Computed tomography can demonstrate both the aneurysm and the presence of gas in the arterial wall (Fig. 17-7), whereas ultrasound may be unable to detect the aneurysm because of degradation of the image due to the mural gas. Like CT, MRI can detect gas in the wall of an aortic aneurysm and any perianeurysmal collections of infected material. The diagnosis of a mycotic aortic aneurysm also can be made by aortography.

## Graft Evaluation

Complications of bypass grafts for abdominal aortic aneurysms include infection, occlusion, hemorrhage, false aneurysm, and graft aneurysm. Because the frequent presence of overlying bowel gas limits the usefulness of ultrasound, CT is the imaging modality of choice in the patient with a suspected graft complication (Fig. 17-8). Unlike ultrasound, in which only a nonspecific periaortic fluid collection may be demonstrated, CT often can identify the specific type of graft complication. Preliminary studies indicate that MRI can demonstrate both the bypass graft and the native aorta without the need for intravenous contrast and (like CT) can identify the specific type of graft complication.

## Overall Imaging Approach

In the patient with a suspected abdominal aortic aneurysm, ultrasound is the initial imaging modality used to verify the clinical diagnosis and as a baseline if repeat studies are needed later to determine whether the aneurysm has enlarged. If the diagnosis of an aneurysm is known and more information is required, CT is performed to reliably demonstrate the extent of the lesion and its effect on surrounding structures, the degree of intraluminal thrombus, involvement of renal and iliac arteries, and complications such as inflammatory fibrosis, and rupture and hematoma. Magnetic resonance imaging may be used in place of CT, especially to differentiate aneurysm rupture and inflammatory fibrosis sur-

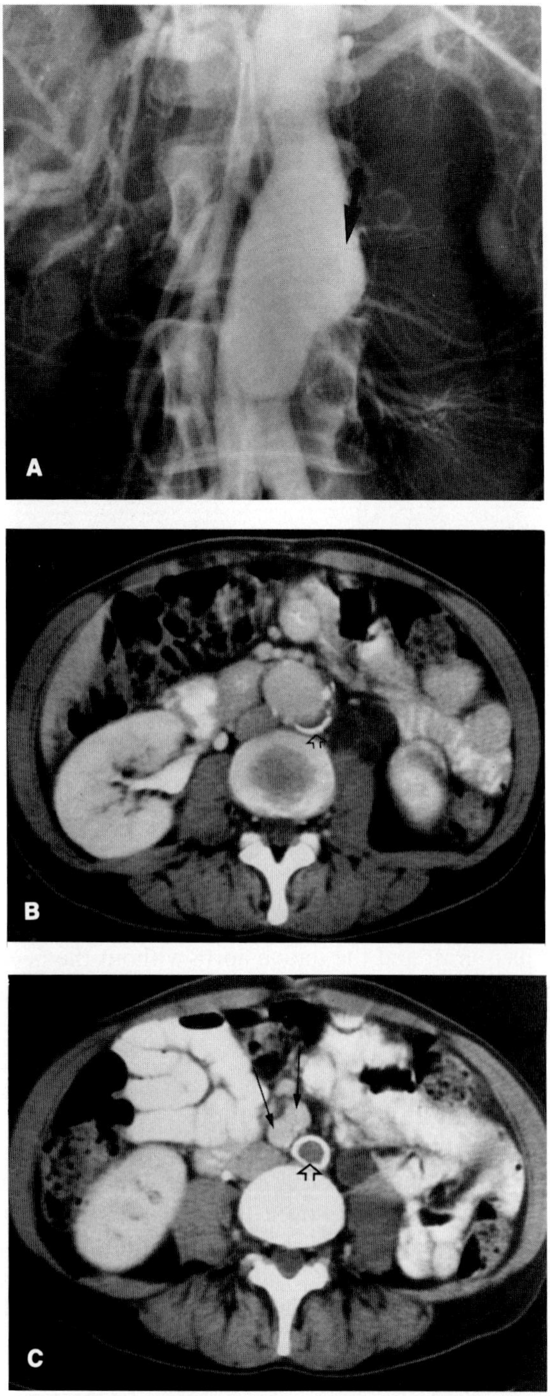

**Figure 17-8.** Bypass graft evaluation. **(A)** Aortogram shows a pseudoaneurysm (*arrow*) at the anastomotic site between the aorta and the end-to-side aortoiliac graft. **(B)** CT scan at the level of the anastomotic pseudoaneurysm demonstrates dense calcification posteriorly (*arrow*) in the native aorta. **(C)** Another CT section shows the densely calcified native aorta (*open arrow*) posterior to the two limbs of the iliac graft (*closed arrows*).

rounding an aneurysm, or in patients in whom intravenous contrast material is contraindicated. Aortography (digital subtraction or conventional) is reserved for patients whose symptoms require demonstration of the renal or visceral arteries or the arterial supply to the lower extremities.

## Bibliography


Amparo EG, Hoddick WK, Hricak H et al: Comparison of MR imaging and ultrasonography in the evaluation of abdominal aortic aneurysms. Radiology 154:451–456, 1985

Anderson JC, Baltaxe HA, Wolf GL: Inability to show clot: One limitation of ultrasonography of the abdominal aorta. Radiology 132:693–696, 1979

Auerbach O, Garfinkel L: Atherosclerosis and aneurysm of aorta in relation to smoking habits and age. Chest 78:805–809, 1980

Axel L: Blood flow effects in magnetic resonance imaging. AJR 143:1157, 1984

Bradley WG, Waluch V: Blood flow: Magnetic resonance imaging. Radiology 154:443, 1985

Braun SD, Illescas FF, Fagert T et al: Measuring abdominal aortic aneurysms on digital subtraction arteriograms. AJR 144:997–998, 1985

Clayton MJ, Walsh JW, Brewer WH: Contained rupture of abdominal aortic aneurysms: Sonographic and CT diagnosis: AJR 138:154–156, 1982

Crawford ES, Cohen ES: Aortic aneurysm: A multifocal disease. Arch Surg 117:1393–1400, 1982

Cullenward MJ, Scanlan KA, Pozniak MA et al: Inflammatory aortic aneurysm (periaortic fibrosis): Radiologic imaging. Radiology 159:75–82, 1986

Dalen JE: Diseases of the aorta. In Petersdorf RG, Adams RD, Braunwald E et al (eds): Harrison's Principles of Internal Medicine, pp 1488–1489. New York, McGraw-Hill, 1983

Eriksson I, Forsberg JO, Hemmingsson A et al: Preoperative evaluation of abdominal aortic aneurysms: Is there a need for aortography? Acta Chir Scand 147:533–537, 1981

Eriksson I, Hemmingsson A, Lindgren PG: Diagnosis of abdominal aortic aneurysms by aortography, computed tomography and ultrasound. Acta Radiol (Diagn) 21:209–214, 1980

Evancho AM, Osbakken M, Weidner W: Comparison of NMR imaging and aortography for preoperative evaluation of abdominal aortic aneurysm. Mag Res Med 2:41–45, 1985

Flak B, Li DK, Ho BB: Magnetic resonance imaging of aneurysms of abdominal aorta. AJR 144: 991–996, 1984

Geisinger MA, Risius B, O'Donnell JA et al: Thoracic aortic dissections: Magnetic resonance imaging. Radiology 155:407–411, 1985

Glazer HS, Gutierrez FT, Levitt RG et al: The thoracic aortic aneurysm studied by magnetic resonance. Radiology 157:149–155, 1987

Godwin JE, Korobkin M: Acute disease of the aorta. Diagnosis by computed tomography and ultrasonography. Radiol Clin North Am 21:551–574, 1983

Gomes MN, Hakkal HG, Schellinger D: Ultrasonography and CT scanning. A comparative study of abdominal aortic aneurysms. CT 2:99–110, 1978

Gomes MN, Schellinger D, Hufnagel CA: Abdominal aortic aneurysms: Diagnostic review and new technique. Ann Thorac Surg 27:480–488, 1979

Gooding GAW: Aneurysms of the abdominal aorta, iliac, and femoral arteries. Semin Ultrasound 3:170–179, 1982

Hadar H, Zelikovski A, Reiss R: Computed tomographic diagnosis of abdominal aortic aneurysm. CT 5:1–7, 1981

Hirsch JH, Thiele BL, Carter SS et al: Aortic and lower extremity arterial aneurysms. J Clin Ultrasound 9:29–31, 1981

Justich E, Amparo EG, Hricak H et al: Infected aortoiliofemoral grafts: Magnetic resonance imaging. Radiology 154:133–136, 1985

Kaufman SL, Chang R, Kadir S et al: Intraarterial digital subtraction angiography in diagnostic arteriography. Radiology 151:323–327, 1984

Larsson EM, Albrechtsson U, Christenson JT: Computed tomography versus aortography for preoperative evaluation of abdominal aortic aneurysm. Acta Radiol (Diagn) 25:98–100, 1984

Lee JKT, Ling D, Heiken JP et al: Magnetic resonance imaging of abdominal aortic aneurysm. AJR 143:1197–1202, 1984

Machida K, Tasaka A: CT patterns of mural thrombus in aortic aneurysms. J Comput Assist Tomogr 4:840–842, 1980

Mark A, Moss AA, Lusby R et al: CT evaluation of complications of abdominal aortic surgery. Radiology 145:409–414, 1982

Pripstein S, Caboto FV, Gerritsen RW: Spontaneous mycotic aneurysm of the abdominal aorta. J Comput Assist Tomogr 3:681–683, 1979

Probst P, Baur HR, Leupi F et al: Postoperative evaluation of composite aortic grafts: Comparison of angiography and CT. Br J Radiol 56:797–804, 1983

Robicsek F: The diagnosis of abdominal aneurysms. Surgery 89:275–276, 1981

Slater EE, DeSantis RW: Diseases of the aorta. In Braunwald E (ed): Heart Disease, pp 1542–1545. Philadelphia, WB Saunders, 1984

Weintraub AM, Gomes MN: Clinical manifestations of abdominal aortic aneurysm and thoracoabdominal aneurysm. In Lindsay J, Hurst J (eds): The Aorta, p 131. New York, Grune & Stratton, 1979

## SUSPECTED ABDOMINAL AORTIC ANEURYSM (AAA)

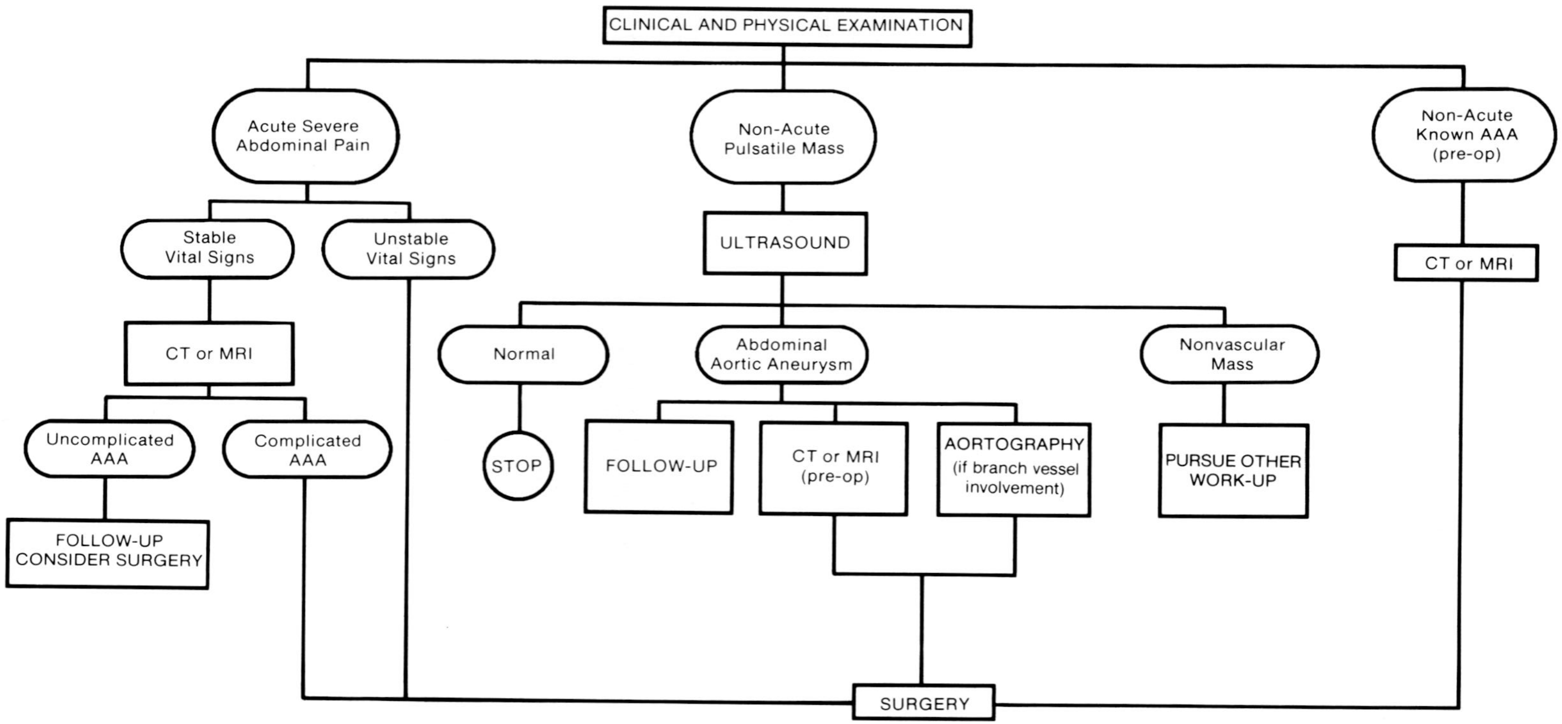

# Chapter 18

# Abdominal Trauma

*Bharat Raval*
*Carl M. Sandler*
*Beth S. Edeiken–Monroe*
*John H. Harris, Jr.*

Trauma is a leading cause of death from ages 1 to 38 years and is also a major cause of disability and loss of productivity. Abdominal trauma accounts for 10% of trauma-related deaths and an even greater proportion of disability. Motor vehicle accidents are the most common cause of abdominal trauma, with penetrating injuries from stab or gunshot wounds also a major cause. Penetrating injuries, especially gunshot wounds to the abdomen, have a very high rate of intra-abdominal organ injury and are explored surgically. The imaging evaluation of patients with this type of injury generally is limited to plain radiographs and excretory urography (if the kidneys are located near the area of injury).

The clinical evaluation may be unreliable in almost half of patients with blunt abdominal injury. These patients present a diagnostic challenge that calls for close cooperation between the trauma surgeon and radiologist to ensure that the appropriate imaging study is performed and to rapidly detect and treat the injury. In general, abdominal trauma is more likely to involve the solid abdominal organs rather than the hollow viscera.

The role of radiographic imaging in the evaluation of the acutely traumatized patient depends on the magnitude of the injury. Polytraumatized patients who remain clinically unstable despite vigorous efforts at resuscitation may not survive the time required for any imaging procedure. In stable patients, whether severely or minimally injured, diagnostic imaging procedures frequently provide information that is valuable to patient management but is neither clinically suspected nor obtainable by any other method.

## DIAGNOSTIC EVALUATION

### *DIAGNOSTIC MODALITIES*

1. Plain radiography
2. Computed tomography
3. Ultrasound
4. Radionuclide scanning
5. Excretory urography
6. Cystography
7. Retrograde urethrography
8. Angiography
9. Magnetic resonance imaging

### Plain Radiography

Although the past decade has seen a remarkable increase in the application of ultrasound, computed tomography (CT), and angiography in evaluating patients with acute abdominal injury, the fundamental radiographic imaging procedure for the initial evaluation of such patients remains the plain abdominal radiograph. In addition to demonstrating the intraperitoneal and extraperitoneal spaces and their contents, plain abdominal radiographs demonstrate the bony pelvis and often-injured soft-tissue structures, such as the urethra, bladder, pelvic vasculature, and rectum. Because the abdomen is inseparable from the chest, trauma to the upper part of the abdomen frequently involves the chest (and vice versa) and thus also requires plain chest radiography.

It is a commonly held, although erroneous, belief that plain abdominal radiographs provide little or no useful information in the evaluation of the acutely traumatized patient because of the poor image quality that often is produced with mobile equipment in the emergency center. Radiographs obtained in this setting are not innately of poor quality but certainly may be suboptimal if neither the technologist nor the radiologist is properly concerned with film quality control. The role of diagnostic imaging in the evaluation and management of patients with acute abdominal trauma is directly proportional to the quality of the radiographic examination. Therefore, the radiologist must be directly involved in ensuring proper patient positioning and radiographic technique, even under the most adverse circumstances.

Blunt abdominal trauma presents diagnostic problems that are completely different from those of penetrating trauma. There is no absolute direct relationship between the mechanism of injury and the magnitude of the blunt trauma and the severity of the resulting abdominal injury. In addition, abdominal injury may be masked by associated injuries to the central nervous system, such as loss of consciousness and paralysis. Because even major abdominal injury may be clinically silent (*e.g.*, the extraperitoneal perivesical hematoma secondary to pelvic-ring disruption), it is necessary for both the clinician and radiologist to have a high index of suspicion, to insist on abdominal images of the highest quality, and to look beyond the usually obvious skeletal injuries for the subtle soft-tissue signs of vascular or lower urinary tract injuries that frequently coexist and often are of more clinical significance.

Although plain abdominal radiographs cannot identify vascular injuries, specific sites of hemorrhage, or subcapsular collections of blood involving the kidneys, liver, or spleen, when compared with other available imaging modalities, the supine radiograph of the abdomen provides the most comprehensive information about all abdominal organ systems in the shortest possible time and with the least patient inconvenience. Therefore, plain abdominal radiography is ideally suited to the initial evaluation of the patient with acute abdominal injury.

The presence of blood in the peritoneal space is indicated by displacement of the colon from the flank stripe. Intraperitoneal fluid also can be demonstrated by CT and ultrasound, although the ultrasound image may be degraded by ileus or patient motion, or even precluded by overlying abdominal dressings.

The clinical significance of pelvic-ring disruption is substantially greater than that of fractures involving only isolated bones of the pelvis (including acetabular fractures). With major pelvic-ring disruption, there is a 30% to 40% incidence of concomitant injury to the lower part of the urinary tract, pelvic vasculature, or sciatic nerve.

Laboratory experiments and clinical experience have established that disruption of the pelvic ring anteriorly must also be associated with disruption of the posterior pelvic arch. This concept is confirmed radiographically by recognition of disruption or asymmetry of the sacral arcuate lines that indicates fracture of the sacral wing. Consequently, there is no validity to the previously accepted notion of an increased association of lower urinary tract injuries with fractures of the "anterior pelvic arch" and/or vascular injuries with fractures of the "posterior arch." Nevertheless, it is generally true that the more distracted the components of the pelvic-ring disruption, the greater likelihood of associated soft-tissue injury to the lower urinary tract, vessels, colon, and nerves.

Injury to the lower urinary tract (bladder and urethra) or vascular injury that results in the accumulation of blood or urine in the extraperitoneal perivesical space is indicated by changes in the radiographic appearance of the soft-tissue structures that normally occupy this region. Localized extraperitoneal pelvic effusion may distort or obliterate the shadow of the obturator internus muscle or its aponeurosis and/or displace the urinary bladder from the midline. A larger effusion may completely obliterate all of the normal soft-tissue planes of the perivesical space and may displace the pelvic peritoneal reflection and the pelvic ileal loops out of the pelvis (Fig. 18-1).

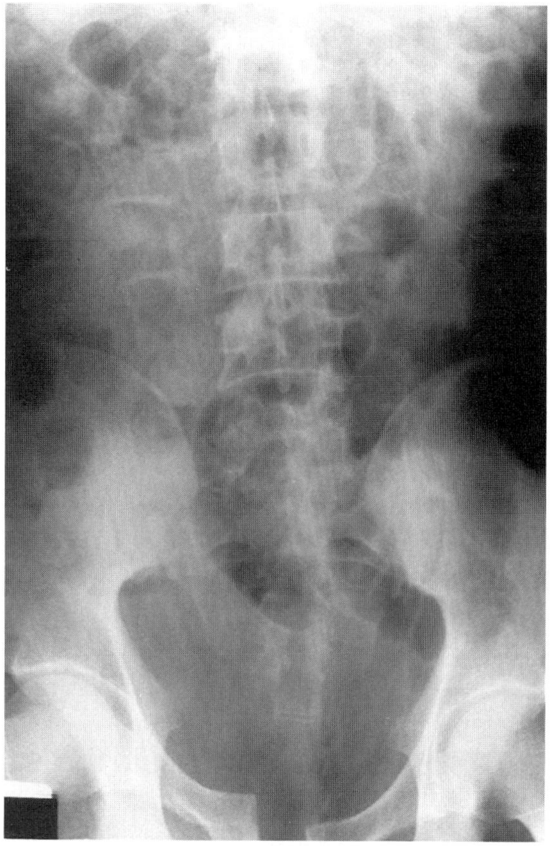

**Figure 18-1.** Plain abdominal radiograph demonstrates a pelvic hematoma displacing loops of bowel out of the pelvis in this patient with diastasis of the symphysis pubis. (Sandler CM, Phillips JM, Harris JD et al: Radiology of the bladder and urethra in blunt pelvic trauma. Radiol Clin North Am 19:195–211, 1981)

## Computed Tomography

Computed tomography is well suited for assessing the abdomen following blunt trauma, because it demonstrates both the intraperitoneal and retroperitoneal compartments and can detect even small amounts of blood in any organ or in the peritoneal cavity. When performing CT in the traumatized patient, careful attention must be paid to technique. Both oral and intravenous contrast should be utilized. The lower abdomen and pelvis should be included so as not to miss small amounts of blood in the peritoneal cavity that may gravitate to the pouch of Douglas. Computed tomography should always be performed before peritoneal lavage.

The hallmark of injury to a solid abdominal organ is a laceration and/or a hematoma. A hematoma may be intraparenchymal or subcapsular, or it may extend around the organ when its capsule is disrupted and lead to hemoperitoneum (Figs. 18-2 and 18-3). A knowledge of the CT appearance of hematomas in various organs, as well as the change in attenuation with time, is essential to ensure reliable detection.

The high sensitivity (92%–100%) and specificity (94%–99%) of CT in detecting splenic, hepatic, and renal injuries has firmly established the important role of this modality in the triage of patients with acute abdominal injury. Computed tomography also can demonstrate hematomas or rupture of the duodenum, pancreatic injuries, and rupture of the diaphragm, although the number of patients reported is small and thus warrants cautious optimism until more data are accumulated.

It is generally agreed that abdominal CT should be performed instead of peritoneal lavage in pediatric patients. In adults, there is a diversity of opinion, with proponents advocating each of these diagnostic techniques. Although peritoneal lavage is reported to have sensitivity and specificity rates of greater than 95% for de-

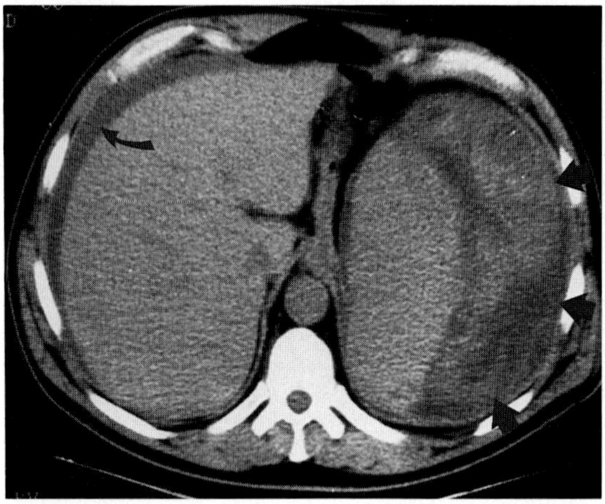

**Figure 18-2.** CT scan shows a perisplenic hematoma with areas of both high and low attenuation (*straight arrows*) displacing the spleen and stomach medially. The curved arrow points to a hemoperitoneum.

tecting bleeding into the peritoneal cavity, a positive lavage occurs in 6% to 25% of patients with trivial injuries that do not require laparotomy. False-positive diagnostic peritoneal lavage may occur in patients with pelvic fractures or as a result of a traumatic peritoneal tap. Unlike CT, diagnostic peritoneal lavage does not assess retroperitoneal structures (kidneys, pancreas, duodenum) and may miss injuries to the small bowel or diaphragm. Although no large comparative study comparing peritoneal lavage with CT has yet appeared, those advocating CT stress that it not only can replace lavage, but when trivial injuries of the spleen, liver, or kidney are detected, CT permits a confident nonoperative management that can reduce the number of laparotomies.

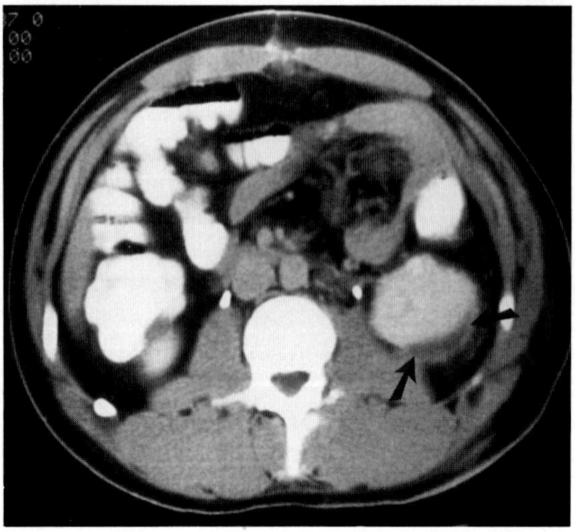

**Figure 18-3.** CT scan shows a subcapsular hematoma (*arrows*) involving the lower pole of the left kidney.

## Ultrasound

Ultrasound is a valuable modality for assessing the abdomen of traumatized patients, because it is noninvasive, does not utilize ionizing radiation, can be performed quickly, and does not need any patient preparation.

The hallmark of abdominal injury on ultrasound is the demonstration of a hematoma in the affected organ and/or blood in the peritoneal cavity. A hematoma can have a variable pattern of echogenicity depending on its age. Acute hematomas have increased internal echoes; with time, the hematoma becomes less echogenic. Hemoperitoneum may appear as fluid in Morison's pouch, the paracolic gutter, or the pouch of Douglas. Ultrasound is less sensitive than CT for detecting injuries to the liver, kidneys, and especially the spleen, although it has a specificity of greater than 95%.

In one study, almost 20% of patients with acute abdominal trauma could not be assessed by ultrasound because of technical difficulties (rib fractures, wounds, obesity). We recommend that ultrasound be used as a primary imaging modality in the traumatized pregnant patient and for follow-up of abdominal injuries when nonoperative management is undertaken.

## Radionuclide Scanning

Prior to the advent of CT and ultrasound, radionuclide scanning was the only noninvasive method available for the diagnosis of upper abdominal injury. At present, the role of radionuclide studies has become more limited because of their inherently poorer spatial resolution.

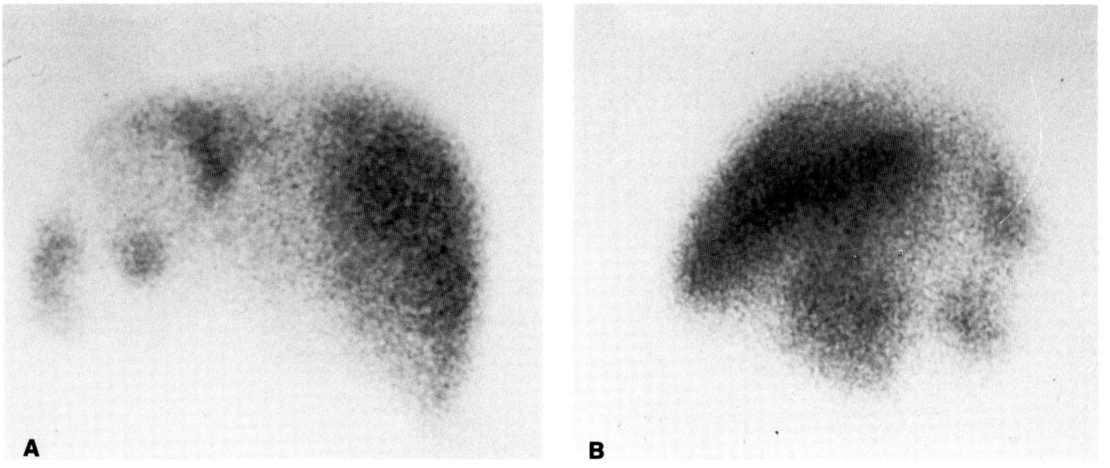


**Figure 18-4.** **(A)** Posterior and **(B)** left lateral views of a radionuclide sulfur colloid scan show multiple photon-deficient areas in the spleen representing splenic lacerations and hematoma.

Nevertheless, radionuclide scanning has a relatively high sensitivity (80%–100%) and specificity (88%–99%) for detecting injury to the liver and spleen and thus may play a valuable role if CT is not available (Fig. 18-4).

Radionuclide scanning requires less patient cooperation (*e.g.*, breath holding) than does CT. In addition, injuries to the liver and spleen that have been managed nonoperatively may be followed using $^{99m}$Tc sulfur colloid liver–spleen scanning, which is less expensive and gives a lower radiation dose than CT. Renal perfusion studies using $^{99m}$Tc diethyltriaminepentaacetic acid ($^{99m}$Tc-DTPA) or glucoheptonate can determine the blood supply to the kidneys following trauma. This technique is of particular value, because it can be performed using mobile scintillation cameras in patients who are too ill to be brought to the radiology department for other imaging studies. Isotopically labeled red blood cells can be used in selected patients to detect continued intraparenchymal organ bleeding.

## Excretory Urography

Despite the advent of newer imaging modalities, excretory urography remains the most widely used procedure for detecting urinary tract injuries following both blunt and penetrating abdominal trauma. The examination may be performed with either bolus or infusion technique. When using a bolus injection, contrast material should be administered in a dose ranging from 0.75 ml to 1 ml per pound of body weight. An initial scout film plus two additional films following contrast administration are sufficient in most patients. Nephrotomography may greatly enhance the study and should be used whenever available.

Indications for excretory urography include hematuria; fractures involving the lower ribs and lumbar vertebral bodies or transverse processes; and the presence of an ecchymosis or soft-tissue mass in the flank. Following penetrating injury, excretory urography is indicated whenever the urinary tract has been in the path of a knife or bullet.

There is controversy about the amount of hematuria that requires further investigation in the absence of other signs of urinary tract injury. In our institution, even a relatively small amount of hematuria (5 to 10 red cells per high-power field on a spontaneously voided specimen) is sufficient to warrant excretory urography. Other authors suggest that significant urinary tract injury is unlikely if the only abnormality is microscopic hematuria that clears within 24 hours. However, it has been shown that major renal injury (including renal artery thrombosis) may

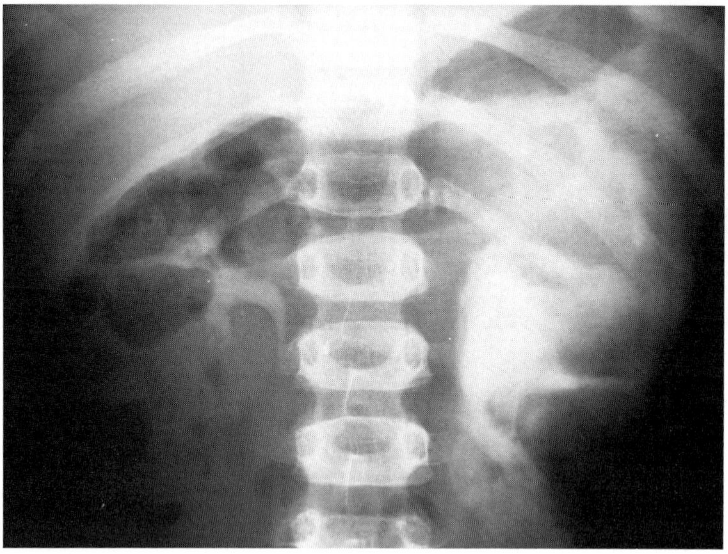

**Figure 18-5.** Excretory urogram in a patient with renal injury shows extravasation of contrast material from the left collecting system.

be present without hematuria and that the degree of hematuria does not correlate with the severity of the injury.

Excretory urography is fairly sensitive in the detection of significant renal trauma and only rarely underestimates the severity of an injury (Fig. 18-5). However, except for contrast extravasation, the findings on excretory urography are relatively nonspecific, and further imaging procedures (including CT and occasionally angiography) are generally required to fully characterize the precise nature of a renal injury. Excretory urography is a very poor screening test for bladder injuries; in one series, only 15% of bladder injuries could be diagnosed on the cystographic phase of excretory urography.

## Cystography

Cystography is the imaging modality of choice for the detection of bladder injuries. Ideally, the procedure is performed under fluoroscopic guidance, although an adequate examination may be obtained using fixed radiographic or even mobile equipment when necessary. Between 300 ml and 400 ml of diluted (15%–30%) contrast material is instilled into the bladder via a Foley catheter (after first excluding urethral injuries in males). Our filming routine consists of an initial scout radiograph followed by a film obtained after approximately 100 ml of contrast material has been introduced. If there is no evidence of gross extravasation, the remainder of the contrast material is instilled and an additional film obtained. A final radiograph is made following drainage of the contrast material from the bladder, so that contrast extravasation that may have been hidden by the distended bladder is not overlooked (Fig. 18-6).

Cystography is indicated in all patients with pelvic-ring disruption and in patients without pelvic fracture who have suffered a blow to the lower abdomen. The procedure also is indicated in patients suffering penetrating injury involving the pelvis, perineum, or buttocks. The vast majority of patients with bladder rupture have gross hematuria.

When properly performed, cystography is a highly accurate technique for detecting rupture of the bladder. False-negative studies usually can be attributed to improper technique, such as inadequate distention and omission of the postdrainage radiograph. Nevertheless, there are occasional reports of false-negative cystograms with both intraperitoneal and extraperitoneal bladder rupture. Most of these cases have involved patients who have suffered penetrating bladder injury secondary to small-caliber bullets. It is presumed that these injuries became

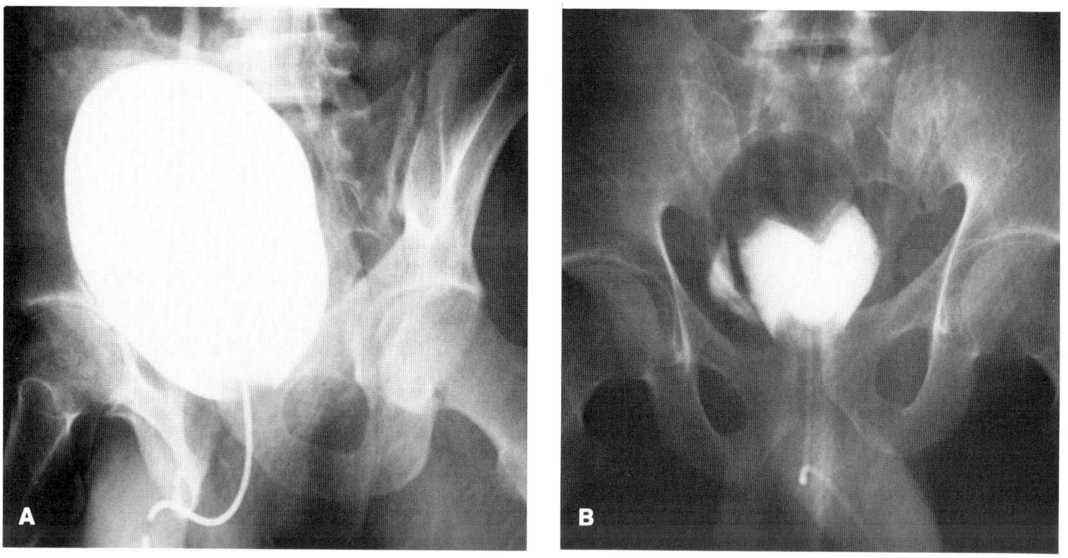


**Figure 18-6.** **(A)** Filled film from a cystogram appears normal. **(B)** Drainage film shows extravasation of contrast material from an extraperitoneal rupture of the bladder. (Sandler CM, Hall JT, Rodriguez MB et al: Bladder injury in blunt pelvic trauma. Radiology 158:633–638, 1986)

sealed by mesenteric or extraperitoneal fat, thereby preventing extravasation of contrast material.

Approximately 10% of males with urethral injuries also have rupture of the bladder. In these patients, cystography should be performed following placement of a suprapubic cystotomy.

## Retrograde Urethrography

Before any attempt at urethral catheterization is made, it is *mandatory* to perform a retrograde urethrogram in all male patients with pelvic-ring disruption, blood at the urethral meatus, or other signs of significant blunt or penetrating penile or perineal injury. Complications of injudicious urethral catheterization include the risk of conversion of a partial urethral rupture into a complete tear, increased hemorrhage, and contamination of a previously sterile hematoma. Urethral injury in the female is extremely rare and need not be considered in the absence of major vaginal laceration.

Ideally, retrograde urethrography is performed using fluoroscopic monitoring. As with cystography, however, an adequate examination may be obtained using only mobile radiographic equipment. A Foley catheter, attached to an irrigating syringe filled with diluted contrast material, is inserted into the penile meatus so that its balloon is placed in the fossa navicularis. Between 1 ml and 2 ml of saline is instilled into the balloon to secure it in place. With the patient in a 25° to 35° oblique position, a radiograph is exposed during the active injection of 25 ml to 30 ml of contrast material (to ensure delineation of the deep bulbar and membranous urethra).

If angiography is to be performed, retrograde urethrography (and cystography) should be deferred until after the vascular examination is completed. This ensures that contrast material extravasated from the lower urinary tract will not obscure small arterial bleeding sites, especially in the pelvis.

Posterior urethral injuries occur in approximately 10% of male patients with pelvic-ring disruption. Unfortunately, the appearance of the fracture is not a reliable predictor of the presence of a urethral injury. Patients with widely diastatic fractures may escape with an intact urethra, whereas those with minimally displaced fractures may have suffered complete urethral disruption (Fig. 18-7). Thus, retrograde ure-

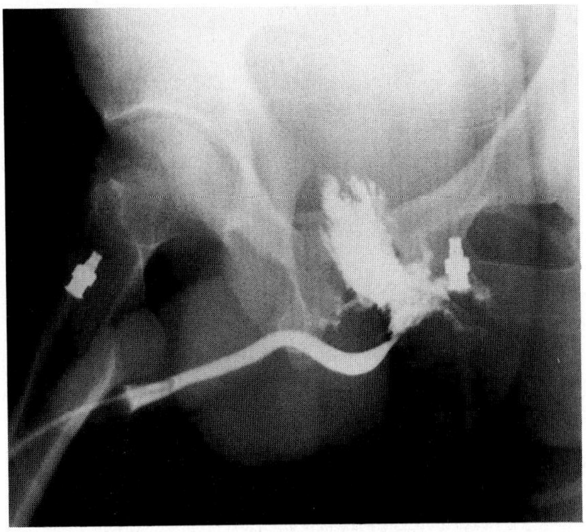

**Figure 18-7.** Retrograde urethrogram in a man with a pelvic fracture demonstrates a complete rupture of the posterior urethra.

thrography to detect urethral injury is essential in all men with pelvic-ring disruption.

## Angiography

In the past, angiography has been utilized in the patient with blunt abdominal trauma to assess vascular patency, organ perfusion, extravasation of contrast material, and hematoma formation within or around an injured organ. At present, angiography should be used in patients with a wide mediastinum suspected of having aortic injury or those with an arterial bleeding site occurring in association with disruption of the pelvic ring. Following evaluation of the mediastinum or pelvis, it is appropriate to investigate the possibility of associated injury to the spleen, liver, and kidneys. This policy permits the patient to be completely studied without the need for transfer to another room or performance of another imaging procedure. Angiographic evaluation of the kidney is indicated whenever urography indicates the unilateral absence of renal excretion. Intra-arterial digital subtraction angiography has been successfully utilized in thoracic aortic rupture and may prove useful in assessing the abdominal organs.

Arteriography is both sensitive and specific for demonstrating splenic, renal (Fig. 18-8), and hepatic injuries. Indeed, primary vascular injuries such as intimal tears, thromboses, pseudoaneurysms, and arteriovenous fistulas are best demonstrated by arteriography. The demonstration of the extent of injury can be helpful in deciding between conservative and operative

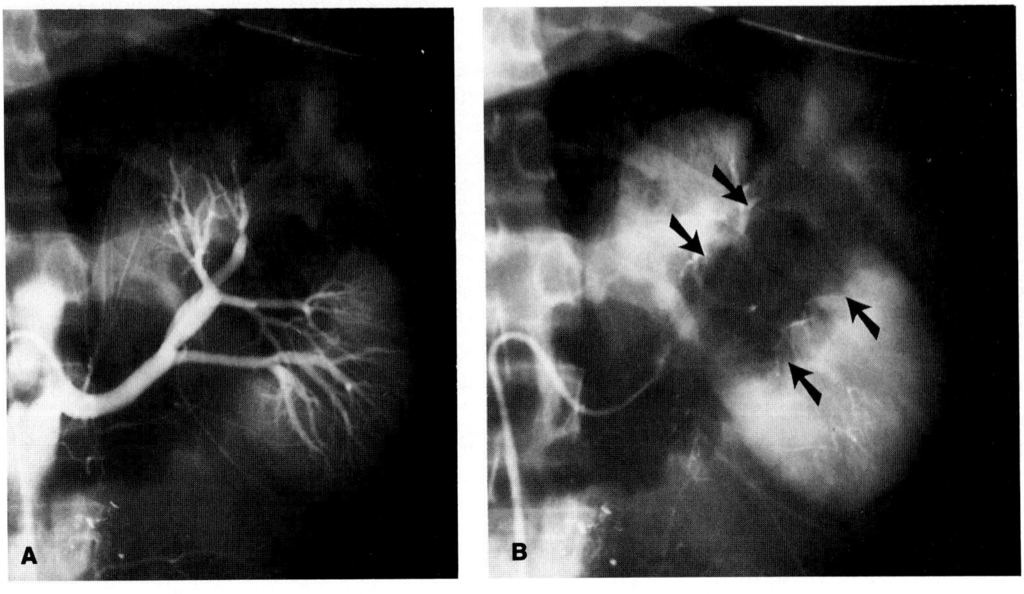


**Figure 18-8.** **(A)** Arterial and **(B)** nephrogram phases of a selective renal arteriogram demonstrate a laceration and intrarenal hematoma (*arrows*) involving the left kidney.

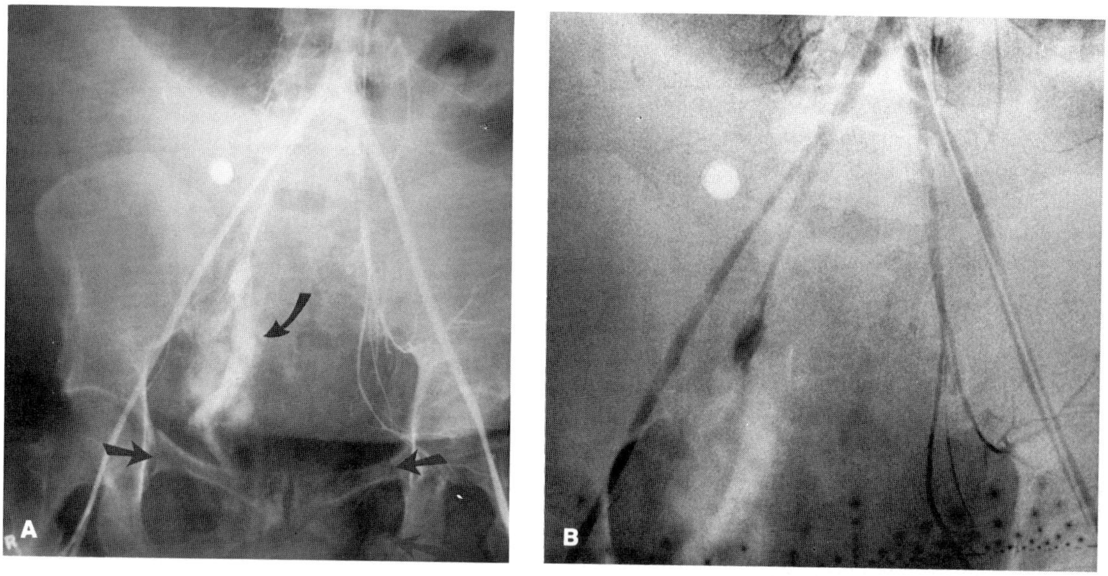


**Figure 18-9.** **(A)** Lower abdominal aortogram demonstrates brisk bleeding from the right internal iliac artery (*curved arrow*). The straight arrows point to disruption of the pelvic ring. **(B)** Following embolization, the bleeding is arrested.

therapy in patients with injuries to the kidneys and, to a lesser extent, the spleen.

Clinical evidence of severe bleeding in a patient with pelvic-ring disruption suggests an arterial bleeding site (Fig. 18-9). Selective internal iliac arteriography can demonstrate extravasation of contrast material from the severed artery (usually the internal pudendal, superior gluteal, lateral sacral, or obturator). Arteriography also can play an important therapeutic role, because embolization of the bleeding artery by autologous blood clot or Gelfoam can produce immediate cessation of the bleeding.

## Magnetic Resonance Imaging

Currently, magnetic resonance imaging (MRI) is not utilized in assessing the abdomen of the traumatized patient. Disadvantages of this modality in such patients include the long acquisition time, lack of reliable identification of the small bowel, patient motion, inability to monitor a critically ill patient without the use of ferromagnetic materials, and the limited availability of the equipment. Nevertheless, the ability of MRI to superbly depict vascular anatomy may permit the noninvasive assessment of vascular patency and flow. Magnetic resonance imaging also can characterize different fluids and thus distinguish among bile, hematoma, and abscess. Therefore, in the future, MRI will probably play some role in the evaluation of stable patients with abdominal trauma.

## Bibliography

Asher WM, Parvin S, Virgilio RW et al: Echographic evaluation of splenic injury after blunt trauma. Radiology 118:411–415, 1976

Blaisdell FW: General assessment, resuscitation and exploration of penetrating and blunt abdominal trauma. In Blaisdell FW, Trunkey DD (eds): Trauma Management. New York, Thieme-Stratton, 1982

Federle MP, Jeffrey RB: Hemoperitoneum studied by computed tomography. Radiology 148:187–192, 1983

Fischer RP, Beverlin BC, Engrav LH et al: Diagnostic peritoneal lavage: Fourteen years and 2586 patients later. Am J Surg 136:701–704, 1978

Gelfand MJ: Scintigraphy in upper abdominal trauma. Semin Roentgenol 19:296–307, 1984

Harris JH, Jr, Harris WH: The Radiology of

Emergency Medicine, 2nd ed. Baltimore, Williams & Wilkins, 1981

Harris JH, Jr: In defense of plain abdominal radiography (Editorial). Ann Emerg Med 11:48–49, 1982

Harris JH, Jr, Loh CK, Perlman HC et al: The roentgen diagnosis of pelvic extraperitoneal effusion. Radiology 125:343–350, 1977

Jackson HJ, Kam J, Harris JH, Jr et al: The sacral arcuate lines in upper sacral fractures. Radiology 145:35–39, 1982

Jones TK, Walsh JW, Maull KI: Diagnostic imaging in blunt trauma of the abdomen. Surg Gynecol Obstet 157:389–398, 1983

Kaufman RA, Towbin R, Babcock DS et al: Upper abdominal trauma in children: Imaging evaluation. AJR 142:449–460, 1984

Lang EK: The role of arteriography in trauma. Radiol Clin North Am 14:353–370, 1976

Mirvis SE, Pais SO, Gens DR: Thoracic aortic rupture: Advantages of intra-arterial digital subtraction angiography. AJR 146:987–991, 1986

Raval B, Lamki N: Computed tomography of the traumatized abdomen. Semin Ultrasound 6: 109–128, 1985

Reuter SR, Redman HC: Gastrointestinal Angiography, 2nd ed. Philadelphia, WB Saunders, 1977

Sandler CM, Hall JT, Rodriguez MB et al: Bladder injury in blunt pelvic trauma. Radiology 158:633–638, 1986

Sandler CM, Harris JH, Jr, Corriere JN et al: Posterior urethral injuries after pelvic fracture. AJR 137:1233–1237, 1981

Sandler CM, Phillips JM, Harris JD et al: Radiology of the bladder and urethra in blunt pelvic trauma. Radiol Clin North Am 19:195–211, 1981

Sandler CM, Toombs BD: Computed tomographic evaluation of blunt renal injuries. Radiology 141:461–466, 1981

Toombs BD, Sandler CM: Computed Tomography in Trauma. Philadelphia, WB Saunders, 1987

Trunkey DD: Trauma. Sci Am 249:28–35, 1983

van Sonnenberg E, Simeone JF, Mueller PR et al: Sonographic appearance of hematoma in liver, spleen and kidney: A clinical, pathologic and animal study. Radiology 147:507–510, 1983

Wicks JD, Silver TM, Bree RL: Gray scale features of hematomas: An ultrasonic spectrum. AJR 131: 977–980, 1978

Wing VW, Federle MD, Morris JA et al: The clinical impact of CT for blunt abdominal trauma. AJR 145:1191–1194, 1985

## BLUNT ABDOMINAL TRAUMA

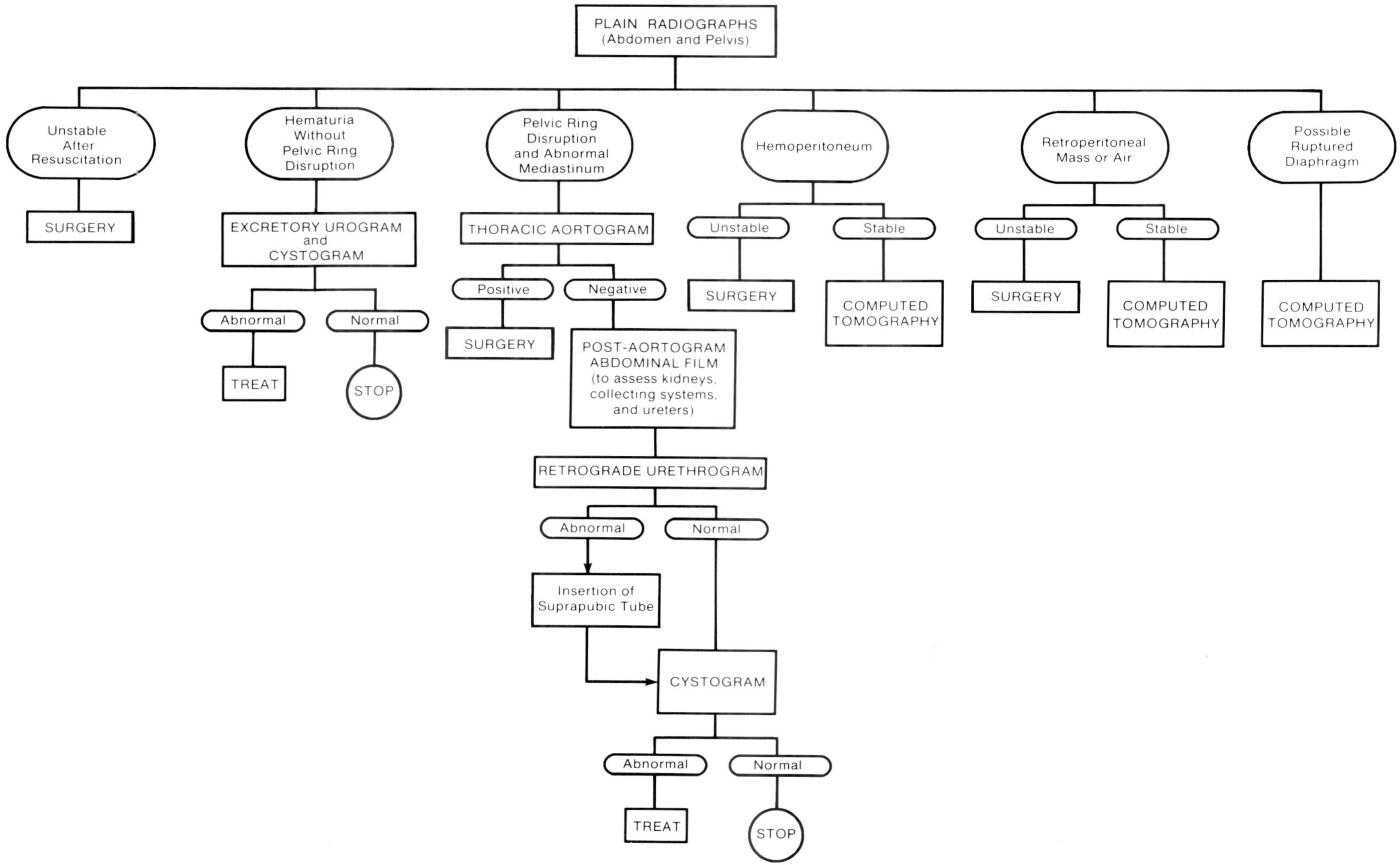

# PART THREE

# Genitourinary Tract

# Chapter 19

# Hypertension

*Donald E. Schwarten*

Hypertension is one of the major risk factors for developing premature cardiovascular disease. Several studies have demonstrated that even minimally elevated blood pressure is associated with a significantly increased risk of coronary, cerebral, and other vascular diseases. Most patients with high blood pressure are characterized as mild hypertensives (persistent diastolic pressures of 90–104 mm Hg). Although the risk per patient in this group is relatively small, since mild hypertensives comprise the majority of the hypertensive population they will suffer most of the premature cardiovascular disease.

An estimated 25 to 35 million Americans have hypertension. Of these, 5% to 10% have a curable cause of their high blood pressure. Underlying conditions include renovascular disease (2%–6%), coarctation of the aorta (1%), primary aldosteronism (0.5%), Cushing's syndrome (0.2%), and pheochromocytoma (0.2%).

It is generally assumed that the excessive and premature cardiovascular disease associated with hypertension may be largely prevented by lowering the blood pressure. Indeed, merely lowering the blood pressure does provide a partial degree of protection, particularly from coronary artery disease. However, the most significant factor is the method by which the blood pressure is lowered. One report showed that among patients whose blood pressure was lowered by drugs, there was no concomitant decrease in the rate of cardiovascular complications when compared with the rate among patients with the same levels of blood pressure who received only placebo therapy. In a landmark study, the long-term results in patients with renovascular hypertension maintained on similar blood pressure control were substantially poorer in patients managed medically than in those who underwent revascularization. After 9 years, 84% of the surgical patients and 43% of those who received only medical therapy were still alive. A review of the outcome of atherosclerotic renovascular disease in patients treated medically and followed by sequential renal angiography noted progressive renal artery obstruction in 44%, including 16% in whom complete renal artery occlusion developed. It has been shown conclusively that in the presence of atherosclerotic renal artery disease, there may be a progressive loss of renal function despite little change in blood pressure or medication requirements. Even fibromuscular dysplasia of the renal arteries has been shown to be progressive, although not usually with as pronounced a tendency to develop complete occlusion and loss of renal function. In summary, revascularization clearly appears to be the treatment of choice in patients with renovascular hypertension. Similarly, surgical correction of the underlying abnormality is preferable to palliation with medical management in other forms of surgically curable hypertension.

Because of the cost and morbidity related to the diagnosis and correction of secondary hypertension, criteria have been established to determine those patients who should be investigated for curable forms of hypertension. Patients with a recognizable clinical syndrome, such as Cushing's syndrome, coarctation of the aorta, or pheochromocytoma, should be further evaluated and appropriately treated for these conditions. In most cases, however, surgically treatable hypertension is related to underlying renovascular disease. Almost 40% of patients with atherosclerotic lesions that cause renovascular hypertension develop elevated blood pressure after the age of 50 years, compared with only 7% of patients with essential hypertension and 3% of patients with fibromuscular disease. Although blacks comprise 30% of patients studied for renovascular hypertension, they represent only 8% of the patients cured by revascularization.

The major clinical indications for investigating a patient for suspected renovascular hypertension include the following:

1. Recent onset of hypertension
2. Change in degree of existing hypertension
3. Poor control of blood pressure with medical therapy
4. Poor patient compliance
5. Complications of medical therapy
6. Deterioration of renal function
7. Onset of hypertension after age 50
8. Females between ages 30 and 50 who have no family history of hypertension
9. Presence of an abdominal or flank bruit
10. Any patient in the pediatric age group

## DIAGNOSTIC EVALUATION

### *DIAGNOSTIC MODALITIES*

1. Digital subtraction angiography
2. Arteriography
3. Rapid-sequence excretory urography
4. Chest radiography
5. Computed tomography
6. Selective renal vein sampling for renin assays
7. Venous sampling
8. Deep duplex ultrasound
9. Magnetic resonance imaging

### Digital Subtraction Angiography

The introduction of digital subtraction angiography (DSA) has significantly enhanced the radiologist's ability to make the diagnosis of renovascular disease with relative ease. In addition, since DSA is much less invasive than conventional arteriography, clinicians are more willing to use this technique to screen their patients for renovascular hypertension.

The accuracy of intravenous digital subtraction angiography (IVDSA) is limited by contrast volumes, motion artifacts, superimposition of vessels, and, occasionally, diminished cardiac output, and it can be enhanced by judicious patient selection. In one prospective study comparing IVDSA with conventional arteriography, IVDSA had a sensitivity of 87.5%, a specificity of 100%, and an accuracy of 95.3% for detecting renal artery stenosis. It should be noted that these results did not include the 6.5% of studies that were eliminated because of inadequate visualization. Intravenous digital subtraction angiography with one or two plain abdominal radiographs for the assessment of renal contour, collecting structures, ureters, and urinary bladder can substitute for a conventional rapid-sequence excretory urogram. In my experience, IVDSA is an acceptable initial imaging modality for those 60% of patients with renovascular hypertension who are likely to have atherosclerosis as the underlying etiology of their renal artery stenosis. Adult patients who are likely to have underlying fibromuscular dysplasia and children

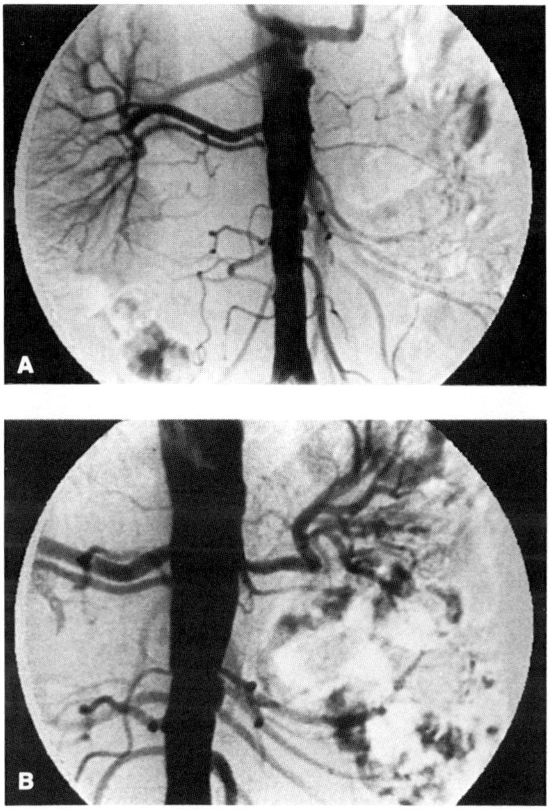

**Figure 19-1.** Intra-arterial DSA in a patient with severe hypertension and mild renal failure. **(A)** Midaortic flush demonstrates occlusion of the left renal artery. **(B)** Repeat midaortic injection following complete lysis and percutaneous transluminal angioplasty shows the previously occluded left renal artery to be widely patent.

with probable branch-artery stenoses should be studied by the intra-arterial route (DSA or conventional arteriography). A major advantage of intra-arterial DSA over conventional arteriography is the ability to use smaller caliber catheters and smaller volumes of contrast, thus making this a lower risk procedure that can easily be performed on an outpatient basis.

An advantage of IVDSA is that renal vein blood samples can be obtained at the same time as the digital study by simply exchanging for the appropriate selective catheter. One report has shown that a combination of IVDSA and properly performed renal vein assays for renin identified all patients with renovascular hypertension.

The use of glucagon and *local* abdominal compression significantly increases the likelihood of obtaining a study of diagnostic quality using DSA. If a single frontal projection fails to detect a renal artery abnormality in the patient with suspected renovascular hypertension, oblique projections are mandatory. In adults with fibromuscular dysplasia or children with branch-vessel lesions, it is necessary to obtain selective oblique examinations in both inspiration and expiration to optimally display the anatomy.

When performing intra-arterial DSA, we use both midaortic flush examinations (catheter placed opposite the orifice of the renal arteries) and selective examinations in the appropriate anteroposterior, oblique, and lateral positions (Fig. 19-1). The use of a 1024 matrix with a 1000-line, high-resolution display permits adequate assessment of even branch lesions in pediatric patients. The rapid exposure rate achievable with large-capacity hard disks, combined with the ability to continuously alter the gray scale, permits an evaluation of flow characteristics in the main renal artery and collateral vessels (Fig. 19-2). At this time, the principal disadvantage of intra-arterial DSA is the inability to consistently and accurately measure the caliber of the renal vessels for the purpose of choosing an appropriate-sized angioplasty catheter to revascularize the kidney. Therefore, prior to angioplasty, conventional arteriography with a known magnification factor must be obtained.

## Arteriography

Screen-film arteriography has been the "gold standard" in the examination of the patient with suspected or known renovascular hypertension. Frontal and oblique abdominal aortograms are highly sensitive and specific for detecting main renal artery lesions. The addition of selective studies with multiple oblique views can demonstrate virtually all arterial abnormalities causing renovascular hypertension and also permits assessment of the distal intrarenal vasculature. Arteriography has been used not only as a diagnostic tool but also as a predictor of the likelihood of achieving a substantial decrease in blood pres-

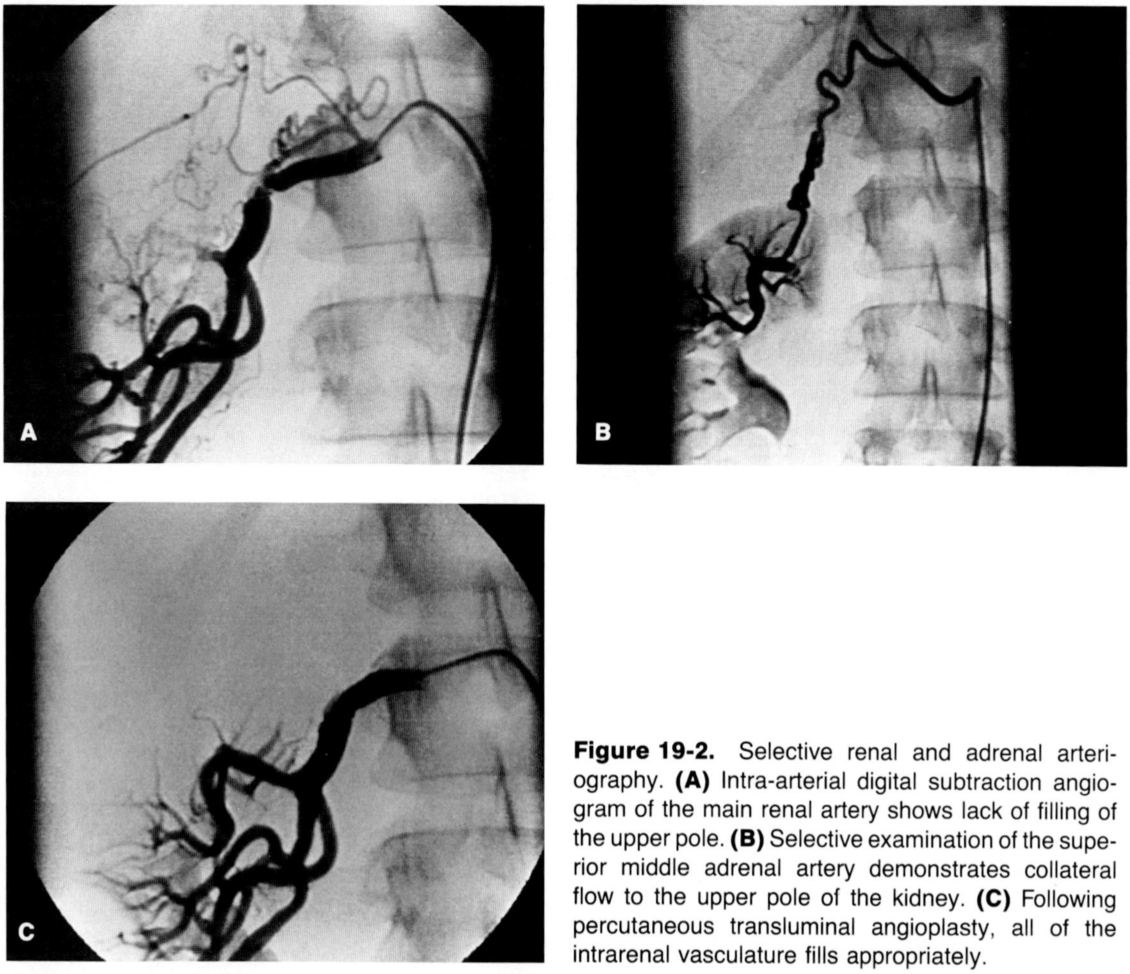


**Figure 19-2.** Selective renal and adrenal arteriography. **(A)** Intra-arterial digital subtraction angiogram of the main renal artery shows lack of filling of the upper pole. **(B)** Selective examination of the superior middle adrenal artery demonstrates collateral flow to the upper pole of the kidney. **(C)** Following percutaneous transluminal angioplasty, all of the intrarenal vasculature fills appropriately.

sure in response to revascularization in the patient with renal artery stenosis and renovascular hypertension.

At present, I seldom use conventional arteriography as a screening procedure for renovascular hypertension. This technique is now reserved for selected difficult cases, primarily certain patients with fibromuscular dysplasia. As noted above, conventional arteriography also is used for calibration purposes.

## Rapid-Sequence Excretory Urography

Excretory urography is a simple, safe, widely available procedure for screening patients with suspected renovascular hypertension. In general, 50 ml to 90 ml of iodinated contrast material is injected through a large-bore needle as rapidly as possible (preferably in less than 10 sec), and rapid-sequence films are obtained at approximately 30 seconds, and 1, 2, 3, and 5 minutes. A delayed film at 15 to 20 minutes should be obtained, and nephrotomography is often used for optimal visualization of the renal outlines.

The major urographic criteria consistent with renovascular hypertension are (1) disparity in kidney length greater than 1.5 cm, (2) difference in calyceal appearance time, and (3) disparity in calyceal and pelvic contrast concentration on late films. A cooperative study showed that a difference in the calyceal appearance time between the two sides is the single most important urographic indicator, having been demonstrated in approximately 60% of patients with renovascular hypertension. Approximately 40% of patients show a significant difference in renal length and/or a disparity in contrast concentration on late films. Other parameters that may be evaluated as indicators of renovascular hypertension include renal outline, opacified urine volume, and ureteropelvic notching (representing large, tortuous collateral blood vessels).

Although its simplicity and wide availability make excretory urography an attractive procedure for screening patients with renovascular hypertension, it is associated with a significant number of false-negative results. In patients with renovascular hypertension who respond favorably to surgical revascularization, only 75% have an abnormal rapid-sequence urogram. Therefore, excretory urography is clearly not the screening test of choice to evaluate patients with renovascular hypertension for potentially curable renal artery stenoses.

## Chest Radiography

Although frequently normal, the chest radiograph may reflect changes related to longstanding and/or severe hypertension, such as left ventricular enlargement and aortic tortuosity. In addition, specific abnormalities on chest radiographs may indicate a possible underlying cause of the elevated blood pressure. Rib notching suggests coarctation of the aorta, especially when seen in conjunction with disproportionate size of the ascending and descending portions of the thoracic aorta or the characteristic reversed-3 sign. A result of the development of collateral vessels, notching most commonly involves the third to eighth ribs. Paramediastinal widening due to increased fat, associated with osteopenia and compression changes in vertebral bodies, suggests Cushing's syndrome. A paravertebral mass in the presence of hypertension suggests a pheochromocytoma, while clavicular erosions may indicate underlying chronic renal disease and secondary hyperparathyroidism.

## Computed Tomography

Computed tomography is the imaging modality of choice for detecting adrenal and extra-adrenal pheochromocytomas. This technique has effectively eliminated the role of arteriography in evaluating patients suspected of having a pheochromocytoma as the underlying cause of their hypertension.

## Selective Renal Vein Sampling for Renin Assays

Properly performed renal vein renin assays are highly predictive of a beneficial blood pressure response to revascularization of an ischemic kidney (if possible) or, if necessary, to nephrectomy. A positive renal vein renin assay indicates a greater than 90% chance of substantially decreasing blood pressure by angioplasty or surgery.

Simple measurement of renal vein renin ratios may not be of sufficient predictive value. Traditionally, the demonstration of a ratio of 1.5 : 1 or greater has been considered indicative of the functional significance of a renal artery stenosis. However, this ratio has at least a 15% false-negative rate in the presence of unilateral renal artery disease, and a false-negative rate of more than 35% in patients with bilateral renovascular disease. Improperly performed assays may lead to a high incidence of false-positive results.

Meticulous standardization of the immunoassay technique in the renin laboratory is required, as is adherence to a strict protocol of examination. Whenever possible, the patient should not have received antihypertensive medication for one week prior to the examination. If this is impossible, it is at least essential to withhold pain medications and to eliminate or control dietary elements known to have an effect on renin output. Some reports suggest the value of administering an angiotensin-converting enzyme inhibitor (captopril) or stimulating renin production with a presampling bolus of Lasix (furosemide).

Contrary to initial reports, it has been shown that it is not necessary to perform arteriography and renal vein renin sampling on separate days, nor does it matter whether the arteriogram is performed prior to or after the renal vein samples are obtained. Nevertheless, it is important to perform these procedures consistently in any specific institution. The sampling catheter should always be placed well into the main renal vein and, on the left, should extend beyond the orifice of the left gonadal vein. If branch renal artery stenoses are present, it is essential that segmental renal samples be obtained. Perhaps the best method is one described by Sos and Laragh, in which samples are sequentially obtained from the right and left renal veins and from the infrarenal and suprarenal portions of the inferior vena cava. The results are tabulated and expressed as ratios, although the most important factor is demonstration of suppressed renin output on the unaffected side in the presence of unilateral disease.

Up to 65% of patients with severe hypertension and a significant renal artery stenosis, but with normal renal vein studies, demonstrate a beneficial blood pressure response to surgical revascularization. In addition, in the presence of atherosclerosis there is likely to be progression of disease with loss of functioning renal parenchyma despite little, if any, change in blood pressure or medication requirements. Therefore, in the presence of atherosclerosis and significant bilateral renal artery disease or significant disease in a single functioning kidney, surgical intervention may be justified for the preservation of renal function regardless of the renin data. An even better case for revascularization despite nonlateralizing renin data in patients with atherosclerosis can now be made because of the availability of low-risk percutaneous transluminal angioplasty.

## Venous Sampling

Aldosterone-producing neoplasms are a rare cause of hypertension. These tumors are frequently small ( < 1 cm in diameter) and may not be detected by CT scanning. Careful adrenal vein sampling during stimulation of adrenocorticotropic hormone (ACTH) can detect and localize approximately 90% of these tumors and is thus the procedure of choice for the preoperative evaluation of the patient with a suspected aldosteronoma. There is no indication, however, for adrenal venography as part of the sampling procedure (Fig. 19-3).

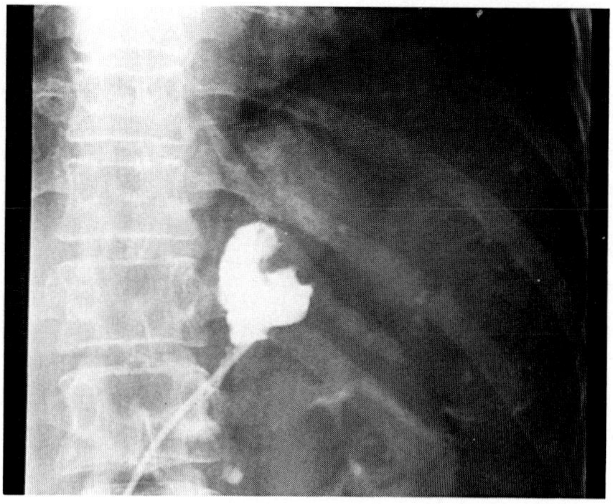

**Figure 19-3.** Rupture of an adrenal gland during adrenal venography in a patient with aldosteronism.

## Deep Duplex Ultrasound

At present, the evaluation of the renal artery with duplex Doppler is a protocol procedure that can obtain adequate studies of the renal artery in approximately 85% of cases. Factors militating against a successful examination include interference with ultrasound transmission from gas in the stomach and duodenum; aortic aneurysm; obesity; and scarring secondary to previous abdominal surgery. Doppler spectra wave forms and corresponding B-mode images obtained from the proximal and distal segments of the renal arteries permit estimation of renal artery stenosis. In addition, signals can be obtained with B-modes images to document the location.

The kidney dimension is measured from real-time images to provide a maximal upper-to-lower pole measurement. With continued improvement in ultrasound equipment, it can be anticipated that in the future more consistent assessment of the renal arteries will be achieved with deep duplex Doppler scanning.

### Magnetic Resonance Imaging

At this time, magnetic resonance imaging (MRI) is rarely used in the evaluation of patients with suspected secondary hypertension. However, this modality has the potential to accurately assess the renal arteries as well as the adrenal gland and the kidney.

## INTERVENTIONAL PROCEDURES

### Percutaneous Transluminal Angioplasty

Multiple low-risk diagnostic imaging modalities are currently available for detecting the cause of renovascular hypertension. The appropriate utilization of these procedures is more important now than in the past because of the availability of percutaneous transluminal angioplasty for the management of renovascular hypertension. Percutaneous transluminal angioplasty is currently the treatment of choice for patients with renovascular hypertension who have renal artery stenosis (Fig. 19-4). The only patients who are not initially considered for revascularization via percutaneous transluminal angioplasty are those with large aortic plaques encompassing the orifice of the renal artery, because these lesions are difficult (if not impossible) to adequately dilate and, even if successfully dilated initially, have a high risk of recurrent stenosis.

Angioplasty is generally performed from either the right or left common femoral artery using the Seldinger technique. For main renal artery lesions, the so-called guide wire exchange technique is generally employed. A 5- or 6-French selective catheter is used to engage the orifice of the renal artery, and a very soft guide wire is employed to cross the stenosis if the catheter tip does not initially pop across it. The initial catheter is exchanged for a catheter containing a balloon equal to the size of the adjacent normal portion of the renal artery or, if this is difficult to assess because of a low flow state, of the same size as the contralateral normal vessel (if the renal arteries are single bilaterally and the kidneys are approximately the same size).

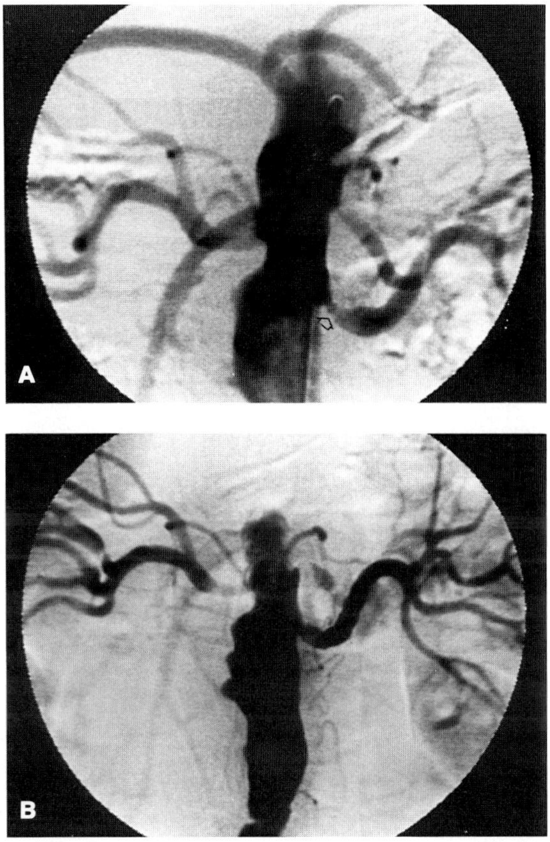


**Figure 19-4.** Nonosteal atherosclerosis. **(A)** Initial intra-arterial digital subtraction angiogram shows the stenotic lesion (*arrow*). **(B)** Repeat examination following percutaneous transluminal angioplasty.

Renal angioplasty procedures are performed in patients who are only lightly premedicated. Narcotic analgesics are not used, because the patient must be able to communicate with the angiographer about the level of discomfort felt during balloon inflation. Severe pain suggests that the balloon is too large; significant pain fol-

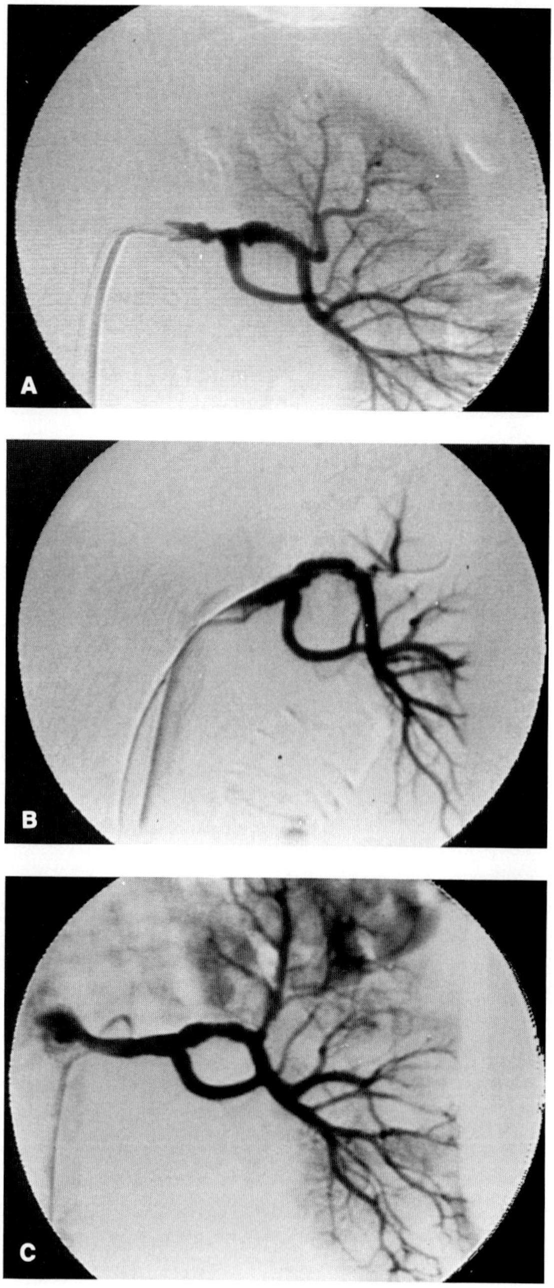

**Figure 19-5.** Medial fibroplasia. **(A)** Initial examination. **(B)** Two catheters are used for the angioplasty because of the involvement of a bifurcation. **(C)** Following percutaneous transluminal angioplasty, severe distal spasm can be managed effectively and rapidly with intra-arterial nitroglycerin.

lowing the procedure suggests renal artery rupture and is an indication for an immediate CT scan. Depending on clinical and radiographic factors, the demonstration of blood around the renal artery on a CT scan following an angioplasty may indicate a need for surgical intervention.

Renal artery spasm is a frequent complication of angioplasty, particularly in patients with fibromuscular disease (Fig. 19-5). This complication can be avoided by the aggressive use of intra-arterial nitroglycerin and oral or sublingual nifedipine. The patient should be carefully hydrated and constantly monitored during the procedure because of the risk of inducing hypotension with vasodilators. Although controversial, I recommend intraprocedure anticoagulation with heparin, especially when dealing with distal disease. Heparin not only serves as an anticoagulant but also reduces the likelihood that vasospasm will develop. Antiplatelet therapy (at a minimum, salicylates) should be employed in all patients with atherosclerosis. Dipyridamole in doses of 50 mg to 75 mg q.i.d. may be of additional benefit.

Following percutaneous transluminal angioplasty, completion arteriograms are obtained. For proximal renal artery lesions, it is preferable to perform an abdominal aortogram rather than risk injecting through an end-hole catheter adjacent to the angioplasty site, which may possibly cause elevation of the intimal–medial cleft and occlusion of the renal artery. For branch renal artery lesions (Fig. 19-6), the completion arteriogram can be obtained via a selective catheter.

Primary anatomic success can be expected in 95% of patients with nonosteal atherosclerotic renal artery stenoses or medial fibroplasia. A beneficial blood pressure response can be anticipated in 85% of patients with atherosclerosis and in 90% to 95% of patients with medial fibroplasia. These results are comparable to those achieved with surgical revascularization procedures and can be obtained by percutaneous transluminal angioplasty without the morbidity and loss of productive time associated with operative intervention. In the hands of an experienced angiographer, the mortality rate of renal angioplasty should be less than 0.5% (operative

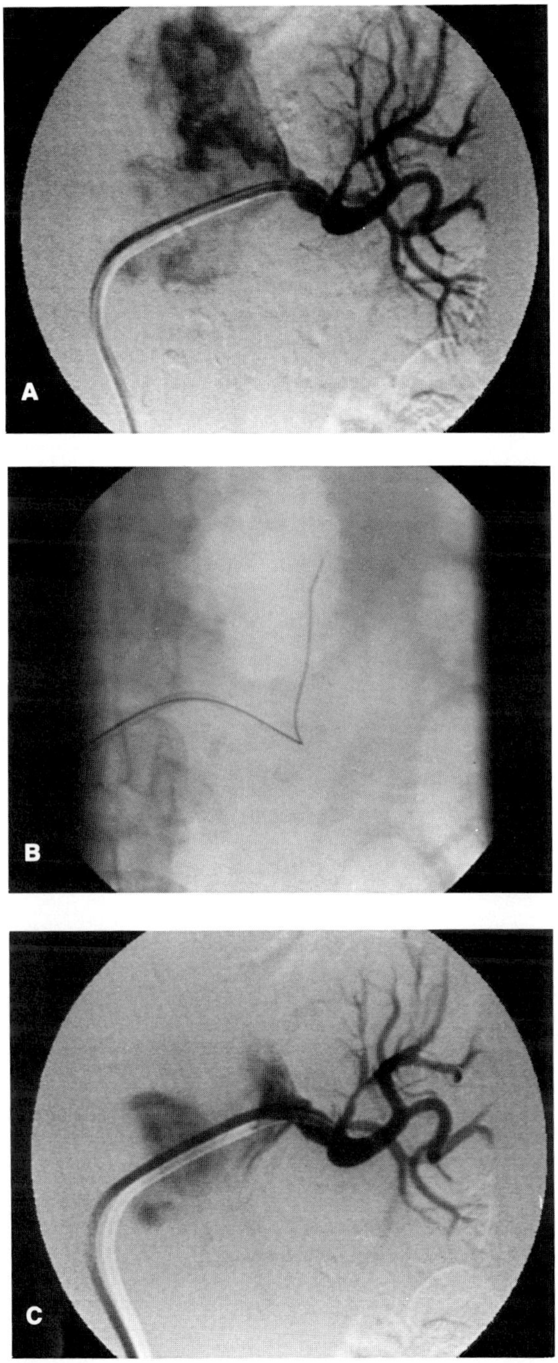

**Figure 19-6.** Distal branch disease. **(A)** Preliminary intra-arterial digital subtraction angiogram. **(B)** A 0.018-inch guide wire has been placed in the branch vessel via an 8-French guiding catheter. **(C)** Post-angioplasty study shows a near-normal-caliber branch vessel. The patient's initial blood pressure of 230/130 mm Hg returned to normal levels following angioplasty.

mortality varies from 1%–9.7% in reported series).

Complications associated with renal angioplasty occur at a rate proportional to the skill and experience of the angiographer performing the procedure. In general, complications requiring surgical intervention should occur at a rate of less than 1%. To date, I have had one patient who required urgent revascularization as a result of a failed angioplasty attempt.

Long-term follow-up data indicate a 5-year patency rate of 80% to 85% in patients treated by angioplasty for atherosclerotic disease of the renal artery. Patients treated with percutaneous transluminal angioplasty for medial fibroplasia rarely develop recurrent stenoses, and the 5-year patency rate is over 95%.

## Bibliography

Atkinson AB, Brown JJ, Cumming A et al: Captopril in the management of hypertension with renal artery stenosis: Its long term effect as a predictor of surgical outcome. Am J Cardiol 49:1460, 1982

Bookstein JJ, Abrams HL, Buenger RE et al: Radiologic aspects of renovascular hypertension. II. The role of urography in unilateral renovascular disease. JAMA 220:1225–1230, 1972

Bookstein JJ, Abrams HL, Buenger RE et al: Radiologic aspects of renovascular hypertension. III. Appraisal of arteriography. JAMA 221:368–374, 1972

Dotter CT, Gruntzig A, Schoop W et al: Percutaneous Transluminal Angioplasty: Technique, Early and Late Results. Berlin, Springer-Verlag, 1983

Gomes AS, Pais SO, Babaric ZO: DSA in the evaluation of hypertension. AJR 140:779, 1983

Grim C, Luft FC, Weinberger MH et al: Sensitivity and specificity of screening tests for renovascular hypertension. Ann Intern Med 91:617, 1979

Hillman BJ, Ovitt TW, Capp MP et al: Potential impact of digital video subtraction angiography on screening for renovascular hypertension. Radiology 142:577, 1982

Hillman BJ, Ovitt TW, Capp MP et al: Renal DSA: 100 cases. Radiology 145:643, 1982

Hunt JC, Strong CG: Renovascular hypertension: Mechanisms, natural history and management. Am J Cardiol 32:562–574, 1973

Illescos FF, Ford KK, Braun SD et al: Intraarterial digital subtraction angiography in hypertensive azotemic patients. AJR 143:1065–1067, 1984

Judson WE, Helmer OM: Diagnostic and prognostic values of renin activity in renal venous plasma in renovascular hypertension. Hypertension 13:79–89, 1965

Kaplan NM: Renin profiles. The unfulfilled promises. JAMA 238:611, 1977

Management Committee of the Australian Therapeutic Trial in Mild Hypertension. Lancet 1:1261, 1980

Marks LS, Maxwell MH: Renal vein renin: Value and limitations in the prediction of operative results. Urol Clin North Am 2:311–325, 1975

Metropolitan Life Insurance Company. Blood pressure: Insurance experience and its implications. New York, 1961

Miller GA, Ford KK, Braun SD et al: P.T.A. versus surgery for renovascular hypertension. AJR 144:447–450, 1985

Schwarten DE: Percutaneous transluminal angioplasty of the renal arteries: Intravenous digital subtraction angiography for follow-up. Radiology 150:369–373, 1984

Schwarten DE: Transluminal angioplasty of renal artery stenosis: 70 experiences. AJR 135:969–974, 1980

Tegtmeyer CT, Elson J, Glass TA et al: P.T.A.: The treatment of choice for renovascular hypertension due to fibromuscular dysplasia. Radiology 143:631, 1982

V.A. Cooperative Study Group on Antihypertensive Agents. Effects of treatment on morbidity in hypertension. II. Results in patients with diastolic blood pressure averaging 90 through 114 millimeters of mercury. JAMA 213:1143, 1970

Weinberger MH, Grim CE, Hollifield TW et al: Primary aldosteronism, diagnosis, localization and treatment. Ann Intern Med 90:386–395, 1979

## HYPERTENSIVE PATIENT

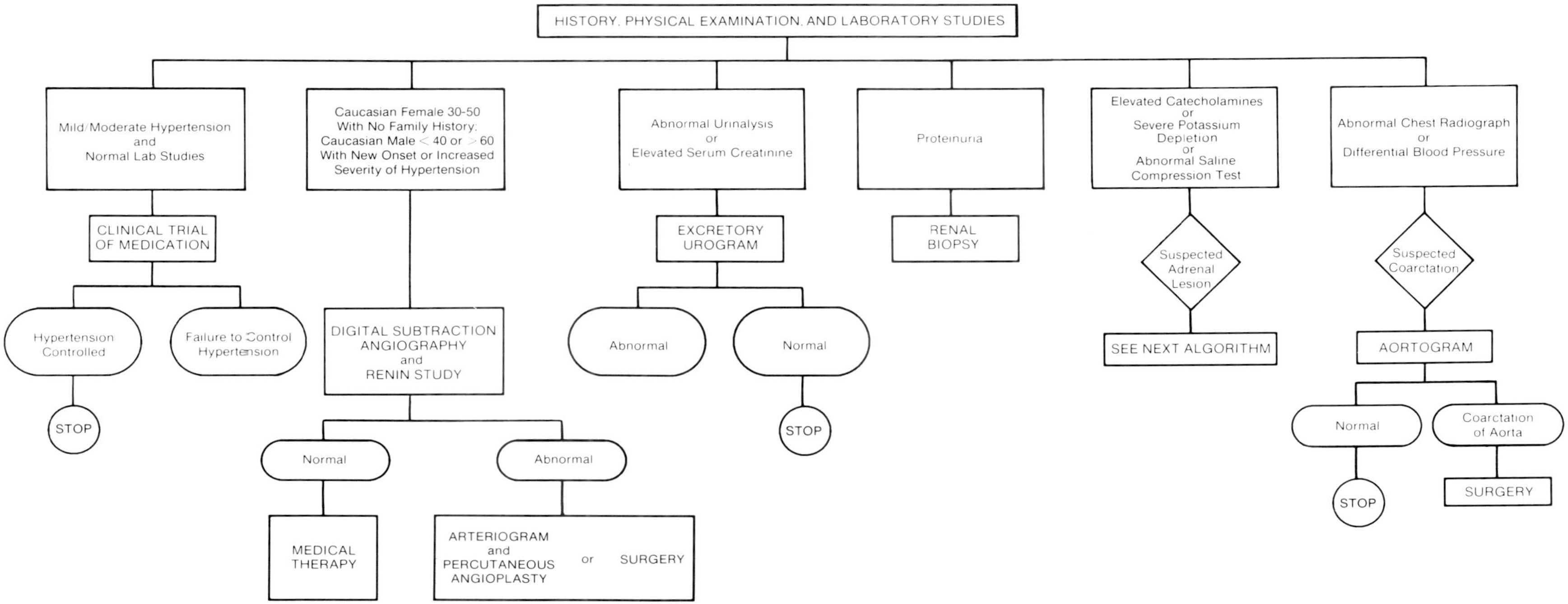

**HYPERTENSIVE PATIENT**

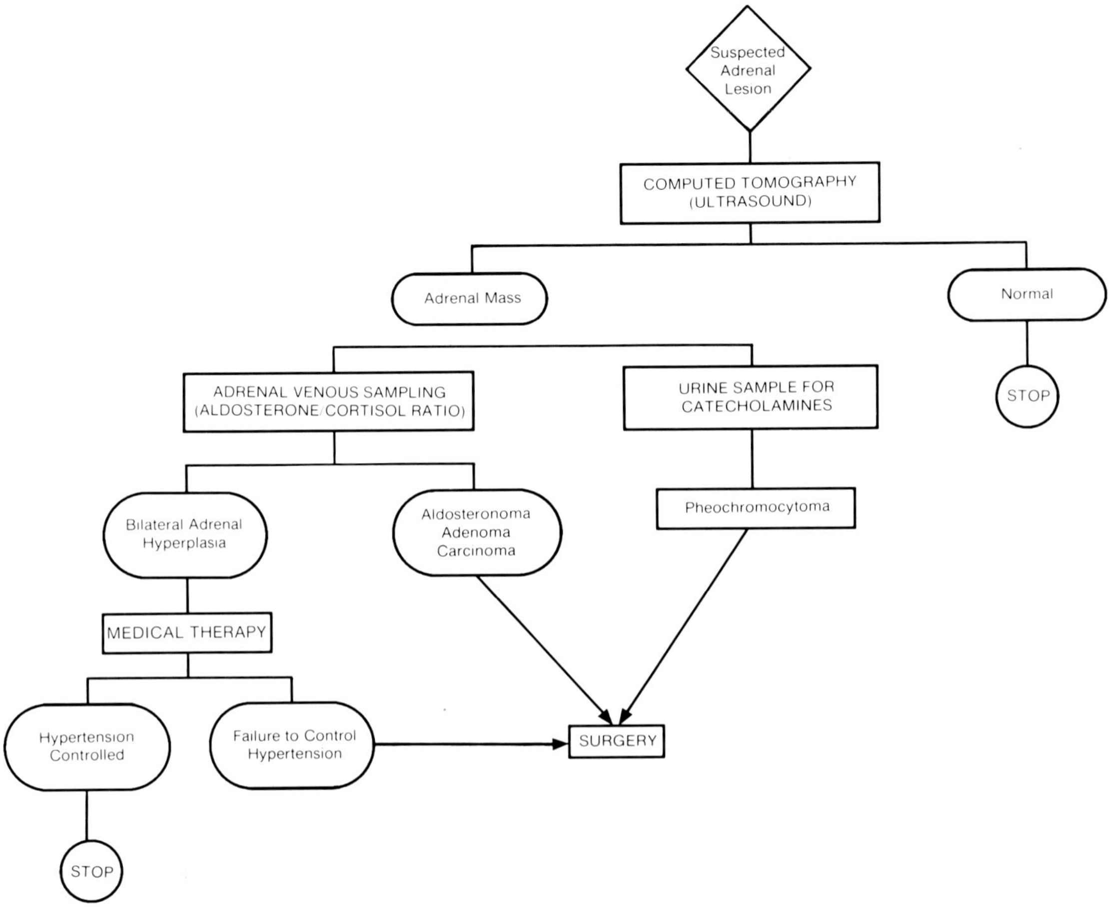

# Chapter 20

# Abnormal Renal Size

*Alan J. Davidson*

The discovery of abnormal renal size may be the unexpected result of an investigation undertaken for symptoms not initially suspected to be of renal origin. Abnormal renal size may be detected by abdominal palpation or by direct anatomic studies of the kidney, such as excretory urography, ultrasound, computed tomography (CT), or even surgical exploration. At times, certain clinical evidence may suggest the presence of a renal disorder that may alter the gross morphology of the kidney, causing it to be detectable by radiographic techniques. Whether through fortuitous discovery or as the result of directed inquiry, knowledge of abnormal renal size is important and leads to logical clinical decision-making. This chapter discusses the ground rules for assessing renal size, the various imaging modalities available for this purpose, and the pathologic implications of abnormalities in the renal size.

## ASSESSMENT OF RENAL SIZE

The renal mass is closely correlated with factors such as body build and age. However, the usefulness of normal values based on these relationships is diminished by geometric distortion in the radiographic method. The standard radiographic image of the kidney tends to be magnified owing to the distance between the kidney and the film, and foreshortened because the kidney *in situ* is not parallel to the plane of the film. In addition, standard radiographs permit measurements of this unusually shaped organ in only two dimensions. To assess the third dimension (thickness), lateral projections and occasionally tomography are needed, resulting in considerable financial cost and radiation exposure. Thus determination of renal volume from standard radiographs is, at best, a difficult task.

Ultrasound and CT eliminate the vagaries of geometric distortion inherent in traditional radiographic technique. These modalities allow precise measurement of organ size that can be related to data for normal organs based on direct anatomic studies. Of the two techniques, ultrasound has the practical advantage of easily generating longitudinal, coronal, or transverse images. Longitudinal CT images, on the other hand, depend on complex, expensive, and time-consuming data reconstruction and are less exact than those derived from ultrasound.

Another problem in the use of renal size as an index of disease is that measurements based on overall length and width assume a constant ratio between functioning renal tissue and the internal structures of the kidney, such as the pelvocalyceal system and peripelvic fat. Data from normal renal volume are invalid in cases of hydronephrosis, cyst, tumor, or peripelvic fat proliferation where mass is preserved at the expense of renal parenchyma.

Despite the weaknesses described previously, a number of studies have attempted to establish a valid quantitative basis for determining normal renal size *in vivo* using data primarily derived from excretory urography. Most formulations are based on the product of the external height and width of the kidney minus the product of the height and width of the collecting structures within the kidney. Other systems measure only maximum renal length and width. Nomograms relating these values to body surface area have also been developed. The technique based on the relationship between kidney length and the height of the second lumbar vertebral body in the adult, while attractive in its simplicity, has no basis in anatomic reality or statistical validity. Data derived from the studies of Moel have the most favorable variance and are based on relatively practical methods (Tables 20-1, 20-2, and 20-3).

Studies of renal volume using cross-sectional techniques have not been based on data derived from normal populations. In addition, they have not taken into account the important variables of age, sex, and body build. Thus, neither ultrasound nor CT offers a practical alternative to excretory urography for measuring renal size, although these modalities do eliminate the problem of geometric distortion.

The wide standard deviations in all available studies make it difficult to apply renal measurement data to the individual patient. Therefore, many radiologists depend on a simple qualitative evaluation of the kidneys in relationship to age, body build, and symmetry. This approach takes into account that the kidney gradually increases in size from birth to the latter part of the second decade, stabilizes until the fifth decade, and then gradually decreases in size. There is also a close, positive correlation between renal size and the overall size of the patient. Furthermore, it is well established that the size, shape, and thickness of the two kidneys in any given person are remarkably symmetric if one allows for the normal tendency of the left kidney to be slightly larger than the right. Any alteration in symmetry, particularly of the renal substance, is therefore another indicator of renal disease.

In any assessment of a person's renal size, the observer must keep in mind not only the variables of body build and age but also the fact that, given the wide range of normal, diseased kidneys with altered renal mass may still remain within normal size limits. Furthermore, the usual progression of events of a pathologic process that initially leads to renal enlargement may well cause subsequent loss of renal mass. During this natural progression, the kidneys pass through a normal range as they change from excessively large to abnormally small.

Despite the imprecisions outlined in this

**Table 20-1** Roentgenographic Length and Width (in cm) of Normal Kidneys, Measured on Plain Roentgenograms of 100 Men and 100 Women, Aged 20–49

| | Men | | | | Women | | | |
|---|---|---|---|---|---|---|---|---|
| | Right | | Left | | Right | | Left | |
| | Length | Width | Length | Width | Length | Width | Length | Width |
| $\bar{x}$ | 12.9 | 6.2 | 13.2 | 6.3 | 12.3 | 5.7 | 12.6 | 5.9 |
| $s$ | 0.8 | 0.4 | 0.8 | 0.5 | 0.8 | 0.5 | 0.8 | 0.4 |

$\bar{x}$ = mean; $s$ = standard deviation
(Moell H: Size of normal kidneys. Acta Radiol (Diagn) 46:640–645, 1956)

**Table 20-2** Roentgenographic Area (Product of Length and Width in cm) of Normal Kidneys Measured on Plain Roentgenograms of 100 Men and 100 Women, Aged 20–49

| | Men | | | Women | | |
|---|---|---|---|---|---|---|
| | Right | Left | Right + Left | Right | Left | Right + Left |
| $\bar{x}$ | 79.6 | 82.7 | 162.3 | 70.1 | 74.1 | 144.2 |
| $s$ | 8.7 | 8.3 | 15.6 | 8.0 | 7.3 | 13.6 |

$\bar{x}$ = mean; $s$ = standard deviation
(Moell H: Size of normal kidneys. Acta Radiol (Diagn) 46:640–645, 1956)

**Table 20-3** Comparison of Roentgenographic Length and Width of Right and Left Kidneys, Measured on Plain Roentgenograms of 100 Men and 100 Women, Aged 20–49

| Relationship Between Right and Left Kidney | Number of Patients | | Significance (0–3+) | |
|---|---|---|---|---|
| | Men | Women | Men | Women |
| Length | | | | |
| Right kidney longer | 27 | 35 | | |
| Both kidneys equal | 1 | 5 | | |
| Left kidney longer | 72 | 60 | | |
| Total number of cases | 100 | 100 | 3+ | 1+ |
| Width | | | | |
| Right kidney wider | 36 | 32 | | |
| Both kidneys equal | 10 | 11 | 0 | 2+ |
| Left kidney wider | 54 | 57 | | |
| Total number of cases | 100 | 100 | | |

(Moell H: Size of normal kidneys. Acta Radiol (Diagn) 46:640–645, 1956)

section, assessment of renal size is important in detecting kidney disease and in formulating an efficient system for the radiographic classification of those diseases that produce structural abnormalities of the kidney.

## DIAGNOSTIC EVALUATION

### *DIAGNOSTIC MODALITIES*

1. Standard radiography and tomography
2. Excretory urography
3. Ultrasound
4. Computed tomography
5. Magnetic resonance imaging

#### Standard Radiography and Tomography

Abnormal renal size is often first suspected on abdominal radiographs performed for an unrelated condition. The standard plain film of the abdomen allows measurement of renal size only when the fat surrounding the kidneys is abundant enough to provide a natural "contrast" material (Fig. 20-1). When the outlines of the kidney are clearly discernible, measurement of renal length and width is easy to perform. Any inaccuracies are only those inherent in the radiographic technique, as discussed in the preceding section.

Plain film radiography may also be accurate in detecting excessive central deposition of radiolucent renal sinus fat. The thickness of the renal parenchyma can be measured as the distance between the margins of the central and perirenal fat lucencies.

The ability to measure renal size without the use of exogenous contrast material is enhanced by tomography. This technique places the renal and perirenal areas in sharp focus by blurring those structures (primarily gas- and fluid-filled bowel) that overlie and often obscure the kidneys (Fig. 20-2).

Both standard radiographs and tomographic studies without contrast material depend on the inherent differences in the radiation absorption properties of fat and "soft tissue" to image the kidneys. The quality of the image will be influenced by technical factors. Since contrast differences between tissues decrease as kilovoltage increases, standard radiographs and tomograms should be exposed in the 60 kVp to 75 kVp range.

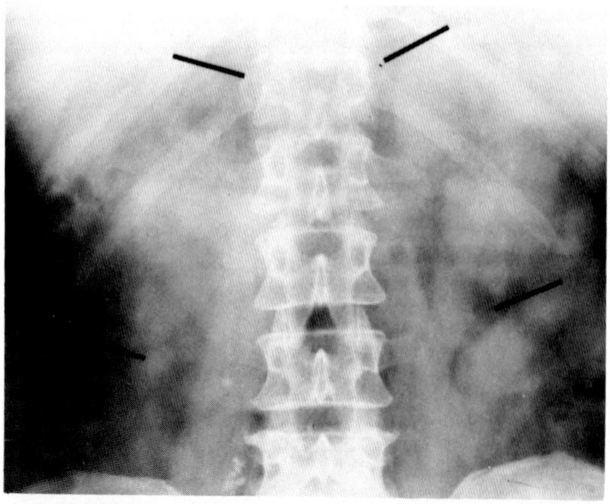

**Figure 20-1.** Standard radiograph. Both kidneys can be outlined, but only with uncertainty.

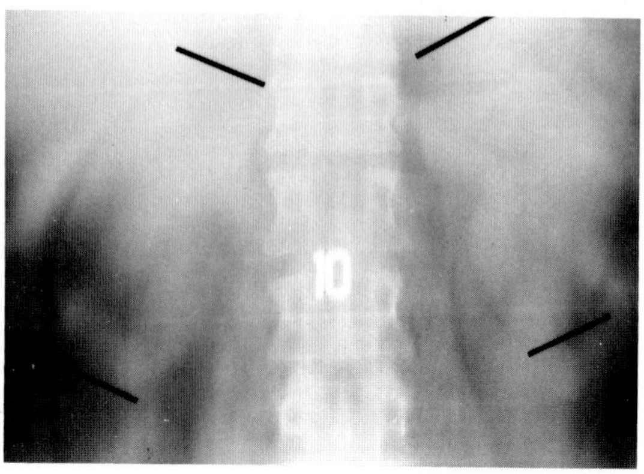

**Figure 20-2.** Tomography of the same patient as in Figure 20-1. The kidney outlines are sharper than in Figure 20-1, despite the absence of radiopaque contrast material.

Standard radiographic techniques fail to accurately outline the kidneys in many patients, particularly those who are young and lean, or cachectic. Furthermore, these methods do not provide any information about the internal structure of the kidney (nephrogram, papillae, calyces) and thus are of limited value in detecting the many processes that change renal bulk in a focal or regional distribution. Therefore, more complex techniques are usually required to adequately assess renal size.

Standard film radiography is the least expensive technique for measuring renal size and requires less exposure than other radiation-dependent modalities. If an abnormality in renal size is suspected, an excretory urogram should be performed. Tomography approximately doubles the cost and requires several times more radiation than does a standard film. Therefore, it is infrequently indicated and should be used only if the plain abdominal radiograph fails to demonstrate the renal margins and excretory urography is contraindicated (*e.g.*, prior history of severe reaction to contrast material).

## Excretory Urography

Radiographic imaging of the kidneys after intravenous injection of iodinated contrast material not only almost always permits accurate assessment of renal length and width but also provides valuable information about renal function and structural integrity. Excretory urography is most reliable when an adequate dose of contrast material is used (15 g–20 g of iodine total dose in patients with normal renal function; 30 g–40 g in those with renal failure). The passage of iodine-bearing contrast molecules through the glomerulus and into the proximal tubules renders the normal renal parenchyma homogeneously white (the "urographic nephrogram") and permits distinction of perfused, functioning, and structurally intact renal tissue from its internal and external surroundings. The number of atoms of iodine filtered into the proximal tubule per unit of time is highest within the first minute following intravenous contrast injection. Because the density of the nephrogram is greatest at this time, a film exposed as soon as possible after a bolus injection of contrast material has become the standard reference for evaluation of renal size, position, and contour, as well as for the functional and structural integrity of the kidney parenchyma (Fig. 20-3). Rapid bolus injection of contrast material results in higher plasma levels than do equal amounts of iodine given as a drip infusion over 10 to 15 minutes. Since optimum opacification depends on plasma levels of contrast material, the rapid bolus technique is preferred for assessing renal size.

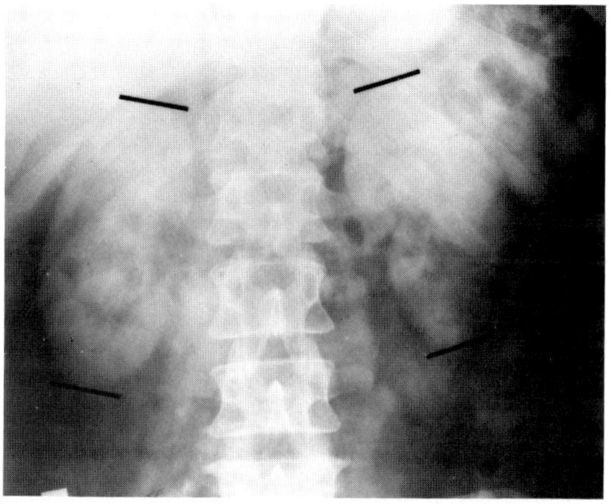

**Figure 20-3.** Same patient as in Figures 20-1 and 20-2. This film was exposed 1 minute after the bolus injection of iodinated contrast material. The renal parenchyma is densely opaque, permitting easy measurement of renal size.

If fluid- and gas-filled loops of bowel obscure the kidneys, or if renal functional impairment is so advanced that the kidneys are only faintly opacified, tomography is required to supplement the excretory urogram (Fig. 20-4).

Because urographic contrast agents are excreted by the kidney, they transiently enlarge renal bulk. This is presumably due to the increase in volume of filtrate caused by the strong osmotic diuretic effect of contrast agents, although increased intrarenal blood volume due to a transient increase in renal blood flow may also contribute to this well-documented phenomenon. Kidney size can increase as much as 10% to 15% over baseline (precontrast) measurements. This may be apparent as early as the

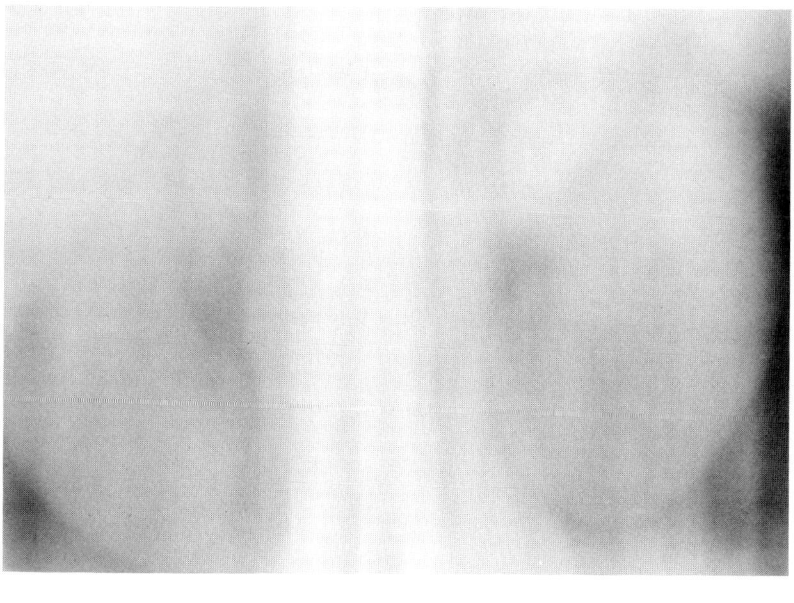

**Figure 20-4.** Rapidly progressive glomerulonephritis in a 42-year-old man. Tomogram obtained 10 minutes after injection of 37.5 g of iodine (125 ml of sodium diatrizoate, 50%). Nephrographic density, although faint, was maximal at this time. (Davidson AJ: Radiology of the Kidney. Philadelphia, WB Saunders, 1985)

"immediate" (approximately 1 minute) film and usually returns to baseline within 15 minutes.

Excretory urography is technically successful in assessing renal size in most cases, although adjunctive use of tomography may be necessary in some. Opacification of the parenchyma provides far more detail than does plain radiography, thus permitting detection of focal or regional changes in renal tissue as well as other features of kidney structure and function. Mild complications (nausea, vomiting, urticarial rash) occur frequently with excretory urography, although serious reactions are unusual.

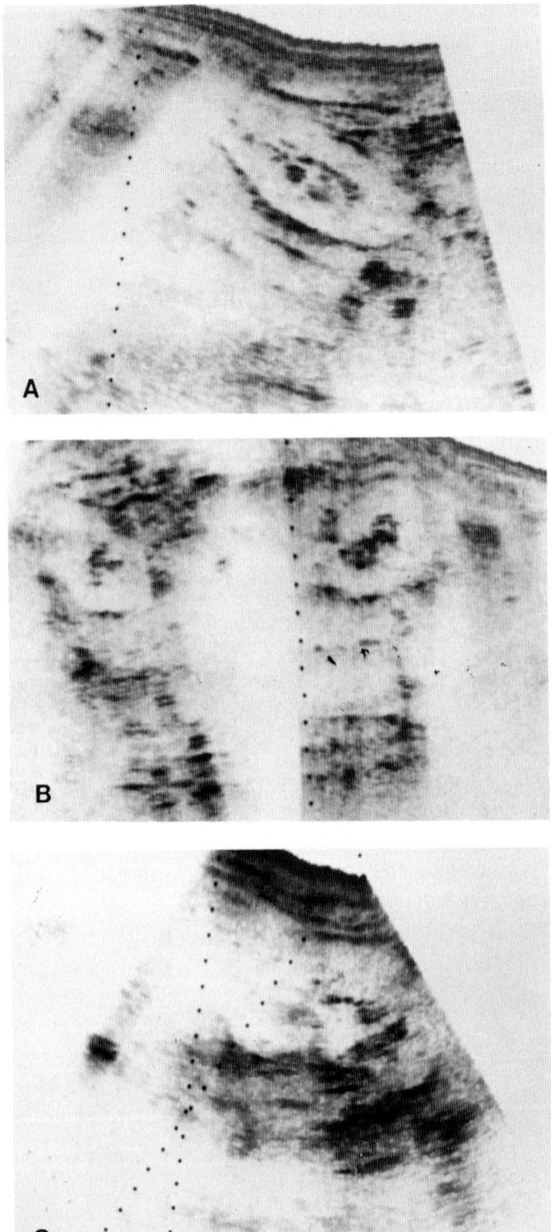

Figure 20-5. Ultrasound images of normal kidney in longitudinal (A), transverse (B), and coronal (C) projections.

### Ultrasound

Ultrasound has been one of the most important innovations in diagnostic radiologic techniques for kidney disease since the development of modern iodinated contrast agents in 1952. Measurement of renal size, definition of the solid or fluid nature of renal masses, determination of the presence or lack of hydronephrosis, and detection of perirenal or pararenal fluid collections are diagnostic tasks superbly performed by ultrasound, even in patients with severely impaired renal function.

Ultrasonic display of the kidney in longitudinal, transverse, or coronal sections permits exact measurement of the external outline of the kidney with none of the geometric distortions associated with standard radiography (Fig. 20-5). Renal parenchyma can be readily distinguished from structures in the renal hilus. Because ultrasound is independent of contrast material excretion, no functional information can be derived from this technique.

No normal standards for renal size based on ultrasonic data that take into account the important variables of age, sex, and body build have been published. Nevertheless, in view of the true representation of renal size by ultrasound, standard anatomic studies relating renal size, body build, and age are a valid reference. However, these do not take into account the effect of hydration on renal size, an important practical consideration in the usual clinical setting. Dehydration will cause a decrease in renal volume, and hydration will produce the opposite effect, just as contrast material or other osmotic diuretics enlarge the kidneys. The extent of water-induced renal enlargement is less than 10%; thus its significance is generally limited to those patients in whom repeated studies are made to determine any changes in kidney size. Such patients should be examined under standardized conditions of hydration.

Ultrasound images of the kidney do not estimate renal sinus volume as well as CT does. Thus, ultrasound is not as accurate in defining the actual thickness of renal parenchyma as it is in imaging the external dimensions of the entire kidney. Similarly, details of small scars or focal enlargements may be lacking in the ultrasound image of the kidney. Another disadvantage of ultrasound compared with other imaging modalities is the occasional technical difficulty of performing the examination in obese patients or when bowel gas or a recent skin incision lie over the area of interest. Furthermore, the quality of ultrasound images is subject to a great deal of variability, because it is so operator dependent.

The lack of ionizing radiation or any known hazards associated with diagnostic ultrasound are clear-cut advantages of this technique over other radiographic methods, including CT. The use of contrast material is avoided, and patients experience no discomfort.

Ultrasound is the procedure of choice in the patient in anuric or oliguric renal failure in whom, in addition to renal size, reliable information regarding chronic ureteral obstruction can also be obtained. A further advantage of ultrasound is its independence of contrast material, the use of which may be nephrotoxic in patients with failed kidneys.

### Computed Tomography

Computed tomography accurately images the kidney in transverse sections (Fig. 20-6). the perirenal and renal sinus structures are sharply defined and easily distinguished from the renal parenchyma. By comparing precontrast scans with those obtained following intravenous contrast injection, assessment of the perfusion, function, and structural integrity of the kidney can be made. No standards for normal size based on CT data have yet been published.

Computed tomography has evolved into the "gold standard" for renal imaging, including the evaluation of renal masses, cystic diseases, perfusion abnormalities, and "medical" diseases. However, because of cost considerations as well as general availability, CT is rarely indicated as a primary modality in assessing abnormalities of renal size, although it is of great adjunctive value in further assessing abnormalities detected by other, simpler techniques. To display a frontal (coronal) or longitudinal CT image of the kidney requires time-consuming and expensive computer reconstruction of data derived from transverse sections. Without these projections, the measurement of renal height and width is impractical. Furthermore, reconstructed images lack spatial resolution.

### Magnetic Resonance Imaging

The use of magnetic resonance imaging in the practical evaluation of abnormal renal size has not yet been established. Potential applications include the assessment of renal vein patency in patients with suspected renal vein thrombosis and the further evaluation of renal masses and retroperitoneal involvement suggested by other imaging modalities.

## DIAGNOSTIC STRATEGIES

For the clinician who needs to know whether kidney size is abnormal, excretory urography and ultrasound are the diagnostic studies of choice. Ultrasound is preferred in patients with oliguric or anuric renal failure, because hydronephrosis can be accurately evaluated at the same time that renal size is measured. Exposure to contrast material and radiation is also avoided. In all other clinical situations, the additional functional information and better anatomic detail make excretory urography the initial procedure of choice.

Once an abnormality of renal size is estab-

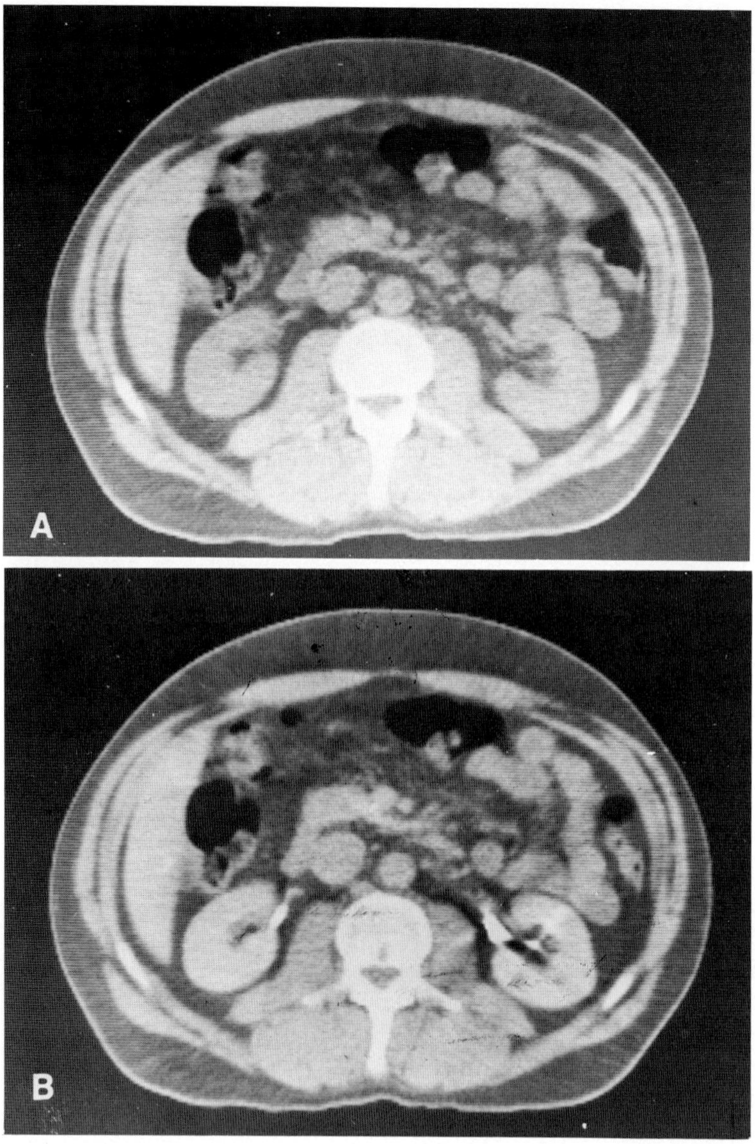

**Figure 20-6.** CT of the kidney prior to the introduction of contrast material **(A)** and after the use of contrast material **(B)** (Redman HC, Fisch AE: Advanced Exercises in Diagnostic Radiology. Philadelphia, WB Saunders, 1979)

lished, the specific cause must be identified as precisely as possible. One organizational approach to this problem considers renal abnormalities according to their effect on renal bulk (increased or decreased size), the distribution of a lesion within the kidney (focal, global, or regional), and whether the lesion inherently affects the total renal mass or is limited to one kidney (bilateral, unilateral). The following diagnostic sets detail this systematic approach.

Assignment of each entity to a given diagnostic set is based on arbitrary considerations such as (1) the most common form of presentation of each entity, (2) the stage at which the radiologist is most likely to encounter the abnormality in the average clinical setting, and (3) the elemental distribution of a specific lesion. The latter consideration acknowledges that some entities, in their simplest form, are focal (reflux nephropathy) or unilateral (renal vein throm-

**_Diagnostic Set: Small, Scarred, Unilateral_**

Reflux nephropathy
Lobar infarction

**_Diagnostic Set: Small, Smooth, Unilateral_**

Ischemia due to focal arterial disease
Chronic infarction
Radiation nephritis
Congenital hypoplasia
Postobstructive atrophy
Postinflammatory atrophy
Reflux atrophy

**_Diagnostic Set: Small, Smooth, Bilateral_**

Generalized arteriosclerosis
Benign and malignant nephrosclerosis
Atheroembolic renal disease
Chronic glomerulonephritis
Papillary necrosis
Hereditary nephropathies
- Hereditary chronic nephritis (Alport's syndrome)
- Medullary cystic disease

Amyloidosis (late)
Arterial hypotension

**_Diagnostic Set: Large, Smooth, Bilateral_**

Proliferative/necrotizing disorders
- Acute glomerulonephritides
- Polyarteritis nodosa (microscopic form)
- Systemic lupus erythematosus
- Wegener's granulomatosus
- Allergic angiitis
- Diabetic glomerulosclerosis
- Lung hemorrhage and glomerulonephritis (Goodpasture's syndrome)
- Anaphylactoid purpura (Schonlein–Henoch syndrome)
- Thrombotic thrombocytopenic purpura
- Focal glomerulonephritis associated with subacute bacterial endocarditis

Amyloidosis
Multiple myeloma
Acute tubular necrosis
Acute cortical necrosis
Leukemia
Acute interstitial nephritis
Acute urate nephropathy
Acromegaly
Physiologic response to contrast material and diuretics
Nephromegaly associated with cirrhosis, hyperalimentation, and diabetes mellitus
Hemophilia
Homozygous S disease
Fabry's disease

bosis) and that it is only a random, chance occurrence when they are more widespread (multiple scars of reflux nephropathy or bilateral renal vein thrombosis).

The correct diagnosis can sometimes be made from the radiologic study alone. Reflux nephropathy and lobar infarction have characteristic features on excretory urography; the ultrasonic pattern of hydronephrosis may be confused with only a few other conditions. In most circumstances, however, the imaging data must be integrated with information from the bedside, the clinical laboratory and, sometimes, microscopic study of biopsy material. Radiologic techniques other than excretory urography or ultrasound are sometimes required to evaluate patients with abnormalities of renal size. These include arteriography and radionuclide scanning

***Diagnostic Set: Large, Smooth, Unilateral***

Renal vein thrombosis
Acute arterial infarction
Obstructive uropathy
Acute bacterial nephritis
Compensatory hypertrophy
Duplicated pelvocalyceal system

***Diagnostic Set: Large, Multifocal, Bilateral***

Adult polycystic disease (Potter Type III)
Hodgkin's disease and malignant lymphoma

***Diagnostic Set: Large, Multifocal, Unilateral***

Xanthogranulomatous pyelonephritis
Multicystic (dysgenetic) kidney disease (Potter Type II)
Malakoplakia

***Diagnostic Set: Large, Unifocal, Unilateral***

- Solid masses
  - Malignant neoplasms
    - Adenocarcinoma
    - Adult nephroblastoma
    - Sarcoma
    - Metastatic deposits
    - Invasive transitional cell carcinoma
  - Benign neoplasms
    - Hamartoma
    - Adenoma
    - Mesenchymal tumor
  - Inflammatory mass
- Fluid-filled masses
  - Simple cyst
  - Focal hydronephrosis
  - Multilocular cystic nephroma
  - Arteriovenous malformation

in the investigation of renal arterial embolization or infarction, venography or CT in the assessment of renal vein thrombosis, and CT in patients with renal masses.

## Bibliography

Amis ES, Jr, Hartman DS: Renal ultrasonography 1984: A practical overview. Radiol Clin North Am 22:315, 1984

Davidson AJ: Radiology of the Kidney. Philadelphia, WB Saunders, 1985

Dunnick NR, Korobkin M: Computed tomography of the kidney. Radiol Clin North Am 22:297, 1984

Griffiths GJ, Cartwright G, McLachlan MSF: Estimation of renal size from radiographs: Is the effort worthwhile? Clin Radiol 26:249–256, 1975

Moell H: Kidney size and its deviation from normal in acute renal failure. A roentgendiagnostic study. Acta Radiol (Diagn) (Suppl) 206(56):5, 1961

Moell H: Size of normal kidneys. Acta Radiol (Diagn) 46:640–645, 1956

Newhouse JH, Markisz JA, Kazam Z: Magnetic resonance imaging of the kidney. Cardiovasc Intervent Radiol 8:351–366, 1986

Siegle RL, Lieberman P: A review of untoward reactions to iodinated contrast material. J Urol 119: 581–587, 1978

Van Zee BE, Hoy W, Talley TE et al: Renal injury associated with intravenous pyelography in nondiabetic and diabetic patients. Ann Itern Med 88: 51, 1978

Vuorinen P, Pyykonen L, Antilla P: A renal cortical index obtained from urography films. Br J Radiol 33:622–626, 1960

Walk H: The weight of normal adult human kidneys and its variability. Arch Pathol 213:493, 1937

## SUSPECTED ABNORMAL RENAL SIZE

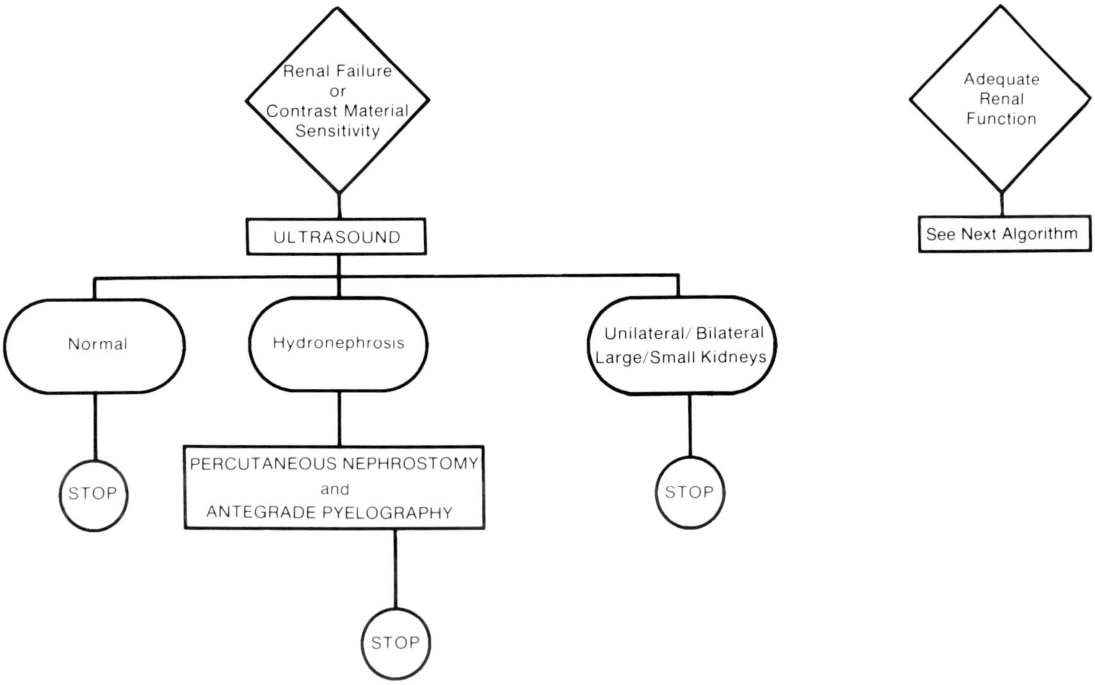


## SUSPECTED ABNORMAL RENAL SIZE

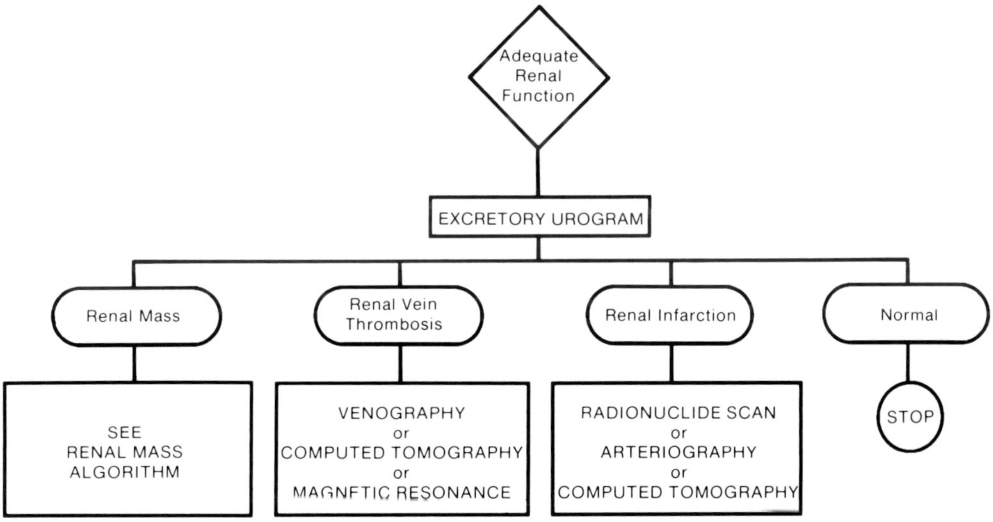

# Chapter 21

# Renal Masses

*Barbara E. Demas*
*Madeleine R. Fisher*

Renal masses may be detected by screening excretory urography or physical examination in the symptomatic patient, or they may be incidentally discovered by urography, ultrasound, or computed tomography (CT) in the patient being evaluated for unrelated abdominal pathology. Most renal masses are benign renal cysts. Of solid masses, however, malignant lesions (primary and metastatic) are more common than benign tumors. The aim of radiographic imaging is to separate cystic from solid lesions and to attempt to characterize and stage solid tumors. Although tissue sampling is required for the definitive diagnosis of many tumors, characteristic imaging appearances have been described for the most frequently encountered neoplasms.

## CLINICAL AND LABORATORY FINDINGS

The kidneys are relatively isolated organs that are surrounded by abundant pararenal fat and invested with dense perirenal fascia. For this reason, both benign and malignant neoplasms may grow to very large size before producing symptoms. Pain may be caused by a tumor stretching the renal capsule or invading adjacent structures, or by bleeding into the lesion. Hematuria frequently develops when tumor invades the pelvocalyceal system, but it may be microscopic and undetected by the patient. Almost a third of patients with renal cell carcinoma have metastatic disease at the time of diagnosis, and the symptoms may be related to the site of metastases.

The laboratory evaluation of patients with benign renal tumors is typically unrewarding. Patients with renal cell carcinoma may demonstrate elevated erythrocyte sedimentation rate (55%), hematuria (40%), anemia (36%), abnormal liver function (14%), and polycythemia (3%). Metastatic disease may produce hypercalcemia.

## DIAGNOSTIC EVALUATION

### *DIAGNOSTIC MODALITIES*

1. Excretory urography and nephrotomography
2. Ultrasound
3. Computed tomography
4. Magnetic resonance imaging
5. Arteriography

6. Renal venography and inferior vena cavography
7. Percutaneous biopsy

### Excretory Urography and Nephrotomography

Excretory urography remains the initial or screening examination in the radiographic evaluation of renal masses. The excretory urogram permits an assessment of the renal contours and the morphology of the collecting system; distortion of these structures by a mass is readily detected if the quality of the examination is optimal. Small intrarenal lesions, masses projecting anteriorly or posteriorly, and tumors that do not affect the pelvocalyceal structures may be difficult or impossible to visualize (Fig. 21-1). Thus, a normal excretory urogram in the patient with hematuria should not preclude further imaging evaluation.

Nephrotomography can improve the characterization of a renal parenchymal mass. The diagnosis of a simple renal cyst is suggested when tomograms reveal a rounded, low-density, thin-walled mass that is sharply delineated from the adjacent contrast-enhanced renal parenchyma. Sonographic confirmation is frequently required, especially if the suspected cyst is entirely intrarenal. The nephrotomographic detection of a renal mass of high or heterogeneous radiographic density that has poorly delineated margins, contains calcium, or distorts the collecting structures suggests a solid renal neoplasm. In this situation, CT is the logical choice for further diagnostic evaluation.

Nephrotomography can provide a detailed view of the morphology of the pelvocalyceal system. Discrete filling defects in the collecting system may be caused by calculi, benign or malignant urothelial neoplasms, inflammatory tissue or debris, sloughed papillae, or blood clots. Suspected radiolucent calculi may be further evaluated by ultrasound or CT. Renal calculi cause posterior shadowing on ultrasound; virtually all renal stones are of high attenuation on noncontrast CT scans (Fig. 21-2). If the diagnosis remains equivocal following ultrasound or CT, retrograde pyelography and cytologic sampling may be necessary to document whether a urothelial tumor is present.

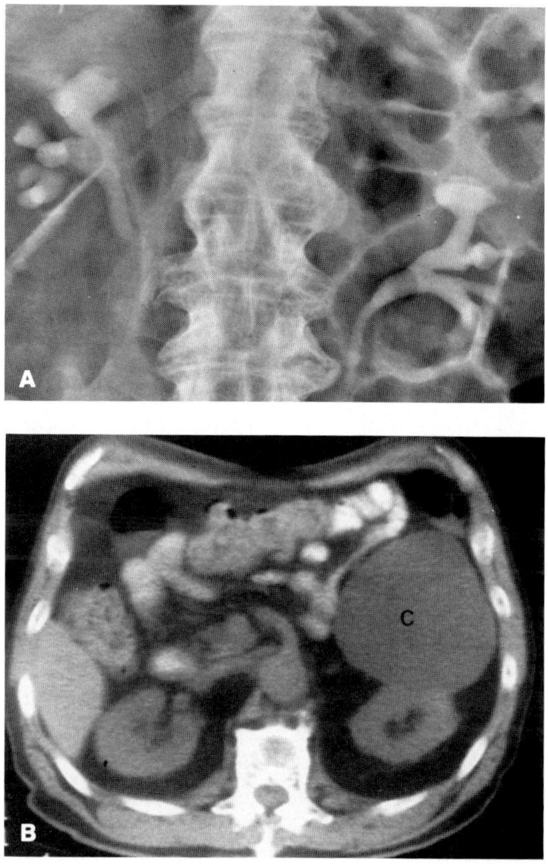


**Figure 21-1.** Renal cyst. **(A)** Excretory urogram demonstrates bilateral hydronephrosis but does not clearly define the renal contours nor show any sign of renal mass. **(B)** CT scan in the same patient shows a large cyst (*C*) arising from the anterior aspect of the left kidney.

Excretory urography is generally a safe procedure, with a mortality rate of approximately 1 in 50,000 examinations. There is a 1% to 2% incidence of morbidity (usually not severe), primarily urticaria, or nausea and vomiting.

### Ultrasound

The distinction of a purely cystic renal mass from a complex or solid lesion is most simply and reliably accomplished by ultrasound. Simple renal cysts appear as smooth-walled, echofree structures with good through sound transmission (Fig. 21-3). Because ultrasound has such a high accuracy in detecting and characterizing simple renal cysts, cyst puncture usually is not required for diagnostic purposes. Cyst puncture may be necessary if there is difficulty in visualizing the entire margin of a cyst or if a large cyst causes pain. Solid masses possess a variable degree of internal echogenicity and do not show posterior wall enhancement. However, because virtually identical sonographic appearances may be produced by hemorrhagic or infected cysts, solid benign and malignant neoplasms, and inflammatory masses, CT or even histologic evaluation may be required to distinguish among these possibilities. Ultrasound permits the noninvasive evaluation of the perirenal soft tissues, renal veins, inferior vena cava, and liver. Thus, ultrasound may be used to stage the abdominal extent of a renal malignancy, although it is less accurate than CT. Utrasound also provides assistance in performing percutaneous renal biopsies.

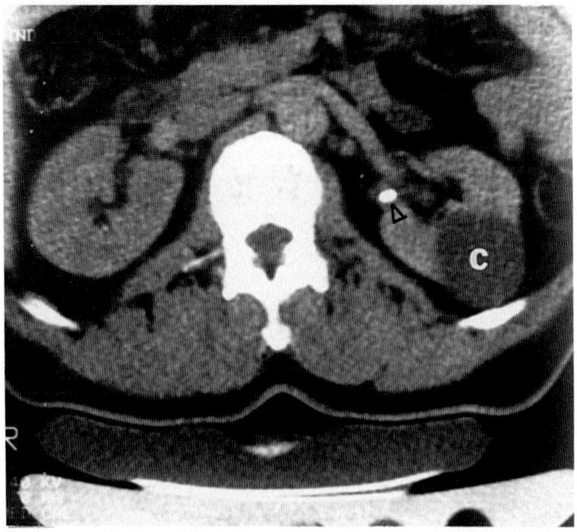

**Figure 21-2.** Renal calculus. CT scan of the kidneys performed without the use of intravenous contrast material shows a high-density calculus (*arrow*) in the left renal pelvis. A left renal cyst (*C*) is also present.

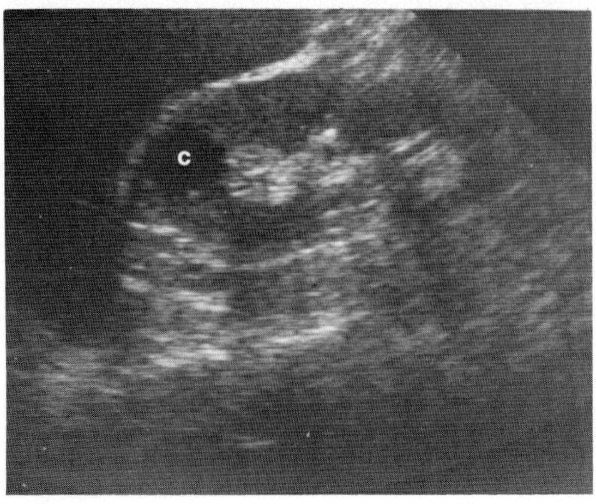

**Figure 21-3.** Renal cyst. Longitudinal sonogram shows a cyst (*C*) in the upper pole of the left kidney. The cyst is free of internal echoes, possesses a smooth posterior wall, and demonstrates good sound transmission into the tissues posterior to the cyst.

Because ultrasound is highly operator dependent, it requires expertise on the part of the technician or physician performing the examination. Images of diagnostic quality may be impossible to achieve in obese patients. Dilated air-filled loops of bowel in the upper abdomen may obscure the perirenal anatomy. However, ultrasound is convenient, cost effective, and completely without biologic risk, and its ability to separate cystic and solid lesions may obviate the need for more expensive and more invasive diagnostic imaging studies.

## Computed Tomography

Computed tomography has become the major imaging procedure for the detection, characterization, and staging of renal masses. Tailored CT examinations designed for evaluating the renal anatomy include the use of thinly collimated contiguous sections, the administration of iodinated contrast material by intravenous bolus injection, and the use of rapid-sequence scanning to allow imaging within the first 1 to 2 minutes following contrast injection (when renal parenchymal enhancement is maximum). Delayed scanning can evaluate the contrast-ladened pelvocalyceal structures. Nonenhanced scans are necessary only if there is suspicion of a calcified lesion (stone, tumor, chronic inflammatory mass).

A small renal mass that does not deform the renal contour may be evident on CT images, because its pattern of enhancement following administration of contrast material differs from that of surrounding normal parenchyma. Most renal tumors are of lower attenuation than normal renal parenchyma on both enhanced and nonenhanced images. Hypertrophied columns of Bertin and fetal renal lobulations, normal variants that may produce contour abnormalities on excretory urograms, enhance in a pattern identical to that of adjacent renal tissue and are not easily mistaken for masses on CT scans.

Renal cysts appear on CT images as nonenhancing masses of water attenuation that have clearly defined margins and thin, nearly indiscernible rims (Fig. 21-4). If all these criteria are met, the diagnosis of a renal cyst can be made with great certainty on the basis of the CT findings. Hemorrhagic or infected cysts may be of high or heterogeneous attenuation and may have irregular outlines or thick walls. Such lesions may be indistinguishable from solid neoplasms, and biopsy may be necessary for diagnosis.

Renal cell carcinomas are the most common solid renal tumors. On CT images, these tumors appear as masses of heterogeneous attenuation (Fig. 21-5). Rapid-sequence scanning immediately following the intravenous injection of a bolus of contrast material may reveal areas of dense enhancement within a predominantly low-attenuation mass. This appearance is caused by the abundant tumor vascularity often present in renal cell carcinomas. Computed tomography has an accuracy rate of greater than 90% for staging the anatomic extent of spread of a renal malignancy. It can clearly evaluate the tumor margins, detect tumor thrombi in the renal veins and the inferior vena cava, delineate retroperitoneal adenopathy, and demonstrate distant metastases.

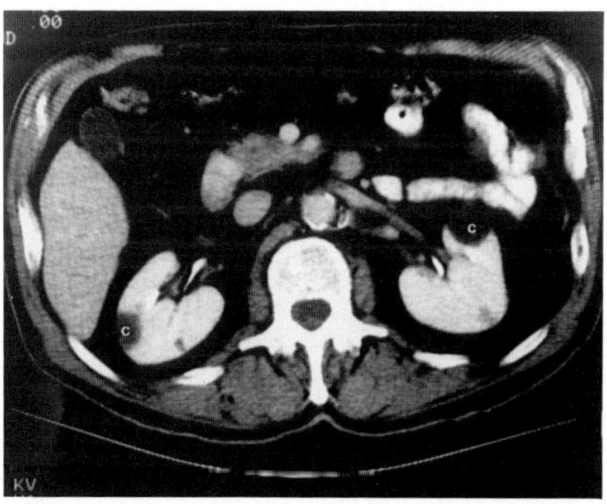

**Figure 21-4.** Multiple renal cysts. CT scan of the kidneys shows the multiple cysts (*C*) to have water-density attenuation, smooth contours, and thin rims. The cysts are not enhanced following the intravenous injection of contrast material.

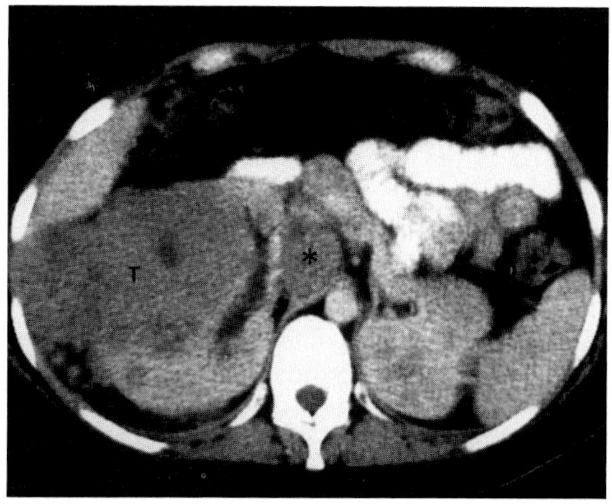

**Figure 21-5.** Renal cell carcinoma. CT scan of the kidneys shows the large tumor (*T*) arising from the right kidney. The mass has a heterogeneous density and an attenuation that is lower than that of the adjacent normal parenchyma. There is also retrocaval lymph node enlargement (*asterisk*).

Metastatic tumors and the majority of benign renal tumors present as masses of variable size and density that remain of lower attenuation than adjacent parenchyma on contrast-enhanced images. The hypervascular appearance associated with renal cell carcinomas is typically absent. The large amount of fat within an angiomyolipoma produces an appearance that is sufficiently characteristic to allow the confident CT diagnosis of this benign renal tumor.

## Magnetic Resonance Imaging

Magnetic resonance imaging (MRI) allows detailed demonstration of the renal anatomy and approaches the accuracy of CT in staging the abdominal extent of tumor in the patient with a previously diagnosed renal cell carcinoma. Advantages of MRI include its ability to clearly demonstrate any perivascular adenopathy or tumor thrombus within a vascular lumen without the need for intravenous contrast material (Fig. 21-6). The multiplanar imaging capability of this modality allows visual discrimination between adrenal tumors and upper pole renal masses and is of value in demonstrating tumor extension into adjacent organs. The spin-echo pulse sequences currently available cannot reliably distinguish hemorrhagic cysts or fatty tumors from solid malignant lesions; in such situations, correlation with CT or ultrasound may be required. The accuracy of MRI in detecting small renal tumors has not yet been established.

## Arteriography

In most medical centers, CT has replaced arteriography in the diagnosis and staging of renal masses. Arteriography is primarily performed to aid in surgical planning, especially in patients in whom parenchyma-sparing surgery is desired (*e.g.*, bilateral renal tumors, mass in a solitary kidney).

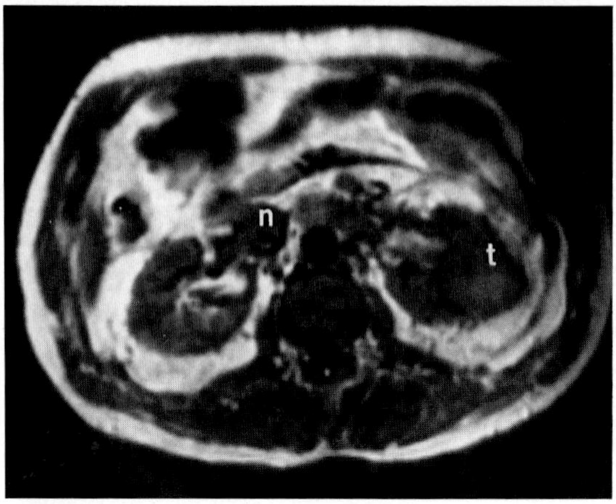


**Figure 21-6.** Renal cell carcinoma. Transverse MRI of the kidneys obtained using spin-echo technique (TR, 800 msec; TE, 25 msec) shows the left renal tumor (*t*) and associated tumor thrombus (*n*) in the inferior vena cava.

Arteriography is nonspecific, and a variety of benign and malignant processes may produce strikingly similar appearances. Although renal cell carcinomas are typically hypervascular, approximately 5% are avascular. Inflammatory masses and benign neoplasms with mild hypervascularity cannot be distinguished from relatively hypovascular renal cell carcinomas. High-dose arteriography may be of value in demonstrating the extension of tumor into the renal vein and inferior vena cava.

## Renal Venography and Inferior Venacavography

Renal venography and inferior vena cavography are most often performed in patients with diagnosed renal cell carcinoma and suspected intravascular tumor thrombi. Because tumor thrombi can usually be detected by ultrasound, CT, MRI, or high-dose arteriography, an additional venous study is not routinely indicated for preoperative tumor staging. Renal venography and inferior venacavography are required only if noninvasive studies produce equivocal results.

## Percutaneous Biopsy

Percutaneous biopsy of renal masses and percutaneous cyst puncture may be performed under ultrasound or CT guidance. Ultrasound guidance is generally preferred, because it provides flexibility in the choice of scanning plane and allows direct visualization of needle placement during real-time scanning. When performed by an experienced radiologist, the fine-needle aspiration technique is associated with an extremely low incidence of complications. Recovery of tissue that is adequate for cytologic evaluation can be accomplished in more than 90% of cases. While the diagnostic accuracy of this technique clearly depends on the skill of the cytologist, accuracy rates of more than 80% have been reported. Of course, percutaneous biopsy and cyst puncture should be performed only in those patients in whom the results are likely to obviate the need for surgical intervention.

## Bibliography


Bosniak MA: Angiomyolipoma (hamartoma) of the kidney: A preoperative diagnosis is possible in virtually every case. Urol Radiol 3:135–142, 1981

Chisholm GD: Nephrogenic ridge tumors and their syndromes. Ann NY Acad Sci 230:403–423, 1974

Elyaderani MR, Gabrielle OF: Ultrasound of renal masses. Semin Ultrasound 2:21–43, 1981

Engelstad B, McClennan BL, Levitt RG: The role of pre-contrast images in CT of the kidney. Radiology 136:153–155, 1980

Hricak H, Demas BE, Williams RD et al: Magnetic resonance imaging in the diagnosis and staging of renal and perirenal neoplasms. Radiology 154: 709–715, 1985

Juul J, Torp–Pedersen S, Gronvall S et al: Ultrasonically guided fine needle aspiration biopsy of renal masses. J Urol 133:579–581, 1985

Kass DA, Hricak H, Davidson AJ: Renal malignancies with normal excretory urograms. AJR 141:731–734, 1983

Lang EK: Angiocomputed tomography and dynamic computed tomography in staging of renal cell carcinoma. Radiology 151:149–155, 1984

Levine E, Maklad NF, Rosenthal SJ et al: Comparison of computed tomography and ultrasound in abdominal staging of renal cell carcinoma. Urology 16:317–322, 1980

Mauro MA, Wadsworth DE, Stanley RJ et al: Renal cell carcinoma: Angiography in the CT era. AJR 139:1135–1138, 1982

McClennan BL, Stanley RJ, Nelson GL et al: CT of the renal cyst: Is cyst aspiration necessary? AJR 133:671–678, 1979

## SUSPECTED RENAL MASS

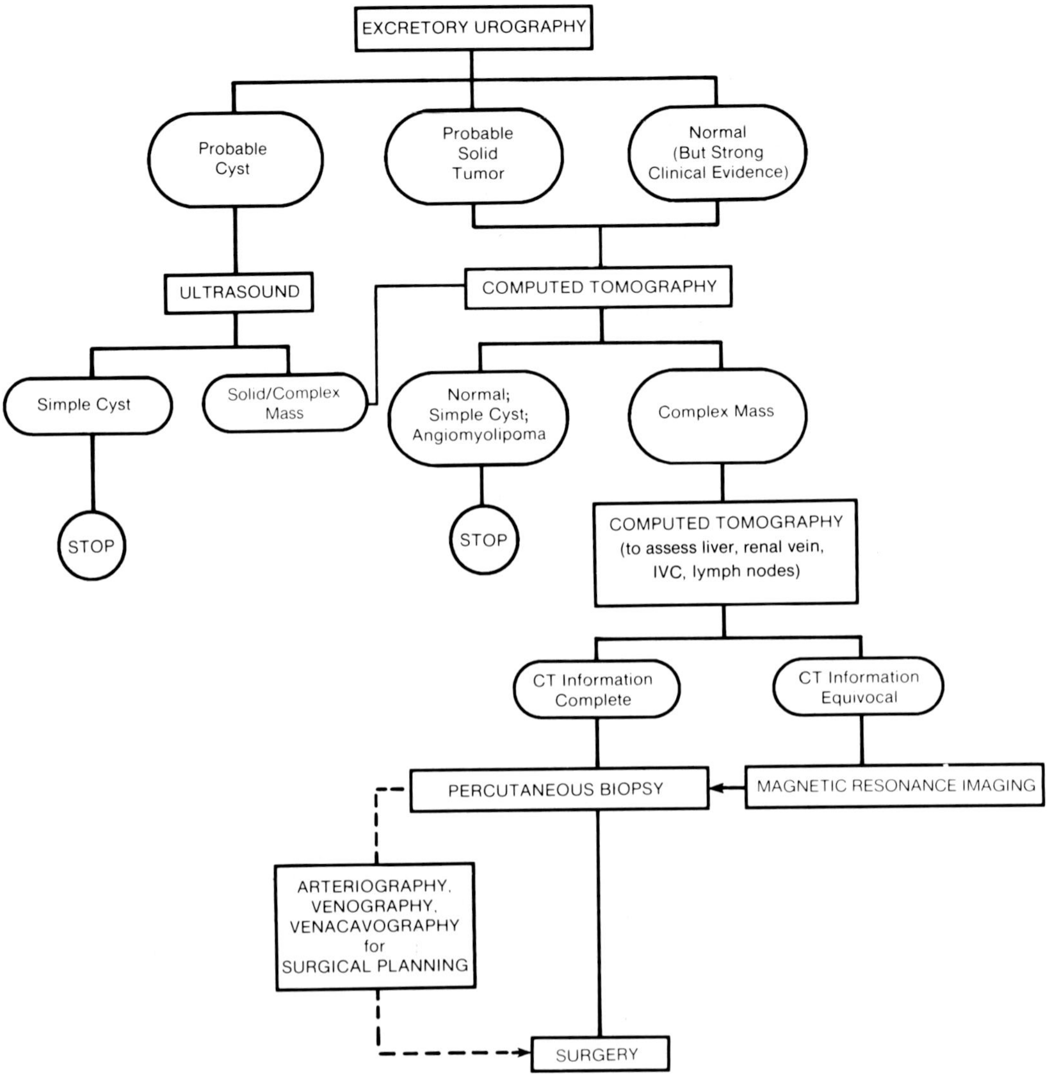

# Chapter 22

# Fever and Flank Pain: Suspected Infection of the Upper Urinary Tract in Adults

*Peter F. Hahn*
*Isabel C. Yoder*

Fever and flank pain are the most important clinical manifestations of a spectrum of serious infections of the upper urinary tract that vary in their implication and therapy. The underlying conditions include the following:

1. Acute pyelonephritis
2. Acute focal bacterial nephritis
3. Subacute multifocal bacterial nephritis
4. Renal abscess
5. Perinephric abscess
6. Pyonephrosis

The decision whether to image a patient with suspected upper urinary tract infection during the acute period is one of clinical judgment. Most patients have simple pyelonephritis that will respond promptly to antibiotic therapy. Indications for obtaining prompt imaging studies of a patient with acute upper urinary tract infection are (1) a sluggish response to appropriate intravenous antibiotics, (2) an immunocompromised patient or one who is difficult to assess clinically, (3) culture of an unusual organism (*e.g.*, anaerobic bacteria), and (4) a severely ill patient.

The use of radiographic imaging following an episode of urinary tract infection is controversial. Urinary tract infections are very common in young women; each year, approximately 6% of the adult female population seeks medical attention for urinary tract symptoms associated with significant bacteriuria. Several studies have demonstrated that the indiscriminate use of imaging procedures in this population detects no more abnormalities that alter therapy than would be expected in the population at large. Conversely, longitudinal studies over several decades suggest that young women hospitalized for severe urinary tract infection suffer a high degree of morbidity, often requiring intervention. Indications for elective imaging of the urinary tract after infection include the following:

1. Infection requiring hospitalization
2. Impaired renal function
3. Relapsing infection
4. Infection in a male

Patients with anatomic or physiologic abnormalities of the urinary tract (*e.g.*, renal calculus, papillary necrosis, neurogenic bladder) will have difficulty in completely clearing their infection. Relapse must be distinguished clinically from the much more common recurrence of simple urinary tract infection.

In elderly patients, the most common cause of bacteremia is pyelonephritis, which has an equal likelihood of developing regardless of whether there is urinary tract obstruction. Nevertheless, imaging is usually indicated, because urinary tract obstruction may have devastating implications in critically ill patients.

Special consideration must be given to the patient with chronic renal failure. As in other immunologically compromised patients, severe urinary tract infection may present in a cryptic fashion with malaise and failure to thrive, or with acute symptoms apparently unrelated to the urinary tract. Infection of an obstructed kidney can occur in these patients and may be the terminal event.

## DIAGNOSTIC EVALUATION

### *DIAGNOSTIC MODALITIES*

1. Excretory urography
2. Ultrasound
3. Radionuclide scanning
4. Angiography
5. Ileography (ileal loopogram)
6. Retrograde pyelography
7. Voiding cystourethrography
8. Computed tomography
9. Magnetic resonance imaging
10. Antegrade pyelography and percutaneous nephrostomy

### Excretory Urography

Excretory urography, usually with nephrotomography, provides an enormous amount of information about both the structure and function of the urinary tract (Fig. 22-1*A*). However, visualization of the kidneys is unlikely when the creatinine level is over 8 mg/100 ml. Relative contraindications include a history of severe contrast reaction and moderate renal failure (especially if associated with multiple myeloma, diabetes mellitus, or oliguria).

A normal excretory urogram in the patient with acute urinary tract infection excludes pyonephrosis and other severe renal infections. However, it does not eliminate the possibility of vesicoureteral reflux, which predisposes to repeated infection but is not believed to be a cause of ongoing renal damage in adults. Excretory urography also may fail to detect a perinephric inflammatory process, particularly if it is of hematogenous origin.

### Ultrasound

Ultrasound has assumed the pre-eminent role in the evaluation of the critically ill patient with suspected upper urinary tract infection. With good portable equipment, the examination can be performed at the bedside. This modality is extremely sensitive to even the slightest dilatation of the intrarenal collecting system. Overall renal size, shape, and echogenicity provide evidence of acute and chronic inflammatory or vascular processes and clues to the presence of renal anomalies. Renal stones, even poorly calcified ones, are usually detected as shadowing echogenic foci. Cysts, rare cystic tumors, and liquefied renal abscesses are readily demonstrated as hypo- or anechoic regions with enhanced through transmission, but these distinct conditions may not be separable on the basis of internal characteristics. Perinephric inflammatory

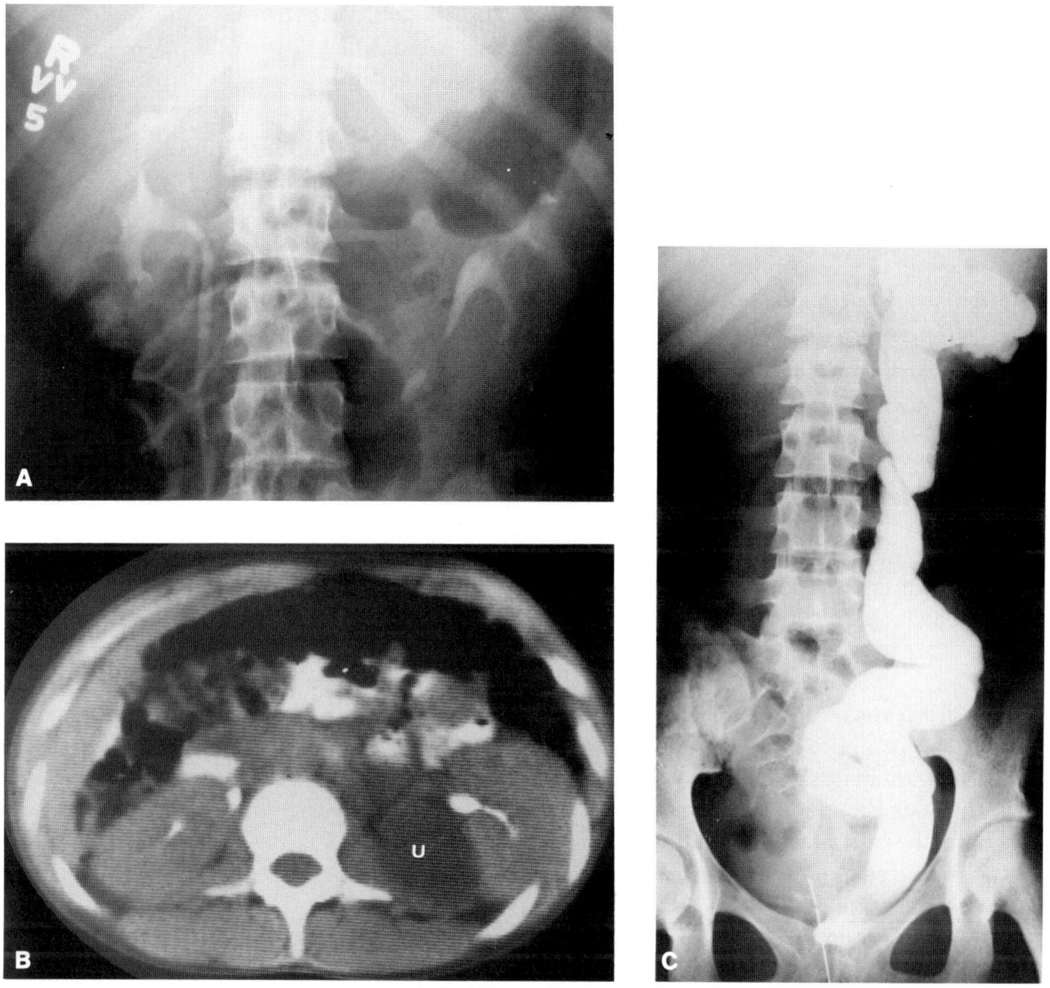


**Figure 22-1.** Duplex left kidney with infected and obstructed upper pole moiety. **(A)** Excretory urogram shows the "drooping lily" sign, with seeming rotation of the collecting system downward because the upper pole calyces are not opacified. **(B)** Contrast-enhanced CT scan shows the pyonephrotic, unopacified upper pole collecting system (*U*) medial to the lower pole moiety. **(C)** Antegrade pyelogram shows severe ectasia of the upper pole collecting system and of the ectopically inserting ureter. The antegrade needle has been removed.

processes can be difficult to detect using ultrasound unless there is liquefaction.

## Radionuclide Scanning

Radionuclide scanning performed with $^{99m}$Tc diethyltriaminepentaacetic acid ($^{99m}$Tc-DTPA) can provide a gross assessment of the morphologic structure of the upper urinary tract. However, the spatial resolution of this modality is so limited that hydronephrosis may be difficult to distinguish from a large extrarenal collecting system. The major value of radionuclide scanning of the urinary tract is that it provides a quantitative assessment of the blood flow and function of each kidney individually, information that can be particularly useful in deciding whether to salvage a severely diseased kidney.

### Angiography

Angiography is usually performed to evaluate a renal mass and occasionally may detect an underlying inflammatory condition, especially xanthogranulomatous pyelonephritis. However, angiography generally is not indicated for the evaluation of a suspected upper urinary tract infection.

### Ileography (Ileal Loopogram)

Ileography is extremely valuable for assessing patients with ileal loop diversions following cystectomy. Unlike colon conduits, which are used almost exclusively in children, ileal conduits normally demonstrate reflux. Because the intrarenal collecting systems may be chronically dilated, ultrasound is less reliable in this population. Contrast material instilled in a retrograde fashion at low pressure into the ileal loop should quickly fill both ureters (if present) and the intrarenal collecting systems of both kidneys. Failure to demonstrate both collecting systems in a patient with an ileal loop and a suspected upper urinary tract infection requires that a procedure be performed (usually percutaneous needle aspiration) to sample urine above the obstruction.

### Voiding Cystourethrography

Voiding cystourethrography and the corresponding radionuclide study are major imaging modalities for evaluating the pediatric patient with urinary tract infection. These procedures are required to exclude and grade vesicoureteral reflux, which is a widespread and dangerous condition in this population. Although reflux may continue into adulthood and predispose to recurrent infections, it does not appear to cause progressive renal damage after childhood. Voiding cystourethrography is the principal modality for detecting urethral abnormalities that may lead to recurrent infection, particularly in males.

### Computed Tomography

Computed tomography (CT) is usually reserved for patients with upper urinary tract infection who are seriously ill or in whom significant pathology is suspected. Contrast-enhanced CT is an excellent technique for detecting and characterizing renal masses and for distinguishing an organizing abscess from inflammatory edema. Computed tomography has revolutionized the evaluation of the perinephric spaces. At times, CT guidance may be necessary to plan an interventional procedure to avoid injury to the bowel or other sensitive structures. Computed tomography is not particularly sensitive to changes in the intrarenal collecting system (*e.g.*, calyceal deformity or mild hydronephrosis).

### Magnetic Resonance Imaging

Magnetic resonance imaging (MRI) has been used to detect and to characterize retroperitoneal masses. Fluid-containing processes in the retroperitoneum are readily visualized, because water is distinctively bright on T2-weighted images (Fig. 22-2). However, abscesses cannot be distinguished from necrotic tumors. Better specificity has been demonstrated in the case of hematomas, which are distinguished by the short T1 (paramagnetic) effect of hemoglobin degradation products. These masses display a bright signal on T1-weighted images, often in a peripheral ring. Hydronephrosis appears on T1-weighted images as a branching region of low signal that appears bright on T2-weighted images. Increased signal arising from the collecting system on T1-weighted images should raise the suspicion of blood or pus (diamagnetic T1 shortening).

### Antegrade Pyelography and Percutaneous Nephrostomy

Antegrade pyelography provides the fastest and most accurate method of diagnosis in the patient suspected of having an infection of an obstructed kidney. The puncture may follow either nephrotomographic or ultrasound demonstration of

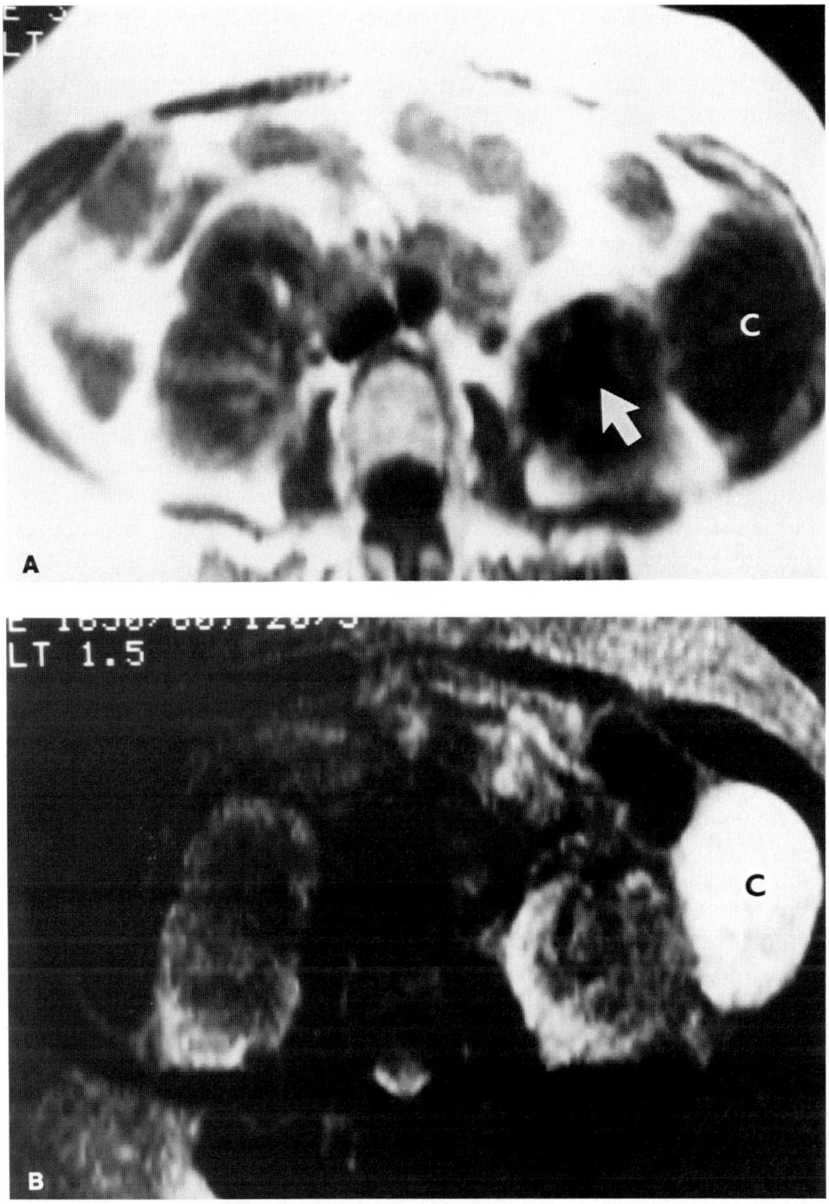


**Figure 22-2.** Perinephric abscess. **(A)** Transverse T1-weighted spin-echo image (TR, 310 msec; TE, 20 msec) shows uniform low signal from a collection (*C*) lateral to the left kidney. A dilated calyx (*arrow*) is visible in the lower pole of the kidney. **(B)** On a T2-weighted image (TR, 1650 msec; TE, 120 msec), the abscess is distinctively bright relative to adjacent structures.

hydronephrosis. Prophylactic antibiotic therapy is suggested in potentially infected patients to minimize the possibility of gram-negative septicemia developing during the interventional procedure.

An antegrade pyelogram is begun by introducing a 22-gauge needle into the kidney via a posterior approach. The aspiration of cloudy or purulent urine confirms the presence of pyonephrosis. Fluid samples are sent for Gram stain, culture, and cytologic examination as required. If the purulent urine is not too thick, the pressure within the collecting system can be measured with a water manometer. Intrarenal pressure is normally below 14 cm of $H_2O$; pressures in an obstructed system range from 14 cm to nearly 50 cm of $H_2O$. Paradoxically, higher pressures predict a better response to decompression. A kidney unable to mount a high pressure in the face of obstruction is "giving up."

Iodinated contrast material is then introduced into the collecting system to demonstrate the degree of calyceal dilatation, the presence of papillary necrosis or filling defects, the level and etiology of the obstruction, and the optimal site for placement of the percutaneous nephrostomy tube (See Fig. 22-1*B*). It is essential that the volume of contrast material introduced always be less than the amount of urine removed from the kidney, so as to avoid pyelorenal backflow or perinephric extravasation of infected urine. If sufficient contrast material cannot be introduced to permit a diagnostic study , a nephrostogram can be obtained later, following placement of the nephrostomy tube and clearing of the infection.

Once purulent urine is detected by fine-needle aspiration, a percutaneous nephrostomy tube should be inserted. This can be achieved by either the Seldinger method or the trocar–cannula technique, in which a long length of pliable 8- to 12-French Silastic catheter is directly inserted into the renal collecting system. In most cases, an 8-French nephrostomy catheter has a large enough lumen to drain thick pus, and the flow of urine helps to keep the tube open. At times, flushing is required to eliminate blood clots.

Patients treated with antibiotics and catheter drainage of infected urine experience prompt relief of symptoms and usually become afebrile within 24 hours. The placement of a nephrostomy catheter also has other diagnostic and therapeutic uses. It can evaluate residual kidney function and, by measuring the creatinine clearance of the affected kidney, can aid in deciding whether to preserve the kidney or to perform a nephrectomy. The nephrostomy catheter can also be used to obtain diagnostic nephrostograms, to perform ureteral perfusion, and for the therapeutic dissolution of stones and long-term drainage of the kidneys. Any concomitant perinephric abscess can be drained at the time of percutaneous nephrostomy.

Major complications (infection, hemorrhage, urine leak, pneumothorax) occur in 4% of all percutaneous nephrostomies. Minor complications, which occur in 15% of procedures, include hematuria, catheter misplacement or dislodgement, and small hematomas. The percutaneous drainage of pyonephrosis is associated with a higher complication rate. Major complications (septic and hemorrhagic shock) occur in 9% of procedures, while minor complications (marked temperature elevation, shaking chills, and transient decrease in blood pressure) occur in 19% of cases.

A severe bleeding diathesis is the only contraindication to percutaneous nephrostomy. Close consultation with a urologist is indispensable, because any significant complications related to the nephrostomy may require an urgent operation. In addition, a large number of patients eventually require surgery to correct obstruction of the urinary tract.

## IMAGING APPROACH TO SPECIFIC INFECTIOUS PROCESSES

### Acute Pyelonephritis

Acute pyelonephritis is the most common infection of the upper urinary tract. Bacteria usually ascend from the lower urinary tract to invade the renal interstitium, resulting in edema, hyperemia, and leukocytic infiltration. Classically, the patient presents with fever and flank pain, and urinalysis reveals pyuria and bacteriuria. The infection usually responds rapidly to antibiotics directed against the organism cultured from the urine, and in otherwise healthy individuals imaging usually can be withheld pending the results of therapy. Three fourths of patients with acute pyelonephritis have normal excretory urograms and sonograms. The remainder show renal enlargement, diminished nephrogram, delayed pyelogram, or collecting system abnormalities such as calyceal compression or attenuation. Acute pyelonephritis does not cause permanent urographic abnormalities.

In at least one third of cases, pyelonephritis presents as a simple urinary tract infection without symptoms or signs directing attention to the kidney. Imaging studies are not helpful in this situation and should not be used for screening purposes. In practice, failure of single-dose antibiotic therapy is taken as evidence of occult upper tract disease and is treated for longer periods—up to 6 weeks. Failure of this extended therapy is associated with anatomic abnormalities and is an indication for urography.

### Acute Focal Bacterial Nephritis

Acute bacterial nephritis (focal pyelonephritis, acute lobar nephronia) is a more severe form of renal interstitial infection than acute pyelonephritis and usually is associated with a positive blood culture. Imaging is indicated in the acute period to exclude urinary obstruction. Excretory urography demonstrates a renal mass simulating a renal abscess or neoplasm. Ultrasound shows a poorly marginated hypoechoic swelling, although there is no drainable pus. Nonenhanced CT fails to demonstrate an area of liquefaction; following the administration of intravenous contrast material, there is a wedge-shaped zone of reduced parenchymal enhancement.

### Subacute Multifocal Bacterial Nephritis

Subacute multifocal bacterial nephritis is a more severe and diffuse form of renal interstitial infection in which the entire kidney is involved by a leukocytic infiltrate. Diabetes is a predisposing condition in half the patients, who frequently are septic. Excretory urography demonstrates the more global abnormality of the involved kidney, which is enlarged and excretes poorly. Contrast-enhanced CT shows multiple wedge-shaped defects in the nephrogram (Fig. 22-3). On ultrasound, multiple ill-defined hypoechoic areas occur within the renal parenchyma. Following medical therapy with intravenous antibiotics and supportive measures, follow-up urography shows a permanent decrease in renal size and often calyceal deformity.

### Renal Abscess

A renal abscess forms from the coalescence of multiple small suppurative foci. Unless therapy is instituted, a fibrous capsule soon forms around the necrotic center. The onset may be insidious, with systemic symptoms predominating, or the patient may be quite sick with pus under pressure. Pyuria is absent in 20% of cases, because the abscess does not communicate with the urinary collecting system. Because excretory urography may or may not demonstrate a mass, the urographic differential diagnosis may include both a necrotic tumor and bacterial nephritis. Ultrasound can identify a hypoechoic zone of liquefaction, although tumor necrosis and occasionally even healing focal nephritis can produce a similar appearance. Contrast-enhanced CT of

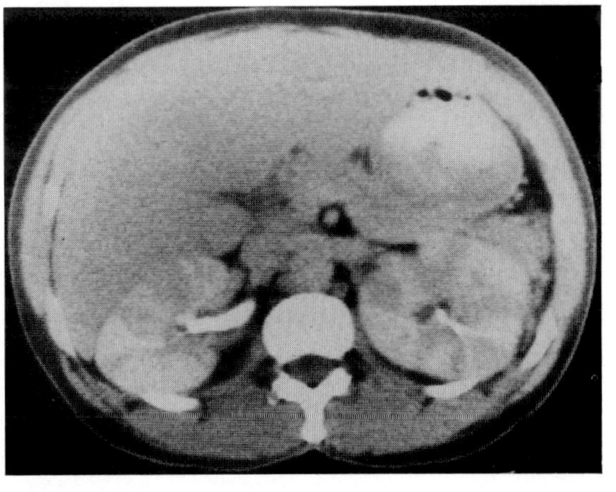

**Figure 22-3.** Subacute multifocal bacterial nephritis. Contrast-enhanced CT scan demonstrates characteristic wedge-shaped nephrographic defects bilaterally.

a well-established renal abscess demonstrates the central low density of liquefaction with the peripheral enhancement pattern of a capsule (which is hypervascular at angiography). Small abscesses can sometimes be managed conservatively with intravenous antibiotics. If a clinical response to antibiotics is delayed, percutaneous fine-needle aspiration can help to confirm the diagnosis and provide material for culture. Most abscesses require either percutaneous or surgical drainage.

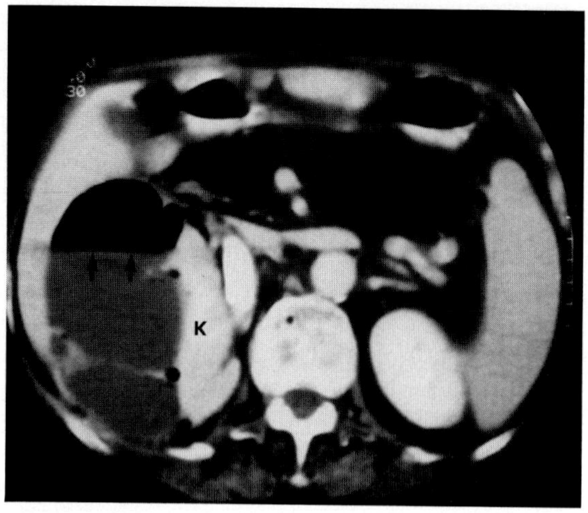


**Figure 22-4.** Perinephric abscess containing gas. Contrast-enhanced CT scan shows a complex collection compressing the right kidney (*K*) medially. The air–fluid level is clearly demonstrated (*arrows*).

## Perinephric Abscess

A perinephric abscess usually results from extrarenal rupture of an intrarenal infection and is often associated with pyonephrosis or diabetes mellitus. Hematogenous spread is implicated in one third of cases, usually by gram-positive organisms from a cutaneous infection or intravenous drug abuse. A patient with a perinephric abscess is usually toxic. However, the source may be difficult to localize, because the pain is often abdominal or referred to the lower extremity by involvement of the psoas muscle.

Although plain abdominal radiographs may show gas within a perinephric abscess and nephrotomography may demonstrate a soft-tissue mass, excretory urography is unreliable in detecting perinephric collections. The ultrasound appearance is nonspecific because of the variable manifestations of perinephric inflammatory processes. CT is the imaging modality of choice in the evaluation of the retroperitoneum. The extent of the inflammatory process and the presence of fluid collections are readily demonstrated (Fig. 22-4). If necessary, enhancement of the renal parenchyma with intravenous contrast material permits the kidney to be distinguished from the perinephric process. A combined approach to treatment (with antibiotics and drainage) is usually necessary.

## Pyonephrosis

Pyonephrosis refers to the presence of pus in a dilated (hydronephrotic) urinary collecting system. Patients with pyonephrosis typically present with fever, chills, and flank pain and are often seriously ill. However, cryptic presentations also occur, and in one series 15% of patients were afebrile. The role of the radiologist is critical both for diagnosis and treatment, because relief of the obstruction and appropriate antibiotic treatment of the infection can produce an excellent response.

Excretory urography in pyonephrosis usually shows obstruction, with a dense nephrogram and delayed excretion of contrast material into a dilated collecting system. At times, the affected kidney does not function. Urography also permits assessment of the function of the contralateral kidney. However, urography cannot distinguish pyonephrosis from uninfected hydronephrosis.

Pyonephrosis is excluded by a normal ultrasound examination, which can be performed at the bedside of a critically ill patient. In pyonephrosis, sonography typically shows the dilated intrarenal collecting system. At times, a large staghorn calculus obscures the dilated collecting system; in such cases, an additional study is required to exclude urinary obstruction. Ultrasound is diagnostic of pyonephrosis when a fluid-level or low-level echoes are detected in the dilated collecting system (Fig. 22-5). However, absence of these specific findings does not ex-

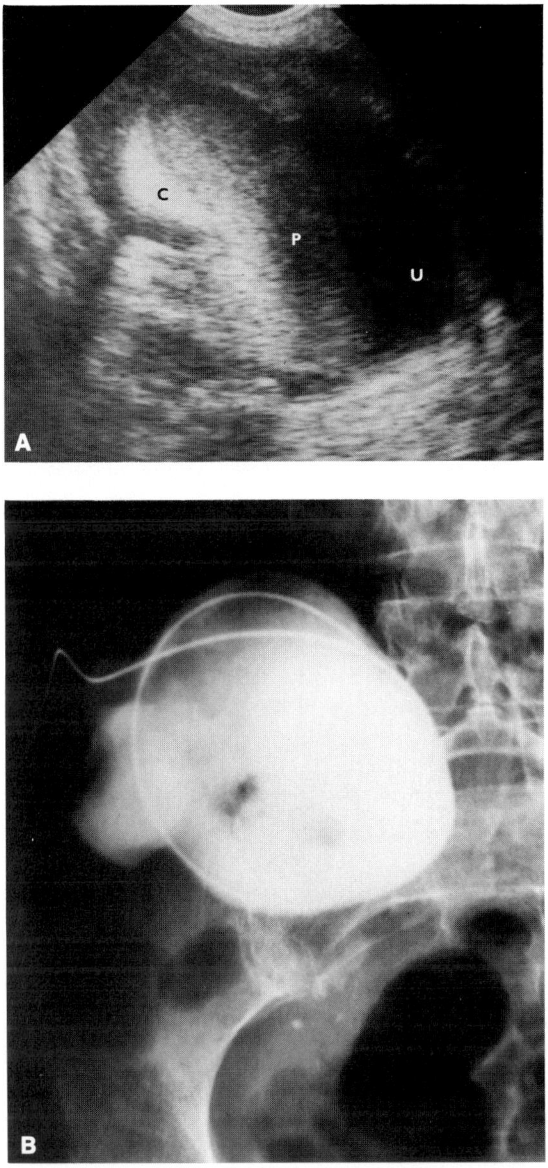


**Figure 22-5.** Pyonephrosis. **(A)** Sonogram reveals a dilated collecting system containing fluid in three layers. The dependent layer consists of uric acid crystals (*C*). The middle layer is pus (*P*), while the supernatant layer is relatively clear urine (*U*). **(B)** After confirmation of the diagnosis by fine-needle aspiration, a percutaneous nephrostomy was performed. The diagnostic nephrostogram shows the massively dilated collecting system secondary to ureteropelvic junction obstruction.

clude pyonephrosis; diagnostic aspiration of a hydronephrotic collecting system is necessary when infection is suspected.

## Bibliography

Coleman BG, Arger PH, Mulhern CB, Jr et al: Pyonephrosis: Sonography in the diagnosis and management. AJR 137:939–943, 1981

Corriere JN, Sandler CM: The diagnosis and immediate therapy of acute renal and perirenal infections. Urol Clin North Am 9:219–228, 1982

Cronan JJ, Amis ES, Dorfman GS: Percutaneous drainage of renal abscesses. AJR 142:351–354, 1984

Cronan JJ, Amis ES, Scola FH, Schepps B: Renal obstruction in patients with ileal loops: US evaluation. Radiology 158:647–648, 1986

DeLange EE, Jones B: Unnecessary intravenous urography in young women with recurrent urinary tract infections. Clin Radiol 34:551–553, 1983

Fairchild TN, Shuman W, Berger RE: Radiologic studies for women with recurrent urinary tract infections. J Urol 128:344–345, 1982

Finn DJ, Palestrant AM, DeWolf WC: Successful percutaneous management of renal abscess. J Urol 127:425–426, 1982

Gerzof SG: Percutaneous drainage of renal and perinephric abscess. Urol Radiol 2:171–179, 1981

Gerzof SG, Gale ME: Computed tomography and ultrasonography for diagnosis and treatment of renal and retroperitoneal abscess. Urol Clin North Am 9:185–193, 1982

Gold RP, McClennan BL, Rottenberg RR: CT appearance of acute inflammatory disease of the renal interstitium. AJR 141:343–349, 1983

Hoddick W, Jeffrey RB, Goldberg HI et al: CT and sonography of severe renal and perirenal infections. AJR 140:517–520, 1983

Hoverman IV, Gentry LO, Jones DW, Guerriero WG: Intrarenal abscess Report of 14 cases. Arch Intern Med 140:914–916, 1980

Jeffrey RB, Laing FC, Wing VW, Hoddick W: Sensitivity of sonography in pyonephrosis: A reevaluation. AJR 144:71–73, 1985

Kuligowska E, Newman B, White SJ, Caldarone A: Interventional ultrasound in detection and treatment of renal inflammatory disease. Radiology 147:521–526, 1983

Kunin CM: Does kidney infection cause renal failure? Ann Rev Med 36:165–176, 1985

Morehouse HT, Weiner SN, Hoffman JC: Imaging in inflammatory disease of the kidney. AJR 143:135–141, 1984

Morehouse HT, Weiner SN, Hoffman–Tretin JC: Inflammatory disease of the kidney. Semin Ultrasound, CT, and MR 7:246–258, 1986

Morgan WR, Nyberg LM: Perinephric and intrarenal abscesses. Urology 26:529–536, 1985

Newhouse JH, Rhea JT, Murphy RX, Pfister RC: Yield of screening urography in young women with urinary tract infections. Urol Radiol 4:187–190, 1982

Papanicolaou N, Hahn PF, Edelman RR et al: Magnetic resonance imaging of the kidney. Urol Radiol 8:139–150, 1986

Rubin RH, Tolkoff–Rubin NE, Cotran RS: Urinary tract infection, pyelonephritis, and reflux nephropathy. In Brenner BM, Rector FC, Jr (eds): The Kidney, 3rd ed, pp 1085–1141. Philadelphia, WB Saunders, 1986

Subramanyam BR, Raghavendra BN, Bosniak MA et al: Sonography of pyonephrosis: A prospective study. AJR 140:991–993, 1983

Yoder IC, Pfister RC, Lindfors KK, Newhouse JH: Pyonephrosis: Imaging and intervention. AJR 141:735–740, 1983

Yoder IC, Lindfors KK, Pfister RC: Diagnosis and treatment of pyonephrosis. Radiol Clin North Am 22:407–414, 1984

Zaontz MR, Pahira JJ, Wolfman M et al: Acute focal bacterial nephritis: A systematic approach to diagnosis and treatment. J Urol 133:752–757, 1984

# FEVER AND FLANK PAIN

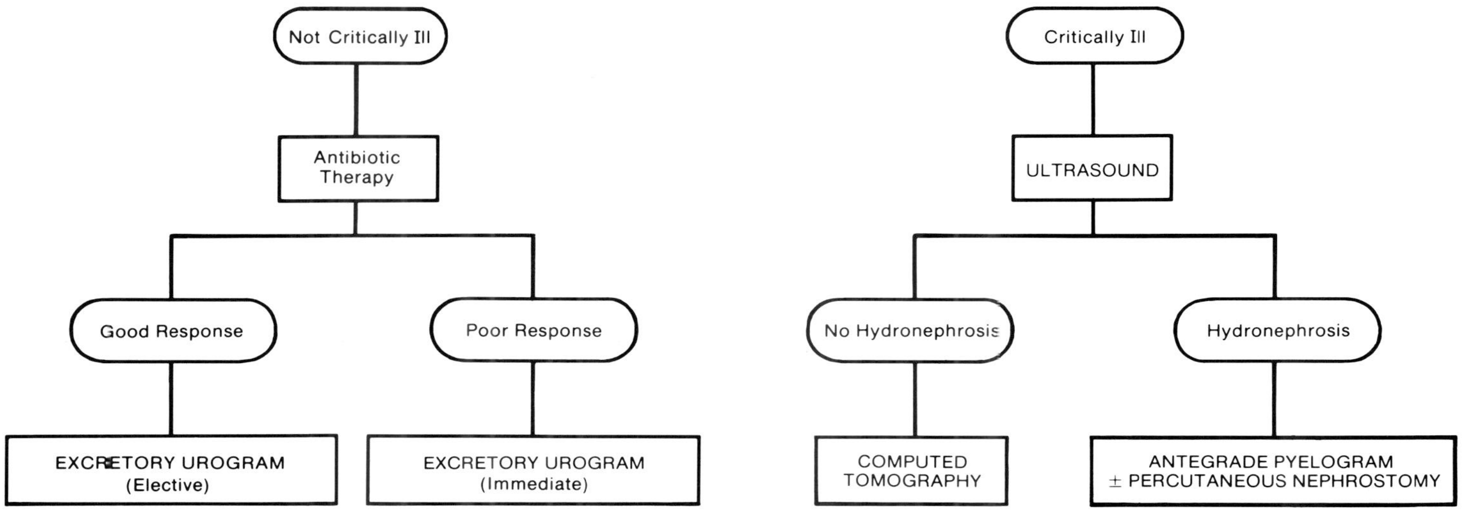

# Chapter 23

# Urinary Tract Infection in Children

*John C. Leonidas*

## CLINICAL CONSIDERATIONS

Urinary tract infection (UTI) is common in infants and children, second in frequency only to infections of the respiratory tract. Although there are differences among various populations and racial groups, 5% to 10% of girls of Northern European origin develop UTI during their school years, and 1% to 2% are found to have asymptomatic bacteriuria. A major contributing factor in the development of UTI is urinary stasis; since an obstructed system will eventually become infected, early detection and prompt treatment of urinary tract obstruction may eliminate recurrent UTI. Thus, an essential part of the diagnostic investigation of the child with UTI is to detect underlying anatomic abnormalities, which may be either structural (ureteropelvic junction obstruction; posterior urethral valves) or functional (neurogenic bladder; detrusor–sphincter incoordination). However, with the exception of young infants and boys, most patients with UTI have no detectable evidence of urinary stasis. Recent studies have suggested that functional urinary stasis may be related to the presence of certain fimbriated bacteria that adhere to the uroepithelium and produce an endotoxin-mediated ureteral aperistalsis.

Vesicoureteral reflux (VUR) has long been considered a major factor in the development of upper urinary tract infections, renal scarring, and progressive loss of renal function. Up to 40% of children with asymptomatic bacteriuria or UTI have VUR. As many as 25% of these children may have renal scarring at the time of their first diagnostic evaluation, and 90% of these scarred kidneys are drained by refluxing ureters. To emphasize the important role of reflux, the clinical complex of UTI, VUR, and chronic atrophic pyelonephritis has been termed "reflux nephropathy."

Although any investigation of childhood UTI should include a search for VUR, it should be emphasized that not all patients with reflux are at risk for developing reflux nephropathy. Reflux nephropathy may be responsible for up to 40% of all patients with end-stage renal disease, but the individual chance for progression from reflux nephropathy to renal failure is estimated to be only about 1:1000. The effect of VUR is highly dependent on its severity (Table 23-1;

**Table 23-1** Grades of Vesicoureteral Reflux (International Classification, 1981)

| | |
|---|---|
| Grade 1 | Reflux into ureter only |
| Grade 2 | Reflux into ureter, pelvis, and calyces. No dilatation; normal calyceal fornices |
| Grade 3 | Reflux as in Grade 2, but with mild or moderate dilatation and/or tortuosity of the ureter; mild or moderate dilatation of the renal pelvis but no (or slight) blunting of the fornices |
| Grade 4 | Reflux as in Grade 2, but with moderate dilatation and tortuosity of the ureter and complete obliteration of the sharp angles of the fornices; maintenance of papillary impressions in the majority of calyces |
| Grade 5 | Reflux as in Grade 2, but with gross dilatation and tortuosity of the ureter; gross dilatation of the renal pelvis and calyces without preservation of the papillary impressions. |

Fig. 23-1); VUR does not directly predispose to infection unless a substantial volume of refluxing urine creates a condition similar to that of urinary stasis. The major cause of VUR is failure of the ureterovesical junction to properly develop so that an adequate length of intramural ureter may act as a flap valve (Fig. 23-2). Unless severe and associated with high grades of VUR, this condition tends to improve and even return to normal with age, so that in most cases VUR ceases spontaneously. Infection per se causing VUR is uncommon, although this situation may occur in a patient with a marginally competent ureterovesical junction.

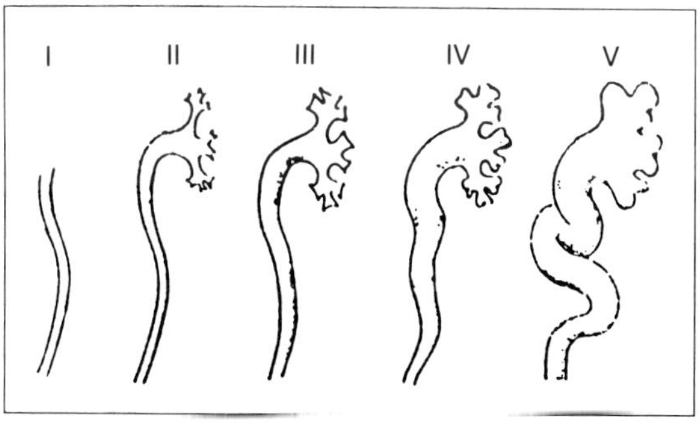


**Figure 23-1.** Grades of vesicoureteral reflux (International classification). (International Reflux Study Committee: Medical versus surgical treatment of primary vesicoureteral reflux. Pediatrics 67:392–400, 1981)

In general, patients with UTI but no VUR are at no risk for renal damage. Patients who have incidental VUR without infection may be at some risk for developing reflux nephropathy if they are young and the reflux is massive. Children with combined UTI and VUR but with normal kidneys are at low risk for developing renal scarring if they are already older than 4 years. Intrarenal reflux, a form of pyelotubular backflow affecting the renal papillae of infants and young children and believed to be responsible for allowing infected urine to reach the renal parenchyma, normally ceases at approximately 4 years of age. Nevertheless, it is prudent to prevent recurrent infections in these patients until VUR disappears. The presence of UTI and VUR in a young infant represents a definite risk for the development of renal scars. If evidence of renal scarring is already present, a patient with VUR and UTI is at high risk for progressive renal damage regardless of age.

## DIAGNOSTIC EVALUATION

### *DIAGNOSTIC MODALITIES*

1. Voiding cystourethrography
2. Excretory urography
3. Ultrasound
4. Radionuclide cystography
5. Renal scintigraphy
6. Computed tomography/magnetic resonance imaging

### Voiding Cystourethrography

Voiding cystourethrography is essential for obtaining good anatomic and, to a degree, functional information about the lower urinary tract of a child with UTI. In the direct method of voiding cystourethrography, the bladder is filled by gravity with relatively dilute contrast material after aseptic catheterization. Both the filling of the bladder and the subsequent voiding are monitored fluoroscopically with intermittent, brief periods of observation, and radiographs are exposed as needed. The degree of any observed reflux is then graded (see Table 23-1; Fig. 23-1). The accuracy and reproducibility of VUR and its grading is not precisely known, nor is it clear how pertinent this information is in the overall management of the child with UTI. For example, VUR may be elusive and detected in one examination but not in a subsequent study performed soon afterward.

The indirect method of voiding cystourethrography is actually part of an excretory urogram and refers to a technique in which the bladder is filled by renal excretion of contrast material injected intravenously. Although this indirect method has the greatest advantage of requiring no catheterization of the bladder, it offers no reliable information about the presence of VUR and therefore is rarely used today. Gross VUR may be suspected with this procedure, although continuous opacification of the ureters from injected contrast material precludes the detection of lesser grades of reflux. In addition, dilution of contrast material in the bladder degrades the degree of visualization of the urethra. The indirect method of voiding cystourethrography occasionally may be used selectively in cooperative children (who may be relied on to be positioned and void on command at the end of an excretory urogram) if there is a contraindication to catheterization of the bladder and if the physician is not interested in detecting a small degree of reflux.

## Excretory Urography

Excretory urography offers both anatomic as well as functional information about the upper urinary tract and has long served as the "gold standard" for the detection of reflux nephropathy. Indeed, the traditional signs of reflux nephropathy (Table 23-2) have been derived mainly from the study of excretory urograms as well as from gross pathologic and histologic material.

Disadvantages of excretory urography include the exposure to ionizing radiation and the need for the intravenous injection of contrast material, which is uncomfortable and occasionally difficult in young infants and may produce an allergic reaction. Renal function must be adequate, but even with good renal function, superimposition of intestinal gas and fecal material

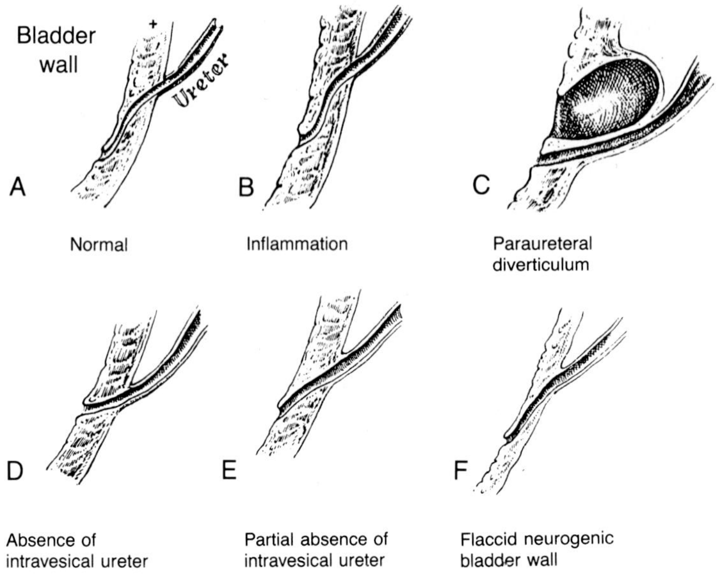


**Figure 23-2.** Diagrammatic presentation of some causes of vesicoureteral reflux. (King LR: Nonobstructive uropathy. In Kelalis PP, King LR, Belman AB (eds): Clinical Pediatric Urology. Philadelphia, WB Saunders, 1976)

**Table 23-2** Forms of Reflux Nephropathy

| |
|---|
| Focal renal parenchymal scar (usually at upper pole); normal renal size |
| Multiple renal parenchymal scars; normal or minimally affected renal size |
| Multiple renal parenchymal scars with renal contraction and distortion of the collecting systems |
| Impairment of renal growth, with or without renal cortical scars |
| Generalized renal hypoplasia |
| Segmental renal hypoplasia (Ask–Upmark kidney) |

There is usually calyceal blunting corresponding to the parenchymal cortical scars.

may make evaluation of the kidneys difficult and may cause focal renal scars to be missed.

## Ultrasound

Ultrasound is now probably the single most frequently used imaging modality in children with UTI. Its simplicity and noninvasiveness and the absence of ionizing radiation make ultrasound the ideal screening technique for detection of underlying anatomic abnormalities and significant renal scarring. Although ultrasound offers no information about the functional status of the kidneys, a normal-appearing kidney on ultrasound in the absence of any clinical or laboratory evidence of renal failure has an extremely low likelihood of being functionally compromised. Ultrasound cannot permit detection of any but the most severe grades of reflux, but this is probably of little consequence, because the treatment of minor degrees of VUR is conservative and there is good evidence that kidneys without scars after the age of 4 or 5 years will remain normal despite continuing low grades of VUR. Focal renal scars detectable on excretory urography occasionally may be missed on ultrasound (Fig. 23-3); in the absence of VUR, however, the clinical value of identifying such localized renal scars is unclear. If repeat sonograms show relatively normal growth of the affected kidney, the presence of small focal scars changes neither the management of the patient nor the prognosis. Ultrasound appears to be more reliable than excretory urography for determination of renal size and may demonstrate focal acute pyelonephritis or renal abscesses not detectable on urography.

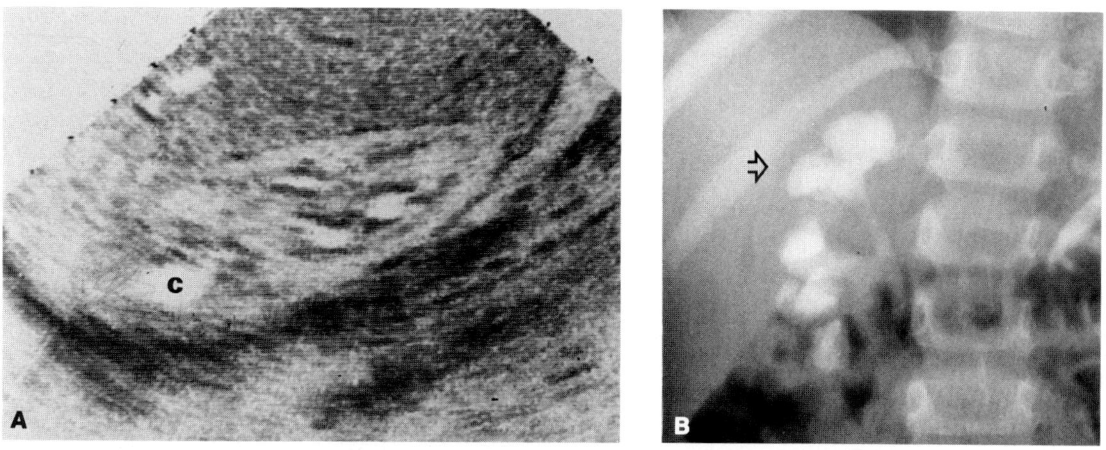


**Figure 23-3.** **(A)** Sagittal sonogram of the right kidney shows dilatation of the upper pole calyx (*c*) and possible scarring of the overlying renal cortex. **(B)** An excretory urogram more clearly shows the loss of cortical thickness (*arrow*) adjacent to the hydronephrotic upper pole calyx. (Leonidas JC, McCauley RGK, Klauber G et al: Sonography as a substitute for excretory urography in children with urinary tract infection. AJR 144:815–819, 1985)

### Radionuclide Cystography

Radionuclide cystography may be performed directly after the introduction of radionuclide (usually $^{99m}$Tc pertechnetate) into the bladder via a catheter or indirectly as part of a functional radionuclide imaging study of the upper urinary tract. As with indirect voiding cystourethrography, indirect radionuclide cystography is also of very limited value.

Radionuclide cystography has an accuracy similar to that of voiding cystourethrography in the detection of VUR and delivers much less radiation to the gonads. However, radionuclide cystography lacks the fine resolution of voiding cystourethrography and thus should not be used as an exclusive imaging modality in boys, a group with relatively higher frequency of structural abnormalities of the lower urinary tract. In contrast, radionuclide cystography may be employed as an exclusive imaging modality (even at the time of the first investigation) in young girls, who are unlikely to have lower urinary tract abnormalities in association with UTI. Because of its lower gonadal radiation dose, radionuclide cystography is an ideal modality for follow-up studies of children with documented VUR.

### Renal Scintigraphy

Dynamic radionuclide imaging of the upper urinary tract with an agent exclusively excreted by glomerular filtration (*e.g.*, $^{99m}$Tc diethyltriamine-pentaacetic acid [DTPA]) offers both anatomic and physiologic information about renal perfusion, glomerular filtration rate, accumulation of radionuclide in the renal pelves, and drainage of isotope from the renal collecting system. Renal scintigraphy using radionuclides concentrated by the renal tubules (*e.g.*, $^{99m}$Tc DMSA, $^{99m}$Tc glucoheptonate) provides superb imaging of the renal parenchyma and occasionally may permit identification of focal renal scars missed on ultrasound or excretory urography. In patients with focal areas of decreased isotope uptake, the demonstration of a high concentration of either $^{67}$Ga citrate or $^{111}$In-labeled white blood cells in the same regions is diagnostic of acute pyelonephritis (Figs. 23-4 and 23-5).

### Computed Tomography/Magnetic Resonance Imaging

Computed tomography and magnetic resonance imaging are currently of limited use in the investigation of children with UTI. Although both modalities can demonstrate underlying anatomic abnormalities, focal renal parenchymal scars, and areas of acute inflammation, in the overwhelming majority of patients the high cost and complexity of these techniques make them much less practical than other equally accurate imaging modalities that are simpler, less expensive, and more readily available.

## OVERALL APPROACH TO THE IMAGING OF CHILDREN WITH UTI

The imaging approach to the child with UTI depends on the age and sex of the child, the clinical symptoms and signs, and the likelihood and expected utility and consequences of possible outcomes. All infants and boys should have a complete investigation of their urinary tracts after an episode of UTI, because the probability of an underlying anatomic abnormality is relatively high. This is best accomplished be performing conventional voiding cystourethrography and a renal sonogram. If either is abnormal, an excretory urogram or renal scintigram should follow. In contrast, it is controversial whether older girls (who constitute the overwhelming majority of those affected) should also be subjected to radiographic imaging after an initial UTI. Up to three quarters are found to have no detectable abnormality, and the risk for the development of reflux nephropathy in older girls with normal urinary tracts at the time of their first UTI is very small. Nevertheless, some imaging information is obviously needed to exclude a significant anatomic abnormality or already established renal scars.

Because it entails no radiation exposure, all

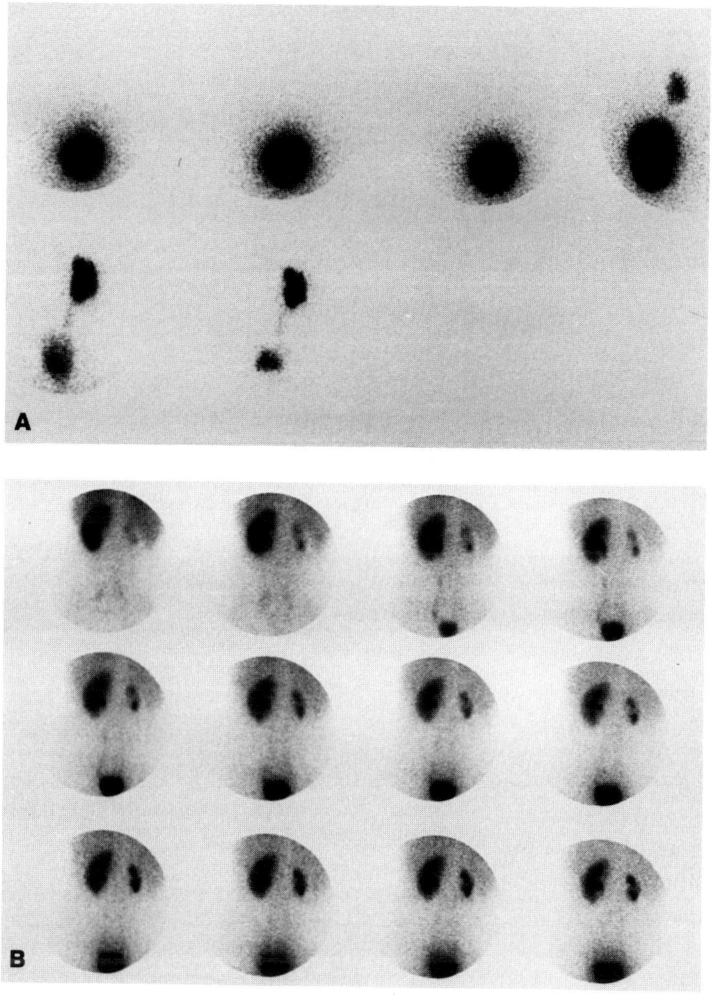

**Figure 23-4. (A)** Radionuclide cystogram (posterior view) in a 10-year-old girl with recurrent UTI shows significant VUR on the right. **(B)** Renal scintigram with $^{99m}$Tc-DTPA (posterior view) shows a small right kidney, indicating reflux nephropathy. (Courtesy of M. Majd, M.D.)

children with symptomatic UTI should undergo sonography immediately. Dilatation of the upper tracts suggests a high grade of VUR and is an indication for conventional or radionuclide cystography to document the degree of reflux. Infants and boys should undergo conventional voiding cystourethrography; for older girls, radionuclide cystography appears to be sufficient. It must be remembered that ultrasound has been reported to be overly sensitive for detecting upper tract dilatation and is likely to yield many false-positive readings of mild hydronephrosis. In a girl older than 4 years who has a normal renal sonogram during her first documented UTI, it might be best to simply repeat the sonogram 6 months and 1 year later to ensure continuing normality of her urinary tract. In this manner a cystogram, with its attendant discomfort and gonadal radiation, may be avoided.

An abnormal sonogram is an indication for cystography, which need not be performed until after the UTI clears, because it may be important to demonstrate whether VUR occurs only during periods of infection (as in children with a marginally competent ureterovesical junction that may permit intermittently infected urine to reflux into the renal parenchyma). In all cases, an abnormal or doubtful sonogram should

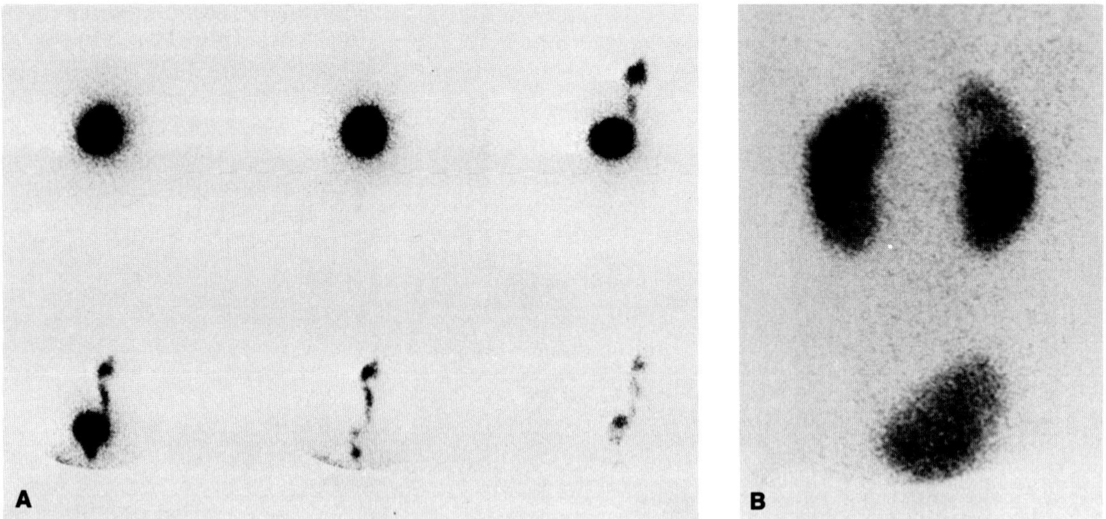


**Figure 23-5.** **(A)** Radionuclide cystogram (posterior view) in a 4-year-old girl with symptoms and signs of acute pyelonephritis demonstrates right VUR. **(B)** Renal scintigram shows the decreased isotope uptake in an area of active inflammation. (Courtesy of M. Majd, M.D.)

be followed by an excretory urogram or renal scintigram. The choice and sequence of these imaging modalities should be based on the type of information required. Excretory urography is better suited for providing excellent anatomic definition of the renal collecting systems, ureters, and bladder and for localizing the level of a possible obstruction. In contrast, a radionuclide scan with $^{99m}$Tc DTPA can evaluate renal function and, in some doubtful cases, may be the best imaging modality for confirming the presence or absence of an obstruction (especially if performed with a diuretic agent such as furosemide).

## Bibliography

Bailey RR: The relationship of vesico-ureteric reflux to urinary tract infection and chronic pyelonephritis—reflux nephropathy. Clin Nephrol 1:137–141, 1974

Belman AB: Genitourinary infections. In Kelalis PP, King LR, Belman AB (eds): Clinical Pediatric Urology. Philadelphia, WB Saunders, 1985

Ben Ami T: The sonographic evaluation of urinary tract infections in children. Semin Ultrasound 5:19–35, 1984

Cardiff–Oxford Bacteriuria Study Group. Sequelae of covert bacteriuria in schoolgirls. Lancet 1:889–893, 1978

Claesson I, Lindberg U: Asymptomatic bacteriuria in schoolgirls. Radiology 124:179–183, 1977

Conway JJ: Radionuclide cystography. In Hudson CJ, Heptinstall RH, Winberg J (eds): Reflux Nephrography Update: 1983. New York, S Karger, 1984

Dinkel E, Ertel M, Dittrich M et al: Kidney size in childhood. Sonographical growth charts for kidney length and volume. Pediatr Radiol 15:38–43, 1985

Friedland GW: The voiding cystourethrogram: An unreliable examination. In Hudson CJ, Kincaid–Smith P (eds): Reflux Nephropathy. New York, Masson Publishing USA, 1979

Jequier S, Forbes PA, Nogrady MB: The value of ultrasonography as a screening procedure in a first documented urinary tract infection in children. J Ultrasound Med 4:393–400, 1985

Kay CJ, Rosenfield AT, Taylor KJW et al: Ultrasonic characteristics of chronic atrophic pyelonephritis. AJR 132:47–49, 1979

Kessler RM, Altman DH: Real time sonographic detection of vesicoureteral reflux in children. AJR 138:1033–1036, 1982

Kincaid–Smith P: Reflux nephropathy. Br Med J 286:2002–2003, 1983

Leonidas JC, McCauley RGK, Klauber G et al: Sonography as a substitute for excretory urography in children with urinary tract infection. AJR 144:815–819, 1985

Majd M: Nuclear medicine. In Kelalis PP, King LR, Belman AB (eds): Clinical Pediatric Urology. Philadelphia, WB Saunders, 1985

Roberts JA: Pathogenesis of pyelonephritis. J Urol 129:1102–1106, 1983

Rosenbaum DM, Korngold E, Teele RL: Sonographic assessment of renal length in normal children. AJR 142:467–468, 1984

Shah KJ, Robins DG, White RHR: Renal scarring and vesicoureteric reflux. Arch Dis Child 53: 210–217, 1978

Smellie JM, Normand ICS: Urinary tract infection: Clinical aspects. In Williams DI, Johnston JH (eds): Paediatric Urology. London, Butterworth, 1982

**INFANTS AND MALE CHILDREN**

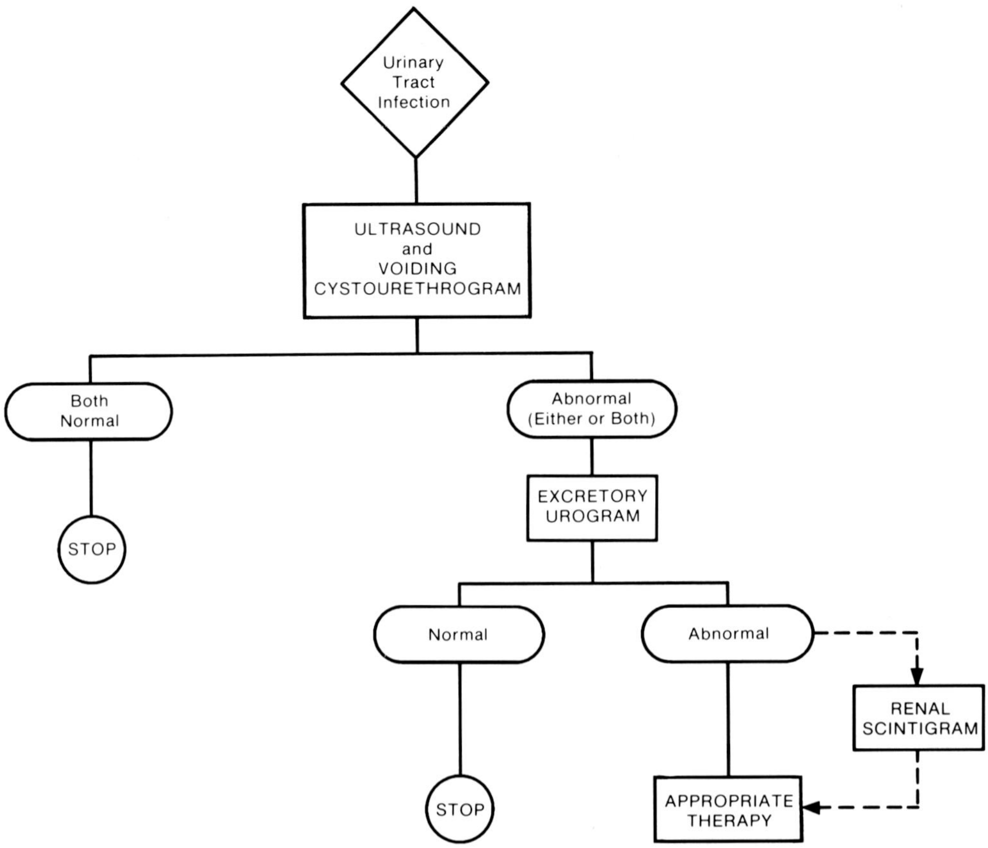

**OLDER FEMALE CHILDREN (Over 4 Years)**

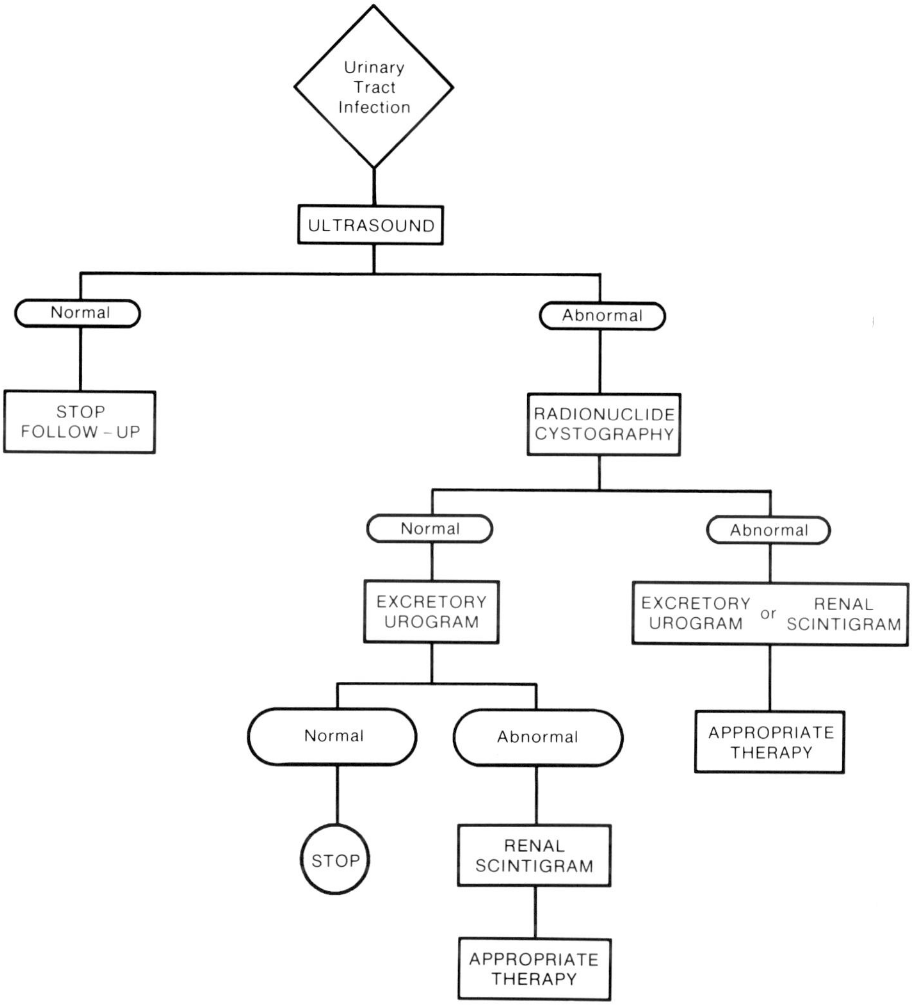

**ALTERNATIVE APPROACH TO ALL CHILDREN WITH UTI**

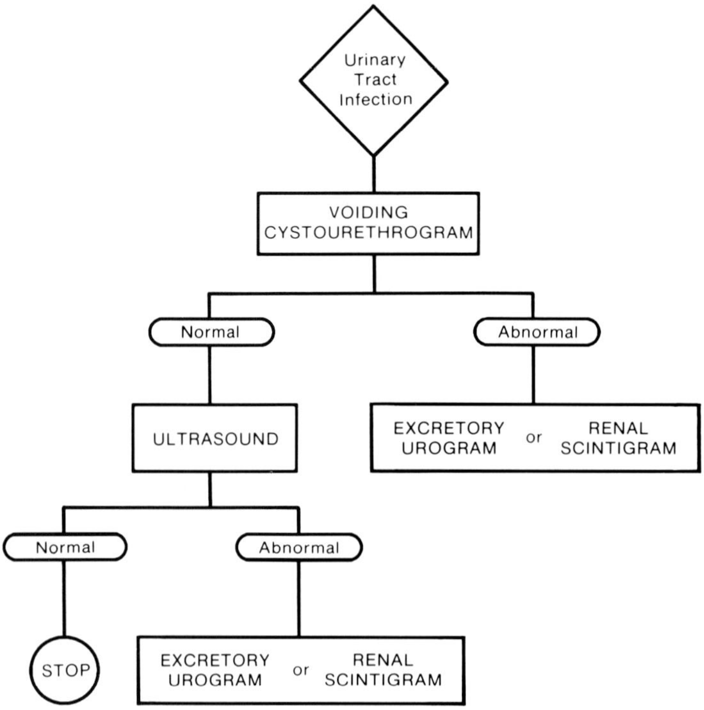

# Chapter 24

# Complications of Renal Transplantation

*Rajendra Kumar*

Renal transplantation has become a well-established therapeutic modality for patients with end-stage renal disease. Improved surgical techniques, tissue typing, and human leukocyte antigen (HLA) matching of the donor and recipient have resulted in 1-year survival rates of 80% from living related donors and 50% for cadaveric donor kidneys. A grafted kidney should begin to function between 2 to 10 minutes after a successful transplant. Failure of a graft to function is primarily reflected by an elevated serum creatinine level and decreased urinary output.

Post-transplantation problems leading to poor graft function can be classified as medical and surgical complications. Medical complications, consisting mainly of acute tubular necrosis and rejection phenomena, require medical management. Most postoperative surgical complications, however, are amenable to radiologic or surgical intervention, and thus early and precise diagnosis of the cause of renal failure is essential to permit appropriate treatment to ensure long-term survival of the graft.

## MEDICAL COMPLICATIONS

Acute tubular necrosis develops in the immediate postoperative period and is usually reversible without treatment within 1 to 4 weeks after transplantation. The most common cause of poor function of cadaveric grafts, acute tubular necrosis is usually related to nonimmunologic factors, such as difficulties in harvesting and preserving the kidney, or ischemic renal injury during transplantation. In acute tubular necrosis, urinary creatinine concentration is decreased and urinary sodium excretion is increased. The opposite may occur with acute rejection.

The rejection phenomena are classified on the basis of the time of development following transplantation surgery. Hyperacute rejection occurs within minutes after surgery and is manifested by anuria and a pale and flaccid appearance of the graft. Believed to be due to preformed antibodies circulating against the graft, this complication is now rarely seen because of improved matching techniques and better preoperative immunologic preparation. Acute rejection, which is mediated by T-cell lymphocytes, is the most common form of graft rejection and generally is reversible with treatment. Although it may occur at any time after transplantation, acute rejection usually develops 1 week or more following surgery and presents with a sudden decrease in urine output, leading to anuria that is associated with fever, graft tenderness, and hypertension. Elevated serum creatinine levels and proteinuria often occur. Accelerated acute rejection, which usually develops within the first 5 postoperative days, is more severe than acute rejection and is often refractory to treatment. Chronic rejection usually develops 1 month or more following surgery and produces a gradual decrease in renal function, often with hypertension and weight gain. The rejection is especially intense if the tissue compatibility between the donor and recipient was poor. Repeated subclinical episodes of rejection result in progressive destruction of the graft.

## SURGICAL (UROLOGIC) COMPLICATIONS

Improvement in surgical techniques, especially meticulous attention to the preservation of ureteral blood supply at the time of harvesting, has decreased the post-transplant urologic complication rate to less than 5%. Early urologic complications, which develop during the first 3 weeks following surgery, include perirenal fluid collections (other than lymphoceles), vascular complications, ureteral obstruction, urinary fistula, and graft rupture. Urinomas are extraperitoneal urine collections secondary to leakage of urine that usually occurs at the site of ureteroneocystostomy. They present with lower abdominal tenderness and distention, decreased urinary output from the urethra, and increased wound drainage. A large urinoma may compress and obstruct the ureter. Compromised blood supply or associated rejection may cause ureteral necrosis and urinary leak. Small hematomas are often seen in the immediate postoperative period. Large hematomas are rare and generally are caused by rupture of the renal vascular pedicle. Postoperative abscesses present with fever, localized tenderness, and leukocytosis and may be an early or late complication. They may develop *de novo* or may be secondary to infection of a urinoma, hematoma, or lymphocele. A perirenal abscess may predispose to renal vein thrombosis or renal artery rupture and may result in graft failure.

Renal artery stenosis, the most common postoperative vascular complication, develops in 10% to 15% of transplanted kidneys and may produce hypertension and an associated bruit. In most cases, the stenosis is distal to the anastomosis and is caused by intimal damage to the renal artery during removal of the kidney or cannulation. Preanastomotic stenosis of the hypogastric artery is usually due to an atheromatous plaque; stenosis at the anastomotic site is most often the result of faulty surgical technique during transplantation. Thrombosis of the major renal artery leads to renal infarction and necessitates removal of the graft. Segmental thrombosis may produce only focal renal infarction. Renal vein thrombosis is a rare but important cause of graft failure and may be associated with perirenal fluid collections (*e.g.,* abscess, lymphocele). Rupture of the renal artery, which is invariably the result of local infection, usually occurs at the site of anastomosis and is often fatal.

Postoperative ureteral obstruction may be due to edema at the site of ureteroneocystostomy, blood clot, stone, periureteral fibrosis, ureteral stenosis, bladder outlet obstruction, or a periureteral fluid collection. Depending on the cause, ureteral obstruction may occur in the early or late postoperative period and may compromise graft function. A urinary fistula involving the ureter, bladder, or a calyx may develop following obstruction, infarction, instrumentation (*e.g.,* renal biopsy), or infection. Early surgical repair is essential to reduce the otherwise high mortality rate from this serious complication. Spontaneous rupture of the transplanted kidney is a rare complication that generally occurs within the first 2 weeks following surgery. It presents with enlargement of the graft, localized pain, anuria, and shock. If detected early, surgical repair can salvage the kidney and result in the resumption of normal renal function within a few hours or days.

The major late postoperative urological complications of renal transplantation are lymphoceles, renal calculi, and neoplasms. Lymphoceles are perirenal fluid collections that develop following interruption of the recipient's lymphatics during transplant surgery (as shown by lower extremity lymphography) or lymphatic leakage from the surface of the graft kidney (as shown by lymphatic typing). Small lymphoceles often are asymptomatic and discovered incidentially, while larger lymphoceles may cause ureteral or venous obstruction with ipsilateral leg edema and decreased graft function. Lymphoceles rarely resorb spontaneously; if large and symptomatic, surgery is indicated for intraperitoneal marsupialization. Postoperative renal calculi may be due to renal tubular acidosis, secondary hyperparathyroidism, steroid therapy, oxalosis, chronic infection, or papillary necrosis. Both ureteral and bladder calculi may occur. Post-transplant patients undergoing immunosuppression therapy have a far higher than normal incidence of renal or uroepithelial tumors. These patients also have a very substantial risk of lymphoma (especially of the central nervous system), as well as squamous cell carcinoma of the skin, leukemia, and Kaposi's sarcoma.

## EXTRARENAL COMPLICATIONS

The administration of steroids and immunosuppressive therapy following transplantation may lead to serious extrarenal complications. Bacterial, viral, and fungal infections, especially with unusual organisms, are relatively common and primarily involve the urinary tract, lungs, gastrointestinal tract, liver, and surgical wounds. Steroid therapy may lead to aseptic necrosis, especially of the femoral heads, and generalized osteoporosis that may result in fractures of the vertebral bodies, ribs, and pelvis. There is also an increased postoperative incidence of peptic ulcer, gastric perforation, gastrointestinal hemorrhage, and pancreatitis.

## DIAGNOSTIC EVALUATION

### *DIAGNOSTIC MODALITIES*

1. Radionuclide scanning
2. Ultrasound
3. Excretory urography
4. Retrograde pyelography and cystography
5. Antegrade pyelography
6. Angiography
7. Magnetic resonance imaging
8. Computed tomography
9. Interventional radiologic procedures

### Radionuclide Scanning

Radionuclide scanning (most commonly using $^{99m}$Tc diethyltriaminepentaacetic acid [DTPA]) should be the initial imaging modality if graft function is compromised. The vascular, excretory, and drainage phases of the examination permit the evaluation of renal perfusion, renal parenchymal function, and the status of the collecting structures. The absence of renal perfusion on a radionuclide scan suggests an occluded renal artery and is an indication for renal arteriography to exclude vascular obstruction as the cause of renal failure. Ureteral obstruction can be demonstrated during the drainage phase of the study (Fig. 24-1). The presence of abnormal periureteral isotope activity (Fig. 24-2) can indicate a urinary leak and urinoma at an earlier stage than can excretory urography. Although a mild to moderate prolongation of aortorenal transit time is generally seen in acute tubular necrosis and a marked prolongation of the transit time (and poor renal uptake of isotope) is characteristic of acute rejection (Fig. 24-3), radionuclide scans have not proved as useful as initially claimed in differentiating these two conditions. Radionuclide studies using $^{67}$Ga or $^{111}$In-labeled white blood cells are effective in demonstrating renal and perirenal abscesses (see Fig. 24-4).

Radionuclide studies are also useful in the follow-up of patients recovering from graft dysfunction.

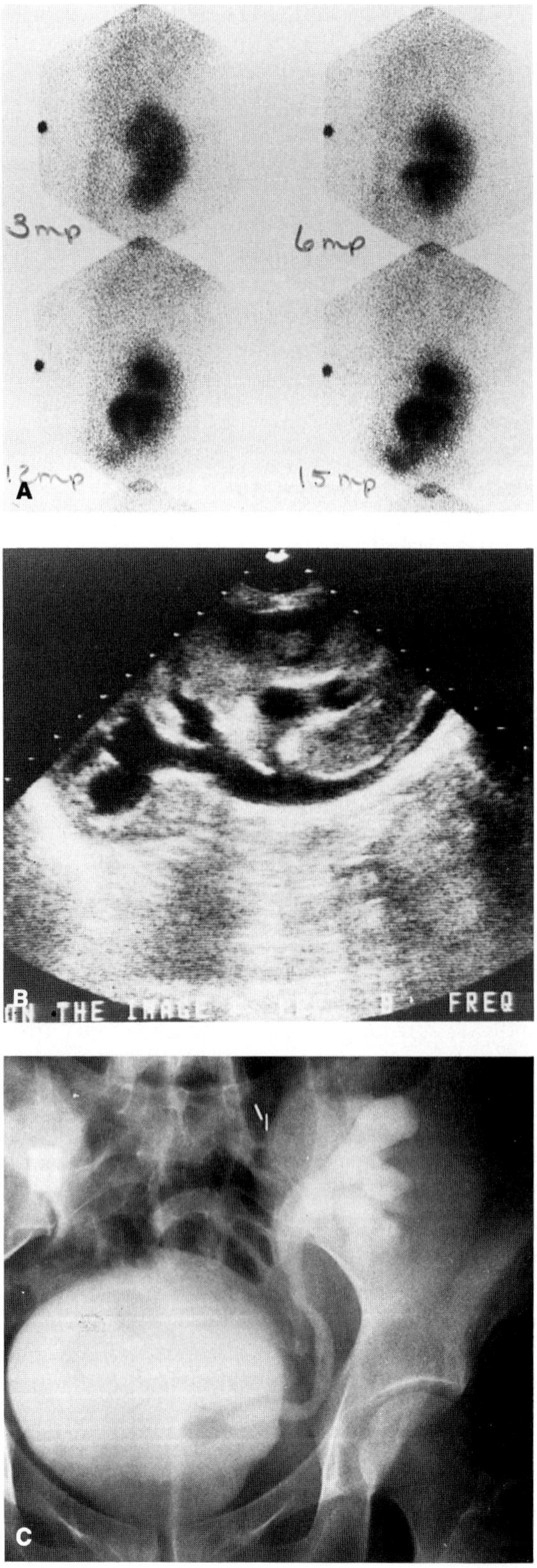

**Figure 24-1.** Ureteral obstruction. **(A)** Radionuclide scan shows dilatation of the collecting structures. **(B)** Ultrasound confirms hydronephrosis and hydroureter. **(C)** Excretory urography shows ureteral obstruction due to edema at the site of the ureteroneocystostomy. (Kumar R, Wilson DD, Santa-Cruz FR: Postoperative urological complications of renal transplantation. RadioGraphics 4:531, 1984)

## Ultrasound

As a noninvasive procedure that does not utilize ionizing radiation and is independent of graft function, ultrasound is an important imaging modality for evaluating complications of renal transplantation. It can assess renal volume and easily demonstrate a hydronephrotic obstructed kidney (see Fig. 24-1*B*). Ultrasound is an excellent screening technique for the patient with a suspected perirenal fluid collection. A urinoma appears as an anechoic fluid collection; the diagnosis can be confirmed by the radionuclide demonstration of a urinary leak (see Fig. 24-2). An abscess has a more complex appearance and may contain a few or many echoes within the fluid-filled structure (Fig. 24-4*A*). In most cases, the diagnosis can be confirmed by radionuclide scanning with $^{67}$Ga or $^{111}$In-labeled white blood cells (Fig. 24-4*B*). The sonographic appearance of a hematoma depends on its age. Recent hematomas tend to be anechoic or hypoechoic, whereas old hematomas are generally more complex masses that contain echogenic and cystic components and simulate an abscess (Fig. 24-5). Lymphoceles are anechoic fluid collections that may contain septations (Fig. 24-6). Whenever a perirenal fluid collection is detected, ultrasound can be used to guide diagnostic and/or therapeutic needle aspiration.

Ultrasound is of great value in diagnosing graft rejection. The most useful sign of rejection is a decrease in the amplitude of the central sinus echoes, which reflects the replacement of normal sinus fat (hyperechoic) by fibrous tissue (hypoechoic) in a rejected graft (Fig. 24-7). Other less specific sonographic findings that suggest graft rejection include increased renal volume, increased cortical thickness, indistinctness of the

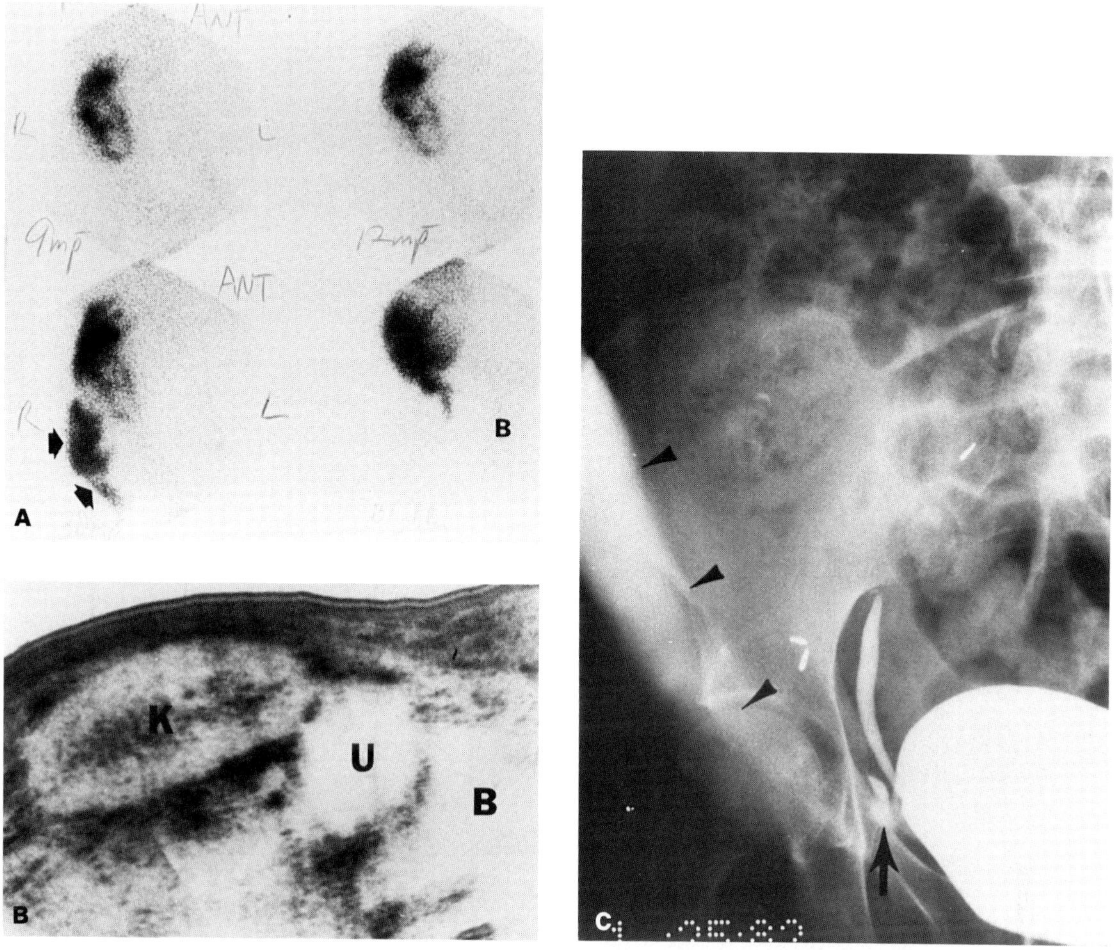


**Figure 24-2.** Ureteral leak and urinoma. **(A)** Radionuclide scan shows abnormal periureteral isotope activity (*arrows*). **(B)** Ultrasound demonstrates a periureteral anechoic fluid collection (*U*) between the kidney (*K*) and bladder (labeled *B*), consistent with a urinoma. **(C)** Retrograde cystography confirms the urinary leak (*arrowheads*) at the site of the ureteroneocystostomy (*arrow*). (Kumar R, Wilson DD, Santa-Cruz FR: Postoperative urological complications of renal transplantation. RadioGraphics 4:531, 1984)

corticomedullary boundary, and enlargement and increased translucency of the medullary region.

Ultrasound is useful in guiding the placement of a needle for renal biopsy, which may be required in some instances to determine the underlying cause of graft failure. Ultrasound guidance also can be employed in percutaneous drainage of an obstructed collecting system and other interventional radiologic procedures performed in the management of postoperative complications of renal transplantation.

## Excretory Urography

Excretory urography has a limited role in the evaluation of a poorly functioning renal graft. The contrast materials used for excretory urography are nephrotoxic and may further damage a

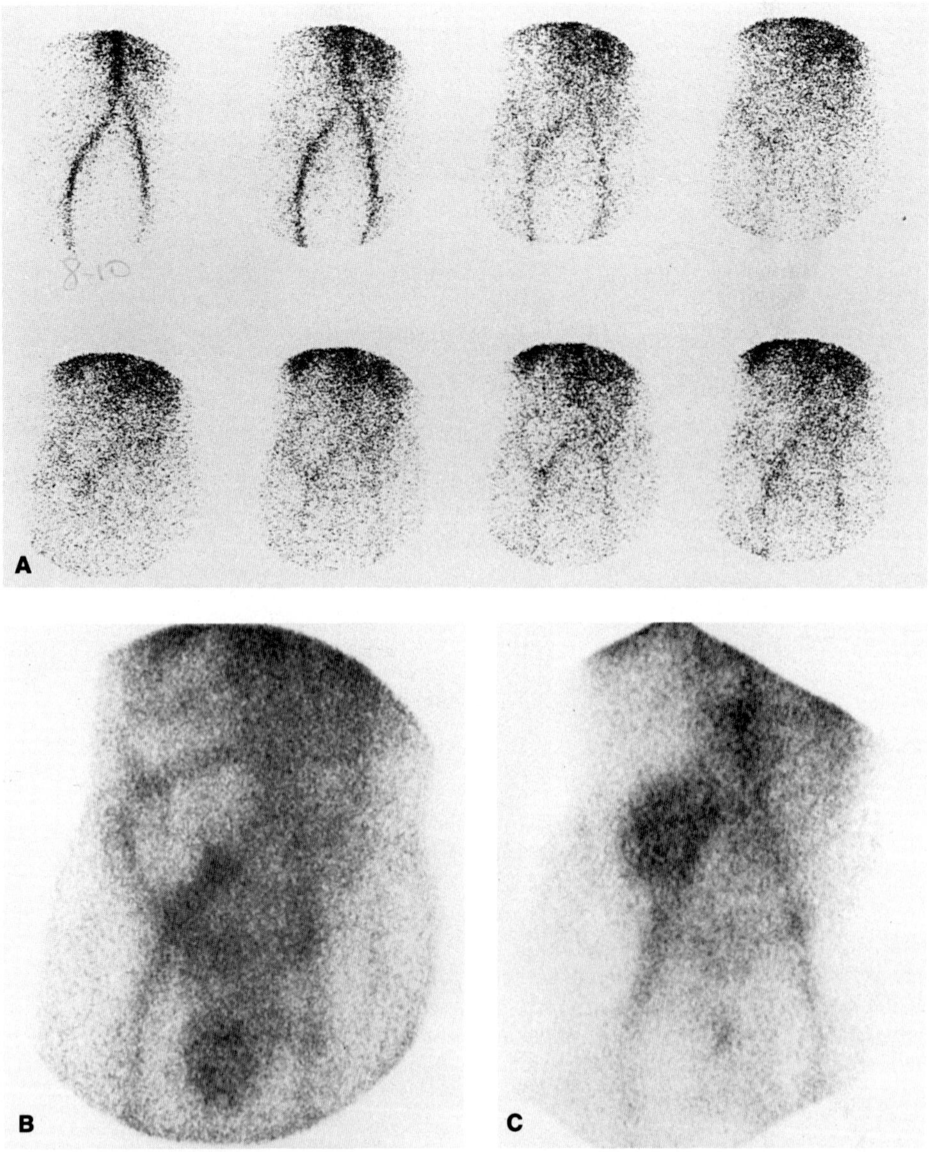

**Figure 24-3.** Graft rejection. **(A)** Perfusion phase of radionuclide study shows a markedly prolonged aortorenal transit time. **(B)** On the static image, the absence of isotope activity in the renal graft is consistent with acute rejection. **(C)** Baseline static scan performed immediately following transplant surgery shows good isotope uptake by the functioning graft.

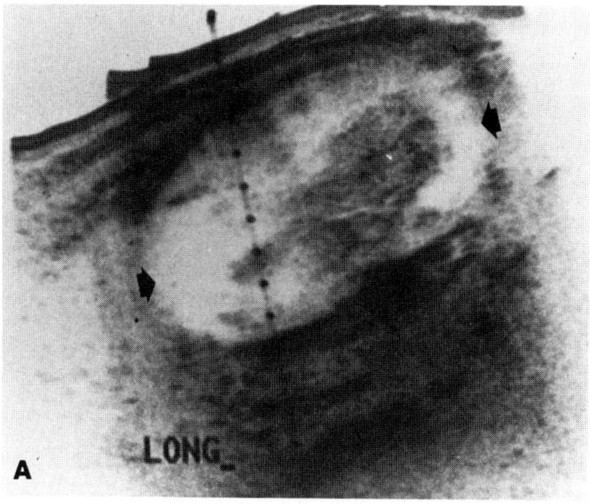


A

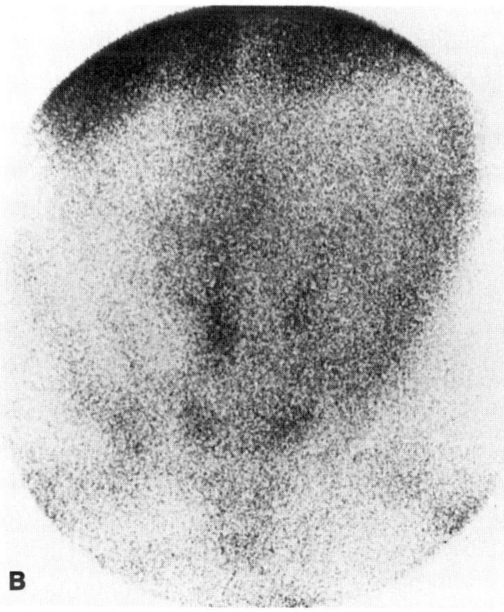

B

**Figure 24-4.** Renal abscess. **(A)** Longitudinal sonogram in a patient with symptoms of infection shows cystic areas (*arrows*) containing a few echoes in a transplanted kidney. **(B)** $^{67}$Ga scan shows increased isotope uptake in the corresponding areas, consistent with abscesses. (Kumar R, Wilson DD, Santa-Cruz FR: Postoperative urological complications of renal transplantation. RadioGraphics 4:531, 1984)

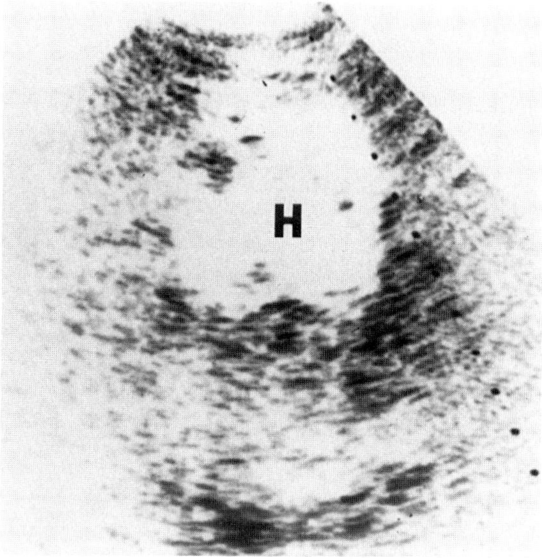


**Figure 24-5.** Hematoma. Real-time sonogram shows a predominantly sonolucent mass containing many echogenic foci. Needle aspiration confirmed the diagnosis. (Kumar R, Wilson DD, Santa-Cruz FR: Postoperative urological complications of renal transplantation. RadioGraphics 4:531, 1984)

transplanted kidney that already has compromised function. In addition, a significant loss of renal function precludes a successful urogram, because the collecting structures do not opacify. Infrequently, excretory urography can be performed to confirm the site of a ureteral leak or obstruction (see Fig. 24-1*C*).

## Retrograde Pyelography and Cystography

Retrograde pyelography may be performed to better demonstrate the site of a ureteral obstruction or leak. However, the retrograde passage of a catheter through an area of ureteral stenosis is difficult, and in most cases it is preferable to use an antegrade approach through a nephrostomy tube. Retrograde cystography is the procedure of choice if evaluation of the bladder is necessary (see Fig. 24-2*C*).

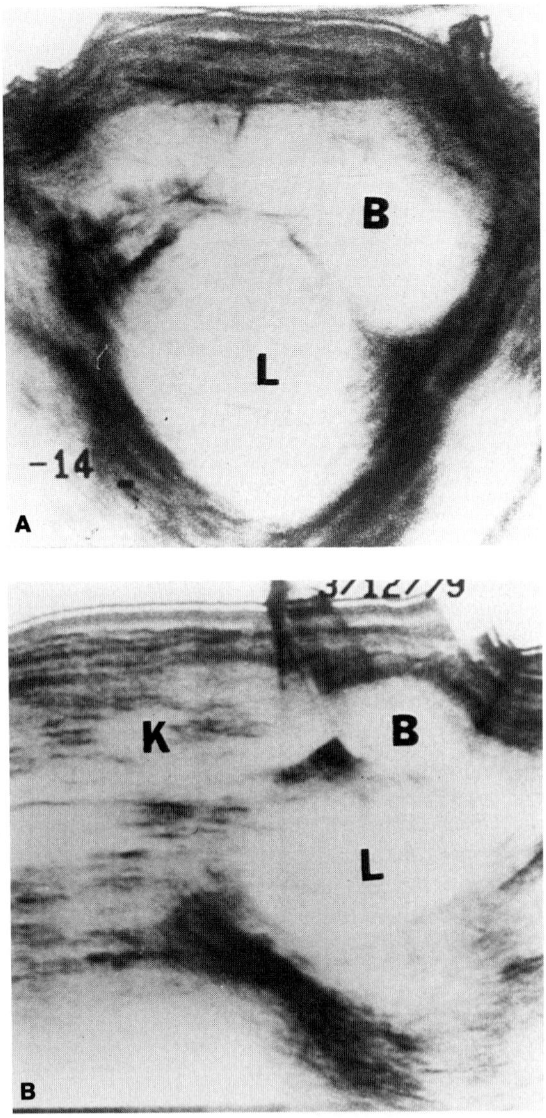


**Figure 24-6.** Lymphocele. **(A)** Transverse and **(B)** longitudinal sonograms show the lymphocele as a large sonolucent mass (*L*) inferior to the kidney (*K*) and compressing the bladder (labeled *B*). (Kumar R, Wilson DD, Santa-Cruz FR: Postoperative urological complications of renal transplantation. RadioGraphics 4:531, 1984)

## Antegrade Pyelography

Antegrade pyelography is a valuable procedure for demonstrating the site of ureteral obstruction or leak (Fig. 24-8). Through use of a percutaneous approach under ultrasound guidance, a catheter is placed in the pelvocalyceal structures of the transplanted kidney and contrast material is injected to fill the collecting system.

## Angiography

Renal arteriography may be indicated to confirm a vascular complication (renal artery stenosis, aneurysm, or rupture) suspected on the perfusion phase of a radionuclide scan. This technique can also demonstrate a traumatic arteriovenous fistula and can provide a route for therapeutic occlusion. Renal venography can confirm the diagnosis of renal or iliac vein thrombosis. Vascular complications of renal transplantation can also be evaluated by digital subtraction angiography and Doppler ultrasound studies.

## Magnetic Resonance Imaging

Although some studies have reported magnetic resonance imaging (MRI) to be of value in assessing complications of renal transplantation (Fig. 24-9), further investigation is necessary before it can be recommended as a routine imaging procedure in these patients.

## Computed Tomography

Computed tomography has a limited role in evaluating the failing renal transplant. It is primarily of value in detecting and staging abdominal lymphoma, which has a far higher than normal incidence following transplant surgery.

## Interventional Radiologic Procedures

Interventional radiologic procedures are being increasingly used as a prelude to or substitute for

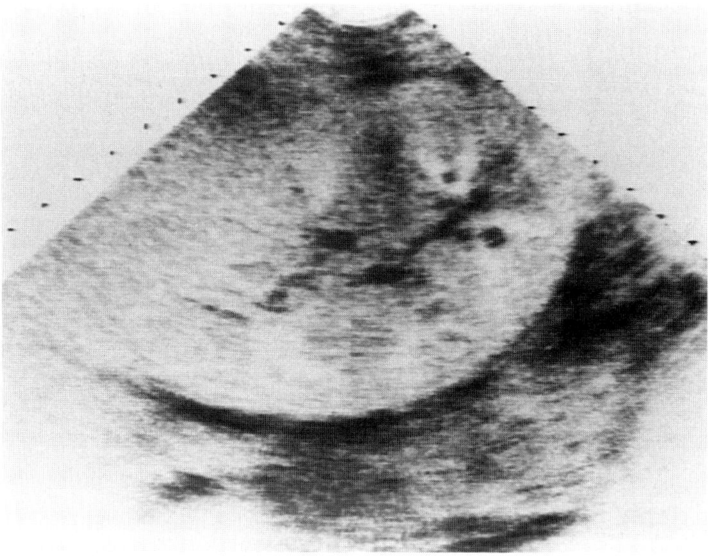

**Figure 24-7.** Acute rejection. Real-time longitudinal sonogram shows the transplanted kidney to be edematous with an indistinct corticomedullary boundary and decrease in central sinus echoes.

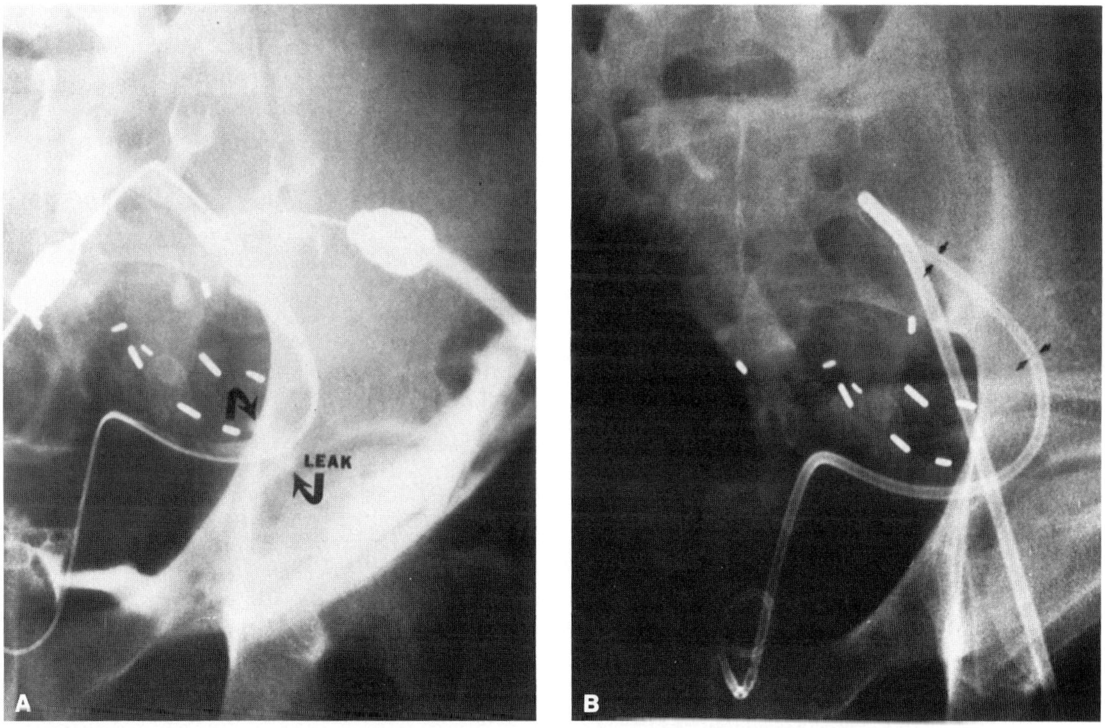


**Figure 24-8.** Urinary leak. **(A)** Antegrade pyelogram via a percutaneously placed catheter shows the leak of contrast material. **(B)** A ureteral stent (*arrows*) is now in place. When the stent was removed 4 weeks later, the leak had sealed. (Kumar R, Wilson DD, Santa-Cruz FR: Postoperative urological complications of renal transplantation. RadioGraphics 4:531, 1984)

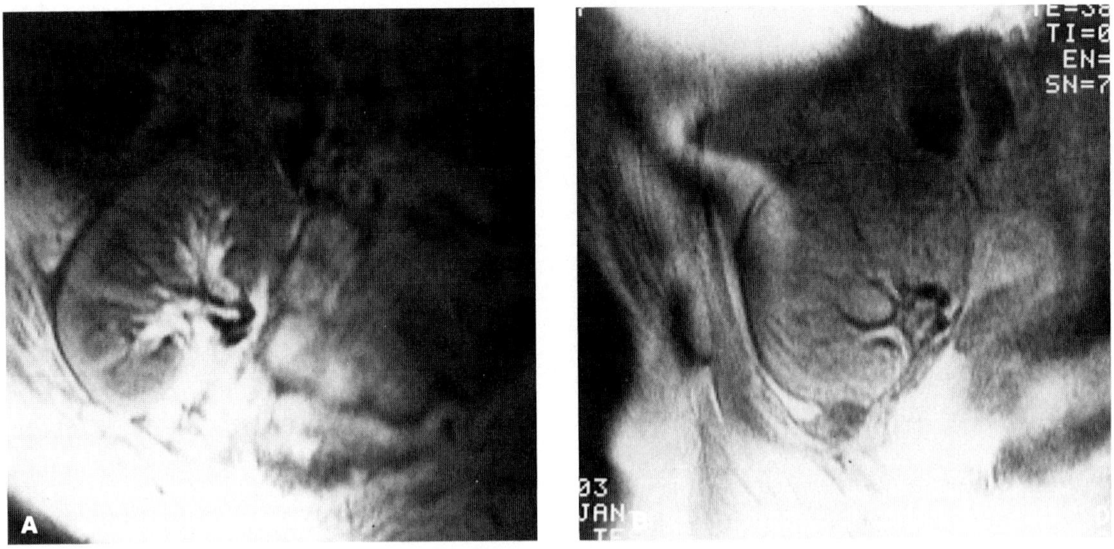


**Figure 24-9.** MRI of renal transplant. **(A)** Normal graft appearance of a well-defined corticomedullary boundary and prominent signal intensity due to normal renal sinus fat. **(B)** In acute rejection, there are poor demarcation of the corticomedullary boundary due to edema and a markedly decreased signal intensity from the renal sinus, reflecting the lack of fat.

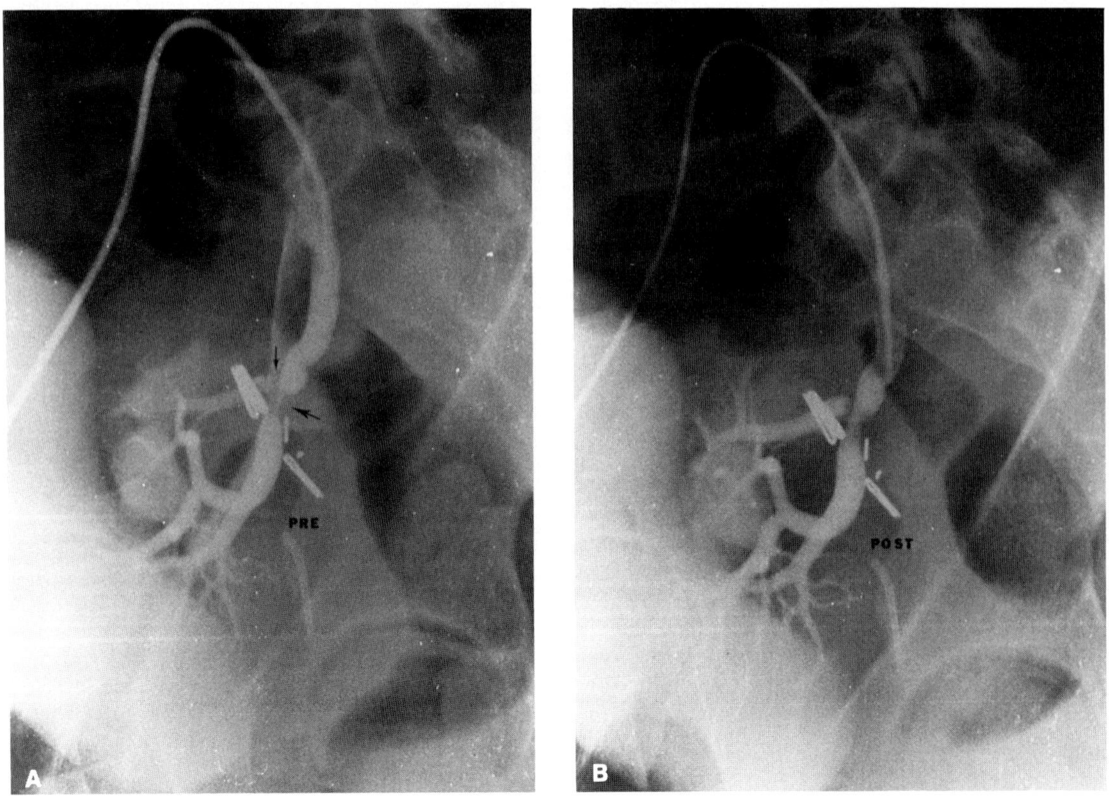

surgery in the diagnosis and management of many post-transplantation urologic complications. Percutaneous nephrostomy provides temporary drainage of an obstructed urinary collecting system. It can also be used for extracting calculi, stenting a ureteral leak, and dilating a ureteral stricture (see Fig. 24-8). Percutaneous transluminal angioplasty offers an alternative to surgery in the management of renal artery stenosis. Because this procedure has a success rate equal to surgery but with much less patient morbidity, percutaneous transluminal angioplasty is now generally considered the procedure of choice for treating the patient with post-transplant renal artery stenosis (Fig. 24-10). In extracorporeal shock wave lithotripsy, ultrasound waves are used to fragment renal calculi without the need for surgery. This procedure may be combined with percutaneous nephrostomy for retrieval of stone fragments.

## Bibliography

Barbaric ZL, Thompson KR: Percutaneous nephrostomy in the management of obstructed renal transplants. Radiology 126:639–642, 1978

Becker JA, Kutcher R: Urologic complications of renal transplantation. Semin Roentgenol 13(4): 341–351, 1978

Coyne SS, Walsh JW, Tisnado J et al: Surgical correctable renal transplant complications: An integrated clinical and radiologic approach. AJR 136: 1113–1119, 1981

Curry NS, Cochran S, Barbaric ZL et al: Interventional radiologic procedures in the renal transplant. Radiology 152:647–653, 1984

Frick MP, Feinberg SB, Sibley R et al: Ultrasound in acute renal transplant rejection. Radiology 138: 657–660, 1981

Frick MP, Salomonowitz E, Hanto DW et al: CT of abdominal lymphoma after renal transplantation. AJR 142:97–99, 1984

Fisher MF, Haaga JR, Persky L et al: Renal stone extraction through a percutaneous nephrostomy in a renal transplant patient. Radiology 144: 95–96, 1982

Geisinger MA, Risius B, Jordan ML et al: Magnetic resonance imaging of renal transplants. AJR 143: 1229–1234, 1984

George EA: Radionuclide diagnosis of allograft rejection. Semin Nucl Med XII(4):379–386, 1982

Gerlock AJ, Jr, MacDonell RC, Smith CW et al: Renal transplant arterial stenosis: Percutaneous transluminal angioplasty. AJR 140:325–331, 1983

Hricak H, Cruz C, Eyler WR et al: Acute post-transplantation renal failure: Differential diagnosis by ultrasound. Radiology 139:441–449, 1981

Hricak H, Romanski RN, Eyler WR: The renal sinus during allograft rejection: Sonographic and histopathologic findings. Radiology 142:693–699, 1982

Hricak H, Terrier F, Demas BE: Renal allografts: Evaluation by MR imaging. Radiology 159: 435–441, 1986

Hunter DW, Castaneda–Zuniga WR, Coleman CC et al: Percutaneous techniques in the management of urological complications in renal transplant patients. Radiology 148:407–412, 1983

Kumar R, Wilson DD, Santa-Cruz FR: Postoperative urological complications of renal transplantation. Radiographics 4(3):531–547, 1984

Lucas BSC, Castro JE: Calculi in renal transplants. Br J Urol 50:302–306, 1978

Maklad NF: Ultrasonic evaluation of renal transplants. Semin Ultrasound II(1):88–96, 1981

Reinig JW, Gordon L, Frey D et al: Glomerular filtration rate in transplantation patients. Estimation of renal function using Tc-99m DTPA. Radiology 156:505–507, 1985

Silver TM, Campbell D, Wicks JD et al: Peritransplant fluid collections. Ultrasound evaluation and clinical significance. Radiology 138: 145–151, 1981

Sniderman KW, Sos TA, Sprayregen S et al: Percutaneous transluminal angioplasty in renal transplant arterial stenosis for relief of hypertension. Radiology 135:23–26, 1980

Spigos DG, Tan W, Pavel DG et al: Diagnosis of urine extravasation after renal transplantation. AJR 129:409–413, 1977

◀ **Figure 24-10.** Renal artery stenosis. **(A)** Arteriogram shows severe postanastomotic renal artery stenosis (*arrows*) following renal transplant in a hypertensive patient. **(B)** Following percutaneous transluminal angioplasty, a repeat arteriogram shows dilatation of the previously stenotic segment. The patient's hypertension substantially decreased. (Kumar R, Wilson DD, Santa-Cruz FR: Postoperative urological complications of renal transplantion. RadioGraphics 4:531, 1984)

**DECREASE IN RENAL GRAFT FUNCTION**
**Medical Complications**

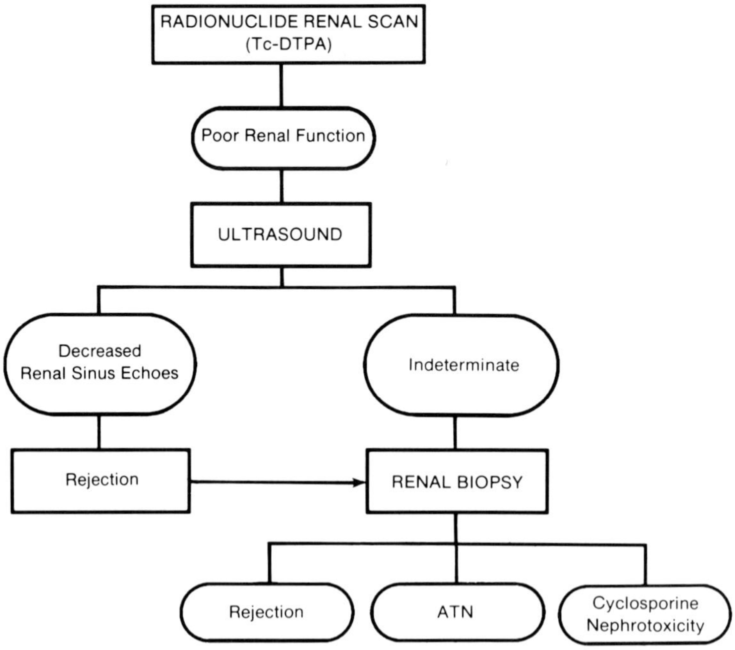

## DECREASE IN RENAL GRAFT FUNCTION
**Early Urological Complications**

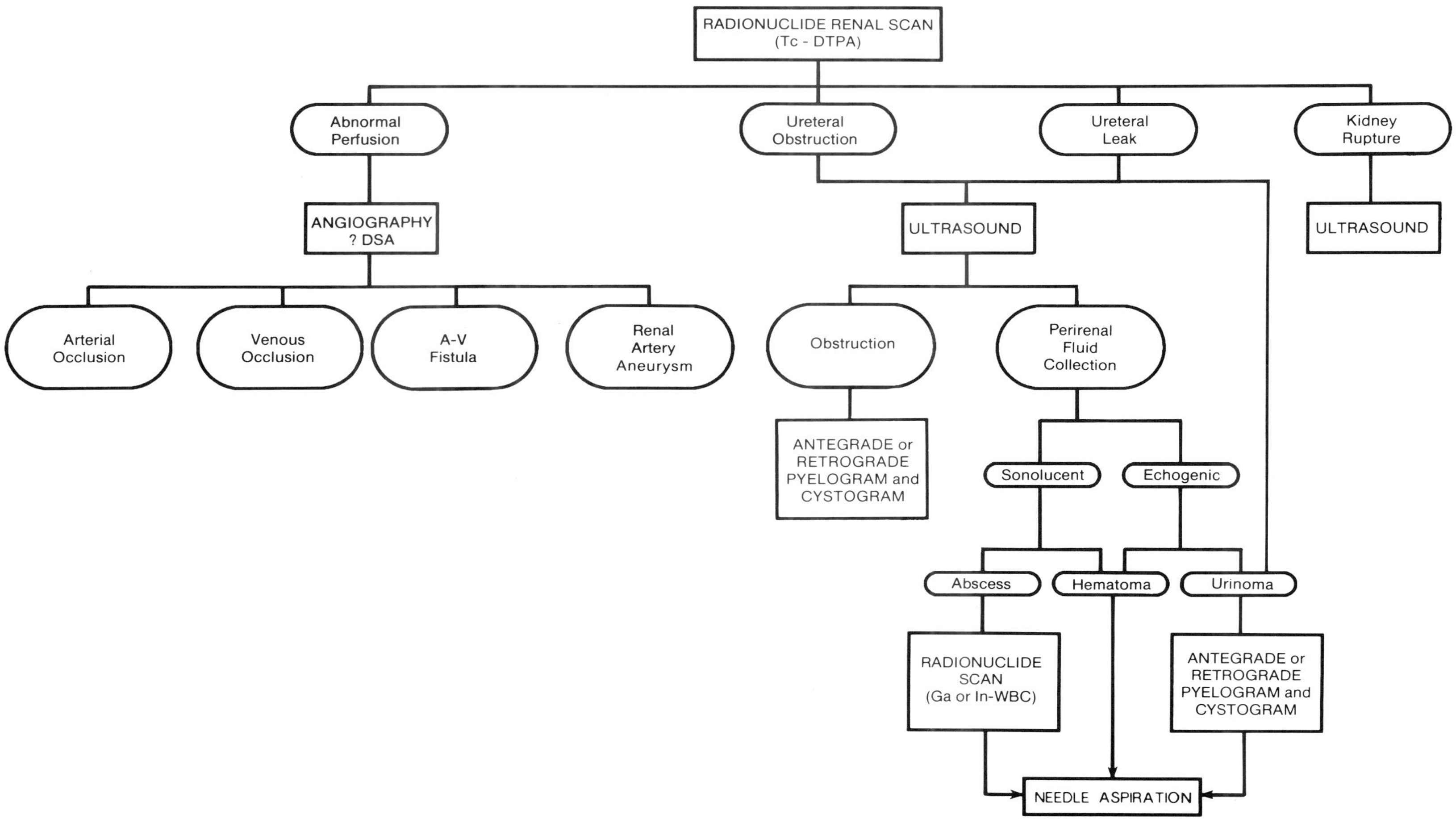

## DECREASE IN RENAL GRAFT FUNCTION
### Late Urologic Complications

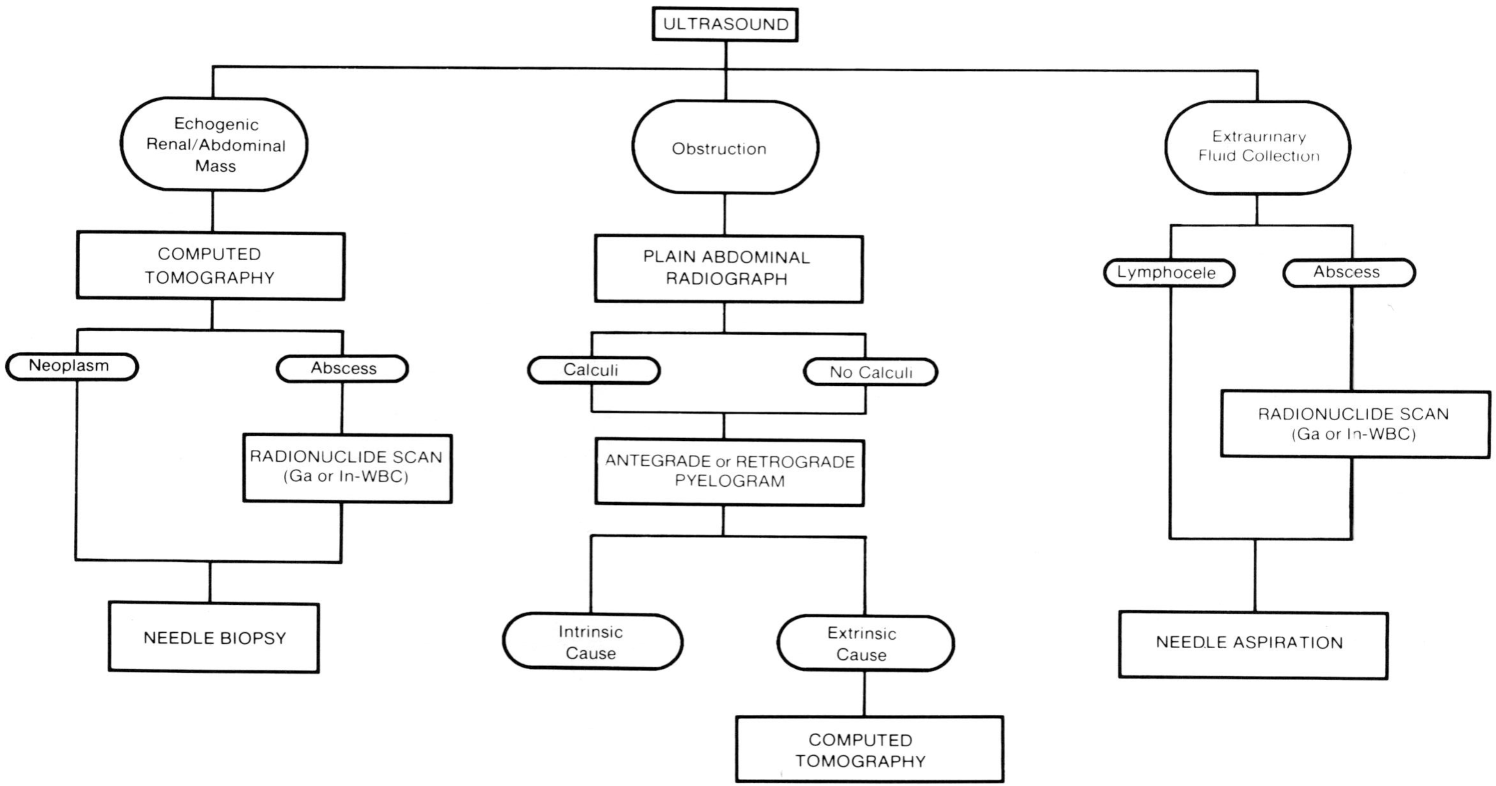

# Chapter 25

# Adrenal Disease

*Harold A. Mitty*

Diagnostic imaging of the adrenal glands primarily involves three groups of patients. Traditionally, radiographic evaluation has been performed on patients who had endocrinopathies suspected to be of adrenal origin. A second group of patients, seen with increasing frequency, present with the incidental discovery on computed tomography (CT) examination of an adrenal mass that is of no apparent clinical significance. A third major group consists of patients with adrenal masses who have a malignancy in another part of the body, and further evaluation is required to determine whether the adrenal lesion represents a metastasis.

## DIAGNOSTIC EVALUATION

### *DIAGNOSTIC MODALITIES*

1. Excretory urography and nephrotomography
2. Computed tomography
3. Ultrasound
4. Radionuclide studies
5. Magnetic resonance imaging
6. Adrenal arteriography and venography
7. Needle aspiration

#### Excretory Urography and Nephrotomography

In the past, excretory urography and nephrotomography have been the basic screening examinations for patients with suspected disease of the adrenal glands. Approximately 80% of adrenal masses (other than aldosteronomas) can be detected by combined excretory urography and nephrotomography. However, small adrenal masses and extra-adrenal pheochromocytomas are difficult to demonstrate using these modalities.

As left-sided adrenal masses enlarge, they displace the kidney downward and rotate the upper pole laterally. Because the left adrenal is anterior and medial relative to the kidney, large left-sided adrenal masses also indent the posterior aspect of the stomach. On the right side, much of the adrenal gland is truly suprarenal in location and enlarging tumors tend to compress the upper pole of the kidney and displace the kidney downward. Large masses that also grow anteriorly and compress and thin the right lobe of the liver may be misdiagnosed as lesions of the right hepatic lobe. On radionuclide scans, the thinned liver can be mistaken for a cold area caused by an intrinsic hepatic neoplasm. This type of diagnostic error can now usually be obviated by the use of the cross-sectional techniques, especially CT or magnetic resonance imaging (MRI).

Plain abdominal radiographs can demonstrate calcifications in the adrenal glands. Bilateral adrenal calcifications in an adult, once believed to reflect healed tuberculosis, are now believed to be most often the result of neonatal adrenal hemorrhage. Approximately 15% of adrenal cysts contain calcification that is usually located at the periphery and is curvilinear in appearance. However, since calcification also occurs in approximately 10% of adrenal tumors, the presence of calcification in an adrenal mass is usually an indication for aspiration and/or surgery. In children, the combination of an adrenal mass and calcification suggests a neuroblastoma.

## Computed Tomography

Computed tomography has become the imaging modality of choice in the evaluation of most patients with suspected adrenal disease. The CT appearance of an adrenal gland depends on the level of the section. Scans through the superior aspect of the gland demonstrate a linear structure that usually is oriented in an anterolateral or posterior direction (Fig. 25-1*A*). This configuration is seen most often on the right, where the adrenal gland is identified between the liver laterally and the crus of the diaphragm medially. In the midportion of the gland, the cross-section image demonstrates an inverted V- or Y-shaped structure that reflects the increasing separation of the limbs of the gland at more caudal levels (Fig. 25-1*B*).

The adrenal glands are surrounded by the perirenal fat, which separates them from the adjacent kidney, aorta, liver, and crus of the diaphragm. The presence of this perinephric fat permits the demonstration of the adrenal glands in more than 95% of cases. In children (or the rare adult) who have diminished retroperitoneal fat, the adrenal glands may not be detectable on CT and ultrasound or venography may be required.

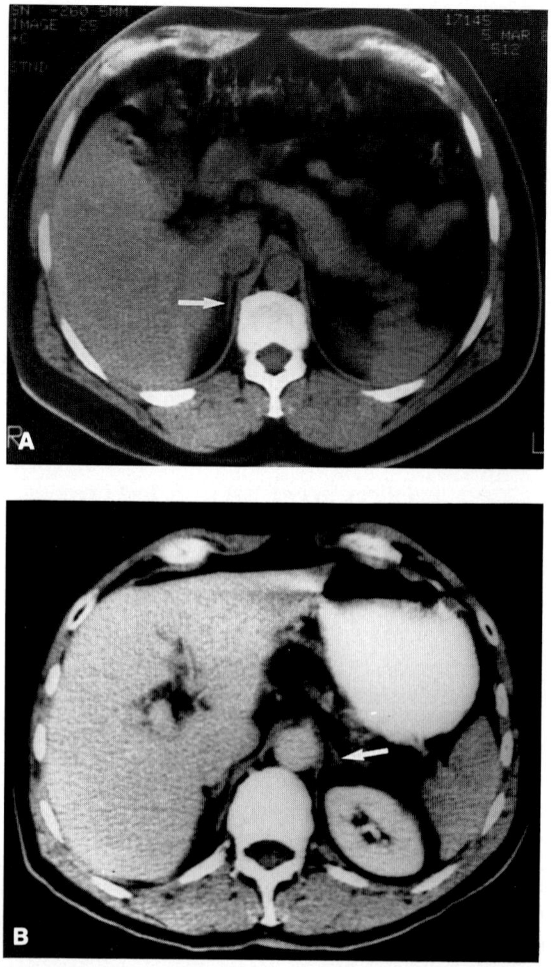


**Figure 25-1.** CT scans of normal adrenal glands. **(A)** A section through the superior aspect of the right adrenal gland demonstrates a thin linear structure (*arrow*) posterior to the vena cava. **(B)** A section of the left adrenal at a level just above the renal hilum reveals the typical inverted-Y shape (*arrow*).

Several adrenal lesions have inherent characteristics that may permit a precise CT diagnosis. Some cortical adenomas associated with Cushing's syndrome or aldosteronism have been reported to have a low attenuation number, although in my experience these tumors have not been confused with low-attenuation retroperitoneal fat. The relatively rare myelolipoma, which contains large amounts of fat in addition to myeloid elements, can be demonstrated by CT with confidence (Fig. 25-2). Pheochromocytomas tend to develop areas of necrosis detectable by CT, although this appearance may also be seen with carcinomas of the adrenal cortex.

## Ultrasound

Ultrasound provides an alternative method for evaluating the adrenal glands. However, because the glands may be partly obscured by overlying gas within abdominal viscera and in the posterior costophrenic angles, the sonographic demonstration of the adrenals is often a challenging task. Nevertheless, careful scanning in the anterior transverse projection, using structures such as the spleen for a sonographic window, permits the detection of the adrenals in 70%–80% of patients.

The major application of adrenal ultrasound is as a screening procedure in patients (particularly children) from families with the multiple endocrine neoplasia syndromes. In addition, ultrasound can be employed in patients who are poor candidates for CT scanning because of a paucity of retroperitoneal fat.

A prospective study comparing the effectiveness of CT and ultrasound in evaluating the adrenal glands showed that the two modalities had a similar sensitivity, but that the specificity and accuracy of CT was far higher than that of ultrasound. This strongly supports the concept that CT should be the procedure of choice for evaluating most types of adrenal disease.

## Radionuclide Studies

Radionuclide scanning for localization of adrenal masses has been seriously limited by the need to perform scans 2 to 14 days after the intravenous administration of the isotope ($^{131}$I-labeled cholesterol derivatives). This prolonged delay is an inherent disadvantage of the method resulting from the need for the radionuclide to be incorporated into adrenal steroid synthesis. In general, repeat scanning is required to identify the time of optimal image production.

Recently, a new agent ($^{131}$I-MIBG [meta-

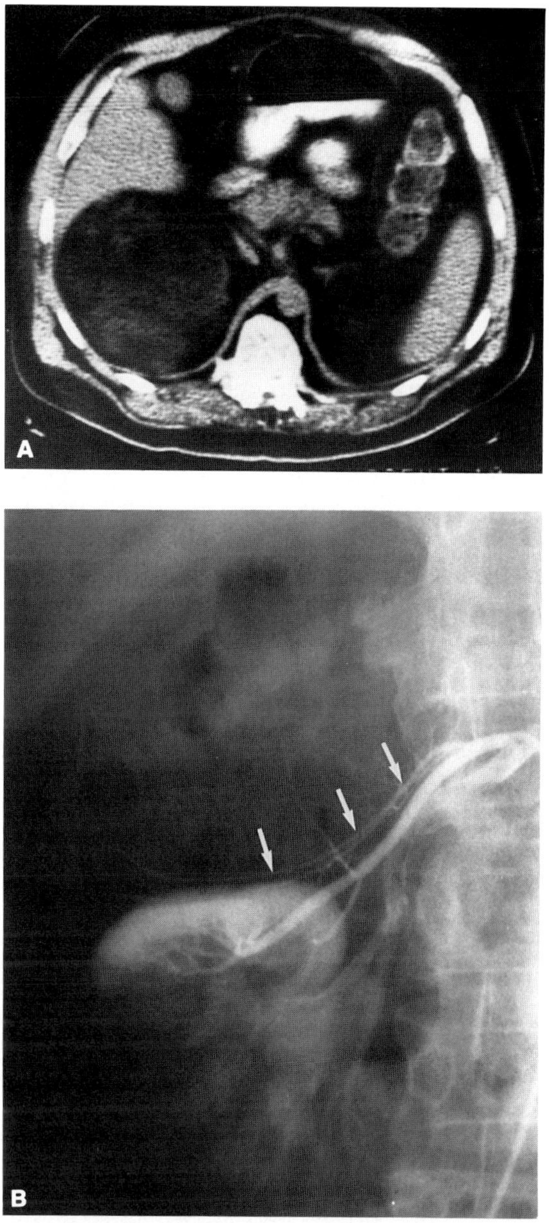

**Figure 25-2.** Myelolipoma of the adrenal. **(A)** CT scan shows a large right-sided mass that compresses the liver and has an attenuation characteristic of fat. **(B)** Renal arteriogram confirms the extrarenal origin of the mass. The inferior adrenal branches are enlarged (*arrows*) and enter the inferior aspect of the mass.

iodobenzylguanadine]) has shown great promise for localizing adrenal medullary lesions and the often elusive extra-adrenal pheochromocytomas.

## Magnetic Resonance Imaging

Several studies have reported that MRI is equal to CT in detecting normal adrenal glands and in identifying a variety of adrenal abnormalities (Fig. 25-3). Initial work indicates that MRI may also be able to characterize an adrenal mass by relating its signal intensity to that of the liver. Using this technique, adenomas could be distinguished from metastases, carcinomas, and pheochromocytomas. Adrenal adenomas have low signal intensity, while pheochromocytomas produce strong signals; carcinomas have intermediate signal strength.

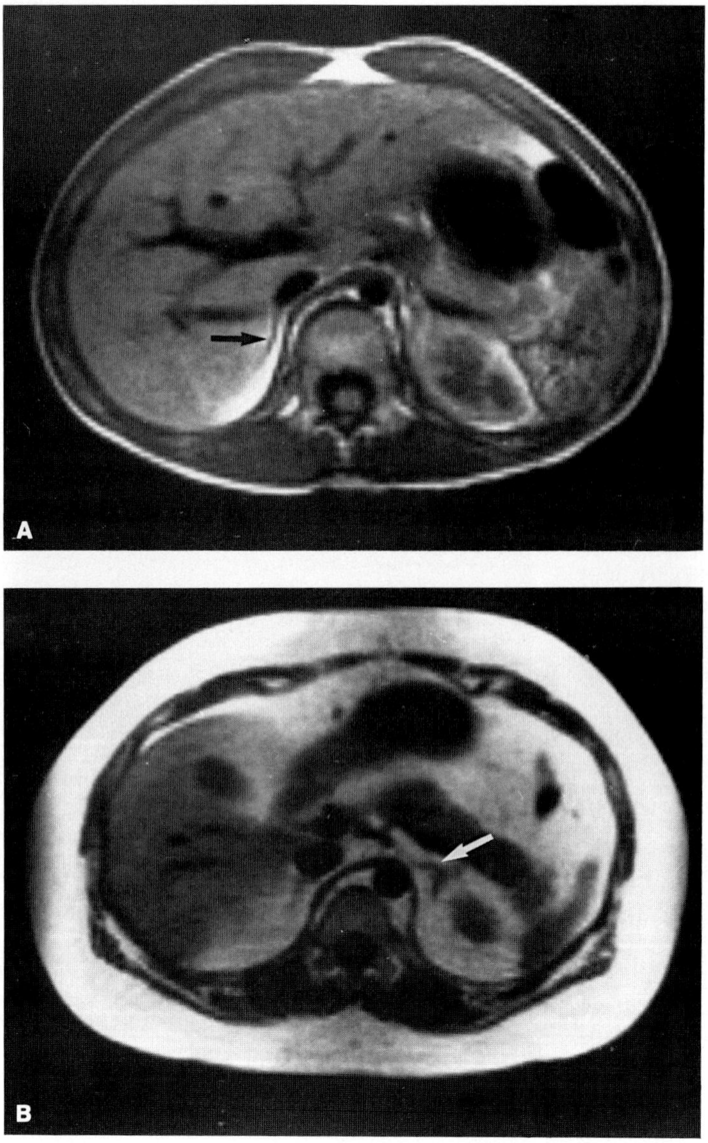


**Figure 25-3.** MR images of normal adrenal glands. **(A)** The right adrenal appears as a linear structure (*arrow*) just posterior to the inferior vena cava. The gland appears relatively dark, because it is surrounded by the strong signal intensity of the perirenal fat. **(B)** The inverted-Y shape of the left adrenal (*arrow*) is seen anteromedial to the kidney. (Courtesy of Jesse Cohen, M.D.)

### Adrenal Arteriography and Venography

Arteriography is rarely indicated in the evaluation of adrenal disease. In patients with extremely large tumors, arteriographic demonstration of the vascular supply may be of value in establishing the adrenal origin, and a preoperative vascular "road map" may be required by the surgeon. In the past, adrenal venography was used to outline the extent of an adrenal mass. However, this role of venography has been eliminated by CT and ultrasound. In some patients with aldosteronism, adrenal venography with venous sampling still remains an important modality for localizing an underlying tumor that may be too small to be detected by CT. To verify the adrenal origin of the sample, it is important to also measure the level of cortisol. The right adrenal vein is small and usually difficult to catheterize. On the left, it is essential to be certain that the sample is not obtained from the inferior phrenic vein, which joins the adrenal vein before entering the renal vein.

### Needle Aspiration

Needle aspiration of the adrenal gland is most often performed under CT guidance. Larger lesions, however, may also be biopsied using either ultrasound or fluoroscopy. The major role of needle aspiration of adrenal masses is to document metastatic disease. In addition, needle aspiration can be used in questionable cases to confirm the diagnosis of an adrenal cyst.

On the right, the adrenal gland is often entirely suprarenal so that a direct posterior approach is possible. Some right-sided lesions may be reached via the transhepatic route (Fig. 25-4). In general, the anterior approach to right-sided masses should be avoided, because this usually necessitates traversing the inferior vena cava. On the left, the anterior approach is more feasible, because the adrenal gland is situated anterior and medial to the kidney. Depending on the location of the mass and the individual patient's anatomy, some left-sided masses may also be reached via a direct posterior route.

## APPROACH TO INDIVIDUAL DISEASE ENTITIES

### Cushing's Syndrome

Appropriate therapy for Cushing's syndrome cannot be initiated until the underlying cause has been determined. Imaging studies are necessary to distinguish patients with Cushing's disease caused by bilateral adrenal hyperfunction due to a pituitary disorder from those with a primary adrenal neoplasm or an ectopic source of adrenocorticotropic hormone (ACTH) production. Clinical history and laboratory studies (*e.g.*, ACTH levels, dexamethasone suppression test) can often point to the correct diagnosis. Patients with an adrenal tumor causing Cushing's syndrome have low ACTH levels, while those with an ectopic source of ACTH have higher levels of this hormone. The administration of dexamethasone suppresses cortical steroid production in patients with bilateral adrenal hyperplasia, while it has no effect on those with primary adrenal tumors or an ectopic source of ACTH.

Adrenal adenomas and micronodular hyperplasia can be cured by appropriate adrenal surgery. In contrast, the results of surgery for adrenal carcinoma are poor. Cushing's disease in children traditionally has been treated by pituitary irradiation, although success has been recently reported with transsphenoidal microadenomectomies. The therapy of choice for adults with Cushing's disease is transsphenoidal resection of the responsible pituitary tumor, which has a cure rate of 70% to 90%. In the event of therapeutic failure, pituitary irradiation can be used. If neither of these forms of therapy is successful, bilateral adrenalectomy can be performed. This cures Cushing's syndrome, but it requires that the patient receive lifelong steroid replacement.

Because transsphenoidal hypophysectomy is the primary treatment for the patient with generalized adrenal hyperfunction due to a pituitary microadenoma, it is vitally important that a discrete adrenal mass be excluded as the cause of

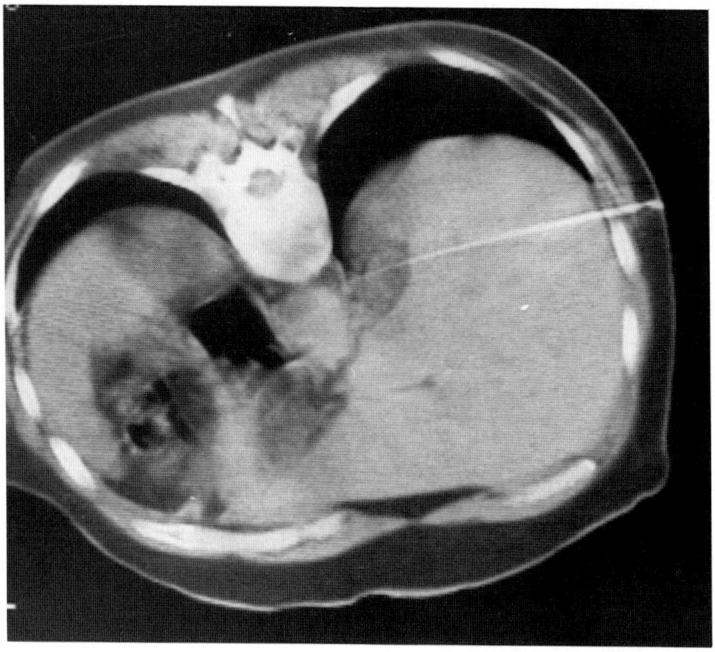

**Figure 25-4.** Right adrenal biopsy (prone position). The transhepatic route was used to reach this right adrenal mass.

Cushing's syndrome. High-resolution CT scanners can detect adrenal adenomas or carcinomas with virtually 100% accuracy. Diagnostic pitfalls on CT scanning may be related to adjacent pseudotumors, such as opacified bowel loops, ectopic spleen, blood vessels, or the gastric fundus. Since preoperative evaluation of the sella turcica by computed or conventional tomography is unreliable in patients with Cushing's disease, negative tomographic examinations do not exclude a microadenoma and will not preclude surgical exploration.

Hyperfunctioning adrenal glands causing Cushing's syndrome may appear on CT to be diffusely enlarged with retention of their basic shape (Fig. 25-5); at times, no enlargement of the glands can be detected. A possible problem is the differentiation of an adrenal adenoma from nodular hyperplasia of the gland. Hyperplastic macronodules are usually less than 2 cm in diameter, are often multiple, and may be found in enlarged glands. In contrast, most adenomas are 2.5 cm or more in size and tend to be solitary when the patient presents clinically with Cushing's syndrome (Fig. 25-6).

Although adrenal venography is a reliable technique for demonstrating an adrenal tumor in a patient with Cushing's syndrome (Fig. 25-7), this modality is rarely necessary if CT and the dexamethasone suppression test are available. Recent studies have indicated the value of venous sampling of the pituitary effluent in the petrosal sinuses to localize the central source of ACTH production in patients with adrenal hyperfunction. Concomitant sampling of other systemic veins also may aid in localizing the source of ectopic ACTH production.

Radionuclide studies in patients with Cushing's syndrome demonstrate bilaterally symmetric uptake of isotope in those with adrenal hyperfunction but unilateral uptake in the presence of a functioning tumor. This modality is also useful in detecting adrenal remnants in the patient who has previously undergone bilateral adrenalectomies and presents with a recurrence of the endocrinopathy.

## Aldosteronism

Hypertension due to primary aldosteronism is associated with persistent hypokalemia, an in-

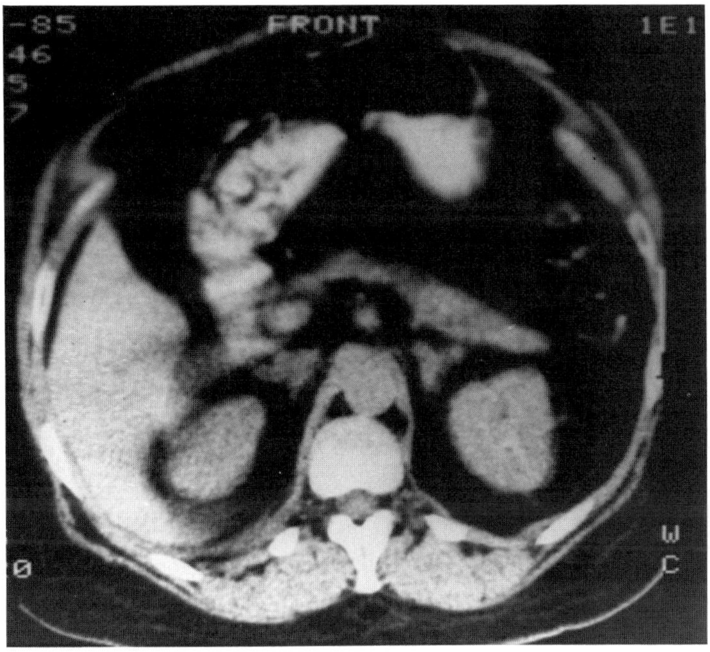


**Figure 25-5.** Cushing's syndrome due to adrenal hyperfunction. Both glands are large, although their basic shapes are intact.

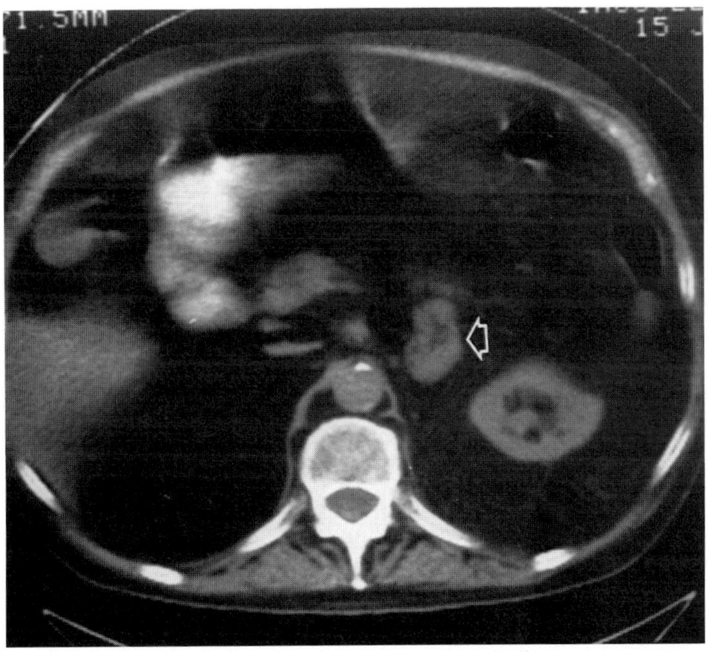

**Figure 25-6.** Cushing's syndrome due to a cortical adenoma. There is a lobulated mass (*arrow*) anterior and medial to the left kidney.

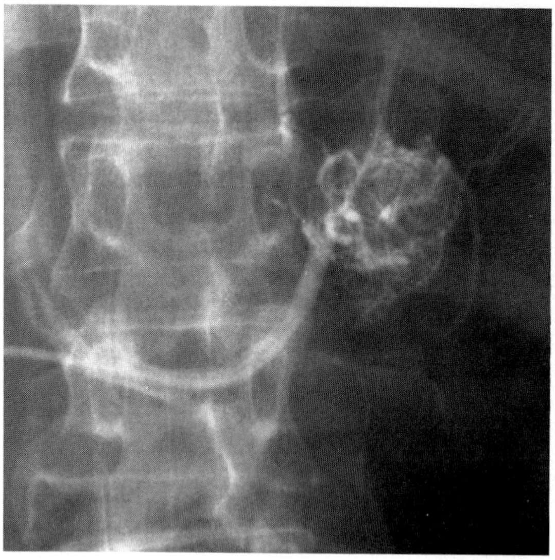

**Figure 25-7.** Cushing's syndrome due to an adenoma. Left adrenal venogram clearly demonstrates the tumor.

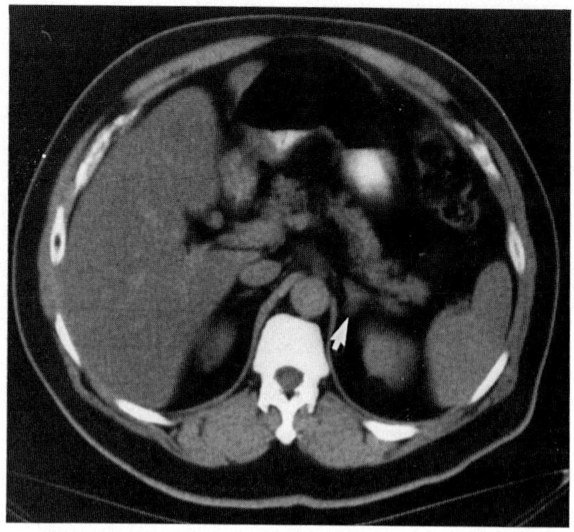

**Figure 25-8.** Aldosteronoma. CT scan shows a questionable area of decreased attenuation (*arrow*) in the medial aspect of the left adrenal gland. Although an adrenal venogram did not show the lesion, venous blood samples localized the adenoma to the left.

crease in plasma and urine aldosterone levels, and suppressed plasma renin activity. Approximately 2% of hypertensives (8% in the black population) have this syndrome. Up to 90% of patients with primary aldosteronism have an adrenal cortical adenoma that is surgically curable. Most of the remaining patients have idiopathic aldosteronism, which is often associated with adrenal cortical hyperplasia and may be related to an underlying pituitary abnormality. It is essential to distinguish hypertensive patients with an adrenal cortical adenoma from those with idiopathic aldosteronism. Resection of an adrenal cortical adenoma cures both hypertension and hypokalemia, whereas adrenalectomy fails to relieve hypertension in a patient with adrenal hyperplasia.

Computed tomography is the imaging modality of choice for evaluating the patient with aldosteronism. Nevertheless, the small size of many aldosterone adenomas (which can be hidden within the contour of a normal-sized gland) makes CT much less sensitive in these patients than in those with cortical adenomas associated with Cushing's syndrome (Fig. 25-8). The CT demonstration of several small adrenal masses suggests the diagnosis of nodular hyperplasia; at times, it may be impossible to distinguish an adenoma from a single prominent nodule associated with nodular hyperplasia.

Adrenal venography with venous sampling can localize virtually all aldosterone adenomas that cannot be detected by CT. Aldosterone levels from the positive side are usually substantially higher than those from the normal side. The major complication of adrenal venography is rupture of the vein, which has been reported in 5% to 8% of patients. For this reason, it is generally good practice to collect the venous sample before attempting to obtain a contrast venogram.

An alternative approach to distinguishing cortical adenomas from adrenal hyperplasia in patients with primary aldosteronism is radionuclide scanning, which has been reported to have high sensitivity and accuracy rates.

## Pheochromocytoma

Pheochromocytomas are found in 0.1% of the hypertensive population. Approximately 10% of pheochromocytomas are malignant, and a similar percentage of tumors are bilateral or arise in an extra-adrenal location. Pheochromocytomas commonly develop in patients with the multiple endocrine neoplasia syndromes and have also been associated with neurofibromatosis and von Hippel–Lindau disease. The laboratory diagnosis of pheochromocytoma requires the demonstration of elevated levels of catecholamines or their metabolites in plasma or urine.

Computed tomography has replaced all previous imaging modalities as the initial examination for the detection and localization of a pheochromocytoma. If the CT scan is negative or equivocal, or demonstrates only a single lesion in a patient in whom there is the suspicion of multiple tumors, ultrasound, adrenal venography and arteriography, or radionuclide scanning may be performed. Recent reports recommend MRI for detecting a pheochromocytoma, especially because with this modality the signal pattern may specify the nature of the tumor, unlike CT, which can merely show the presence of a soft-tissue mass.

Arteriography is rarely used today in evaluating adrenal or extra-adrenal pheochromocytomas. Occasionally, a very large lesion may be studied by arteriography to provide a road map of the vascular supply as an aid to the surgeon. Because of the severe hypertensive reactions that may develop during the injection of contrast material, it is essential that a patient with a suspected pheochromocytoma be premedicated with an α-adrenergic blocking agent. An intravenous drip of phentolamine hydrochloride should be running, and careful monitoring of the electrocardiogram and blood pressure is mandatory. In the past, venography was used to localize pheochromocytomas, because the adrenal has only one draining vein requiring contrast injection as opposed to the multiple injections required to visualize the several arteries supplying the gland. However, venography requires the same precautions as arteriography and is now rarely used.

### Nonfunctioning Adrenal Adenomas

With the increasing use of CT scanning and its superb visualization of the adrenal gland, incidental adrenal adenomas are being discovered in almost 1% of cases. The management of patients with incidentally detected, nonfunctioning adrenal adenomas has become an important issue. If the patient has no clinical or biochemical evidence of adrenal hyperfunction and no history of malignant disease, the lesion can be followed without surgery. Computed tomographic criteria that support the diagnosis of an incidental adrenal adenoma include smooth, round or oval contours; a mass less than 5 cm in diameter; clear separation of the tumor margins from adjacent structures; and no growth of the lesion on serial CT scans performed at 3-, 6-, and 12-month intervals. This last point usually permits differentiation of incidental adenomas from adrenal carcinomas, which often exhibit significant growth within a year. Adrenal carcinomas occasionally present as nonfunctioning tumors, but in such cases they typically have irregular contours, are larger than 8 cm at the time of diagnosis, and often invade adjacent structures or show evidence of distant metastases. Calcifications and differences in tissue attenuation on CT are unreliable in differentiating benign from malignant adrenal masses.

### Metastatic Disease

The adrenal gland is a frequent site of metastases, especially from carcinomas of the lung. As a result, it has become standard practice to include CT scans of the adrenal glands in the preoperative assessment of patients with lung tumors (Fig. 25-9). Other malignancies that tend to metastasize to the adrenal gland are breast and thyroid carcinomas, gastrointestinal tumors, lymphoma, and melanoma. Unfortunately, CT cannot distinguish adrenal metastases from other masses within the gland. In the absence of adrenal hyperfunction, bilateral adrenal masses in a patient with a known primary tumor are highly suggestive of metastatic disease. In contrast, a solitary nonfunctioning adrenal tumor in a patient with a known malignancy is not considered pathognomonic for metastatic disease. In two series, only about half of the adrenal masses detected in patients with known primary

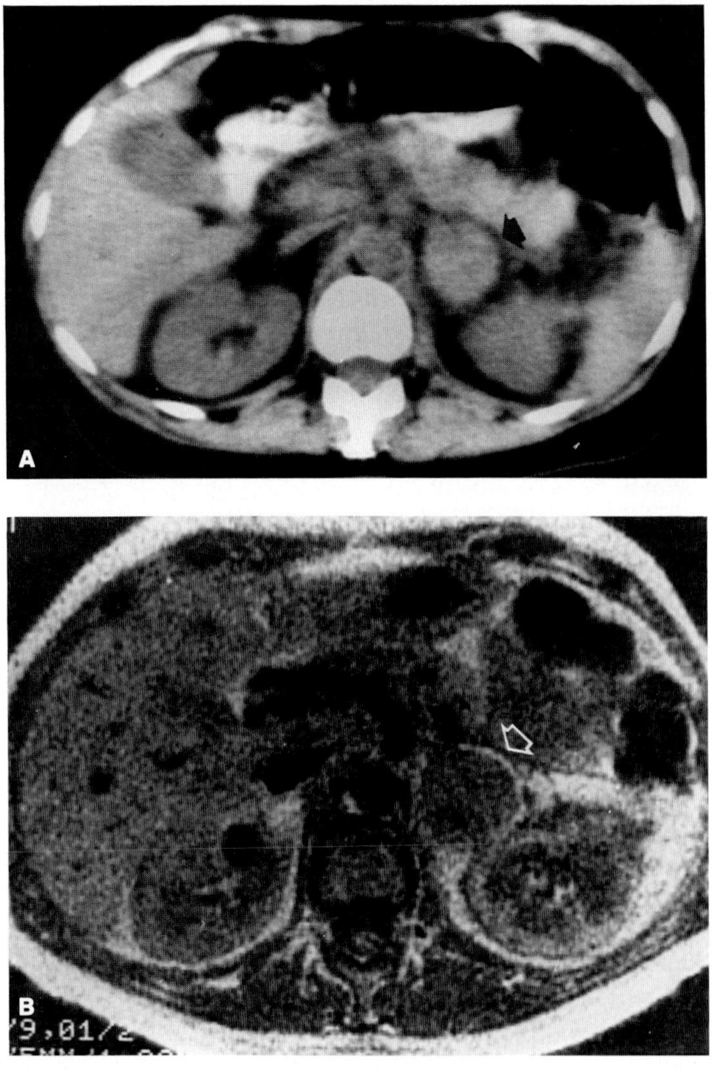

**Figure 25-9.** Left adrenal metastases from carcinoma of the lung. **(A)** CT scan clearly defines a left adrenal mass (*arrow*) anteromedial to the kidney. **(B)** MRI using spin-echo technique (TR, 610 msec; TE, 28 msec) shows the adrenal mass to be of somewhat less signal intensity than the normal hepatic parenchyma.

tumors proved to be malignant when biopsied. Therefore, percutaneous aspiration biopsy with CT, ultrasound, or fluoroscopic guidance should be performed in these patients to distinguish metastases from an incidental adenoma or a primary adrenal carcinoma.

## Bibliography


Abrams HL, Siegelman SS, Adams DF et al: Computed tomography versus ultrasound of the adrenal gland: A prospective study. Radiology 143: 121–128, 1982

Bennett AH, Harrison JH, Thorn GW: Neoplasms of the adrenal gland. J Urol 106:607, 1971

Bernadino ME, McClellan MW, Phillips VM et al: CT-guided adrenal biopsy. Accuracy, safety, and indications. AJR 144:67–69, 1985

Bravo EL, Gifford RW Jr: Pheochromocytoma: Diagnosis, localization, and management. N Engl J Med 311:1298–1303, 1984

Brunt LM, Wells SA: The multiple endocrine neoplasia syndromes. Invest Radiol 20:916–927, 1985

Carey RM, Sin S, Dolan LM et al: Idiopathic hyperaldosteronism: A possible role for aldosterone-stimulating factor. N Engl J Med 311:94–99, 1984

Dunnick NR, Doppman JL, Gill JR et al: Localization of functional adrenal tumors by computed tomography and venous sampling. Radiology 142: 429–433, 1983

Franco-Saenz R, Mulrow PJ, Kim K: Idiopathic aldosteronism: A possible disease of the intermediate lobe of the pituitary. JAMA 251: 2555–2558, 1984

Ganguly A, Donohue JP: Primary aldosteronism: Pathophysiology, diagnosis and treatment. J Urol 129:241–247, 1983

Ganguly A, Weinberger MH: Preoperative distinction of adenoma from hyperplasia in primary aldosteronism. J Nucl Med 20:7, 1979

Glazer HS, Weyman PJ, Sagel SS et al: Nonfunctioning adrenal masses: Incidental discovery on computed tomography. AJR 139:81–85, 1982

Glazer GM, Woolsey EJ, Borrello J et al: Adrenal tissue characterization using MR Imaging. Radiology 158:73–79, 1986

Gross MD, Thompson NW, Beierwaltes WH: Scintigraphic approach to the localization of adrenal lesions causing hypertension. Urol Radiol 3: 241–244, 1982

Ishikawa H, Tachibana M, Hata M et al: Myelolipoma of the adrenal gland. J Urol 126:733–739, 1981

Karstaedt N, Sagel SS, Stanley RJ et al: Computed tomography of the adrenal gland. Radiology 129: 723–730, 1978

Katz RL, Shirkhoda A: Diagnostic approach to incidental adrenal nodules in the cancer patient: Results of a clinical, radiologic and fine needle aspiration study. Cancer 55:1995–2000, 1985

Khuri FJ, Alton DJ, Hardy BE et al: Adrenal hemorrhage in neonates: Report of 5 cases and review of the literature. J Urol 124:684, 1980

Mitnick JS, Bosniak MA, Megibow AJ: Nonfunctioning adrenal adenomas discovered incidentally on computed tomography. Radiology 148:495–499, 1983

Mitty HA, Gabrilove JL, Nicolis GL: Non-tumorous adrenal hyperfunction: Problems in angiographic–clinical correlation. Radiology 122:89, 1977

Mitty HA, Yeh HC: Radiology of the Adrenals with Sonography and CT. Philadelphia, WB Saunders, 1982

Moon KL, Hricak H, Crooks LE et al: Nuclear magnetic resonance imaging of the adrenal gland: A preliminary report. Radiology 147:155–160, 1983

Oldfield EH, Chrousos GP, Schulte HM et al: Preoperative lateralization of ACTH-secreting pituitary microadenomas by bilateral and simultaneous inferior petrosal venous sinus sampling. N Engl J Med 312:100–103, 1985

Reinig JW, Doppman JL, Dwyer AJ et al: Adrenal masses differentiated by MR. Radiology 158: 81–84, 1986

Schultz CL, Haaga JR, Fletcher BD et al: Magnetic resonance imaging of the adrenal gland: A comparison with computed tomography. AJR 143: 1235–1240, 1984

Sisson JC, Shapiro B, Beierwaltes WWH et al: Localizing pheochromocytomas by scintigraphy using $^{131}$I-Metaiochobenzylguanidine. Cancer 34: 86–92, 1984

Sommers SC: Adrenal glands. In Anderson WAD, Kissane JM (eds): Pathology, pp 1658–1679. St. Louis, CV Mosby, 1977

Styne DM, Grumbach MM, Kaplan SL et al: Treatment of Cushing's disease in childhood and adolescence by transsphenoidal microadenomectomy. N Engl J Med 310:889–893, 1983

Tyrrell JB, Brooks RM, Fitzgerald PA et al: Cushing's disease. Selective transsphenoidal resection of pituitary microadenomas. N Engl J Med 298:753, 1978

Welch TJ, Sheedy PF, van Heerden JA et al: Pheochromocytoma: Value of computed tomography. Radiology 148:501–503, 1983

White EA, Schambelan M, Rost CR et al: Use of computed tomography in diagnosing the cause of primary aldosteronism. N Engl J Med 303: 1503–1507, 1980

Yeh HC, Mitty HA, Rose J et al: Ultrasonography of adrenal masses—usual features. Radiology 127: 467–474, 1978

## CUSHING'S SYNDROME

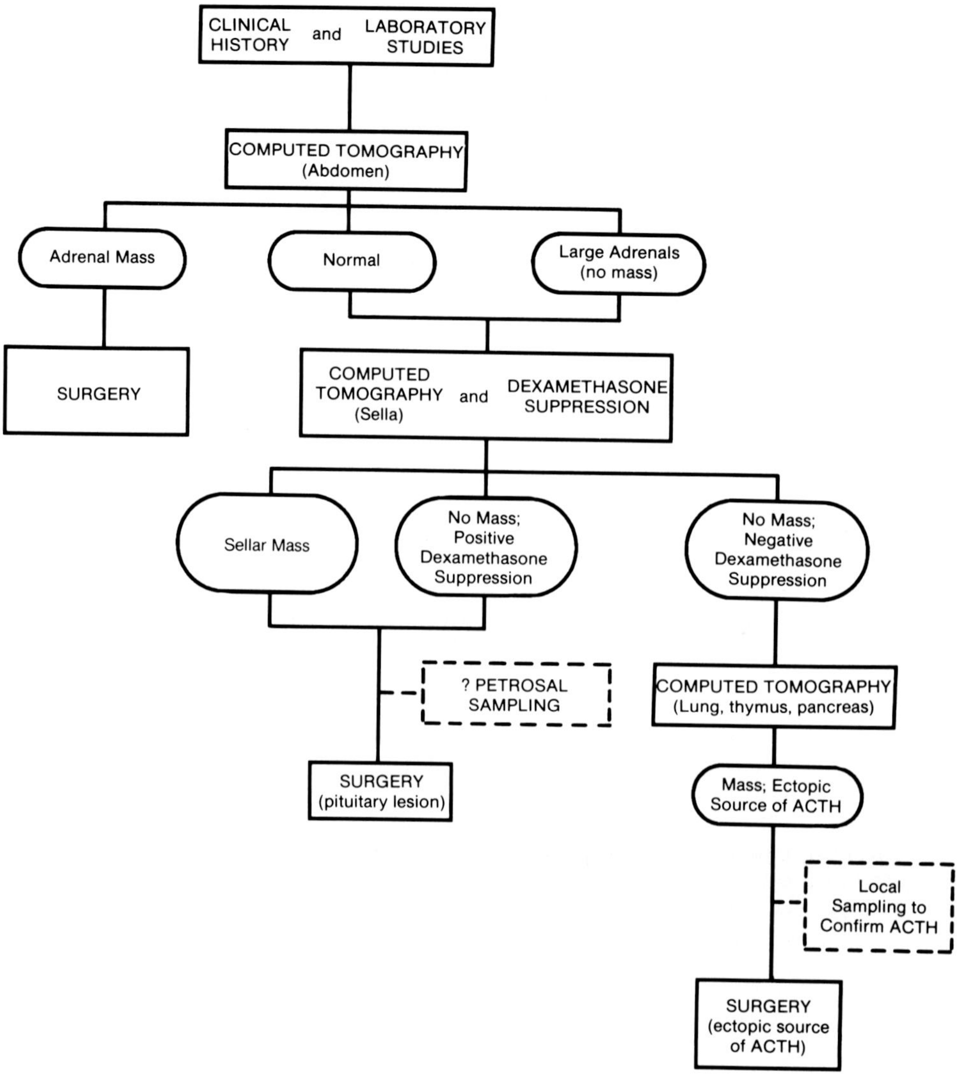

## SUSPECTED ALDOSTERONISM

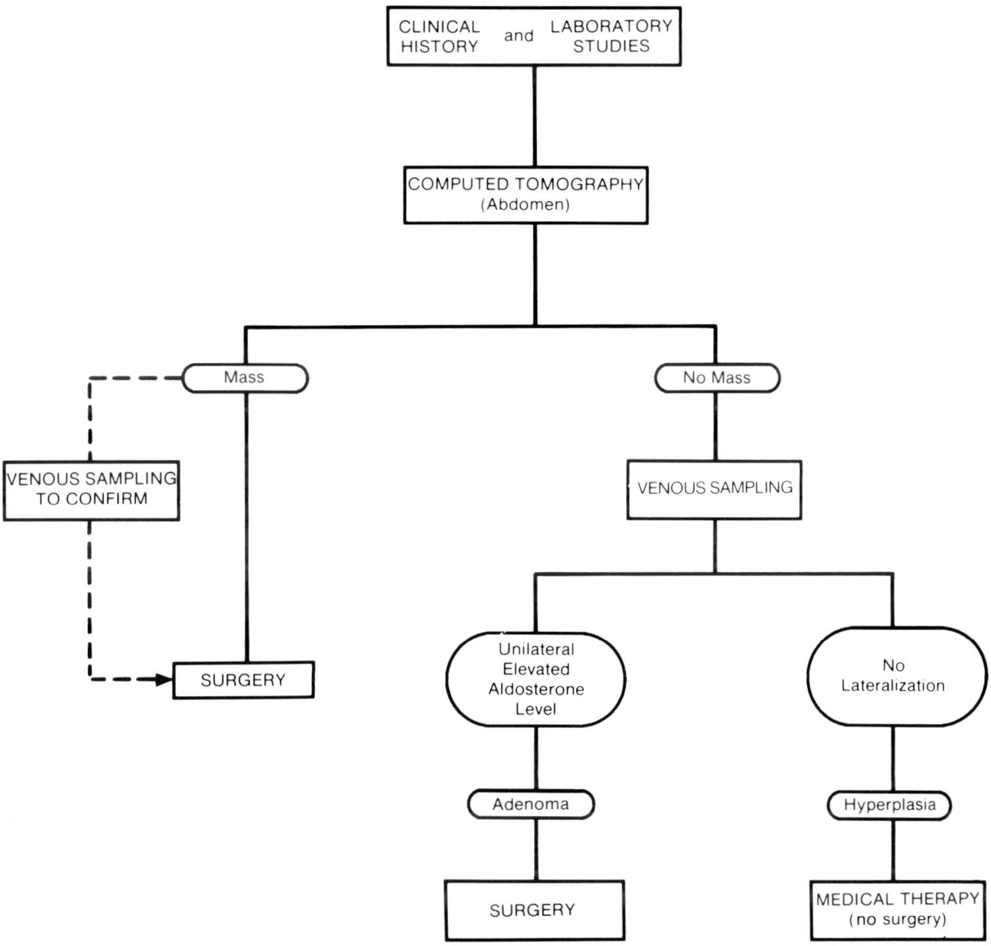

**PHEOCHROMOCYTOMA**

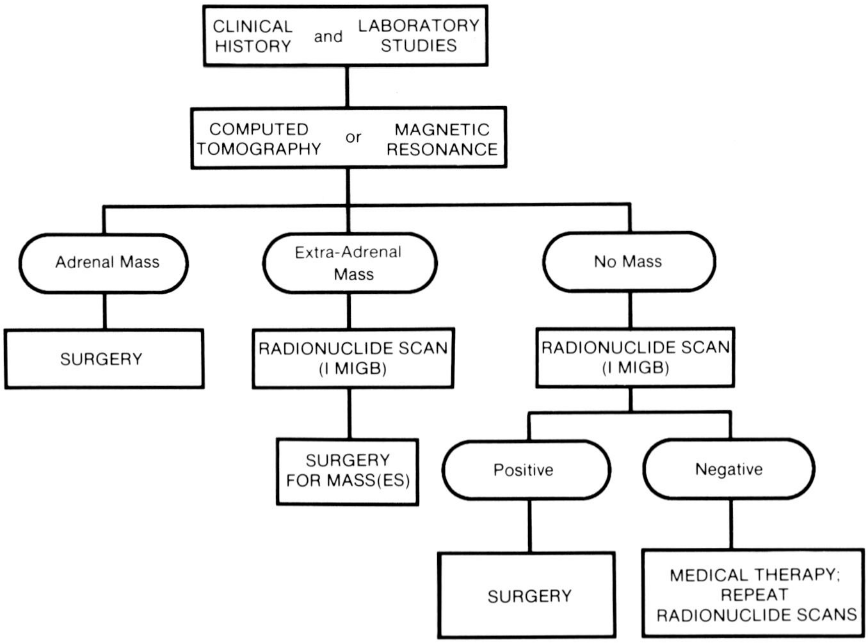

# Chapter 26

# Pelvic Masses

*Arthur C. Fleischer*
*Max I. Shaff*
*Leo F. Drolshagen*
*Faye C. Laing*

A variety of diagnostic studies can be performed to evaluate the patient with a pelvic mass. The selection of the initial imaging modality depends on factors such as the age of the patient, the most likely diagnosis based on clinical and laboratory evaluation, and the accessibility of the diagnostic procedure requested.

## CLINICALLY IMPORTANT PARAMETERS

Regardless of the diagnostic modality utilized, it is essential to obtain certain information that is vital to the appropriate clinical management of the patient. Once a clinically suspected or palpable pelvic mass is documented, it is important to delineate its size, internal consistency, and contour as well as its origin and anatomic relation to other structures. Imaging studies must also demonstrate any evidence of ascites, invasion of neighboring organs, or other signs of metastatic disease.

## DIAGNOSTIC EVALUATION

### *DIAGNOSTIC MODALITIES*

1. Ultrasound
2. Computed tomography
3. Magnetic resonance imaging
4. Excretory urography
5. Barium enema
6. Plain radiography

### Ultrasound

Ultrasound is the modality of choice for evaluating the patient with a pelvic mass that is clinically suspected to be benign or due to an infectious process. It can establish the presence of a mass, its organ of origin, and its internal consistency. The variety of scanning planes that can be obtained with real-time sonography can demonstrate the anatomic relation of a mass relative to the pelvic organs. The entire ultrasound examination can be performed in 20 to 30 minutes once the patient has an adequately distended urinary bladder, and the cost is substantially less than that of computed tomography (CT) or magnetic resonance imaging (MRI).

In diagnosing a pelvic mass, sonography relies on its ability to delineate normal and abnormal structures. The ovaries and uterus can be identified in most patients, although occasionally it may be difficult to show the relatively small ovaries in the postmenopausal patient or an ovary that is surrounded by bowel loops (Fig. 26-1*A*). Indeed, the detailed depiction of the ovary obtainable with sonography is utilized for monitoring ovarian follicular development in patients undergoing ovulation induction. This modality has even been evaluated as a screening test for ovarian carcinoma.

Once a pelvic mass has been documented, the sonographic approach to differential diagnosis involves assessment of the internal consistency of the mass and its organ of origin (Table 26-1). Although the sensitivity of ultrasound in identifying pelvic masses larger than 2 cm is more than 90%, the specificity is substantially lower because of the overlap in the sonographic appearance of various pelvic masses. Certain sonographic findings are highly specific, such as the focal echogenic areas (corresponding to fat and calcification) within a dermoid cyst, and the thin and regular septations within a cystadenoma.

Completely cystic masses have smooth walls, enhanced through transmission, and no internal echoes. The most common pelvic mass with this appearance is the physiologic (follicular or luteal) cyst (Fig. 26-1*B*). A large hydrosalpinx or paraovarian cyst may have a similar appearance. Endometriomas typically contain low-level internal echoes (corresponding to clotted blood), and their borders tend to be more irregular than those of physiologic cysts because of the fibrotic reaction surrounding the mass.

Some types of cystic masses contain septations or small solid areas. Ovarian epithelial tumors produce the quite distinct sonographic appearance of predominantly cystic masses containing thin internal septations (Fig. 26-2). The more irregular and solid the components contained within a predominantly cystic mass, the greater the chance of malignancy. In addition to showing the primary tumor, ultrasound can demonstrate ascites, liver metastases, and even peritoneal or omental metastases.

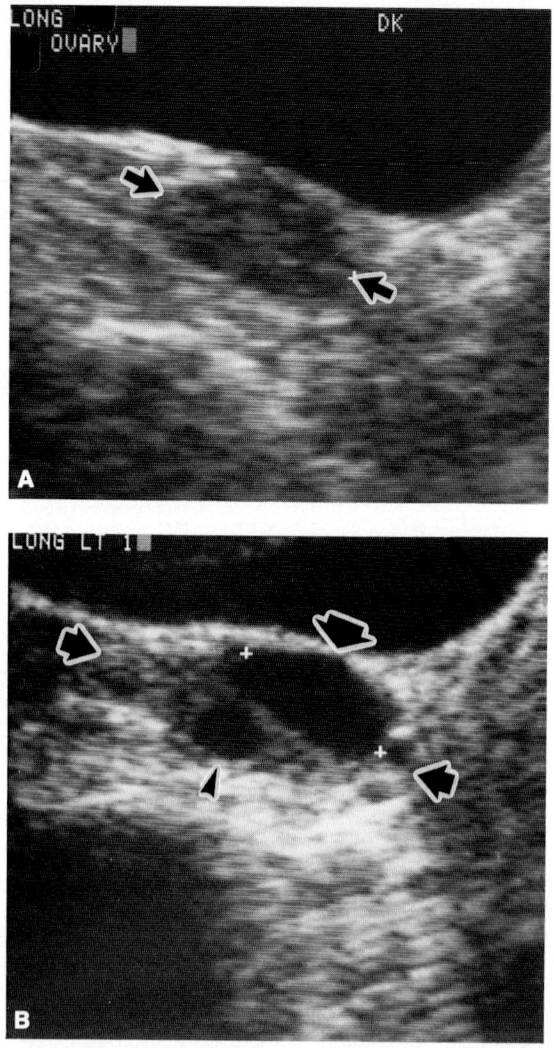


**Figure 26-1.** Longitudinal magnified sonograms of a normal left ovary (*between arrows*). **(A)** "Quiescent" state without follicles (menstrual phase). **(B)** The ovary contains a mature follicle (*large arrow*) and an immature follicle (*arrowhead*) in the late follicular phase.

Complex masses contain both anechoic (fluid) and echoic (solid) areas. The most common pelvic mass with this appearance is the dermoid cyst (Fig. 26-3), which contains high-level

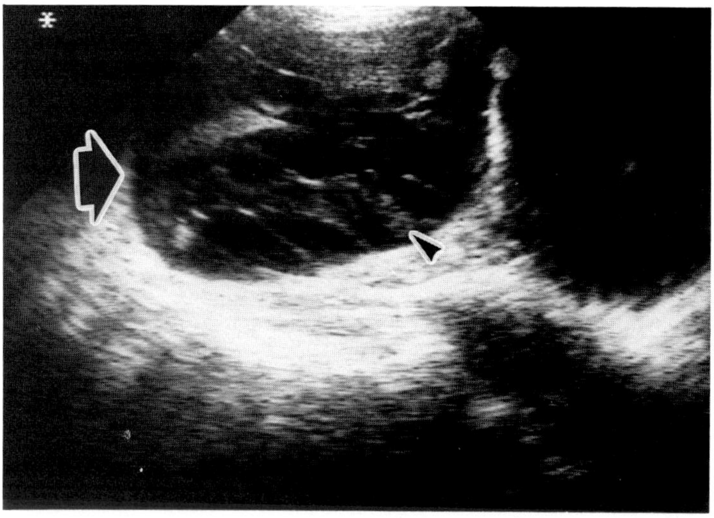

**Figure 26-2.** Mucinous cystadenocarcinoma. Longitudinal pelvic sonogram shows a complex, predominantly cystic mass (*large arrow*), which contains several irregular septations (*arrowhead*).

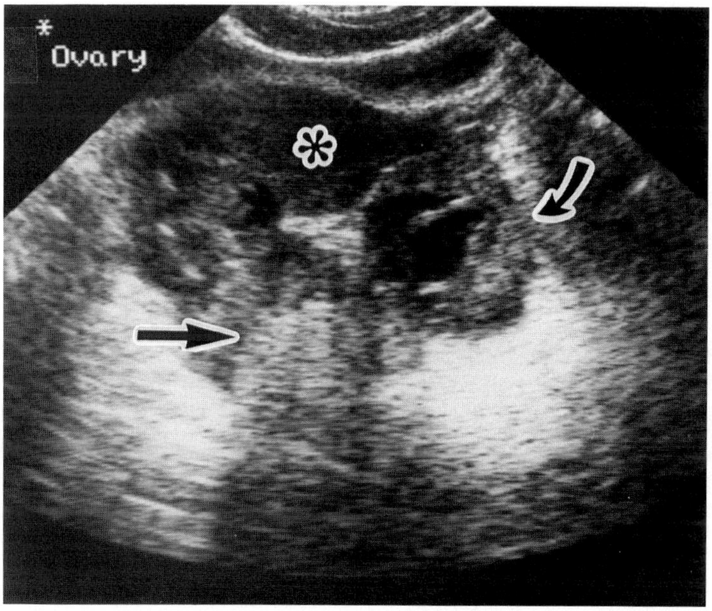


**Figure 26-3.** Transverse pelvic sonogram shows bilateral adnexal masses on either side of the uterus (*asterisk*). The mass on the right contains a focal echogenic area (*straight arrow*) arising from fat within a dermoid cyst. The complex left adnexal mass (*curved arrow*) represents a tubo-ovarian abscess.

echoes related to fat and/or calcification within the mass. Other complex masses include hemorrhagic corpus luteum (Fig. 26-4), ruptured ectopic pregnancy (Figs. 26-5 and 26-6), and tubo-ovarian abscess (Fig. 26-6). Intraovarian masses usually can be distinguished from extraovarian masses by demonstrating the rim of ovarian tissue that surrounds an intraovarian mass.

Ultrasound is the imaging modality of choice for evaluating the patient with a suspected ectopic pregnancy, because it can demonstrate the adnexal mass and confirm the lack of an intrauterine pregnancy (Fig. 26-6). The size and consistency of the mass associated with an ectopic pregnancy depends on the gestational age of the pregnancy and whether or not rupture has occurred (see Fig. 26-4). Ultrasound alone can de-

(*Text continues on p. 392.*)

**Table 26-1** Sonographic Differential Diagnoses of Pelvic Masses*

| Cystic | Complex | Solid |
|---|---|---|
| Completely Cystic | Predominantly Cystic | Uterine |
| Physiologic ovarian cyst<br>Cystadenoma<br>Hydrosalpinx<br>Endometrioma | Cystadenoma<br>Tubo-ovarian abscess<br>Ectopic pregnancy<br>Cystic teratoma | Leiomyoma (sarcoma)<br>Endometrial carcinoma, sarcoma |
| Multiple | Predominantly Solid | Extra-uterine |
| Endometriomas | Cystadenoma (carcinoma)<br>Germ cell tumor | Solid ovarian tumor |
| Septated | | |
| Cystadenoma (carcinoma)<br>Mucinous<br>Serous<br>Papillary | | |

* Based on most common appearance

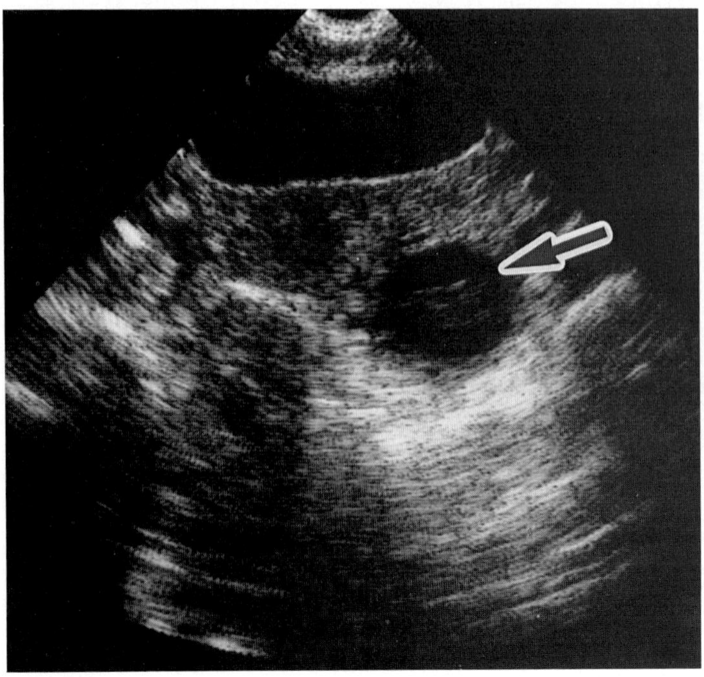

**Figure 26-4.** Hemorrhagic corpus luteum. Transverse pelvic sonogram shows a complex left adnexal mass containing a layer of echogenic material (*arrow*) arising from organized clot.

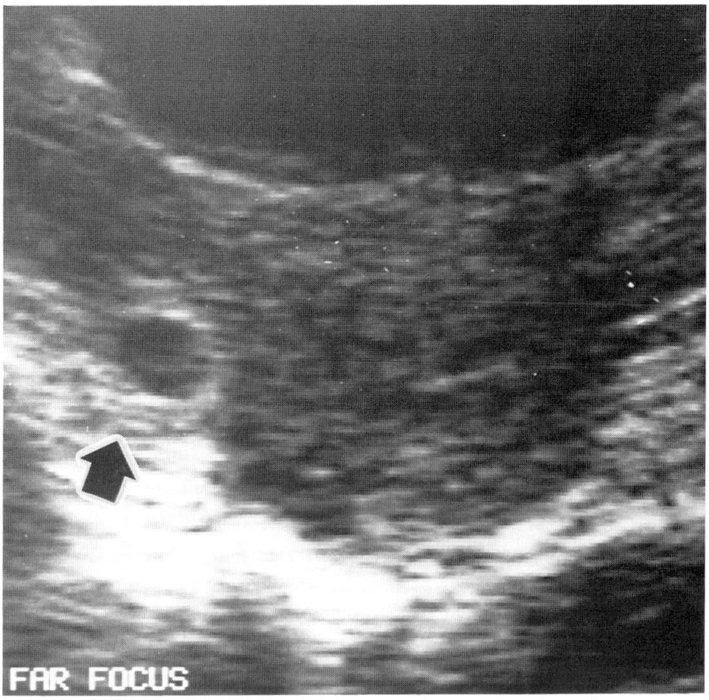


**Figure 26-5.** Sonogram shows an unruptured right tubal ectopic pregnancy (*arrow*) as a rounded mass with an echogenic rim and a hypoechoic center.

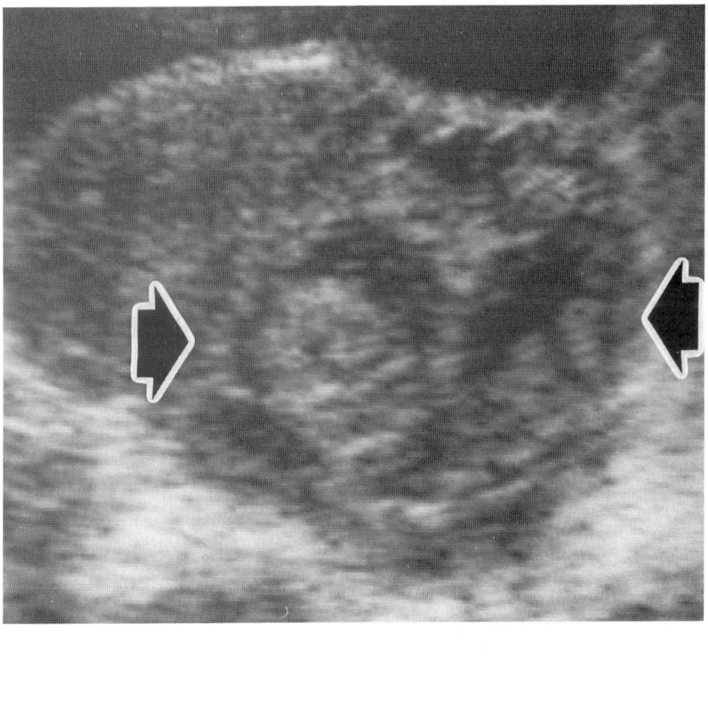

**Figure 26-6.** Magnified transverse pelvic sonogram demonstrates a solid left adnexal mass (*arrows*), which represents an irregularly shaped hematoma resulting from a ruptured ectopic pregnancy.

tect approximately 80% of ectopic pregnancies; when combined with the results of a sensitive pregnancy test (β-hCG), ultrasound is approximately 90% accurate in establishing the diagnosis of ectopic pregnancy. An ectopic pregnancy may coexist with a corpus luteum, and the sonographic appearance of these two masses can be similar.

Solid pelvic masses have an echogenic texture, and their differential diagnosis depends largely on their organ of origin. Most solid pelvic masses arise from the uterus and represent leiomyomas (Fig. 26-7). Except for pedunculated subserosal fibroids, the contiguity of leiomyomas to the uterus usually can be demonstrated. Other solid masses in the pelvis include uncommmon types of ovarian tumors (dysgerminoma, adenocarcinoma), chronic ectopic pregnancies, pelvic hematomas, and enlarged ovaries resulting from intermittent ovarian torsion.

A large bulky uterus resulting from uterine malignancy (*e.g.*, sarcoma) occasionally presents as a pelvic mass contiguous with the uterus. Recent studies have suggested that sonography can be used to evaluate the depth of myometrial invasion in patients with endometrial carcinoma, and thus potentially affect their pre- and postsurgical management.

Ultrasound plays an important role in evaluating the pregnant patient who presents with a pelvic mass. Completely cystic masses (luteal cysts, benign epithelial tumors) can be distinguished from complex or solid masses (dermoid cysts, leiomyomas). Ultrasound provides an objective means to assess growth or regression of the mass during pregnancy, as well as any evidence of torsion or other complications.

The major limitations of the sonographic evaluation of pelvic masses involve problems with surrounding bowel gas obscuring delineation of lesions in the lower abdomen or retroperitoneum. In the lower pelvis and cul-de-sac, bowel gas can be displaced by using a water enema during the sonographic evaluation. In the lower abdomen and pelvis, most pelvic masses displace bowel loops to a sufficient degree that

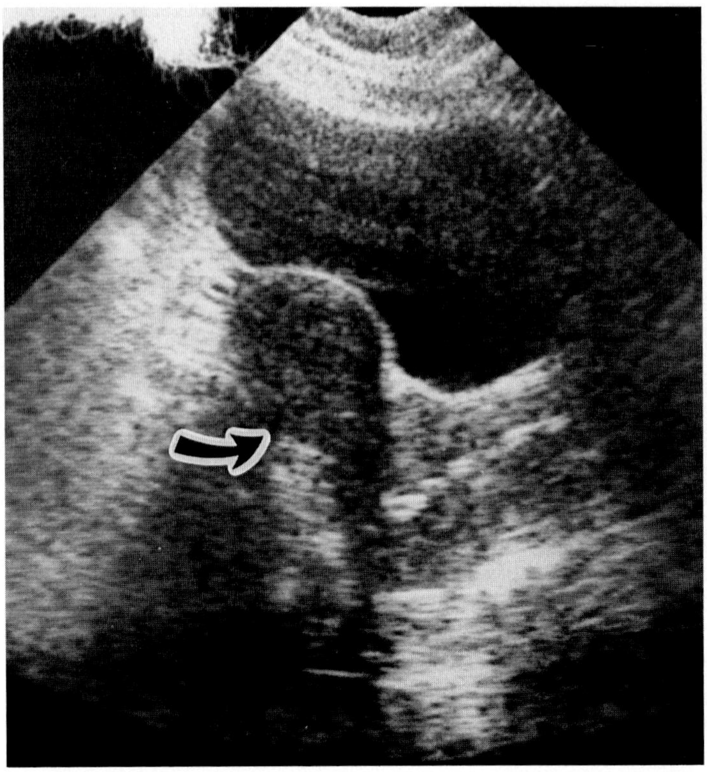

**Figure 26-7.** Fibroid in a retroflexed uterus. Long-axis sonogram shows the fibroid as a relatively hypoechoic area (*arrow*) contiguous with the uterine outline.

they can be adequately imaged. Tumor extension and the presence of lymphadenopathy are difficult to demonstrate on ultrasound and are better depicted by CT.

New developments in gynecologic sonography include transducers that can be placed intravaginally and some that can scan radially when placed within the lumen of the uterus. The endovaginal approach permits better demonstration of the area of the cervix and pelvic sidewalls. Endovaginal scanning also may improve imaging of the ovaries or masses that are located deep within the pelvis or cul-de-sac, because the transducer can be placed closer to these structures. The intraluminal uterine scanner is being evaluated in some centers as a means to evaluate the depth of myometrial invasion of uterine tumors.

## Computed Tomography

The major role of CT in the examination of the pelvis is to evaluate and stage neoplastic processes. It can clearly delineate normal and pathologic anatomy, and it can readily differentiate soft-tissue structures, fat planes, bone, and bowel gas. Indeed, the inherent contrast provided by fat and air contained in normal pelvic structures increases the contrast resolution of CT in this region. The administration of oral, rectal, and intravenous iodinated contrast material accentuates attenuation differences between normal and diseased tissue and can delineate the rectum, small and large bowel, ureters, and bladder. Oral contrast material should be used liberally in the examination of the female pelvis to permit differentiation of bowel loops from true masses with attenuation properties similar to those of fluid-filled bowel.

Narrow contiguous sections (2 mm–4 mm) or narrow overlapped slices are obtained when multiplanar reconstruction is contemplated. Unlike MRI, multiplanar reconstructed CT images have inferior spatial resolution compared with axial sections. The quality of the reconstructed images can be improved by obtaining multiple overlapped sections through the area of interest. Sections 8 mm to 10 mm apart are sufficient to evaluate large lesions or for scanning the pelvis in a patient in whom there is little suspicion of a mass lesion.

Computed tomography can demonstrate the size and volume of tumor, its internal characteristics (fat or calcium content), and evidence of contiguous spread or direct invasion of neighboring structures, such as bowel, ureter, and pelvic sidewalls. It also can reliably identify distant metastases (Fig. 26-8). A routine abdominal

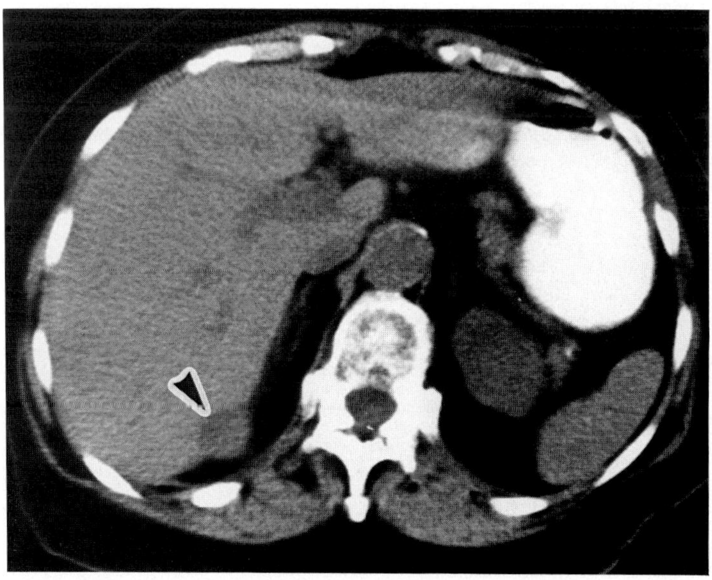

**Figure 26-8.** Serosal liver metastases (*arrowhead*) from ovarian carcinoma. These tumors typically spread to the serosal surface of the liver rather than metastasizing within the parenchyma.

scan may detect tumor spread to cutaneous, subcutaneous, intra-abdominal, and retroperitoneal structures. If clinically warranted, scans of the head, chest, or extremities can be obtained. Computed tomography is inferior only to radionuclide scintigraphy in detecting bone metastases.

Computed tomography is very sensitive in identifying small volumes of ascites. It is occasionally more accurate than ultrasound, which may fail to detect small amounts of peritoneal fluid that are concealed from the probe by bowel gas, bone, or surgical dressings. In general, exudative ascites has a higher CT attenuation value than transudative ascites (Fig. 26-9). Sedimentation of proteinaceous material often produces a fluid–fluid layer that reflects the different densities. Serosal and omental "cake" metastases can be easily identified, especially on contrast-enhanced scans.

Computed tomography can evaluate the kidneys, bladder, and ureters. Hydronephrosis, urinomas, and urinary leaks are easily identified. The entire course of the ureters can be followed even without contrast opacification, because unopacified urine in a hydroureter provides sufficient contrast for detection. The precise site of ureteral obstruction usually can be demonstrated (Fig. 26-10). Ureteral or extraureteral masses can be differentiated from fibrosis. Computed tomography can demonstrate invasion of the bladder with greater accuracy than excretory urography.

Computed tomography can identify lymph node enlargement (>1.5 cm) at or remote from the site of a primary tumor (Fig. 26-11). However, this modality may be unable to differentiate inflammatory from neoplastic lymphadenopathy. In the pelvis, lymph nodes may be difficult to differentiate from blood vessels and redundant loops of bowel. Therefore, patients may have to be rescanned after additional oral contrast or with dynamic rapid sequential scans following bolus intravenous contrast enhancement to conclusively differentiate lymphadenopathy from normal vascular or intestinal structures. Lymph node aspiration under CT guidance can be extremely useful. In experienced hands, marginally enlarged lymph nodes can be successfully aspirated.

Computed tomography can aid in differentiating benign cystic disease from malignancy by demonstrating a homogeneous fluid-filled mass without internal solid elements or septations and enclosed by a thin cyst wall. Because CT numbers are unreliable for tissue characterization, equivocal masses should be evaluated by ultrasound. Benign cysts occasionally are multilocular, septated, or contain high-density internal elements due to hemorrhage; if these features

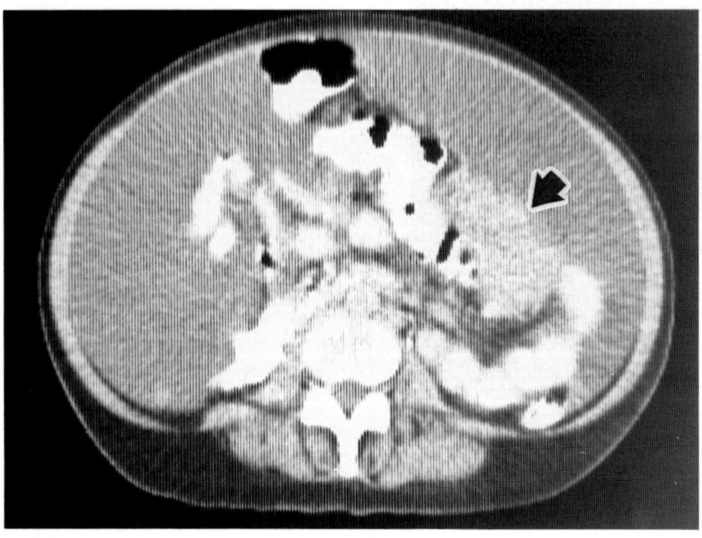

**Figure 26-9.** CT scan shows ascites and omental metastases (*arrow*) associated with ovarian malignancy.

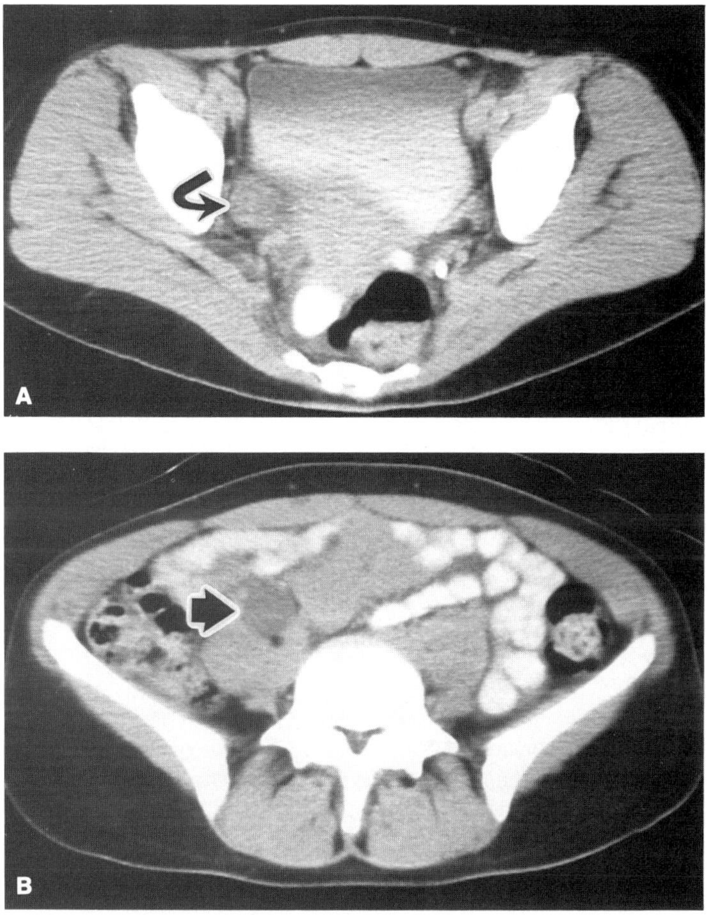

**Figure 26-10.** Advanced cervical carcinoma. **(A)** Cervical carcinoma (*arrow*) extending to the right pelvic sidewall. **(B)** Right hydroureter (*arrow*).

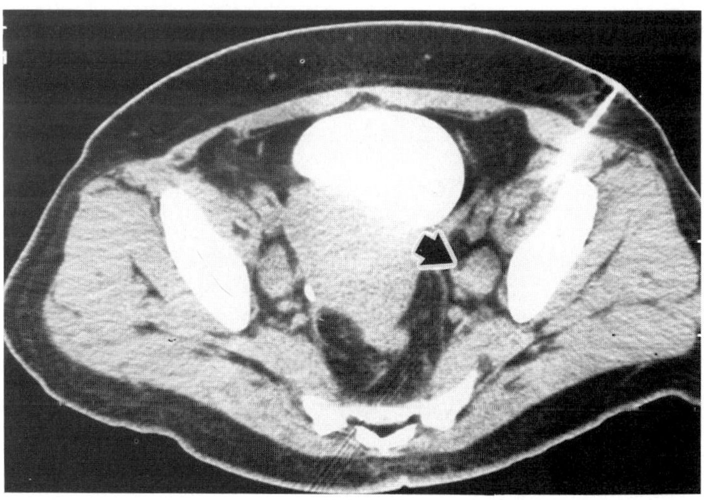

**Figure 26-11.** Metastatic cervical carcinoma. The biopsy needle is seen traversing the left iliopsoas muscle into the left obturator nodes (*arrow*). The biopsy was positive for metastatic involvement.

are present, percutaneous biopsy or surgical intervention is necessary to exclude malignancy.

Percutaneous fine-needle biopsy can be performed under CT guidance to obtain cytologic evaluation of malignancy (Fig. 26-11). Pathologic tissue can even be obtained from small and remote retroperitoneal deposits, thus often saving the cancer patient from exploratory surgery. Computed tomographic guidance also can be used for the aspiration and drainage of pelvic abscesses and other fluid collections.

Because CT can clearly show the relation of a tumor to surrounding structures, it has become an important aid in determining the appropriate surgical strategy (complete respectability, amenability to debulking procedures, inoperability). Computed tomography can be used to design the boundaries of radiation ports. After the insertion of radiation applicators, CT can permit accurate dosimetric determination and can detect unsuspected uterine perforation.

Computed tomography is the imaging modality of choice for detecting recurrent tumor from a pelvic malignancy. However, postoperative and irradiation changes may be indistinguishable from recurrent tumor.

## Magnetic Resonance Imaging

Because of its cost effectiveness, ultrasound will probably continue as the screening modality of choice for most pelvic disorders. However, MRI will compete with CT as the major imaging procedure for assessing and staging pelvic masses. Magnetic resonance imaging provides superior soft-tissue contrast and demonstration of pelvic vasculature than CT, and it can demonstrate pelvic organs in axial and nonaxial planes. Since MRI utilizes no ionizing radiation, it is of special value in the imaging of children. However, MRI and CT require sedation whereas most ultrasound studies can be performed without it.

Certain pelvic malignancies (*e.g.*, uterus, urinary bladder) may be better staged with MRI than with CT. Pulse sequences with long TE and TR parameters are of value in determining the extent of myometrial invasion by endometrial carcinoma. The markedly increased signal intensity of endometrial cancer on T2-weighted images can be easily distinguished from the decreased signal intensity of normal myometrium and the junctional zone (Figs. 26-12 and 26-13).

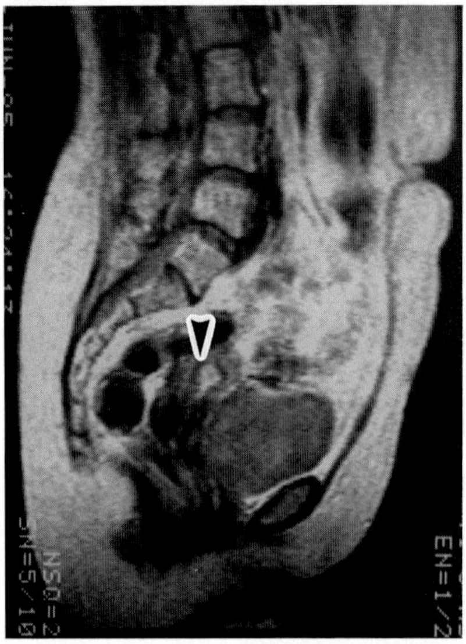

**Figure 26-12.** Noninvasive endometrial carcinoma. T2-weighted MRI shows good definition of the intact, low-signal subendometrial layer (*arrowhead*) consistent with lack of neoplastic invasion.

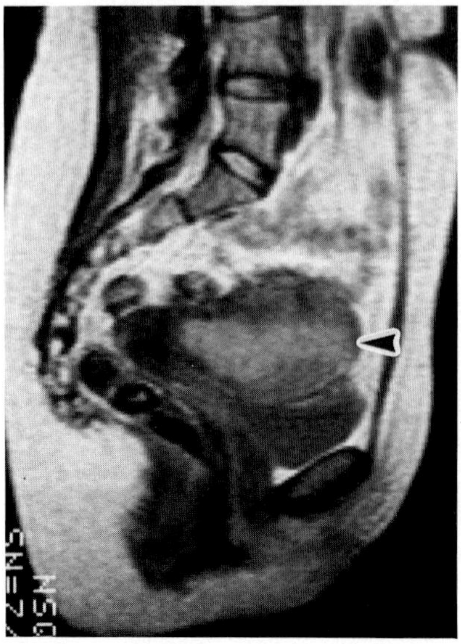

**Figure 26-13.** Invasive endometrial carcinoma. T2-weighted MRI shows invasion extending to the fundal serosa (*arrowhead*).

The junctional zone represents an area of well-perfused and compact inner myometrium, which lies immediately beneath the endometrium. In premenopausal women it is readily apparent, and any discontinuity in this zone may be considered an indication of myometrial invasion. In postmenopausal women, however, the appearance of the junctional zone is variable, and the demonstration of a discontinuity cannot be used as a definite sign of tumor invasion.

The sagittal imaging capabilities of MRI permit improved assessment of the relation of cervical cancer to the vagina, rectum, and urinary bladder. On T1-weighted images, pelvic sidewall extension can be demonstrated, because the parametrial fat has bright signal intensity whereas cervical cancer usually has a signal of intermediate intensity. The intermediate signal intensity of lymph nodes on T2-weighted images can be clearly distinguished from the low-signal intensity of pelvic vessels without the use of intravenous contrast material.

Magnetic resonance imaging can demonstrate ascites and bone metastases, although peritoneal and omental spread may be difficult to evaluate due to bowel peristalsis and respiratory artifact.

Tissue characterization of ovarian tumors may be difficult, because both benign and malignant lesions have varying signal intensities on MRI. Dermoid cysts may show a triple intensity due to fat, fluid, and bone; however, this appearance has been reported in only one third of cases.

Uterine leiomyomas typically have a signal intensity either decreased or equal to that of the uterus on T2-weighted images. Necrotic foci within the tumor produce an increased signal intensity; calcification causes decreased signal.

Magnetic resonance imaging can accurately evaluate the depth of invasion of bladder cancer and can distinguish superficial and deep muscle invasion (T2, T3a) from invasion through the bladder wall (T3b). However, it cannot differentiate superficial and deep muscle invasion from no invasion of the lamina propria (T1). Bladder cancer cannot be unequivocally distinguished from inflammation on signal characteristics alone, because both conditions have increased signal intensity on both T1- and T2-weighted images. Short echo time (TE) pulses can identify papillary components of the mass. Sagittal planes best evaluate the base of the bladder, the posterior and posterolateral walls, and any extravesical spread.

There are several limitations to the use of MRI for imaging pelvic masses. Equipment expenditures and start-up costs are far higher than those of CT, with consequent increased patient charges. Although respiratory motion does not adversely affect pelvic MR images the way it does those in the upper abdomen, bowel peristalsis can reduce image quality. The use of glucagon and bowel preparation may significantly diminish this problem. The spatial resolution of current MRI systems remains slightly less than that of CT or ultrasound. Contraindications to the use of MRI include ferromagnetic intracranial aneurysm clips, implanted cardiac pacemakers, and prosthetic valves.

## Excretory Urography

Conventional excretory urography is indicated in patients with pelvic masses to evaluate the function of the upper urinary tract, to look for hydronephrosis, and to observe the position of the ureters. The presence and degree of hydronephrosis can be established by either ultrasound or CT. Occasionally, a pelvic "mass" may be shown to be a pelvic kidney. Bladder displacement or invasion may also be evaluated by excretory urography. Lateral displacement of the bladder is almost always significant, but the differential diagnosis is quite extensive and includes diverse entities such as hematoma formation, abscess, lymphadenopathy, bladder diverticulum, and sacral myelomeningocele. In most instances, the contrast study does not assist in ascertaining the specific cause of the displaced bladder. On the other hand, the bladder can occasionally have a teardrop configuration, raising the possibility of pelvic lipomatosis. Computed tomography can be diagnostic for this benign condition.

Ultrasound or CT often not only provide information similar to that of excretory urography, but both can simultaneously evaluate the mass that is causing the hydronephrosis, ureteral obstruction, or bladder displacement. Because both CT and urography employ contrast material, both studies can also demonstrate the presence or absence of contrast excretion by the kidneys and the path of the ureters. This is not meant to imply that CT should be performed as a substitute for excretory urography. However, if CT must be performed to stage a pelvic malignancy, the function and appearance of the urinary tract should be simultaneously studied so that a conventional excretory urogram may not be required. Because ultrasound is not a functional study and does not routinely visualize the ureters, it is usually necessary to perform excretory urography in addition to a sonographic examination.

It cannot be overly stressed that the patient's clinical presentation frequently dictates the choice and order of diagnostic studies. If hematuria and pelvic mass are present, the urinary tract should first be evaluated by an excretory urogram. Should a bladder mass be discovered, the most logical and direct approach would be to perform a cystoscopic examination and biopsy. If the biopsy is positive for malignancy, CT may then be performed for staging. On the other hand, if a patient presents with renal failure, ultrasound should be performed to look for hydronephrosis and the possibility of a pelvic or bladder mass causing the obstruction.

## Barium Enema

A barium enema examination of the colon should be performed in only a select group of patients with pelvic masses. It is of value if the clinical history suggests gastrointestinal pathology such as a neoplasm or inflammatory process, if hematochezia is present, or if the proctoscopic examination reveals a mass. It can also be useful in evaluating patients for possible appendicitis. Prior to ultrasound and CT, a barium enema examination was routinely used to evaluate possible masses that were too small in size or too masked by obesity to be palpable on abdominal examination. Large pelvic masses tend to displace, straighten, or flatten the rectum and sigmoid colon. Smaller masses may be more readily visible on postevacuation views. The sensitivity, and particularly the specificity, of barium enema studies in these patients is so low that this examination should no longer be considered as a primary diagnostic modality. Only about 50% of patients with pelvic masses have positive barium enema examinations. As with displacement of a contrast-filled urinary bladder, the presence of a pelvic mass may only be inferred from indirect evidence.

## Plain Radiography

Detection of a pelvic mass by plain film examination is often difficult unless the lesion is large enough to produce an abnormal increase in soft-tissue density. At times, a mass may be detected because it displaces normal viscera, particularly the small bowel, or because it obliterates or distorts normal fat planes. Phleboliths, which are commonly bilateral and symmetric, are visible on pelvic radiographs in 25% to 48% of adults; their displacement is an indirect sign of a pelvic mass. Plain film findings are most often nonspecific regarding an etiologic diagnosis or even the organ of origin. Occasionally, a pelvic mass may appear to be radiolucent, indicating an abnormal collection of either fat (benign cystic teratoma, pelvic lipomatosis) or air (abscess formation, vaginitis emphysematosa). The most radiographically visible pelvic masses are those associated with calcification, such as uterine leiomyoma or, rarely, certain types of ovarian neoplasm.

Because plain film examination of the pelvis has no complications and is noninvasive, safe, relatively inexpensive, and widely available, it is frequently performed as part of the workup of the patient with a pelvic mass. Because it lacks specificity and has a low sensitivity, most plain radiographs of the pelvis are unrewarding. Indeed, since the advent of other noninvasive techniques with much higher diagnostic accuracy, there is serous question about the routine need for obtaining the study. In patients suspected of having calcified, fat, or air-containing masses, the findings on plain film examination may occasionally be pathognomonic.

## COMMENT

Ultrasound is generally considered the initial imaging procedure of choice in the patient with a suspected benign pelvic mass because of its cost effectiveness; portability; and real-time capability to document the mass, its size and consistency, and usually its origin. If a pelvic malignancy is suspected, however, CT frequently is the initial imaging procedure because of its ability to show the size of the tumor, its internal characteristics, and evidence of contiguous spread, direct invasion of neighboring structures, or distant metastases. The eventual role of MRI is unclear, although the improved spatial resolution promised by the use of surface coils and its inherent superior soft-tissue contrast may permit MRI to supplant CT in the staging of some pelvic neoplasms. The development of paramagnetic contrast agents combined with bowel preparation and the use of glucagon will improve the effectiveness of MRI for demonstrating bowel involvement by malignant pelvic tumors.

## Bibliography

Campbell S, Geossens L, Goswamy R: Real-time ultrasonography for determination of ovarian morphology and volume. A possible early screening test for ovarian cancer? Lancet 1:425, 1982

Fleischer A, Boehm F, James AE: Sonography and radiology of pelvic masses and other maternal disorders. Semin Roentgenol 18:172, 1982

Fleischer A, Dudley S, Entman S et al: Sonographic detection of myometrial invasion. Radiology 162:307–311, 1987

Fleischer A, James AE, Millis J: Differential diagnosis of pelvic masses by gray-scale sonography. AJR 131:469, 1978

Fleischer A, Jones H, Shaff M et al: Sonographic evaluation of gynecologic masses: Techniques and role of sonography relative to other imaging modalities. Radiol Clin North Am 20:397–412, 1982

Gross B, Moss A, Mihara K et al: Computed tomography of gynecologic diseases. AJR 141:765–773, 1983

Hricak H: MRI of the female pelvis: A review. AJR 146:1115, 1986

Lupetin A, Dash N, Beckman I et al: Magnetic resonance appearance of the pelvic dermoid. Magnetic Resonance Imaging 4:135, 1986

Mahoney B, Filly R, Nyberg D et al: Sonographic evaluation of ectopic pregnancy. J Ultrasound Med 4:231–238, 1985

Meire J, Ferant P, Guha T: Distinction of benign from malignant ovarian cysts by ultrasound. Br J Obstet Gynaecol 85:893, 1978

Walsh J, Amendola M, Konerding K et al: Computed tomographic detection of pelvic and inguinal lymph node metastases from primary and recurrent pelvic malignant disease. Radiology 137:157–166, 1980

Warner M, Fleischer A, Bundy A et al: Adnexal torsion: Sonographic findings and clinical implications. Radiology 154:773, 1985

Weckstein D, Boucher M, Tacher H: Accurate diagnosis of early ectopic pregnancy. Obstet Gynecol 65:393, 1985

Winkler M, Hricak H: Pelvic imaging with MR: Technique for improvement. Radiology 158:848–849, 1985

Worthington J, Balfe D, Lee J et al: Uterine neoplasms: MR imaging. Radiology 159:725–730, 1986

# PELVIC MASS

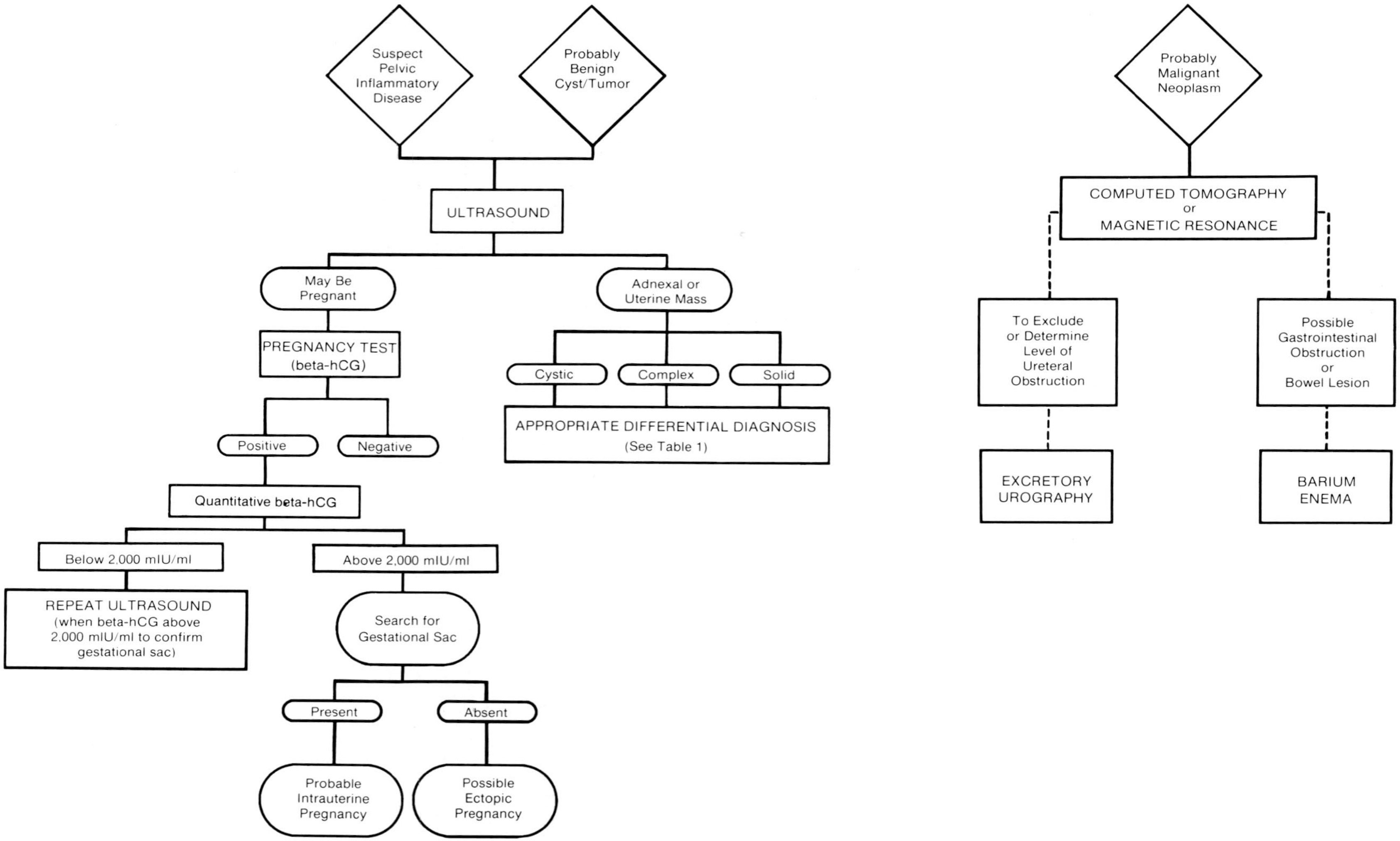
Suspect
Pelvic
Inflammatory
Disease
Probably
Benign
Cyst/Tumor
ULTRASOUND
May Be
Pregnant
PREGNANCY TEST
(beta-hCG)
Positive
Negative
Quantitative beta-hCG
Below 2,000 mIU/ml
REPEAT ULTRASOUND
(when beta-hCG above
2,000 mIU/ml to confirm
gestational sac)
Above 2,000 mIU/ml
Search for
Gestational Sac
Present
Absent
Probable
Intrauterine
Pregnancy
Possible
Ectopic
Pregnancy
Adnexal or
Uterine Mass
Cystic
Complex
Solid
APPROPRIATE DIFFERENTIAL DIAGNOSIS
(See Table 1)
Probably
Malignant
Neoplasm
COMPUTED TOMOGRAPHY
or
MAGNETIC RESONANCE
To Exclude
or Determine
Level of
Ureteral
Obstruction
EXCRETORY
UROGRAPHY
Possible
Gastrointestinal
Obstruction
or
Bowel Lesion
BARIUM
ENEMA

# Chapter 27

# Scrotal Masses

*Leonard A. Wald*
*Matthew D. Rifkin*

Scrotal enlargement or a scrotal mass is usually detected initially by the patient on self-examination or during a routine medical checkup. The clinical presentation, which may vary from a previously undetected painless mass to the acute onset of pain and/or tenderness, is of diagnostic importance and usually defines the most appropriate initial imaging study. A broad spectrum of conditions may result in a focal scrotal mass or enlargement of the scrotum (or hemiscrotum). These include primary and metastatic tumors of or to the testis, epididymis, or other intrascrotal structures; fluid collections (hydroceles, varicoceles, cysts); torsion, trauma; and inflammatory or postinflammatory processes.

Current imaging modalities allow for extensive analysis of the scrotum and its contents and often permit an accurate diagnosis. Ultrasound has become the primary imaging technique for evaluation of the scrotum. Radionuclide scanning, previously the only examination to successfully image the scrotal contents, has become a complementary procedure to ultrasound in most clinical situations. However, it is still the imaging study of choice to confirm certain conditions, such as torsion of the spermatic cord.

## NORMAL ANATOMY

During embryologic development, the normal testicle descends from the abdomen into the scrotum via the processus vaginalis. In the postpubescent male, the testis is ovoid and measures about 4.0 cm × 3.5 cm × 2.5 cm in size. Spermatogenesis takes place in the lobules, pie-shaped structures that are separated from one another by fibrous septa that join at the mediastinum testis. The testis is encased by a dense fibrous capsule, the tunica albuginea. The appendix testis is situated at the superior margin. The epididymis lies along the superior and posterior aspects of the testis and is composed of the head, body, and tail. The epididymal head is round or triangular-shaped, 6 mm to 15 mm thick, and is connected to the testis via the vasa efferens. The body of the epididymis courses along the dorsal aspect of the testis, extends to form the epididymal tail, and angles acutely cephalad as the vas deferens (Fig. 27-1). The body and tail of the epididymis are smaller than the head and measure approximately 2 mm to 4 mm in diameter. A small protuberance, the appendix of the epididymis, may arise from the

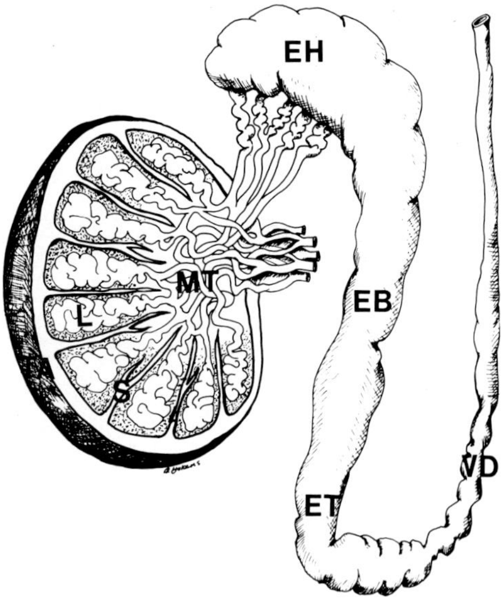


**Figure 27-1.** Normal scrotum. Line diagram of a sagittally oriented transected normal scrotum demonstrates the lobules (*L*), septa (*S*), mediastinum testis (*MT*), and the normal epididymis and vas deferens (*VD*). (*TA,* tunica albuginea; *EH,* epididymal head; *EB,* epididymal body; *ET,* epididymal tail)

head. The testes are covered by a thin double membrane, the tunica vaginalis, which is a remnant of peritoneum.

The lifeline of the testis is the spermatic cord, which courses through the inguinal canal to reach the scrotal contents. It is connected to the testis at the mediastinum testis and contains the single artery supplying the testis (testicular artery), the draining testicular veins (pampiniform plexus), the sperm-transporting vas deferens, and lymphatics and nerves.

## DIAGNOSTIC EVALUATION

### *DIAGNOSTIC MODALITIES*

1. Ultrasound
2. Radionuclide scanning
3. Computed tomography
4. Plain radiography
5. Angiography
6. Magnetic resonance imaging

#### Ultrasound

Ultrasound has become the primary imaging modality for evaluation of the scrotum. It is best performed with a short-focused, high-resolution 7.5 MHz or 10.0 MHz transducer, although a 5.0 MHz transducer may be acceptable if it is superficially focused. Although direct contact scanning may be successful, it may be necessary to perform the examination by placing a water-filled latex glove between the transducer and the scrotum. Synthetic water delay systems in the form of the gel mattress have been developed that simplify use of the traditional water path.

The normal testicle demonstrates a homogeneous, low-to-medium level of echogenicity (Fig. 27-2). Individual testicular lobules cannot be routinely defined. The mediastinum testis, produced by the junction of the fibrous septa with the tunica albuginea that invaginates into the posterior aspect of the testis, may be identified as a bright, thick echogenic band. The appendix testis, situated at the superior aspect, is usually not well visualized unless a hydrocele is present (Fig. 27-3). The head of the epididymis demonstrates an echogenicity that is similar to or slightly increased relative to that of the testicle and epididymal body (which is normally equal to or slightly less echogenic than the normal testis). The tail of the epididymis often is not well seen.

In patients with cryptorchidism who have an absent or small testicle on palpation, ultrasound can demonstrate approximately 70% of the aberrant testicles situated in the inguinal canal. If the testicle is not found in the inguinal canal, computed tomography (CT) or testicular angiography is the imaging procedure of choice to identify the position of an undescended or ectopically placed testis (Fig. 27-4).

Scrotal masses found on routine physical examination warrant further evaluation by ultrasound. Ultrasound can clearly delineate whether the mass is testicular or extratesticular, solid or fluid; in some cases, it may permit differentiation of a benign from a malignant mass.

Testicular neoplasms develop between ages 18 and 40 and are the most common tumors in men aged 25 to 35. Most primary testicular neoplasms are germ cell tumors (seminoma, embryonal cell carcinoma, teratoma, choriocarcinoma,

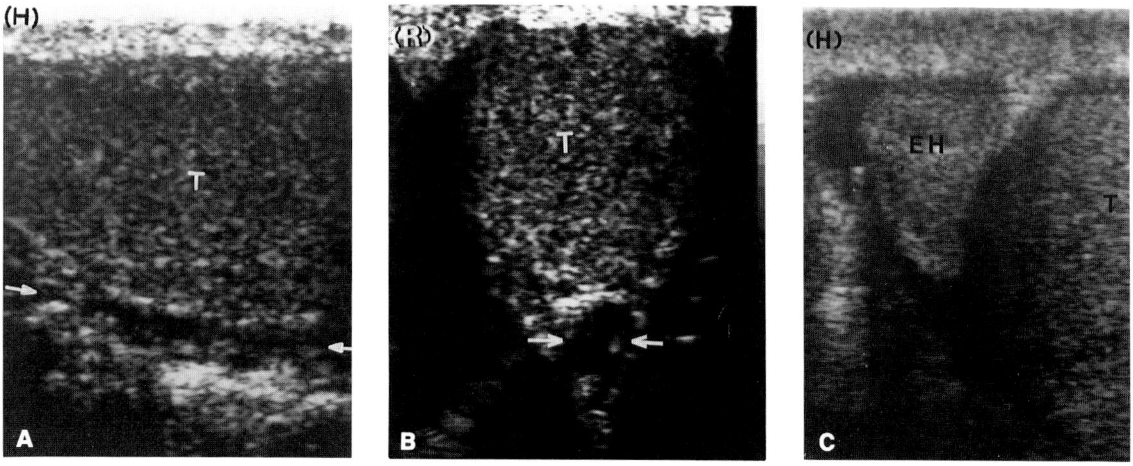


**Figure 27-2.** Ultrasound of normal testis. **(A)** Longitudinal and **(B)** transverse images of the normal scrotum show the testis (*T*) and epididymis (*arrows*). **(C)** Longitudinal section of the superior aspect of the normal testis (*T*) demonstrates a normal-sized (1.5 cm) epididymal head.

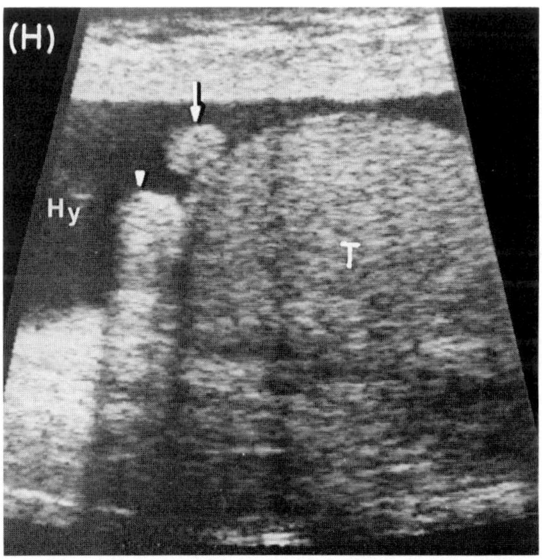


**Figure 27-3.** Ultrasound of normal testis. Longitudinal real-time scan clearly shows the epididymal head (*arrowhead*) and appendix of the testis (*arrow*) because of the associated hydrocele (*Hy*).

or of mixed germ cell elements). The most common metastatic lesions involving the testes are lymphomatous and leukemic infiltration. Scrotal neoplasms present clinically as nontender focal masses or as diffusely enlarged testes, often with erythema or induration. The tumor distorts the normal homogeneous architecture of the testis and may extend beyond the fibrous capsule. The echogenicity of testicular tumors varies widely (Fig. 27-5), and overlapping sonographic findings may make it difficult to distinguish a neoplasm from missed torsion and certain inflammatory processes. Solid extratesticular neoplasms are relatively rare and predominantly involve the epididymis. Most are benign (*e.g.*, adenomatoid tumors and sperm cell granulomas), although metastatic lesions have been reported.

Various types of fluid collections may present as painless scrotal masses or generalized enlargement. Hydroceles are the most common type of fluid collection and result from an abnormal collection of fluid between the layers of the tunica vaginalis. They may be congenital (persistent communication with the abdominal cavity), primary (idiopathic), or secondary (reactive) to inflammation, neoplasm, or trauma. Although often small, hydroceles may attain substantial size. Transillumination of the scrotal contents can clinically confirm an acute hydrocele, but thickening of the tunica vaginalis in chronic hydroceles does not permit transmission of light. Ultrasound can demonstrate the anechoic mass without septations (Fig. 27-6), thus confirming the fluid contents and excluding other diagnoses.

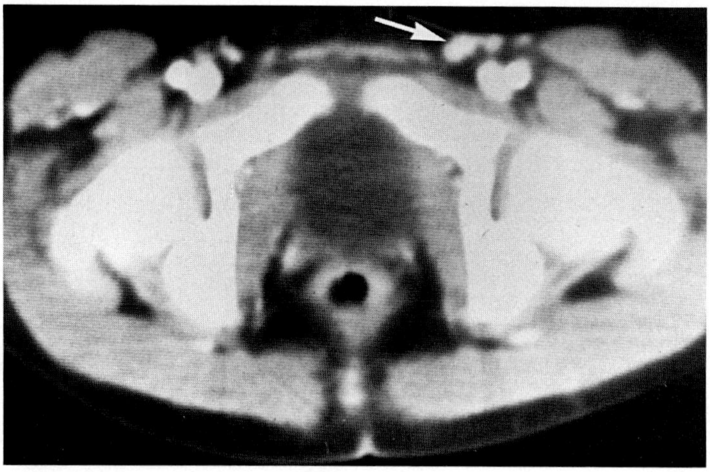

**Figure 27-4.** Undescended testis. CT scan shows the aberrant gonad in the inguinal region on the left (*arrow*). The spermatic cord, but not the testicle, is seen on the left.

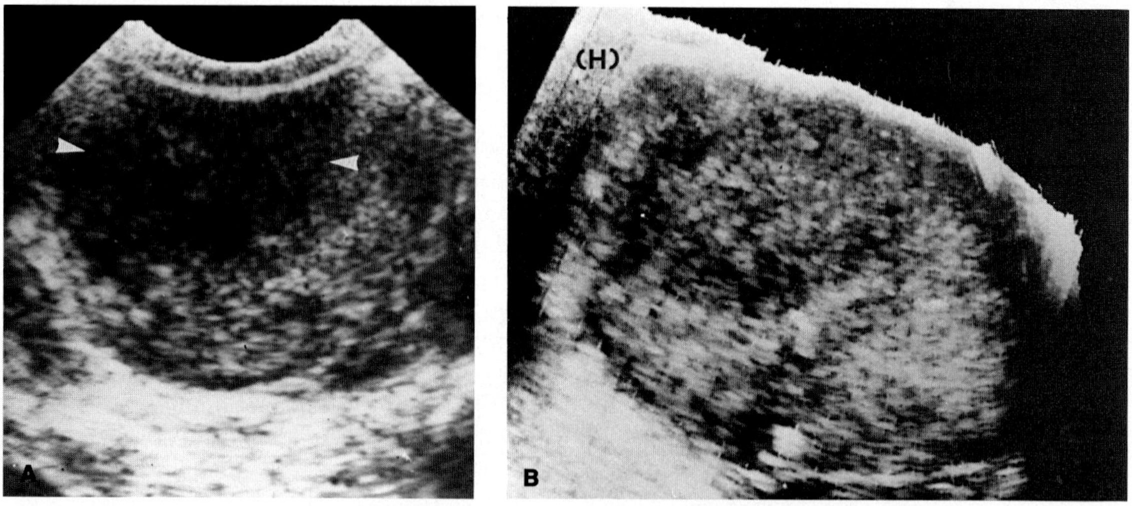


**Figure 27-5.** Testicular seminomas. **(A)** Hypoechoic neoplasm (*arrowhead*) in the anterior portion of the testis. **(B)** More echogenic tumor seen posteriorly in another patient.

Hemorrhage or infection (hematocele or pyocele) may produce internal debris within the mass, although at times the sonographic appearance may be indistinguishable from simple fluid.

Varicoceles represent dilatation of the veins of the pampiniform plexus (draining the testes) or, less commonly, of the cremasteric plexus draining the scrotal skin and epididymis. A large varicocele may present as a palpable extratesticular mass. Because of the indirect drainage of the left side into the inferior vena cava, unilateral varicoceles are more common on the left than the right. Approximately 40% of infertile males have varicoceles, compared with 8% to 15% of the normal male population. Ultrasound demonstrates varicoceles as tubular, round or serpiginous, fluid-filled structures (Fig. 27-7). Unlike normal vessels, the abnormal veins of a varicocele dilate when the patient stands erect or performs a Valsalva maneuver. High-resolution, real-time scanning may show reversal of blood flow. Doppler studies of the engorged plexi may confirm the venous nature of the dilated vessels and can be used to assess venous reflux.

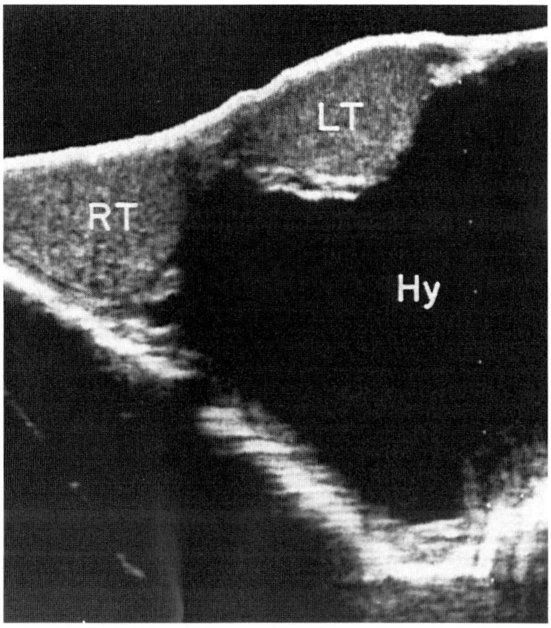


**Figure 27-6.** Hydrocele. Ultrasound shows the left-sided hydrocele (*Hy*) to be posterior to the normal left testis (*LT*) and lateral to the normal right testis (*RT*).

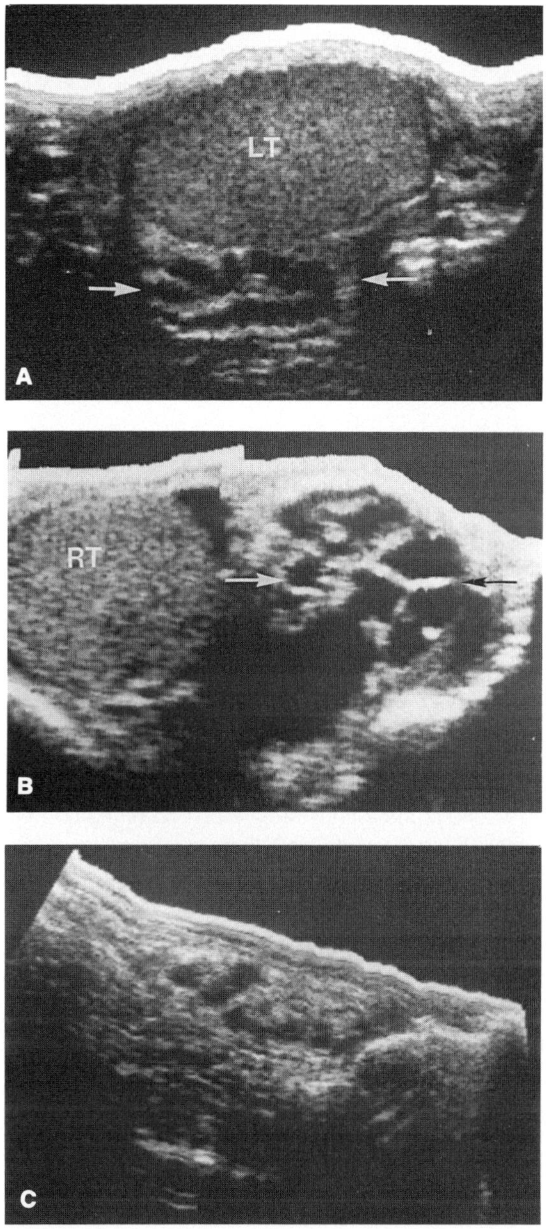


**Figure 27-7.** Varicocele. **(A)** Longitudinal and **(B)** transverse scans of the scrotum demonstrate normal left (*LT*) and right (*RT*) testes. The left-sided varicocele produces dilated tortuous vessels (*arrows*) that are superior to the left testicle on the longitudinal scan and posterior to the left testicle on the transverse view. **(C)** Sonogram of the area of the spermatic cord shows the dilated vessels within it.

Extratesticular cysts (*e.g.*, spermatoceles, epididymal cysts) present as well-defined scrotal masses that usually are palpable and obviously extratesticular in nature. Spermatoceles represent cystic dilatations of the epididymis that are due to tubular obstruction and are filled with creamy, sperm-filled fluid. True epididymal cysts are secondary to intrinsic cystic dilatation of the epididymal tubules and are filled with serous fluid. Ultrasound can demonstrate the cystic nature of these lesions (Fig. 27-8), but it cannot distinguish among them.

Testicular cysts are more common than previous data indicate. They may be congenital or post-traumatic, although the precise etiology is unclear. Peripheral testicular cysts present clinically as nonpainful masses, while small and centrally placed cysts are generally detected as incidental findings on ultrasound. Testicular cysts appear as anechoic, well-defined structures with sharp walls and good through transmission of sound.

Scrotal hernia is usually a clinical diagnosis. In the patient with acute symptoms in whom

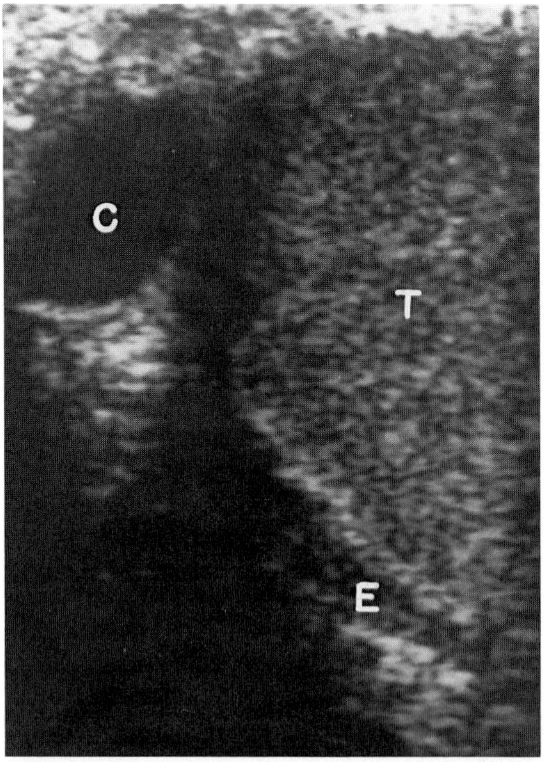


**Figure 27-8.** Epididymal cyst. Longitudinal real-time sonogram demonstrates a portion of the normal testis (*T*) and a well-defined, 2-cm epididymal cyst (*C*) involving the adjacent head of the epididymis. (*E*, normal epididymal body)

physical examination is difficult, ultrasound may demonstrate a complex mass within the scrotum that represents loops of bowel and omentum. A similar pattern on scans of the inguinal canal confirms the diagnosis. Real-time imaging may show intestinal peristalsis. The testes should be seen separately, although this may be difficult due to bowel gas and omental fat in the scrotal sac.

A painful, swollen, tender scrotum associated with fever and leukocytosis suggests an inflammatory process. Due to extreme tenderness, in up to 50% of cases it may be difficult, on physical examination, to differentiate an inflammatory process from torsion of the spermatic cord. Occasionally, a tumor may clinically mimic an acute inflammatory process. Although radionuclide scanning is the imaging procedure of choice to diagnose an acute torsion requiring emergency surgery (see Radionuclide Scanning), when an inflammatory process other than torsion is clinically suspected, ultrasound can be of value to help delineate its nature and the structures involved.

The most common inflammatory process of the scrotum is epididymitis, which affects all age groups although most commonly adolescents and middle-aged men. The acutely enlarged epididymis produces decreased echogenicity, with a heterogeneous pattern often secondary to edema (Fig. 27-9). The presence of fluid containing internal echoes suggests hemorrhage, a grave sequela of epididymitis. Chronic epididymitis may produce increased epididymal echogenicity. Approximately 20% of patients with epididymitis develop an associated orchitis, in which the testis appears sonographically normal or slightly enlarged with decreased or heterogeneous echo-

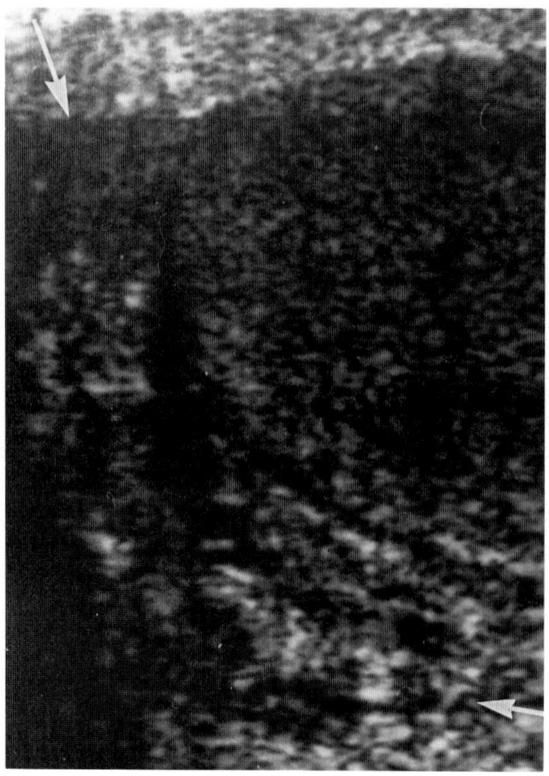

**Figure 27-9.** Epididymitis. Longitudinal real-time sonogram demonstrates the classic appearance of an enlarged and swollen epididymis (*arrows*). The testicle is normal.

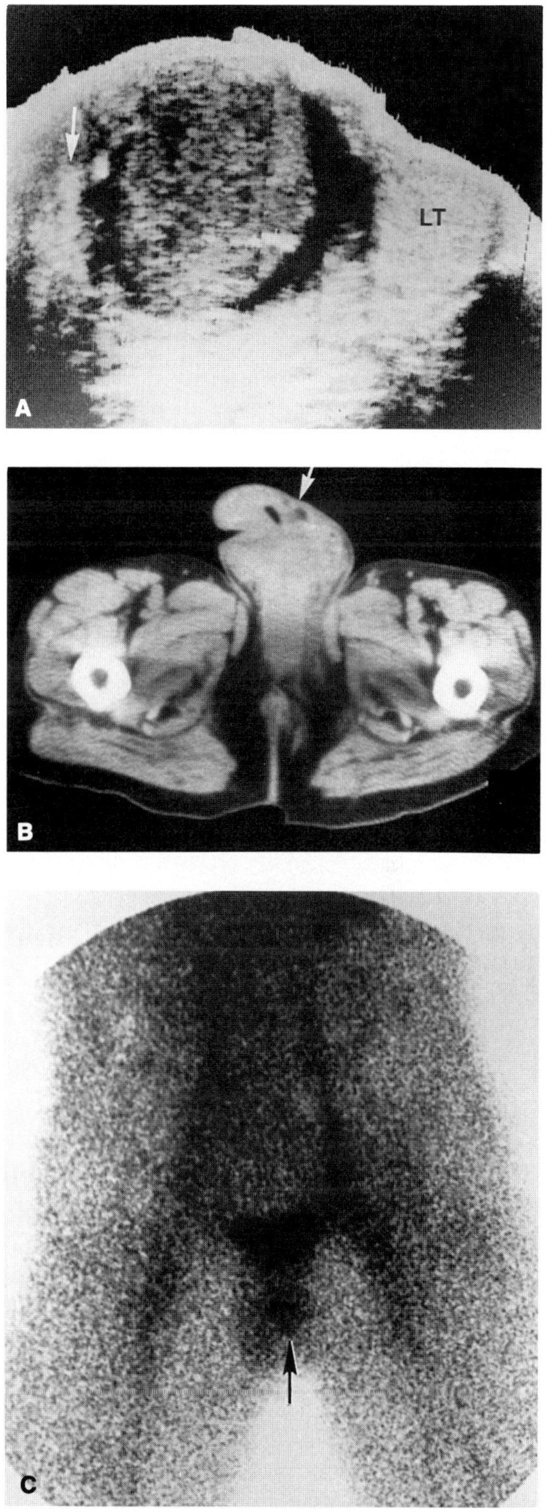


**Figure 27-10.** Orchitis and scrotal abscess. **(A)** Transverse sonogram shows the diffusely abnormal right testis containing a gas-forming abscess. The fluid (due to purulent material) and air (*arrow*) cause acoustic shadowing. The left testicle (*LT*) is normal. **(B)** In another patient, CT scan shows a gas-forming scrotal abscess. The arrow points to air within the superior aspect of the scrotal contents. **(C)** Radionuclide scan in a patient with left-sided orchitis shows a hot left testis (*arrow*).

genicity. Although this pattern may mimic a testicular neoplasm, the clinical findings of epididymitis and associated scrotal skin thickening should suggest an inflammatory process.

Inflammatory processes involving the epididymis and testis may form discrete or diffuse scrotal abscesses that present sonographically as hypoechoic or complex scrotal masses. Anaerobic infections may produce gas that causes echogenic foci with "dirty" acoustic shadowing (Fig. 27-10).

Spermatic cord torsion, usually secondary to congenital laxity of the supporting ligaments, presents as acute scrotal pain and swelling in young or adolescent boys. Associated clinical findings include nausea and vomiting, fever, and pyuria. Extensive edema may prevent an adequate physical examination and preclude clinical differentiation of spermatic cord torsion from acute epididymitis. Because the twisted spermatic cord compromises the vascular supply to the testis and must be surgically repaired within 6 hours to maximize testicular survival, accurate and early diagnosis is essential. Although radionuclide imaging is the study of choice in the evaluation of acute spermatic cord torsion (see Radionuclide Scanning), ultrasound may provide complementary information. During the first 24 hours, the testis and epididymis are enlarged with decreased (occasionally increased) echogenicity. Doppler examination at this time reveals no arterial flow in the proximal portion of the spermatic cord. During the subacute phase (1–10 days), the testis and epididymis remain enlarged and their normal sonographic architecture is disrupted due to edema and hemorrhage (Fig. 27-11). In the late stage (after 10 days),

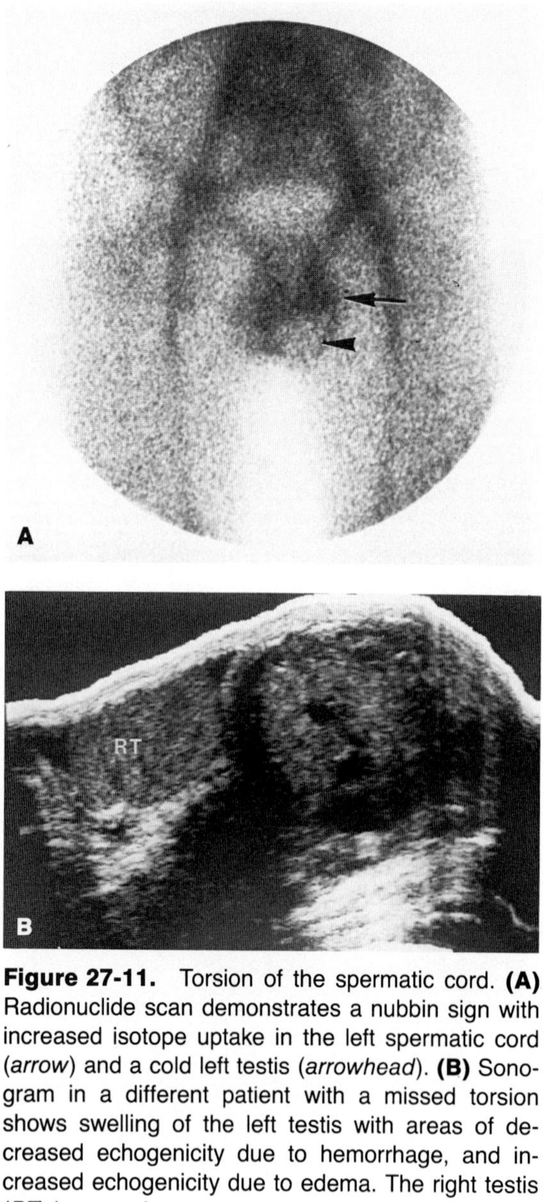


**Figure 27-11.** Torsion of the spermatic cord. **(A)** Radionuclide scan demonstrates a nubbin sign with increased isotope uptake in the left spermatic cord (*arrow*) and a cold left testis (*arrowhead*). **(B)** Sonogram in a different patient with a missed torsion shows swelling of the left testis with areas of decreased echogenicity due to hemorrhage, and increased echogenicity due to edema. The right testis (*RT*) is normal.

ultrasound demonstrates a small testis with either increased or decreased echogenicity secondary to fibrous infiltration or atrophy (Fig. 27-12), respectively.

Blunt trauma to the scrotum may cause testicular contusion, rupture, or peritesticular hematoma. A poorly marginated testis with surrounding fluid suggests rupture of the tunica albuginea, which requires immediate surgical intervention. Contusions without rupture produce testicular echogenicity that is either increased or decreased (due to edema and/or hemorrhage) and lacks associated fluid.

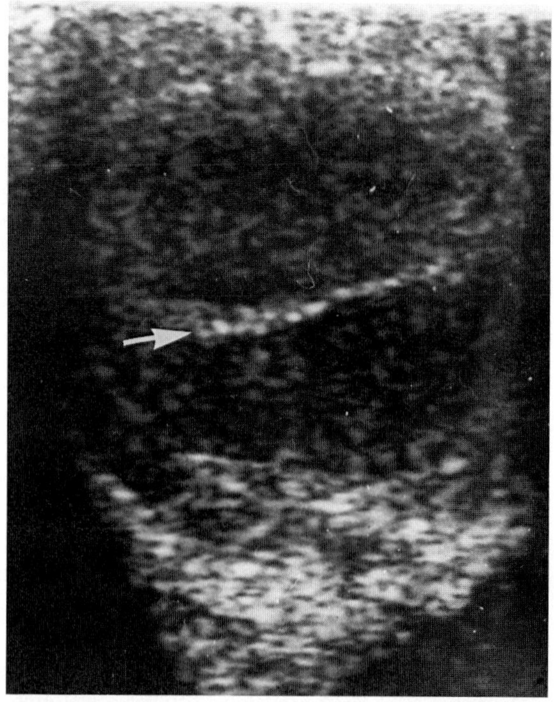

**Figure 27-12.** Atrophy. Real-time ultrasound image shows the testis to be small (2 cm x 2 cm) with diffusely decreased echogenicity. A linear band (*arrow*) represents thickening of a septum as it courses toward the mediastinum testis.

## Radionuclide Scanning

Radionuclide scanning evaluates the vascular perfusion to the scrotum and its contents. It provides an accurate technique for imaging the acutely painful and swollen scrotum and is extremely valuable in differentiating epididymo-orchitis from acute torsion of the spermatic cord. Between 15 and 20 millicuries of $^{99m}$Tc pertechnetate is administered intravenously after pretreatment with oral perchlorate. Dynamic images (radionuclide angiography) are obtained as the bolus passes through the scrotal area, and static images (high-resolution tissue phase) are acquired before the isotope accumulates in the urinary bladder. The iliofemoral arteries are normally well visualized, and the testes appear as focal hot spots, although with no greater activity than the soft tissues of the thigh.

Acute epididymo-orchitis produces increased blood flow and isotope uptake in the dynamic and static phases, respectively (see Fig. 27-10). If only the epididymis is involved, the increased isotope uptake may appear eccentric and curvilinear, conforming to the contour of the inflamed epididymis. If an abscess has formed, the dynamic phase shows increased flow, while the static images may reveal a relatively cool area due to the abscess itself.

Radionuclide scanning is the imaging procedure of choice in patients with suspected torsion of the spermatic cord. This technique has a 90% sensitivity for detecting a torsion and a 98% specificity for excluding this surgical emergency. In the acute stage, there is an abrupt cutoff of perfusion at the iliac artery on the affected side ("nubbin" sign). Static images demonstrate a cold testis (see Fig. 27-11). In the subacute phase, there also may be the development of a "halo" sign, representing concentric arterial flow to the dartos fascia. In the late phase ("missed torsion"), the "nubbin" and "halo" signs persist and the testis continues to appear cold. Torsion of the appendix testis and epididymis may present with similar, but milder, clinical findings. Radionuclide scanning is usually normal, although minimal hyperemia may occur.

Testicular neoplasms may demonstrate mild isotope uptake on the affected side. Hydroceles, hematoceles, spermatoceles, and cysts appear as cold areas, while varicoceles (especially large ones) are usually hot. Radionuclide imaging in these entities is of little clinical value, and ultrasound remains the modality of choice for these and other conditions in which tissue delineation is required.

## Computed Tomography

Computed tomography can identify the scrotal sac and testes, but it is ineffective in evaluating underlying pathology. Computed tomography is the major imaging modality for detecting undescended testes, which appear as ovoid, asymmetric soft-tissue structures along the normal course of testicular descent. The undescended testis is usually smaller than the normally situated gonad (see Fig. 27-4). If both gonads appear normal in size, malignant degeneration of the undescended testis should be suspected.

Computed tomography is of value in assessing the local and distant (retroperitoneal and mediastinal nodes) spread of primary testicular neoplasms. It also can determine the extent of lymphomatous metastases to the testes.

## Plain Radiography

Plain radiography may delineate abnormal opacities or lucencies within the scrotal sac. Calcifications may be secondary to dystrophic changes from meconium peritonitis, hematoma, or an inflammatory process such as tuberculosis. Gas-producing organisms may result in air density within the scrotal sac. Radiopaque foreign bodies may be detected following trauma. Plain chest radiography can evaluate the mediastinum for metastatic spread of primary testicular malignancy.

## Angiography

Spermatic venography may be employed to further evaluate varicoceles in infertile men. The diagnosis is established by demonstrating abnormal retrograde flow via the inferior vena cava or left renal vein into the internal spermatic vein. Retrograde filling of the testicular vein and the pampiniform plexus, as well as any collateral vessels, may be visualized prior to surgery. Embolization, sclerotherapy, or balloon occlusion may be used as therapeutic procedures.

Venography or arteriography may be performed in the patient with cryptorchidism if ultrasound and CT fail to demonstrate the undescended testis. Retrograde venography of the internal spermatic vein may delineate the testicular vein and pampiniform plexus and may produce a mild testicular blush. Arteriography may yield similar results, but it is more invasive.

Venous sampling of the gonadal veins has

been performed in some patients with occult endocrine tumors.

## Magnetic Resonance Imaging

Magnetic resonance imaging (MRI), utilizing a surface coil, has the ability to clearly delineate the anatomy of the scrotal contents. Different signal intensities are obtained from the testes, epididymis, tunica albuginea, fluid, fat, and spermatic cord. Magnetic resonance imaging can demonstrate testicular and extratesticular disease processes, although its cost-effectiveness is still a shortcoming and significant merits of MRI over ultrasound have not been clearly demonstrated.

## Bibliography

Baker LB, Hajek PC et al: MR imaging of the scrotum: Normal anatomy. Radiology 163:89–92, 1987

Baker LB, Hajek PC et al: MR imaging of the scrotum: Pathologic conditions. Radiology 163:93–98, 1987

Becker JM, Ritchie WGM, Goldenberg NJ: Ultrasound of the scrotum and its contents. Semin Ultrasound 3:348–355, 1982

Bird K, Rosenfeld AT, Taylor KJW: Ultrasonography of testicular torsion. Radiology 147:527–534, 1983

Burney BT, Klatte EC: Ultrasound and computed tomography of the abdomen in the staging and management of testicular carcinoma. Radiology 132:415–419, 1979

Chen DC, Holder LE, Melloul M: Radionuclide scrotal imaging: Further experience with 210 patients. Part I: Anatomy, pathophysiology and methods. J Nucl Med 24:735–742, 1983

Chen DC, Holder LE, Melloul M: Radionuclide scrotal imaging: Further experience with 210 patients. Part II: Results and discussion. J Nucl Med 24:841–853, 1983

Foy PM, Rifkin MD: Hydroceles: Acoustic characterization and diagnosis. J Ultrasound Med 7:91–94, 1983

Holder LE, Martire JR, Holmes ER et al: Testicular radionuclide angiograpy and static imaging. Anatomy, scintigraphic interpretation, and clinical indications. Radiology 125:739–752, 1977

Holder LE, Melloul M, Chen D: Current status of radionuclide imaging. Semin Nucl Med 11: 232–249, 1981

Hricak H: Genitourinary ultrasound. Clin Diagn Ultrasound, vol 18, 1986

Leopold GR, Woo VL, Scheible FW et al: High resolution ultrasonography of scrotal pathology. Radiology 131:719–722, 1979

Levitt SB, Kogan SJ et al: The impalpable testis: A rational approach to management. J Urol 120: 515–520, 1978

Lupetin AR, King W et al: The traumatized scrotum. Radiology 148:203–207, 1983

Margulis AR, Kaufman L, Crooks LE: Clinical Magnetic Resonance Imaging. San Francisco, University of California Press, 1983

Mishkin FS, Freeman LM: Freeman and Johnson's Clinical Radionuclide Imaging, 3rd ed, pp 1437–1441, New York, Grune & Stratton, 1984

Nachtsheim DA, Scheible FW: Ultrasonography of testis tumors. J Urol 129:978–981, 1983

Rifkin MD: Diagnostic Imaging of the Lower Genitourinary Tract. New York, Raven Press, 1985

Rifkin MD, Roy PM, Kurtz AB et al: The role of diagnostic ultrasound in varicocele evaluation. J Ultrasound Med 2:271–275, 1983

Rodriguez DD, Rodriguez WC, Rivera JJ et al: Doppler ultrasound versus testicular scanning: The evaluation of the acute scrotum. J Urol 125: 343–346, 1981

Vick CW, Bird KI, Rosenfield AT et al: Scrotal masses with a uniformly hypoechoic pattern. Radiology 148:209–211, 1983

## PALPABLE SCROTAL MASS OR GENERALIZED SCROTAL ENLARGEMENT

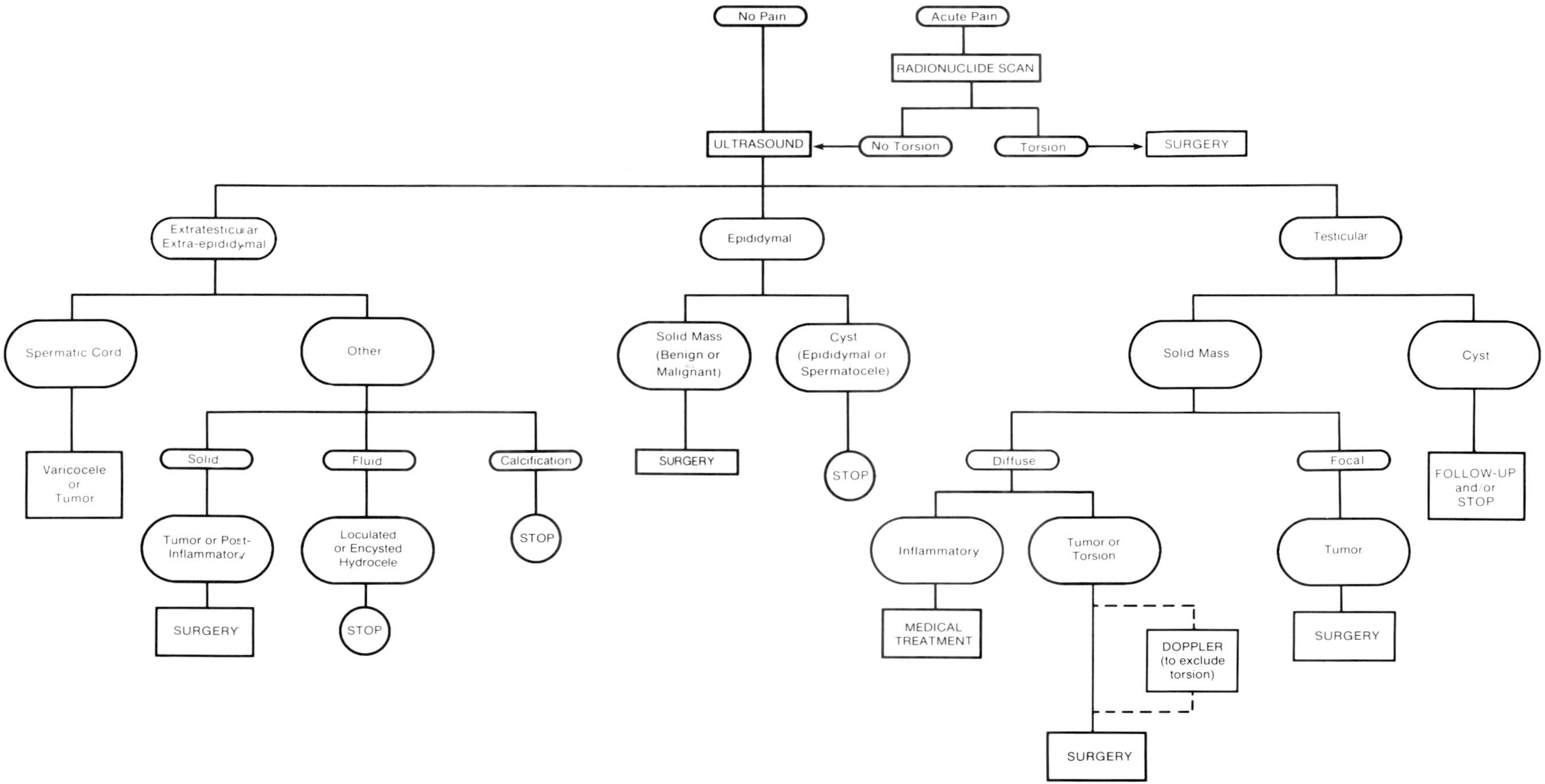

# PART FOUR

# Musculoskeletal System

# Chapter 28

## Back Pain

*John C. Brown*
*D. M. Forrester*

Back pain is a common disorder. Fortunately, less than 1% of patients complaining of back pain have a serious underlying cause for their malady. The radiologist plays the key role in distinguishing serious causes of back pain from benign (biomechanical) ones.

Three rare categories of disease (infection, tumor, ankylosing spondylitis) constitute most of the serious causes for back pain. These conditions are, in most instances, easily visualized using plain film radiography. Therefore, a screening plain film examination is mandatory for every patient complaining of back pain.

### DIAGNOSTIC EVALUATION

#### *DIAGNOSTIC MODALITIES*

1. Plain film radiography
2. Tomography: linear, computed, magnetic resonance imaging
3. Radionuclide bone scan: $^{99m}$Tc phosphate, $^{67}$Ga citrate
4. Contrast examination: myelography, epidural venography
5. Diagnostic block: facet block, epidural block
6. Tissue examination: needle aspiration, bone biopsy

#### Plain Film Radiography

- *Indication:* Primary radiologic investigation in the patient with back pain
- *Advantage:* Low cost; lower radiation; high yield in diagnosis of infection, tumor, and spondylitis
- *Disadvantage:* Inability to outline intraspinal lesions (encroachment on spinal canal)

Plain film examination still has a higher diagnostic yield than other radiologic techniques and is therefore mandatory in patients with back pain. Other modalities such as myelography, scintigraphy, and CT support and refine the plain film and clinical diagnosis. The following are the major plain film radiographic signs suggesting a serious cause of back pain.

##### *Radiographic Signs of Infection*

1. Paravertebral mass (Fig. 28-1)
2. Destruction of vertebral end plate (Fig. 28-2)

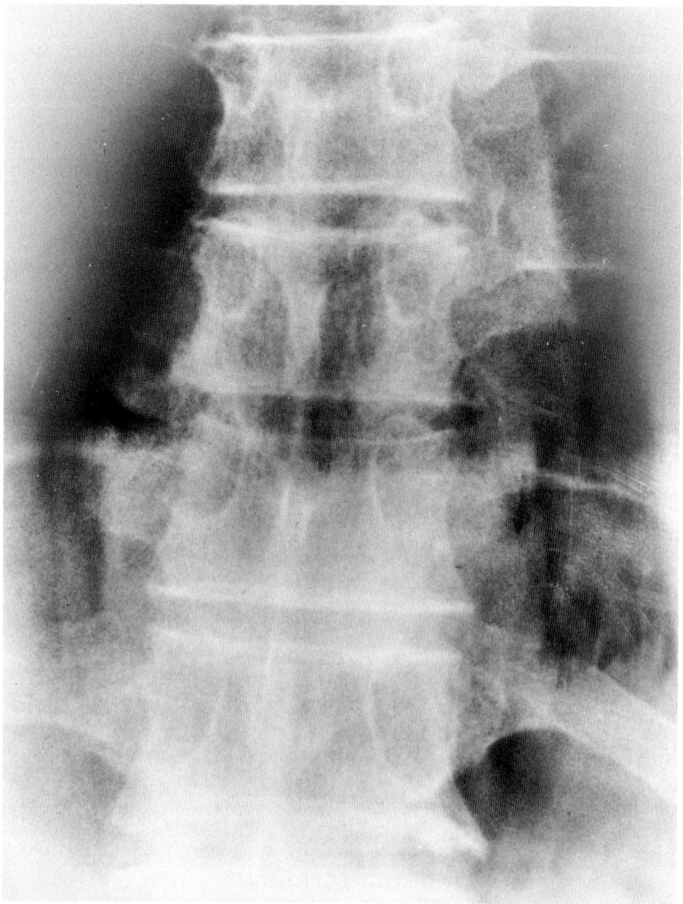

**Figure 28-1.** Paravertebral mass. The only radiographic abnormality is a soft-tissue density adjacent to T11. Aspiration yielded *Staphylococcus aureus* in this abscess.

3. Isolated intervertebral disc space narrowing in the absence of signs of degenerative disc disease

*Radiographic Signs of Ankylosing Spondylitis*

1. Sacroiliitis
2. Ankylosis of apophyseal joints (Fig. 28-3)
3. Presence of syndesmophytes (Fig. 28-3)

*Radiographic Signs of Vertebral Neoplasm*

1. Bone destruction (Fig. 28-4)
2. Osteoblastic lesions (Fig. 28-5)
3. Severe diffuse osteoporosis

The plain film signs of benign biomechanical spinal disorders are

*Anterior Signs (Disc and Vertebral Body) (Fig. 28-6)*

1. Disc narrowing
2. Vertebral body osteophytes
3. Vacuum disc
4. Degenerative spondylolisthesis

Age, everyday life, and particularly posture stress the shock-absorbing system of the spine, especially in areas of excessive lordosis. Thus, C4, C5, and C6 in the cervical spine and L4, L5 and S1 in the lumbar region are prone to disc degeneration and osteophyte formation.

*Posterior Signs (Facet Joint) (Fig. 28-7)*

1. Joint space narrowing
2. Reactive sclerosis

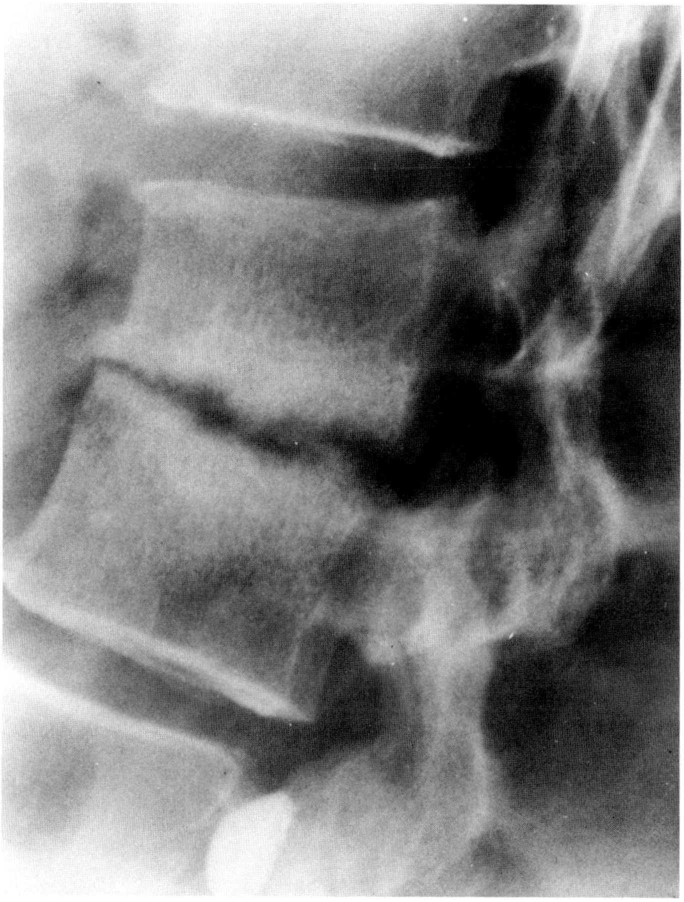

**Figure 28-2.** Destruction of vertebral end plate and disc space narrowing. Note the irregularity of the two adjacent end plates and reactive sclerosis of the bodies. Aspiration of the disc space yielded *Escherichia coli.*

3. Osteophytes
4. Foraminal encroachment

The four signs of facet joint abnormalities are all components of osteoarthrosis. Because of the fixed relationship of the two posterior facet joints to the disc, abnormalities of any of these articulations necessarily result in strain on the other two. It is common to see degenerative changes of the facet joints in conjunction with similar signs of degenerative disease in the associated disc spaces.

## Tomography

Conventional tomography is used to evaluate lesions that are seen, but poorly defined, on plain film examination. It confirms the presence of an abnormality and better defines the extent of the lesion. Conventional tomography is a valuable technique for distinguishing between vertebral destruction caused by infection and tumor. Computed tomography (CT) is more useful in evaluating the extraosseous extent of a lesion, defining the anatomy of the posterior elements, demonstrating a narrowed spinal canal in the rare spinal or intervertebral foramen stenosis, and, on occasion, specifying the tissue type of the radiographic abnormality. In addition, CT defines extradural compression from soft-tissue encroachment due to herniated disc or tumor (Fig. 28-8).

One problem with the cross-sectional slices of CT is the possibility of creating artifacts re-

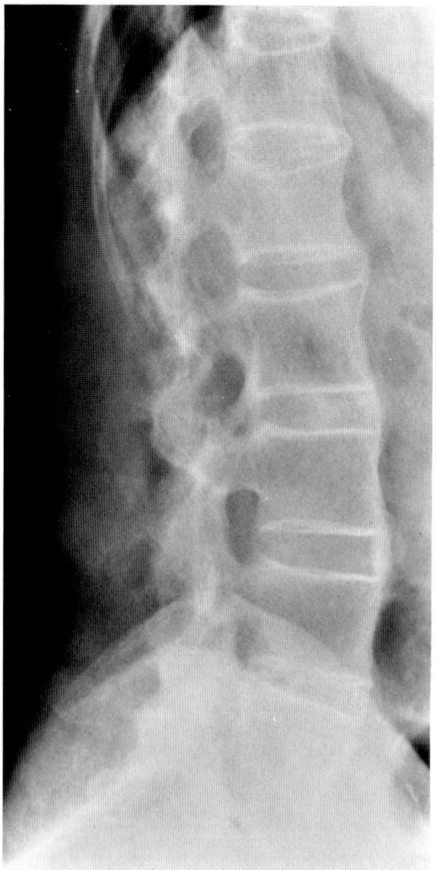

**Figure 28-3.** Apophyseal joint ankylosis and syndesmophytes. Fusion of the posterior facet joints and the vertebral bodies documents the presence of ankylosing spondylitis.

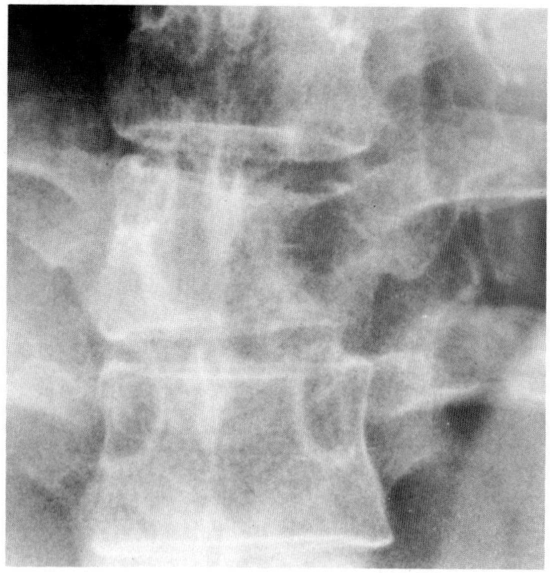

**Figure 28-4.** Bone destruction. There is loss of the pedicle and left side of the vertebral body of T11 secondary to breast carcinoma metastatic to bone.

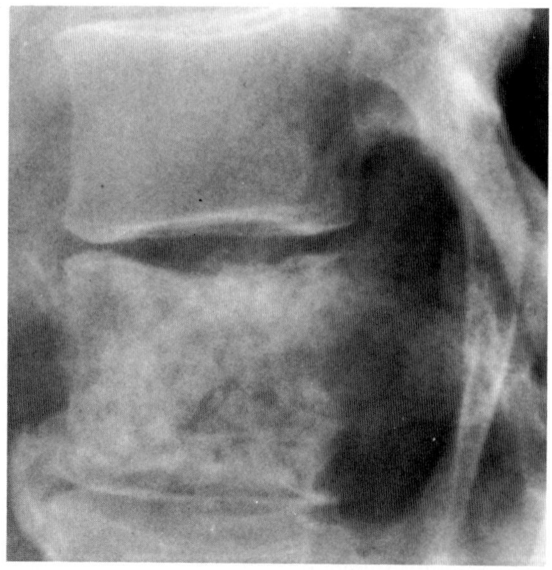

**Figure 28-5.** Osteoblastic lesions. A mottled increase in density involves a solitary vertebral body. In addition, there is lytic destruction of the associated pedicle in this patient with breast carcinoma who was undergoing chemotherapy.

lated to tomographic cuts made tangential to the normal curvature of the spine. Unless compensation is made for the angle of the vertebral body, artifactual "blastic lesions" and "destructive processes" may be seen on isolated tomographic cuts of a normal vertebral body.

Magnetic resonance imaging (MRI) is the most sensitive imaging modality for detecting degenerative disc disease, herniated nucleus pulposis, or disc space infection. The normal, well-hydrated disc has a bright signal on the T2-weighted image; the signal intensity decreases as the patient ages. The sagittal and coronal images produced by MRI are of higher technical quality than the reconstruction images of CT. Thus, herniation of disc material into the spinal canal can be easily detected using MRI (Fig. 28-9).

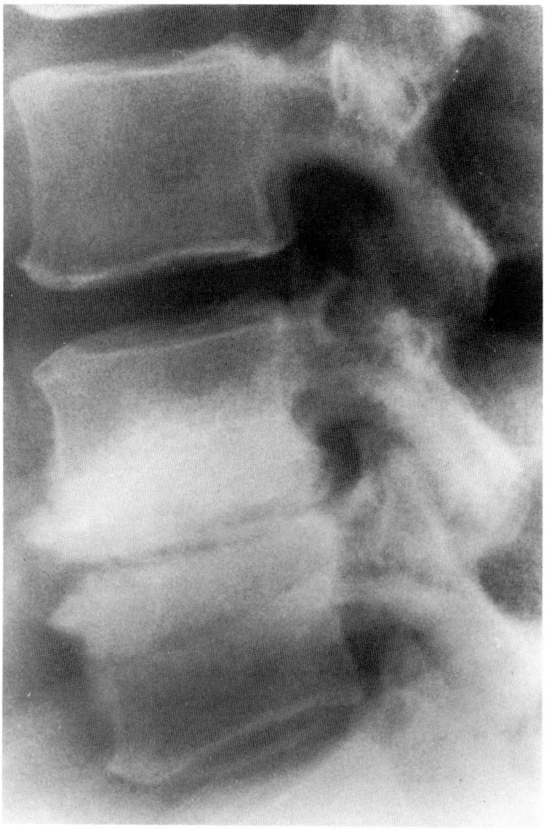

**Figure 28-6.** Degenerative disc disease. Disc space narrowing, reactive sclerosis of the adjacent vertebral bodies, and the formation of anterior and lateral osteophytes typify the productive changes of degenerative disc disease.

The high signal of normal marrow allows easy detection of marrow-destroying diseases, such as infection and tumor (Fig. 28-10). Magnetic resonance imaging has demonstrated the presence of metastases when plain radiographs and radionuclide bone scans were normal.

Neither linear nor computed tomography or MRI should ever be used merely to solve physician frustration in the presence of a patient with pain who has a normal plain film and physical examination. Furthermore, even though osteophytic encroachment on an intervertebral foramen may be better demonstrated on CT, this finding is often irrelevant and no relationship to the patient's pain.

### Lincar Tomography

- *Indication:*
  - Precise visualization of intraosseous lesions
  - Measurement of diameter of osseous spinal canal
- *Advantage:*
  - Low cost, moderate irradiation
- *Disadvantage:*
  - No detail of soft-tissue structures

### Computed Tomography

- *Indication:*
  - Measurement of diameter of osseous spinal canal
  - Definition of soft-tissue and bony encroachment on the contents of the spinal canal
  - Observation of individual nerve roots and lateral spinal stenosis
- *Advantage:*
  - Precise anatomy demonstrated
- *Disadvantage:*
  - High cost and high irradiation

### Magnetic Resonance Imaging

- *Indication:*
  - Evaluation of marrow cavity for metastases

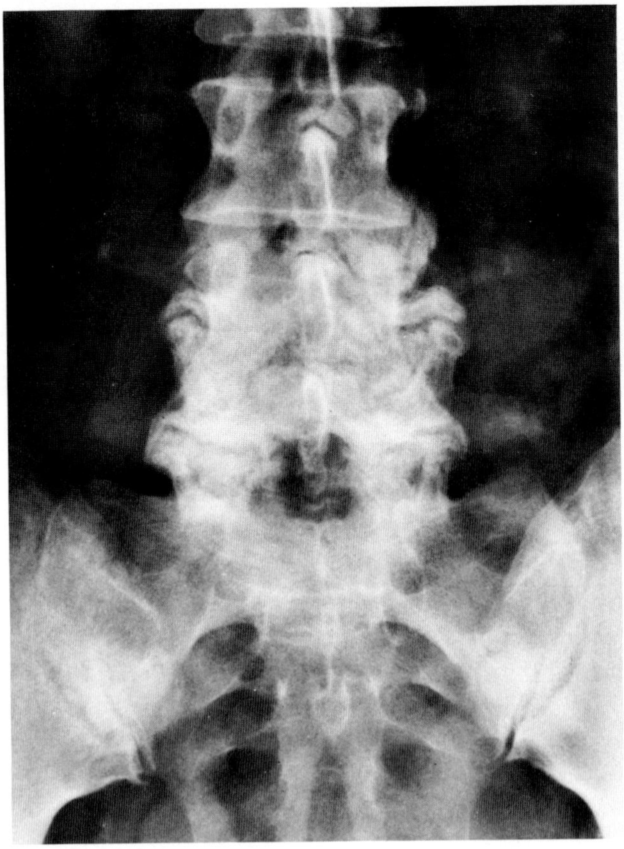

**Figure 28-7.** Facet joint osteoarthrosis. Narrowing of the joint space, sclerosis of the articular facets, and osteophyte formation appear as marked deformities of the L3–L4, L4–L5, and L5–S1 facet joints on this anteroposterior view of the lumbar spine.

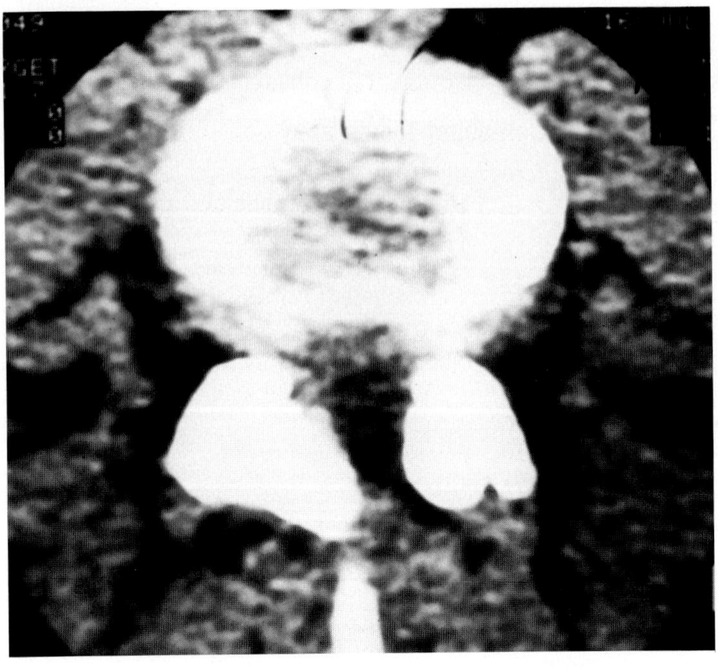

**Figure 28-8.** CT scan of herniated disc. An axial section through the disc space at the L4–L5 level demonstrates posterior and lateral bulging of a herniated disc, which compromises both intervertebral foramina as well as the spinal canal. Hypertrophy of the facet joints further encroaches on the spinal canal.

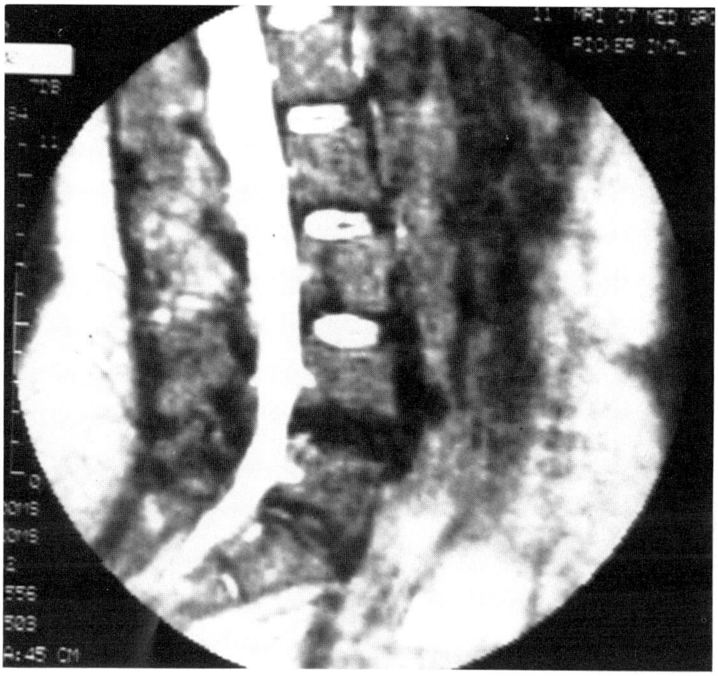

**Figure 28-9.** MRI of herniated disc. The decreased signal intensity of the L4–L5 and L5–S1 discs denotes dehydration and degenerative changes. There is a posterior bulge of the L4–L5 disc. (See Fig. 28-8 for the CT scan in the same patient.)

Most sensitive technique for detecting degenerative disc disease, disc herniation, and infectious spondylitis

- *Advantage:*

  Noninvasive, no irradiation

  Distinguishes nuclear characteristics of adjacent soft tissues that are isodense on CT scan

- *Disadvantage:*

  High cost

## Radionuclide Bone Scan

- *Indication:*

  Suspected osseous lesion that is ill-defined by plain film radiography

  Suspected osteomyelitis (particularly in intravenous drug addicts) or metastasis in a patient whose plain films are normal

- *Advantage:*

  Noninvasive procedure, moderate cost

- *Disadvantage:*

  Sensitive, but nonspecific, for bony reaction (degenerative changes also display activity)

In contrast to tomography, which confirms and more precisely defines the anatomy of a lesion suspected from plain films, scintigraphy is useful in establishing the presence of abnormal bone uptake when plain films are normal (Fig. 28-11).

Radionuclide imaging with $^{99m}$Tc methylene diphosphonate (MDP) is the most sensitive method for assessment of bone pathophysiology. Focal increased uptake of the isotope reflects increased blood flow and reparative or reactive bone formation. Its nonspecificity, however, does not allow discrimination of benign from serious disease. The response of bone to degenerative cartilage, metabolic diseases, fracture, tumor, and infection are all reflected as increased radionuclide uptake on a technetium phosphate scan.

Gallium-67 citrate is another useful scanning agent in the diagnosis of back pain. Its mechanism of uptake is believed to be secondary to the *in vivo* labeling of leukocytes. Gallium-67 offers a specificity not available with $^{99m}$Tc-MDP. Its major value is in helping to determine whether destructive and reparative changes seen on the plain film examination (narrowing of the intervertebral disc space and reactive bony

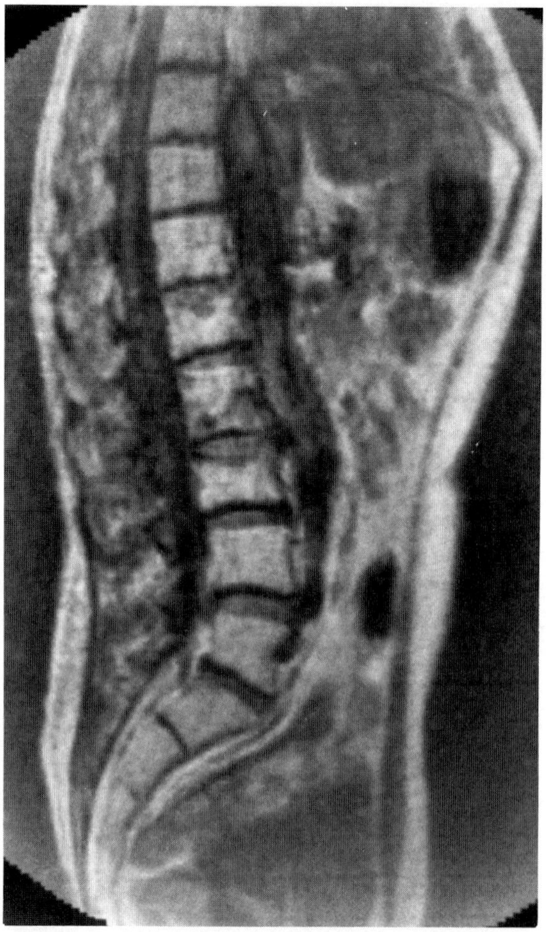

**Figure 28-10.** MRI of metastases. The patchy decreased signal intensity of L1 and L2 represents bone marrow replacement by metastases.

changes) are due to infection or degenerative disc disease. Furthermore, lack of uptake of $^{67}$Ga differentiates a healed infectious spondylitis from active disease. In addition to increased uptake in focal areas of infection, a few tumors (Hodgkin's disease; non-Hodgkin's lymphoma; and metastatic lung, breast, prostate, and renal carcinoma) may also accumulate $^{67}$Ga citrate.

## Contrast Examination

Contrast examinations are useful in detecting intrathecal space-occupying lesions. They are performed only to evaluate a progressive neurologic deficit for which surgery is contemplated; they should never be used as a diagnostic tool for pain alone! Myelography (Pantopaque or metrizamide) and epidural venography identify lesions encroaching on the contents of the spinal canal. Epidural venography is limited to the identification of mass lesions suspected in the lower lumbar region, and its use has been virtually eliminated by CT.

Ideally, the initial evaluation of the low back for suspected herniated disc utilizes unenhanced CT without metrizamide. For the patient with persistent back pain following surgery, the addition of intravenous contrast material may be of value, because scar tissue enhances and can thus be differentiated from an extruded disc.

### Myelography, Oil-Soluble Contrast (Fig. 28-12)

- *Indication:*

  Progressive neurologic deficit (never for pain alone!) indicating spinal cord or cauda equina compression

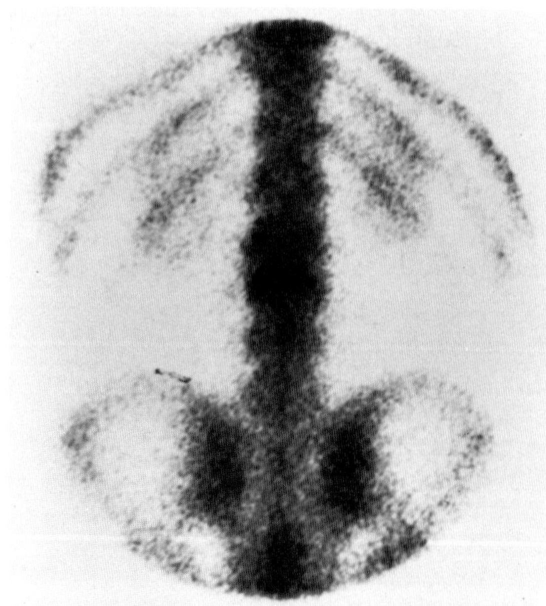

**Figure 28-11.** Tc-MDP scan. Increased radionuclide uptake at L2 and L3 is seen in a patient with a history of heroin addiction and back pain. The plain films were normal. Aspiration yielded *Staphylococcus aureus.*

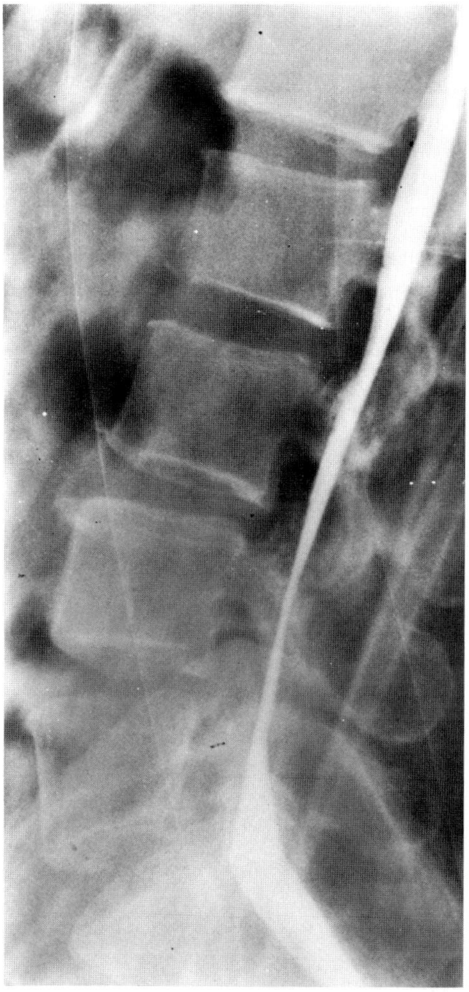

**Figure 28-12.** Pantopaque myelogram demonstrates an extradural mass from L2 to the sacrum in a heroin addict with a normal plain film examination and progressive lower extremity weakness. Aspiration and culture documented infection as the cause of the mass.

- *Advantage:*
  Good outline of extramedullary compression
- *Disadvantage:*
  Invasive technique. Side-effects of contrast in subdural space include the following:
  a. Immediate—headache and contrast reaction
  b. Long-term—arachnoiditis

### Myelography, Water-Soluble Contrast

- *Indication:* Same as for oil contrast
- *Advantage:* Better definition of fine structures (*i.e.*, nerve roots, lateral canal); no long-term arachnoiditis
- *Disadvantage:* Contrast reactions and seizures (rare)

### Epidural Venography

- *Indication:* Suspicion of herniated disc in lumbar region
- *Advantage:* May diagnose lateral disc herniation following false-negative myelogram
- *Disadvantage:*
  Invasive technique, time-consuming procedure
  Limited to lumbar spine
  Cannot demonstrate lesions of subarachnoid space
  High cost, high irradiation

## Diagnostic Block

- *Indication:*
  When possibility of infection, tumor, or spondylitis has been eliminated
  To relieve acute inflammation around facet joint or in epidural space around a prolapsed disc
  To diagnose posterior (facet joint) or anterior (disc prolapse) pain syndrome
- *Disadvantage:* Invasive procedure with moderate discomfort, side-effects of corticosteroids, and rarely lidocaine reaction

The injection of diluted steroid and lidocaine into precise areas in the back is of significant value in localizing the site of pain production. A correctly placed injection often alleviates pain in the same way that tennis elbow improves following steroid injection. However, it should be stressed that local block does not differentiate serious lesions from benign ones.

### Facet Block

The majority of patients over the age of 50 years who experience low back pain will gain immediate relief following a facet block. This supports the notion that most chronic back pain originates from the facet joints. The six lumbar facet joints, from L3–L4 to L5–S1, are injected simultaneously with 3 ml of a mixture of lidocaine and steroid. The joints are localized by metal grids placed over the facets on a posteroanterior film. Injected steroid may sometimes produce intermittent glycosuria in an unstable diabetic; the only other side-effect is an occasional lidocaine reaction.

### Epidural Block

Using a caudal approach to the epidural canal, 60 ml (5 ml of lidocaine diluted with 50 ml saline, 5 ml of Solu-Medrol) are injected into the caudal sac. The epidural block is of special value in differentiating an anterior (disc) lesion from the facet syndrome. The pain caused by an acutely inflamed disc responds well to this technique. Acute and severe pain of short duration often accompanies an epidural injection in the presence of a "hot" disc.

## Tissue Biopsy (Fig. 28-13)

- *Indication:* When precise diagnosis of tumor or infection is required
- *Advantage:* Positive cellular or bacterial diagnosis
- *Disadvantage:*
  Invasive technique
  Immaculate localization required for positive diagnosis

When radiographic procedures have demonstrated a destructive lesion caused by malignancy or infection, it is mandatory to define the organism causing the infection or the specific cell type of the tumor.

If the classic radiographic features of infectious spondylitis are present (destructive lesion involving the vertebral body and end plate), aspiration of the disc space is the most expeditious procedure. Remember, however, that the infection is blood borne and arises in the vertebral body rather than the avascular disc, which is infected only by contiguous spread of the organism. Failure to isolate the offending culprit by disc aspiration or blood culture necessitates bone biopsy.

Bone biopsy is required to determine the nature of a destructive lesion when primary tumor or metastatic disease without a known primary is suspected. It is also necessary in the presence of infectious spondylitis, where disc aspi-

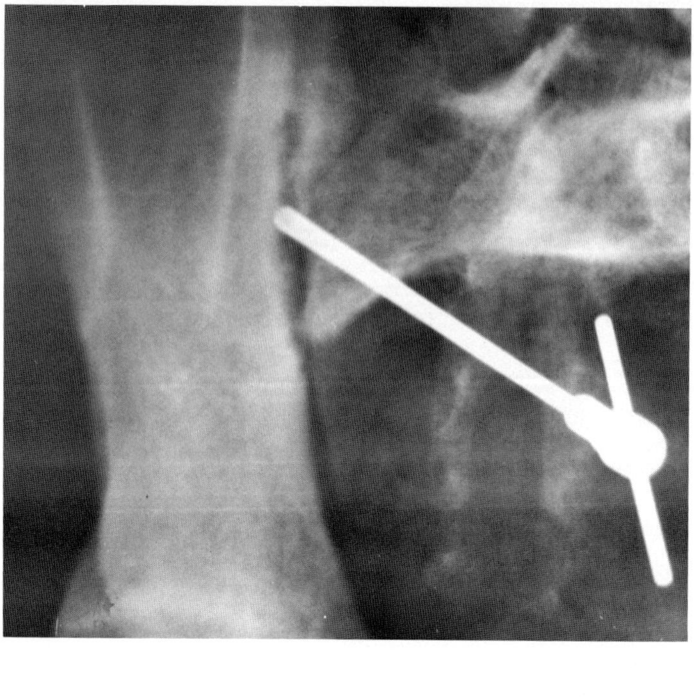

**Figure 28-13.** Tissue biopsy. Precise localization of the biopsy needle can be done using fluoroscopy or CT scanning. Biopsy of this unilateral sacroiliitis demonstrated *Klebsiella.*

ration and blood cultures have failed to grow the organism.

Correct placement of the needle requires either fluoroscopic or CT guidance.

## USE OF THE ALGORITHM

The spine reacts to a variety of insults with similar symptoms of pain, spasm, and resultant difficulty of movement. When nerve or spinal cord impingement occurs, neurologic deficit results. These clinical findings can be caused by superimposed abnormal stress on a normal back or by normal stress on a back compromised by infection, tumor, or spondylitis.

The initial radiographic study of the patient with back pain is the plain film examination.

### STEP I. Do the Radiographic Signs Reflect Serious Disease, Benign Disease, Spinal Stenosis, or a Normal Plain Film?

#### Signs of a Serious Disorder

Paravertebral Mass. The presence of a paravertebral mass suggests abscess or tumor tissue. A paravertebral mass increases the width of the prevertebral soft tissues in the cervical region and displaces the posterior medastinal stripe in the thoracic region. Displacement of bowel gas away from the vertebral body indicates a mass on the lateral projection of the lumbosacral region, and enlargement of the psoas muscle shadow on an anteroposterior projection indicates a psoas abscess associated with infectious spondylitis.

Destruction of Bone. Loss of the normal organized trabecular pattern, a lytic lesion within the vertebral body, or absence of a portion of the posterior elements (pedicle, transverse process, lamina, spinous process) signals a destructive process. Infection, primary bone neoplasm, and metastatic disease may affect the vertebral bodies. In contrast, infection rarely presents as destruction of the posterior elements.

Destruction of Vertebral End Plate. Cartilage acts as a barrier to the extension of tumor. Thus, when one sees destruction of the sharp, well-defined white vertebral end plate, the diagnosis of infection is established. Because of Batson's plexus, the offending organism readily spreads to the adjacent vertebral body. The classic radiographic picture of spondylitis is the destruction of two adjacent vertebral end plates and narrowing of the intervertebral disc space.

Pathologic Fracture (Fig. 28-14). Structural weakening of the vertebral body may result in a compression fracture after only minor stress. This occurs with tumor, infection, or severe osteoporosis.

Isolated Intervertebral Disc Space Narrowing. Most commonly, disc space narrowing is a consequence of degenerative changes of the cartilaginous disc and thus is accompanied by the other radiographic signs of degenerative disease (reactive sclerosis of the subchondral bone and osteophyte formation). In the absence of these reassuring findings, one must always be alert for the presence of an underlying infectious spondylitis. Destructive changes of the vertebral body and end plate may be too small to be detected by plain film examination, and more sensitive tests (*i.e.*, bone scan, MRI) are necessary to establish the presence of a serious underlying disorder. This phenomenon of isolated disc space narrowing is seen more frequently in children than in adults.

Blastic Lesion (Fig. 28-15). Focal or diffuse increased density of the vertebral body or posterior elements implies reactive or reparative changes. Paget's disease, lymphoma, chronic granulomatous infection, and blastic metastases affect the vertebral body. Increased density of a pedicle may be due to blastic metastases or a primary bone tumor (*e.g.*, Ewing's sarcoma)

Sacroiliitis. Inflammatory changes of a sacroiliac joint are manifested by irregularity of the cartilage space and loss of the sharply defined white subchondral line. Reactive sclerosis

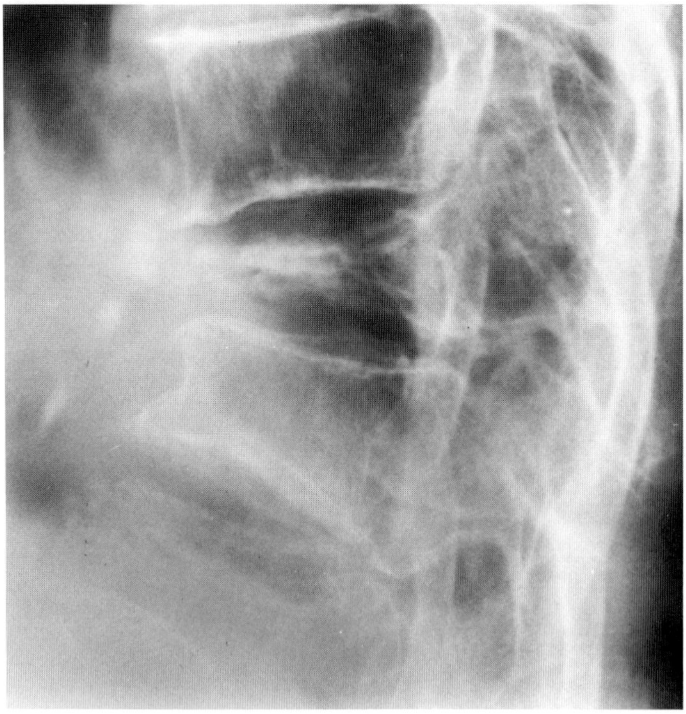

**Figure 28-14.** Pathologic fracture. Complete collapse of one vertebral body and partial collapse of a second occurred in a patient with a history of breast carcinoma.

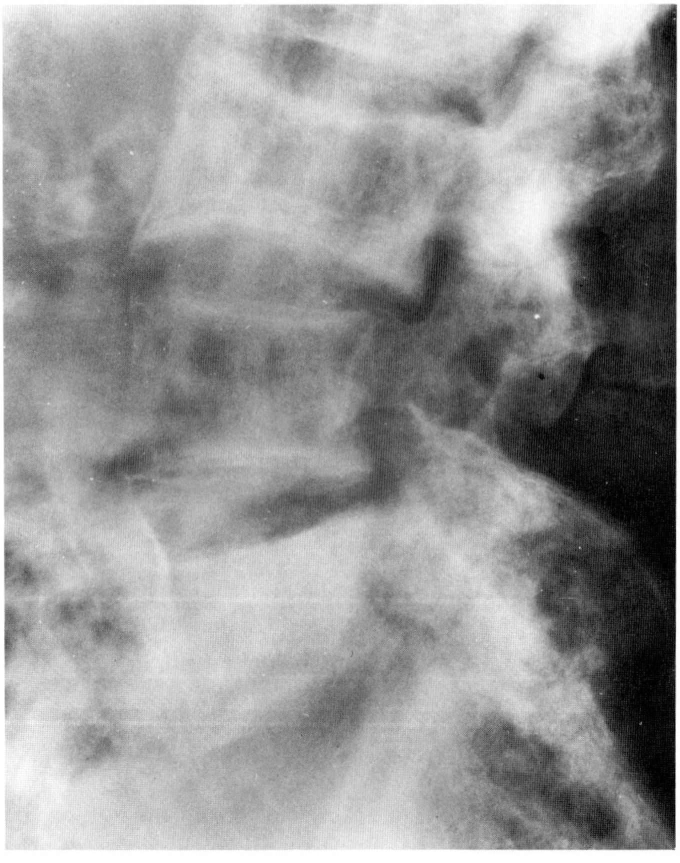

**Figure 28-15.** Blastic lesion. Increased density of several vertebral bodies and posterior elements are seen in a patient with back pain. The increased size and coarsened trabecular pattern are typical of Paget's disease.

and bony ankylosis are signs of healing. Any of the four rheumatoid variants (ankylosing spondylitis, psoriatic arthritis, Reiter's syndrome, arthritis associated with inflammatory bowel disease) affect the sacroiliac joints; in psoriatic arthritis and Reiter's syndrome, sacroiliac changes may precede any evidence of peripheral arthritis. If the sacroiliitis is unilateral, infection must also be added to the list of diagnostic possibilities (Fig. 28-16).

Apophyseal Joint Ankylosis. Because the apophyseal joint is a synovial joint, inflammatory changes occur in the rheumatoid variants. When the apophyseal joints are affected, the sacroiliac joints are also involved. Early signs of narrowing and erosion are difficult to detect. Eventually, bony ankylosis occurs and is easily recognized on anteroposterior or oblique views of the lumbar region and lateral views of the cervical spine.

Syndesmophytes. A predominant component of the disease process of the rheumatoid variants is the inflammatory involvement of ligaments. Stimulation of osteoblastic activity beneath the anterior longitudinal ligament results in the formation of bridging bone called syndesmophytes. Occasionally, osteophytes may be thin and vertical, and may affect multiple levels and mimic syndesmophytes. Since sacroiliitis is always present when axial skeletal involvement occurs in the rheumatoid variants, radiographs of the sacroiliac joints clarify this occasionally confusing picture.

### Signs of Benign Disease

Degeneration of a disc segment narrows the intervertebral space and secondarily wears out the apophyseal joints. The severity of the degenerative process is often totally unrelated to the patient's symptoms. Because degenerative changes are common, one must always be alert to the possible coincidence of an occult, dangerous lesion in the presence of benign radiographic signs.

### Signs of Congenital Spinal Stenosis

Congenital spinal stenosis is rare compared with acquired spinal stenosis from osteophyte formation of the vertebral body and facet joints. The shape and anteroposterior diameter of the spinal canal can be easily evaluated on the axial

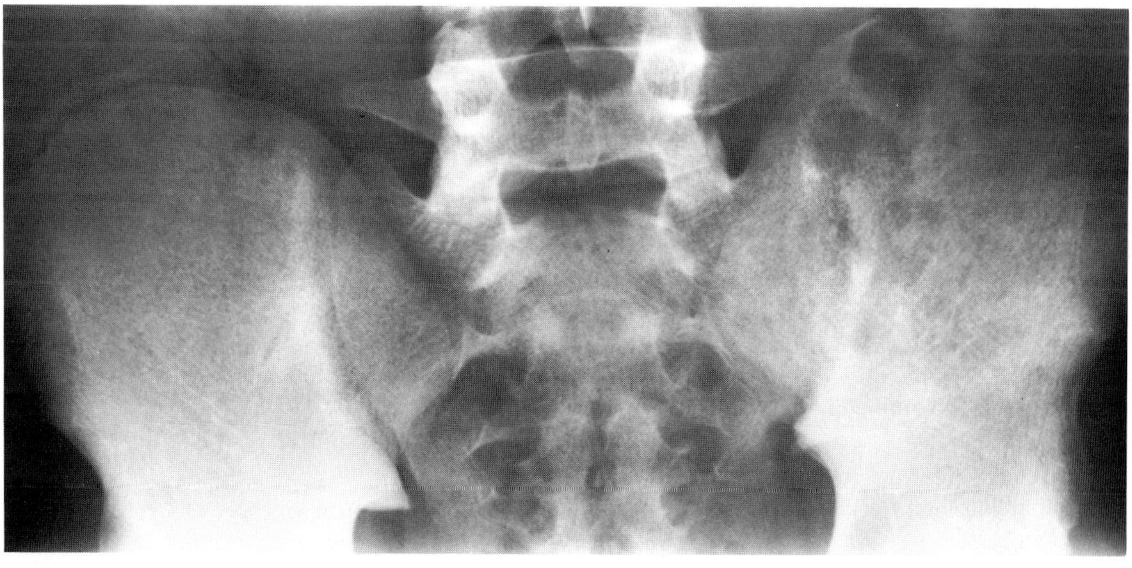

**Figure 28-16.** Sacroiliitis. Irregularity, widening, and reactive sclerosis of the left sacroiliac joint are the classic features of inflammatory disease. In this case, biopsy demonstrated infection.

sections of CT. An anteroposterior diameter of less than 12 mm severely compromises the space for the thecal sac.

Achondroplasia, although a rare condition, is associated with severe spinal stenosis secondary to impaired enchondral ossification. Because the condition can lead to neurologic deficit and paraplegia, it cannot be disregarded in an algorithm on back pain. The radiographic signs of achondroplasia are

1. Progressive reduction of the interpedicular distance from L1 to L5
2. Posterior vertebral body scalloping
3. Champagne-glass shape of the pelvic cavity
4. Marked spinal stenosis on CT scan

### No Radiologic Signs

A normal plain film should simply be reported as such. There is no justification for hedging the report with meaningless equivocal phrases. However, if there is high clinical suspicion that a dangerous lesion exists in the face of normal plain films, a series of further steps will uncover the lesion.

## STEPS II and III. Radiographic Signs of a Serious Underlying Disorder—Infection? Tumor? Ankylosing Spondylitis?

If signs of infection are present on plain radiographs, aspiration of the lesion and culture are the next steps. Problems arise when the aspirating needle is incorrectly placed or when the lesion is missed on open biopsy (particularly in the thoracic spine). Therefore, it is imperative that the lesion be precisely localized by intraoperative radiography, fluoroscopy, or CT.

When signs of neoplasm are present on plain films, the radionuclide bone scan will define whether the neoplasm is solitary or metastatic. If metastases are present, biopsy of the most accessible lesion will lead to the histologic diagnosis. If the neoplasm is solitary, CT may be required for further definition of soft-tissue involvement of the spinal canal.

Ankylosing spondylitis is usually obvious on the plain film. Questionable findings may be confirmed by oblique films of the sacroiliac joints or an anteroposterior view of the pelvis with the tube angled 25° cephalad (Ferguson view). If the patient carries the HLA-B27 gene, this is further evidence for ankylosing spondylitis (90% of patients with ankylosing spondylitis are HLA-B27 positive, compared with only 5% of the normal population).

## STEPS II and III. Radiographic Signs of Benign Disease—Degenerative Disc Disease? Facet Joint Osteoarthrosis? Degenerative Disease with Neurologic Signs?

It first must be decided whether one, two, or three of the above pathologic conditions are present. Acute inflammation secondary to disc protrusion or facet joint irritation can be confirmed by local block and eased with the addition of corticosteroids. Neurologic impairment implies cauda equina, nerve root, or spinal cord compression. Further delineation in the presence of neurologic deficit requires CT, myelography, or MRI.

## STEPS II and III. No Radiographic Signs in the Presence of Back Pain—Pain Only? Neurologic Signs Present? Suspicion of Occult Tumor or Infection?

The clinical suspicion of occult tumor or infection requires a radionuclide bone scan or MRI. Patients with suspected spinal cord compression are evaluated in the same manner as those with signs of degenerative disease and neurologic deficit. A normal plain film in the presence of pain is common in the younger person with intervertebral disc disease. Diagnosis and treatment may require epidural or facet block. When clinical signs and symptoms do not coincide, there may be a multitude of emotional reasons for the patient's back pain.

## Bibliography

Ayres J et al: An improved method for sacroiliac joint imaging: A study of normal subjects, patients with sacroiliitis and patients with low back pain. Clin Radiol 32:441, 1981

Borlaza GS et al: Computed tomography in the evaluation of sacroiliac arthritis. Radiology 139:437, 1981

Boyd WR, Gardiner GA: Metrizamide myelography. AJR 129:481–484, 1977

Brant–Zawadzki M, Burke VD, Jeffrey RB: CT in the evaluation of spine infection. Spine 8:358–365, 1983

Byrd SE, Cohn ML, Biggers SL et al: The radiographic evaluation of the symptomatic postoperative lumbar spine patient. Spine 10:652–662, 1985

Carrera GF: Computed tomography in sacroiliitis. Clin Rheum Dis 9:403–417, 1983

Dyck P, Pheasant HG, Doyle JB et al: Intermittent cauda equina compression syndrome: Its recognition and treatment. Spine 2:75–82, 1977

Forrester DM, Brown JC: The Radiology of Joint Disease, 3rd ed. Philadelphia, WB Saunders, 1986

Gershater R, Holgate RC: Lumbar epidural venography in the diagnosis of disc herniations. AJR 126:992–1002, 1976

Helms CA, Vogler JB: Computed tomography of spinal stenosis and arthroses. Clin Rheum Dis 9: 417–443, 1983

Helms CA, Vogler JB III: Spinal stenosis and degenerative lesions. In Newton TH, Potts DG (eds): Modern Neuroradiology. San Anselmo, CA, Clavadel Press, 1983

Hollingsworth PN, Dawkins RL, Forrester DM: Difficulties in the radiographic diagnosis of sacroiliitis. Clin Rheum Dis 9:323–333, 1983

Joshi KB, Brinker RA: Fine needle diagnosis in lumbar osteomyelitis. Skeletal Radiol 10:173–176, 1983

Kerr R, Resnick D: Radiology of the seronegative spondyloarthropathies. Clin Rheum Dis 11: 113–147, 1985

Miller MH, Handel SF, Coan JD: Transfemoral lumbar epidural venography. AJR 126:1003–1009, 1976

Mooney V, Robertson J: The facet syndrome. Clin Orthop 115:149–156, 1976

Nachemson AL: The lumbar spine. An orthopedic challenge. Spine 1:59–71, 1976

Nance EP, Jr, Kaye JJ: The rheumatoid variants. Semin Roentgenol 17:16–25, 1982

Park WM: The place of radiology in the investigation of low back pain. Clin Rheum Dis 6:93–133, 1980

Resnick D: Degenerative diseases of the vertebral column. Radiology 156:3–14, 1985

Resnick D, Niwayama G: Radiographic and pathologic features of spinal involvement in diffuse idiopathic skeletal hyperostosis (DISH). Radiology 119:559–568, 1976

Resnick D, Shaul SR, Robins JM: Diffuse idiopathic skeletal hyperostosis (DISH): Forestier's disease with extraspinal manifestations. Radiology 115: 513–524, 1975

Schutte HE, Park WM: The diagnostic value of bone scintigraphy in patients with low back pain. Skeletal Radiol 10:1–5, 1983

**A RADIOLOGIC APPROACH TO THE DIFFERENTIAL DIAGNOSIS OF BACK PAIN***

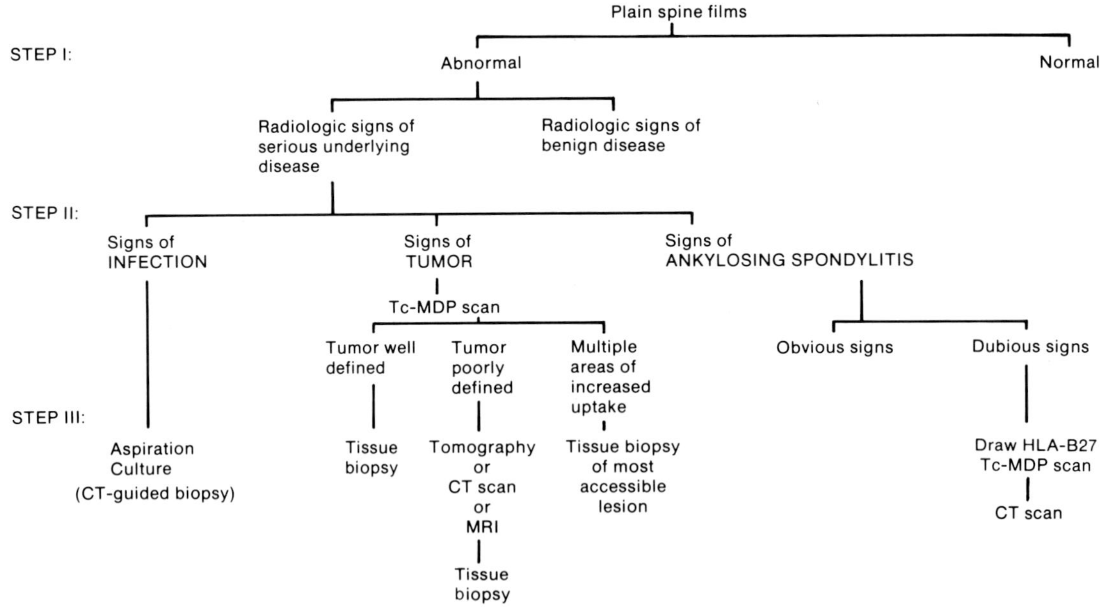


*If medicolegal implication, obtain a CT scan

Modified from Forrester DM, Brown JC, Nesson JW: The Radiology of Joint Disease, 3rd ed., Philadelphia, WB Saunders, 1986.

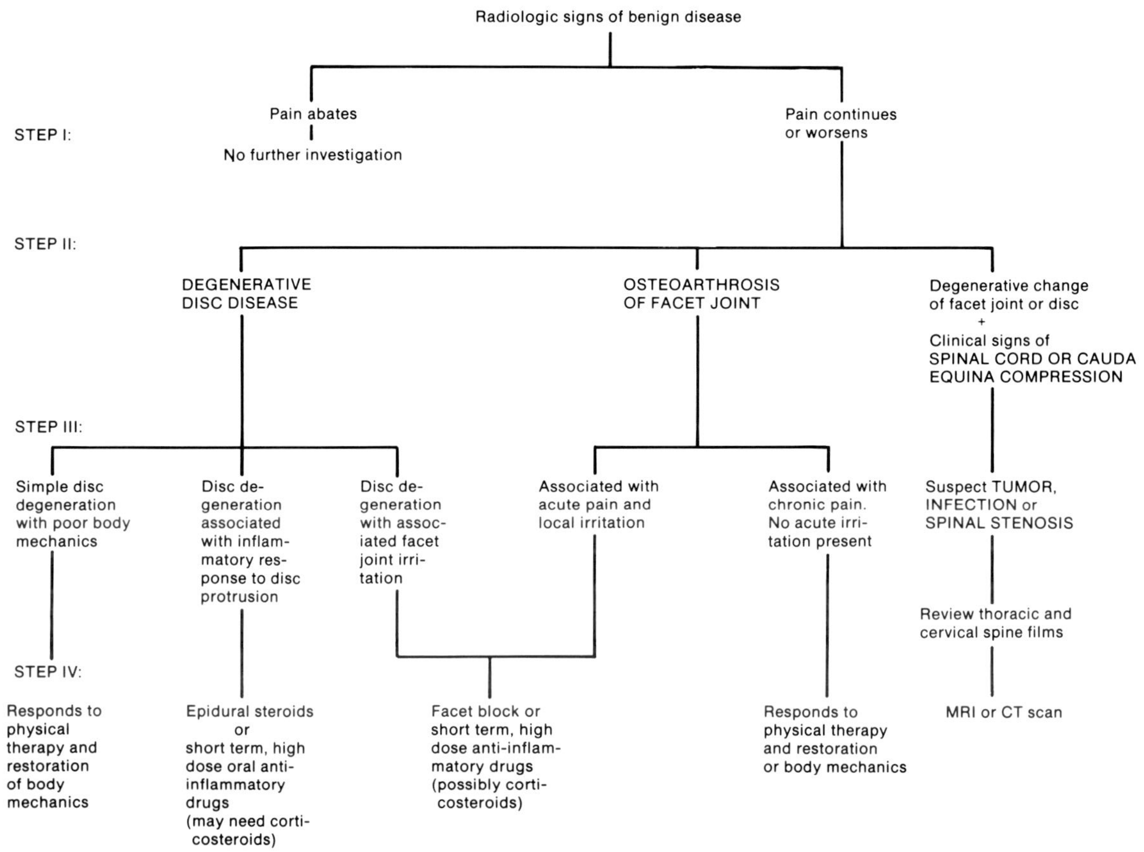
Radiologic signs of benign disease
STEP I:
Pain abates
No further investigation
Pain continues or worsens
STEP II:
DEGENERATIVE DISC DISEASE
OSTEOARTHROSIS OF FACET JOINT
Degenerative change of facet joint or disc
+
Clinical signs of SPINAL CORD OR CAUDA EQUINA COMPRESSION
STEP III:
Simple disc degeneration with poor body mechanics
Disc degeneration associated with inflammatory response to disc protrusion
Disc degeneration with associated facet joint irritation
Associated with acute pain and local irritation
Associated with chronic pain. No acute irritation present
Suspect TUMOR, INFECTION or SPINAL STENOSIS
Review thoracic and cervical spine films
STEP IV:
Responds to physical therapy and restoration of body mechanics
Epidural steroids or short term, high dose oral anti-inflammatory drugs (may need corticosteroids)
Facet block or short term, high dose anti-inflammatory drugs (possibly corticosteroids)
Responds to physical therapy and restoration or body mechanics
MRI or CT scan

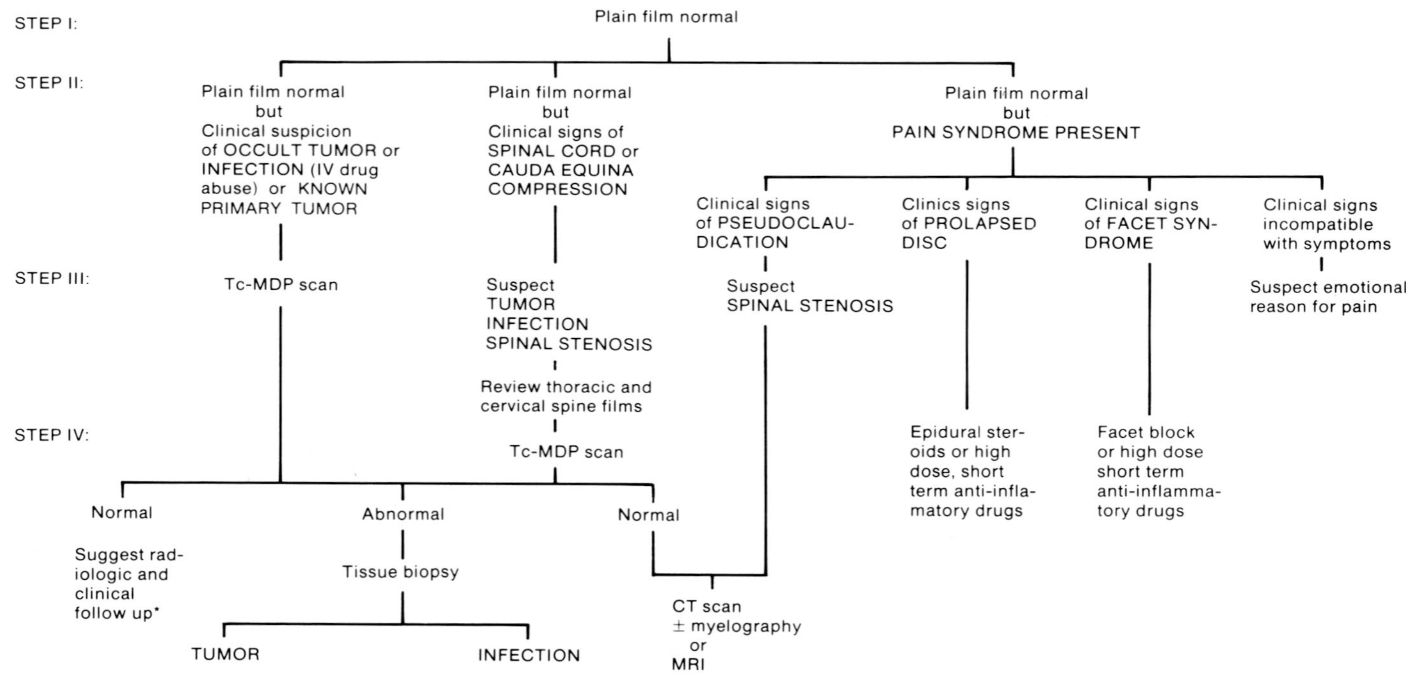


*Multiple myeloma is the one tumor which can suppress osteoblastic activity and give a negative Tc—MDP scan.

# Chapter 29

# Arthritis

John C. Brown
D. M. Forrester

People the world over complain of aches and pains, but comparatively few suffer from "true" arthritis. Strict clinical and radiologic criteria are required to determine whether pain is secondary to a pathologic condition of the joint itself or arises from something around a normal joint.

## CLINICAL FINDINGS

The clinical findings for arthritis include the following:

- Pain or tenderness to palpation
- Swelling
- Deformity or loss of motion

## DIAGNOSTIC EVALUATION

The radiographic criteria for the diagnosis of arthritis are more complicated than the clinical criteria, because a physical examination is usually not available to the radiologist and the clinical history is most often abbreviated at best. Despite the sophisticated techniques listed below, plain radiography remains the primary imaging procedure.

### *DIAGNOSTIC MODALITIES*

1. Radionuclide scans
2. Arthrography
3. Computed tomography
4. Magnetic resonance imaging
5. Thermography
6. Plain radiography

### Radionuclide Scans

The technetium phosphate bone scan is an exquisitely sensitive, but nonspecific, imaging modality. Its major value is in localizing the site of musculoskeletal complaints to joints that are difficult to examine and in establishing a specific joint as the etiology of pain in a patient with focal musculoskeletal complaints and a normal plain radiograph. Typically, the isotope uptake in acute arthritis localizes to both articular bones, thus indicating that the primary site of disease is the joint rather than bone or surrounding soft tissues (Fig. 29-1*A*).

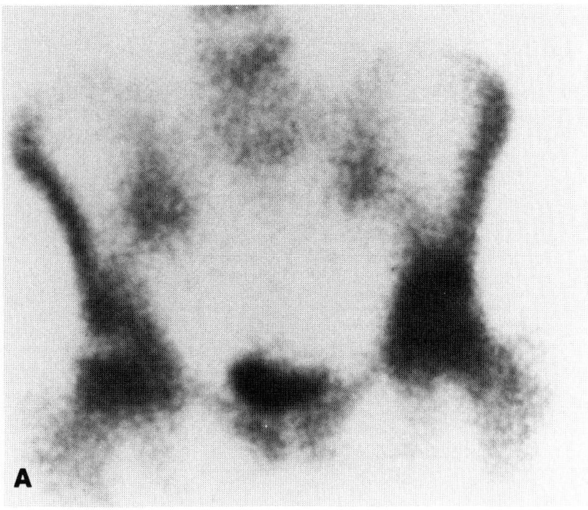


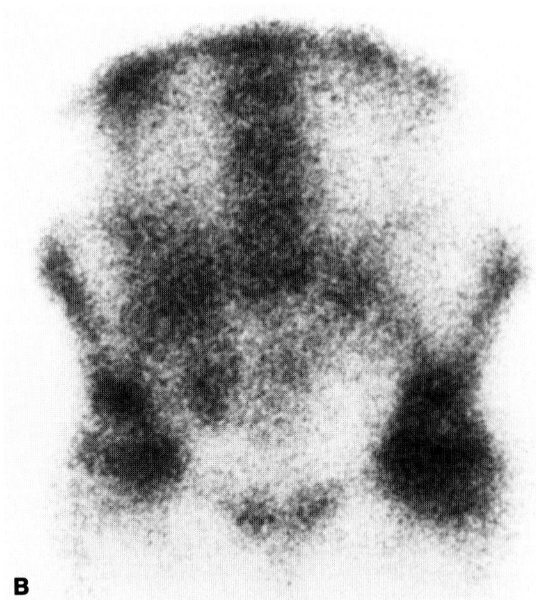


**Figure 29-1.** Infectious arthritis. **(A)** Marked increased uptake of $^{99m}$Tc-MDP in the left hip documents the presence of a monarticular arthritis. **(B)** $^{67}$Ga citrate collects in the left hip joint, corresponding to the bone scan and diagnostic of an active infectious arthritis.

Scans using $^{99m}$Tc pertechnetate or $^{99m}$Tc-methylene diphosphonate (MDP) can verify a questionably inflamed joint. Immediate scanning following injection of the radionuclide demonstrates the blood flow, resulting in a blood pool image. Increased activity around the joint indicates hyperemia and an active inflammatory arthritis. To diagnose the cause of inflammation, however, requires joint aspiration (arthrocentesis) and assessment of the synovial fluid.

The conventional delayed $^{99m}$Tc-MDP scan establishes the distribution of the arthritis. Whereas the blood pool scan (immediate scan) reveals the hyperemic areas, the delayed scan demonstrates involved joints, including ones that may be difficult to visualize (*e.g.*, the sternomanubrial and temporomandibular joints). Since evaluation of a radionuclide scan is based on a comparison with the uptake of the normal contralateral side, symmetric involvement may be difficult to assess by this technique.

The $^{67}$Ga citrate scan is a useful adjunct to the technetium phosphate bone scan. Because the isotope tags to white blood cells and plasma proteins, it tends to localize in areas of infections. The focal uptake of gallium in the region of the joint is evidence of a pyarthrosis (Fig. 29-1*B*).

## Arthrography

Arthrography has no role in the determination of the type of arthritis. Although synovial hypertrophy may be detected as a filling defect on arthrography, it is diagnosed more inexpensively by a physical examination or plain radiography. In the presence of severe unexplained secondary osteoarthrosis, arthrography is occasionally useful in detecting osteochondral fragments within the joint capsule from previous episodes of trauma.

The most common use of arthrography is to verify the intra-articular position of a needle following attempted aspiration of a difficult or inaccessible joint. A small amount of water-soluble contrast material injected after aspiration can outline the joint capsule and establish the proper placement of the needle.

## Computed Tomography

Rarely, computed tomography (CT)may be necessary to verify destructive changes of a large joint that are suspected clinically but not seen on plain films (Fig. 29-2). Chronic synovial hyper-

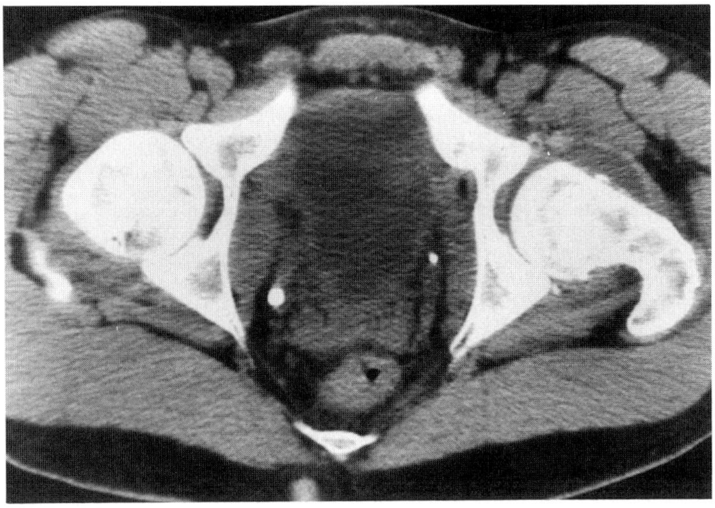

**Figure 29-2.** CT scan of hip joint. Soft-tissue window demonstrates decreased attenuation around the femoral head and displacement of the joint capsule, representing an effusion. Small intra-articular bone fragments are seen, as well as asymmetric narrowing of the joint space. The secondary osteoarthrosis developed during the year following a posterior dislocation of the hip with retained fracture fragments.

trophy may result in erosion of the articular bone, but CT plays no role in determining the cause of the synovitis. If the "hypertrophied" synovium is discovered to be a malignant tumor, CT should be used to determine whether there has been invasion of the underlying bone.

Evaluation of the sacroiliac joints is notoriously difficult during the earliest stages of disease. If the diagnosis of a rheumatoid variant rests on the determination of axial skeletal involvement, CT might be considered as a supplementary diagnostic tool. Similarly, although the sternoclavicular joints are impossible to evaluate with plain films, CT scans can easily identify degenerative or inflammatory changes involving these joints.

### Magnetic Resonance Imaging

Magnetic resonance imaging (MRI) was initially believed to be most suited for imaging the brain and spinal cord. With greater experience, however, MRI has been found to have many applications in the evaluation of musculoskeletal disorders. Because tendons, muscles, cartilage, and joint fluid have different signal intensities, MRI provides a unique noninterventional method for assessing joints. Although the application of this modality to problems of arthritis is in its infancy, the high signal intensity of a joint effusion makes MRI a useful tool for assessing early arthritis when plain films are normal (Fig. 29-3). Meniscal tears, ligamentous ruptures, and rotator cuff tears may also be evaluated with this technique.

### Thermography

Like the radionuclide blood pool image, thermography may be useful in establishing the location of inflamed joints. Increased blood flow results in increased temperature, which is easily detected by thermography. It is debatable, however, whether thermography or radionuclide scanning adds more than a careful physical examination by an experienced observer.

## RADIOPATHOLOGY OF JOINT DISEASE

There are three categories of arthritis:

- Inflammatory joint disease
- Degenerative joint disease (osteoarthrosis)
- Metabolic deposition disease

### Inflammatory Joint Disease

Of the three compartments of a synovial joint—bone, cartilage, and synovium—the last bears the brunt in inflammatory joint disease. Because

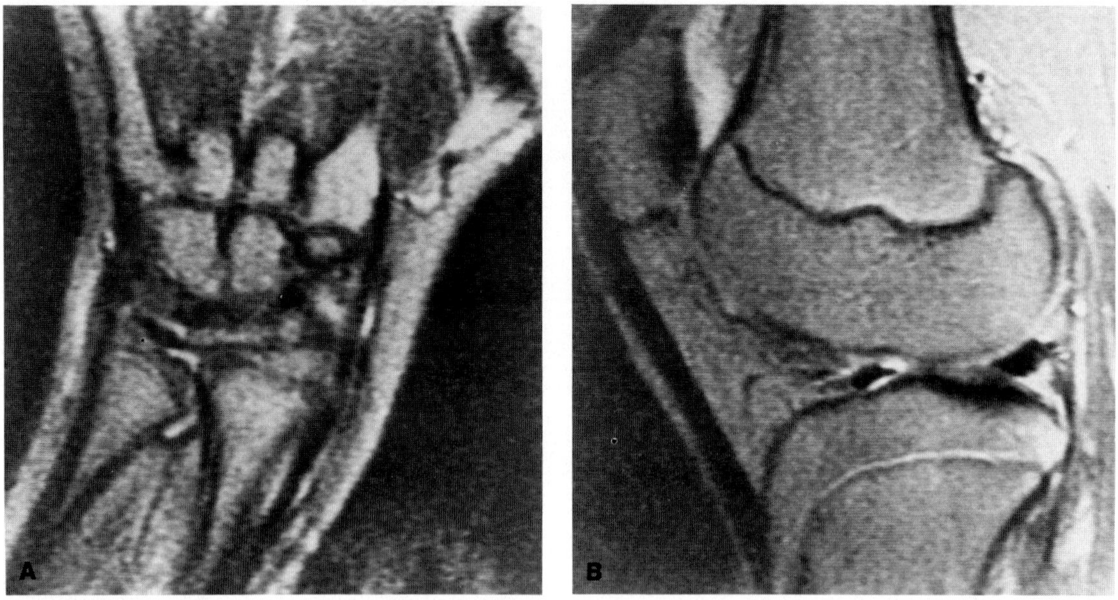

**Figure 29-3.** MRI in rheumatoid arthritis. **(A)** The increased signal within the flexor carpi radialis tendon and the radio-ulnar and radiocarpal joints indicates excess synovial fluid. **(B)** A joint effusion appears as a high-intensity signal that fills the suprapatellar recess, surrounds the triangular low-signal intensity menisci, and outlines the posterior femoral condyle. (Courtesy of David Stoller, M.D.)

of its vascularity and phagocytic potential, the synovium reacts to any irritant (whether bacteria, urate crystal, or immune complex) with inflammatory swelling and exudation of inflammatory fluid. Later the synovium hypertrophies and contains a large number of inflammatory cells. If the inflammatory disease continues, the prolonged destructive action of both the inflammatory fluid and the creeping, invasive hypertrophied synovium (pannus) dissolves away the cartilage cap. The cartilage thins, and joint fluid forces its way into the unyielding bony substructure (bony erosion).

The radiographic signs of inflammatory joint disease are

- Soft-tissue swelling (often synovial effusion and synovial hypertrophy)
- Uniform loss of cartilage space
- Bony erosions

The seronegative spondyloarthropathies (rheumatoid variants) frequently produce a pronounced inflammation of tendons and ligaments in addition to arthritis. This leads to periosteal reaction around an inflamed joint and syndesmophyte formation about the vertebral bodies.

## Degenerative Joint Disease (Osteoarthrosis)

Excessive wearing of hyaline cartilage causes the formation of osteophytes, a bony reaction to buttress the articulation. The cause may be idiopathic (primary osteoarthrosis) or secondary to disease of bone and cartilage (see Secondary Osteoarthrosis).

The radiographic signs are similar in both primary and secondary disease. The biomechanical wear and tear produces uneven loss of cartilage space (joint space narrowing) and the development of osteophytes. When calcification of cartilage predisposes to premature wear, chondrocalcinosis occurs. The combination of osteoarthrosis and chondrocalcinosis suggests the presence of secondary osteoarthrosis.

### Metabolic Deposition Disease

The deposition of substances within the synovial joints and their surrounding structures occurs in various diseases, most notably gout. The deposit manifests itself as a soft-tissue lump that eventually may invade the cartilage and bony structures. The radiographic criteria of metabolic deposition diseases are asymmetric para-articular soft-tissue swelling and associated periarticular erosion.

## MAJOR AND MINOR RADIOGRAPHIC CRITERIA OF ARTHRITIS

The plain firm radiographic criteria of arthritis are

*Major Criteria*
- Joint effusion (Fig. 29-4)
- Joint space narrowing (Fig. 29-5)
- Erosion (Fig. 29-6)
- Chondrocalcinosis (Fig. 29-7)
- Osteophytes (Fig. 29-8)

*Minor Criteria*
- Alignment changes (Fig. 29-9)
- Juxta-articular demineralization (Fig. 29-10)
- Periosteal reaction (Fig. 29-11)
- Diffusely swollen digit (cocktail sausage digit) (Fig. 29-11)

The major radiographic criteria of arthritis are reliable indicators of true joint pathology. There is one note of caution. The presence of an osteophyte at the articular margin of a joint indicates underlying degenerative cartilage and the presence of osteoarthrosis. However, response to the pull of tendons and ligaments around joints may also cause formation of bony spurs (*i.e.*, olecranon, patellar, and calcaneal spurs) without underlying arthritis. In one group of patients, spur formation along the anterior longitudinal ligament of the spine or in peripheral tendons is common even without underlying cartilage degeneration or pain. The condition is known by several names—Forestier's disease, diffuse idiopathic skeletal hyperostosis (DISH), and ankylosing vertebral hyperostosis.

The four minor radiographic criteria may be seen in conditions other than arthritis and thus do not by themselves establish the presence of joint disease. Alignment abnormalities of the large joints or small joints of the hands and feet may indicate an underlying arthritis and may be due to uneven wear of cartilage or to inflammatory involvement of the joint capsule and surrounding tendons and ligaments. Nonarthritic conditions, however, may also cause alignment abnormalities. Neuromuscular imbalance from an underlying neurologic or muscle disorder may cause deformity around a joint. For example, dorsal contraction of the toes is a common radiographic finding. It usually signifies biomechanical imbalance with dorsal subluxation and only rarely signals an underlying inflammatory arthritis.

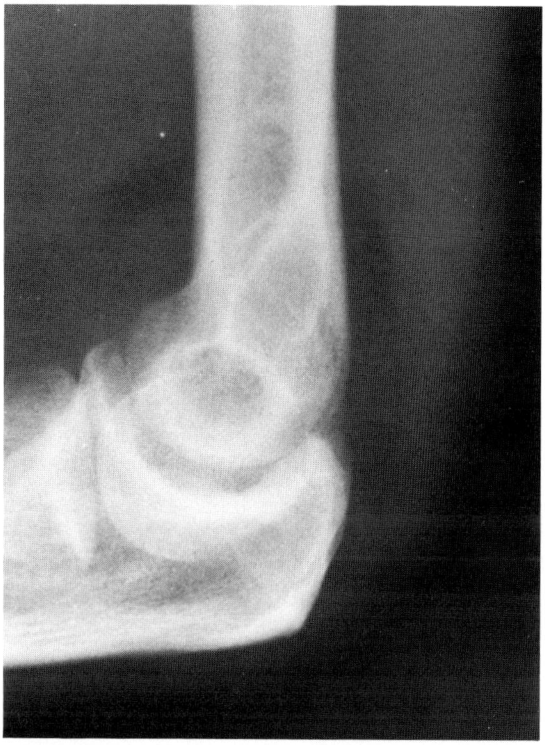

**Figure 29-4.** Joint effusion. Displacement of the anterior and posterior fat pads documents distention of the capsule of the elbow joint.

Hyperemia associated with inflammatory arthritis quickly leads to juxta-articular demineralization about the individual joints. This find-

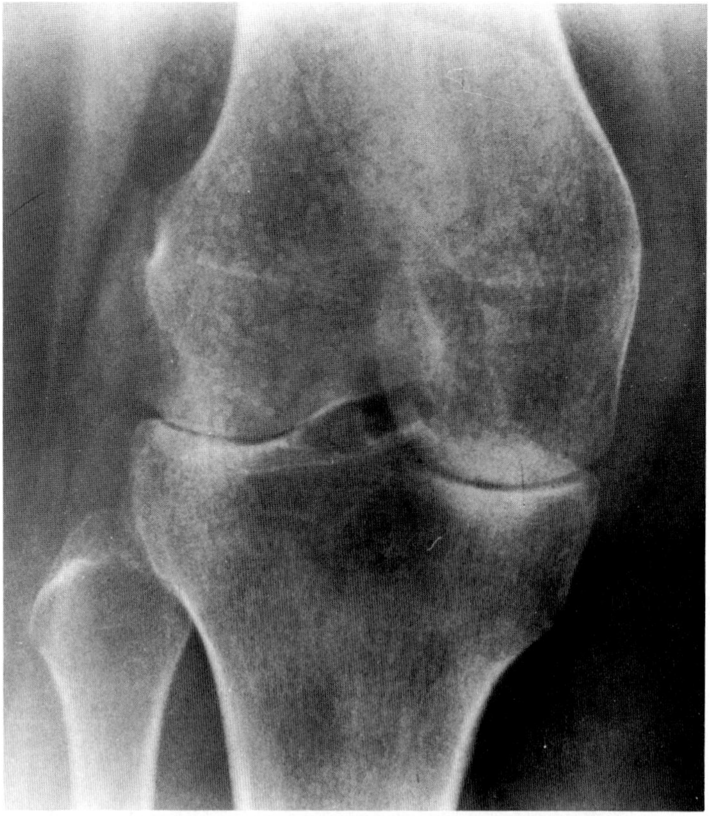

**Figure 29-5.** Joint space narrowing. Uniform joint space narrowing between the femur and tibia indicates inflammatory arthritis with destruction of cartilage.

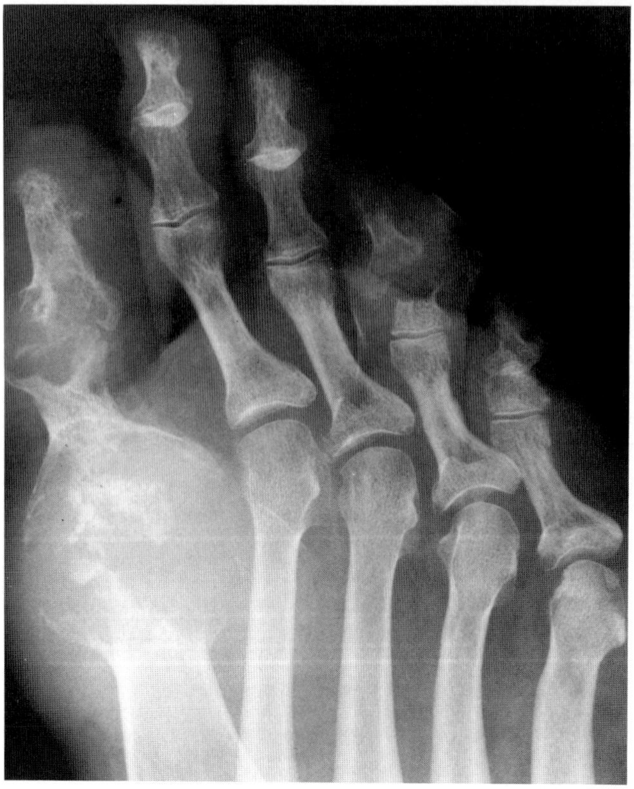

**Figure 29-6.** Erosion. Huge erosions of the first metatarsophalangeal joint, the interphalangeal joint of the great toe, and the distal interphalangeal joint of the fourth toe document a destructive joint disease.

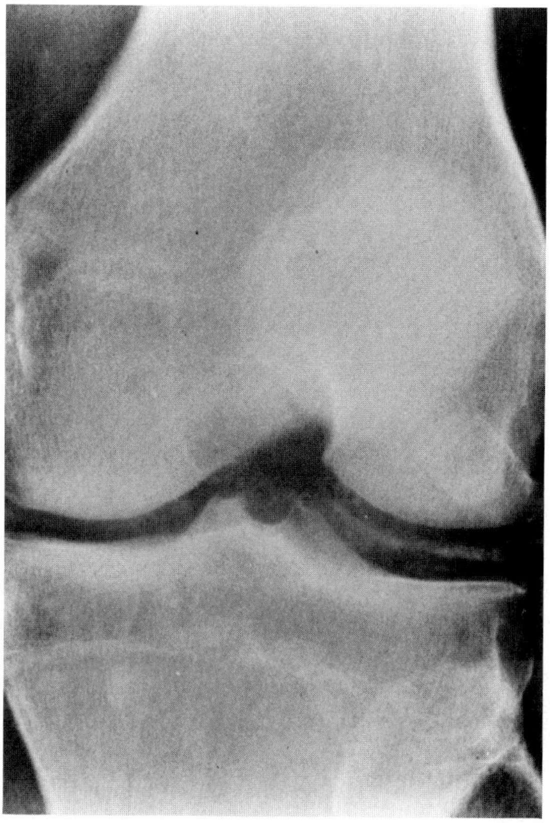

**Figure 29-7.** Chondrocalcinosis. Faint outlines of the meniscal and hyaline articular cartilage can be seen, with no associated wear and tear of the joint.

ing is very nonspecific, however, and may be seen with disuse, Sudeck's atrophy (reflex sympathetic dystrophy syndrome), and systemic corticosteroid use.

Periosteal reaction is associated with both infectious arthritis and the inflammatory arthritis of the rheumatoid variants. It may also be seen with underlying osteomyelitis or tumor. Generalized periosteal reaction occurs in hypertrophic osteoarthropathy and idiopathic osteoarthropathy. In these two conditions, an arthritis may be present clinically but generally is not a predominant clinical complaint.

A diffusely swollen digit may reflect the arthritis and tendinitis of a rheumatoid variant. The generalized soft-tissue response, however, may also be seen with osteomyelitis or cellulitis.

## SOFT-TISSUE SYNDROMES MIMICKING ARTHRITIS

Pain often arises from structures around joints—bursae, tendons, and ligaments. At the shoulder, for instance, pain commonly occurs at the site of insertion of the rotator cuff muscles and both heads of the biceps. At the knee, unbalanced mechanics stress the medial ligament and in-

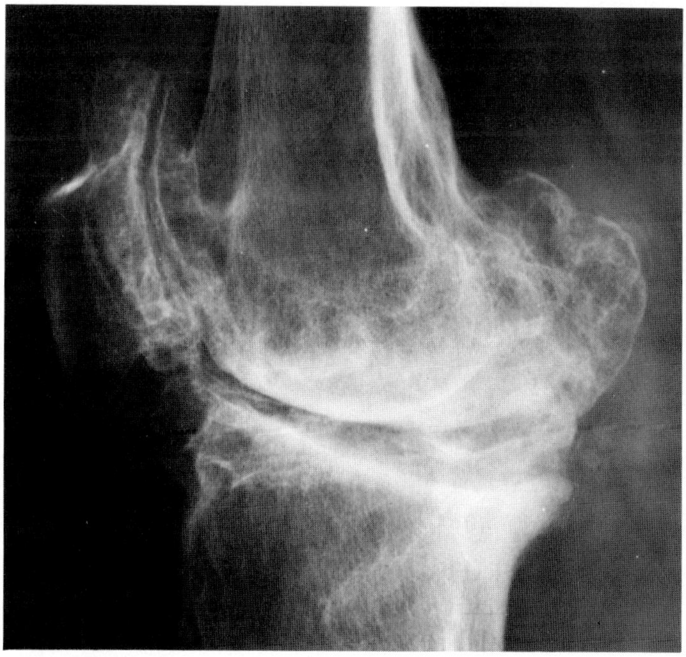

**Figure 29-8.** Osteophytes. Huge osteophytes deform the patellofemoral and femorotibial joints of the knee.

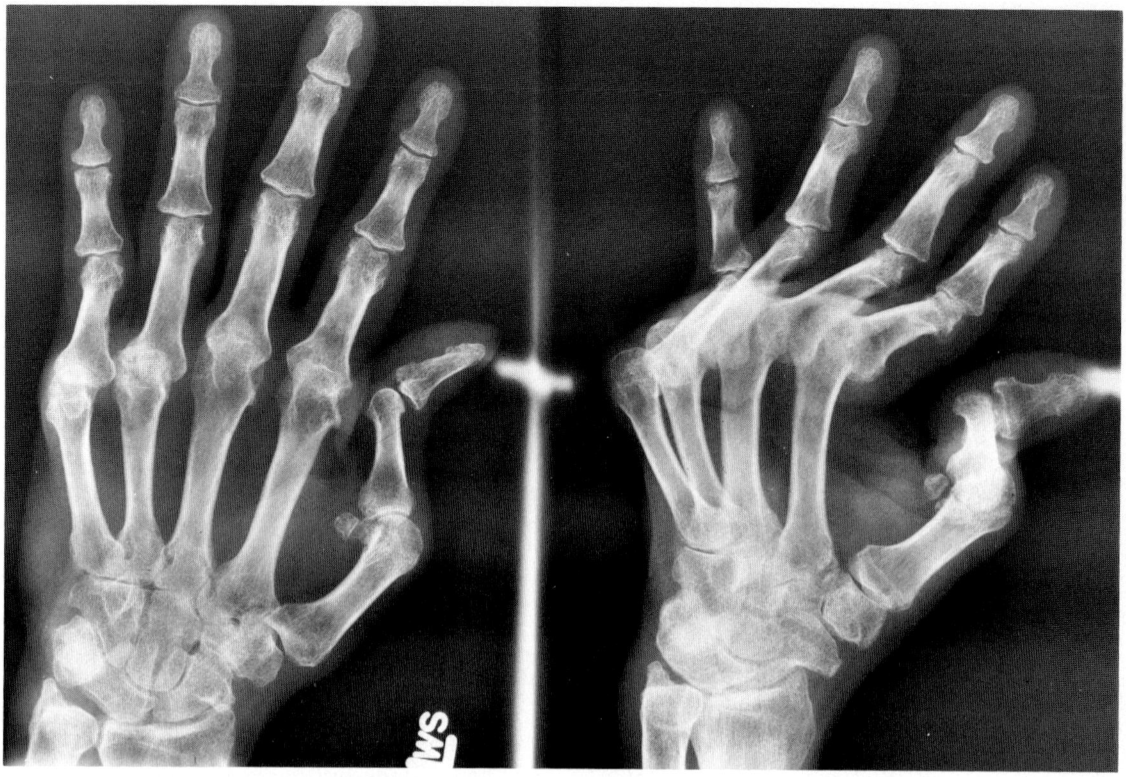

**Figure 29-9.** Alignment changes. Subluxation of the phalanges at the metacarpal articulation and hyperextension of the proximal interphalangeal joints indicate inflammatory arthritis.

flame the anserine bursa, one of the three characteristic sites for knee pain.

In the athlete, no diagnostic confusion arises, because this soft-tissue pain is usually associated with a normal radiograph. In the older patient, however, similar pain often occurs in the presence of osteoarthrosis. The source of pain may then be incorrectly attributed to the radiographic findings.

Atrophy and poor use of tendons (shoulder, elbow, hip, and knee) may result in intratendinous calcification. Rupture of these deposits acutely inflames neighboring bursae and also mimics "acute arthritis" (Fig. 29-12). One must be wary, however, of assuming that the source of pain is from an adjacent calcified tendon; pain may originate from tendons that do not contain a calcified focus. Correlation with the physical examination is essential to localize correctly the involved tendon during an acute episode of pain.

Accurate diagnosis of the soft-tissue syndromes is important, because these conditions respond to simple therapeutic methods.

## THE RADIOGRAPHIC EXAMINATION

There is no such thing as an "arthritis survey." Ideally, the radiographic assessment of arthritis includes a comparison view of the opposite extremity. Initial films include all symptomatic joints. Most radiology departments are accustomed to obtaining standard views for suspected trauma, but generally the diagnosis of arthritis requires fewer projections.

The following views are essential:

- *Hands (including wrists):* anteroposterior
- *Elbow:* anteroposterior and lateral
- *Shoulders:* anteroposterior in neutral position and internal rotation; axillary view

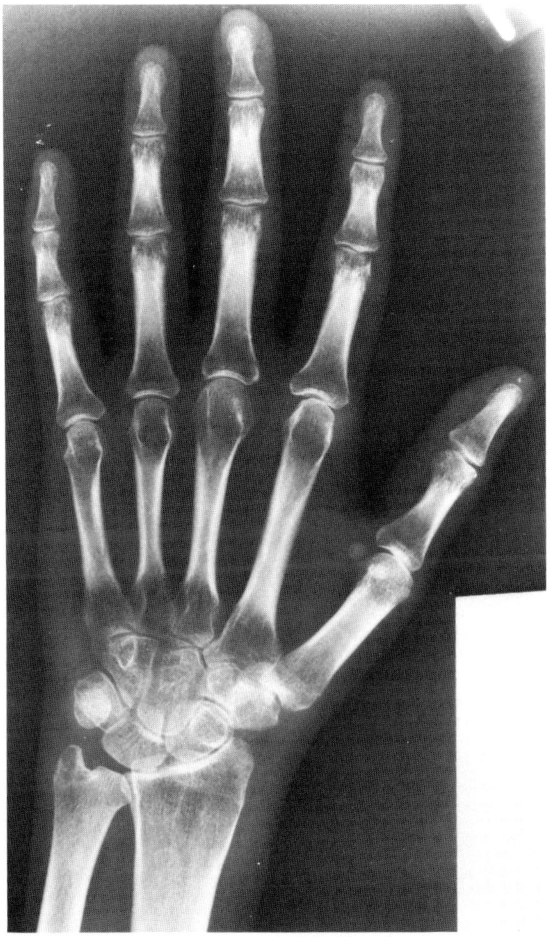

**Figure 29-10.** Juxta-articular demineralization. All bones of the hand demonstrate marked osteoporosis limited to the region of the joint capsules.

- *Neck:* anteroposterior and lateral cervical spine
- *Pelvis:* anteroposterior, including hips and sacroiliac joints
- *Sacroiliac joints:* anteroposterior or posteroanterior view of the pelvis (oblique views or Ferguson view if abnormality questioned on pelvic radiograph)
- *Hips:* anteroposterior pelvis; frogleg view of symptomatic hip
- *Knees:* anteroposterior and lateral
- *Ankle:* anteroposterior and lateral
- *Feet:* anteroposterior and lateral

A patient with arthritis of the small joints of the hands or feet frequently has involvement of both extremities. Since the pattern of distribution is as important as the specific radiographic changes, both hands or both feet should be included in the initial assessment. For example, a patient with a painful wrist should have anteroposterior films of both hands. Similarly, examination of the foot

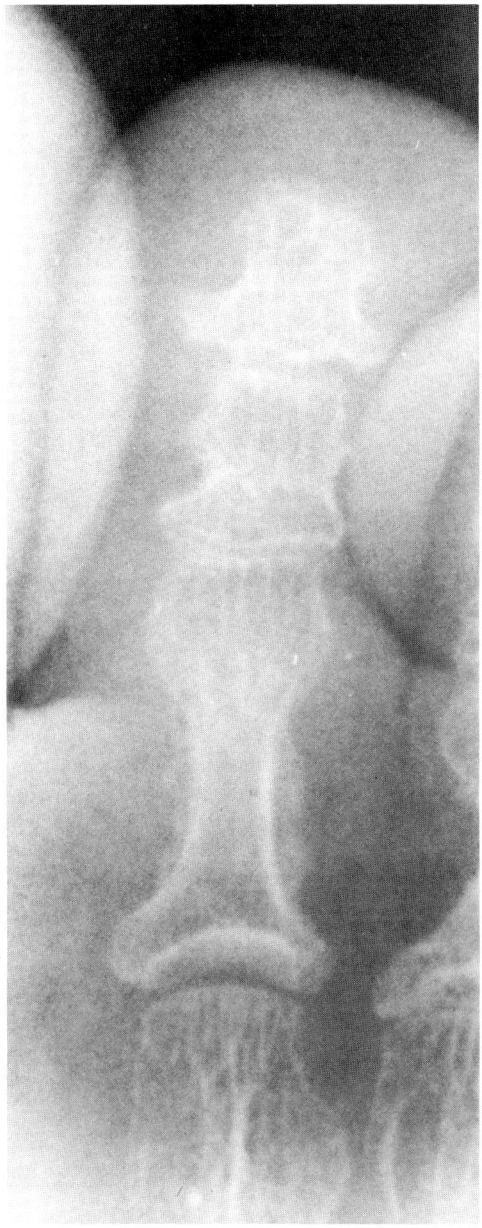

**Figure 29-11.** Periosteal reaction accompanying a diffusely swollen digit. Fluffy periosteal new bone surrounds the proximal phalanx in this diffusely swollen toe.

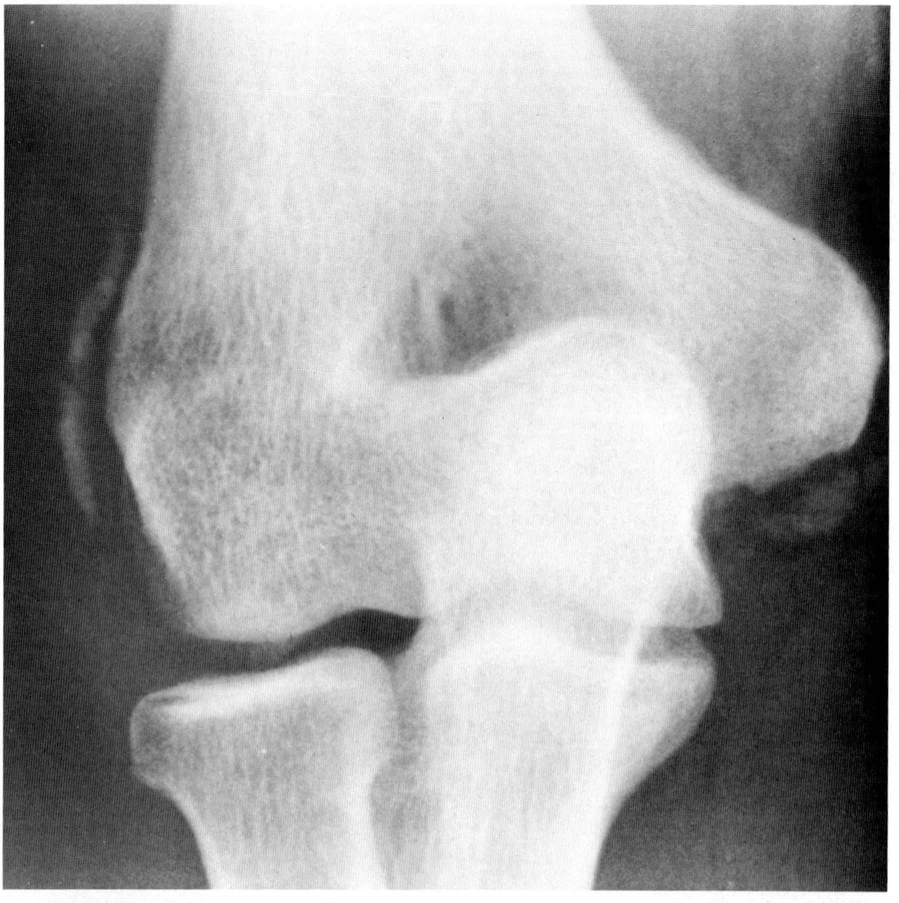

**Figure 29-12.** Calcific tendinitis. There is amorphous calcification in the region of the extensor and flexor tendons. No radiographic evidence of arthritis is present.

must include the opposite foot as well as a lateral projection in order to assess the joints of the midfoot and hindfoot.

Effusions of the knee, ankle, and elbow are best visualized on a lateral projection. The initial screening examination of these joints requires anteroposterior and lateral views.

The vast majority of patients with shoulder pain have one of the soft-tissue syndromes. Two anteroposterior views, using different degrees of rotation of the humerus, maximize the ability to detect subtle calcifications of the rotator cuff, which may be superimposed on the humeral head on a single projection. The axillary view projects the tendons of the rotator cuff anterior and posterior to the humeral head, thus localizing the site of increased density to bone or soft tissue.

Because of variations in width and appearance of the hip joint, an anteroposterior view of the pelvis allows comparison with the patient's asymptomatic joint. Furthermore, pain from sacroiliitis and facet joints, as well as the pubic rami and symphysis joint, is frequently referred to the hip; inclusion of the sacroiliac joints and lower lumbar spine on the pelvic radiograph is important in the assessment of hip pain. By adding a frogleg projection, early signs of avascular necrosis may be detected, and a second look at the soft tissues may demonstrate previously undetected calcification.

Because of the obliquity of the sacroiliac joints, it may be impossible to assess them from a single frontal projection. It is reassuring to recognize that a normal-appearing sacroiliac joint on an anteroposterior projection will appear normal on other views. However, if the sacroiliac joint is abnormal on the anteroposterior projection (narrowed, eroded, or sclerotic), it is necessary to obtain additional projections in order to view the joint tangentially. Either 30° oblique views, a posteroanterior (prone) view, or a Ferguson view (anteroposterior, with the tube angled 25° toward the head), which visually elongates the joint, offers a more precise method for evaluating the joint space. Rarely, one must resort to CT to delineate the joint space and the articular margins of the sacrum and iliac bones.

## HOW TO USE THE ALGORITHM

### STEP I. Are Major or Minor Criteria Present?

Using the major and minor criteria of joint disease, the first step is to decide whether arthritis is present. If no major or minor criteria are present, the radiologic report should state, "No radiographic evidence of arthritis." Further follow-up films are indicated if clinically required.

### STEP II. Are Minor and Major Criteria Fulfilled?

If only minor criteria are present, be suspicious of underlying joint pathology. Periosteal reaction with or without a diffusely swollen digit (cocktail sausage digit) indicates a possible rheumatoid variant or osteomyelitis. Juxta-articular demineralization or alignment abnormalities signify a possible inflammatory polyarthritis.

The presence of one or more major criteria means that joint pathology is present.

### STEP III. Monarticular Arthritis or Polyarthritic Disease?

Occasionally, only one joint is available for review. In these instances, the patient should be viewed as having monarticular disease unless other information becomes available. The presence of monarticular or polyarticular disease should be decided according to the major criteria.

### STEP IV. Monarticular Disease

If signs of osteoarthrosis are present and there is no effusion, be suspicious that only a symptomatic joint was examined, because osteoarthrosis is a polyarticular disease.

In the presence of effusion, there are four causes of monarticular arthritis:

- Trauma
- Infection
- Crystal-induced (gout or pseudogout)
- Rheumatoid arthritis

Of these four conditions, trauma is the most common cause and monarticular rheumatoid arthritis is the rarest. Immediate diagnosis of the cause of the monarticular arthritis is aimed at the early detection of infection, because rapid destruction of articular cartilage in bone will occur if correct antibiotic therapy is delayed. The plain film study rarely reveals the exact diagnosis. Traumatic effusions may develop even without a visible fracture, because excessive strain or soft-tissue injury may result in a noninflammatory joint effusion. The presence of chondrocalcinosis is required to suggest the diagnosis of crystal-induced inflammatory arthritis. This may occur in gout and pseudogout, and a specific diagnosis requires further diagnostic steps. Ancillary imaging procedures, such as technetium phosphate scanning, document the presence of increased metabolic activity of the articular bone but may lead no closer to a precise diagnosis. Therefore, once monarticular arthritis is established by the previously described criteria, diagnosis is made by aspiration of the joint and examination of the fluid for blood, white cells, bacteria, and crystals. An inflammatory arthritis that remains undiagnosed after aspiration necessitates a synovial biopsy. Chronic granulomatous infection (tuberculosis, coccidioidomycosis, and blastomycosis) and rheumatoid arthritis may be demonstrated on biopsy and microscopy. In tuberculous arthritis, synovial fluid cultures may occasionally be negative even though synovial tissue is positive for acid-fast bacilli on microscopy. Synovial tumors (pigmented villonodular synovitis, synovial chrondromatosis, hemangioma, sarcoma) are rare and also can be accurately diagnosed by biopsy. Therefore, if this scheme of diagnostic procedures for monarticular arthritis is followed, no cause, rare or common, will escape detection.

It is important to note that because the hip and shoulder joints are surrounded by large muscle masses, these two joints should be aspirated using fluoroscopic guidance. If no fluid is obtained, a small amount of contrast material is then injected to verify the intra-articular position of the needle. The sacroiliac joints should be aspirated or biopsied using CT guidance for correct needle placement.

## STEP V. Polyarthritis—Inflammatory? Osteoarthrosis? Metabolic Deposition Disease?

### Inflammatory Arthritis

To establish the diagnosis of inflammatory arthritis, one must see either joint effusion or uniform joint space narrowing. Erosions of the articular surfaces may not be present in early or minimal inflammatory polyarthritis.

### Osteoarthrosis

In contrast to the destructive change of inflammatory arthritis, osteoarthrosis is characterized by uneven loss of cartilage space, the production of osteophytes, and subchondral sclerosis. The cause may be primary or secondary.

### Metabolic Deposition Disease

Three characteristic radiographic findings indicate metabolic deposition disease: soft-tissue masses, periarticular erosions, and preservation of the cartilage space. In advanced deposition disease, cartilage may also be worn down (joint space narrowing) secondary to the infiltrating deposit.

## STEP V. Inflammatory Polyarthritis—Rheumatoid Type or Rheumatoid Variant?

### The Rheumatoid Type

The *distribution* of involved joints distinguishes the rheumatoid types from the rheumatoid variants. There are four rheumatoid types:

- Rheumatoid arthritis
- Systemic lupus erythematosus
- Progressive systemic sclerosis (scleroderma)
- Dermatomyositis (polymyositis)

All four are characterized by inflammatory arthritis of the small joints of the hands and feet (wrists, metacarpophalangeal joints, proximal interphalangeal joints, and metatarsophalangeal joints), sparing the distal interphalangeal joints. Of the four rheumatoid types, only rheumatoid arthritis is characterized by severe inflammation and consequent destructive changes. Lupus, scleroderma, and polymyositis are mild inflammatory disorders in which radiographic findings are subtle. Joint effusions are small and frequently are radiographically undetectable, and there is generally no destruction of cartilage or articular bone. Vasculitis may occur in rheumatoid arthritis, lupus, and scleroderma and is reflected in loss of soft tissue of the distal digits and resorption of the underlying phalangeal tufts. Subcutaneous calcification occurs in scleroderma.

### The Seronegative Spondyloarthropathies (Rheumatoid Variants)

There are four rheumatoid variants:

- Ankylosing spondylitis
- Psoriatic arthritis
- Reiter's syndrome
- Inflammatory bowel disease (ulcerative colitis and Crohn's disease)

The rheumatoid variants are distinguished from the rheumatoid types by the following criteria:

1. Asymmetric or random involvement of the small joints of the hands and feet

2. Diffuse soft-tissue swelling of a finger or toe (cocktail sausage digit)
3. Large joint involvement only
4. Sacroiliac and spine involvement

When a digit is involved, there is diffuse soft-tissue swelling, in contrast to the localized capsular swelling of rheumatoid arthritis. If the condition has persisted for longer than 2 weeks, periosteal reaction is frequently severe enough that fluffy periosteal new bone can be seen along the diaphysis of the metacarpals, metatarsals, or phalanges. Inflammatory spur formation and periosteal reaction at the heels are also characteristic of the rheumatoid variants.

The radiographic changes reflect the intensity and duration of the inflammation and are identical for all four of the rheumatoid variants. The specific diagnosis depends on additional clinical information. Inflammatory bowel disease is documented by a barium enema or small bowel study. Psoriatic arthritis and Reiter's syndrome are distinguished from the two other causes by the demonstration of skin and mucocutaneous rashes. Ankylosing spondylitis primarily involves the sacroiliac joints and spine and is diagnosed by excluding gastrointestinal, skin, and mucocutaneous lesions.

## STEP V. Osteoarthrosis—Primary or Secondary?

### Primary Osteoarthrosis

Osteoarthrosis (uneven cartilage wear and osteophyte formation) of the distal interphalangeal joints, proximal interphalangeal joints, and the first carpometacarpal joint of the wrist, without chondrocalcinosis, defines primary osteoarthrosis (Kellgren's disease). Some patients react with a low-grade inflammatory response that results in painful swelling and erosion of articular bone (erosive osteoarthrosis). In addition to small joints, weight-bearing joints such as the hips, knees, and first metatarsophalangeal joints may suffer the same changes in this disease.

### Secondary Osteoarthrosis

A specific underlying etiology of degenerative joint disease must always be considered when any of the following four criteria are present:

1. Effusion
2. Presence of osteoarthrosis in a joint other than those involved in primary osteoarthrosis
3. Chondrocalcinosis
4. Deformity of epiphysis

Although primary osteoarthrosis of the knee occasionally may be associated with transient, noninflammatory effusions, the presence of a joint effusion in association with degenerative changes forces the radiologist to search for an underlying cause of the arthritis. Both gout and pseudogout may produce acute attacks of inflammatory arthritis, particularly involving the knee. When secondary degenerative changes occur, a pattern of acute inflammatory arthritis superimposed on osteoarthrosis will be seen.

A neuropathic joint may be identified before major fragmentation and disorganization make the diagnosis obvious. The presence of a *chronic* effusion associated with mild degenerative changes should arouse suspicion of a Charcot joint. Aspiration of bloody or noninflammatory fluid commits one to search for evidence of a neuropathy.

The combination of uniform joint space narrowing (signaling inflammatory arthritis) with osteophytes and eburnation may represent an osteoarthrosis secondary to a process that destroys articular cartilage in a generalized manner. This pattern should suggest pseudogout or, if occurring in a *weight-bearing joint,* underlying inflammatory arthritis (infection, rheumatoid arthritis, or a rheumatoid variant).

When osteoarthrosis appears to affect unusual joints (radiocarpals, elbows, shoulders, and hips), secondary osteoarthrosis should be suspected. If chondrocalcinosis is present, the osteoarthrosis is clearly secondary.

Secondary osteoarthrosis may be caused by lesions of cartilage or underlying bone. Infiltration associated with certain metabolic diseases causes the hyaline cartilage to become brittle and thus prone to premature wear. The principal causes are chondrocalcinosis due to:

1. Unknown cause, the so-called calcium pyrophosphate dihydrate (CPPD) deposition disease
2. The presence of an excess of some cations, such as *calcium* in hyperparathyroidism, *iron* in hemochromatosis, and *copper* in Wilson's disease
3. Chronic gout

The degenerative changes may sometimes obliterate the joint space completely so that chondrocalcinosis becomes difficult to see. In such instances, review of other typical sites (hyaline and meniscal cartilage of the knee, triangular cartilage of the wrist, symphysis pubis, and hips) may reveal underlying chondrocalcinosis. Therefore, screening films for this condition should include anteroposterior views of the pelvis and hands and anteroposterior and lateral views of the knees.

Whenever articular surfaces are improperly formed, the normally smooth motion between two surfaces is altered, and wear and tear of the cartilage leads to secondary osteoarthrosis. Deformity of an articular surface may be secondary to avascular necrosis, epiphyseal fracture, or dysplastic changes of the epiphysis. In the hip, congenital dislocation or slipped capital femoral epiphysis may result in dysplastic changes of articular bone and the onset of osteoarthrosis at a young age.

In summary, a secondary cause of osteoarthrosis should be suspected if joints not usually involved in primary osteoarthrosis show excessive wear and tear, if chondrocalcinosis is present, or if osteoarthrosis is present at a young age.

### STEP V. Metabolic Deposition Disease—Gout or a Rare Cause?

There are four metabolic deposition diseases:

- Chronic tophaceous gout
- Amyloidosis
- Hyperlipidemia
- Multicentric reticulohistiocytosis (lipoid dermatoarthritis)

The radiographic findings are identical in all four diseases. However, two additional radiographic findings, if present, allow for the differentiation of gout from the three rare conditions. Of the four, only gout is associated with chondrocalcinosis. Furthermore, the accumulation of calcium urate within the soft-tissue masses results in a cloudlike increased density compared with the homogeneous water-density masses of the other three metabolic arthritides. In the absence of these two distinctive features, the precise diagnosis must be made by aspiration of a lump or joint effusion and subsequent examination for crystals. If no crystals are identified, the lump must be biopsied and the specimen examined with special stains for lipid and amyloid.

## Bibliography


Aho K, Leirigalo–Repo M, Repo H: Reactive arthritis. Clin Rheum Dis 11:25–41, 1985

Ansell BM: Chronic arthritis in childhood. Ann Rheum Dis 37-107, 1978

Ansell BM: Juvenile arthritis. Clin Rheum Dis 10: 657–673, 1984

Bonavita JA, Dalinka MK, Schumacher HR, Jr: Hydroxyapatite deposition disease. Radiology 134: 621, 1980

Brower AC, Allman RM: Pathogenesis of the neurotrophic joint: Neurotraumatic vs. neurovascular. Radiology 139:349, 1981

Dalinka MK, Reginato AJ, Golden DA: Calcium deposition disease. Semin Roentgenol 17:39, 1982

Edeiken J: Radiologic approach to arthritis. Semin Roentgenol 17:8–16, 1982

Fam AG et al: Clinical and roentgenographic aspects of pseudogout: A study of 50 cases and a review. Can Med Assoc J 124:545, 1981

Forrester DM, Brown JC: The radiographic assessment of arthritis: The plain film. Clin Rheum Dis 9:281–307, 1983

Forrester DM, Brown JC: The Radiology of Joint Disease, 3rd ed. Philadelphia, WB Saunders, 1986

Genant HK: Roentgenographic aspects of calcium pyrophosphate dihydrate crystal deposition disease (pseudogout). Arthritis Rheum (Suppl) 19:307, 1976

Goldman AB: Some miscellaneous joint diseases. Semin Roentgenol 17:60, 1982

Greyson, ND: Radionuclide bone and joint imaging in

rheumatology. Bull Rheum Dis 30:1034–1039, 1980

Hatfield MK, Gross BH, Glazer GM et al: Computed tomography of the sternum and its articulations. Skeletal Radiol 11:197–204, 1984

Hellmann DB, Helms CA, Genant HK: Chronic repetitive trauma: A cause of atypical degenerative joint disease. Skeletal Radiol 10:236–243, 1983

Hoffer PB, Genant HK: Radionuclide joint imaging. Semin Nucl Med 6:121–137, 1976

Hoffman GS: Polyarthritis: The differential diagnosis of rheumatoid arthritis. Semin Arthritis Rheum 8:115–141, 1978

Jajic I et al: Primary hypertrophic osteoarthropathy (PHO) and changes in the joints. Clinical, X-ray, scintigraphic, arteriographic and histologic examination of 19 patients. Scand J. Rheumatol 9:89, 1980

Laurent MR: Psoriatic arthritis. Clin Rheum Dis 11: 61–87, 1985

Lawson JP: The joint manifestations of the connective tissue diseases. Semin Roentgenol 17:25–39, 1982

Kingston S: The role of technetium and gallium imaging in musculoskeletal disorders. Clin Rheum Dis 9:347–387, 1983

Lee P, Rooney PJ, Sturrock RD et al: The etiology and pathogenesis of osteoarthrosis: A review. Semin Arthritis Rheum 3:189–218, 1974

Lisbona R, Rosenthal L: Observations on the sequential use of $^{99m}$Tc-phosphate complex and $^{67}$Ga imaging in osteomyelitis, cellulitis, and septic arthritis. Radiology 123:123–129, 1977

Martel W, Braunstein EM, Brolaza G et al: Radiologic features of Reiter's disease. Radiology 132: 1–10, 1979

Martel W, Stuck KJ, Dworin AM et al: Erosive osteoarthritis and psoriatic arthritis: A radiologic comparison in the hand, wrist and foot. AJR 134: 125–137, 1980

McCarthy DJ, Halverson PB, Carrera GF et al: "Milwaukee shoulder"—association of microspheroids containing hydroxyapatite crystals, active collagenase, and neutral protease with rotator cuff defects. Arthritis Rheum 24:464–473, 1981

Meachim G et al: An investigation of radiological, clinical and pathological correlations in osteoarthrosis of the hip. Clin Radiol 31:565, 1980

Moon KL, Jr, Genant HK, Helms CA et al: Musculoskeletal applications of nuclear magnetic resonance. Radiology 147:161, 1983

Norgaard F, Odont D: A follow-up study of the earliest radiological changes in rheumatoid polyarthritis. Br J Radiol 53:63–73, 1980

Pavlov H, Goldman AB, Arnold WO: Haemophilic arthropathy in the joints of the hands and feet. Br J Radiol 52:173–180, 1979

Resnick D: Infectious arthritis. Semin Roentgenol 17:49, 1982

Resnick D, Niwayama G, Goergen TG: Comparison of radiographic abnormalities of the sacroiliac joint in degenerative disease and ankylosing spondylitis. AJR 128:189–196, 1977

Resnick D, Niwayama G, Goergen TG et al: Clinical radiographic and pathologic abnormalities in calcium pyrophosphate dihydrate deposition disease (CPPD): Pseudogout. Radiology 122:1–15, 1977

Resnick D, Shaul SR, Robins JM: Diffuse idiopathic skeletal hyperostosis (DISH): Forestier's disease with extraspinal manifestations. Radiology 115: 513, 1975

Rosenthal L, Hawkins D: Radionuclide joint imaging in the diagnosis of synovial disease. Semin Arthritis Rheum 7:49–61, 1977

Sherman J, Esdaile J, Hawkins D et al: Predictive value of radionuclide joint scintigrams. Arthritis Rheum 25:83–86, 1982

Smith DL, Bennet RM, Regan MG: Reiter's disease in women. Arthritis Rheum 23:335–340, 1980

## A RADIOLOGIC APPROACH TO THE DIFFERENTIAL DIAGNOSIS OF ARTHRITIS*

STEP I:

- Plain film examination
  - No radiographic criteria of arthritis
  - Radiographic criteria of arthritis (Go to Step II)

STEP II:

- Radiographic criteria of arthritis
  - Major criteria (effusion joint space narrowing erosion chrondrocalcinosis osteophytes) (Go to Step III)
  - Minor criteria
    - Juxtaarticular demineralization
      - Alignment abnormalities
        - → SUSPECT INFLAMMATORY ARTHRITIS
    - Periosteal reaction
      - Diffusely swollen digit
        - → SUSPECT RHEUMATOID VARIANT or INFECTION

*Modified from Forrester DM, Brown JC, Nesson JW: The Radiology of Joint Disease, 3rd ed. Philadelphia, WB Saunders, 1986.

STEP III:

- Major criteria of arthritis present
  - Monarticular disease (Go to Step IV)
  - Polyarticular disease (Go to Step V:A)

STEP IV:

- Monarticular disease
  - Effusion present
    - TRAUMA<br>CRYSTAL INDUCED<br>INFECTION<br>RHEUMATOID ARTHRITIS<br>SYNOVIAL TUMOR
      - Chondrocalcinosis
        - GOUT<br>PSEUDOGOUT
      - Uniform joint space narrowing
        - INFECTION<br>RHEUMATOID ARTHRITIS
      - Uneven joint space narrowing
        - OSTEOARTHROSIS<br>CHARCOT JOINT
  - Effusion absent
    - OSTEOARTHROSIS (Go to Steps V:B,C)

STEP V:A

- Polyarticular disease
  - Effusion / Uniform joint space narrowing
    - INFLAMMATORY ARTHRITIS
      - Asymmetric small joint involvement / Large joint only / Sacroiliac joints and spine
        - RHEUMATOID VARIANT
      - Symmetrical small joint involvement
        - RHEUMATOID TYPE
          - Effusion / Alignment abnorm. / Juxtaarticular demineralization
            - RHEUMATOID ARTHRITIS / LUPUS / SCLERODERMA / DERMATOMYOSITIS
          - Erosions / Joint space narrowing
            - RHEUMATOID ARTHRITIS
          - Subcutaneous calcifications
            - SCLERODERMA
  - Osteophytes / Uneven joint space narrowing
    - OSTEOARTHROSIS
      - Hands (Go to Step V:B)
      - Large joints (Go to StepV:C)
  - Soft tissue masses / Normal joint space / Periarticular erosions
    - METABOLIC DEPOSITION DISEASE
      - Chondrocalcinosis / Calcification in soft tissue mass
        - GOUT

STEP V:B

- OSTEOARTHROSIS
  - Hands
    - Chondrocalcinosis
      - PSEUDOGOUT (CPPD disease)
    - Isolated joint
      - TRAUMA / PSEUDOGOUT
    - DIP, PIP / 1st carpal-metacarpal
      - No erosions
        - PRIMARY OSTEOARTHROSIS (Kellgren's)
      - Erosions
        - EROSIVE OSTEOARTHROSIS

STEP V:C

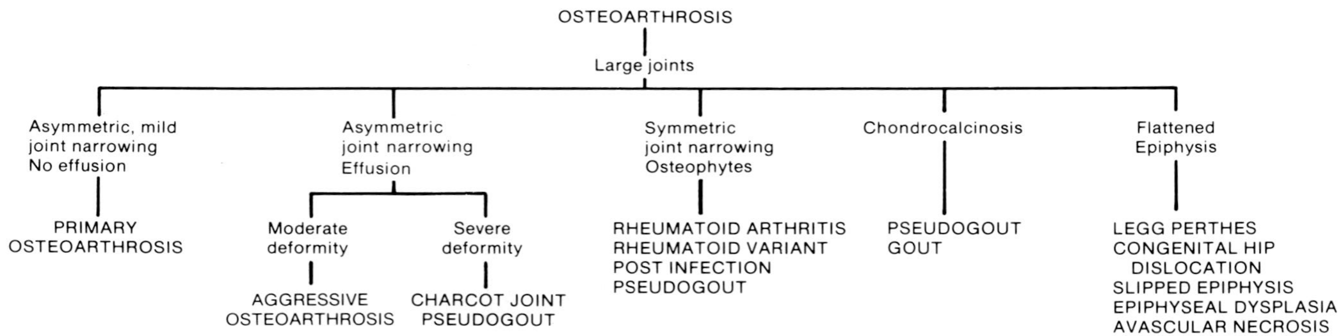
OSTEOARTHROSIS
Large joints
Asymmetric, mild joint narrowing No effusion
PRIMARY OSTEOARTHROSIS
Asymmetric joint narrowing Effusion
Moderate deformity
AGGRESSIVE OSTEOARTHROSIS
Severe deformity
CHARCOT JOINT
PSEUDOGOUT
Symmetric joint narrowing Osteophytes
RHEUMATOID ARTHRITIS
RHEUMATOID VARIANT
POST INFECTION
PSEUDOGOUT
Chondrocalcinosis
PSEUDOGOUT
GOUT
Flattened Epiphysis
LEGG PERTHES
CONGENITAL HIP DISLOCATION
SLIPPED EPIPHYSIS
EPIPHYSEAL DYSPLASIA
AVASCULAR NECROSIS

# Chapter 30

# Cervical Spine Trauma

*Beth S. Edeiken–Monroe*
*John H. Harris, Jr.*

Patients requiring radiographic examination of the cervical spine following trauma fall into two large groups: the severely injured and the less severely injured. In this chapter, the severely injured patient is one who is unconscious, has obvious clinical signs of craniocervical trauma or a myelopathy, or is polytraumatized (multiple areas of injury). The less severely injured patient is one who is conscious, may have a radiculopathy rather than a myelopathy if any neurologic deficit is present, and is ambulatory or at least stable enough to be transported.

## DIAGNOSTIC EVALUATION

### *DIAGNOSTIC MODALITIES*

1. Plain radiography
2. Conventional tomography
   a. Rectilinear tomography
   b. Polydirectional tomography
3. Computed tomography
4. Metrizamide-enhanced CT myelography
5. Ultrasound
6. Magnetic resonance imaging

#### Plain Radiography

Plain radiography is the basic imaging technique for examining the patient with acute cervical spine trauma. The radiographic dictum "one view is no view" is nowhere more applicable than in the radiographic evaluation of acute cervical spine injury. A minimum of two views, preferably obtained in perpendicular planes, is essential.

The initial radiographic examination of the cervical spine depends on the patient's clinical condition, neurologic status, and, to a lesser degree, the type and magnitude of the causative force. It is essential to include the entire area from the base of the skull to the seventh cervical vertebra. The cervical spine is not completely evaluated unless the seventh cervical vertebra is adequately visualized. To do so frequently requires conventional or computed tomography.

The need for a high-quality radiographic examination cannot be emphasized too strongly. In addition, to optimally demonstrate both soft tissue and bone, the cervical spine series must be free of motion or grid artifacts that could prevent detection of a fracture. Superimposition of the shoulders may obscure the cervicothoracic segments of the spine, and it is frequently necessary to employ special radiographic projections and techniques to ensure adequate visualization of these spinal segments.

The initial plain radiographic examination of the cervical spine must be evaluated by a radiologist or other appropriately qualified physician prior to obtaining any additional projections or using other imaging techniques.

### The Severely Injured Patient

In the severely injured patient, a limited cervical spine examination consisting of horizontal-beam lateral and anteroposterior projections usually is sufficient for evaluation of the acute problem. If possible, an "open-mouth" view should be performed to visualize the atlanto-axial articulation in frontal projection. However, this often is impossible to obtain because of unconsciousness, transnasal or transoral intubation, or associated facial or mandibular fractures. The horizontal-beam lateral projection is especially important and, ideally, should be obtained prior to the application of head and upper extremity traction so as to preclude distraction of an existing skeletal or soft-tissue injury.

If the lower cervical segments are not seen on the initial lateral radiograph, and if no abnormalities are present in those portions of the cervical spine visualized in the anteroposterior and lateral projections, various techniques may be employed to eliminate the obscuring density of the superimposed shoulders. The simplest method is to apply traction to the cervical spine simultaneously via the scalp the upper extremities, unless other injuries to these areas preclude this maneuver. As has been emphasized previously, the use of cervical traction for diagnostic radiographic purposes is specifically contraindicated in the presence of a known cervical spine injury.

In addition to clearly demonstrating the bony structures, the radiographic technique used for the lateral projection must demonstrate the prevertebral soft tissues. Abnormal prevertebral soft-tissue swelling seen in lateral projection may be the most prominent sign of a subtle, minimally displaced Jefferson bursting fracture, dens fracture, or traumatic spondylolisthesis. Diffuse prevertebral soft-tissue swelling throughout the cervical area, in conjunction with normally aligned cervical vertebrae, is a constant sign of hyperextension-dislocation of the cervical spine and may be the only indication of this injury in approximately one third of patients. Prior endotracheal or nasogastric intubation usually diminishes the value of the prevertebral soft tissues as an indicator of cervical spine injury. Swallowing or apnea during the time of exposure of the horizontal-beam lateral radiograph may produce changes that mimic cervical prevertebral soft-tissue swelling. If the patient is able to cooperate and has not been intubated, a horizontal-beam lateral radiograph obtained during inspiration provides optimal delineation of the prevertebral soft tissues.

The anteroposterior radiograph of the cervical spine does not routinely include the atlanto-axial articulation, because these segments are usually obscured by the superimposed densities of the mandible, maxilla, skull base, and occipital bone. Consequently, an open-mouth projection of the atlanto-axial articulation must be obtained whenever clinically possible to provide a complete frontal examination of the cervical spine. Despite this deficiency, the anteroposterior projection of the remainder of the cervical spine is extremely valuable, because it provides a frontal view of the anterior column (vertebral bodies) and posterior column (articular masses, laminae, and spinous processes) of the cervical spine. The vertical fracture of a vertebral body that is characteristic of a bursting (axial-loading) fracture of the lower cervical spine usually is clearly visible in the anteroposterior projection, as is the infrequent fracture of the uncinate process. Disruption of the "lateral column" (the articular masses) indicates a unilateral or bilateral interfacetal dislocation, pillar fracture, or hyperextension fracture-dislocation. Displacement of the spinous processes form the midline is indicative of a rotational component of the mechanism of injury, as occurs in unilateral interfacetal dislocation in which the spinous processes point to the side of dislocation. Widening of the interspinous distance is indicative of disruption of the posterior column, a characteristic of hyperflexion injury.

To evaluate the cervicothoracic region, supine oblique projections of each side of the cervical spine are recommended. Even though image blurring will result from the magnification associated with a short-target film distance, the supine oblique projection is much more likely to be of diagnostic quality and to provide useful information than the "swimmer's" (Twining) projection. A major advantage of the supine oblique projection is that it does not require any additional motion of the patient's head or neck. The posterolateral aspects of the vertebral bodies and the pedicles are clearly seen in oblique projection, as are the laminae that project through the articular masses. When analyzed in conjunction with the anteroposterior radiograph, the composite image of the lower cervical spine derived from the supine oblique and anteroposterior projections usually is adequate to establish or exclude a major lower cervical or cervicothoracic injury. If the supine oblique projections are nondiagnostic or equivocal, the cervical spine must remain immobilized until either conventional or computed tomography can be performed.

The initial radiographic examination of the cervical spine in a severely injured patient usually is obtained in the trauma center. Although the condition of the patient may dictate a limited study or one with less-than-optimum positioning, as well as the use of mobile equipment, these factors are neither an excuse nor justification for radiographs of routinely inferior quality. Indeed, optimum quality must be the rule rather than the exception when using radiography to assess the massively injured patient under adverse conditions.

### The Less Severely Injured Patient

The less severely injured patient generally is ambulatory or at least stable enough to be transported and therefore is best examined in the radiology department with standard views and techniques. If possible, the patient should be examined in a standing or sitting position and a target-film distance of 6 feet should be used to eliminate magnification distortion. If the patient's condition precludes an erect examination, studies of good diagnostic quality may be obtained with the patient supine and using a target-film distance as short as 40 inches.

The basic examination in the less severely injured patient should include anteroposterior, lateral, open-mouth, and both oblique projections. Oblique projections are included to visualize the intervertebral foraminae, to provide a view of the uncinate processes of the vertebral bodies different from that seen in the anteroposterior projection, and to evaluate the integrity and orientation of the articular masses and laminae. Normally, the lamina of the upper vertebra is located posterior to the lamina of the immediately lower segment. A line extending from the vertical axis of the upper lamina should project behind that of the lower lamina, producing a configuration resembling that of shingles on a roof.

The "basic" examination of the cervical spine should be reviewed by a radiologist or other qualified physician before obtaining additional plain films or employing other imaging techniques. This is especially important with respect to lateral flexion and extension views, which should be reserved *only* for those patients in whom there is historic or clinical evidence of a flexion or a combined flexion-extension (whiplash) injury, or in whom radiographic signs on the basic study suggest anterior subluxation (hyperflexion sprain).

Other authors contend that the five-film examination described above is inadequate and advocate inclusion of a "pillar" view (specifically designed to visualize the cervical articular masses *en face*) in the routine evaluation of all patients with acute cervical spine injuries. However, it is generally agreed that the pillar view should be reserved for those patients who are either clinically or radiographically suspected of having articular mass fractures. The pillar view is obtained by rotating the patient's head in one direction, off-centering the x-ray tube approximately 2 cm from the midline in the opposite direction, and with the central beam angled approximately 30° caudad and centered at the level of the superior margin of the thyroid cartilage. Because of the normal cervical lordosis, the caudally angled central beam is in tangent to the plane of the apophyseal joints only in the middle and lower cervical regions. Rotation of the head is essential to eliminate superimposition of the mandible on the articular masses. Because the patient must be able to rotate the head on command, it is essential that an upper cervical spine injury by previously excluded on the basis of the original plain radiographs.

The "swimmer's" (Twining) projection is designed to visualize the cervicothoracic junction in those patients in whom the density of the superimposed shoulders obscures the lower cervical segments in lateral projection. Optimal positioning for this view requires that the patient be rotated slightly from true lateral, with one upper extremity abducted 180° and extended cranially while the other extremity is extended posterocaudally. Because of the relatively large amount of patient motion required to obtain the swimmer's view, it may be difficult, if not impossible, to obtain in the severely injured patient and may be frankly contraindicated in patients in whom there is a high suspicion of injury to the cervicothoracic junction.

## Tomography

Conventional or computed tomography (CT) is *not* mandatory to ensure a complete radiographic evaluation of *all* types of acute spinal injury. However, any institution intending to provide definitive management of acute spinal trauma *requires* tomographic capability to be available on a timely basis. Computed tomography now is considered essential for the comprehensive assessment and management of patients with acute spinal trauma.

Although the inclusion of thin-section plain-film tomography has been advocated as part of the "routine" initial radiographic examination of acute cervical injuries, it has not been commonly adopted. Polydirectional tomography is superior to rectilinear tomography, because its better resolution provides sharper image definition. However, polydirectional tomography is not widely available because of the cost of the equipment, the complexity and sophistication of its operation, and its relatively limited application compared with CT. On the other hand, rectilinear tomography is widely available, because it is considerably less expensive and simple to operate and usually is a component of a general diagnostic radiographic unit. Although inferior to polydirectional tomography, rectilinear tomography is a reasonable alternative when polydirectional tomography is not available and plain-film tomography is indicated in the radiographic evaluation of acute cervical spine trauma.

Plain-film tomography (rectilinear or polydirectional) can provide multisegmental spatial display in either coronal or sagittal plane with sharper resolution than coronal and sagittal reformatted CT images. Because plain-film tomography is traditionally oriented parallel to the longitudinal axis of the spinal column, it can demonstrate axially oriented fractures (*e.g.*, high [type II] dens fracture, horizontally oriented avulsion fracture of the anterior arch of the atlas, anterior or posterior arch component of Jefferson bursting fracture of C1) more clearly and reliably than CT. A fracture may be missed if the axial plane of the CT section randomly falls above or below the plane of the fracture or coincides with the plane of an axially oriented fracture (as described above). Conversely, plain film tomography is unable to provide axial sections, and patient movement is required to obtain images in any plane other than the coronal.

Computed tomography is the *tomographic* technique of choice for evaluating the patient with acute cervical spine trauma because of its inherent axial display and because images in sagittal and coronal planes can be reformatted without additional patient motion or radiation exposure. The overall patient radiation dose is less with CT than with plain-film tomography. Disadvantages of CT include cost, somewhat limited availability, relatively poor resolution of the reformatted images, and the possible failure to detect axially oriented fractures. However, the advantages of CT far outweigh its disadvantages, and plain-film radiography combined with CT (with indicated) is the imaging technique of choice for the evaluation of acute cervical spine injury.

Although tomography is not required for every type of acute spinal trauma, it is reasonably indicated in any injury producing a neurologic deficit, in fractures of the posterior arch of the spinal canal, and in every burst fracture with retropulsion of the posterior vertebral body fragments. Within these general guidelines, Table 30-1 lists the specific types of cervical spine injuries for which tomography (plain film or computed) can be expected to provide new or additional data (*e.g.*, extent of bony injury, position of fragments, integrity of the spinal canal) relative to plain radiographs. Table 30-2 lists those injuries for which tomography should *not* be expected to provide new or additional data beyond that available from the plain film studies. It cannot be emphasized too strongly that these tables are not to be construed as lists of injuries for which tomography is either "indicated" or "contraindicated."

## Metrizamide-Enhanced CT Myelography

Metrizamide-enhanced CT myelography has largely replaced plain film myelography in the evaluation of acute cervical cord trauma, because the enhanced CT myelogram provides all the information obtainable with plain film myelography in addition to the advantages inherent with CT. The indications for post-traumatic CT myelography are varied and controversial, as is its role as a guide to patient management. Computed tomography following the intrathecal administration of water-soluble contrast material (metrizamide) provides direct visualization of the spinal cord, the cauda equina, and the nerve roots, thereby permitting the distinction between intramedullary and extramedullary cord or nerve root injuries and demonstrating root avulsion, dural tear, or post-traumatic syringomyelia. Small amounts (4 ml–6 ml) of 170 mg/dl water-soluble contrast material are commonly used. Although this may be introduced using traditional myelographic technique, the patient motion required usually precludes this approach. The contrast material may be instilled into the lumbar subarachnoid space with the patient prone (with or without fluoroscopic guidance). When CT myelography is indicated for cervical or upper thoracic injuries, the contrast material may be introduced via a lateral C1–C2 approach with the patient supine and after the application of traction. Actual CT scanning should be delayed approximately 4 hours to permit reduction in the density of the metrizamide by redistribution and resorption.

**Table 30-1** Cervical Spine Injuries for Which Tomography Does Generally Provide Additional Useful Information

| |
|---|
| Flexion teardrop fracture |
| Pillar fracture |
| Jefferson bursting fracture of atlas |
| Burst fracture of lower cervical spine |
| Laminar fracture |
| Hyperextension fracture-dislocation |

**Table 30-2** Cervical Spine Injuries for Which Tomography Does Not Generally Provide Additional Useful Information

| |
|---|
| Anterior subluxation (hyperflexion sprain) |
| Bilateral interfacetal dislocation |
| Simple wedge (compression) fracture |
| Clay shoveler's fracture |
| Unilateral interfacetal dislocation |
| Hyperextension dislocation |
| Extension teardrop fracture |
| Avulsion fracture of anterior arch of atlas |
| Isolated fracture of posterior arch of atlas |
| Traumatic spondylolisthesis |
| Dens fracture |

## Ultrasound

Ultrasound has no role in the initial evaluation of acute injuries of the cervical spine. This technique has been reported to be useful in intraoperative monitoring of the position of fragments during reduction of thoracolumbar and lumbar spine fractures.

## Magnetic Resonance Imaging

Contrary to initial impressions, preliminary studies indicate that high-field strength magnetic resonance imaging (MRI) will play a major role in the initial evaluation of acute cervical spine injuries. Indeed, it now seems probable that MRI may even become the imaging technique that provides the most comprehensive information in patients with acute spinal trauma.

Factors earlier thought to limit the use of MRI in acute spinal trauma, particularly of the cervical spine, included the lack of MRI-compatible life-support or monitoring systems and the inability of MRI to record cortical bone. Life-support and patient monitoring systems that are MRI-compatible have now been developed, as have techniques for maintaining cervical traction during MRI examinations of the cervical spine.

High-field-strength MRI can provide direct images of individual vertebrae, including small (although not tiny) fragments, and of the entire spinal column with greater resolution and definition than even high-resolution CT sagittal and coronal reformations (Fig. 30-1). The ability of MRI to directly demonstrate pathology within the spinal cord itself as well as its surrounding structures should allow this technique to replace metrizamide CT myelography in the evaluation of post-traumatic cord compression and obstructing intraspinal lesions. Sequential MRI provides a qualitative assessment of cord injury not previously available by any other diagnostic technique.

Magnetic resonance imaging can clearly demonstrate edema and/or hemorrhage of the paraspinal soft tissues. At the appropriate sagittal levels, the vertebral arteries can be shown by MRI without the need for contrast injection. This is particularly valuable in the patient whose fracture and/or dislocation involves the transverse processes or the course of the vertebral arteries themselves.

At present, MRI is neither necessary nor indicated in the evaluation of the cervical spine injuries listed in Table 30-1 and probably should be reserved for acute cervical spine injuries known to be characterized by spinal canal involvement or to have produced a clinical neurologic deficit.

The principal disadvantages of MRI are its inability to detect small cortical fragments, its limited availability, and the relative unavailability of MRI-compatible support and monitoring systems.

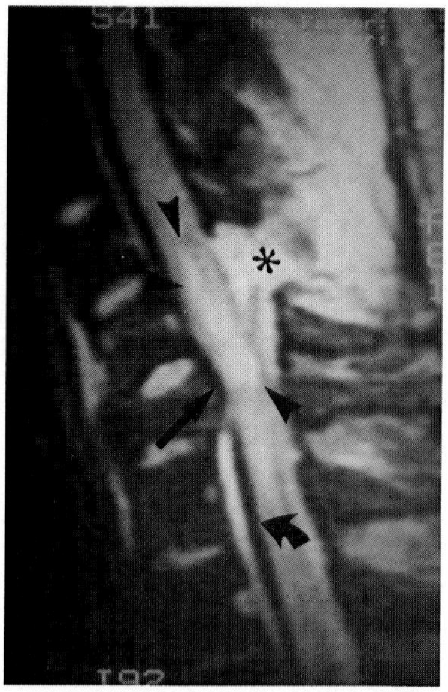

**Figure 30-1.** Bursting fracture. T2-weighted sagittal MRI clearly shows impingement of the retropulsed vertebral body fragments on the ventral surface of the spinal cord (*straight arrow*). The arrowheads indicate the high-intensity signal localizing the area and extent of cord damage. The high-intensity signal in the posterior column (*asterisk*) indicates edema or hemorrhage associated with tear of the posterior ligament complex. The posterior longitudinal ligament (*curved arrow*) has been lifted away from the posterior cortical margins of the subjacent vertebrae by edema or hemorrhage that is indicated by the high-intensity signal interposed between the vertebral bodies and the posterior longitudinal ligament.

## Bibliography

Bailey RW, Sherk HH, Dunn EJ et al (eds): The Cervical Spine. Philadelphia, JB Lippincott, 1983

Harris JH, Jr: Radiographic evaluation of spinal trauma. Orthop Clin North Am 17:75–86, 1986

Harris JH, Jr: The Radiology of Acute Cervical Spine Trauma. Baltimore, Williams & Wilkins, 1978

Harris JH, Jr, Harris WH: The Radiology of Emergency Medicine. Baltimore, Williams & Wilkins, 1981

Kaufman HH, Harris JH, Jr, Spencer JA et al: Danger of traction during radiography for cervical trauma. JAMA 247:2369, 1982

Keene JS, Goletz TH, Lilleas F et al: Diagnosis of vertebral fractures: A comparison of conventional radiography, conventional tomography and computed axial tomography. J Bone Joint Surg 64A:586–595, 1982

Leo JS, Bergeron RT, Kricheff II et al: Metrizamide myelography for cervical spinal cord injuries. Radiology 129:707–711, 1978

Maravilla KR, Cooper PR, Sklar FH: The influence of thin-section tomography on the treatment of cervical spine injuries. Radiology 127:131–139, 1978

McGahan JP, Benson D et al: Intraoperative sonographic monitoring of reduction of spinal fractures. Abstract presented at Radiological Society of North America Scientific Assembly, Washington, DC, 1984

Post MJD: Radiographic Evaluation of the Spine: Current Advances with Emphasis on Computed Tomography. New York, Masson, 1980

Yeakley J, Edeiken-Monroe B, Harris JH, Jr: Computed tomography of spinal trauma and degenerative disease. American Academy of Orthopaedic Surgeons Instructional Course Lectures, Vol XXXIV, pp 85–97. St. Louis, CV Mosby, 1985

# ACUTE CERVICAL SPINE INJURY

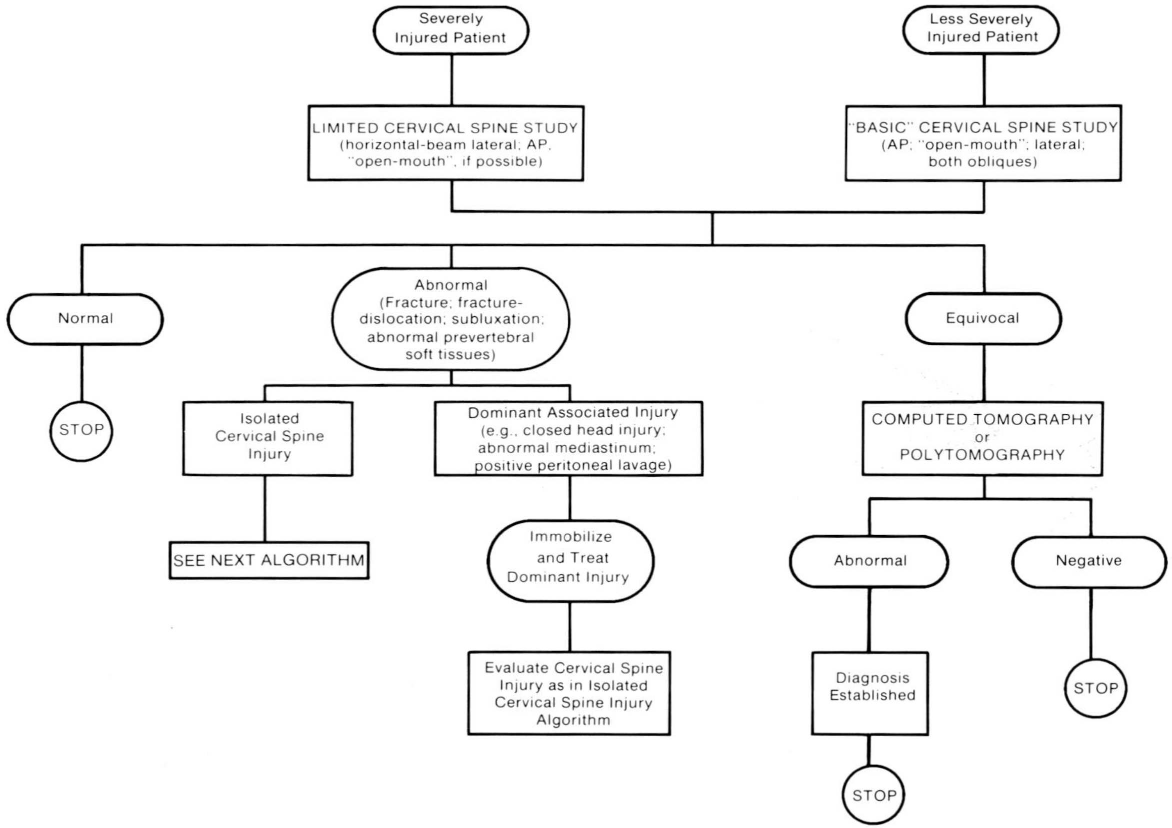

## ACUTE CERVICAL SPINE INJURY (continued)

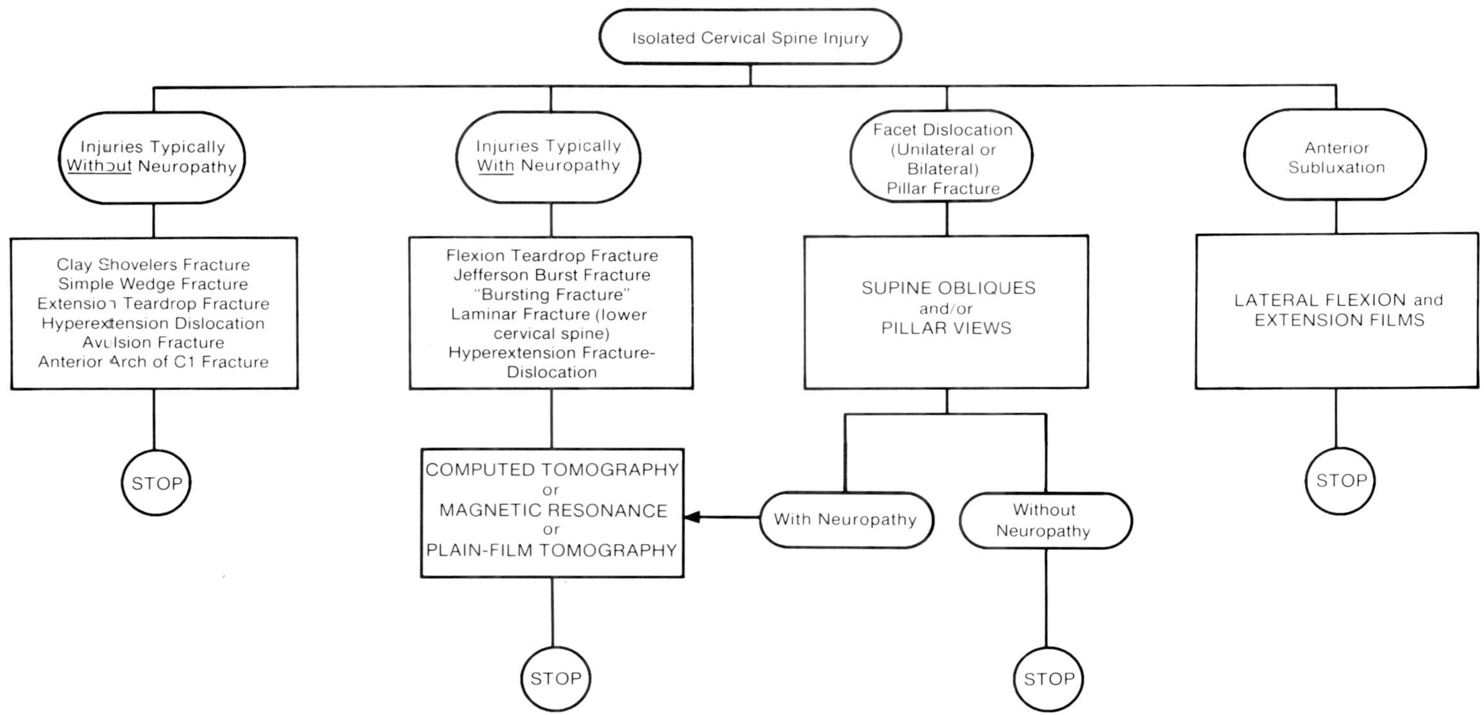

# PART FIVE

# Head and Neck

# Chapter 31

# Head Trauma

*Barry D. Pressman*

Computed tomography (CT) is now firmly established as the primary imaging examination for patients who have sustained acute head trauma. Computed tomography provides more diagnostic information on the general spectrum of intracranial disease than any other single neuroradiologic examination. It permits the early diagnosis of injuries requiring surgical intervention, which may improve the outcome. Although more invasive diagnostic procedures may have a complementary role in a limited number of cases, in the vast majority CT is the only imaging procedure required initially and for follow-up of head trauma. It is, however, important to be aware of the limitations of CT and the specific conditions for which other neuroradiologic procedures may be of diagnostic value.

## DIAGNOSTIC EVALUATION

### *DIAGNOSTIC MODALITIES*

1. Plain skull radiography
2. Computed tomography
3. Radionuclide brain scanning
4. Magnetic resonance imaging
5. Cerebral arteriography

#### Plain Skull Radiography

Post-traumatic skull radiographs have been obtained to detect fractures, to define their relationship to vascular grooves, to delineate depressed fractures, and to examine deep open wounds with possible contamination or foreign body. Plain skull films are also often requested by referring physicians for "medicolegal" reasons or simply out of habit.

The indications and efficacy of plain skull radiographs in the evaluation and subsequent treatment of a patient with head trauma have been extensively discussed and debated in the literature. In an effort to reduce the number of unnecessary post-traumatic skull radiographs with associated reduction in radiation exposure and expense, Bell and Loop and other authors have developed lists of high-yield clinical findings that are significantly associated with the presence of a skull fracture. If the presence or absence of a skull fracture were an adequate indicator of the likelihood of significant intracranial injury, the use of plain skull radiographs would be a valuable screening technique for patients with head trauma who demonstrated any of the high-yield clinical findings. However, it has been clearly shown that the mere presence of a skull fracture is of little significance in itself and correlates poorly with the effect and sequelae of head trauma on the cranial contents. Indeed, a break in the calvarium may actually protect the intracranial contents by absorbing much of the impact force. Conversely, severe intracranial abnormalities can exist with no detectable fracture.

The detection of a skull fracture on plain radiographs generally has little effect on the subsequent medical management. Although depressed or open fractures may require specific treatment and penetrating injuries or basilar fractures are often treated with antibiotics, CT can not only define these lesions but also can delineate any accompanying abnormality in the underlying brain. Computed tomography is far more accurate than plain skull radiographs for showing the depth of depressed fractures and the location of foreign bodies. Therefore, unless CT is not available, plain skull radiographs are of almost no value in patients with head trauma. In rare instances, skull radiographs may be useful for clarifying equivocal CT findings or for excluding a depressed fracture high on the convexity of the calvarium that was clinically suspected but not demonstrated on CT.

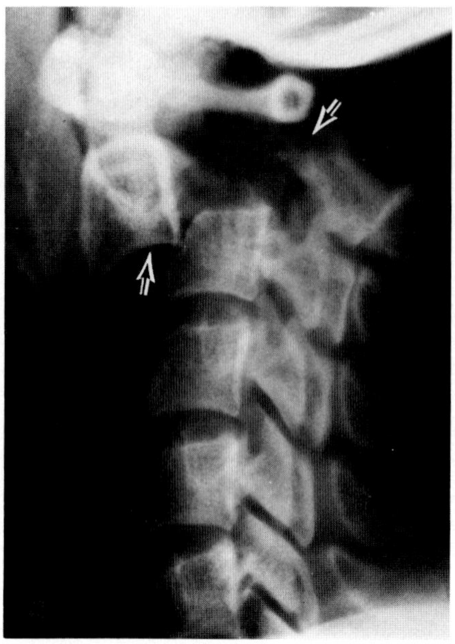

**Figure 31-1.** Plain lateral radiograph of cervical spine shows a hangman's fracture with complete C2–C3 anterior subluxation. The patient became quadriplegic when her neck was flexed for CT head study. Review of the pre-CT lateral skull film showed the cervical fracture but no subluxation.

Although plain radiographs of the skull are rarely indicated in patients with acute head trauma, plain films of the cervical spine frequently are required. Cervical spine injuries are relatively frequent concomitants of severe head injury; odontoid fractures are often present in patients who die from acute head trauma. Therefore, it is advisable to obtain at least a cross-table lateral view of the cervical spine in all patients with moderate or severe craniocervical injury (especially of the axial loading type) before a CT scan is performed, because positioning of the patient on the CT table may exacerbate an unsuspected neck injury (Fig. 31-1). If the cross-table lateral or complete cervical spine series demonstrates an abnormality or is equivocal, the cervical spine may be evaluated by CT after the head examination has been completed.

## Computed Tomography

Computed tomography is clearly the initial imaging procedure of choice for evaluating the patient with acute head trauma. Short scanning times and rapid reconstruction allow a complete noncontrast head examination to be performed and available for interpretation within 15 minutes, even in patients who are not fully cooperative. Limited examinations can be performed even more quickly if there is a clinical suspicion of a life-threatening hemorrhage requiring immediate surgery. General anesthesia may be administered within the CT suite, whereas this may be difficult or impossible to accomplish with magnetic resonance imaging (MRI).

### Skull Fractures

High-resolution CT is extremely sensitive for detecting skull fractures (Fig. 31-2). In addition to the routine brain images, bone window images should be obtained in all patients with head trauma, because they permit much better delin-

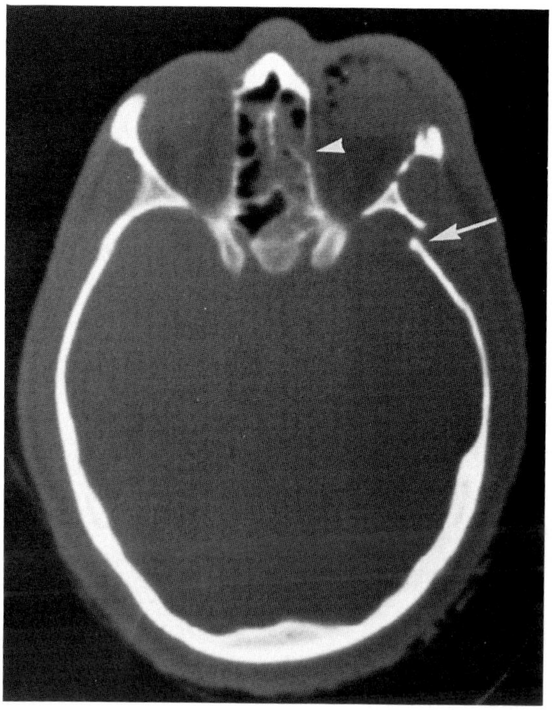

**Figure 31-2.** CT bone window image demonstrates depressed temporal fracture (*arrow*), lateral orbital wall fracture, medial orbital wall fracture (*arrowhead*), and ethmoid opacification (hemorrhage). Note the air in the orbital soft tissues secondary to medial fracture into the ethmoids.

eation of skull fractures. Fluid in the sinuses or mastoids and, occasionally, pneumocephalus may be more easily detected on bone window images.

Almost all depressed skull fractures are readily apparent on axial sections. The only exception is a depressed fracture situated high on the convexity, which is parallel to the plane of section and may require coronal sections or plain skull radiographs for delineation. Basal skull fractures may be imaged directly or may be suggested by secondary signs, such as fluid levels in the sphenoid sinuses, opacified mastoid air cells or tympanic cavities, and intracranial air. If a basal skull fracture is of particular clinical concern, thin sections (3 mm or 5 mm) and bone algorithm studies may be required.

Linear skull fractures are often seen on axial images using bone windows. Linear skull fractures also may be detected on the high-quality frontal and lateral digital localizing radiographs that are available on most present-day scanners (Fig. 31-3). Because the orbits and facial bones are at least partially included on most head CT examinations, facial and orbital fractures as well as gross displacement of the globes may also be demonstrated.

### Edema

Post-traumatic edema may produce a focal or diffuse area of decreased attenuation on CT of the head, although it may be too slight to be appreciated in the immediate post-traumatic period. Thus, on initial scans the only indication of cerebral edema may be a local mass effect or compression of the ventricles, cisterns, or sulci that are normally bilaterally symmetric. It is important to evaluate the size of the ventricles and sulci in relation to the patient's age. Because the basal ganglia, brain stem, and cerebellum are often spared in traumatic edema, these structures may serve as a natural contrast agent for improving the detection of diffuse cerebral edema (Fig. 31-4).

Special attention should be given to the perimesencephalic and quadrigeminal plate cisterns, which may be distorted or obliterated as a result of primary brain stem swelling or secondary to cerebral edema with or without secondary brain stem compression (Fig. 31-5). Cisternal compression due to cerebral edema typically produces a relatively featureless appearance in the midbrain area. The detection of brain stem injury or compression is important, because it has a significant adverse effect on the prognosis.

Post-traumatic diffuse cerebral edema is more common in children than adults. In addition to compression of the ventricles and cisterns, diffuse cerebral edema in children may even present as a generalized increase in brain attenuation caused by increased cerebral blood flow.

### Intracranial Hemorrhage

Computed tomography is the best imaging modality for establishing the presence or absence of intracranial blood, whether intracerebral, in-

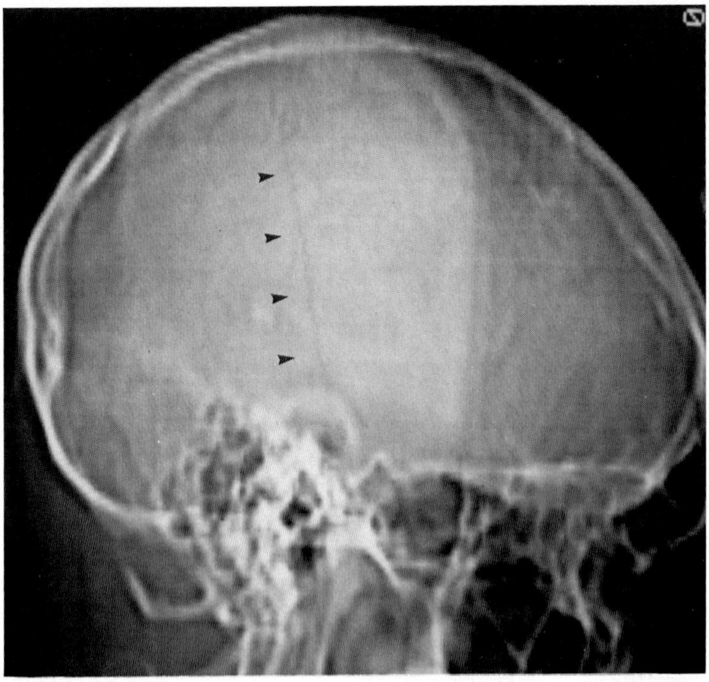

**Figure 31-3.** Linear fracture (*arrowheads*) well demonstrated on lateral localizing digital radiographs performed using CT scanner.

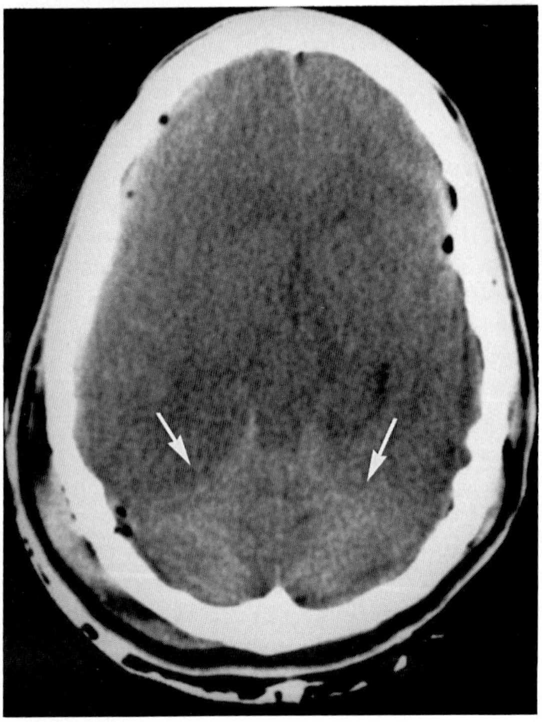

**Figure 31-4.** Diffuse cerebral edema indicated by marked compression of the ventricles and a reduced density of the cerebrum compared with that of the cerebellum (*arrows*). Note the scattered pneumocephalus.

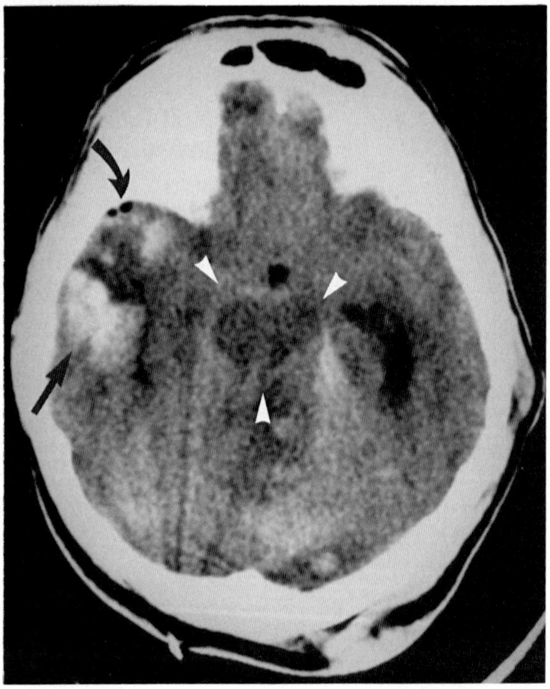

**Figure 31-5.** Severe head trauma with basal skull fracture. The brain stem (*arrowheads*) is distorted and the perimesencephalic cisterns are not visible because of cerebral edema. There is also a right temporal lobe hematoma (*straight arrow*), pneumocephalus (*curved arrow*), and hydrocephalus.

traventricular, subarachnoid, subdural, or epidural, and it has effectively replaced cerebral arteriography in evaluating these patients. The attenuation of intracranial hemorrhage is directly proportional to the hemoglobin level. Acute hemorrhages are usually hyperdense, and their density decreases with time as a result of red blood cell lysis and hemoglobin degradation. Depending on the size and location of the bleeding, intracranial hemorrhages generally become isodense within 2 to 4 weeks. Because a hemoglobin level of 8 g to 11 g is approximately isodense with the normal brain, an acute hemorrhage may be isodense in anemic patients, in whom its recognition depends on the presence of associated edema or mass effect. Eventually, intracranial hemorrhages become hypodense, so that intra-axial hematomas may appear as cystic masses while extra-axial hematomas may be difficult to differentiate from hygromas (collections of fluid similar to cerebrospinal fluid), atrophy (widening of the subarachnoid space), or arachnoid cysts (Fig. 31-6).

### Contusions

Contusions consist of petechial hemorrhages within an edematous area and thus appear on CT as lesions of mixed high and low attenuation. Contusions may be isolated, may surround parenchymal hematomas, or may abut extra-axial hemorrhages. A common cause of cerebral contusion is the coup-contrecoup type of injury, in which the contusion develops directly opposite to the site of extracranial soft-tissue swelling. Because of this mechanism, contusions most frequently develop in the anterior portions of the temporal and frontal lobes and in the occipital poles (Fig. 31-7).

### Parenchymal Hemorrhage

Parenchymal hemorrhages vary in size and may arise in subpial, cortical, subcortical, or deep locations (Fig. 31-8). Unlike the heterogeneity of contusions, parenchymal hemorrhages have relatively homogeneous attenuation values on CT scans. In contrast to extra-axial hematomas, cortical and subcortical hematomas are frequently associated with surrounding edema. Most traumatic subcortical and corpus callosum hemorrhages are believed to be secondary to shearing injuries developed from the transmission of the forces of impact across the gray–white junction. Since the gray and white matter are of different density, shearing forces occur at this junction, and arteries or veins may be ruptured. Intracerebral hematomas can occur at any age; in older patients, they may develop with only moderate head truama. Intracerebral hematomas often have associated edema or contusion surrounding them and are generally larger than cortical hematomas.

Delayed post-traumatic intracerebral hematoma is important clinically. It may develop hours to days after the initial injury. Predisposing factors to this complication include hypoxia, hypercapnia, venous congestion, and loss of autoregulation. Surgical decompression of the tamponade effect of an extra-axial lesion (*e.g.*, subdural hematoma) may precipitate the development of intracerebral hemorrhage (Fig. 31-9). Therefore, if the condition of a patient with severe head injury deteriorates, a repeat CT should be performed even if the initial study was normal.

### Extra-Axial Hematoma

Post-traumatic extra-axial hemorrhage occurs in the subdural or extradural compartments. Because the dura adheres tightly to the skull, extradural hematomas are usually confined to a relatively small area, most commonly in the temporal fossa or at the lower portion of the convexity. The much more common subdural hematomas tend to spread over a more extensive area and generally are less well defined. Most extradural hematomas are associated with skull fractures and are convex, whereas subdural hematomas usually occur without an associated fracture and tend to be medially concave. Only about 15% of subdural hematomas assume a biconvex shape as they become chronic.

As discussed previously, acute intracranial hematomas are hyperdense unless the patient is anemic. "Hyperacute" (very shortly after injury) extra-axial hematomas also may be of mixed density. This is believed to be secondary to rapid bleeding with clot formation and retraction, although the exact mechanism is not definitely known. This appearance may be a sign of a coag-

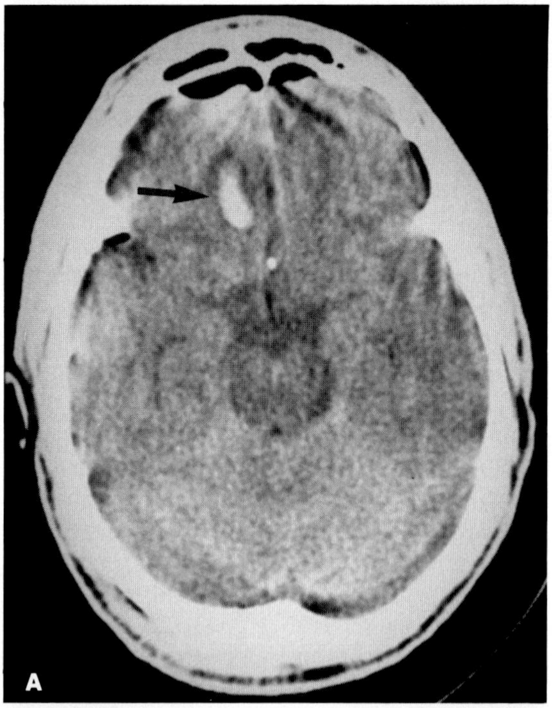

**Figure 31-6.** Intracranial hemorrhage. **(A)** CT scan shows acute hyperdense collection (*arrow*) representing a post-traumatic right frontal hemorrhage. **(B)** Ten weeks later, the hematoma is now hypodense. **(C)** MRI obtained at the same time as *B* shows the hyperintense right frontal hematoma. There are bilateral occipital areas of hyperintensity (*arrows*), which presumably represent resolving hemorrhagic contusions that were not demonstrated by CT.

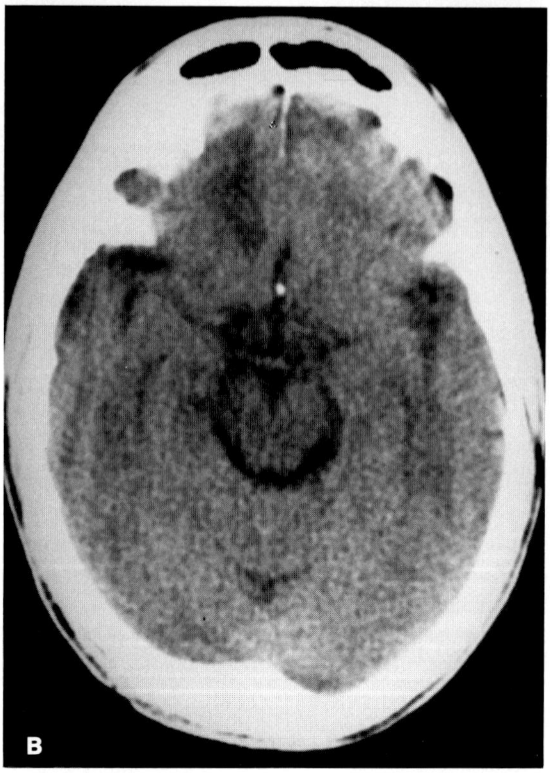

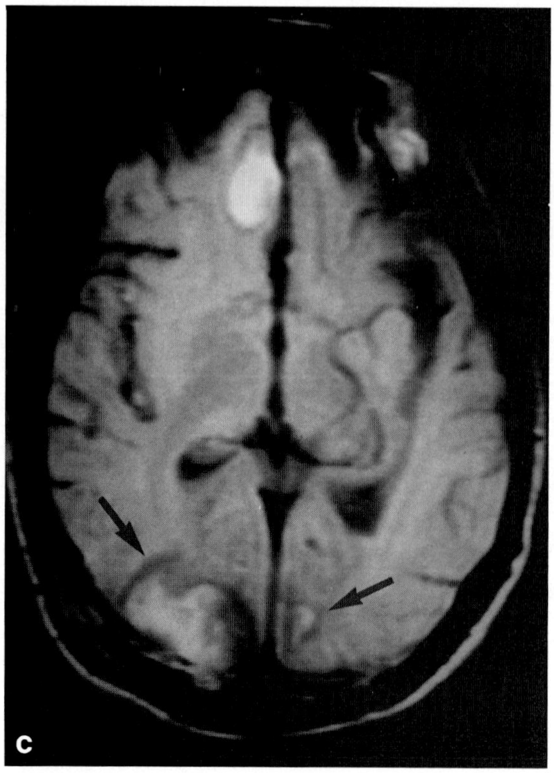

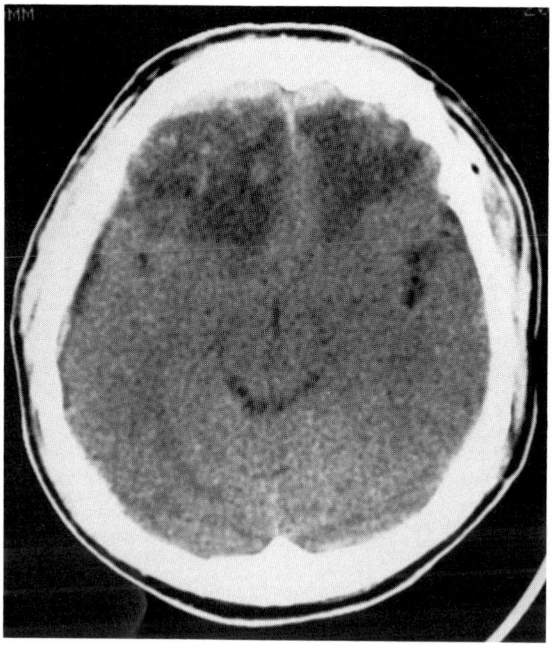

**Figure 31-7.** Acute bifrontal contusions. CT scan shows small punctate hemorrhages (high density) within extensive areas of edema (low density).

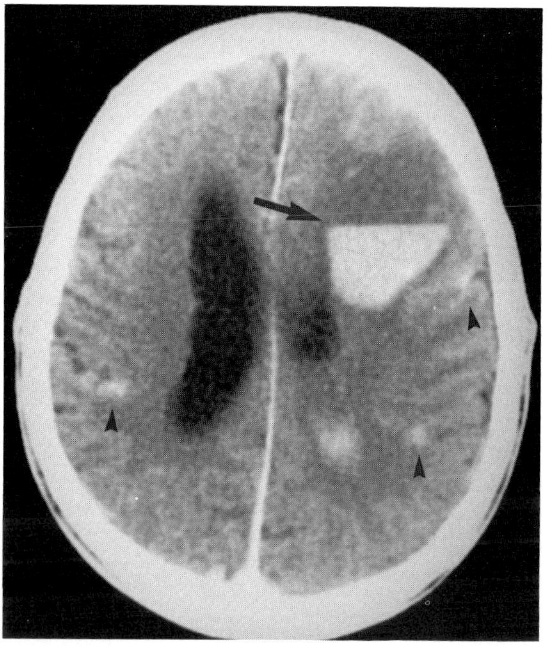

**Figure 31-8.** Acute head trauma has resulted in cortical hemorrhages in subpial and subcortical locations (*arrowheads*). There is a large hematoma containing a fluid level (*arrow*) secondary to settling of hemoglobin-laden red cells.

ulation abnormality resulting in ongoing hemorrhage (Fig. 31-10). A similar CT appearance may be seen with chronic hematomas, particularly subdural hematomas with recurrent bleeding from capillaries in granulation tissue or secondary to repeat trauma.

Extra-axial hematomas (and, less commonly, parenchymal hemorrhage) may produce a fluid–fluid level on CT scans, with higher density hemglobin-filled red blood cells in the dependent portion and lower density serum above. Extradural hematomas usually have associated mass effect, whereas the mass effect with subdural hematomas is more variable and depends on their volume and distribution.

Thin subdural hematomas, even those of high attenuation, may be obscured by overlying bone, especially if they are located high on the convexity. If there is a mass effect or ventricular or sulcal asymmetry suggestive of a subdural hematoma, wider window-width images should be obtained so as not to miss a subtle subdural hematoma obscured by overlying bone density. Coronal MRI may be of value if CT fails to demonstrate the hematoma (see Figs. 31-11 and 31-12).

Subfrontal or subtemporal extra-axial hematomas may be difficult to detect on axial views and may require coronal reformation or direct coronal imaging. These additional procedures may also be needed in patients with tentorial subdural hematomas, which frequently are associated with subdural hematomas in the posterior interhemispheric space and must be differentiated from cerebellar or occipital parenchymal hemorrhages (Fig. 31-11). Again, MRI may be diagnostic or confirmatory in difficult cases.

Isodense subdural hematomas may be difficult to recognize on CT scans. Most are seen several weeks after head trauma and apparently represent subdural hematomas in which the hemoglobin level has dropped to a level such that the degree of attenuation of the hematoma is equivalent to that of normal brain parenchyma. In anemic patients, even acute subdural hematomas may be isodense. The demonstration of an

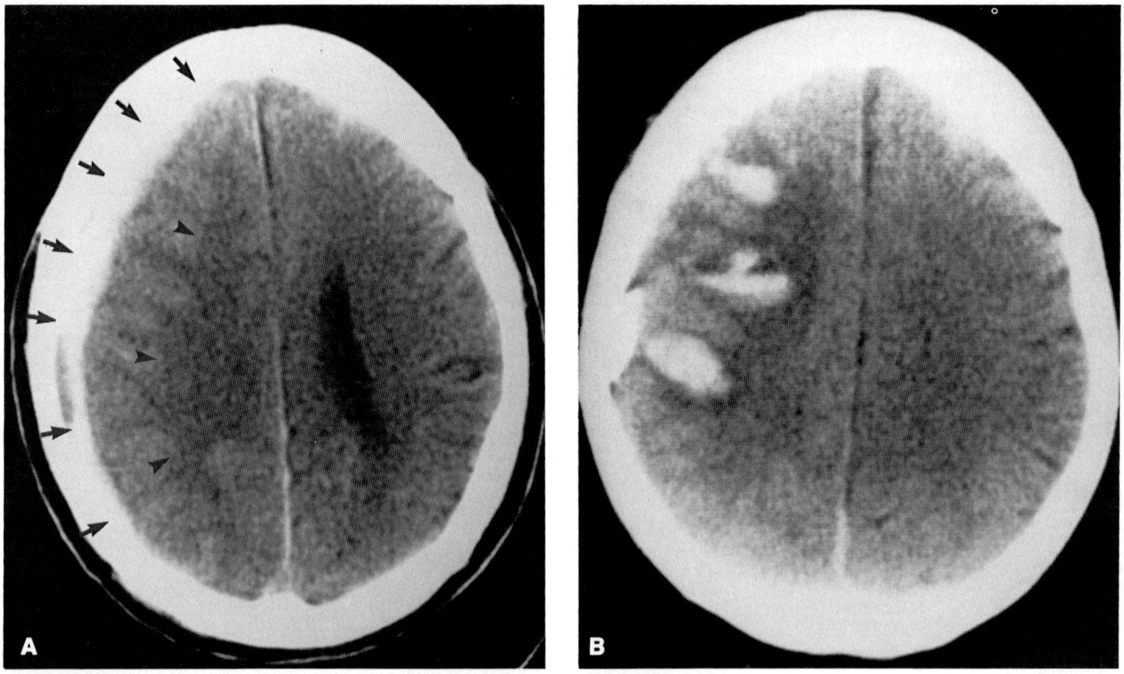


**Figure 31-9.** **(A)** Acute right subdural hematoma with hyperdensity (*arrows*), medial displacement of gray–white junction (*arrowheads*), and ventricular compression. **(B)** Several hours after surgical removal of the subdural hematoma, the patient showed clinical deterioration. Repeat CT scan shows multiple parenchymal hemorrhages and edema deep to the previous subdural hematoma.

isodense subdural hematoma requires an appreciation of the resulting mass effect, which may produce no more than subtle differences in the size of the ventricular system and in sulcal size and distribution (Fig. 31-12). Another sign of isodense subdural hematoma is medial displacement of the gray–white matter junction with buckling of the white matter (unlike parenchymal lesions, which often expand the white matter due to associated edema).

Bilateral isodense subdural hematomas may be especially difficult to recognize on CT scans. Signs that suggest this condition include an absence of sulci, narrowing and elongation of the ventricles, medial displacement of the gray–white junction with thickening of the cortical "rind," and narrowing of the white matter. Contrast enhancement may be needed to define the cortical edge, to enhance the subdural membranes or stretched bridging veins, or to opacify the subdural collection itself (Figs. 31-12 and 31-13). At times, MRI or arteriography is necessary to confirm the diagnosis of bilateral isodense subdural hematomas.

Chronic low-attenuation subdural hematomas are generally easy to detect on CT scans, although occasionally they may be difficult or impossible to differentiate from hygromas or atrophy with widening of the subarachnoid space. Signs that suggest atrophy include a fluid density equal to that of cerebrospinal fluid, interdigitation of the fluid with the cerebrospinal fluid in the sulci, and absence of any mass effect. It may be necessary to view narrow window (20 Hounsfield units [HU]) images to determine the attenuation of the fluid collection relative to that of cerebrospinal fluid (Fig. 31-14). If the attenuation of the fluid is clearly different from that of cerebrospinal fluid, a chronic subdural hematoma should be suspected. The use of intravenous contrast material may result in opacification of the hematoma. The true nature of a subdural collection is best established by MRI.

Delayed post-traumatic extra-axial fluid col-

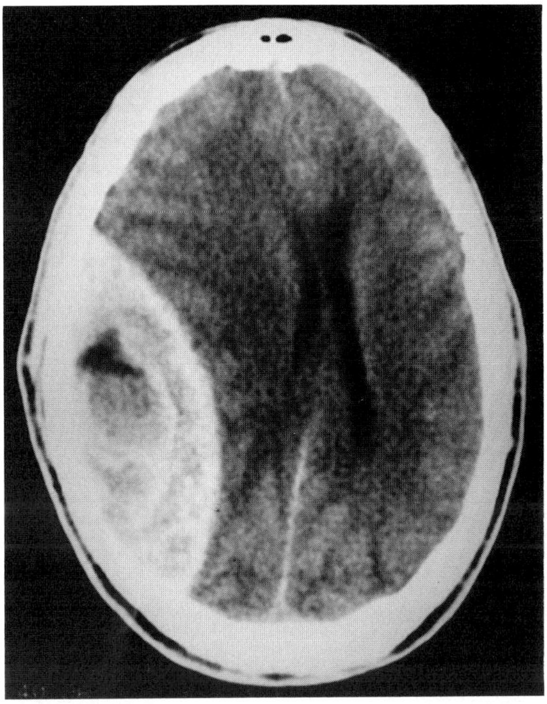

**Figure 31-10.** Huge acute right epidural hematoma. The lesion is sharply defined and produces a marked mass effect. Note the medial convexity of the epidural hematoma, in contrast to the subdural hematoma seen in Figure 31-9*A*. The central heterogeneity, which also can occur in subdural hematomas, is presumably explained by rapid continued bleeding in this patient with a coagulopathy.

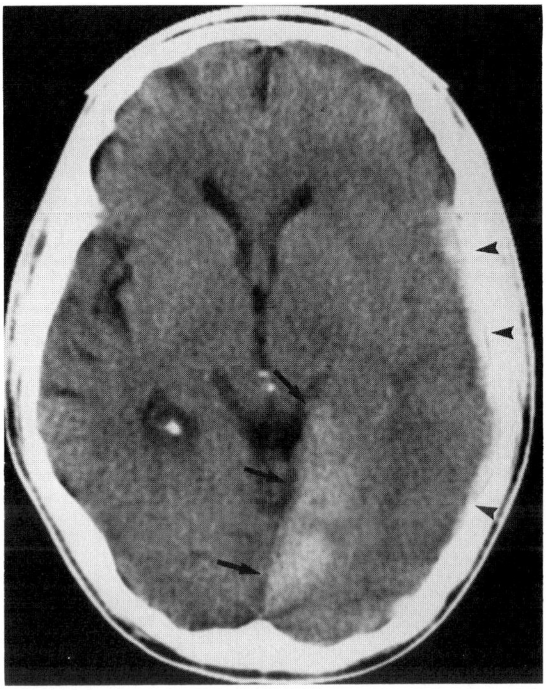

**Figure 31-11.** Subdural hematoma on superior surface of tentorium (*arrows*). The medial margin is sharp because the incisura and tentorial surface abut the hematoma at this point in the axial image. It is important not to confuse this appearance with a parenchymal hemorrhage. Note also the thin peripheral subdural hematoma (*arrowheads*).

lections are almost always hygromas, which develop secondary to arachnoid tears and extravasation of cerbrospinal fluid into the subdural space. They are usually of low attenuation, are associated with severe head injury, and most often develop within 14 days of trauma.

Recurrent subdural hematomas may occur after surgical drainage, as may pneumocephalus (Fig. 31-15). A repeat CT should be performed if the patient's clinical condition does not improve or deteriorates following drainage of a subdural hematoma.

## Other Intracranial Hemorrhage

Intraventricular hemorrhage may occur as a primary post-traumatic event or may be secondary to extension of a parenchymal hematoma. Subarachnoid hemorrhage also may occur without other evidence of trauma, although it is frequently associated with parenchymal or extra-axial bleeding. It is commonly present in abused children, but frequently it is not recognized. The CT demonstration of increased attenuation along the posterior interhemispheric fissure may be the only evidence of subarachnoid blood. A similar appearance may be produced by a specious increase in attenuation due to surrounding cerebral edema or falx calcification, or may reflect an interhemispheric subdural hematoma. The latter condition typically has sharp medial and convex lateral margins and often extends to the tentorial surface.

## Contrast Enhancement in CT

The CT evaluation of the patient with acute head trauma does not require contrast enhancement to determine the presence of a lesion amenable

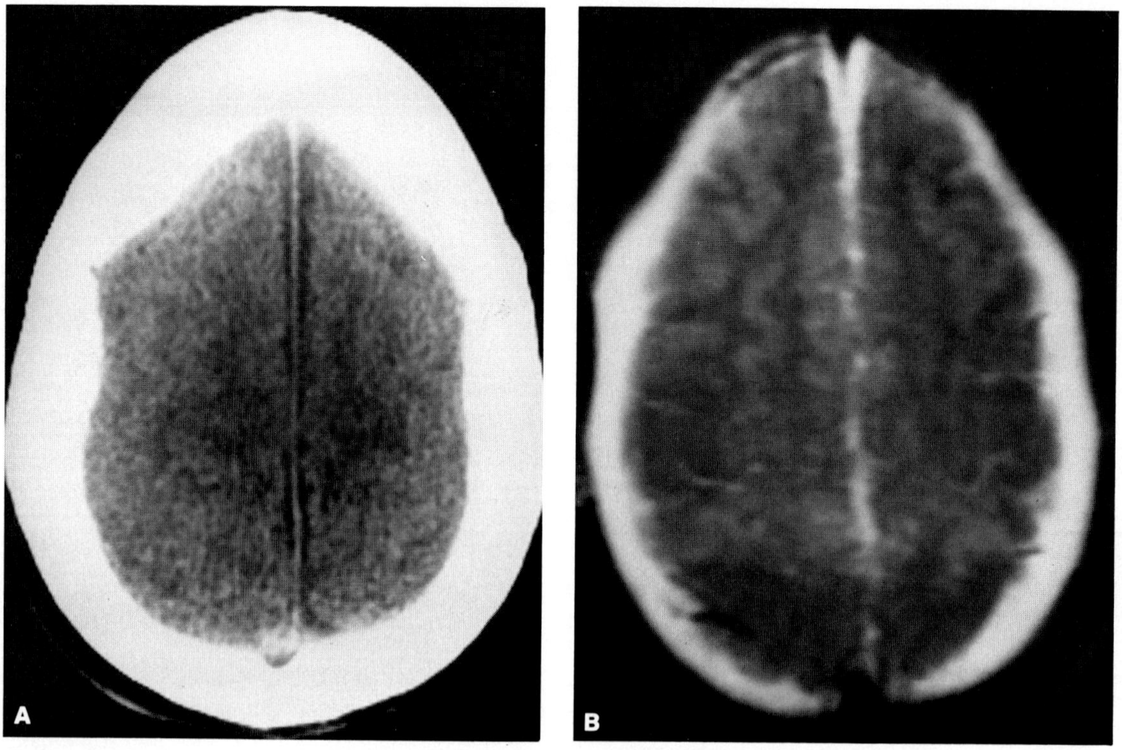


**Figure 31-12.** Seventy-five-year-old man with continued headache weeks after head trauma. **(A)** CT fails to show the prominent cortical sulci expected in a patient of this age. No definite subdural hematoma is seen. **(B)** MRI clearly demonstrates bilateral hyperintense extra-axial fluid collections (consistent with subdural hematomas) that were isodense on CT.

to surgery. Contrast enhancement may aid in differentiating an extradural hematoma from a subdural hematoma by demonstrating dural sinus displacement in the former, but this is rarely necessary. The major value of contrast enhancement is in patients whose signs and symptoms are not explained on unenhanced CT scans. In such cases, contrast enhancement may develop in areas of edema or contusion, thus indicating the site of an otherwise unrecognized injury. As described previously, contrast enhancement may also be helpful in the evaluation of isodense or hypodense subdural hematomas (see Fig. 31-13).

### Radionuclide Brain Scanning

Radionuclide brain scanning no longer has a role in the evaluation of patients with acute head trauma. This modality may rarely be of value to confirm a subacute or chronic extra-axial hemorrhage that is equivocal on CT, or to demonstrate a clinically suspected but undetected isodense-balanced subdural hematoma. Nevertheless, even in these conditions, radionuclide brain scanning should be performed only if MRI is unavailable.

### Magnetic Resonance Imaging

Magnetic resonance imaging is considerably less satisfactory than CT in the evaluation of acute head trauma. Fractures are not adequately demonstrated using this technique. Acute hemorrhage, both parenchymal and extra-axial, may appear isointense for 1 to 3 days and thus go unrecognized. The time required to perform MRI is far too long for patients with head trauma who are acutely ill and may require intense monitoring or may be uncooperative. In addition,

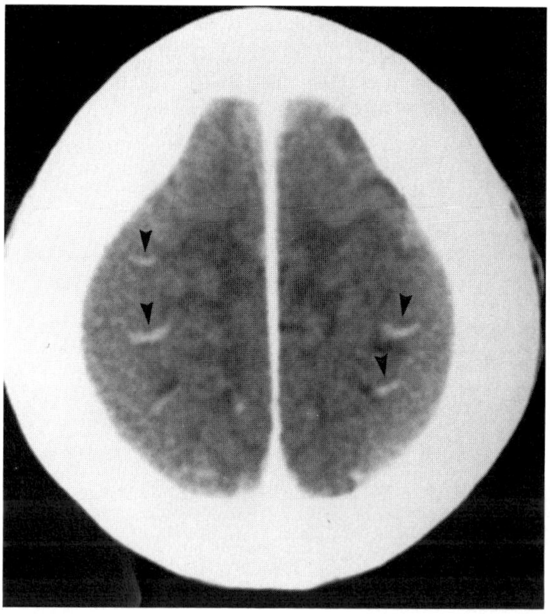

**Figure 31-13.** Contrast-enhanced CT scan shows opacification of bridging veins (*arrowheads*) that are medially displaced and indicate the presence of isodense subdural hematomas.

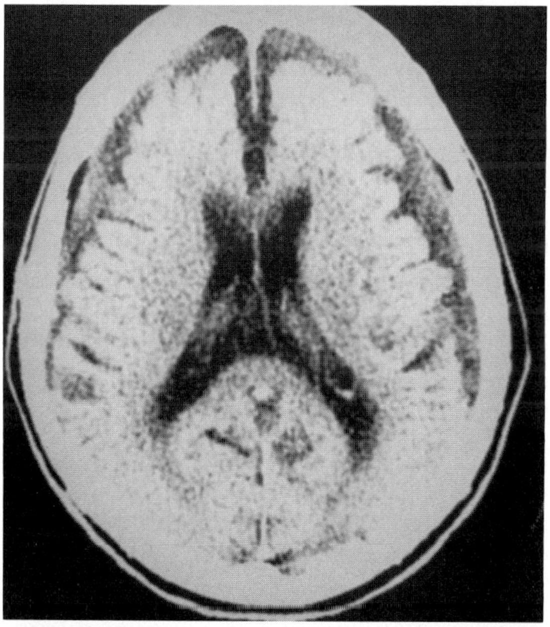

**Figure 31-14.** CT with narrow windows (20 HU) shows bilateral hypodense chronic subdural hematomas in an elderly man. The subdural collections are obviously of higher attenuation than the cerebrospinal fluid within the ventricles. This was difficult to discern at the routine brain window levels (80 HU–100 HU).

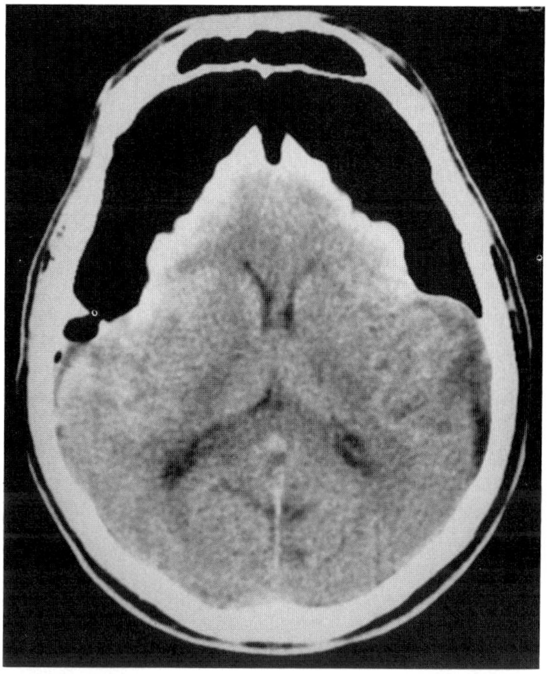

**Figure 31-15.** CT scan in a patient who deteriorated rapidly several hours after drainage of the bilateral subdural hematomas seen in Figure 31-14. There is severe bilateral tension pneumocephalus with marked compression of the ventricles.

monitors and anesthesia equipment usually cannot be brought into the scanner room.

Magnetic resonance imaging is exquisitely sensitive to hemorrhages that are more than a few days old, because they are hyperintense on both T1- and T2-weighted images (see Figs. 31-6 and 31-12). Unlike CT scans, on which hemorrhage becomes isodense after several weeks and then becomes hypodense, on MRI intracranial hemorrhage remains hyperintense for a year or more and thus remains easily detectable. Because MRI is also very sensitive to abnormalities such as edema, post-traumatic gliosis, and encephalomalacia, it is of particular use in evaluating patients in whom CT has not demonstrated lesions sufficient to explain the clinical signs and symptoms. Magnetic resonance imaging is of particular value in patients with suspected posterior fossa lesions or subdural hematomas extending to the high convexity, since these areas are difficult to evaluate by CT because of bone artifacts (see Fig. 31-12).

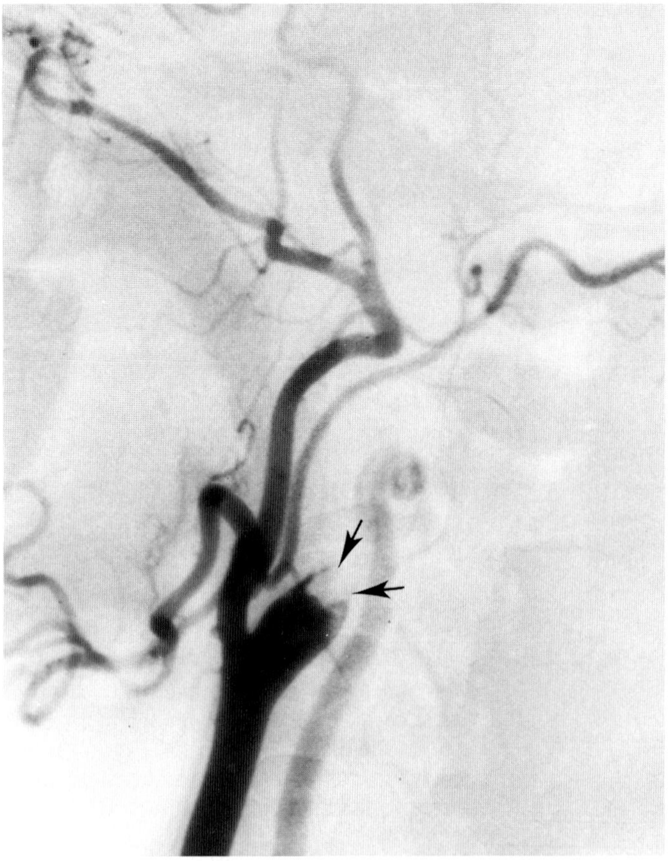

**Figure 31-16.** Lateral view from a left common carotid arteriogram in a patient with blunt cervical injury shows thrombosis of the internal carotid artery (*arrows*).

Magnetic resonance imaging should be the primary imaging modality in patients with chronic post-truamatic symptoms, because it is more sensitive than CT for detecting parenchymal lesions and chronic hemorrhages and can show equally well the size and shape of the ventricles. If MRI is negative in these patients, no other imaging is required unless bony injury is suspected.

## Cerebral Arteriography

Cerebral arteriography is now rarely required in the evaluation of a patient with acute head trauma. In rare cases of penetrating trauma with suspected vascular injury, arteriography may be used to demonstrate the site of meningeal or pial arterial bleeding; this information may be important to the neurosurgeon, especially if there is recurrent hemorrhage for which a second surgical procedure is required. If MRI is unavailable, arteriography occasionally may be needed to confirm the presence of an isodense subdural hematoma. In such cases, digital subtraction angiography (intravenous or reduced-dose intra-arterial) can be performed.

The cervical or intraosseous portions of the carotid artery may be injured at the time of trauma, especially in patients with acute deceleration injuries, skull fractures, and penetrating wounds. Dissection of the cervical carotid artery may occur following hyperextension injuries to the neck (with or without external evidence) and may lead to embolism, occlusion, or false aneurysm formation. Because the cerebral manifestations of carotid artery injury may be delayed for hours or even days following trauma, arteriography should be considered whenever neurologic deficits or deterioration occurs fol-

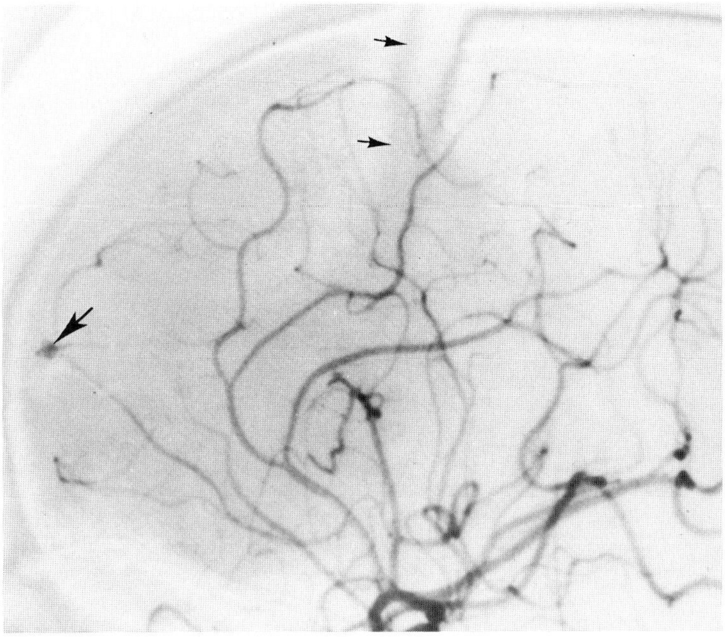

**Figure 31-17.** Lateral view from a left internal carotid arteriogram shows a severe diastatic fracture of the coronal suture (*small arrows*) and a post-traumatic frontopolar aneurysm (*large arrow*). Displacement of the cortical vessels away from the inner table was caused by a large epidural hematoma.

lowing head injury and whenever the CT scan is either normal or demonstrates findings that suggest vascular injury (*e.g.*, enlarging hematoma, acute infarction) (Fig. 31-16).

Post-traumatic cerebral aneurysms that develop secondary to blunt or penetrating injuries may require arteriography for diagnosis. The most common sites of post-traumatic cerebral aneurysm include meningeal or cortical vessels caught instantaneously within a fracture line, the middle cerebral artery injured by the sphenoid ridge, and the pericallosal artery traumatized by the falx (Fig. 31-17).

## Bibliography


Bell RS, Loop JW: The utility and futility of radiographic skull examination for trauma. N Engl J Med 284:236–239, 1971

Brunctti J, Zingcsscr L, Dunn J et al: Delayed intra cerebral hemorrhage as demonstrated by CT scanning. Neuroradiology 18:43–46, 1979

Danziger A, Price H: The evaluation of head trauma by computed tomography. J Trauma 19:1–5, 1979

DeSmet AA, Fryback DG, Thornbury JR: A second look at the utility of radiographic skull examination for trauma. AJR 132:95–97, 1979

Eyes B: Post-traumatic skull radiographs: Time for a reappraisal. Lancet 85–89, 1978

Freed HA: Skull x-ray criteria endorsed by the Food and Drug Administration: Some flaws and proposed modifications. Neurosurgery 7:636–638, 1980

George AE, Russell EJ, Kricheff II: White matter buckling: CT sign of extraaxial intracranial mass. AJR 135:1031–1036, 1980

Gomori JM, Grossman RI, Goldberg HI et al: Intracranial hematomas: Imaging by high-field MR. Radiology 157:87–93, 1985

Greenhouse AH, Barr JW: The bilateral isodense subdural hematoma on computerized tomographic scan. Arch Neurol 36:305–307, 1979

Harwood–Nash DC, Hendrick EB, Hudson AR: The significance of skull fractures in children. Radiology 101:151–155, 1971

Jennet B: Skull x-rays after recent head injury. Clin Radiol 31:463–469, 1980

Kishore PRS, Lipper MH, Becker DP et al: Significance of CT in head injury: Correlation with in tracranial pressure. Am J Neuroradiol 2:307–311, 1981

Koo AH, LaRoque RL: Evaluation of head trauma by computed tomography. Radiology 123:345–350, 1977

Larsen KT, Koziol DF: High yield criteria in emergency department skull radiography. JACEP 8: 393–395, 1979

Lipper MH, Kishore PRS, Enas GG et al: Computed tomography in the prediction of outcome in head injury. Am J Neuroradiol 6:7–10, 1985

Lipper MH, Rad FF, Kishore PRS et al: Delayed intracranial hematoma patients with severe head injury. Neuroradiology 133:645–650, 1979

Masters SJ: Evaluation of head trauma: Efficacy of skull films. Am J Neuroradiol 1:329–337, 1980

Merino–DeVillasante J, Taveras JM: Computerized tomography (CT) in acute head trauma. AJR 126:765–778, 1976

Moon KL, Brant–Zawadzki M, Pitts LH et al: Nuclear magnetic resonance imaging of CT-isodense subdural hematomas. Am J Neuroradiol 5: 319–322, 1984

Nokes SR, Silbiger ML: Referral criteria pare down skull x-rays' clinical waste. Diagn Imaging 68–71, September 1985

Osborn AG: Head trauma. In Eisenberg RL, Amberg JR (eds): Critical Diagnostic Pathways in Radiology: An Algorithmic Approach. Philadelphia, JB Lippincott, 1981

Parkinson D, West M: Traumatic intracranial aneurysms. J Neurosurg 52:11–20, 1980

Radcliffe WB, Guinto FC, Adcock DE et al: Subdural hematoma shape; a new look at an old concept. AJR 115:72–77, 1972

Scatliff JH, Williams AL, Krigman MR et al: CT recognition of subcortical hematomas. Am J Neuroradiol 2:49–53, 1981

Seelig JM, Becker DP, Miller D et al: Traumatic acute subdural hematoma: Major mortality reduction in comatose patients treated within four hours. N Engl J Med 304:1511–1518, 1981

Sipponen JT, Sepponen RE, Sivula A: Chronic subdural hematoma: Demonstration by magnetic resonance. Radiology 150:79–85, 1984

Smith WP, Batnitzky S, Rengachary SS: Acute isodense subdural hematomas. Am J Neuroradiol 2:37–40, 1981

Thornbury JR, Campbell JA, Masters SJ et al: Skull fracture and the low risk of intracranial sequelae in minor head trauma. AJR 143:661–664, 1984

Tsai FY, Teal JS, Itabashi HH et al: Computed tomography of posterior fossa trauma. J Comput Assist Tomogr 4:291–305, 1980

Tsai FY, Teal JS, Quinn MF et al: CT of brain stem injury. AJR 134:717–723, 1980

Zimmerman RA, Bilaniuk LT, Gennarelli T et al: Cranial computed tomography in diagnosis and management of acute head truama. AJR 131: 27–34, 1978

# ACUTE HEAD TRAUMA

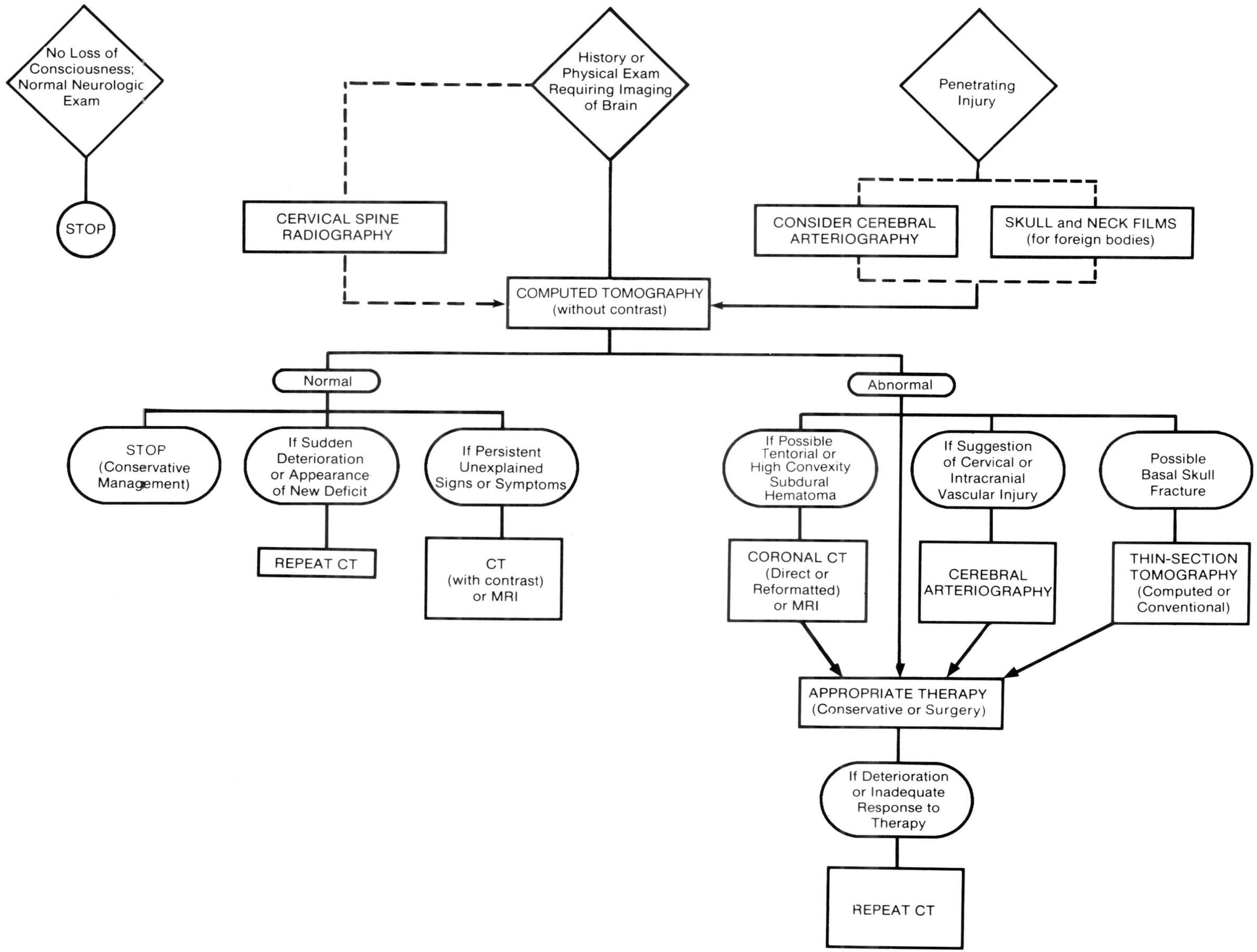

# Chapter 32

# Headache

*Robert L. DeLaPaz*
*Clark H. Millikan*

Headache is one of the most common pain problems, estimated to affect 90% of the population. Headache results in 16,000,000 visits to physicians every year (the 14th most common reason to consult a doctor). In contrast to this large figure, only approximately 6300 persons die each year from both malignant and benign intracranial tumors.

Most pain identified as headache arises from structures outside the cranial cavity. Common extracranial causes include paranasal sinus, ocular, dental, ear, and cervical spine disorders. Thus, proper clinical screening of the large group of patients with headache is vital, not only to determine whether imaging studies are appropriate but also to choose which studies are needed.

## CLINICAL CONSIDERATIONS

Six high-priority clinical questions must be answered before the physician can formulate a rational radiographic approach to the patient with headache. These are listed below.

### Age of the Patient

Mild headache arising after a blow to the head in a teenager may require only observation. In a patient 50 years of age or older, however, the chance of a headache being the result of a subdural hematoma increases, and appropriate imaging studies should be performed. Similarly, an intermittent headache arising in the second or third decade of life frequently represents migraine, for which additional studies are unnecessary. However, if this same type of headache begins in the sixth decade of life, imaging studies to exclude or identify intracranial lesions are indicated.

### How Long Had Headache Been a Problem?

It is important to ascertain whether the patient's headache has significantly changed his behavior, such as forcing him to miss work or to cancel recreation plans. If the headache is of recent onset, is worsening, and prevents the patient from pursuing his usual activities, imaging studies are usually required. A long history of headaches, with normal activity pattern and normal neurologic examination, is usually not an indication for further imaging evaluation.

## Are There Associated General or Focal Neurologic Abnormalities?

In patients with headaches who experience speech, vision, motor, or sensory dysfunction, or abnormalities in mentation, imaging studies should be obtained.

## Is There Evidence of a Systemic Illness?

In patients with phenomena suggesting systemic illness (malaise, fever, fatigue, anorexia, weight loss), an abnormal neurologic examination is an indication for magnetic resonance imaging (MRI) or computed tomography (CT); if the neurologic examination is normal, imaging studies are optional.

## Character of the Pain

Tension headaches are bilateral, commonly cervical-occipital, and nonthrobbing, with a feeling of tightness in the neck and scalp muscles. In patients with subarachnoid hemorrhage, the onset of headache is usually rapid and very severe, causing the person to stop or change what he was doing. Cluster headache is a blurring pain, in or adjacent to an orbit, that lasts for few minutes. Classic migraine is throbbing, unilateral, and severe enough to interfere with activities. Unfortunately, in many patients with chronic headache the character of the discomfort is nondescript and gives little indication about the etiology. Serious causes of such chronic headache include subdural hematoma, brain tumor, chronic inflammations (cryptococcosis, infectious mononucleosis), renal failure, hypertensive vascular disease, intracranial arteriovenous abnormalities, and unruptured aneurysm.

## Is the Headache Continuous or Intermittent?

### Continuous Headache

Short Duration (Minutes, Hours, or a Few Days). If the headache is severe enough to change the patient's behavior and is associated with a stiff neck or any other neurologic abnormality, the cause may be trauma, infection, primary subarachnoid hemorrhage, or neoplasm. Such a patient requires MRI or CT; after the results of these examinations are available, a decision may be made about the possibility of examining the cerebrospinal fluid or performing an angiographic procedure.

Medium Duration (Days to Weeks). If the headache has been severe enough to begin to change the patient's behavior and is associated with an abnormal neurologic examination, MRI or CT should be performed. If the neurologic examination is normal, additional clinical evaluation is necessary to identify the etiology of the headache. If entities such as infectious mononucleosis, hepatitis, or renal disease are identified, additional imaging studies are not required. However, if the clinical workup is normal or suggests a cause such as intracranial infection, neoplasm, or collagen disorder, MRI or CT should be performed.

Long Duration (Many Months or Years). If the patient has an abnormal neurologic examination, MRI or CT is essential. If the neurologic examination is normal, these imaging procedures are optional and usually unnecessary.

### Intermittent Headache (Mostly Migraine)

Recent Onset. If the patient has an abnormal neurologic examination, MRI or CT should be performed; if the neurologic examination and other nonimaging tests are normal, imaging evaluation is optional.

Ancient Onset. If the patient has an abnormal neurologic examination between attacks or focal neurologic phenomena during attacks,

MRI or CT should be performed. Once these results are available, a decision regarding angiography can be made. On the other hand, if the patient has a normal neurologic examination during and between attacks, there is no need for an imaging procedure. In those patients in whom the severity of attacks is significantly increasing, MRI or CT should probably be performed.

## DIAGNOSTIC EVALUATION

### *DIAGNOSTIC MODALITIES*

1. Plain radiography (skull, cervical spine)
2. Computed tomography
3. Magnetic resonance imaging
4. Cerebral arteriography
5. Radionuclide brain scan
6. Pneumoencephalography
7. Surgery

### Plain Radiography (Skull, Cervical Spine)

A large proportion of patients with symptoms of headaches do not actually have intracranial disease. For this reason, plain radiographs, which are easily obtained and inexpensive, are a useful initial step in the imaging evaluation of headache and may indicate an extracranial etiology for the patient's pain. For example, plain skull radiographs may demonstrate the presence of sinusitis. Similarly, plain films of the cervical spine may demonstrate degenerative facet disease, a common cause of pain at the base of the skull. Computed tomography also can demonstrate extracranial disease, but at most centers (due to the expense) facial and cervical scans are not performed unless specific attention is drawn to these areas. High-resolution CT scans of bony lesions of the paranasal sinuses and temporal bone are often useful if an abnormality is suggested by the plain radiographs.

Plain skull radiographs occasionally demonstrate the presence of intracranial pathology. There may be hyperostosis associated with meningioma or enlargement of the sella turcica and thinning of the dorsum sellae caused by a pituitary tumor. However, plain skull radiographs are very insensitive to intracranial pathology thus should not be used as a screening modality for excluding intracranial lesions.

In the patient with headache in whom there is the clinical suspicion of an intracranial lesion (*e.g.*, focal neurologic deficit), plain radiographs are unlikely to be helpful and the patient should be studied with MRI or CT scanning. Because MRI is more sensitive than CT for detecting cerebral pathology, MRI (if available) should be the initial study for screening patients with headache and suspected intracranial pathology.

### Computed Tomography

Computed tomography is now widely available and is currently the most common imaging modality for screening patients with headache for suspected structural intracranial pathology. Computed tomographic scanning is far superior to plain radiography because of its sensitivity to small differences in x-ray attenuation (electron density) between tissues and because of its ability to demonstrate anatomy in three dimensions. Following the intravenous administration of iodinated contrast material, CT also can show physiologic processes, such as a breakdown in the blood–brain barrier ("enhancement") and patency of large vascular structures ("time-density profiles"). Computed tomography is less sensitive than MRI to subtle increases in tissue-water content and thus to early changes produced by cerebral disease processes. Nevertheless, CT has a high overall sensitivity to intracranial abnormalities, as demonstrated in one study of 366 patient with proven intracranial neoplasms in which CT detected 98% of lesions. The sensitivity of CT for detecting enhancing lesions can be maximized in individual cases by the use of "double dose" intravenous contrast material (74 g of iodine).

The major diagnostic problem with CT is its lack of specificity. Attenuation values do not permit the accurate differentiation of neoplasm from nonneoplastic processes, benign from malignant, or cystic from solid lesions. This lack of specificity is seen commonly with lesions that are less dense than normal brain. One example of this problem is the small acute ischemic infarct with edema, which may be indistinguishable on CT scan from a low-grade astrocytoma that also shows no evidence of enhancement. Similarly, a lucent lesion of cerebrospinal fluid density in the central posterior fossa may represent a cystic tumor (*e.g.*, cystic astrocytoma), an obstructed fourth ventricle (*e.g.*, from basal meningitis), an arachnoid cyst, or an intraventricular epidermoid tumor. Contrast enhancement, which reflects the extravascular accumulation of contrast material via abnormal ischemic, neoplastic, or inflammatory vessel walls, cannot clearly differentiate ischemic, malignant, or "active" inflammatory processes. An example of this lack of specificity is "ring enhancement," which may be found in primary or metastatic tumor, abscess, subacute infarction, or resolving hematoma (Fig. 32-1). At times, a specific CT diagnosis can be made by the typical location and appearance of a lesion (*e.g.*, colloid cyst of the third ventricle) (Fig. 32-2). However, correlation with other imaging procedures, laboratory studies, patient age, and clinical information is usually required for a precise diagnosis.

Complications of CT scanning are infrequent and are related to the need for intravenous infusion of iodinated contrast material in most cases. The small, but predictable, risk of serious morbidity with ionic contrast infusion is approximately 1 in 14,000; the mortality rate is approximately 1 in 40,000. These risks are increased in patients with renal failure and allergic conditions.

Computed tomography has gained widespread clinical application as a screening procedure for patients with headache. However, because MRI is more sensitive for detecting

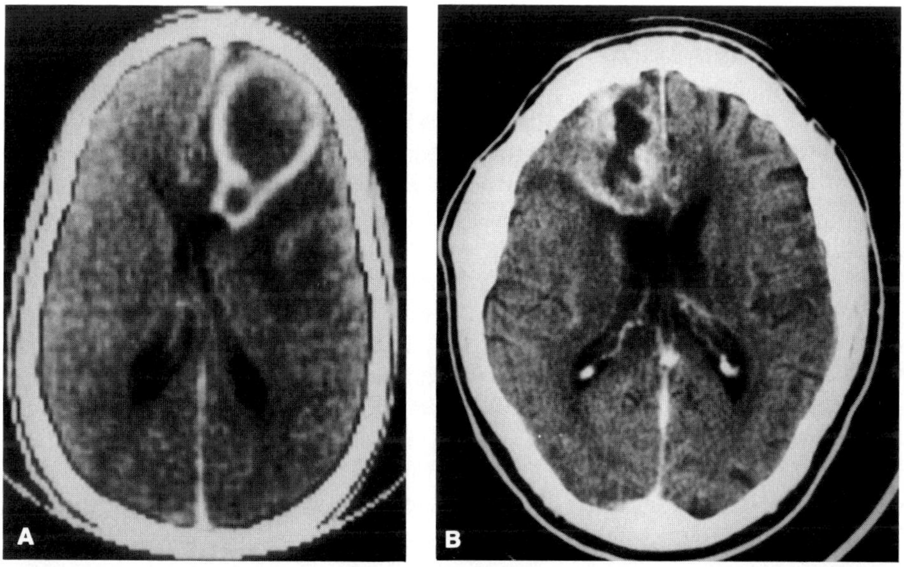


**Figure 32-1.** "Ring" enhancement on CT. **(A)** A thin, smooth ring of enhancement is present at the margin of a postoperative left frontal lobe bacterial abscess. A smaller diameter ring, which appears to be "budding" from the posterior aspect of the lesion, represents a "daughter" abscess. There is also white matter edema and mass effect with a midline shift to the right. The smooth ring of enhancement is most characteristic of cerebral bacterial abscess, but it may also be produced by primary or metastatic neoplasm, subacute infarction, or resolving hematoma. **(B)** Thick, irregular ring of enhancement following resection of a right frontal lobe astrocytoma. This represents recurrence of tumor and is a typical appearance of anaplastic astrocytoma (glioblastoma). However, metastases, early cerebritis/abscess, subacute infarction, or resolving hematoma may also produce this pattern of enhancement.

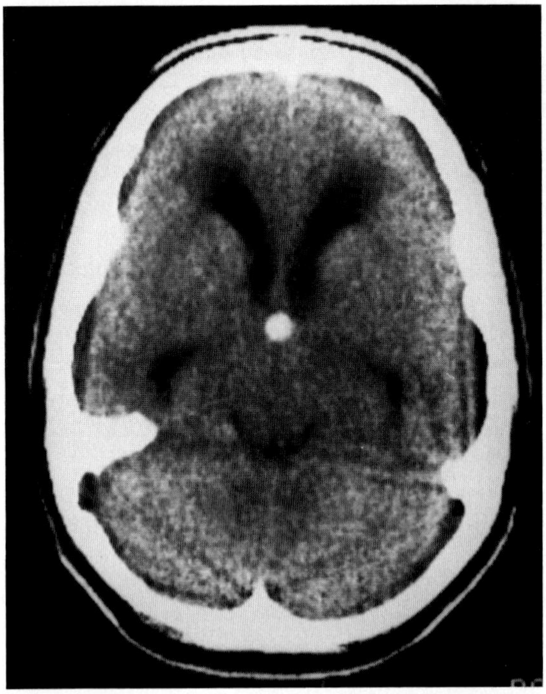

**Figure 32-2.** Colloid cyst of the third ventricle. Nonenhanced CT scan at the level of the foramina of Monro shows a 1-cm, uniformly dense lesion in the anterior portion of the third ventricle. No increase in density was noted on the contrast-enhanced scan. Enlargement of the frontal and temporal horns of the lateral ventricles with low attenuation in the periventricular white matter indicates obstructive hydrocephalus produced by the lesion. This CT pattern is virtually diagnostic of colloid cyst.

parenchymal cerebral lesions, a negative CT study must be considered inconclusive. Conversely, the contrast enhancement of extra-axial lesions and meningeal abnormalities on CT is one of its current advantages over MRI. Experimental studies have demonstrated MRI enhancement (similar to that of CT) using an intravenous paramagnetic contrast agent (Gadolinium diethyltriaminepentaacetic acid [Gd-DTPA]), but this material is not routinely available at the time of this writing. Computed tomography is superior to MRI for detecting calcification, which may be of value in identifying specific neoplastic (*e.g.*, oligodendroglioma) or infectious (*e.g.*, cysticercosis) lesions. Therefore, in screening the patient with headache, MRI (if available) should be used as the initial study, with CT employed for further characterization of detected lesions if needed (*e.g.*, contrast enhancement or calcification) (Fig. 32-3). Computed tomography may be performed as the initial study for suspected extra-axial lesions or meningeal processes which may enhance, at least until a contrast agent becomes routinely available for MRI. Currently CT is less expensive per study than MRI, although this cost differential is likely to be substantially reduced as MRI becomes more widely available.

## Magnetic Resonance Imaging

Magnetic resonance imaging is the most sensitive imaging technique available for detecting cerebral lesions in patients complaining of headache. Magnetic resonance imaging utilizes low-energy, nonionizing radio-frequency signals and magnetic fields to produce images of protons (hydrogen nuclei in water) in tissues. Image contrast is produced by differences in the proton density and the "relaxation times" (T1 and T2) between tissues. Because MRI is exquisitely sensitive to the water content of tissue, this modality can demonstrate cerebral abnormalities caused by such varied pathologic conditions as neoplasm, edema, ischemia, infection, inflammation, and demyelination at a much earlier stage than can CT (*i.e.,* before low attenuation or contrast enhancement develops) (Fig. 32-3). Magnetic resonance imaging also is superior to CT for demonstrating cerebral anatomy, especially in the posterior fossa (Fig. 32-4), and can clearly delineate gray matter, white matter, and vascular structures.

Although extremely sensitive to cerebral pathology, MRI, like CT, is nonspecific. Various pathologic processes in the brain are expressed through a "final common pathway" of increased tissue-water content that results in the nonspecific appearance of high signal on T2-weighted images and low signal T1-weighted images. For example, it is difficult on MRI to differentiate ischemic lesions (*e.g.*, focal subcortical ischemic encephalopathy) from demyelinating white matter lesions such as multiple sclerosis (Fig.

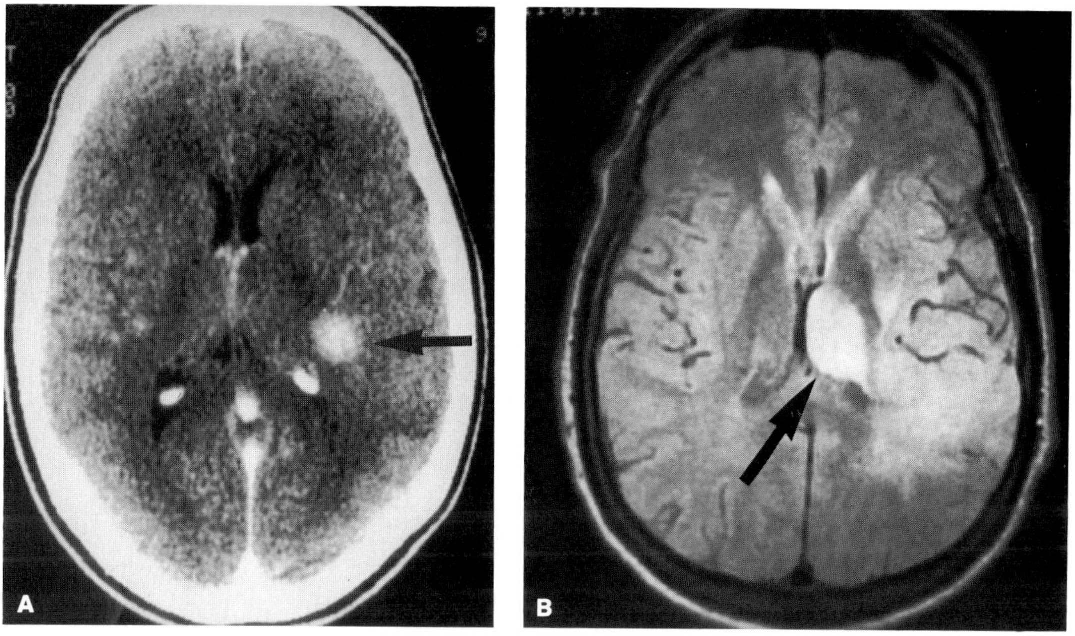


**Figure 32-3.** Cerebral neoplasm. **(A)** Contrast-enhanced CT scan shows a high-density lesion (*arrow*) just lateral to the left thalamus, which represents calcification and enhancement in a primary brain tumor (astrocytoma). Brain calcification and enhancement (indicating a breakdown of the blood–brain barrier) are well seen on CT, but poorly or not at all on MRI. **(B)** T2-weighted MRI in the same patient does not clearly show the region of calcification and enhancement seen on CT. However, MRI does show an abnormal high signal in the left thalamus (*arrow*) and throughout the left temporal lobe in areas that appeared normal on the CT scan. MRI is much more sensitive than CT to the early changes in brain-water content produced not only by neoplasms but also in the early stages of cerebral ischemia, infection, and demyelination.

32-5). Similarly, cerebral tumor may be impossible to differentiate from surrounding edema. In such cases, CT may be of value, because higher grade primary tumors (astrocytoma) and metastases tend to show contrast enhancement that distinguishes them from surrounding cerebral edema. A specific diagnosis sometimes can be made with MRI because of the typical appearance of a lesion (*e.g.*, subacute or chronic hematoma), but correlation with other imaging procedures, laboratory studies, patient age, and clinical information is usually required.

Magnetic resonance imaging is very sensitive to the presence of subacute or chronic hemorrhage in the brain, demonstrating it as a characteristic pattern of high signal on both T1- and T2-weighted images. This appearance may be demonstrated in regions that appear normal or show only nonspecific low attenuation on CT. This identification of subacute or chronic hemorrhage is of value in characterizing small vascular malformations that often show only nonspecific calcification on CT scanning and negative angiography. Acute hemorrhage (less than 1 week old) has a variable appearance on MRI; in most cases the pattern is distinct and specific, although it may be isointense with normal brain (especially small areas of petechial hemorrhage that are partial-volume averaged with brain). Because MRI is not completely reliable in excluding acute hemorrhage, CT should be employed when this diagnosis is an important consideration, especially in patients with possible subarachnoid hemorrhage.

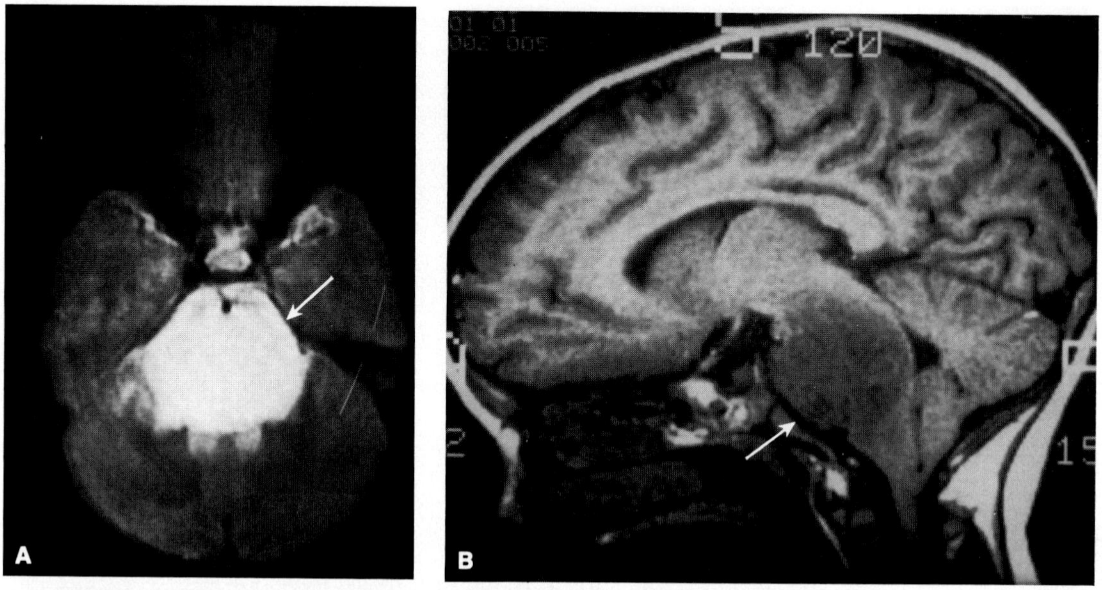


**Figure 32-4.** MRI of the posterior fossa. **(A)** T2-weighted axial MRI of the posterior fossa shows marked enlargement of the pons (*arrow*) with abnormal high signal (infiltrating astrocytoma of the brain stem). **(B)** T1-weighted sagittal MRI in the same patient shows abnormal low signal in the markedly enlarged pons (*arrow*). The sagittal plane is often useful for confirming the intra- or extra-axial location of lesions in the posterior fossa. In general, MRI is more useful than CT for demonstrating abnormalities in the posterior fossa because of the absence of reconstruction artifacts and the ability to image directly in multiple orientations without repositioning the patient.

Sensitivity to fluid motion is a significant qualitative advantage of MRI over CT. The identification of linear flow in blood vessels or pulsatile motion of cerebrospinal fluid adds a new dimension of analysis previously not available on the static views of anatomy obtained with CT scanning (Fig. 32-6). In many cases, MRI can replace angiography for determining the patency or occlusion of major cerebral vessels. For example, flow-sensitive MRI can identify the lack of blood flow and characteristic appearance of luminal thrombus in a patient with thrombosis of a major dural sinus (*e.g.*, superior sagittal sinus). Similarly, MRI can demonstrate patency of the aqueduct of Sylvius (oscillatory motion of cerebrospinal fluid normally occurs in time with cardiac pulsation) to exclude aqueductal obstruction in patients with enlargement of the third and lateral ventricles. Magnetic resonance imaging techniques currently under development (*e.g.*, phase-contrast projection imaging, which produces angiogram-like projection images of vessels rather than planar sections through them) promise to noninvasively duplicate the angiographic demonstration of large-vessel anatomy. At present, however, angiography remains the best imaging technique for demonstrating the detailed contour of large-vessel walls and small-vessel anatomy.

## Cerebral Arteriography

Prior to the development of CT, cerebral arteriography was frequently performed as the initial imaging study in patients with headaches suspected of being caused by an intracranial mass or a traumatic abnormality such as subdural hematoma. The use of angiography (intravenous or intra-arterial digital subtraction angiography, conventional arteriography) is now largely limited to the diagnosis of intrinsic lesions of the cerebrovascular system, whereas CT and MRI are performed to evaluate the brain paren-

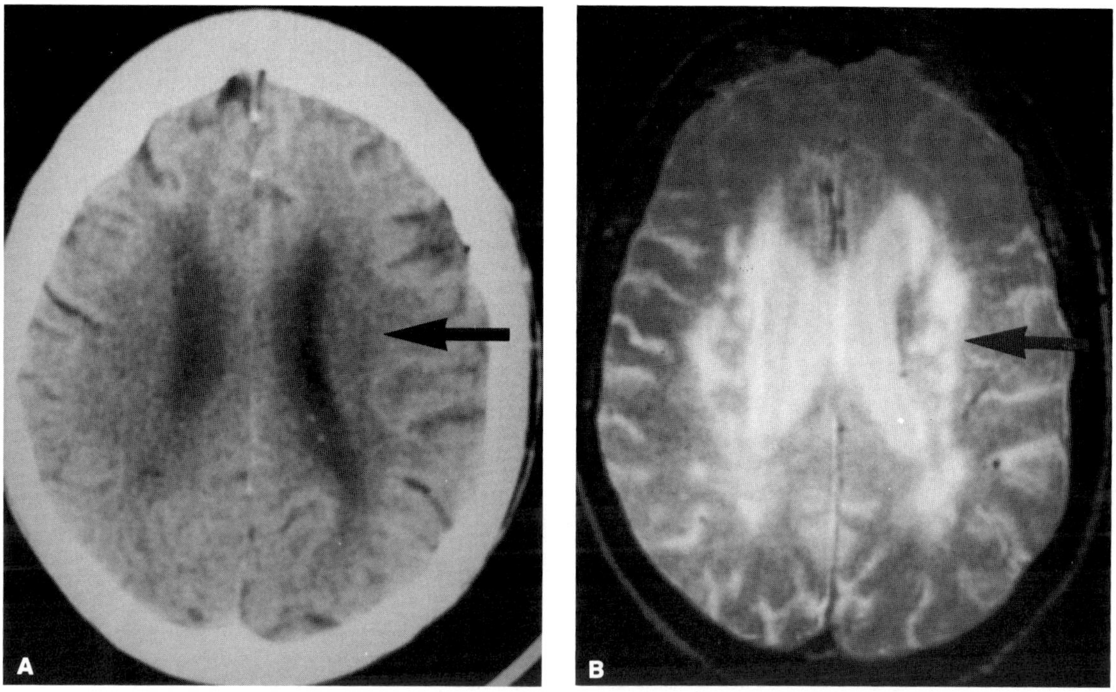


**Figure 32-5.** Subcortical ischemic encephalopathy. **(A)** Nonenhanced CT scan of a 73-year-old man shows minimally reduced attenuation in the white matter of the centrum semiovale (*arrow*) and cortical atrophy. No change was seen on the enhanced scan. **(B)** T2-weighted MRI in the same patient shows a striking pattern of patchy abnormal high signal in the white matter (*arrow*) with cortical atrophy. MRI is consistently more sensitive than CT scanning to this white matter pathology in the elderly, which probably represents the effect of chronic vascular insufficiency and may be associated with dementia. A similar appearance, with more discrete lesions localized primarily to the posterior periventricular regions, may also occur in younger patients with advanced multiple sclerosis.

chyma, ventricles, and extra-axial spaces. Although CT and MRI may demonstrate vascular structures and their patency, cerebral angiography remains the procedure of choice for detailed delineation of vascular lesions. For example, angiography may be required to identify the blood supply and "vascularity" of a tumor or the precise anatomy of a vascular malformation prior to surgery.

An important clinical scenario involves the patient with the sudden onset of severe headache associated with a stiff neck, a pattern of symptoms that strongly suggests the diagnosis of intracranial subarachnoid hemorrhage. This is an emergency situation, in which it is necessary to rapidly confirm the diagnosis of subarachnoid hemorrhage and to identify the source of bleeding. Computed tomography is the most sensitive and reliable modality for detecting subarachnoid hemorrhage. In some cases, small amounts of intraventricular or subarachnoid high-density blood may be identified on CT in a patient in whom the cerebrospinal fluid sampled from lumbar puncture is normal or uninterpretable due to a traumatic puncture. Once an acute subarachnoid hemorrhage is detected, angiography is indicated to demonstrate the precise source of bleeding (aneurysm or vascular malformation). Another reason for performing CT prior to angiography in all patients with suspected subarachnoid hemorrhage is that a knowledge of the distribution of the hemorrhage and identification of any associated parenchymal hematoma often is of value in planning the angiographic

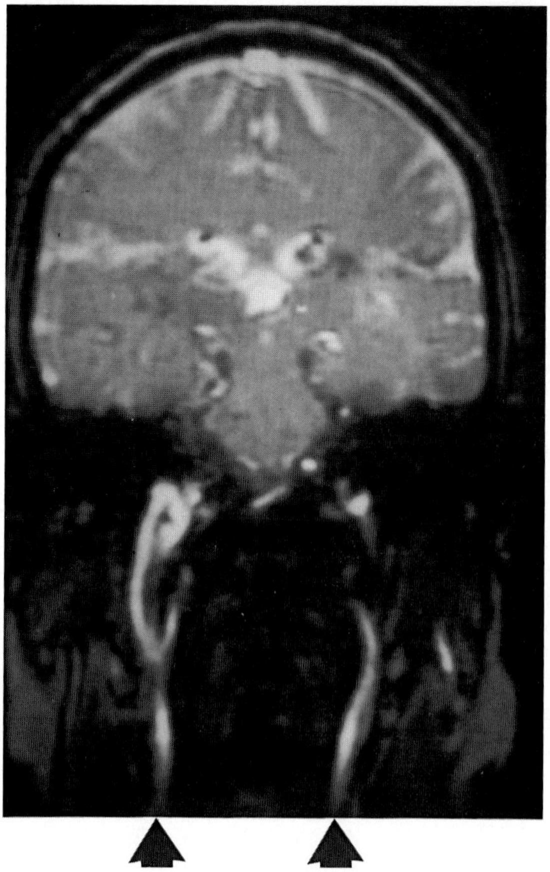

**Figure 32-6.** MRI of vascular anatomy. A specialized, flow-sensitive pulse sequence demonstrates flowing blood in the carotid arteries as high signal (*arrows*). Several MRI techniques currently under development promise to produce highly detailed images of cerebrovascular anatomy and quantitation of vascular flow rates.

procedure (*e.g.*, which vessel to study first and which area to concentrate on with multiple views).

## Radionuclide Brain Scan and Pneumoencephalography

Radionuclide brain scanning and pneumoencephalography are imaging techniques that have been used in the past to study patients with headache, but they are no longer of practical clinical value. Any information provided by these modalities can be obtained less invasively and with more anatomic specificity on MRI or CT. Positron emission tomography (PET), single photon emission tomography (SPECT), and xenon-enhanced CT studies of cerebral metabolism and blood flow are highly specialized studies that have limited availability and generally are not used in the clinical evaluation of headache.

## Surgery

When one or more imaging studies demonstrates an intracranial abnormality in a patient with headache, surgery is often required to make a final diagnosis. Although surgery is potentially the most definitive method available for determining the precise nature of intracranial disease, incomplete diagnosis can occur. Operating through a traditional craniotomy, the surgeon may fail to obtain tissue from a small lesion or may obtain a tissue sample that is not representative of the histologic grade of the majority or most malignant part of a neoplastic lesion. This problem usually can be solved using CT- or MRI-guided stereotaxic biopsy procedures. Extremely accurate probe placement is possible using stereotaxic head frames, which are worn by the patient in the CT scanner or MR imager, and computerized calculation of probe positioning coordinates. Even with accurate probe placement, there remains the fundamental problem of precisely identifying tissue characteristics on imaging studies. For example, although contrast enhancement on CT often indicates malignant tissue or active infection or inflammation, biopsy in these areas does not always yield clinically useful tissue samples. Similarly, at present MRI cannot clearly differentiate malignant or infected tissue from necrosis or edema. New MRI techniques under development may improve the identification of tissue types by the use of computerized image analysis or localized spectroscopic evaluation of tissue metabolism.

## Bibliography

Baker HL, Houser OW, Campbell JR: National Cancer Institute Study: Evaluation of computed tomography in the diagnosis of intracranial neoplasms. I. Overall results. Radiology 136:91–96, 1980

Bradley WG, Waluch V, Yadley RA et al: Comparison of CT and MR in 400 patients with suspected disease of the brain and cervical spinal cord. Radiology 152:695–702, 1984

Brismar, Stromblad LG, Salford LG: Impact of CT in the neurosurgical management of intracranial tumors. Neuroradiology 16:506–509, 1978

Bydder GM, Steiner RE, Young IR et al: Clinical NMR imaging of the brain: 140 cases. AJR 139: 215–236, 1982

DeLaPaz RL, New PFJ, Buonanno FS et al: NMR imaging of intracranial hemorrhage. J Comput Assist Tomogr 8:599–607, 1984

Dumoulin CL, Hart HR: Magnetic resonance angiography. Radiology 161:7–20, 1986

Gomori JM, Grossman RI, Goldberg HI et al: Intracranial hematomas: Imaging by high field MR. Radiology 157:87–93, 1985

Hayman LA, Evans RA, Hinck VC: Delayed high iodine dose contrast computed tomography. Cranial neoplasms. Radiology 136:677–684, 1980

Johnson MA, Pennock JM, Bydder GM et al: Clinical NMR imaging of the brain in children: Normal and neurologic disease. Am J Neuroradiol 4:1013–1026, 1983

Kandalaft N, Diehl J, Neuwelt EA: Non-neoplastic intracranial lesions simulating neoplasms on computed tomographic scan. Excellent sensitivity with limited specificity. JAMA 284:2166–2168, 1982

Lance JW: Mechanism and Management of Headache, 4th ed. London, Butterworths, 1982

Latchaw RE, Gold LHA, Moore JS et al: The nonspecificity of absorption coefficients in the differentiation of solid tumors and cystic lesions. Radiology 125:141–144, 1977

Rothner AD: Headaches in children: A review. Headache 18:169–175, 1978

Zimmerman RA, Bilaniuk LT, Johnson MH et al: MRI of the central nervous system: Early clinical results at 1.5 Tesla. Am J Neuroradiol 7:587–594, 1986

**HEADACHE**

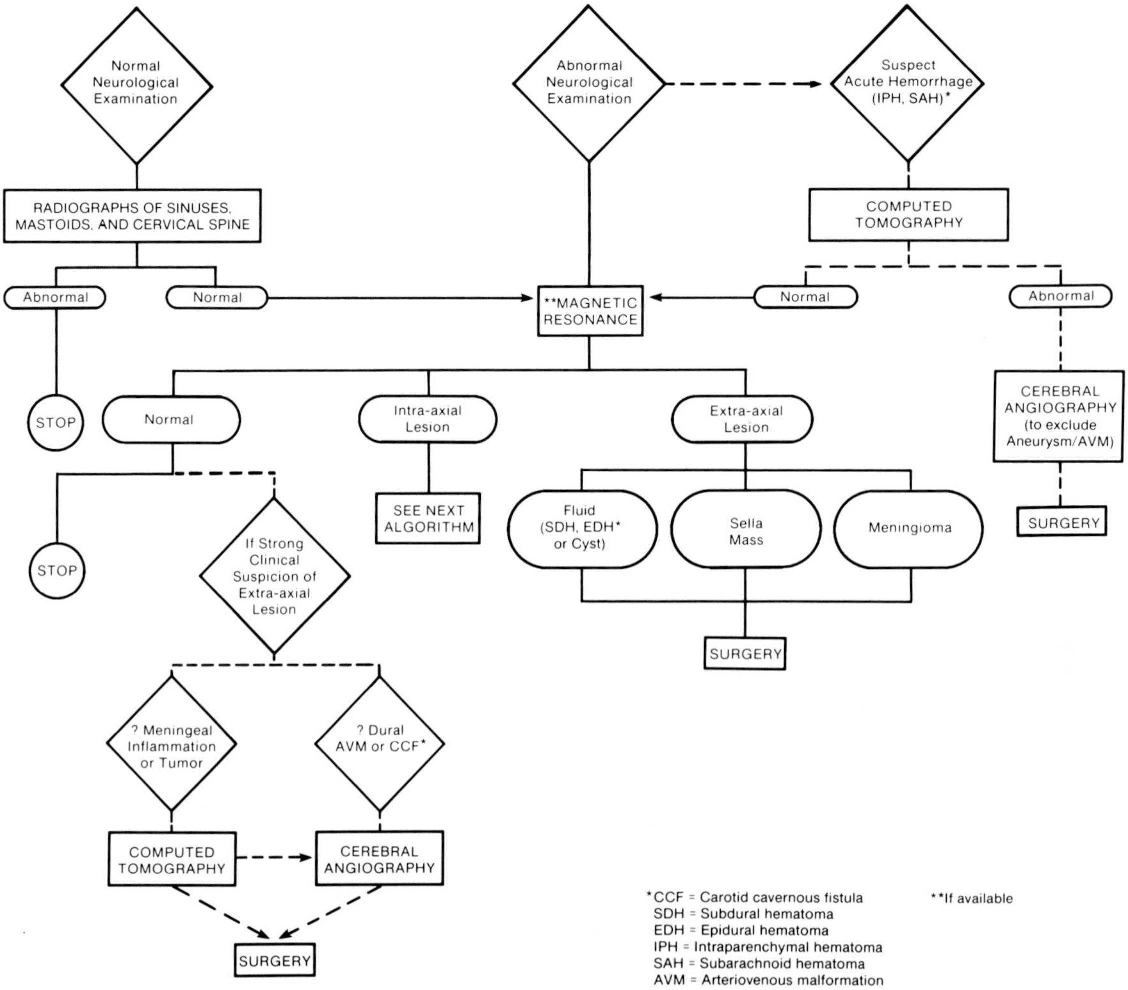


*CCF = Carotid cavernous fistula
SDH = Subdural hematoma
EDH = Epidural hematoma
IPH = Intraparenchymal hematoma
SAH = Subarachnoid hematoma
AVM = Arteriovenous malformation

**If available

## INTRA-AXIAL LESION

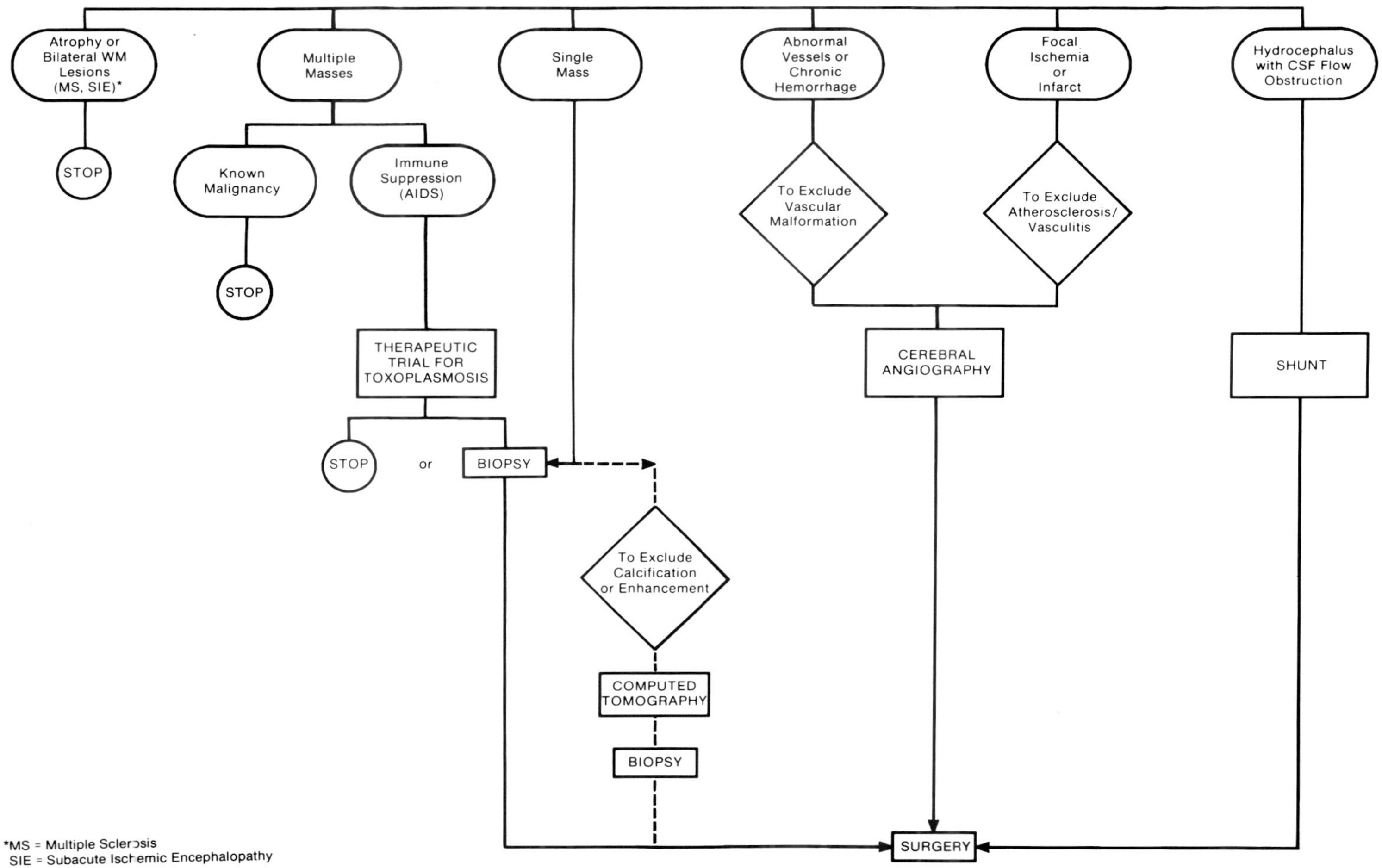


*MS = Multiple Sclerosis
SIE = Subacute Ischemic Encephalopathy

# Chapter 33

# Extracerebral Vascular Disease

*Barbara A. Carroll*

Strokes caused by atherosclerotic disease of the extracranial carotid arteries are the third leading cause of death (more than 250,000 per year) in the United States. About half of these strokes result from atherosclerotic disease located within 2 cm of the carotid bifurcation. For many years, the diagnostic evaluation of extracranial carotid artery disease consisted primarily of physical examination and conventional biplane arteriography. More recently, the development of less invasive, less expensive imaging techniques has significantly changed the diagnostic approach to the patient with suspected extracerebral carotid occlusive disease.

## DIAGNOSTIC EVALUATION

### *DIAGNOSTIC MODALITIES*

1. Indirect noninvasive tests
   a. Oculoplethysmography
   b. Bidirectional periorbital Doppler ultrasound
2. Direct noninvasive tests
   a. Continuous-wave Doppler ultrasound
   b. Pulsed Doppler ultrasound
3. High-frequency real-time ultrasound
4. Duplex carotid ultrasound
5. Digital subtraction angiography
   a. Intravenous subtraction angiography
   b. Intra-arterial subtraction angiography
6. Conventional carotid arteriography

### Indirect Noninvasive Tests

Indirect noninvasive tests are designed to measure blood flow in the orbital and ophthalmic vessels as a means for evaluating occlusive disease of the internal carotid artery. The most popular of the indirect tests are oculoplethysmography (OPG) and bidirectional periorbital Doppler ultrasound. Oculoplethysmography measures the arterial systolic pressure in the ophthalmic arteries and analyzes differences in systolic pressures and pulse arrival times. The

OPG is frequently performed and interpreted in conjunction with carotid phonoangiography, in which a hand-held microphone is used to produce oscilloscope recordings of cervical bruits. The significance of a bruit depends on its origin, length, and time in the cardiac cycle. To perform the OPG, suction-applied eye cups are placed on the corneas, and ophthalmic artery pressure and wave forms as well as pulse arrival times are evaluated simultaneously for each globe. Asymmetry of flow or a significant delay in systolic pulse arrival time indicates a flow-limiting occlusive lesion. Oculoplethysmography (with or without carotid phonoangiography) has a sensitivity rate ranging from 60% to 95% for detecting greater than 60% diameter stenoses; the specificity of this noninvasive test is approximately 90%. However, with this technique it is difficult to evaluate the location, extent, or number of occlusive lesions, plaque characteristics (including ulceration and minimal disease), and bilateral carotid arterial involvement.

Bidirectional periorbital Doppler ultrasound uses continuous-wave Doppler instrumentation to evaluate flow in the posterior orbital, supraorbital and supratrochlear vessels to detect severe occlusive disease and the development of collateral blood flow. Compression of facial or preauricular arteries resulting in either cessation or reversal of the direction of flow in the supraorbital or supratrochlear arteries is diagnostic of carotid occlusive disease. Like the OPG technique, bidirectional periorbital Doppler ultrasound cannot localize the site, extent, or number of flow-limiting lesions nor define minimal plaque or plaque ulceration or hemorrhage.

Indirect noninvasive tests are of limited value in assessing patients with stroke or transient ischemic attacks, because only half of these patients have flow-limiting stenoses. Even in patients with amaurosis fugax, only 75% have flow-limiting narrowing in the internal carotid artery. Indirect noninvasive tests lack both the sensitivity and specificity required for a screening test designed to detect the wide spectrum of carotid arterial plaque disease that potentially could be responsible for ischemic symptoms. Thus, although indirect noninvasive tests may be useful in ambiguous or confusing clinical settings, or if direct noninvasive tests are inconclusive, they are best employed in conjunction with direct noninvasive procedures.

### Direct Noninvasive Tests

Direct noninvasive tests (continuous-wave Doppler ultrasound with spectral analysis, pulsed Doppler ultrasound imaging) use the Doppler detection of frequency shifts within the carotid vessels to produce a flow image in a projectional format that reflects the patent vessel lumen. Continuous-wave Doppler ultrasound is of particular value in defining blood flow characteristics with a wide range of frequencies. Continuous-wave systems also can produce synthesized images that recreate a projectional vascular image based on flow velocity sampled throughout the vessel. Both continuous-wave and pulsed Doppler imaging techniques can quantify the degree of stenosis as a function of the peak frequency shift produced in the area of narrowing. Pulsed Doppler imaging permits the sampling of discrete locations within the vessel and thus provides better depth resolution than continuous-wave systems. Conversely, continuous-wave Doppler units, which utilize two separate transducers (one as a transmitter and one as a receiver), are easier to use and are capable of detecting a much wider range of frequency shifts. In pulsed Doppler units, the highest detectable frequency shift is limited to one half of the Doppler pulse repetition frequency. Thus, if frequency shifts in high-grade stenoses are in the range of 8 kHz to 12 kHz, aliasing may occur that masks the relative degree of frequency shift produced by the stenotic lesion.

Both continuous-wave and pulsed Doppler imaging can be subjected to spectral analysis, although this is more effective using the superior range resolution with pulsed Doppler ultrasound. The amount of turbulence producing spectral broadening can be correlated with the percentage of diameter reduction in a carotid artery. Minimal spectral broadening occurring only in systole is associated with a 15% stenosis. Broadening of frequency spectra throughout systole, but with no evidence of peak systolic frequency elevation, reflects a 16% to 49% stenosis. Pansystolic turbulence associated with an elevated peak systolic frequency corresponds to a stenosis of more than 50%. Other flow parameters, such as the pulsatility index, wave form shape, systolic and diastolic slope and rise times, and velocity ratios also can be correlated with the degree of vascular stenosis. Overall, direct noninvasive tests can detect greater than 50% to 60% carotid arterial stenoses with a sensitivity of 90% to 95%. As with indirect noninvasive studies, however, lesser degrees of atherosclerotic plaque may be missed and Doppler imaging studies lack the ability to define plaque morphology.

### High-Frequency Real-Time Ultrasound

Direct imaging of the carotid bifurcation and extracranial carotid vessels using high-frequency (5 mHz–10 mHz) real-time ultrasound provides essential morphologic vascular information that was previously obtainable only by arteriography. The anatomic detail provided by high-frequency real-time ultrasound permits demonstration of early atherosclerotic plaque and intimal medial hyperplasia. The normal vascular intimal surface echo and the vascular media are imaged routinely as a composite intimal–medial line paralleling the outer wall of the vessel. The intimal surface is an echogenic line overlying the hypoechoic media (Fig. 33-1). Unlike the previously described modalities, high-frequency real-time ultrasound can determine the number of atherosclerotic lesions as well as their location and extent, their structural composition, and the presence or absence of surface irregularities and ulceration. Adequate visualization of the carotid bifurcation and proximal 2 cm of the internal carotid artery can be achieved in 90% to 95% of patients. The remaining patients have carotid bifurcations that are difficult to image due to anatomic variation. False-negative ultrasound examinations may result from acute thrombus being isoechogenic with flowing blood (and thus difficult to detect using imaging alone) or plaque calcifications that obscure portions of the vessel lumen. Nevertheless, high-frequency ultrasound imaging without Doppler has been consistently reported to have a diagnostic accuracy rate of 85% relative to conventional arteriography for detection of greater than 50% to 60% diameter stenoses.

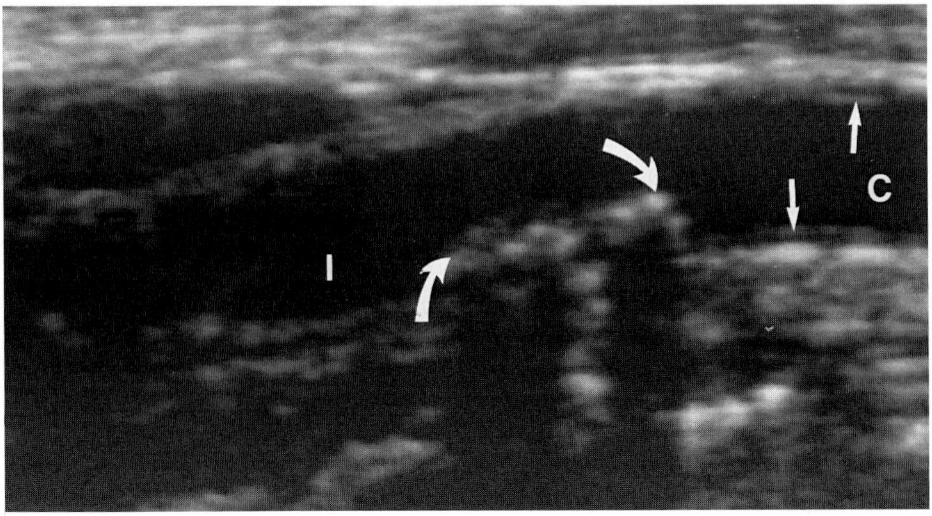


**Figure 33-1.** Longitudinal sonogram through the region of the common carotid artery (*C*), carotid bulb, and origin of the internal carotid artery (*I*) demonstrates the normal intimal–medial line (*arrows*) on both the anterior and posterior aspects of the vessel just proximal to a heterogeneous plaque (*curved arrows*) located at the origin of the internal carotid artery.

Real-time ultrasound can evaluate the surface characteristics and internal composition of atherosclerotic plaque. A heterogeneous plaque with cystic or hypoechoic areas reflects intraplaque hemorrhage (Fig. 33-2). Anechoic or hypoechoic homogeneous plaque represents predominantly lipid disease, while homogeneous plaque with intermediate echogenicity is predominantly fibrous-collagen plaque. Echogenic plaque with posterior acoustic shadowing usually signifies the presence of calcification. The ultrasound detection of plaque ulceration has been reported to have only 43% sensitivity and 95% specificity. However, these initial series primarily compared the ultrasound findings with conventional or digital subtraction angiography (often unreliable for detecting plaque ulceration) rather than with surgical findings. Thus, studies directly correlating ultrasound and surgical findings are essential to properly define the accuracy of ultrasound for detecting plaque ulceration.

Ulcerations must be at least 2 mm deep to be consistently detected on arteriography. In vessels with only minimal plaque formation, ulceration is even more difficult to detect. Several studies indicate that sonography can detect minimal plaque disease more accurately than arteriography. This suggests a potential role for ultrasound in evaluating minimal plaque ulceration in patients with less than 50% to 60% stenoses. Detection of homogeneous, smooth-surfaced, minimal plaque disease would be considered nonsurgical disease (unlikely to be a surgically correctable cause of symptoms), while detection of inhomogeneous plaque with multiple surface irregularities in less than 50% to 60% stenoses might be deemed surgical disease if considered a potential source of embolic phenomena.

## Duplex Carotid Ultrasound

"Duplex" ultrasound is the most accurate noninvasive test and combines high-resolution real-time imaging of the carotid vessels with hemodynamic information about blood flow velocity provided by the Doppler technique. The addition of Doppler information about the presence of blood flow and quantification of spectral data can clarify confusing ultrasound images in which plaque calcification obscures a portion of the vascular lumen or there is acute thrombus that is isoechogenic with flowing blood (Fig. 33-3). One limitation of duplex sonography is in the diagnosis of complete occlusion. Although the negative predictive value of this technique exceeds 99%, approximately 20% of carotid vessels considered to be completely occluded will have some lumen patency. Thus, if duplex ultrasound suggests an occlusion, intra-arterial digital subtraction angiography (DSA) (or conventional arteriography) is usually required to confirm the ultrasound findings before any surgical intervention. "Color flow" instruments may significantly improve the accuracy in diagnosing occlusions.

In approximately 90% to 95% of cases, duplex ultrasound equals conventional arteriography in the detection of extracranial carotid occlusive disease. Additional information obtained from other noninvasive techniques can make duplex sonography even more accurate in its interpretation of flow and imaging data. Some institutions advocate a battery of noninvasive tests based on studies that have indicated that accuracy is increased when two noninvasive tests concur in the diagnosis. However, in view of the cost and known limitations of noninvasive testing, it may be most prudent to use the highly accurate duplex ultrasound examination as the only noninvasive test, with angiographic procedures used to clarify confusing situations and to provide preoperative anatomic information. In some instances, surgery can be performed solely on the basis of duplex ultrasound findings. However, the majority of surgeons prefer an intra-arterial DSA study to demonstrate the intracranial circulation, unless there is a contraindication to angiography.

In patients undergoing endarterectomy, direct intraoperative sonographic vascular imaging has proven more accurate than intraoperative arteriography for detecting intimal flap dissection. The postoperative patency of the carotid vessels can be similarly monitored by ultrasound examinations.

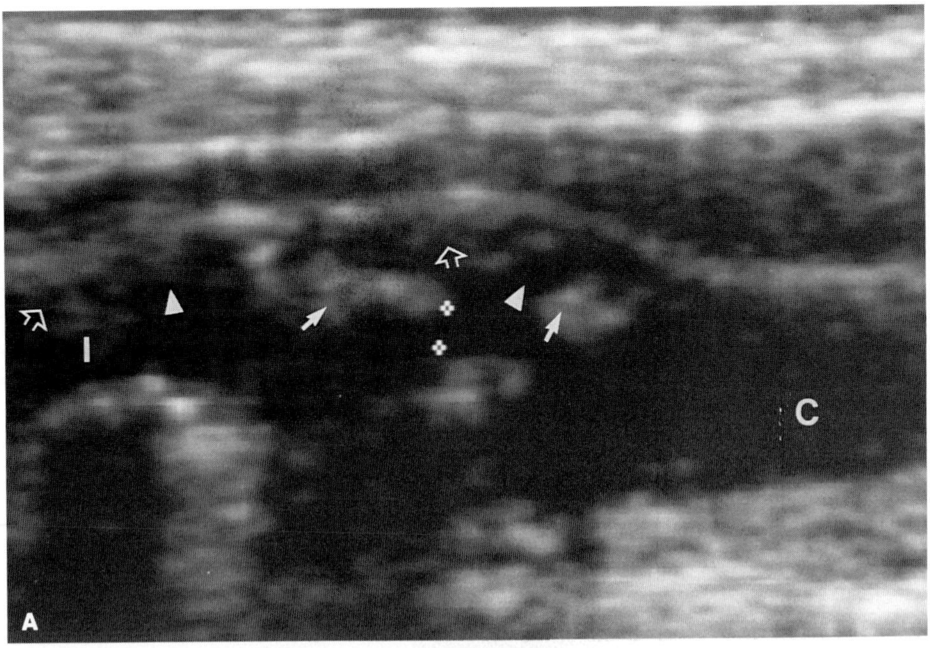


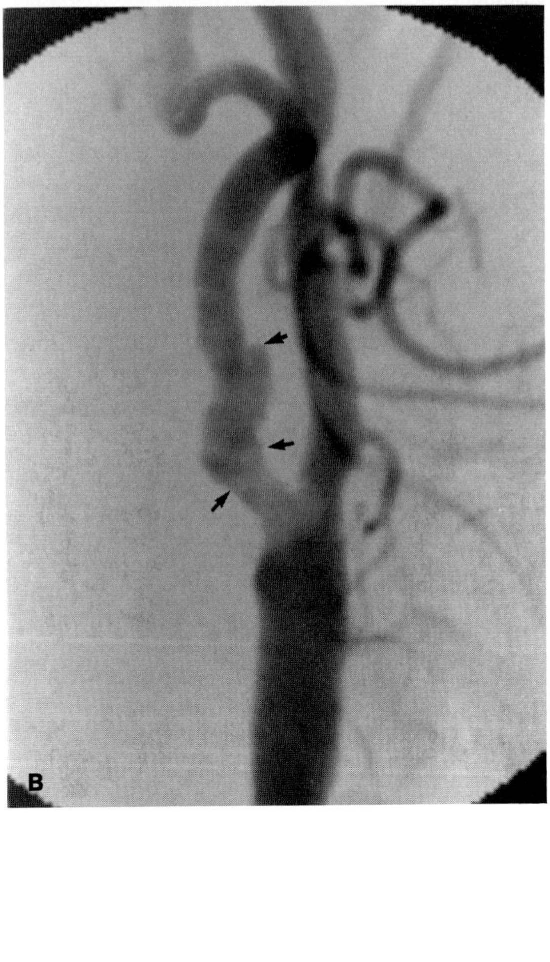


**Figure 33-2. (A)** Longitudinal sonogram through the region of the carotid bifurcation demonstrates a 60% to 70% stenosis of the internal carotid artery (*crossmarks*). The plaque composition is heterogeneous with areas of increased (*closed arrows*) and decreased (*open arrows*) echogenicity within the plaque. Areas of surface ulceration and irregularity are noted (*arrowheads*) (*C*, common carotid artery; I, internal carotid artery). **(B)** Intra-arterial DSA study confirms the stenotic ulcerated lesion (*arrows*) in the internal carotid artery.

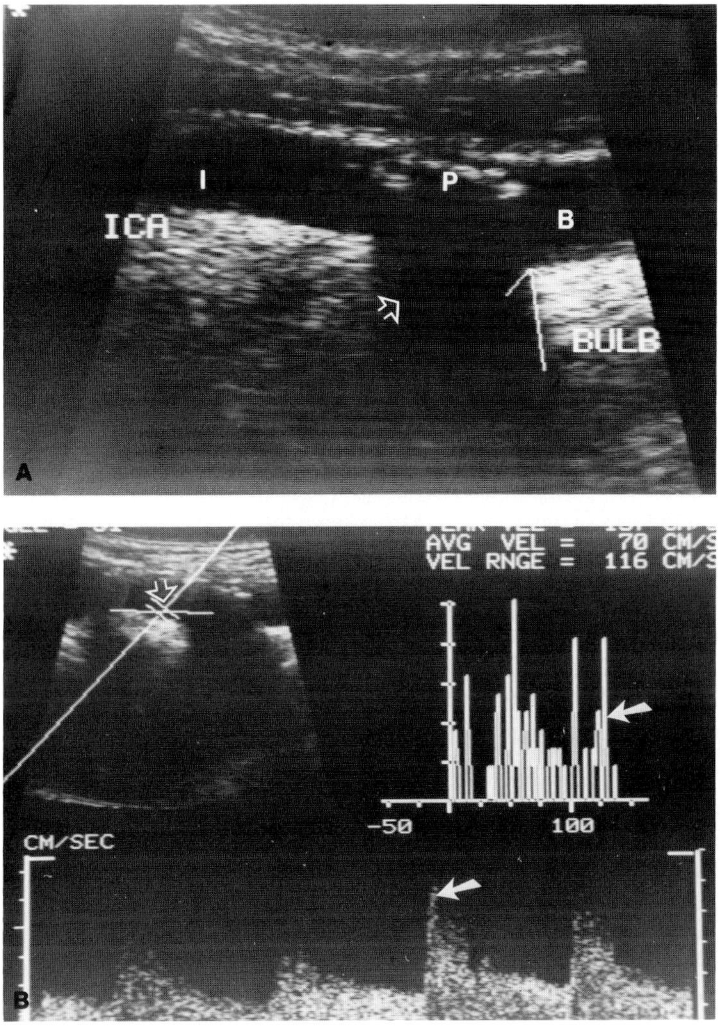


**Figure 33-3. (A)** Longitudinal sonogram through the region of the carotid bifurcation demonstrates the carotid bulb (*B*) and the origin of the internal carotid artery (*I*). A densely calcified plaque (*P*) produces a strong posterior acoustic shadow (*open arrow*), which obscures direct visualization of the vessel lumen and thus makes it impossible to estimate the degree of stenosis produced by the plaque. **(B)** Doppler flow tracing obtained just distal to the plaque (*open arrow*) demonstrates high velocity, turbulent flow compatible with a stenosis of 60% or more. The frequency spectra (*closed arrows*) demonstrate these flow abnormalities, which correspond to a high-degree stenosis but a patent residual lumen.

Doppler color flow imaging of the carotid arteries is still in its infancy. Nevertheless, real-time images of flow combined with real-time anatomic information may facilitate more rapid duplex examinations and clarify ambiguous spectral data.

## Angiography

Conventional biplane arteriography provides the highest resolution images of intraluminal vascular pathology that are currently available. However, the expense of this technique, as well as the associated morbidity and mortality, limits the use of conventional arteriography to a relatively few patients with suspected extracranial carotid occlusive disease. Arteriography has been used to evaluate the intracranial and extracranial collateral circulation in patients with suspected complete occlusion of the internal carotid artery who were being considered for bypass surgery of the external and internal carotid arteries. However, this procedure is no longer indicated in view of the recent studies demonstrating the lack of efficacy of bypass grafting between the internal carotid and external carotid systems. In a few select patients with suspected posterior circulation disease, conventional arteriography may be needed to evaluate the intracranial posterior fossa circulation.

Intravenous digital subtraction angiography (IVDSA) uses a central venous injection of contrast material to demonstrate the carotid bifurcation, aortic arch, carotid siphon, and intracranial circulation. However, the initial enthusiasm for this "poor man's arteriogram" has been dampened as the limitations of IVDSA relative to conventional arteriography have become more apparent. Although less invasive than a conventional arteriogram, IVDSA requires a large contrast load and is associated with catheter trauma and renal function abnormalities. Up to 15% of studies are suboptimal due to such factors as patient motion, vessel overlap or calcification, poor cardiac output and cardiac dysfunction, and substandard system performance (Fig. 33-4). Intravenous DSA is more expensive than duplex ultrasound, and numerous reports have failed to demonstrate any major difference between the sensitivity or specificity of duplex ultrasound and IVDSA for the detection of stenosis, occlusion, or plaque ulceration.

Compared with IVDSA, intra-arterial digital subtraction angiography (IADSA) has superior resolution and has supplanted the intravenous technique in most institutions. Intra-arterial DSA is a safer examination because of the smaller volume and lower concentration of contrast material and the shorter procedure time. A common carotid injection is usually sufficient for evaluating the bifurcation and intracranial vessels, making IADSA less risky than conventional arteriography, in which extensive catheter and guide wire manipulation increases the likelihood of dislodging emboli from diseased vessels. Thc volume of contrast and film cost are substantially less than that required for conventional arteriography, and IADSA often can be performed on an outpatient basis. Because it can provide image quality comparable to conventional arteriography at a lower cost and with less patient risk, it is likely that in most instances IADSA will replace IVDSA and conventional arteriorgraphy in the evaluation of carotid occlusive disease (Fig. 33-5).

## SCREENING PROCEDURES

Patients with hemispheric neurologic symptoms or amaurosis fugax who are considered operative candidates can be evaluated in either of two ways. In an institution where noninvasive testing is well established, duplex ultrasound is a valuable screening test to determine those patients with suspected extracranial carotid artery disease who require angiographic studies. If sonography demonstrates a high-grade stenosis ("surgical" lesion) or complete occlusion, an IADSA is the only other imaging study required prior to surgical intervention. If noninvasive studies are not available or well established, DSA can be used as the screening study for patients with suspected extracranial carotid occlusive disease. Intra-arterial DSA is the procedure of choice, because it can be performed on an outpatient basis, is far more accurate, and requires a lower volume and concentration of contrast material than intravenous DSA.

Patients with asymptomatic bruits or atypical nonhemispheric neurologic symptoms, or those who are at high risk for the development of atherosclerotic disease (diabetes, hypertension, hypercholesterolemia, strong family history of stroke and atherosclerotic disease), are candidates for screening noninvasive duplex sonography to evaluate their extracranial carotid systems. The relatively low cost, high accuracy, and noninvasive nature of duplex ultrasound make it the examination of choice in these patients, because a normal sonogram, or one demonstrating only minimal atherosclerotic plaque disease, may be the sole imaging test required. Even though there may be no need for further imaging of the extracranial carotid arteries, additional imaging procedures are often required to further investigate the cause of the patient's symptoms. For example, computed tomography or magnetic resonance imaging of the intracranial contents may be necessary to exclude a neoplasm or lacunar infarcts. Noninvasive ultrasound imaging also can be of value in patients with a cervical bruit who are scheduled to undergo major vascular surgery. The demonstration of more than 80% stenosis in the extracranial carotid supply of these patients may put them at higher risk for

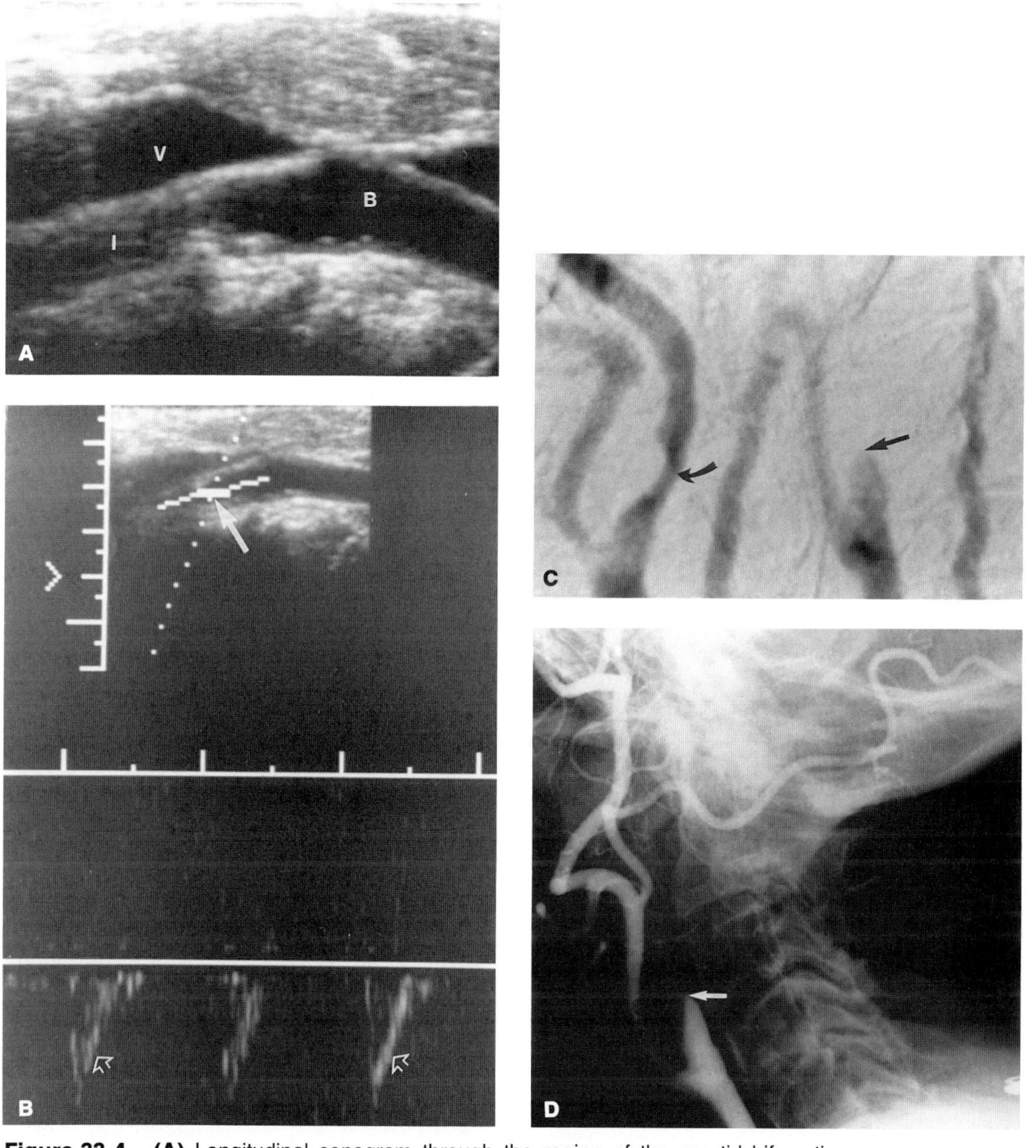


**Figure 33-4. (A)** Longitudinal sonogram through the region of the carotid bifurcation demonstrates a patent carotid bulb (*B*). Echogenic material completely fills the lumen of the proximal internal carotid artery (*I*) (*V,* jugular vein). **(B)** Doppler sampling in the internal carotid artery just proximal to the echogenic intraluminal material (*closed arrow*) demonstrates reversal of normal vascular flow (*open arrows*). No evidence of flow is detected in the internal carotid artery distal to this point. **(C)** Intravenous DSA suggests the presence of a left internal carotid artery occlusion (*straight arrow*). There also is an irregular ulcerated plaque with stenosis at the origin of the right internal carotid artery (*curved arrow*). Because of motion artifacts and reduced cardiac output, a selective injection of the left common carotid artery was performed **(D)** to confirm the complete occlusion of the left internal carotid artery (*arrow*).

suffering transient ischemic attacks or strokes during surgery. Duplex ultrasound is also the ideal screening procedure for imaging the patient with classic hemispheric symptoms but with a medical contraindication to radiographic contrast material. It also can be used to evaluate confusing or equivocal angiographic studies.

## BIBLIOGRAPHY

Ackerman RH, D'Alton JG, Davis KR et al: Complementary roles of a noninvasive test battery and DSA in evaluating carotid artery disease. Am J Neuroradiol 4:757, 1983

Belkin M, Buckman CA, Ginea JE et al: Combined OPG duplex scan: Use in the noninvasive cerebrovascular laboratory examination. Arch Surg 120:809–811, 1985

Blackshear WM, Phillips BJ, Chikes PM et al: Carotid artery velocity patterns in normal and stenotic vessels. Stroke 11:67–71, 1980

Blackshear WM, Phillips BJ, Thiele BL et al: Detection of carotid occlusive diseases by ultrasonic imaging and pulsed Doppler spectrum analysis. Surgery 86:698–706, 1979

Bluth EI, Kay D, Merritt CRB et al: Sonographic characterization of carotid plaque: Detection of hemorrhage. AJR 146:1061–1065, 1986

Brant–Zawadski M, Gould R, Norman D et al: Digital subtraction cerebral angiography by intraarterial injection: Comparison with conventional angiography. Am J Neuroradiol 3:593, 1982

Chilcote WA, Modic MT, Pavlicek WA et al: Digital subtraction angiography of the carotid arteries: A comparative study in 100 patients. Radiology 139:287, 1981

Comerota AJ, Cranley JJ, Katz M et al: Real-time B-mode carotid imaging: A three-year multicenter experience. J Vasc Surg 1:84, 1984

Cooperberg PL, Robertson WD, Fry P et al: High-resolution real-time ultrasound of the carotid bifurcation. J Clin Ultrasound 7:13, 1979

Dreisbach JN, Seibert CA, Smazal SF et al: Duplex sonography in the evaluation of carotid artery disease. Am J Neuroradiol 4:678, 1983

The EC/IC Bypass Study Group: Failure of extracranial–intracranial arterial bypass to reduce the risk of ischemic stroke. N Engl J Med 313: 1191–1200, 1985

Edwards JH, Kricheff II, Rules T et al: Angiographically undetected ulceration of the carotid bifurcation as a cause of embolic stroke. Radiology 132:369, 1979

Eikelboom BC, Ackerstaff RGA, Ludwig JW et al: Digital video subtraction angiography and duplex scanning in assessment of carotid artery disease: Comparison with conventional angiography. Surgery 94:821, 1983

Flanigan DP, Schuler JJ, Vogel M et al: The role of carotid duplex scanning in surgical decision making. J Vasc Surg 2:15, 1985

Garth KE, Carroll BA, Sommer FG et al: Duplex ultrasound scanning of the carotids with spectrum analysis. Radiology 147:823, 1983

Ginsburg MD, Greenwood SA, Goldberg HL: Invasive diagnosis of extracranial disease: Oculoplethysmography, phonoangiography, and directional Doppler ultrasonography. Neurology 29:623–631, 1979

Hoffman MG, Gomes AS, Pair SO: Limitations in the interpretation of intravenous carotid digital subtraction angiography. AJR 142:261, 1984

James EM, Earnest F, Forbes GS et al: High resolution dynamic ultrasound imaging of the carotid bifurcation: A prospective evaluation. Radiology 144:853, 1982

Johnson JM, Ansel AL, Morgan S et al: Ultrasonographic screening for evaluation and follow-up of carotid artery ulceration: A new basis for assessing risk. Am J Surg 144:614, 1982

Meaney TF, Weinstein MA, Buonocore E et al: Digital subtraction angiography of the human cardiovascular system. AJR 135:1153, 1980

O'Leary DH: Vascular ultrasonography. Symposium on ultrasonography of small parts. Radiol Clin North Am 23:40, 1985

O'Leary DH, Clouse ME, Potter JE et al: The influence of non-invasive tests on the selection of patients for carotid angiography. Stroke 16: 264, 1985

O'Leary DH, Gibbons GW, Pinel DF: Limitations of noninvasive testing in assessing the "occluded" carotid artery. Am J Neuroradiol 4:759, 1983

O'Leary DH, Pensson AV, Clouse ME: Noninvasive testing for carotid artery stenosis. I. Prospective analysis of three methods. Am J Neuroradiol 2:437–442, 1981

Reilly LM, Lusby RJ, Hughes L et al: Carotid plaque histology using real-time ultrasonography: Clinical and therapeutic implications. Am J Surg 146:188, 1983

Russell JB, Watson TM, Modi JR: Digital subtraction angiography for evaluation of extracranial carotid occlusive disease: Comparison with conventional arteriography. Surgery 94:604, 1983

Samples JR, Trautman JC, Sundt TM: Interpretation of results of compression ophthalmodynamometry. Stroke 13:655, 1982

Wetzner SM, Kiser LC, Bezreh JS: Duplex ultrasound imaging: Vascular applications. Radiology 150: 507, 1984

Wolverson MK, Heiberg E, Sundaram M et al: Carotid atherosclerosis: High resolution real-time sonography correlated with angiography. Am J Neuroradiol 3:601, 1982

Wood GW, Lukin RR, Tomsick TA et al: Digital subtraction angiography with intravenous injection: Assessment of 100 carotid bifurcations. AJR 140: 855, 1983

Zweibel WJ, Strother CM, Austin CW et al: Comparison of ultrasound and IVDSA for carotid evaluation. Stroke 16:633, 1985

**EXTRACRANIAL CEREBROVASCULAR DISEASE**

**HEMISPHERIC SYMPTOMS/AMAUROSIS FUGAX**

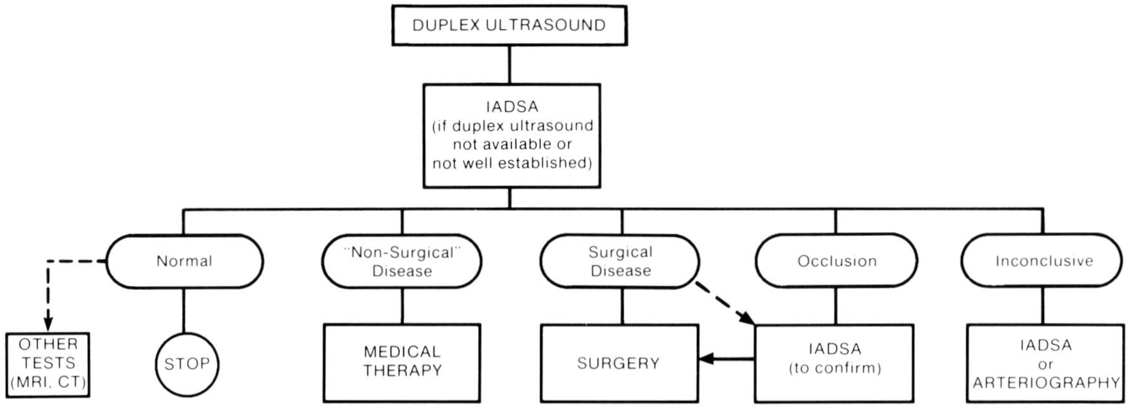


**ASYMPTOMATIC/NON – HEMISPHERIC SYMPTOMS**

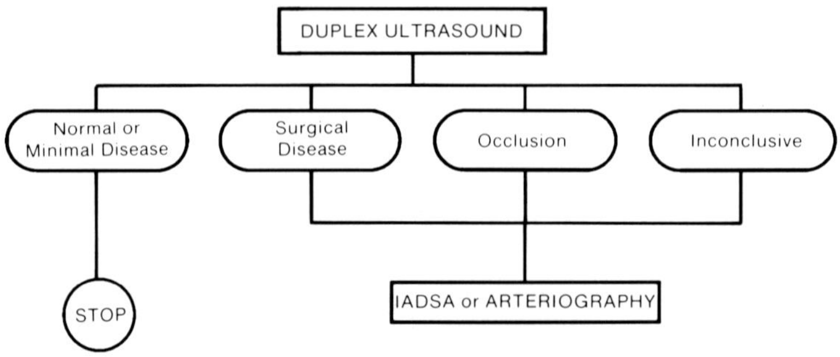

# Chapter 34

# Visual Loss

*Charles M. Strother*
*Richard E. Appen*

Formulating a logical approach to the radiographic investigation of patients with loss of vision is dependent on the findings of the ophthalmologic examination. This chapter describes the common signs and symptoms of patients experiencing visual loss, with emphasis on their value as localizers of visual system dysfunction. In addition, it offers a rationale for the radiographic evaluation of those patients who are considered likely to harbor a mass lesion that is impairing the function of their visual pathways.

## INITIAL CLINICAL EVALUATION

Before planning a logical sequence of radiographic examinations, it must be determined whether the visual deficit can be localized to the prechiasmal (45%), chiasmal (10%), or postchiasmal (45%) segments of the visual pathways (Fig. 34-1). Therefore, the following information should be obtained during the initial clinical assessment of the patient who has experienced visual loss:

1. Were the signs and symptoms monocular or binocular?
2. Was the visual deficit continuous or intermittent?
3. Did the visual impairment have an abrupt or a gradual onset?

The answers to these questions often give valuable clues to the likely etiology of the abnormality and to its location in the visual system. For example, in the face of a normal ocular examination, purely monocular visual loss indicates disease restricted to the optic nerve. On the other hand, binocular involvement indicates either two separate optic nerve lesions or, much more commonly, involvement of the visual system by one lesion either at the optic chiasm or in the postchiasmatic region. The distinction between the optic chiasm and postchiasmatic location is made on the basis of visual field testing. Optic chiasm lesions are generally characterized by temporal visual field defects and impairment of visual acuity in at least one eye; postchiasmatic lesions typically cause homonymous visual field defects without reduction of visual acuity.

Visual symptoms that are intermittent suggest a vascular abnormality. In such patients, the cervical carotid arteries should be carefully investigated as a possible source of the visual defi-

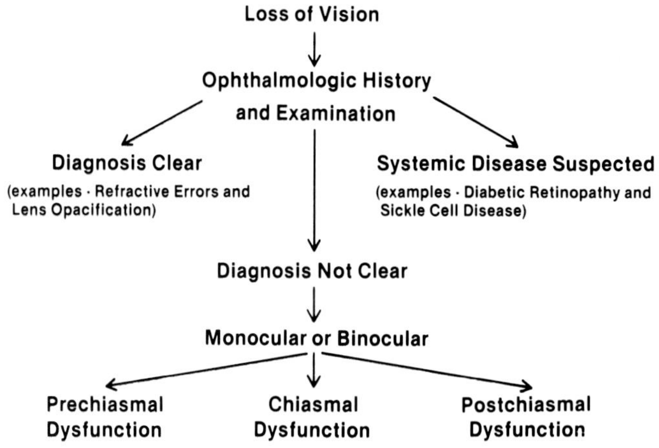


**Figure 34-1.** Diagram of the method of categorizing patients with loss of vision. The radiographic evaluation of patients with prechiasmal, chiasmal, and postchiasmal visual dysfunction differs significantly. The details of these differences are discussed in the text.

cit. Persistent visual loss indicates a definite focal lesion. An abrupt onset of visual loss is characteristic of a vascular disorder, while tumors are more likely to result in a gradually progressive deficit. It must be emphasized, however, that intracranial masses, whether of neoplastic, inflammatory, or vascular (*i.e.*, aneurysm) origin, may at times undergo hemorrhage or thrombosis and cause the sudden loss of visual function. Nevertheless, whether the onset of visual impairment was acute or gradual, the history of slow, progressive worsening of symptoms is the hallmark of mass lesions involving the visual pathways.

The ophthalmologic examination may permit a diagnosis to be made without the need for further investigation. Common examples include patients with refractive errors, lens opacities, and a variety of other diseases that are confined to the retina. At other times, the ocular examination may indicate a systemic disease that secondarily affects the function of the visual system (endocrine ophthalmopathy and the retinopathies of diabetes mellitus, sarcoidosis, and sickle-cell disease). A normal ocular examination or one showing only optic atrophy in a patient with impaired vision strongly suggests the possibility of an orbital or intracranial mass lesion.

Careful assessment of the visual acuity, pupillary response, optic disc appearance, and visual fields almost always indicates whether the portion of the visual pathway that is abnormal is the optic nerve, the optic chiasm, or the postchiasmatic optic tract or radiation.

## UNILATERAL OPTIC NERVE IMPAIRMENT

If the patient with unilateral visual loss has a normal ocular examination (or only optic atrophy) of both the symptomatic and asymptomatic eye, a lesion directly affecting the optic nerve is suggested. Conditions that produce unilateral optic nerve dysfunction include optic neuritis, ischemic optic neuropathy, and a variety of mass lesions that either infiltrate or compress the nerve as it passes from the optic chiasm into the orbit.

The time course of the visual loss is a good indicator for predicting which of these three categories of abnormalities is responsible. In optic neuritis, vision typically deteriorates relatively abruptly over a period of several days. With ischemic optic neuropathy, the visual deficit generally occurs suddenly with the maximum loss of vision arising within a few minutes. In the compressive–infiltrative conditions, visual impairment continues relentlessly over a period of weeks, months, or even years.

### OPTIC NEURITIS

Optic neuritis affects women twice as often as men and occurs predominantly in patients less than 50 years old. Although usually unilateral, optic neuritis is bilateral in up to 25% of patients. Many of these patients have associated tenderness of the eye or pain worsened by eye movement. Abnormality of the optic nerve head (either edema or atrophy) often occurs at some stage of the disease. More than 70% of patients with optic neuritis will regain good vision within several months of the onset of the visual deficit.

In the patient with typical signs and symptoms of optic neuritis, there is initially no need for radiographic studies. However, if the patient has atypical features or if vision continues to deteriorate or, just as importantly, fails to improve, compressive or infiltrative lesions of the optic nerve must be excluded.

## ISCHEMIC OPTIC NEUROPATHY

Ischemic optic neuropathy occurs predominantly in older patients and is a variant of optic neuritis caused by compromise of the small arteries supplying the optic nerve head. The diagnosis is based on the abrupt onset of imparied vision associated with an altitudinal or nerve fiber bundle visual field defect, a sluggish pupil, and in the acute phase of the illness, a swollen optic nerve head. Although visual acuity is normal in 30% of such patients, it may be markedly impaired. Ischemic optic neuropathy may be a manifestation of temporal arteritis but more commonly appears to be secondary to arteriosclerotic vascular disease. It is generally believed that there is no definite need for radiographic diagnostic procedures in ischemic optic neuropathy.

## COMPRESSIVE–INFILTRATIVE OPTIC NEUROPATHIES

The location of the optic nerves renders them susceptible to pressure from many benign and malignant tumors originating either within the orbit or along the margins of the anterior and middle cranial fossae. The nerve may also be directly involved by tumor (*i.e.,* optic nerve glioma) and, because of its unique continuity with the subarachnoid space, may be infiltrated by a number of neoplastic or inflammatory conditions that tend to occur in this location (leukemia, lymphoma, sarcoidosis).

Often the ocular examination indicates whether or not the process affecting the optic nerve is intra-orbital in location. Orbital masses frequently cause exophthalmos, abnormal orbital resiliency, limitation of eye movement, retinal striae, or swelling of the optic disc. Recognition of these signs is important, because the radiographic evaluation of patients with compressive–infiltrative lesions situated within the orbit is different from those with primary intracranial abnormalities.

## DIAGNOSTIC EVALUATION

Some radiographic procedures permit direct visualization of the optic nerve itself. Other techniques demonstrate the bony structures through which the optic nerve passes, thus allowing inferences to be made about the integrity of the nerve.

### *DIAGNOSTIC MODALITIES*

1. Plain radiographs of the orbits, optic canals, and skull
2. Computed tomography
3. Conventional tomography of the orbits, optic canals, and skull
4. Arteriography
5. Pneumoencephalography
6. Ultrasound (both A and B modes)
7. Magnetic resonance imaging

Methods other than those related to ultrasound, computed tomography (CT), and magnetic resonance imaging (MRI) have little place in the definitive evaluation of most patients with compressive or infiltrative lesions of the optic nerve.

### Plain Radiographs of the Orbit, Optic Foramen, and Skull

Although radiographic examinations of the orbit, optic foramen, and skull are inexpensive, almost risk free, and produce a relatively small radiation dose, the information gained from these studies is severely limited. Plain films have a low sensitivity for detecting most diseases that affect the optic nerve. Even when an abnormality is identified, the specificity of this examination is low and a precise diagnosis can seldom be made on the basis of plain film findings alone. In no case is plain radiography the definitive procedure. Therefore, it is our opinion that plain radiography is of no value in the assessment of patients suspected of having a compressive or infiltrative lesion of the optic nerve.

## Computed Tomography

Because of its ability to demonstrate orbital contents with clarity never before possible, CT has rapidly become the most useful method for evaluating patients suspected of having a compressive or infiltrative lesion of the optic nerve. Computed tomography does not require hospitalization and is completely safe, except for the radiation exposure (4–12 rad) and the uncommon serious reaction to iodinated contrast media given as part of most CT studies. The current generation of scanners permits visualization of the full extent of the optic nerve, with the following exceptions:

1. The short segment from the retina to the back of the sclera
2. The extreme apex of the orbit where the nerve is adjacent to the extra-ocular muscles
3. The 6-mm to 9-mm portion of the nerve that is enclosed within the optic canal. The optic canal itself may be visualized on thin slices at a precisely determined location, but the nerve within the canal cannot be demonstrated (Fig. 34-2).

The intracranial segment of the optic nerve can be seen consistently on high-resolution CT, but is usually not demonstrated as clearly as is the orbital segment of the nerve.

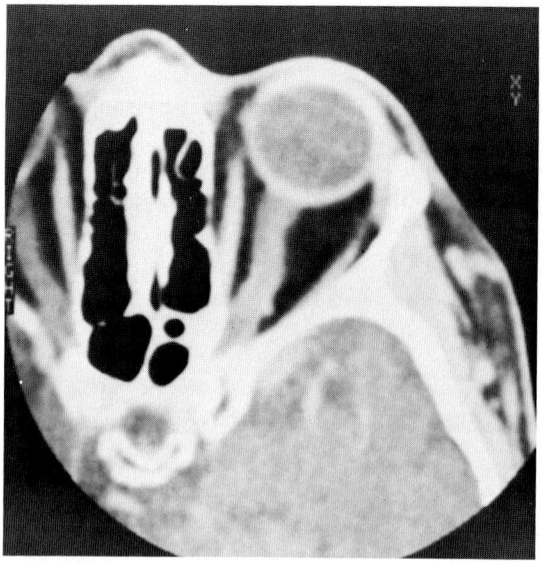

**Figure 34-2.** CT scan of a normal right orbit. The optic nerve is seen from the sclera to the point where it enters the optic canal. The gentle undulation of the curve is normal. At a wider window, the optic canal itself is visible, but the nerve passing through the canal cannot be discerned. (Courtesy of Victor Haughton, M.D.)

## Conventional Tomography

Thin-section tomography performed with pleuridirectional motion enables the bones of the skull and orbit to be visualized in exquisite detail. Conventional tomography is relatively inexpensive and, as with plain radiography, the only risk involved is that of radiation exposure. However, the exposure with conventional tomography is of significantly greater magntiude (10–12 rad to the lens of the eye). The radiation dose varies greatly with different projections and can be substantially reduced if lead glases are used to shield the lens. Prior to the advent of high-resolution CT, thin-section, complex-motion tomography played an important role in evaluating patients suspected of having compressive lesions of the optic nerve, especially those with optic nerve sheath meningiomas or optic gliomas. However, this technique demonstrates only secondary radiographic changes and gives no information about the size or extent of the associated soft-tissue abnormality. Computed tomography, on the other hand, can clearly demonstrate the optic nerve throughout most of its course. Like plain film radiography, complex-motion tomography no longer has a role in the evaluation of these patients.

## Arteriography

Modern arteriography demonstrates the vascular anatomy of the orbit better than any other available modality. However, the examination is expensive and is not ordinarily performed on an outpatient basis. The risks include both the radiation exposure (10–15 rad) and a small (<1%) but definite incidence of mortality and serious morbidity.

Prior to the development of CT, arteriography was performed in patients with suspected compressive lesions of the optic nerve either to establish the presence of a mass adjacent to the nerve or, if an abnormality was known to exist, to demonstrate its extent and vascular supply. Since the advent of CT, the role of arteriography in evaluating these patients has dramatically decreased. Arteriography is rarely indicated for diagnostic exploration of the orbit and is only occasionally used as a preoperative measure. The role of arteriography in evaluating the intracranial portion of the optic nerve will be discussed in the section on chiasmal lesions.

### Pneumoencephalography

Pneumoencephalography has no role in the evaluation of patients suspected of having a compressive or infiltrative lesion of the optic nerve.

### Ultrasound

Although ultrasonic techniques are superior to radiographic procedures in evaluating mass lesions involving the globe and anterior portion of the orbit, in our experience these methods are of limited value in the initial evaluation of the patient suspected of having a compressive or infiltrative lesion of the optic nerve. However, the full potential of ultrasonic techniques has not yet been realized, and there is the future possibility that precise histologic diagnoses ("tissue signature" information) may be generated from analysis of ultrasonic data. One major limitation of ultrasound is its strong dependence on operator proficiency and the need for considerable training and experience to perform an adequate study.

### Magnetic Resonance Imaging

Although experience with MRI is limited, it is clear that this technique will assume increasing importance in the evaluation of the patient suspected of having a compressive lesion of the optic nerve. Using this modality, the full extent of the optic nerve can be easily visualized in multiple projections (Fig. 34-3).

### COMMENT

In our practice, patients suspected of having a compressive or infiltrative lesion of the optic nerve are studied first by CT. Sections are rou-

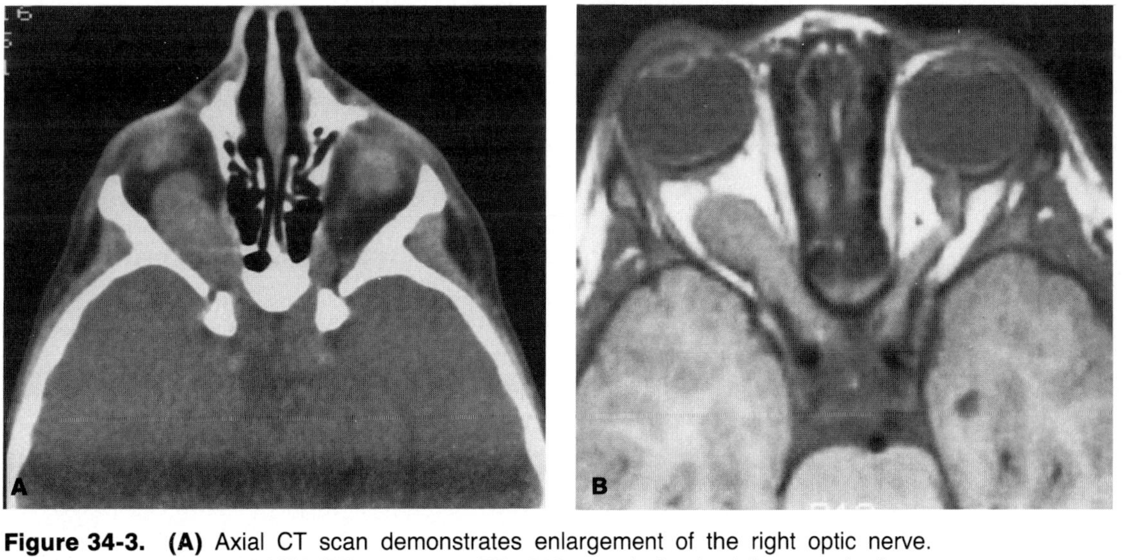

**Figure 34-3.** **(A)** Axial CT scan demonstrates enlargement of the right optic nerve. **(B)** Corresponding axial MRI (TE, 25 msec; TR, 600 msec) clearly delineates the intracanalicular tumor.

tinely taken at both 0° and 35° to Reid's baseline; coronal sections are also extremely useful. When the CT scan is abnormal, there is no need for other diagnostic examinations (Fig. 34-4).

When there is a strong clinical suspicion of a compressive or infiltrative lesion of the optic nerve but a normal CT scan, the next step is MRI.

## OPTIC CHIASM IMPAIRMENT

Loss of vision in both eyes suggests two major considerations. There may be two lesions affecting both optic nerves simultaneously (a rare occurrence) or, far more likely, a single lesion causing dysfunction of either the optic chiasm or a portion of the postchiasmal visual pathway. Visual field testing can usually distinguish between chiasmal and postchiasmal dysfunction. Chiasmal lesions generally cause bitemporal visual field defects, whereas postchiasmal lesions produce defects in the homonymous visual fields. On rare occasions, chiasmal compression can result in defects in the nasal field of vision as well as the more common temporal impairments. Although equal impairment of the temporal visual fields of both eyes might be anticipated with compression of the optic chiasm, in most instances the deficit is substantially greater in one eye than in the other.

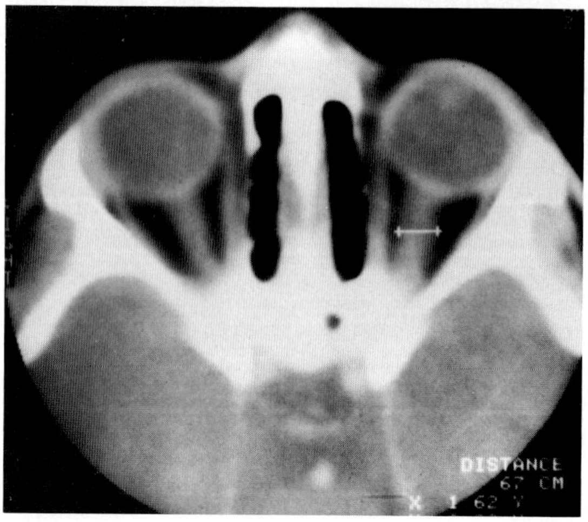

**Figure 34-4.** CT scan of the orbit demonstrates an enlarged optic nerve. Additional CT sections revealed the optic chiasm to be normal. No additional radiographic evaluation is necessary in such cases. (Courtesy of Victor Haughton, M.D.)

Optic chiasmal compression is usually caused by pituitary tumors, meningiomas, craniopharyngiomas, or aneurysms, all of which enlarge gradually and cause insidiously progressive visual loss. However, either spontaneous hemorrhage into a pituitary tumor or craniopharyngioma, or rupture or thrombosis of an aneurysm may produce sudden deterioration of vision, which is often associated with severe headache, obtundation, and ophthalmoplegia.

Recognition of chiasmal dysfunction is important, because both the causes of visual loss and their radiographic evaluation differ from those of either optic nerve abnormalities or postchiasmal dysfunction. The close proximity of neural, vascular, endocrine, and bony structures makes the juxtasellar area unique. These relationships cause the radiographic exploration of this area to be a particularly difficult challenge that demands precise technique.

### DIAGNOSTIC EVALUATION

*DIAGNOSTIC MODALITIES*

1. Plain radiographs of the skull
2. Computed tomography
3. Conventional tomography
4. Arteriography
5. Pneumoencephalography
6. Ultrasound
7. Magnetic resonance imaging

#### Plain Radiographs of the Skull

Limitations similar to those encountered when using plain radiographs to examine the orbit and optic canal also apply to evaluation of the juxtasellar area. Despite the fact that plain skull radiographs often show an abnormality in patients with lesions causing optic chiasm compression, they are too insensitive to be used as a screening test and do not provide sufficient information to allow for appropriate management decisions.

Because plain skull radiographs almost always must be followed by a more definitive examination (CT or MRI), they have little usefulness in these patients.

## Computed Tomography

As with lesions of the optic nerve, CT has rapidly become the procedure of choice for the radiographic evaluation of patients suspected of having a mass compressing the optic chiasm. However, it is essential that each examination be closely supervised to ensure that the correct sections are obtained. We have seen numerous examples of "normal" CT scans which, on critical evaluation, proved to be nondiagnostic either because the full extent of the suprasellar cisterns had not been examined or because the plane of section used was incorrect.

The normal suprasellar cistern has a pentagonal configuration seen most clearly on scans of +35°, or 15° to 20° to Reid's baseline. Coronal sections are superior to axial sections, because the relationship of the juxtasellar cisterns to the pituitary fossa and the base of the brain can be easily determined on this projection (Figs. 34-5 and 34-6). However, some of the older CT scanners cannot readily perform coronal sections nor provide the relatively thin slices required to obtain accurate attenuation values. When working with such scanners, it is advisable to obtain multiple thin overlapping sections through the area of interest so as to achieve images as free of partial volume effects as possible. Ideally, sections that pass solely through either the pituitary fossa or the suprasellar cistern should be obtained so that the data can be reconstructed subsequently in a variety of anatomic planes.

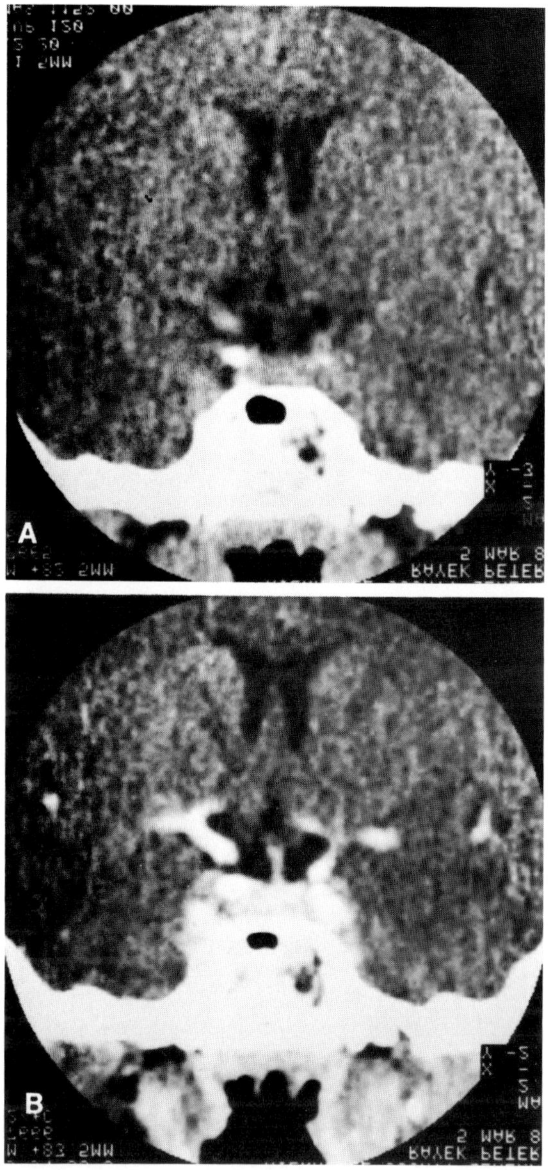


**Figure 34-5.** **(A)** Nonenhanced and **(B)** enhanced coronal CT scans clearly visualize the frontal horns of the lateral ventricles, third ventricle, and suprasellar cisterns. Even on the nonenhanced scans, the supraclinoid carotid arteries may be seen passing through the cerebrospinal fluid density of the supraseller cisterns. After contrast administration, these vascular structures are more clearly demonstrated. There is normal enhancement of the infundibular stalk. (Courtesy of Victor Haughton, M.D.)

## Conventional Tomography

Thin-section, complex-motion tomography can demonstrate the bony structures of the juxtasellar area with precise detail. This technique can identify many osseous and soft-tissue changes that are not apparent on plain film examinations. However, tomographic findings in patients with

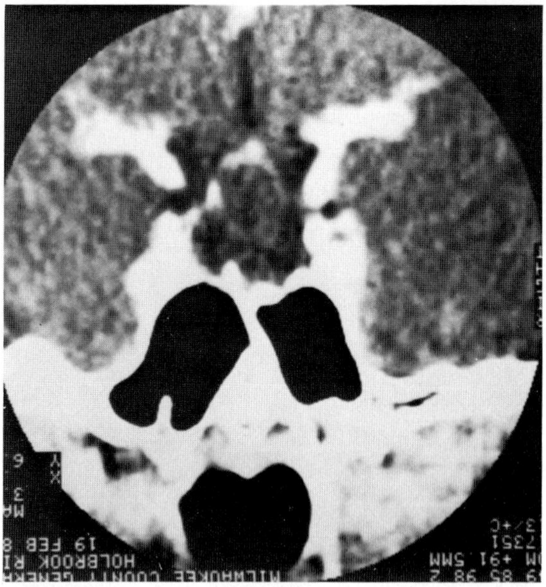

**Figure 34-6.** Contrast-enhanced coronal CT scan demonstrates a suprasellar mass that has a small rim of calcium about its margin. The supraclinoid carotid arteries and proximal middle cerebral arteries are clearly shown. The mass (craniopharyngioma) does not displace the third ventricle. The patient was operated on without any additional studies. (Courtesy of Victor Haughton, M.D.)

evidence of chiasmal compression rarely influence the choice of further diagnostic or therapeutic procedures and are therefore seldom (if ever) indicated.

## Arteriography

Arteriography of the juxtasellar area is an expensive inpatient procedure with a risk of serious morbidity (primarily embolic cerebrovascular accidents) of less than 1%. Although historically performed at an early stage in the evaluation of patients with suspected chiasmal compression, arteriography is now seldom indicated before CT, if at all.

Arteriography will rarely add significant diagnostic information if excellent CT is available (Figs. 34-5 and 34-6). When high-resolution CT detects an abnormality in the juxtasellar region, it is usually also possible to assess both the full extent of the lesion and whether it is of vascular origin, thereby obviating the need for arteriography. When such assessment is not possible on CT, arteriography is indicated. Arteriography may also be necessary to plan the optimal surgical approach. When there is a strong clinical suspicion of chiasmal compression in the face of a normal CT scan, arteriography should be performed with the hope of demonstrating some vascular abnormality (aneurysm, arteriovenous malformation) that is producing symptoms but is not yet visible on CT.

## Pneumoencephalography

Pneumoencephalography no longer has a role in the evaluation of patients suspected of having a compressive lesion of the optic chiasm.

## Ultrasound

Ultrasonic methods currently play no role in the evaluation of patients suspected of having a compression lesion of the optic chiasm.

## Magnetic Resonance Imaging

Magnetic resonance imaging is an ideal modality for evaluating the optic chiasm, because the multiplanar capabilities of this technique are especially useful in examining the juxtasellar area. Even though experience is quite limited, it seems likely that MRI will replace CT as the imaging modality of choice for evaluating patients with a compressive lesion of the optic chiasm.

# POSTCHIASMAL VISUAL SYSTEM DYSFUNCTION

When loss of vision is bilateral and the ophthalmologic examination reveals visual field defects on the same side of the vertical meridian for each eye (a homonymous hemianopia) and normal visual acuity, pupillary reflexes, and ophthalmoscopy, the responsible lesion lies posterior to the optic chiasm. The more posteriorly the lesion is located, the more similar (congruous) are the visual field defects. Thus, the most incongruous field defects are produced by optic tract lesions while the most congruous ones are the result of occipital pole abnormalities. Topographic retinal relationships are maintained in the postchiasmal visual pathways. Fibers from the superior portion of the retina pass through the parietal lobe and end on the upper bank of the calcarine fissure, while those from the inferior portion of the retina pass through the temporal lobe to terminate on the inferior bank of the calcarine fissure. Hence, lesions of these lobes produce, respectively, inferior or superior homonymous quadrantanopic defects. Separate lesions occurring in both cerebral hemispheres can produce bilateral homonymous visual field defects.

Tumors or vascular accidents primarily involving the optic tract are rare. Although the optic radiations are affected by a variety of disease processes, vascular accidents are the most common cause of dysfunction of this portion of the visual system, often resulting in homonymous field defects with no other neurologic impairment. Tumors, either primary or metastatic, and arteriovenous malformations are other relatively common structural lesions that cause dysfunction of the optic radiations.

## DIAGNOSTIC EVALUATION

### *DIAGNOSTIC MODALITIES*

1. Plain radiographs of the skull
2. Computed tomography
3. Conventional tomography
4. Arteriography
5. Pneumoencephalography
6. Ultrasound
7. Magnetic resonance imaging

#### Plain Radiographs of the Skull

Although calcifications related to tumors or arteriovenous malformations may occasionally be recognized on plain skull radiographs and can be localized to portions of the brain containing the visual radiations, it is our opinion that plain skull films have such low sensitivity and specificity as to be useless in evaluating patients suspected of having postchiasmal visual system dysfunction.

#### Computed Tomography

As in the case of patients with suspected abnormalities of the optic nerve or the optic chiasm, CT has become the procedure of choice for the radiographic evaluation of patients with postchiasmal visual system dysfunction. Computed tomography permits such superb visualization of the substance of the cerebral hemispheres that almost all structural lesions that are of sufficient size to cause clinically apparent postchiasmal visual system dysfunction can be detected. An exception is a small cerebral infarct that may be undetectable by CT yet produces visual deficits because of its strategic position in an area in which the visual fibers are very compact. The major limitation of CT in this as well as other areas is its relative lack of specificity. By combining clinical and CT findings, it is generally possible to offer a clinically useful differential diagnosis. It is often impossible to predict the exact nature of a demonstrated abnormality on the basis of a single CT examination. If this is attempted, serious mistakes may result. For example, at the stage in their evolution when mass effect and enhancement are present, the CT appearances of infarcts and tumors may be identical. In such instances, a repeat CT scan performed 4 to 6 weeks later will almost always permit these two conditions to be distinguished. We have also seen several arteriovenous malformations of the occipital lobe that simulated the findings of cerebral infarction on CT performed both with and without intravenous contrast.

#### Conventional Tomography

Conventional tomography plays no role in the evaluation of patients with postchiasmal visual system dysfunction.

### Arteriography

Arteriography remains an important tool for the evaluation of patients with postchiasmal visual system dysfunction. It is usually necessary to perform both carotid and vertebral artery examinations to demonstrate fully the vascular supply to the postchiasmal portion of the visual pathways. When vascular occlusive disease is a consideration, the origins and cervical portions of the carotid and vertebral arteries should be studied. Before arteriography is performed, CT should be obtained. A normal CT scan greatly reduces the chance of finding an arteriographic abnormality, a fact that should weigh against performing the more invasive procedure.

It must be remembered that small infarcts capable of causing a partial homonymous hemianopia may be occult on CT. Although arteriography may not demonstrate such an infarct per se, it may occasionally show vascular changes that can be assumed to be responsible for the clinical deficit. Arteriography may also add specificity to CT findings, such as in the demonstration of deep medullary veins that distinguish primary from metastatic tumors.

### Pneumoencephalography

Prior to the development of CT, pneumoencephalography combined with thin-section tomography was the only method available for radiographic visualization of the optic tracts. Although the optic tracts themselves could not be seen with this technique, the cisternal spaces around them could be demonstrated with sufficient clarity to identify mass lesions. However, the development of CT and the rarity of lesions confined to this area have effectively eliminated the need for pneumoencephalography in the evaluation of patients with postchiasmal visual system dysfunction.

### Ultrasound

Ultrasonic procedures currently play no role in the evaluation of patients with suspected abnormality of the postchiasmal portion of the visual system.

### Magnetic Resonance Imaging

As in other areas of the visual system, MRI is an excellent technique for evaluating the optic tracts, optic radiations, and visual cortex. The multiplanar capability of this method, as well as its increased sensitivity relative to CT for many conditions, should soon make MRI the imaging modality of choice for evaluating patients with suspected abnormality of the postchiasmal visual system.

## COMMENT

In our practice, CT is the initial procedure for investigating the patient with suspected postchiasmal visual system dysfunction. If the CT scan is abnormal, arteriography is frequently performed either to increase the specificity of the CT findings or to plan a surgical approach. If the CT scan is normal, the clinical findings are reassessed; if a strong suspicion of postchiasmal lesion persists, the patient is subjected to arteriography. Magnetic resonance imaging is assuming an increasingly important role in the evaluation of patients with visual loss.

## BIBLIOGRAPHY


Cogan DG: Neurology of the Visual System. Springfield, IL, Charles C Thomas, 1966

Dallow RL: Reliability of orbital diagnostic tests: Ultrasonography, computerized tomography, and radiography. Ophthalmology 85:1218–1228, 1978

Hodes BL, Weinberg P: A combined approach for the diagnosis of orbital disease. Arch Ophthalmol 95:781–788, 1977

Knight CL, Hoyt WF, Wilson CB: Syndrome of incipient pre-chiasmal optic nerve compression. Progress toward early diagnosis and surgical management. Arch Ophthalmol 87:1–11, 1972

Lessel S: Current concepts in ophthalmology. N Engl J Med 299:533–536, 1978

Lloyd GA: The impact of CT scanning and ultrasonography on orbital diagnosis. Clin Radiol 28: 583–593, 1977

Salvolini U, Cabanis EA, Rodallec A et al: Computed tomography of the optic nerve: Part I. Normal results. J Comput Assist Tomogr 2:141–149, 1978

Strother CM, Hoyt WF, Appen RE et al: Meningiomatous changes in the optic canal. Radiology 135:109–114, 1980

Susac JO, Smith L, Walsh FA: The impossible meningioma. Arch Neurol 34:36–38, 1977

Walsh FB, Hoyt WF: Clinical Neuro-ophthalmology, 3rd ed. Baltimore, Williams & Wilkins, 1969

Wende S, Aulich A, Nover A et al: Computed tomography of orbital lesions. A cooperative study of 210 cases. Neuroradiology 13:123–134, 1977

**UNILATERAL OPTIC NERVE IMPAIRMENT**

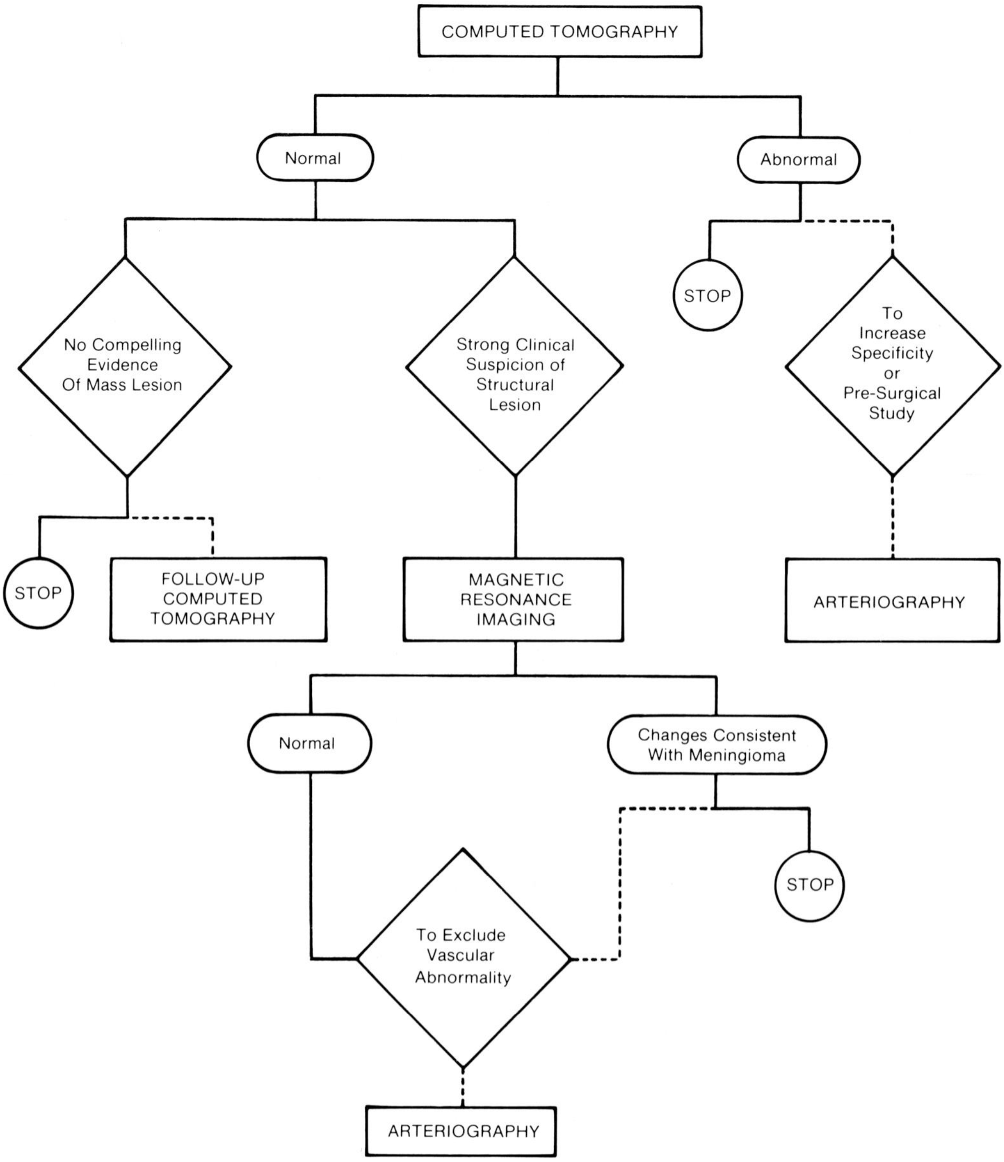

## OPTIC CHIASM IMPAIRMENT

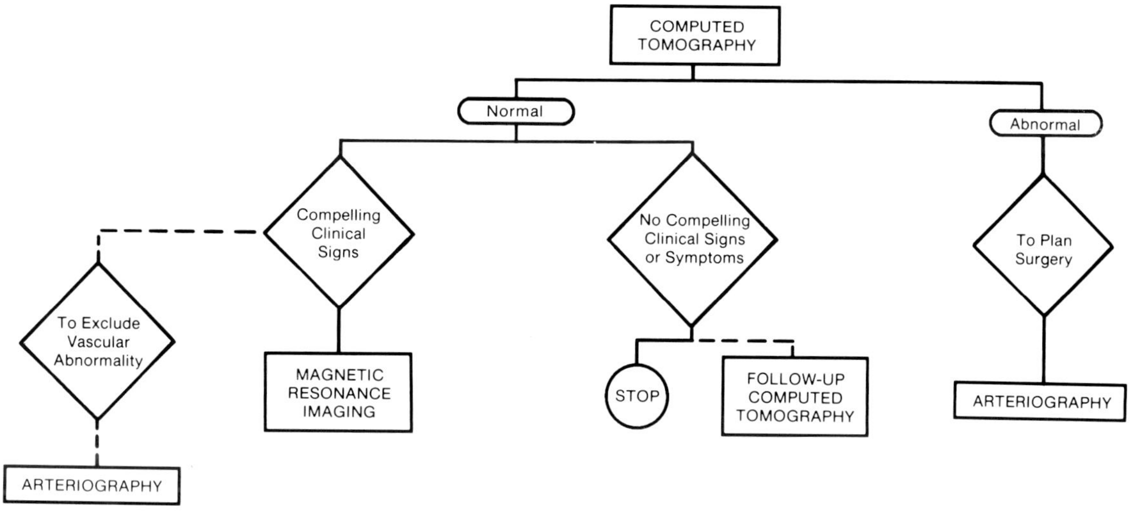


## POST-CHIASMAL VISUAL SYSTEM DYSFUNCTION

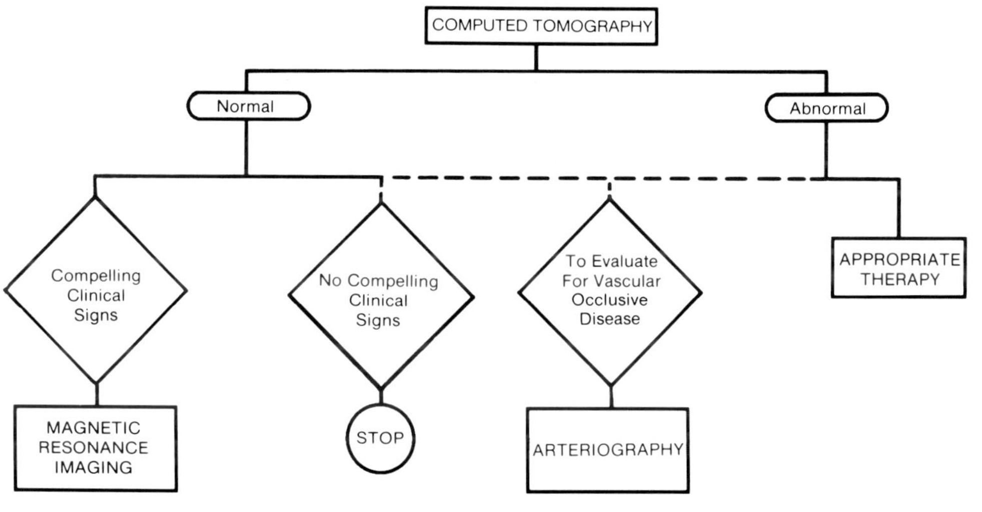

# Chapter 35

# Neck Masses

*Gretchen A. W. Gooding*

Because masses in the neck tend to be superficial, the patient is often the first to notice the abnormality and specifically presents himself to the physician for further evaluation. On other occasions, a mass may be discovered during palpation of the neck as part of a routine physical examination, or following laboratory studies demonstrating elevated serum calcium or thyroid hormone levels.

## DIFFERENTIAL DIAGNOSIS

The differential diagnosis of neck masses includes the following:

1. Lesions of the thyroid
   a. Diffuse or nodular goiter
   b. Thyroiditis, abscess
   c. Thyroid cysts
   d. Solid thyroid lesions (adenoma, carcinoma, metastases, lymphoma)
2. Nonthyroid masses
   a. Congenital lesions (thyroglossal duct cysts, branchial cysts, cystic hygromas)
   b. Inflammatory masses
   c. Neoplastic processes
   d. Vascular lesions
   e. Salivary gland lesions
   f. Parathyroid lesions

## CLINICAL AND LABORATORY FINDINGS

The prime clinical consideration is whether the mass represents a lesion of the thyroid gland or is related to other structures in the neck. Once this initial determination is made, a logical diagnostic approach may be pursued.

In most cases, simple palpation is sufficient to decide whether a mass is of thyroid origin. At times, however, it may be difficult to distinguish between thyroid masses or lesions arising immediately adjacent to the gland. In such cases, either radionuclide scanning or ultrasound can make this critical distinction. Most adult patients with a solitary thyroid nodule should have a thyroid scan ($^{123}$I). Although both modalities accurately determine whether the mass represents thyroid or nonthyroid tissue, they each yield different kinds of information. On ultrasound, the normal thyroid gland has a typical homogeneous echogenic appearance; masses within or adjacent to the gland tend to be discrete, with a sonic pattern different from normal glandular tissue. The radionuclide scan defines thyroid tissue, even in ectopic locations such as the lingual area, and detects both functioning and nonfunctioning nodules within the gland. In the presence of a neck mass, a normal thyroid radionuclide scan suggests an extrathyroidal origin.

Neck masses are usually asymptomatic; pain and tenderness are most commonly associated with hemorrhage into a thyroid adenoma or subacute thyroiditis.

In determining the etiology of a thyroid mass, thyroid function studies are helpful in assessing problems such as Graves' disease or hypothyroid states; however, they may be nonspecific because the patient with a goiter may be hyperthyroid, hypothyroid, or euthyroid. Nevertheless, baseline thyroid function studies are necessary for estimating thyroid replacement doses when thyroidectomy is contemplated. Antimicrosomal and antithyroglobulin antibody titers are essential in patients in whom Hashimoto's disease is suspected.

Of nonthyroidal neck masses, 80% are neoplastic. Of these, 80% are malignant, with the vast majority metastatic and arising from primary tumors above the clavicle (the most common site being the tongue). Only 20% of metastases to the neck arise from primary neoplasms below the clavicle; the lung is the most common source. Therefore, patients with neck masses not related to the thyroid gland should have a thorough examination of the ear, nose, and throat. Metastases to the thyroid gland most commonly originate from carcinomas of the breast, lung, and kidney, or from malignant melanoma.

The combination of a neck mass and elevated serum calcium (and elevated parathyroid hormone) is excellent evidence that the mass represents a lesion of the parathyroid gland. However, most parathyroid tumors are not palpable; present clinically with hypercalcemia and hypophosphatemia; and are often associated with nephrolithiasis, peptic ulcers, excessive bone resorption, and mental changes. An *in vitro* radioimmunoassay technique showing a high circulating concentration of parathyroid hormone can document hyperparathyroidism as the cause for elevated levels of serum calcium and can eliminate other causes of hypercalcemia (sarcoidosis, malignancy, multiple myeloma, vitamin D toxicity); the latter conditions have a low or undetectable concentration of parathyroid hormone, because the hypercalcemia suppresses parathyroid hormone secretion. Most cases of primary hyperparathyroidism (>80%) are caused by neoplasms, almost all of which are benign adenomas. Approximately 15% of cases result from generalized hyperplasia of the parathyroid glands; hyperparathyroidism can also be a manifestation of the multiple endocrine neoplastic syndromes. A rare cause of clinical hyperparathyroidism is parathyroid carcinoma, which usually cannot be distinguished from a benign adenoma unless it has frankly invaded adjacent structures. Secondary hyperparathyroidism, most often due to chronic renal disease, usually produces hyperplasia and generalized enlargement of all the parathyroid glands.

In some clinical situations, the patients with a palpable neck mass does not require any radiographic investigation. For example, in the patient with known Hodgkin's disease, the appearance of a neck mass is presumptive evidence of further lymph node involvement. Similarly, if a patient with a known thoracic or abdominal malignancy develops an enlarged supraclavicular node, a biopsy would be indicated only if confirmation of metastasis is needed.

## DIAGNOSTIC EVALUATION OF THYROID MASSES

### *DIAGNOSTIC MODALITIES*

1. Plain radiography with or without conventional tomography
2. Radionuclide scanning
3. Ultrasound
4. Computed tomography
5. Magnetic resonance imaging
6. Arteriography
7. Biopsy and cyst aspiration

## Plain Radiography With or Without Conventional Tomography

Plain radiography is of no value in the radiographic investigation of the paitent was a mass arising in the thyroid gland. Although plain films may demonstrate calcification in the lesion, this is a nonspecific finding that may occur in both benign and malignant disease.

## Radionuclide Scanning

Radionuclide scanning is the major modality for evaluating the morphology and function of the thyroid gland. Diffuse enlargement of the thyroid suggests the presence of a goiter. The nonfunctioning thyroid nodule, however, is a diagnostic puzzle and a cause for concern because of the risk of thyroid cancer in these patients. A history of neck irradiation in childhood should be carefully sought, because 7% of these patients eventually develop carcinoma of the thyroid gland. There is a 30% probability of malignancy when patients irradiated in the early years of life present with a solitary cold nodule, and a 40% risk if multiple cold nodules are present.

Although 15% to 25% of hypofunctioning "cold" thyroid nodules in patients without a history of prior irradiation to the neck represent carcinoma, the most common cause for this finding is adenomatous hyperplasia (solid or cystic), rather than a malignancy. Therefore, although radionuclide scanning is vital in the identification of thyroid lesions, it cannot discriminate benign from malignant processes, and further diagnostic studies are usually required.

After total thyroidectomy for differentiated thyroid carcinoma, $^{131}$I radionuclide scanning is the modality of choice for detecting thyroid metastases in the chest and neck.

## Ultrasound

Ultrasound is a safe and painless modality for expanding the morphologic information obtained from radionuclide studies of the thyroid gland. Its major value is in determining whether a nonfunctioning lesion on a radionuclide scan is cystic or solid. Thyroid cysts (Fig. 35-1) are demonstrated by ultrasound as smooth, round, fluid collections that appear as nonfunctioning nodules on radionuclide scans. Lesions determined to be solid by ultrasound may include goiter, carcinoma, adenoma, metastases, thyroiditis, or adenomatous hyperplasia. Thyroid adenomas typically have a sonolucent rim surrounding them.

Malignancy in a completely cystic mass is very unusual but occasionally occurs in partly solid, partly fluid lesions. Cystic lesions larger than 4 cm or mixed lesions that are aspirated and recur, especially if they contain hemorrhagic fluid or atypical cells, should be viewed with suspicion for malignancy, even though these changes are nonspecific and may occur in both benign and malignant disease. Hyperechoic masses are virtually never malignant, whereas hypoechoic lesions may be either benign or malignant. Ultrasonically detected calcification is commonly seen in solid thyroid masses. This finding is also nonspecific, and both benign adenomas and malignant papillary follicular carcinomas (Fig. 35-2) may present with eggshell-rim calcification, sometimes dense enough to obscure the lesion itself because of a strong acoustic shadow. Diffuse or nodular enlargement of the thyroid is seen with goiters (Fig. 35-3); enlargement of an affected lobe or lobes with a homogeneous low-amplitude echo pattern is characteristic of subacute thyroiditis. In this self-limited disease, ultrasound can be used to document recovery as the thyroid gland returns to its normal size and echogenic pattern.

Ultrasound is of specific value in patients in whom exogenous iodine contamination from prior contrast studies precludes a radionuclide scan. In addition, thyroid lobes that have been suppressed by hyperfunctioning nodules and therefore are not visible on isotopic scanning may be easily detected by ultrasound.

If a nonfunctioning nodule is unequivocally demonstrated to be cystic by ultrasound, cyst aspiration is indicated. If the mass is solid (Fig. 35-4), surgery or suppression therapy are considerations. Surgery is preferred for those who are

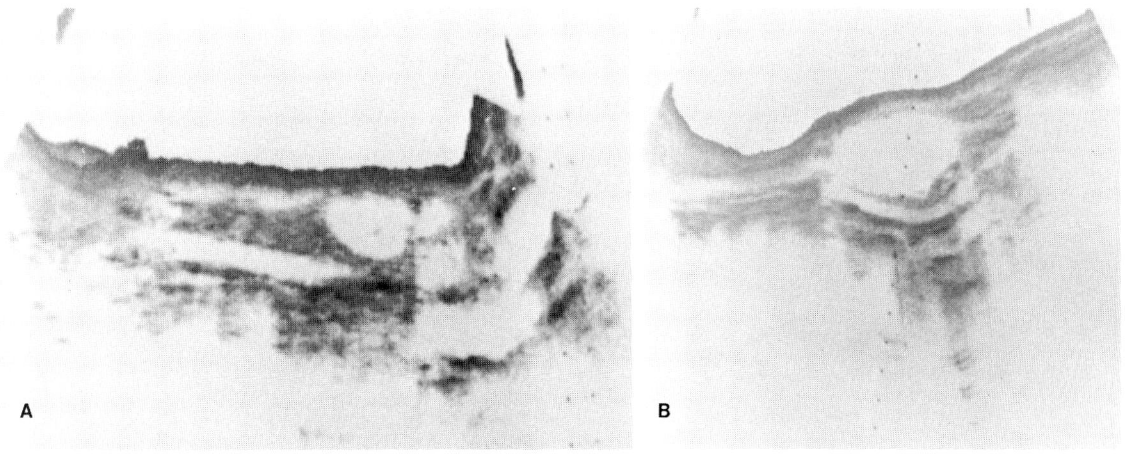

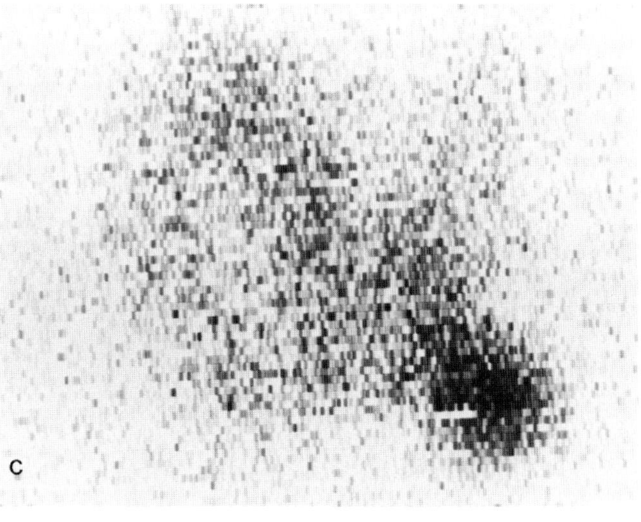

**Figure 35-1.** **(A)** Longitudinal and **(B)** transverse sonograms of the thyroid show several small cysts on the right and one large cyst on the left. **(C)** The radionuclide scan shows the bilateral cold areas of the cysts.

at the greatest risk for carcinoma—younger patients with single cold nodules; men; and patients with a history of head or neck irradiation as children, rapidly growing lesions, or symptoms of pressure in the neck and hoarseness. Suppression therapy is the use of exogenous thyroid hormone to suppress the endogenous excess of thyroid-stimulating hormone that has induced hyperplasia of the gland. It is considered in patients with a small likelihood of carcinoma in the cold nodule, such as the middle-aged woman who lives in an iodine-deficient area, who is suspected of having multinodular goiter, and who has a family history of thyroid disease, patchy radionuclide uptake, and no history of irradiation.

## Computed Tomography

Computed tomography (CT) is less sensitive than high-resolution ultrasound in detecting thyroid abnormalities. The bright enhancement of the thyroid following the intravenous injection of contrast material often obscures small lesions on CT. Computed tomography is of value in demonstrating a substernal thyroid that cannot be detected by ultrasound because of overlying

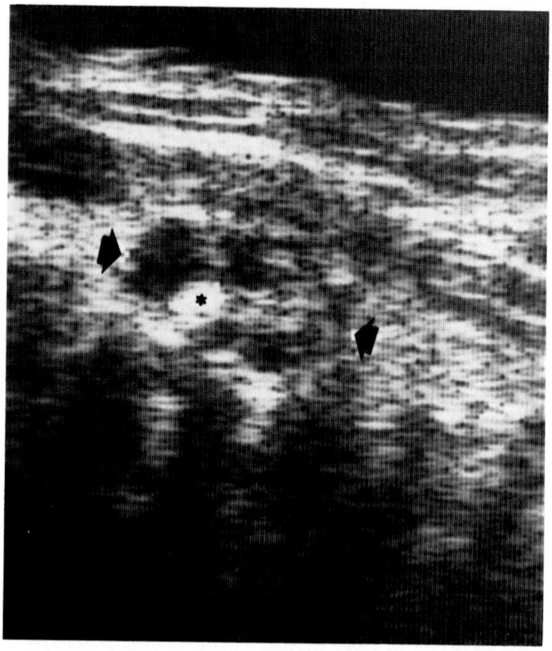

**Figure 35-2.** Longitudinal sonogram shows a papillary follicular carcinoma of the isthmus of the thyroid (*arrows*) containing a bright hyperechoic fleck of calcification within it (*asterisk*).

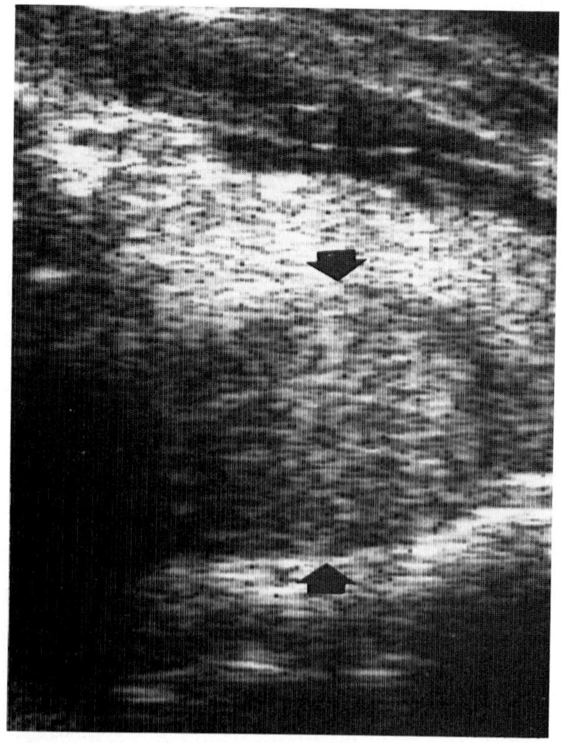

**Figure 35-3.** Transverse sonogram shows a large hyperechoic lesion (adenomatous goiter) in the posterior portion of the thyroid gland.

bone, or by radionuclide scanning when $^{131}I$ uptake is level within the gland. As with ultrasound, CT can demonstrate portions of the thyroid that are suppressed by hyperfunctioning nodules and therefore are not visible on radionuclide scans. Computed tomography may also be of value in determining the extent of thyroid metastases, because ultrasound is limited by air-containing structures and bone, with the former scattering the acoustic beam and the latter attenuating it.

## Magnetic Resonance Imaging

Although the experience with magentic resonance imaging (MRI) is limited, this modality can be of value in defining the substernal extent of the thyroid gland. Differences in T1 and T2 values can be used to accurately assess the presence of cystic components within a thyroid mass. Nevertheless, the resolution of MRI at the present time is far less than that of high-resolution ultrasound.

## Arteriography

In patients with masses of the thyroid gland, arteriography is rarely indicated. Time-consuming, expensive, and more hazardous than other procedures, this modality is unlikely to add any significant diagnostic information.

## Biopsy and Cyst Aspiration

Thyroid masses that are demonstrated to be cystic by ultrasound should usually be subjected to fine-needle aspiration under ultrasonic guidance.

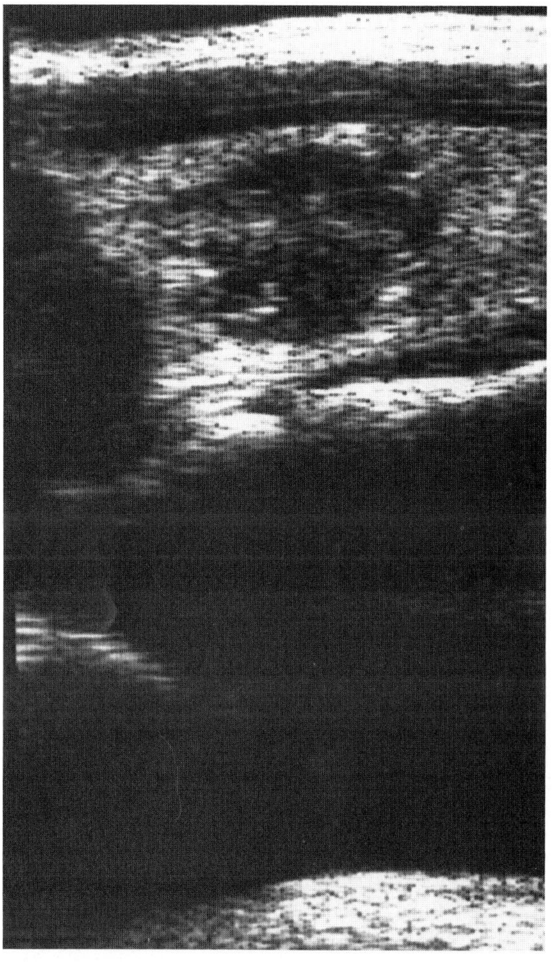

**Figure 35-4.** Longitudinal sonogram shows a well-circumscribed hypoechoic lesion (follicular nodule) surrounded by the hyperechoic thyroid gland.

The fluid in thyroid cysts may be straw-colored, dark brown, or hemorrhagic; even in euthyroid patients, the fluid contains elevated levels of thyroid hormones. The fluid aspirated from cystic thyroid masses should always be sent for cytologic investigation. Following aspiration, cysts may totally disappear. If regression after aspiration does not occur, or if the cyst contents have cellular atypia, surgical removal is mandated.

Because solid lesions of the thyroid cannot be differentiated categorically by ultrasonic or CT characteristics, fine-needle biopsy aspiration has gained favor as a relatively innocuous way to make the preliminary diagnosis before any definitive therapy is begun. Ultrasound is used to define the exact depth and size of the lesion. Fine-needle aspiration and cytologic examination have been reported to have an 88% to 95% accuracy rate in assessing hypofunctioning thyroid nodules.

## DIAGNOSTIC EVALUATION OF NONTHYROID MASSES

### *DIAGNOSTIC MODALITIES*

1. Plain radiography with or without conventional tomography
2. Ultrasound
3. Computed tomography
4. Radionuclide scanning
5. Magnetic resonance imaging
6. Arteriography/venography
7. Barium studies of the pharynx/esophagus
8. Laryngography
9. Sialography
10. Biopsy and cyst aspiration

#### Plain Radiography With or Without Conventional Tomography

Except in rare cases (*e.g.*, stridor suggestive of airway impingement due to infection or postoperative complications), plain radiography of the neck is not indicated in the evaluation of the patient with a neck mass. Although plain films may demonstrate calcification within the lesion, this is nonspecific and can occur in both benign and malignant disease. Phleboliths in a hemangioma have a typical oval calcified appearance (Fig. 35-5).

The extent of bone erosion or destruction also may be identified on plain radiographs, but this is better evaluated by radionuclide scanning or CT. The chest film, however, is an important screening tool in the patient with a neck mass, because tumors of the lung are the most important infraclavicular source of cervical lymphadenopathy.

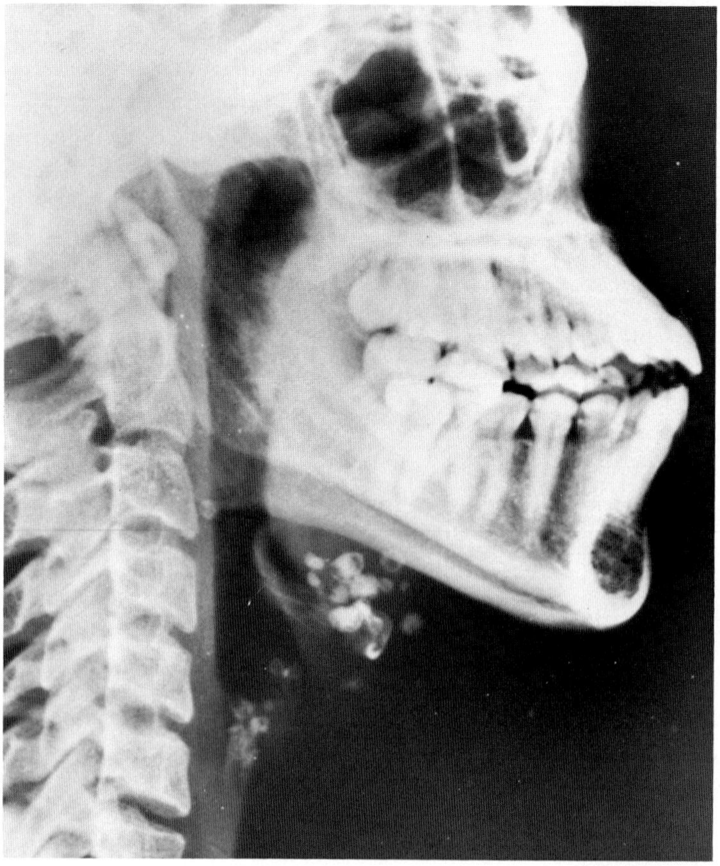

**Figure 35-5.** Plain radiograph demonstrates typical oval calcifications in a hemangioma of the neck.

## Ultrasound

In addition to delineating whether a neck mass is solid or cystic, discrete or irregular, ultrasound can also define the size of the mass and the distance from the skin surface. This modality is of value in assessing a wide spectrum of neck masses, including congenital, inflammatory, neoplastic, and vascular lesions.

Congenital masses in the neck (thyroglossal duct cysts, branchial cysts, cystic hygromas) tend to appear cystic on ultrasound, although they may present as complex masses. Ultrasound may be helpful in discriminating a discrete abscess or lymphadenitis from the diffuse edema of cellulitis, in which no definite fluid collection or mass is identified. The ultrasound pattern, however, is not pathognomonic and it is usually impossible to differentiate neoplastic adenopathy from the appearance of bacterial, viral, or fungal infection. Both with infection and cervical malignancies, the major use of ultrasound is to initially evaluate the size of the lesion, localize a site for biopsy, and then follow the subsequent response to therapy.

Ultrasound can define the relationship of a mass to the large vessels in the neck (carotid artery, jugular vein) (Fig. 35-6) and can differentiate whether a tumor is adjacent to or invading the vessel wall. This modality can identify the origin of the vertebral artery and the proximal portion of the external carotid artery before it branches. Real-time scanning, which instantly displays the dynamics of venous distention during a Valsalva maneuver, can differentiate with precision the transmitted pulsation in a solid mass from that arising in a pulsatile artery.

High-resolution, real-time scanning to map

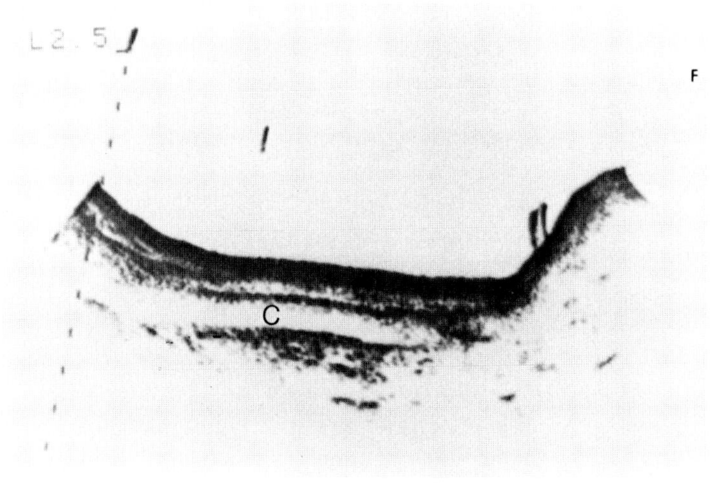


**Figure 35-6.** Longitudinal sonogram (10 MHz) shows a normal carotid artery (*C*).

the carotid vessels, in conjunction with Doppler techniques to monitor flow, is an important screening method for the noninvasive assessment of the carotid artery. After vascular surgery, ultrasound can detect aneurysmal dilatation of a vascular graft as well as delineate false aneurysm formation at the anastomotic site. Intraoperative ultrasound can define intimal flaps or other irregularities in the vessel wall that may have occurred prior to closure of the wound. Hematomas following carotid endarterectomy can be easily identified and followed by ultrasound, as can other postoperative fluid collections (chyloma or seroma) that may follow radical neck dissection.

Ultrasound can be used to assess masses related to the salivary glands, especially the parotid and the submandibular glands. Intraparenchymal masses can be differentiated from extraparenchymal ones, and the discrete, well-demarcated mass of a salivary neoplasm can be distinguished from the diffuse glandular enlargement caused by acute inflammation. The marked sialectasis of Sjogren's syndrome also can be demonstrated.

Since ultrasound does not use ionizing radiation, it can be performed safely in children and pregnant women. Painless and relatively inexpensive, ultrasound is ideal for localizing a lesion for aspiration biopsy; it also permits the clinician to follow a mass for changes in its size or character. One limitation of the technique is the difficulty in demonstrating extension of neck masses into the mediastinum because of air in the lungs, which prevents sound transmission. Open wounds or fistulous tracts are also not amenable to ultrasound imaging.

## Computed Tomography

Although more expensive than ultasound and requiring irradiation of the patient, CT affords exquisite detail of soft-tissue and bony structures that is not readily available by other means (Fig. 35-7). The major advantages of CT in the neck include demonstration of the extent of osseous involvement, definition of soft-tissue limits, and the position of a mass relative to the major cervical vessels. The relationship of a neck mass to the spinal canal or extension of a tumor to the base of the skull or into the mediastinum can be appreciated by CT, but not by ultrasound. Computed tomography is ideal for investigating infections in which extensive bone destruction occurs (*e.g.*, chronic osteomyelitis, lethal midline granuloma) or in identifying postoperative complications (hematoma, seroma, abscess). Computed tomography also can demonstrate the presence of lipomatous tissue within tumor masses. When performed immediately after a sialogram, CT can define the extension of a salivary gland tu-

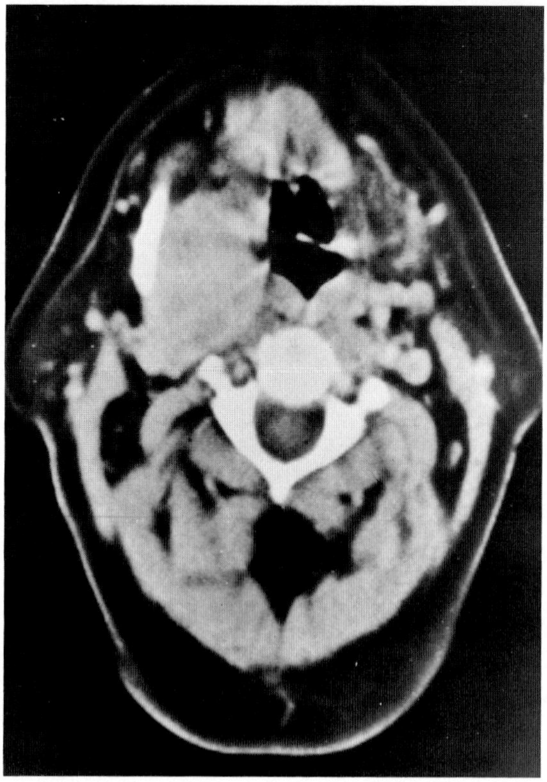

**Figure 35-7.** CT scan of the neck delineates a soft-tissue mass (chemodectoma) on the right.

mor to the base of the skull or infratemporal fossa (not appreciated by other modalities). After the bolus injection of contrast material, CT can identify major cervical arteries, although without the superb resolution of arteriography.

### Radionuclide Scanning

If bone destruction secondary to a neck mass is suspected, radionuclide scanning is the procedure of choice because of the exquisite sensitivity of this modality for detecting bone involvement. Although isotopic studies of the neck may be used to detect highly vascular lesions and to discriminate these masses (*e.g.*, hemangioma) from avascular cystic hygromas, the limited resolution of radionuclide scanning when compared with ultrasound or CT severely limits its use in this area. Double-tracer scintigraphy using thallium and technetium pertechnetate is a sensitive technique for detecting parathyroid adenomas.

### Magnetic Resonance Imaging

Magnetic resonance imaging offers superb soft-tissue discrimination and excellent detail of the cervical cord and orbital compartments. The modality is superior to CT in depicting tumors, syrinxes, and post-traumatic cord lesions, but it is of less value than CT in detecting bony foraminal disease or densely calcified lesions in the area. The use of surface coil techniques has made MRI the imaging procedure of choice for staging tumors of the oropharynx, nasopharynx, hypopharynx, and larynx, because its superior soft-tissue definition provides a better illustration of the extent of disease than does CT.

### Arteriography/Venography

Digital techniques have replaced much of the traditional arteriographic and venographic studies in the evaluation of neck masses. However, in most patients with cystic or solid tumors of the neck, a vascular study is not indicated. If the mass is extremely large, an arteriogram may be an indispensable guide for the surgeon or radiotherapist in assessing the extent and surgical resectability of a lesion (Fig. 35-8). Venography can provide ancillary information about obstruction of venous return (Fig. 35-9).

Arteriography is indicated when ultrasound demonstrates a solid, pulsatile mass suggestive of a chemodectoma. A circumscribed vascular blush at the carotid bifurcation is pathognomonic of this lesion. Bilateral arteriography should be performed in these patients because of the high incidence (26%) of dual tumors in those with a positive family history.

### Barium Studies of the Pharynx and Esophagus

In the patient with a palpable neck mass that is believed to be a metastasis from squamous carcinoma of the head and neck, direct visualization

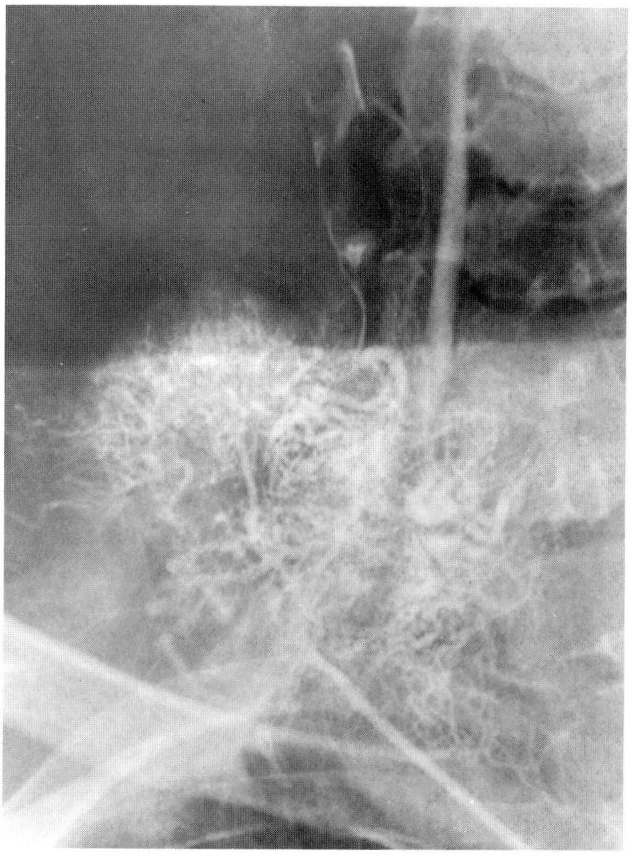

**Figure 35-8.** Arteriogram of a malignant schwannoma demonstrates the vascularity of the lesion and deviation of the trachea due to the mass effect.

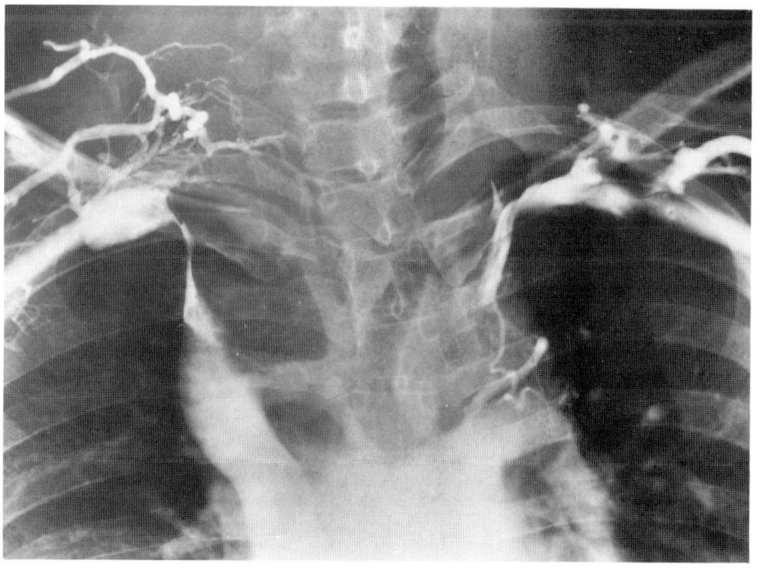

**Figure 35-9.** Venogram of the same patient as in Figure 35-7 shows obstruction of the brachiocephalic veins in the area of the tumor.

of the pharynx and larynx is mandatory. Barium studies of the pharynx may also demonstrate the primary malignancy. In addition, barium examination of the esophagus is essential because of the associated increased frequency of carcinoma of the esophagus in these patients.

### Laryngography

Laryngography is no longer considered the primary technique for detecting or defining the extension of carcinoma in this region. Computed tomography is better than laryngography for showing deep infiltration of tumor, invasion of cartilage, and extension into soft tissues of the neck, and evidence is mounting that surface coil MRI is superior to both modalities. Although CT is now the examination of choice in assessing laryngeal injury and concomitant soft-tissue swelling, MRI may well supplant it.

### Sialography

Sialography is of value in differentiating diffuse inflammatory enlargement of a salivary gland (usually secondary to a stone in the duct) from a discrete tumor mass. The procedure is best performed under fluoroscopic control, and the addition of CT permits the definition of lesions that are small or deep in the center of the gland. However, differentiation of benign from malignant tumors is usually not possible with this technique, and biopsy is required.

### Biopsy and Cyst Aspiration

Cystic masses in the neck should be aspirated and the fluid sent for cytologic investigation. If regression of the cyst following aspiration does not occur, or if the cyst has cellular atypia, surgical removal is mandatory. Most solid lesions in the neck require fine-needle or open biopsy. The fine-needle technique affords a relatively innocuous means for making a preliminary diagnosis before any definitive therapy is contemplated. If the results of the needle biopsy indicate that the mass is a metastasis, the need for an open biopsy may be obviated.

## DIAGNOSTIC EVALUATION OF PARATHYROID MASSES

*DIAGNOSTIC MODALITIES*

1. Ultrasound
2. Double-tracer scintigraphy
3. Computed tomography
4. Arteriography/venous sampling
5. Magnetic resonance imaging
6. Aspiration biopsy

### Ultrasound

Ultrasound using a high-resolution, 10 MHz transducer is the imaging modality of choice for the detection of a parathyroid adenoma (Fig. 35-10). The normal parathyroid gland is only occasionally demonstrated by ultrasound. It can be differentiated from a hyperplastic or adenomatous gland merely on the basis of size (normal, less than 5 mm × 3 mm × 1 mm).

Transverse and parasagittal scans obtained over the anterior neck show a parathyroid adenoma as an anechoic to hypoechoic mass, which is never of greater echogenicity than the thyroid tissue and typically lies posterior to the thyroid, usually oriented in a cranial-caudal direction. Ultrasound can detect almost 80% of parathyroid adenomas; the sensitivity of this modality is substantially less for generalized hyperplasia (50%–75%) because of the relative smallness of the hyperplastic glands. The accurate and noninvasive preoperative localization of a parathyroid adenoma permits decreased surgical dissection and subsequent morbidity, allows for unilateral neck dissection in selected cases, and may reduce the number of patients with persistent or recurrent disease. Ultrasound may be unsuccessful in localizing a parathyroid tumor if the lesion is deep below the surface or is located in a retropharyngeal, retrotracheal,

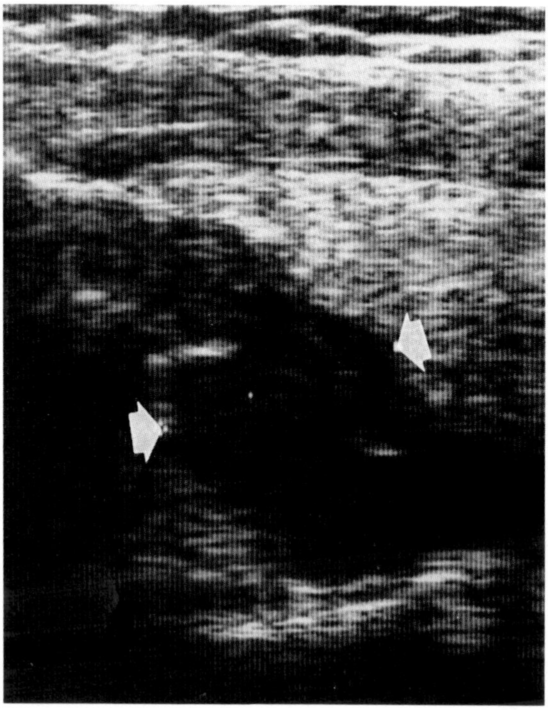

**Figure 35-10.** Longitudinal sonogram demonstrates a hypoechoic, lobulated parathyroid adenoma (*arrows*) situated superior and posterior to the thyroid gland.

retroesophageal, thymic, or mediastinal location. In patients who have had prior parathyroid surgery and have recurrent or persistent disease, ultrasound can be used to localize residual parathyroid tissue, which can then be confirmed by aspiration biopsy with cytology and radioimmunoassay for parathyroid hormone. It should be stressed that the major use of ultrasound (and other imaging modalities for localizing parathyroid adenomas) is in patients who have previously undergone neck surgery for hyperparathyroidism and in whom the surgical success rate for parathyroid re-exploration is less than 65%. Preoperative parathyroid localization often is not required prior to the initial surgical procedure, because in patients who have not had previous neck surgery a standard bilateral neck dissection performed by an experienced parathyroid surgeon can be expected to have a 95% success rate in controlling hyperparathyroidism.

## Double-Tracer Scintigraphy

Double-tracer scintigraphy using $^{201}$Tl followed by $^{99m}$Tc pertechnetate is a sensitive technique for detecting a parathyroid adenoma (Fig. 35-11). It has completely replaced the previously used and now outdated selenomethionine scanning, which also had the disadvantage of a high radiation dose. The normal parathyroid gland is not detected by double-tracer scintigraphy. A parathyroid adenoma appears as a focal extrathyroidal or intrathyroidal collection of thallium activity in an area of absent or diminished technetium activity. A high ratio of thallium intensity to pertechnetate results in a red color typical for parathyroid adenoma, whereas a low ratio appears blue. A possible source of error is the accumulation of thallium in focally abnormal thyroid tissue (*e.g.*, goiter, chronic thyroiditis, lymphoma), areas that usually appear cold on routine technetium scanning. The combination of ultrasound and double-tracer scintigraphy can detect approximately 90% of parathyroid lesions; ei-

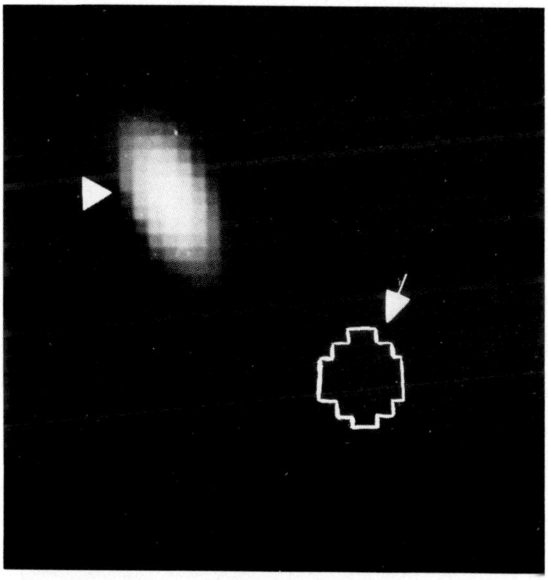

**Figure 35-11.** Double tracer scintigram demonstrates a parathyroid adenoma (*arrow*), which appeared bright red on the original image. The arrowhead points to normal thyroid tissue, which appeared bright blue.

ther imaging modality alone has an overall detection rate of approximately 75%.

### Computed Tomography

Computed tomography is primarily of value as a complement to ultrasound and can aid in increasing the overall accuracy of localization of a parathyroid mass. It is especially valuable in demonstrating aberrantly located parathyroid adenomas in the superior mediastinum. The patient should be placed in a special positioning device to hyperextend the neck and lower the shoulders. Multiple axial slices from the hyoid bone to the left innominate vein are obtained during an intravenous bolus injection of contrast material. The appearance of parathyroid tumors following the intravenous injection of contrast material varies widely from intense enhancement of the lesion to no enhancement at all. The effectiveness of CT may be decreased by artifacts, and small tumors may be impossible to detect.

### Arteriography With Venous Sampling

Digital subtraction arteriography and venography with venous sampling are reserved for those patients with persistent or recurrent hyperparathyroidism in whom ultrasound, scintigraphy, and CT produce conflicting results. These procedures are technically difficult, expensive, and involve some risk. Thus, arteriography and venography with venous sampling should never be considered a routine study for the localization of a parathyroid adenoma.

### Magnetic Resonance Imaging

Initial studies are now under way to determine how effective MRI with surface coil techniques will be in detecting and characterizing parathyroid lesions.

### Aspiration Biopsy

Preoperative fine-needle aspiration biopsy under ultrasound or CT guidance can increase the specificity in localizing and confirming the exact site of a parathyroid adenoma, especially in patients who have undergone previous neck dissection. When a successful aspiration biopsy of the neck is positive for parathyroid cells, there is no doubt that abnormal parathyroid tissue is situated at this site, and this obviates the need for extensive dissection.

## Bibliography

Behan M, Kazam E: The echographic characteristics of fatty tissues and tumors. Radiology 129: 143–151, 1978

Blei CL, Gooding GAW, Rector W: Ultrasonic and fluorescent scanning: A combined noninvasive diagnostic approach to extrathyroid neck lesions. Am J Surg 124:369–374, 1977

Blum M, Goldman AB, Herskovic A et al: Clinical applications of thyroid echography. N Engl J Med 187:1164–1169, 1972

Carter BL, Karmody CS: Computed tomography of the face and neck. Semin Roentgenol 13:257–266, 1978

Clark OH, Okerlund MD, Cavalieri RR et al: Diagnosis and treatment of thyroid, parathyroid and thyroglossal duct cysts. Clin Endocrinol Metab 48:983–988, 1979

Clark OH, Stark DD, Gooding GAW et al: Localization procedures in patients requiring reoperation for hyperparathyroidism. World Surg 8:509–521, 1984

Goldman L, Gordan GS, Roof BS: The parathyroids: Progress, problems and practice. Curr Probl Surg 8:1–64, 1971

Goldstein HM, Zornoza J: Association of squamous cell carcinoma of the head and neck with cancer of the esophagus. AJR 131:791–794, 1978

Gooding GAW: Gray-scale ultrasound detection of carotid body tumors. Radiology 132:409–410, 1979

Gooding GAW, Clark OH, Stark DD et al: Parathyroid aspiration biopsy under ultrasound guidance in the postoperative hyperparathyroid patient. Radiology 155:193–196, 1985

Gooding GAW, Herzog KA, Laing FC et al: Ultrasonic assessment of neck masses. J Clin Ultrasound 5:248–252, 1977

Gooding GAW, Okerlund MD, Stark DD et al: Parathyroid imaging: Comparison of double tracer scintigraphy and high-resolution sonography. Radiology 161:57–64, 1986

Gray SW, Skandalakis JE: Embryology for Surgeons, pp 15–62. Philadelphia, WB Saunders, 1972

Kushner DC, Weber AL: Sialography of salivary gland tumors with fluoroscopy and tomography. AJR 130:941–944, 1978

Lufkin RB, Hanafee WN, Wortham D et al: Larynx and hypopharynx: MR imaging with surface coils. Radiology 158:747–754, 1956

Mancuso AA, Calcaterra TC, Hanafee WN: Computed tomography of the larynx. Radiol Clin North Am 16:195–208, 1978

Miller EM, Norman D: The role of computed tomography in the evaluation of neck masses. Radiology 133:145–149, 1979

Okerlund MD, Sheldon K, Corpuz BSS et al: A new method with high sensitivity and specificity for localization of abnormal parathyroid glands. Ann Surg 381–388, 1984

Reading CC, Charboneau JWE, James EM et al: High-resolution parathyroid sonography. AJR 139:539–546, 1982

Sample WF, Mitchell SP, Bledsoe RC: Parathyroid ultrasonography. Radiology 127:485–490, 1978

Solbiati L, Bolterrani L, Rizzatto G et al: The thyroid gland with low uptake lesions: Evaluation by ultrasound. Radiology 155:187–191, 1985

Stark DD, Clark OH, Gooding GAW et al: High-resolution ultrasonography and computed tomography of thyroid lesions in patients with hyperparathyroidism. Surgery 94:863–868, 1983

Stark DD, Gooding GAW, Clark OH: Noninvasive parathyroid imaging. Semin Ultrasound, CT, MR 6:310–317, 1985

Stark DD, Gooding GAW, Moss AA et al: Parathyroid imaging: Comparison of high-resolution CT and high-resolution sonography. AJR 141: 633–638, 1983

Walfish PF, Hazani E, Strawbridge HTG et al: Combined ultrasound and needle aspiration cytology in the assessment and management of hypofunctioning thyroid nodule. Ann Intern Med 87: 270–274, 1977

Wiley AL, Zagzebski JA, Tolbert DD et al: Ultrasound B-scans for clinical evaluation of neoplastic neck nodes. Arch Otolaryngol 101:509–511, 1975

Winzelberg GG, Hydovitz JD, O'Hara KR et al: Parathyroid adenomas evaluated by TL-201/Tc-99m pertechnetate subtraction scintigraphy and high-resolution ultrasonography. Radiology 155: 231–235, 1985

## NECK MASS

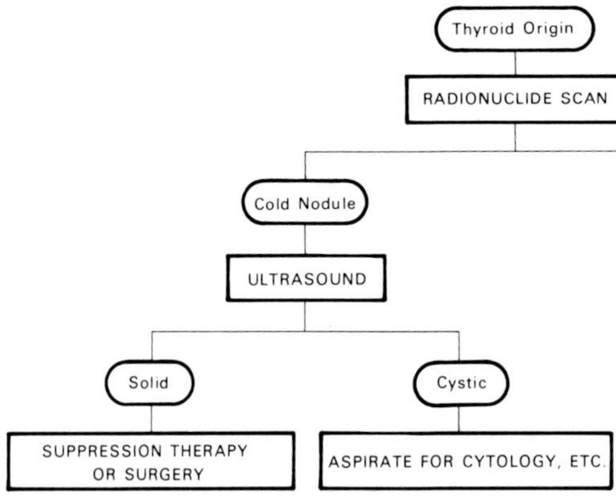


## NECK MASS

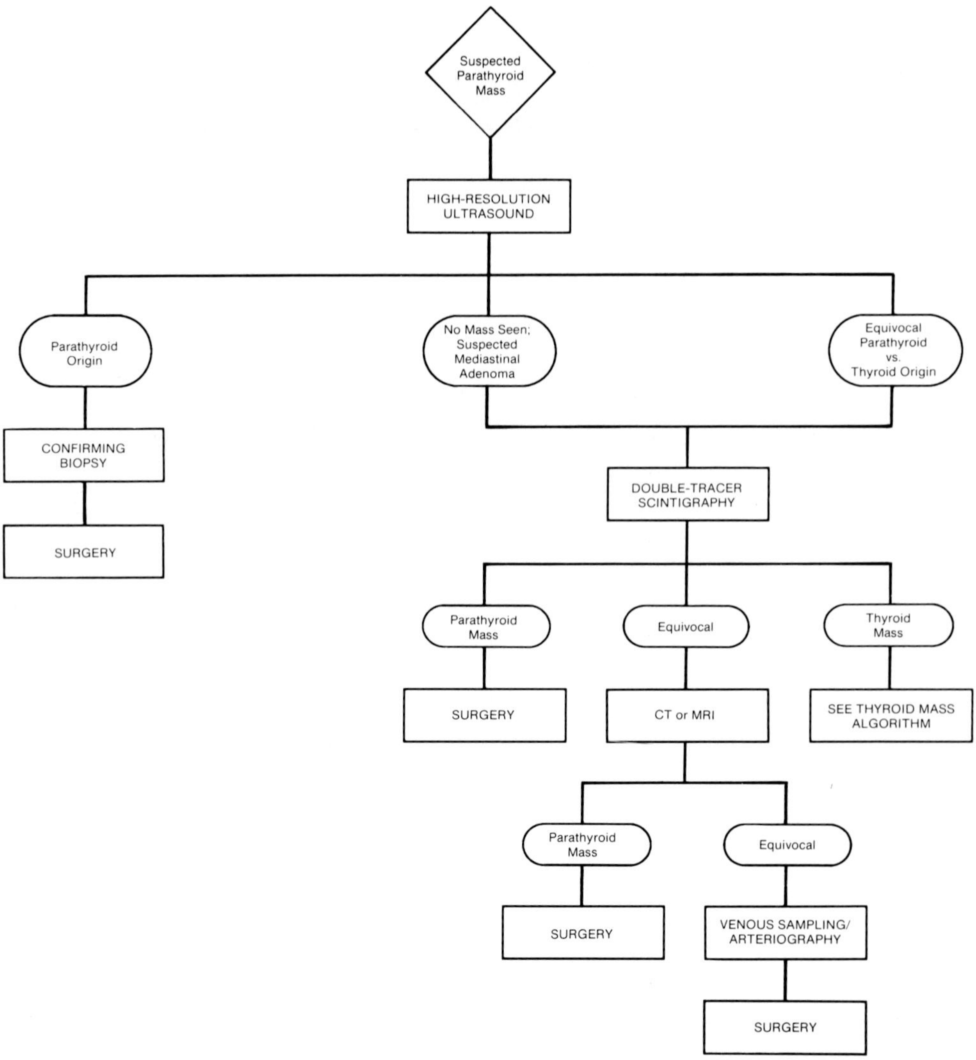

# PART SIX

# Cancer Staging and Detection of Metastases

# Chapter 36

# Biopsy-Proven Peripheral Malignancy—Where Is the Primary?

*Stephen I. Marglin*
*Joanne E. Mortimer*
*Ronald A. Castellino*

Radiologic testing of patients with newly diagnosed cancer usually is directed toward obtaining information required for staging as well as toward accurately delineating those sites of involvement perceived to be most relevant to successful treatment planning and/or follow-up. For patients whose malignancy is first brought to medical attention because of signs and symptoms specifically referable to their metastases, and for whom the primary tumor (*i.e.*, the site from which the neoplasm arose) is not readily apparent, radiologic imaging traditionally has been utilized in an attempt to discover the primary tumor.

The issue of how best to evaluate a patient with a tumor of unknown origin is significant, because 3% to 15% of patients with newly diagnosed solid tumors present in this fashion. These patients are commonly subjected to an extensive array of diagnostic procedures in the belief that the primary tumor can and will be found. Before acceding to the "wisdom" of this conventional approach, it is important to consider carefully two crucial questions. First, what is the likelihood that an exhaustive search will actually demonstrate the primary site of tumor? Second, even if the primary lesion is detected, what is the likelihood that this discovery will improve either the patient's survival or quality of life?

Extensive testing in search of an occult primary tumor most commonly occurs in patients with metastases from adenocarcinomas or undifferentiated neoplasms. With tumors of squamous cell origin, especially those metastatic to upper and middle cervical lymph nodes, the primary lesion can often be found within the head and neck region. In these patients, a meticulous examination of the ears, nose, and throat should be performed, supplemented (when necessary) by endoscopy. Even if the primary tumor is not detected, chemotherapy and radiation therapy (presumably because the hidden tumor may be encompassed within the therapeutic portal) have the potential of producing 5-year survival rates in excess of 30%.

Because the discovery of metastatic undifferentiated carcinoma or adenocarcinoma is so often the prelude to a lengthy and expensive radiographic investigation, the formulation of a logical approach to patients with this condition will be the primary focus of this chapter.

## GENERAL DIAGNOSTIC STRATEGIES

Five strategies may potentially be considered in the imaging approach to the patient with metastases from a tumor of unknown origin:

1. Investigation based on the anticipated pattern of metastatic spread
2. Investigation based on the prevalence of different neoplasms (*i.e.*, attempt to find the most common tumors)
3. Unlimited search
4. Search for treatable disease
5. Maximization of utility

### Investigation Based on the Anticipated Pattern of Metastatic Spread

This strategy is based on the assumption (not always correct) that tumors of occult origin "behave" in a fashion similar to tumors whose primary site is readily apparent. The term "behave" is meant to imply that tumors of unknown origin, were their primary sites known, would metastasize to the same organs with essentially the same frequency as do tumors whose primary sites are identifiable. An example of this line of reasoning is the plan to "run the GI tract" of every patient who presents with hepatic metastases, based on the acknowledged propensity of colon cancers to metastasize to the liver. Without specifically addressing the merits of such a plan, the data in Table 36-1 suggest that significant differences exist in the biologic behavior of the two groups of tumors (best illustrated in the shaded areas of the table). Although the data for tumors of unknown origin are based on small numbers and are not yet statistically significant, it would appear that the approach of "working backwards" may, in certain instances, be based on an invalid assumption and may therefore be ineffective in detecting the primary cancer site. The expected yield from this strategy will be further discussed in the section "Unlimited Search."

### Investigation Based on Prevalence of Different Neoplasms

Radiologic imaging based on knowledge of disease prevalence can be applied to the evaluation of tumors of unknown origin in at least two ways. The first approach assumes that the prevalence of primary sites for initially occult tumors approximates the prevalence of primary sites for tumors whose site of origin can be easily discerned. Thus, radiographic imaging is directed toward finding those tumors that are most common in the general population. The second approach is based on imaging those organs that are most commonly identified as the primary sites of initially occult tumors.

Table 36-2 shows the distribution of primary sites for all patients with cancer and for those patients whose primary site is initially occult. Carcinomas of the lung, colon, breast, and prostate, which account for more than 50% of tumors in the general population, account for only 33% of initially occult tumors. On the other hand, tumors that are relatively uncommon in the general population (*e.g.*, primary pancreatic and liver tumors) have a consideraby greater prevalence in patients whose primary cancer site is initially unknown. Therefore, the pursuit of those tumors that are "most common" in the general population may not be rewarding.

The second, more direct approach evaluates

**Table 36-1** Percent Metastatic Involvement at Presentation

| | Bone | | Lung | | Liver | | Brain | |
|---|---|---|---|---|---|---|---|---|
| Primary Site | A | B | A | B | A | B | A | B |
| Lung | 30–50 | 4 | 34 | 90 | 30–50 | 36 | 15—30 | 21 |
| Pancreas | 5–10 | 28 | 25–10 | 31 | 50–70 | 72 | 1–4 | 3 |
| Colorectal | 5–10 | 13 | 25–40 | 40 | 71 | 87 | 1 | 0 |
| Liver | 8 | 31 | 20 | 19 | — | 100 | 0 | 6 |
| Prostate | 50–75 | 25 | 13–53 | 75 | 13 | 50 | 2 | 25 |

A = carcinoma with evident primary site
B = occult carcinoma
(Modified from Nystrom JS et al: Metastatic and histologic presentations is unknown primary cancer. Semin Oncol 4:53–58, 1977)

**Table 36-2** Distribution of Primary Cancer Sites

| | General Population | | Patients with Occult Primary Cancer Site | |
|---|---|---|---|---|
| Lung | 15% | 52% (Lung, Colorectal, Breast, Prostate) | 18% | 33% (Lung, Colorectal, Breast, Prostate) |
| Colorectal | 15% | | 10% | |
| Breast | 14% | | 2% | |
| Prostate | 8% | | 3% | |
| Pancreas | 3% | | 20% | |
| Stomach | 3% | | 8% | |
| Liver* | 2% | | 11% | |
| Kidney | 2% | | 6% | |

* Includes primary hepatocellular carcinoma, intra- or extra-hepatic bile duct carcinoma, gallbladder carcinoma
(Modified from Nystrom JS et al: Metastatic and histologic presentations in unknown primary cancer. Semin Oncol 4:53–58, 1977)

those organs that are the most common sites of primary tumor in patients with initially occult tumors. Data concerning these tumors can be derived from Table 36-2. Whether investigation of this subset of tumors is likely to be rewarding depends in large part on the adequacy of current imaging techniques (see Unlimited Search).

### Unlimited Search

For a considerable number of years, the strategy of "unlimited search" has generally been the most common approach to the evaluation of patients with initially occult tumors. This approach involves the performance of an extensive number of examinations (upper gastrointestinal series, barium enema examination, excretory urogram, ultrasound), the sequencing of which is more often determined by time pressure and scheduling considerations than by any attempt at rational selection. The "logical extension" of this strategy is to continue testing until the primary cancer site is found.

The merits of this strategy of unlimited search (at least as it relates to conventional, or analog, imaging) were evaluated in a retrospective analysis of 266 patients with tumors initially believed to be "occult." Unlimited search was successful in revealing the true site of origin antemortem in only 22 patients (8%). The accuracies achieved by the individual imaging modalities are summarized in Table 36-3. Although the overall "diagnostic" accuracy rate of 94% appears at first glance to be excellent, it is important to clarify a potential source of confusion. In the process of constructing the percentages tabulated in Table 36-3, examinations that were believed to be neither true positive, false positive, nor false negative were "coded" as true negatives. Because more than half of the patients were never examined postmortem, the true negative category was clearly considerably inflated. Similarly, since examinations were not considered to be false positive unless the radiologist was emphatic about the malignant nature of the abnormality, the category "false positive" was underestimated. Even without these clarifica-

**Table 36-3** Radiologic Testing in Search of Occult Tumors

| | Upper Gastrointestinal Series | Barium Enema | Excretory Urogram | Combined |
|---|---|---|---|---|
| Sensitivity | 67% | 60% | 56% | 61% |
| Specificity | 97% | 96% | 94% | 96% |
| Accuracy of positive diagnosis | 57% | 53% | 31% | 47% |
| Accuracy of negative diagnosis | 98% | 97% | 98% | 97% |
| Overall accuracy | 95% | 93% | 92% | 94% |

(Modified from Nystrom JS et al: Identifying the primary site of metastatic cancer of unknown origin. JAMA 241:381–383, 1979; copyright 1979, American Medical Association)

tions, it should be noted that the ability to detect tumor (*i.e.*, the sensitivity of all the tests combined) was a disappointing 61%. In light of these results, a strategy of unlimited search using conventional imaging modalities is difficult to defend in either medical or monetary terms. Moreover, since this unlimited approach can be viewed as unsuccessful, it can be assumed that the more limited, albeit targeted, imaging approaches described in the two preceding sections are also relatively fruitless.

Two recent publications have addressed the potential contributions that newer cross-sectional imaging techniques (particularly computed tomography) might make to the evaluation of patients with tumors of unknown origin. In both reports, computed tomography (CT) permitted identification of the primary neoplasm in approximately one third of cases. Although far from "ideal," this success rate in detecting occult neoplasms is 3 to 4 times the detection rate achieved by conventional imaging techniques. Considering the fact that in both these reports the examinations were performed with equipment that currently would be regarded as less than "state of the art," the potential detection rate is probably even somewhat higher. In addition to detecting the primary neoplasms, CT provided valuable information regarding additional and often unsuspected metastases in approximately 65% of the patients studied.

The efficacy of ultrasound was briefly addressed in one of the two reports. Although no rigorous attempt was made to prospectively evaluate ultrasound and CT, in those patients examined by both modalities, CT was felt to be superior to ultrasound in both diagnostic accuracy and the ability to define the true extent of metastic involvement.

## Identification of Treatable Disease

Even if radiographic investigation were successful in demonstrating the site of an unknown primary, does such a discovery contribute to improved patient survival or quality of life? The question that is central to all search strategies is whether tumors of unknown origin are more likely to be palliated or controlled if their sites of origin are ultimately identified. Although therapy of certain metastatic tumors may lead to cures (*e.g.*, tumors of germ cell origin, ovarian and trophoblastic tumors, Hodgkin's and non-Hodgkin's lymphomas, and certain soft-tissue sarcomas), and although other tumors (*e.g.*, breast tumors, ovarian tumors, multiple myeloma, small cell lung cancers, and certain sarcomas) may be palliated with prolonged survival, for most metastatic tumors no statistical difference can be demonstrated in median survival time between those patients in whom the primary cancer site was identified during life and those in whom it was not (Fig. 36-1). Although patients who responded to chemotherapy lived longer than those who did not, response rates to

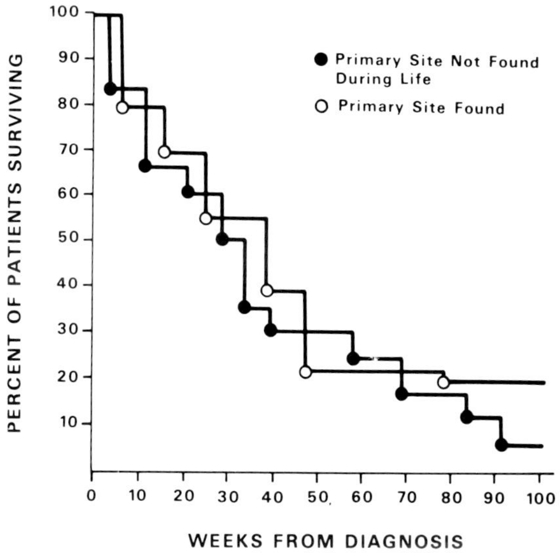


**Figure 36-1.** Survival from time of diagnosis of patients with unknown primary cancer with respect to whether or not the primary cancer site was found during life. (Modified from Stewart JF, Tattersall MHN, Woods RL et al: Unknown primary adenocarcinoma: Incidence of overinvestigation and natural history. Br Med J 1:1530–1533, 1979)

chemotherapy were uniformly low. Because carcinomas of the pancreas and lung are the most common primary sites of initially occult tumors (see Table 36-2), it is easy to understand why chemotherapy so seldom has an impact on the overall survival. Detection of the primary site, at least in statistical terms, may therefore not be "worth the trouble."

A decision about which tumors are treatable is to some degree both subjective and variable: subjective in that certain physician–patient combinations might be inclined to test more agressively, looking for a tumor with a finite, albeit low, rate of response; variable in that the rate of responsiveness of tumors is constantly changing. As newer therapeutic regimes are evaluated, tumors that were previously characterized as having an abysmal prognosis become more successfully treatable. Physicians who deal with such patients must remain current with recent oncologic literature or refer these patients to those who specialize in their evaluation and care.

## Maximization of Utility

This strategy employs a mathematical concept (borrowed from the fields of psychology and economics) that evaluates radiographic testing in terms of all potential outcomes, good and bad, and attempts to rank potential examinations in such a way as to maximize "the utility" (well-being) to the patient. To employ this approach, one must know the probabilities of all possible test outcomes (*i.e.*, true positive, true negative, false positive, and false negative). Of equal importance, it is essential to "know" how a given patient values these outcomes. Even if a primary lesion can be correctly identified, consideration must be given to the following: (1) the likelihood that the demonstrated lesion will respond to treatment, (2) the possibility that diagnostic studies might cause morbidity or even result in fatal complications; and (3) the fact that radiographic testing is often expensive or may require sophisticated equipment not universally available.

In this approach, the patient becomes an active participant in the decision-making process. The "cost" (see Appendix at the end of this chapter) and impact of various tests are determined, and the patient (with appropriate assistance) selects choices that maximize his "utility" or well-being. Since this method considers the differing sensitivities and specificities of all relevant examinations and also considers the patient's expressed preferences regarding possible outcomes, it is reasonable to sequence "least cost" examinations before examinations that "cost" more. By employing this approach we, as physicians, would theoretically be pursuing the patient's expressed objectives (*i.e.*, attempting to maximize the patient's "utility").

This strategy is perhaps the most detailed and logical of any of those discussed. Unfortunately, at present this approach is neither practical nor realistic. The true sensitivity and specificity of many radiographic procedures are not well established, and a rigorous and accepted system for obtaining patient assessment of possible outcomes has not yet been developed. Although maximization of utility may be an approach for the future, at present this strategy has little or no practical application.

## RECOMMENDED DIAGNOSTIC APPROACH

Five strategies have been considered, none of which is entirely satisfactory. Our current approach to this problem is to begin with a meticulously performed history and physical examination. Any potential primary cancer sites suggested by the results of the history and physical examination (*e.g.*, pain, palpable mass, change in bowel or bladder function, hemoptysis, hematuria, gastrointestinal bleeding) are further evaluated.

A review of the pathologic specimen can often provide meaningful clues about the potential primary cancer site. The pathologist should be specifically questioned about the adequacy of the tissues submitted; if necessary, additional tissues should be obtained and, in women, hormone receptor assays should be performed. If the tumor is of breast origin, and if the estrogen receptor assay is positive, the patient would be expected to have a response rate to hormonal maneuvers of approximately 60% to 70% (depending on the site of disease). If the receptor assay is negative, the response rate to hormonal manipulation would only be approximately 5%. It is reasonable to evaluate potential primary sites suggested by the pathologist, especially if documentation of these sites is likely to make a contribution to the patient's management or sense of well-being.

Clues to the probable primary site may potentially be derived from serologic measurement of α-fetoprotein and the β subunit of human chorionic gonadotropin (hCG), one or both of which is elevated in 70% of tumors of germ cell origin. Chemotherapy alone is curative in 70% of testicular germ cell cancers and in 45% of those arising from extragonadal sites. Carcinoembryonic antegen (CEA) is a nonspecific marker in a number of cancers, but its elevation does not suggest a specific site of tumor origin.

Advances in immunocytochemical staining have aided in the identification of primary tumor sites. The diagnosis of prostate cancer is suggested by antiprostate-specific acid phosphatase staining, while the diagnosis of thyroid cancer is supported by antithyroglobulin staining. Despite normal serum levels of α-fetoprotein and β-hCG, some germ cell malignancies can be confirmed by immunocytochemical staining of the tumor with antibodies to these substances. Antibodies to serotonin, bombesin, and chromogranin can be found in neuroendocrine tumors.

Immunocytologic staining of intermediate-sized filaments is the most recent contribution to the pathologic workup. All mammalian cells contain a cytoskeletal system of three major filaments (thin, thick, or intermediate-sized) that can be identified on light microscopy. Intermediate filaments are the integrators of the cytoplasm and display biochemical variations. Vimentin and desmin are present in all mesenchymal cells; however, desmin is found only in differentiated subsets such as skeletal, smooth, and cardiac muscles. Cytokeratin, the best known of the intermediate filaments, is contained in all epithelial cells containing keratin. Three specific cytokeratins have been identified that permit the distinction of cholangiocarcinomas from hepatomas, and renal cell carcinomas from pancreatic tumors. The antiglial fibrillary acid protein can be identified in primary gliomas but not in meningiomas or lymphomas of the central nervous system. Further pathologic workup using this battery of substances may aid in the identification of the primary site in the patient with a tumor of unknown origin.

Electron microscopy, although extremely expensive, may be of value in identifying the premelanosomes of melanomas or the neurosecretory granules in tumors of endocrine origin.

Even if the history, physical, and laboratory data are not contributory, certain radiographic studies may still be indicated. We feel that mammography is warranted in any woman who presents with a tumor of unknown origin, because hormonal manipulation and/or chemotherapy so often achieves remarkable palliation. Although far from ideal, we currently utilize CT in the patient with an occult primary tumor, because it provides a comprehensive overview of the abdomen and pelvis with a sensitivity at least 3 to 4 times better than conventional imaging modalities. In the past, we recommended that radionuclide thyroid scans be performed routinely, because differentiated thyroid malignancies are among the most responsive of all metastatic cancers. However, the low likelihood of this tumor being an occult primary site and the recent advances in immunocytochemistry have caused us to reconsider this recommendation.

## COMMENT

In the patient with metastatic cancer in the absence of a known primary lesions, there is little justification for "routine" extensive radiographic investigations such as barium studies, excretory urography, arteriography, or ultrasound. The radiographic search for an unknown primary tumor should be restricted to those screening procedures designed (1) to detect the most treatable occult primaries; (2) to investigate those patients who have historical, physical, or laboratory evidence of specific organ dysfunction; and (3) to pursue those potential primary sites suggested by newer forms of pathologic testing. The determination of which tumors are "most treatable" must be continually reassessed. Many tumors previously regarded as hopeless are today known to be highly treatable and, in some cases, even curable. Even though at present the quest to identify the primary tumor site has proven frustrating, there is no reason to assume that it will always continue to be so.

## APPENDIX

The term "cost" is meant to encompass both financial as well as physical and psychological costs. The patient might, for example, be asked to estimate on a numerical scale his assessment of the "cost" or impact of the outcomes previously listed. If the probabilities of the various outcomes were known, the average cost of the examination could be calculated using the following equation:

- $C = C_O + C_{TP}P_{TP} + C_{TN}P_{TN} + C_{FP}T_{FP} + C_{FN}P_{FN}$
- $C$ = average cost of examination
- $C_O$ = dollar cost
- $C_X$ = "cost" of outcome $_X$
- $P_X$ = probability of outcome $_X$
- TP = true positive
- TN = true negative
- FP = false positive
- FN = false negative

Cost C is the sum of the actual dollar cost of the examination $C_O$ plus an amalgam of the patient's stated evaluations of the possible outcomes multiplied by the probability of achieving these outcomes. It should be emphasized that while the financial cost of the examination ($C_O$) is a given, and while the probabilities of outcome are derived from experimental data, the "cost" of the outcome is an expression of the patient's preferences and is *individually* determined.

## Bibliography


Comess MS, Beahrs OH, Dockerty MD: Cervical metastases from occult carcinoma. Surg Gynecol Obstet 104:607–617, 1957

Didolkar MS, Fanous N, Elias EG et al: Metastatic carcinoma from occult primary tumors. Ann Surg 186:625–630, 1977

Fitzpatrick PJ, Kiltalik JF: Cervical metasis from an unknown primary tumor. Radiology 110:659–663, 1974

France CJ, Lucas R: The management and prognosis of metastatic neoplasms of the neck with an unknown primary. Am J Surg 106:835–839, 1963

Goldberg RM, Smith FP, Ueno W et al: 5-Fluorouracil, Adriamycin and Mitomycin in the treatment of adenocarcinoma of unknown primary. J Clin Oncol 4:395–399, 1986

Golomb HM, Thomson S: Estrogen receptor—Therapeutic guide in undifferentiated metastatic carcinoma in women. Arch Intern Med 135: 942–945, 1975

Gown AM, Gabbiani G: Intermediate-sized (10-nm) filaments in human tumors. In DeLellis RA (ed): Advances in Immunochemistry. New York, Masson Publishing, 1984

Greco FA, Oldham RK, Fer MF: The extragonadal gem cell cancer syndrome. Semin Oncol 9: 448–455, 1982

Greco FA, Vaughn WK, Hainsworth JD: Advanced poorly differentiated carcinoma of unknown primary site: Recognition of a treatable syndrome. Ann Intern Med 104:547–553, 1986

Holmes FF, Fouts TL: Metastatic cancer of unknown primary site. Cancer 26:816–820, 1970

Jesse RH, Neff LE: Metastatic carcinoma in cervical nodes with an unknown primary site. Am J Surg 112:547–553, 1966

Jesse RH, Perez CA, Fletcher GH: Cervical lymph node metastasis: Unknown primary cancer. Cancer 31:854–859, 1973

Kiang DT, Kennedy BJ: Estrogen receptor assay in the differential diagnosis of adenocarcinomas. JAMA 238:32–34, 1977

Krementz ET, Cerisse EJ: Metastatic lesions of undetermined source. Hosp Med 6:91–112, 1970

MacComb WS: Diagnosis and treatment of metastatic cancerous nodes from an unknown primary site. Am J Surg 124:441–449, 1972

Marchetta FC, Mruphy WT, Kovaric JJ: Carcinoma of the neck. Am J Surg 106:974–979, 1963

Martin H, Morfit HM: Cervical lymph node metastasis as the first symptom of cancer. Surg Gynecol Obstet 78:133–159, 1944

Martin H, Romieu C: The diagnostic significance of a "lump in the neck." Postgrad Med 11:491–500, 1952

Metz CE: Basic principles of ROC analysis. Semin Nucl Med 8:283–298, 1978

Moertel CG: Adenocarcinoma of unknown origin. Ann Intern Med 91:646–647, 1979

Moertel CG, Reitermeir RJ, Schutt AJ et al: Treatment of the patient with adenocarcinoma of unknown origin. Cancer 30:1469–1479, 1972

Nystrom JS, Weiner JM, Heffelfinger–Juttner J et al: Metastatic and histologic presentations in unknown primary cancer. Semin Oncol 4:53–58, 1977

Nystrom JS, Weiner JM, Wolf RM et al: Identifying the primary site of metastatic cancer of unknown origin. JAMA 241:381–383, 1979

Osteen RT, Kopf G, Wilson RE: In pursuit of the unknown primary. Am J Surg 135:494–498, 1978

Steckel RJ, Kagan AR: Diagnostic persistence in working up metastatic cancer with an unknown primary site. Radiology 134:367–369, 1980

Stewart JF, Tattersall MHW, Woods RL et al: Unknown primary adenocarcinoma: Incidence of overinvestigation and natural history. Br Med J 1:1530–1533, 1979

Woods RL, Fox RM, Tattersall MHN, et al: Metastatic adenocarcinomas of unknown primary site. N Engl J Med 303:87–89, 1980

## WHERE IS THE PRIMARY?

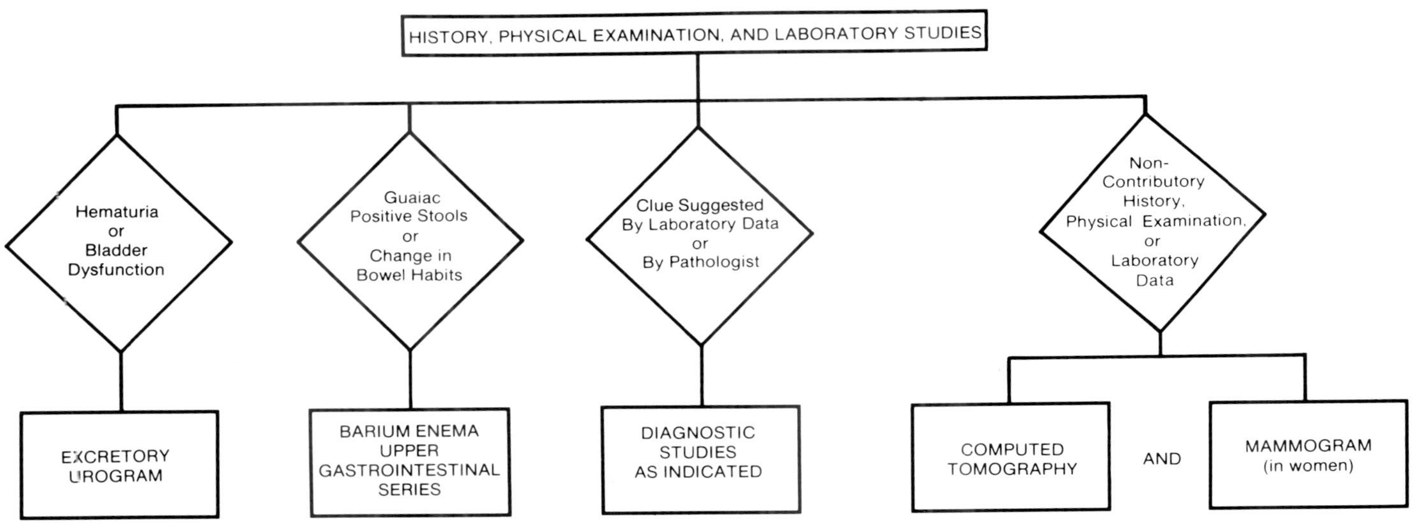

# Chapter 37

# Pulmonary Metastases

*Dixie J. Anderson*
*Stuart S. Sagel*

As cancer therapies have become increasingly successful and sophisticated, defining the extent of malignant disease has become increasingly important. Establishing the presence of metastases in the lung often has tremendous clinical implication, because it may dictate some modification of treatment or management. Up to 30% of patients with cancer will develop pulmonary metastases; in approximately half, the only demonstrable metastases will be confined to the lungs. In some patients, pulmonary metastases are the initial sign of an underlying malignancy; occasionally, they may be the only indicator of recurrent disease. Yet, only about 30% of patients with isolated pulmonary metastases have any symptoms, and these are usually nonspecific. Sputum cytology is generally of little value, because it is positive in only about 5% of patients with metastatic disease. Bronchoscopy with biopsy and brush cytology has been reported to be positive in almost 75% of cases. Nevertheless, conventional chest radiography (along with ancillary conventional techniques, computed tomography, and radionuclide studies) continues to play the major role in detection of lung metastases.

The development of lung metastases depends on the escape of malignant cells from the primary tumor. This most commonly occurs by venous or lymphatic drainage; unusual routes of lung dissemination include endobronchial spread (especially in bronchoalveolar carcinoma) and spread from intermediary hepatic metastases. Most sarcomas and some carcinomas gain access to the pulmonary circulation from venous channels draining the tumor site, while most carcinomas initially spread by efferent lymphatics. Tumors continuously shed malignant cells but are more likely to seed the lung with metastases when the cells are released in clumps. In addition, the larger the tumor emboli, the greater the number of pulmonary nodules eventually present in the lung parenchyma.

Metastatic foci ultimately spread hematogenously to the pulmonary parenchyma and thus are usually distributed peripherally in the lung, especially in a subpleural location. The successfully implanted malignant cells proliferate in the pulmonary capillary bed to produce the typical (more than 75% of cases) radiographic appearance of multiple pulmonary nodules in a peripheral and bibasilar distribution. Most pulmonary metastases are round and well-circumscribed, although some immediately subpleural nodules may have plaquelike, stellate, or "hairy" shapes on computed tomography (CT). Other presenting patterns of metastatic disease on chest radiographs (Fig. 37-1) include a solitary pulmonary nodule, interstitial lung infiltrate, and spontaneous pneumothorax.

Cavitation occurs in approximately 2% of pulmonary metastases (6% in primary bronchogenic carcinoma). Those primary tumors whose metastases are most likely to cavitate are epidermoid lesions of the head and neck, cervix, or lung. Occasionally, metastases from primary adenocarcinomas of the colon, breast, or pancreas may cavitate. Cavitary metastases usually have smooth outer margins, in contrast to cavitary primary lesions whose borders are generally irregular. The presence of cavitation in pulmonary metastases has no prognostic significance, except for the often thin-walled cavitary metastases from sarcomas that may lead to spontaneous pneumothorax following the rupture of a peripheral lesion.

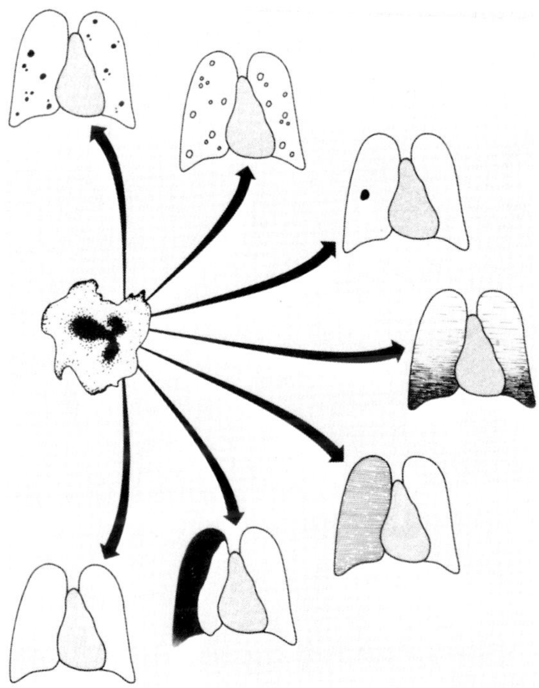

**Figure 37-1.** Metastatic involvement of the lungs may produce one of several chest radiographic patterns as represented by these diagrams (beginning at the top and proceeding clockwise): multiple nodules, multiple cavitary nodules, solitary pulmonary nodule, diffuse infiltrate, unilateral infiltrate, pneumothorax, and a normal chest image. The first two patterns are by far the most common.

Although calcification is usually a sign of benign disease, it can occur in metastases from osteosarcoma; chondrosarcoma; synovial cell sarcoma; giant cell tumor of bone; hemangiopericytoma; and mucinous carcinoma of the colon, ovary, breast, and thyroid. In addition, some metastases may calcify after chemotherapy.

Although up to 20% of patients with lymphangitic metastases have normal chest radiographs, this type of spread typically produces a unilateral or bilateral reticulonodular pulmonary infiltrate that may be associated with septal line thickening. This appearance, which most often results from the hematogenous dissemination of adenocarcinoma, is usually due to neoplastic cells within interstitial spaces and a surrounding connective tissue reaction. Carcinoma of the breast is the most common primary neoplasm producing the lymphangitic pattern of metastatic disease. Carcinomas of the stomach, pancreas, and thyroid may lead to a similar appearance. Unilateral involvement or an associated large lung mass suggests underlying bronchogenic carcinoma. Regardless of the primary site, concomitant involvement of hilar lymph nodes and the pleura is frequently seen. Although lymphangitic pulmonary metastases may be the only indication of tumor spread, they are most often seen in widely disseminated disease and are associated with a much poorer prognosis than the more common appearance of multiple pulmonary nodules. For example, the mean survival of patients with melanoma who have evidence of lymphangitic spread is usually measured in weeks or months, compared with a mean survival of several years for patients with multiple or solitary nodular metastases.

## DIAGNOSTIC EVALUATION

The detection of pulmonary metastases, potentially one of the most significant contributions of chest radiology, is generally straightforward. In an adult, demonstration of new multiple pulmonary nodules, typically of varying sizes and with a basilar predominance, is virtually diagnostic of pulmonary metastases. Other causes to be considered include septic pulmonary emboli, granulomatous disease, rheumatoid nodules, Wegener's granulomatosis, sarcoidosis, multiple arteriovenous malformations, multiple hamartomas, juvenile laryngeal papillomatosis, malakoplakia, and pulmonary dirofilariasis. The radiographic evaluation of suspected pulmonary metastases focuses on (1) identifying pulmonary nodules on plain chest radiography or, when necessary, computed (or conventional) tomography, (2) confirming the new onset of lesions by comparing current films to a previous baseline study, and (3) monitoring biopsy procedures to confirm malignancy or to provide pathologic support for an alternative diagnosis.

### *DIAGNOSTIC MODALITIES*

1. Plain chest radiography
2. Ancillary plain radiographic techniques
3. Computed tomography
4. Magnetic resonance imaging
5. Radionuclide scanning
6. Percutaneous needle biopsy

## Plain Chest Radiography

Plain chest radiography, consisting of posteroanterior and lateral views, is a simple, universally available, relatively inexpensive, and reasonably sensitive screening tool for the detection of pulmonary metastases. In many instances, it is the only imaging study required to identify and document metastatic disease.

It has been well established that lesions smaller than 3 mm in diameter usually are not seen on standard chest radiographs. Almost all lesions larger than 15 mm in diameter should be clearly detectable. In the intermediate size range (3 mm–15 mm), the detectability of a nodule is influenced by several factors. The complexity of surrounding anatomic structures has a substantial influence on the ability to visualize a metastatic nodule. Overlying ribs or blood vessels tend to obscure the outline of a metastatic lesion. In general, lung nodules 6 mm in diameter or smaller are only seen when they are projected directly over rib interspaces. Certain unfavorable locations tend to mask nodules until they are relatively large. Such sites include the lung apices, the inferior recesses just above the dome of the diaphragm, and the subpleural regions.

The best technique for detecting pulmonary metastases utilizes a fixed, relatively high (120–140) kilovoltage combined with a low range of milliampere-seconds (mAs). A method of automatic film exposure is strongly recommended. The high-kilovoltage technique is preferable not only because it permits decreased exposure times but also because this energy range decreases interference from overlying osseous structures that might obscure a nodule. We use a 110 fine-line stationary grid of 10 : 1 ratio; the use of an air gap rather than a grid to decrease scattered radiation may result in slightly better detectability, but is associated with such disadvantages as increased magnification (frequently requiring two frontal films to encompass the entire thorax) and the need for a larger room for the chest unit and a higher x-ray tube output. Although in the past a very high-kilovoltage (350 kVp) technique using a field-emission x-ray generating tube has been implemented with some success for the sole purpose of screening for pulmonary metastases, this method is no longer used.

Even with optimal chest radiographs, the detection of pulmonary metastases is limited by errors in interpretation. It has been shown, for example, that approximately 50% of radiologists will overlook a 1 cm pulmonary nodule. Two or three readings of each film diminish the likelihood of missing small lesions but are generally impractical.

## Ancillary Plain Radiographic Techniques

When the plain chest radiograph is equivocal, fluoroscopy with spot films, conventional tomography, or alternative views such as the apical lordotic or oblique projections may be helpful in assessing the presence of one or more pulmonary nodules. These techniques are of special value for demonstrating the true nature of a lesion that simulates a metastatic nodule. For example, although a pleural plaque may be mistakenly identified as a possible pulmonary nodule on standard chest radiographs, it usually can be correctly diagnosed on oblique or fluoroscopic spot views. Similarly, healing rib fractures, pleural loculations or masses, and other chest wall lesions can be more precisely characterized using these ancillary techniques. However, if the abnormalities on a chest radiograph are believed to be secondary to multiple poorly defined pulmonary nodules, CT should be the next imaging modality of choice.

Whole lung tomography is more sensitive than plain chest radiography and may be valuable in detecting and characterizing pulmonary metastases when CT is either unavailable or not easily accessible. Whole lung tomography usually demonstrates those pulmonary metastases in the 5 mm to 15 mm range that are not visible on standard chest radiographs. Although some reports in the literature cite a 20% additional yield in demonstrating such otherwise undetectable lesions, in our experience this rate has been substantially less. Recent investigations have indicated that whole lung tomography has a diagnostic yield that is no better than plain chest radiography in detecting pulmonary metastases in patients with breast cancer, germ cell tumors, and gynecologic malignancies. Nevertheless, in the cancer patient at high risk for pulmonary metastases, especially if such an individual is stout, whole lung tomography may disclose lesions not detectable on plain radiographs. The demonstration of these otherwise occult lesions is attributable to the elimination of overlying obscuring structures (ribs, heart, diaphragm, pulmonary vessels).

Whole lung tomography is generally performed with linear motion, using a 30° to 40° arc at 70 kVp to 80 kVp in the anteroposterior projection only. Phantom images caused by linear motion are usually not a serious problem in the thorax because of the horizontal orientation of the overlying ribs. Linear tomography can be accomplished using a relatively short exposure time (usually 0.5–1 sec), significantly reducing the unsharpness created by vascular and respiratory motion when pleuridirectional tomography requiring 2 to 6 seconds of exposure time is used. Although hypocycloidal tube movement has been advocated by some, its practicality is limited by equipment availability and the long tube-cooling period sometimes necessary between exposures. The use of an aluminum trough filter in patients with usual body habitus enables better demonstration of both the lungs and the mediastinum on a single exposure. Tomography should be performed so that both posterior and anterior ribs are demonstrated to ensure complete evaluation of the pulmonary parenchyma. Tomographic sections are usually obtained at 1-cm intervals; intervening slices may be obtained to better define equivocal areas. If a questionable nodule is seen, or if a specific area is poorly imaged on whole lung tomography, coned-down tomographic views may be helpful (Fig. 37-2). At the completion of the study, a 35 cm × 43 cm film centered at the level of the diaphragm and oriented transversely should be obtained to demonstrate an otherwise occult lesion in the posterior costophrenic sulci.

To distinguish stable, healed, noncalcified granulomas from neoplastic metastases, repeat tomography after a suitable interval (*e.g.*, 6 weeks) may be advisable. It should be emphasized that lesions smaller than 5 mm in diameter usually are not demonstrable on whole lung tomograms. Also, the pleural margins of the lungs, especially anteriorly and posteriorly, are not optimally imaged on tomograms performed in the frontal plane. Because this is an area prone to metastatic seeding, it is another potential source of false-negative results.

## Computed Tomography

Computed tomography provides a more sensitive imaging modality for discovering small pulmonary metastases that are undetectable or poorly seen on standard chest radiography or whole lung tomography. Used either as a screening examination or as a problem-solving study, this relatively noninvasive technique has a high sensitivity for detecting the multiple peripheral pulmonary nodules of varying sizes that are characteristic of pulmonary metastases.

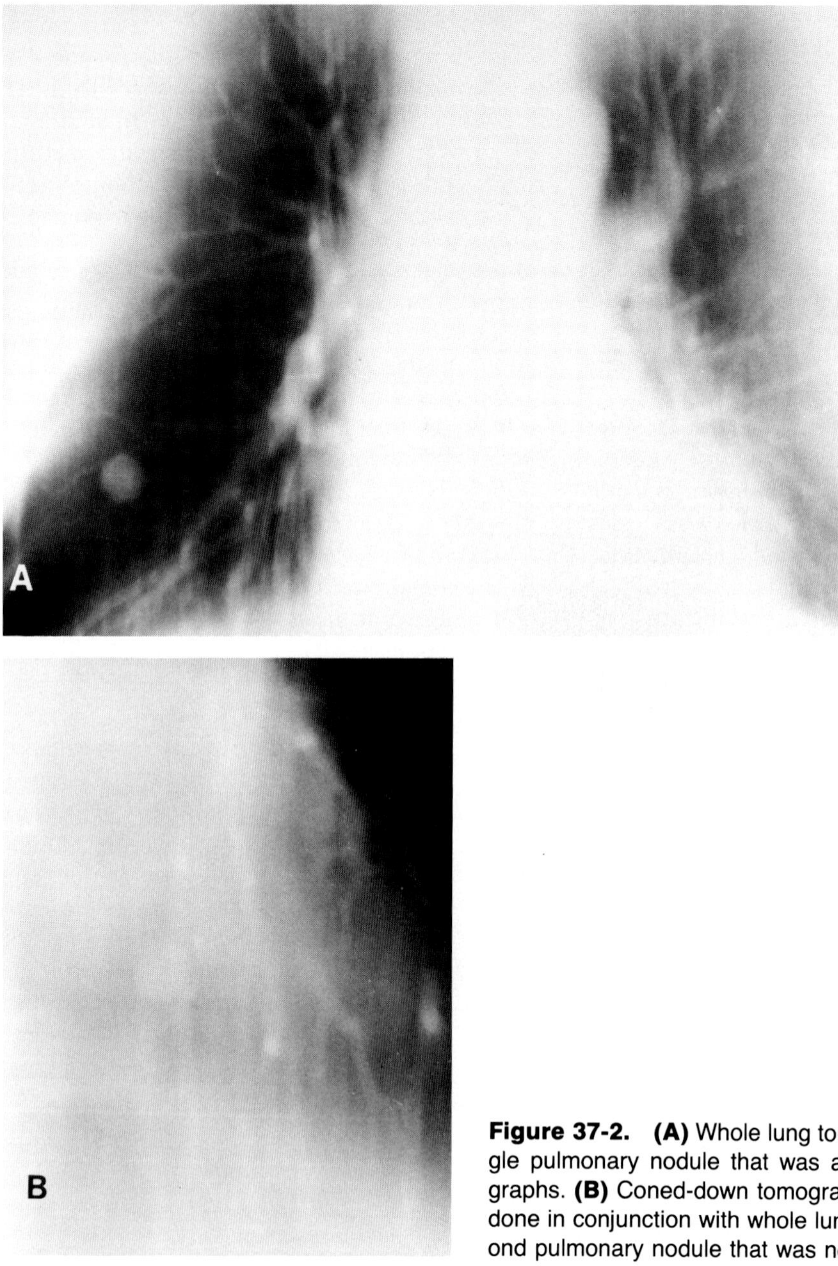


**Figure 37-2.** **(A)** Whole lung tomogram demonstrates a single pulmonary nodule that was also present on chest radiographs. **(B)** Coned-down tomogram of the retrocardiac region done in conjunction with whole lung tomography shows a second pulmonary nodule that was not visible on chest films.

The added yield of CT in detecting otherwise occult small nodules (usually 3 mm–10 mm in diameter) is largely attributable to elimination of obscuring and confusing superimposed bony or vascular structures. The transverse orientation of CT scans is particularly suited for the demonstration of peripheral subpleural lesions, as well as metastases in the costophrenic angles; retrosternal, perihilar, and retrocardiac regions; and in the extreme lung apices. In addition, observer error frequently accounts for pulmonary nodules being overlooked on conventional chest films or whole lung tomograms due to the lack of contrast with the surrounding lung. The increased contrast sensitivity of CT and the ability to displace such nodules as white dots against a black background, thus enhancing their density differences, improves the detectability of metastatic lesions (Fig. 37-3).

Computed tomography of the chest for metastatic disease may be performed on any current third- or fourth-generation scanner. Using a scan time of 3–5 seconds, sections should be obtained from the lung apex to the diaphragm at contiguous 10-mm intervals using 8-mm to 10-mm collimation during suspended full inspiration.

For most primary tumors, CT is the most sensitive imaging modality available for the detection of pulmonary metastases, especially those in a peripheral subpleural location. In addition, CT also images the mediastinum, the pleural space, and the upper abdomen, sometimes providing valuable information that is not available using any other imaging technique.

The major limitation of CT is the frequent inability to differentiate small metastatic nodules

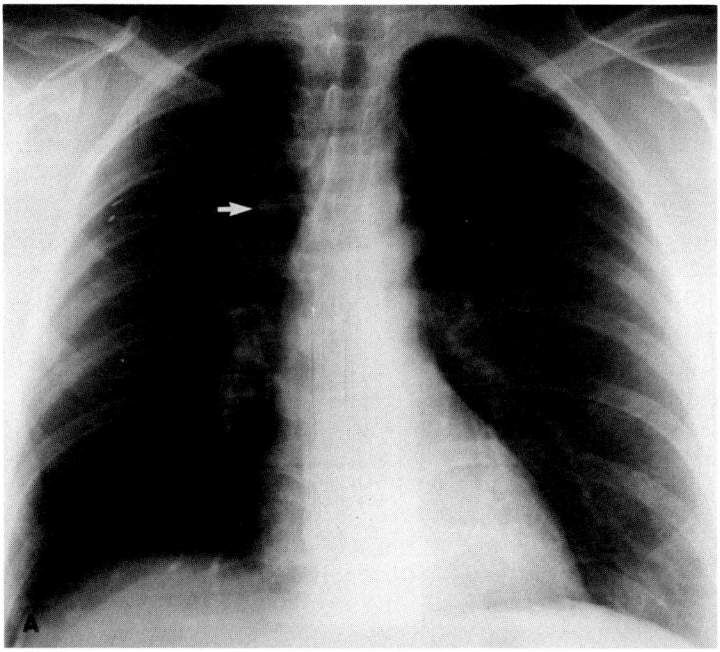

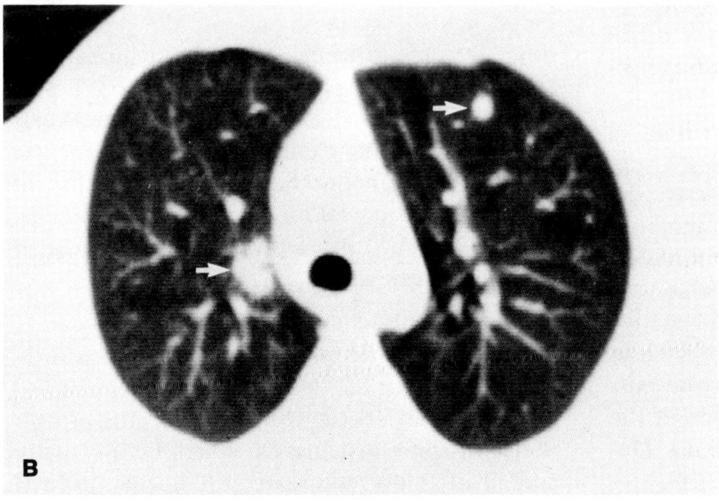

**Figure 37-3.** **(A)** Chest radiograph in a woman with a prior mastectomy demonstrates a questionable nodule in the right suprahilar region (*arrow*) that was not seen on the lateral view. No other lesions are seen. **(B)** CT scan demonstrates two metastatic lesions (*arrows*) at this level and several additional pulmonary nodules on other sections.

from noncalcified benign healed granulomas. In areas where histoplasmosis is endemic, approximately 20% to 45% of pulmonary nodules are benign even in patients with documented primary neoplasms. However, European studies from areas in which granulomatous disease is rare have shown a much higher specificity for neoplasm when CT demonstrates multiple nodules.

Although no single criterion or combination of criteria are absolutely reliable, several factors (number, size, density, and roundness of nodules) have been identified as being of value in predicting malignancy. The demonstration of multiple noncalcified nodular densities is presumptive evidence for metastatic disease. If the presence of pulmonary metastases would alter therapy, more definitive corroboration can be achieved by follow-up CT studies (to look for interval growth) or by histologic sampling. The latter, unfortunately, often requires local limited thoracotomy, because fiberoptic bronchoscopy may have a low yield and percutaneous needle aspiration may not be definitive.

Pulmonary metastases may be missed on CT examination for several reasons. A lesion may go unnoticed because it lies in a "skip area" produced by inconsistency in the depth of suspended respiration, which may vary up to 8 mm near the diaphragm even in cooperative patients. Patient movement in the scanner may result in exclusion of a section of lung from the study. Thus, some authors have advocated performing CT at end tidal volume if the primary objective of the study is to search for pulmonary metastases. Pulmonary nodules may be indistinguishable from pulmonary vessels on CT. Although 3 mm has been established as a lower limit of detectability for peripheral lesions, more centrally located nodules must be 6 mm in size to be consistently detected. Prone scans sometimes may aid in differentiating vessels from nodules. Partial-volume averaging of small nodules with adjacent lung accounts for some false-negative CT studies. At times, normal structures such as the anterior portion of the first rib may be mistakenly identified as a pulmonary nodule if the observer is unacquainted with such pitfalls. Despite all of these theoretical problems, CT remains the most sensitive imaging procedure for defining pulmonary metastases.

In the patient with suspected pulmonary metastases who has a normal chest radiograph, the decision to obtain CT is based on the following three questions:

1. Would the presence of pulmonary metastases alter the clinical management of the patient's primary tumor?
2. What is the propensity of the specific type of tumor to metastasize to the lungs?
3. Is there effective therapy available for metastatic disease of this tumor type?

In selected primary malignancies, an accurate assessment of the extent of metastatic disease may be crucial in reaching a therapeutic decision. It is essential when a major operation is being considered (*e.g.*, amputation for osteosarcoma, extensive node dissection for melanoma, lobectomy for presumed solitary metastasis). In such circumstances, imaging evaluation beyond the standard chest radiograph is clearly indicated, and CT is usually the next examination performed.

## Magnetic Resonance Imaging

The use of magnetic resonance imaging (MRI) for pulmonary nodule detection has not yet been well investigated. Although one early study reported that MRI could show pulmonary nodules undetected by CT because of close proximity to blood vessels, in most patients the pulmonary nodules were visible on both imaging modalities. In addition, the spatial resolution of CT permitted better detection of nodules situated close to the diaphragm, pleura, or to each other. At present, CT remains the imaging modality of choice for the detection of pulmonary nodules; MRI is reserved for a problem-solving role in selected cases.

## Radionuclide Scanning

Radionuclide perfusion lung scanning has proven useful in some instances in which lymphangitic spread of tumor is suspected clinically even if there is no evidence of an interstitial infiltrate on chest radiographs. Lymphangitic carcinomatosis produces a relatively specific peripheral photopenia or a large number of small, peripherally located perfusion defects that are distributed throughout the lungs and often "map" pulmonary segments (Fig. 37-4). Although this pattern may be seen with other entities (vasculitis, primary pulmonary hypertension, drug abuse, multiple chronic or recurrent pulmonary emboli, fat emboli), in the proper setting it is considered reasonably sensitive and specific for lymphangitic metastases.

In the patient with suspected metastases from thyroid carcinoma, $^{131}$I total body scanning is an alternative radiographic detection method. This technique is somewhat more sensitive than the chest radiograph in identifying functioning thyroid carcinoma metastases to the lung and, of course, is quite specific. Radionuclide imaging with $^{131}$I can be used to screen for metastases in the post-thyroidectomy patient with well-differentiated follicular or papillary thyroid carcinoma. To increase the yield of this technique, the procedure should not be performed until at least 6 weeks after thyroid ablation so that thyroid-stimulating hormone levels and subsequent uptake of isotope are maximized. Radionuclide imaging with $^{131}$I for the detection of thyroid metastases is usually performed 24 hours after oral administration of the isotope. Total body images are routinely obtained as well as specific images of the neck and lungs, the two most common sites of recurrent disease.

Radionuclide imaging with $^{99m}$Tc diphosphonate has been used for the detection of pulmonary metastases from osteosarcoma. However, this technique has a very limited role (if any), because it can identify only about 5% of pulmonary metastases detected by CT.

Tumor imaging with radiolabeled monoclonal antibodies (or antibody fragments) directed against single human antigenic determinants holds promise for the future. Several reports have demonstrated success in detecting a variety of metastatic lesions (1.5 cm–8 cm in size), but imaging inconsistency has prevented practical application of this fascinating research tool.

### Percutaneous Needle Biopsy

Percutaneous biopsy using fine-needle aspiration technique coupled with cytologic evaluation is invaluable for the confirmation of malignant disease. Diagnostic yields of 85% to 95% are common, and the predictive value of a positive result is almost 100%. False-positive diagnoses have been reported in patients with tuberculosis, actinomycosis, and other chronic inflammatory lesions. The predictive value of a negative result, however, is much lower (50%–90%). In general, the accuracy rates of percutaneous biopsy in metastatic disease do not differ significantly from those with primary tumors. One limitation of this technique is the not infrequent inability to assign a cell type with certainty. In the patient with suspected pulmonary metastases, however, simple confirmation of malignancy is generally sufficient to permit the institution of potentially high-risk treatment.

Fine-needle aspiration biopsy is advocated by some for the evaluation of a solitary pulmonary nodule in a patient with a known primary tumor. If the specimen proves compatible with metastatic disease, appropriate treatment may be instituted without further evaluation. On the other hand, if inflammatory disease or some other neoplasm is found, a substantially different management approach can be pursued.

Most percutaneous lung biopsies are performed with fluoroscopic guidance. Occasionally, CT guidance may be required to reliably sample lesions that are small or difficult to reach.

Metastatic pulmonary nodules infrequently may persist unchanged in size following chemotherapy. This generally represents residual scar tissue rather than a persistent focus of malignancy. If required, percutaneous needle biopsy can clarify the situation.

## IMPORTANT CLINICAL FACTORS IN THE SELECTION OF IMAGING MODALITIES

### Characteristics of Specific Neoplasms

The propensity of a given primary tumor to metastasize to the lungs and the various patterns of metastatic spread often influence the extent of

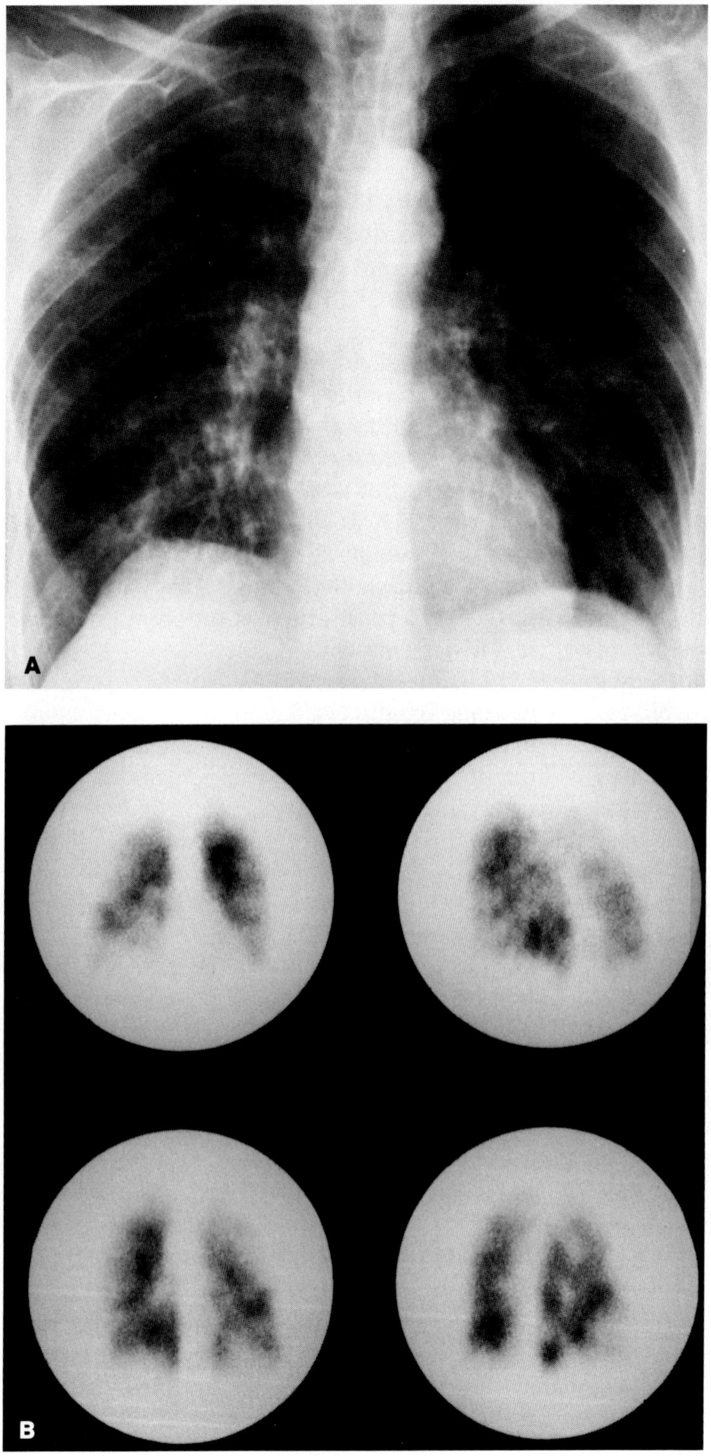

**Figure 37-4.** **(A)** Chest radiograph shows new diffuse, patchy infiltrates. **(B)** Radionuclide lung scan shows multiple small peripheral perfusion defects. Transbronchial biopsy confirmed the diagnosis of lymphangitic carcinomatosis.

the imaging evaluation. Statistics based solely on plain chest radiography are likely to underestimate the true incidence of pulmonary metastases. However, in a relative way these figures can provide guidance in developing appropriate and efficient algorithms for patient care.

Tumors that initially drain into the systemic venous system (melanoma, osteosarcoma, head and neck tumors) are more likely to spread first to the pulmonary bed. These primary tumors have a higher incidence of pulmonary metastases than those that initially drain to the liver (colon, pancreas, stomach) or even than tumors arising in organs that are rich in lymphatics (prostate).

### Melanoma

Approximately 70% of patients with melanoma have localized disease at the time of presentation and a 5-year survival rate of 80%. Regional or distant spread of tumor is associated with a sharp reduction in survival. It is almost impossible to predict which organ system will be invaded by a melanoma from a given primary site. Nevertheless, pulmonary metastases can be detected at the time of presentation in approximately 5% of patients with malignant melanoma. After wide local excision with lymph node dissection, if indicated, up to 45% of patients with melanoma will develop lung metastases during the first year. In patients dying from the disease, metastases to the lungs can be demonstrated at autopsy in approximately 80% of patients; only 2% have pulmonary involvement without other sites being affected.

In patients with localized disease, the Clark level provides some guidance for determining the intensity of the search for pulmonary metastases. Primary melanoma lesions less than 0.76 mm thick (Clark level I) metastasize rarely, whereas metastases are almost invariable if the initial lesion is more than 4 mm thick (Clark level V). Once regional metastases have occurred, however, the depth of local invasion is no longer an important prognostic parameter.

The metastatic spread of melanoma to the lungs usually produces pulmonary nodules. Diffuse infiltrates, which are much less frequently seen, are associated with a poor prognosis.

Plain chest radiography is probably inadequate for detecting early melanoma metastases amenable to surgical resection. This modality also is not sufficiently definitive for making management decisions regarding immunotherapy. Chest CT may reveal pulmonary nodules undetected on plain chest radiographs. It also can demonstrate additional nodules in approximately 30% of patients presenting with advanced melanoma (Clark levels IV or V). Conventional whole lung tomography is of little clinical value.

### Testicular Carcinoma

Up to 20% of patients with testicular carcinoma have pulmonary metastases at the time of presentation. The lung is a common site for metastatic involvement, and pulmonary metastases are frequently associated with lymph node enlargement. Whole lung tomography is of little value in patients with either seminomatous or nonseminomatous germ cell tumors. The role of CT has not yet been clarified.

### Osteosarcoma

Pulmonary metastases are usually the first sign of metastatic spread in patients with osteosarcoma. The detection of these metastases is of vital importance, not only with regard to prognosis but also because chemotherapy and surgery can successfully treat metastatic disease. Chest CT is positive in approximately 30% of patients with osteosarcoma who have normal plain chest radiographs. Because chest CT can define additional pulmonary nodules not seen on chest radiography, it is mandatory before any contemplated surgical resection of presumed pulmonary metastases.

### Head and Neck Carcinoma

Cancers of the head and neck metastasize to the lungs in approximately 10% of patients. Nasopharyngeal carcinomas have a somewhat higher incidence (approximately 20%). Nevertheless, the presence of pulmonary metastases rarely affects patient management, and thus a compulsive search for lung metastases is probably not indicated in this patient population.

To offer the best chance for cure, any new solitary pulmonary lesion in the patient with head and neck carcinoma should be regarded as though it represents a second primary (*i.e.*, bronchogenic carcinoma), unless there is good evidence to the contrary.

### Prostate Carcinoma

Pulmonary metastases, sometimes in the form of lymphangitic carcinomatosis, usually occur only late in the course of patients with prostatic carcinoma. They almost always are preceded or accompanied by bone metastases. On plain chest radiographs, pulmonary nodules and reticulonodular opacities are reasonably specific (>90% true positive) for metastatic disease. However, a nonspecific reticular pattern is just as likely to represent nonmetastatic disease.

### Thyroid Carcinoma

The pulmonary metastases of differentiated thyroid carcinoma generally are micronodular (<1 cm) and often require radionuclide scanning or CT imaging for detection. Radionuclide scanning is especially valuable in this specific clinical setting, because CT scans may be particularly difficult to interpret in the central or perihilar region in which metastatic nodules may have to be quite large to be distinguished from pulmonary vessels.

Iodine-131 is an established technique for treating well-differentiated thyroid carcinoma. Ablation of lung metastases (along with ablation of the primary tumor) that is maintained for 3 years makes the development of recurrent tumor very unlikely. Because recurrent thyroid carcinoma can virtually always be diagnosed by radionuclide imaging, regular monitoring with this procedure is recommended in these patients.

### Colon Carcinoma

Pulmonary metastases develop in only 4% of patients with colon carcinoma who do not manifest hepatic involvement. Thus, a negative chest radiograph in the absence of liver metastases is a highly reliable indicator that there are no pulmonary metastases.

### Breast Carcinoma

Pulmonary lesions are the initial manifestation of metastatic disease in only about 6% of patients with breast carcinoma. In most cases, the standard chest radiograph remains an adequate screening method for the detection of metastases. If the plain chest radiograph is normal, there is no indication for whole lung tomography.

### Endometrial Carcinoma

Pulmonary metastases occur in only about 3% of patients with endometrial cancer. Most patients with spread to the lungs also have concomitant metastatic disease in the abdomen and pelvis.

### Cervical Carcinoma

Most patients with intrathoracic metastases from cervical carcinoma have evidence of locally extensive disease. Pulmonary metastases develop in approximately 5% of patients with stage I carcinoma of the cervix, 16% in stage II, 24% in stage III, and 75% in stage IV. Nevertheless, approximately 25% of patients with pulmonary metastases have no other evidence of malignant spread.

The incidence of pulmonary metastases is higher for adenocarcinoma of the cervix (20%) than for squamous call carcinoma (4%). Both cell types produce the radiographic appearance of single or multiple nodules.

The detection of pulmonary metastases indicates a grim prognosis in the patient with carcinoma of the cervix or endometrium. Approximately 80% of patients with pulmonary involvement are dead within 1 year.

### Ovarian Carcinoma

Peritoneal carcinomatosis is almost always present when pulmonary metastases develop in patients with ovarian carcinoma. Lung metastases usually occur in patients with clinically obvious widespread dissemination and often herald imminent death.

### Bronchogenic Carcinoma

Pulmonary metastases from carcinoma of the lung are unusual at the time of diagnosis. They generally occur only with very undifferentiated tumors, especially of the small cell variety. In autopsy studies, however, lung to lung metastases are common in all types of bronchogenic carcinoma.

Bronchoalveolar carcinoma occasionally presents as multiple regional foci simulating metastases. Lymphangitic obstruction with reversal of lymphatic flow is believed to be the basis for this phenomenon.

## Modifying Factors in the Search for Pulmonary Metastases

In addition to the predilection of a given tumor to metastasize to the lung, the extent of the primary tumor and other evidence of distant spread at the time of diagnosis is often useful in predicting the likelihood of the development of metastases and, consequently, the need for and nature of a search for lung metastases. Melanoma is a classic example of how the depth of the primary tumor influences the probability of metastases to the lung. Other evidence of distant metastatic involvement (*e.g.*, positive bone marrow biopsy) may preclude a vigorous search for possible new pulmonary metastases.

The treatment available for any given tumor also is an important consideration in determining the value of a search for metastatic disease. If there is no effective treatment for metastases, as in renal or transitional cell carcinoma, the detection of pulmonary metastases is of no clinical significance. Conversely, the availability of a highly efficacious treatment for metastatic disease provides strong incentive for early detection and treatment of dissemination of tumor to the lungs. Unfortunately, the list of primary malignancies with potentially curable pulmonary metastases—either by chemotherapy, radiotherapy, or surgery—is quite short and is currently limited to osteogenic sarcoma, choriocarcinoma, testicular carcinoma, and certain functioning thyroid carcinomas. Some solitary or focal lung metastases may be amenable to surgical resection. Metastatic breast cancer also is potentially curable, although pulmonary lesions are rarely the initial manifestation of metastases in this disease.

Aggressive surgical resection of pulmonary metastases has been rewarding in tumors (osteosarcomas, nonseminomatous testicular tumors, renal cell carcinomas) that commonly metastasize first to the lungs. Factors that increase the likelihood of survival following surgical resection of pulmonary metastases include a relatively long interval (at least 12 months) between treatment of the primary neoplasm and the detection of pulmonary metastases, fewer than five pulmonary lesions, and a slow doubling time (>40 days). On the other hand, the presence of bilateral lesions, more than five nodules in both lungs, or multiple nodules in a single lobe adversely affects the prognosis, as does the demonstration of concomitant enlargement of mediastinal lymph nodes.

### Solitary Pulmonary Metastasis

Although a solitary pulmonary lesion in a patient with a known extrathoracic primary malignancy may represent metastatic disease, a second primary or a benign lesion also must be considered. In a patient without a previous history of cancer, a solitary pulmonary nodule has about a 1% chance of representing a metastatic focus. The risk of metastatic disease dramatically increases if the patient with a new solitary pulmonary nodule has a prior or concomitant history of malignant neoplasm (up to 80%, depending on the origin and cell type of the primary). In general, a new pulmonary nodule in a patient with a previous squamous cell carcinoma is more likely to represent a new primary, whereas a metastatic focus would be more likely in the patient with a previous melanoma or sarcoma. Patients with pre-existing adenocarcinomas tend to have an equal likelihood of developing a new primary or a metastatic lesion. With certain primary carcinomas (head, neck, stomach, prostate, breast) that have a higher association with metachronous or synchronous development of bronchogenic carcinoma, a solitary pulmonary nodule has a greater chance of being a new primary than representing a single metastatic focus.

## COMMENT

In the initial evaluation and follow-up of most patients with common primary neoplasms (*e.g.*, lung, breast, colon), standard posteroanterior and lateral chest radiographs are the only imaging examinations required for the detection of pulmonary metastases. This diagnostic approach is dictated by the low cost and high sensitivity of plain chest radiography combined with the difficulty of treating lung metastases.

Computed tomography has become invaluable both for metastasis screening and for problem-solving in patients with abnormal chest radiographs. However, the impact of CT depends largely upon proper patient selection for the study. If the overall incidence of lung metastases from a given primary tumor is very low (*e.g.*, stage I carcinoma of the cervix), the extra cost and effort to detect occult pulmonary nodules is probably not justified. Conversely, CT is indicated in patients with primary tumors that have a high propensity for lung metastases (osteosarcoma, localized melanoma of Clark level IV or V), or in those in whom the importance of detecting additional lesions is great (presumed solitary lung metastasis or several nodules localized to one lobe). Computed tomography also is justified in patients in whom the detection of lung nodules would alter the course of treatment, usually by the cancellation of planned extensive surgery (*e.g.*, radical amputation or retroperitoneal lymph node dissection).

## Bibliography

Apple JS, Paulson DF, Baber C et al: Advanced prostatic carcinoma: Pulmonary manifestations. Radiology 154:601–604, 1985

Chang AE: Flexible fiberoptic bronchoscopy in metastatic cancer to the lungs. Cancer 52:1949–1951, 1983

Chaudary MA, Maisey MN, Shaw PJ et al: Sequential bone scans and chest radiographs in the postoperative management of early breast cancer. Br J Surg 70:517–518, 1983

Chiles C, Ravin C: Intrathoracic metastasis from an extrathoracic malignancy: A radiographic approach to patient evaluation. Radiol Clin North Am 23:427–438, 1985

Crane R, Rudd TG, Dail D: Tumor microembolism: Pulmonary perfusion pattern. J Nucl Med 25: 877–880, 1984

Crow J, Slavin G, Kreel L: Pulmonary metastasis: A pathologic and radiologic study. Cancer 47: 2595–2602, 1981

Curtis AM, Ravin CE, Collier RE et al: Detection of metastatic disease from carcinoma of the breast: Limited value of full lung tomography. AJR 134:254–255, 1980

Dwyer AJ, Reichert CM, Woltering EA et al: Diffuse pulmonary metastasis in melanoma: Radiographic-pathologic correlation. AJR 143: 983–984, 1984

Gordon RE, Mettler FA, Jr, Wicks JD et al: Chest x-rays and full lung tomograms in gynecologic malignancy. Cancer 52:559–562, 1983

Gross BH, Glazer GM, Bookstein F: Multiple pulmonary nodules detected by computed tomography: Diagnostic implications. J Comput Assist Tomogr 9:880–885, 1985

Heaston DK, Putman CE, Rodan BA et al: Solitary pulmonary metastases in high-risk melanoma patients: A prospective comparison of conventional and computed tomography. AJR 141:169–174, 1983

Heitzman R, Markarian A, Raasch BN et al: Pathways of tumor spread through the lung: Radiologic correlations with anatomy and pathology. Radiology 144:3–14, 1982

Hidalgo H, Korobkin M, Finney TR et al: The problem of benign pulmonary nodules in children receiving cytotoxic chemotherapy. AJR 140:21–24, 1983

Jochelson MS, Garnick MB, Balikian JP et al: The efficacy of routine whole lung tomography in germ cell tumors. Cancer 54:1007–1009, 1984

Johnson RD, Gobien RP, Valicenti JF, Jr: Current status of radiologically directed pulmonary thin needle aspiration biopsy. An analysis of 200 consecutive biopsies and review of the literature. Ann Clin Lab Sci 13:225–239, 1983

Libshitz HI, Jing B-S, Wallace S et al: Sterilized metastases: A diagnostic and therapeutic dilemma. AJR 140:15–19, 1983

Libshitz HI, North LB: Pulmonary metastases. Radiol Clin North Am 20:437–451, 1982

Lefor AT, Bredenberg CE, Kellman RM et al: Multiple malignancies of the lung and head and neck. Arch Surg 121:265–270, 1986

Lund G, Heilo A: Computed tomography of pulmonary metastases. Acta Radiol (Diagn) 23: 617–620, 1982

Malefatto JP, Kasimis BS, Moran EM et al: The clinical significance of radiographically detected pulmonary neoplastic lesions in patients with head and neck cancer. J Clin Oncol 2:625–630, 1984

Moldofsky PJ, Powe J, Mulhern CB Jr et al: Metastatic colon carcinoma detected with radiolabeled F(ab′)2 monoclonal antibody fragments. Radiology 149:549–555, 1983

Muller NL, Gamsu G, Webb WR: Pulmonary nodules: Detection using magnetic resonance and computed tomography. Radiology 155:687–690, 1985

Piekarski JD, Schlumberger M, Leclere J et al: Chest computed tomography (CT) in patients with micronodular lung metastases of differentiated thyroid carcinoma. Int J Radiat Oncol Biol Phys 11:1023–1027, 1985

Pilotti S, Rilke F, Gribaudi G et al: Transthoracic fine needle aspiration biopsy in pulmonary lesions. Updated results. Acta Cytol 28:225–232, 1984

Poe RH, Ortiz C, Israel RH et al: Sensitivity, specificity, and predictive values of bronchoscopy in neoplasm metastatic to lung. Chest 88:84–88, 1985

Putnam JB, Jr, Roth JA, Wesley NM et al: Analysis of prognostic factors in patients undergoing resection of pulmonary metastases from soft tissue sarcomas. J Thorac Cardiovasc Surg 87:260–268, 1984

Schaner EG, Chang AE, Doppman JL et al: A comparison of computed and conventional whole lung tomography in detecting pulmonary nodules: A prospective radiologic-pathologic study. AJR 131:51–54, 1978

Sinner WN: Fine needle biopsy of solitary pulmonary metastasis. Eur J Radiol 4:9–13, 1984

Sostman HD, Brown M, Toole A et al: Perfusion scan in pulmonary vascular/lymphangitic carcinomatosis: The segmental contour pattern. AJR 137: 1072–1074, 1981

Sostman HD, Matthey RA: Thoracic metastases from cervical carcinoma: Current status. Invest Radiol 15:113–119, 1980

Tellis CJ, Beechler CR: Pulmonary metastasis of carcinoma of the cervix. Cancer 49:1705–1709, 1982

Vanel D, Henry AM, Lumbroso J et al: Pulmonary evaluation of patients with osteosarcoma: Roles of standard radiography, tomography, CT, scintigraphy, and tomoscintigraphy. AJR 143: 519–523, 1984

## SUSPECTED PULMONARY METASTASES

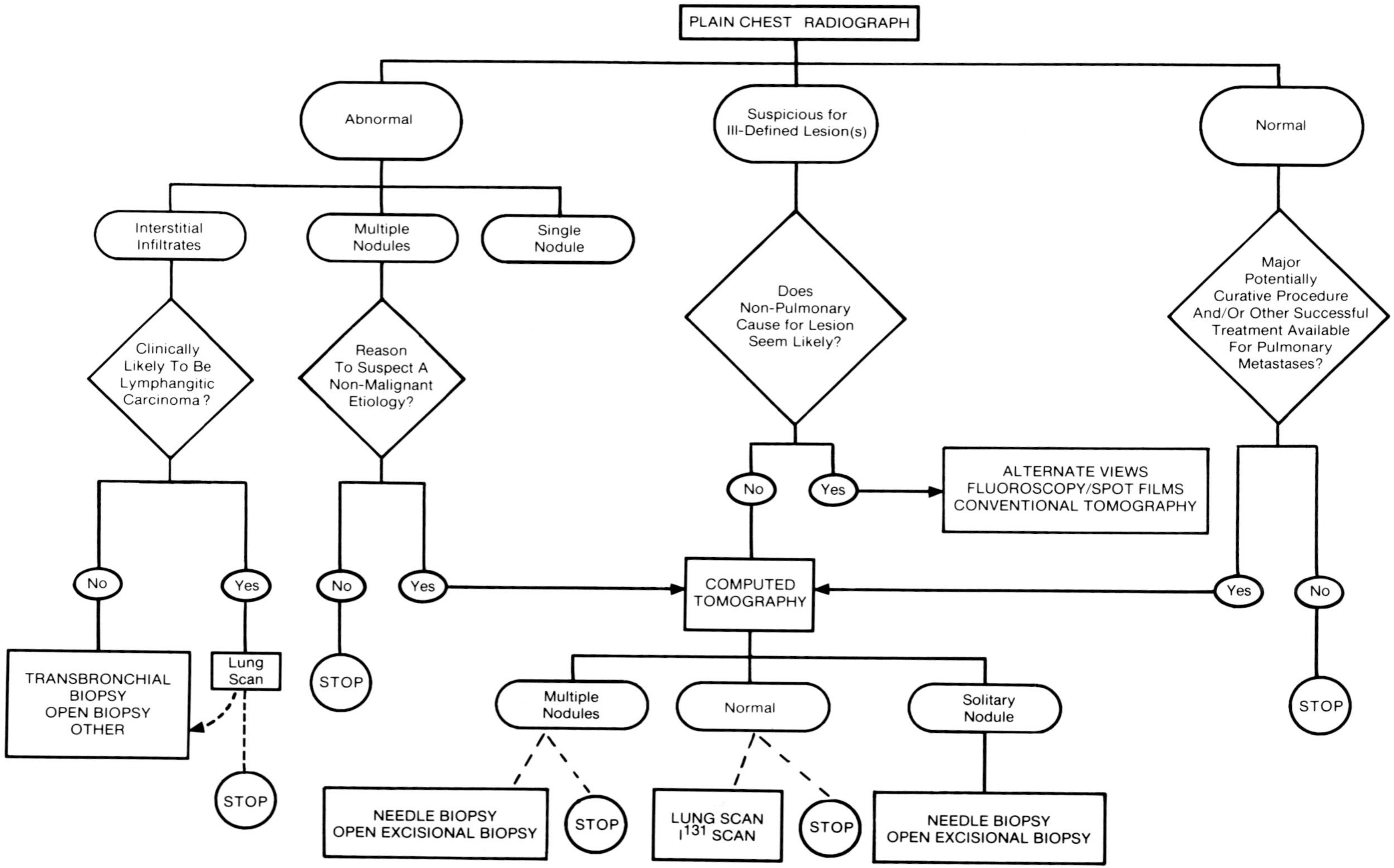

# Chapter 38

## Skeletal Metastases

*Jay C. Mall*
*Neil I. Chafetz*
*Stephen R. Bunker*

The incidence of metastases to bone varies with the type of primary neoplasm and duration of disease (Table 38-1). Nevertheless, skeletal metastases are present in a significant number of patients at the time of initial staging, especially those with breast, lung, and prostate carcinoma and with lymphoma. Therefore, detection of skeletal metastases in patients with known or suspected neoplastic disease is critical for proper management, both at the time of initial staging and during the period of continuing follow-up care. The presence of metastases may exclude some patients from receiving the radical "curative" therapy that is offered to those without disseminated disease, thus sparing these patients from fruitless, high-morbidity procedures for a nonremediable condition.

### CLINICAL AND LABORATORY FINDINGS

The majority of skeletal metastases are "silent." Pain is the main clinical symptom, but it occurs in only a small percentage of lesions and usually not until bone destruction is quite advanced.

Although various laboratory studies are usually performed to screen for possible metastases, all are insensitive and usually not positive until later in the course of metastatic disease. For example, serum alkaline phosphatase (bone fraction) becomes elevated when skeletal metastases are widespread but is only rarely increased when there is early or minimal involvement. Serum calcium is also very insensitive, although it may be elevated when there is extensive skeletal destruction, especially with breast carcinoma or myeloma. Extracapsular spread of prostate carcinoma may result in increased levels of serum acid phosphatase, although this does not necessarily imply skeletal involvement and rarely occurs in patients with minimal disease spread.

### DIAGNOSTIC EVALUATION

#### *DIAGNOSTIC MODALITIES*

1. Radionuclide bone scan
2. Conventional radiography
3. Computed tomography
4. Magnetic resonance imaging
5. Needle biopsy
6. Surgical biopsy

**Table 38-1** Incidence of Bone Metastases at Autopsy in Selected Malignant Diseases

| Primary Site | Percentage Involvement |
|---|---|
| Breast | 50–85 |
| Lung | 30–50 |
| Prostate | 50–70 |
| Hodgkin's | 50–70 |
| Kidney | 30–50 |
| Bladder | 12–25 |
| Thyroid | 40 |
| Melanoma | 30–40 |

(Modified from McNeil BJ: Rationale for the use of bone scans in selected metastatic and primary bone tumors. Semin Nucl Med 8:336–345, 1978)

## Radionuclide Bone Scan

The best screening examination for detection of asymptomatic skeletal metastases is the radionuclide bone scan performed with $^{99m}$Tc-labeled phosphate compounds. Comparative studies have consistently demonstrated that the radionuclide bone scan is far more sensitive than the radiographic "skeletal survey." Various series have reported detection rates of 99% to 100% for skeletal metastases from breast, lung, and prostate carcinoma and from lymphoma, malignancies that have a high incidence of bone involvement. In addition, the radionuclide bone scan is also the best examination for following the course of patients with known skeletal metastases from any source. The most common abnormal finding is a focal area of increased labeling (hot spot), due to local alteration of blood flow

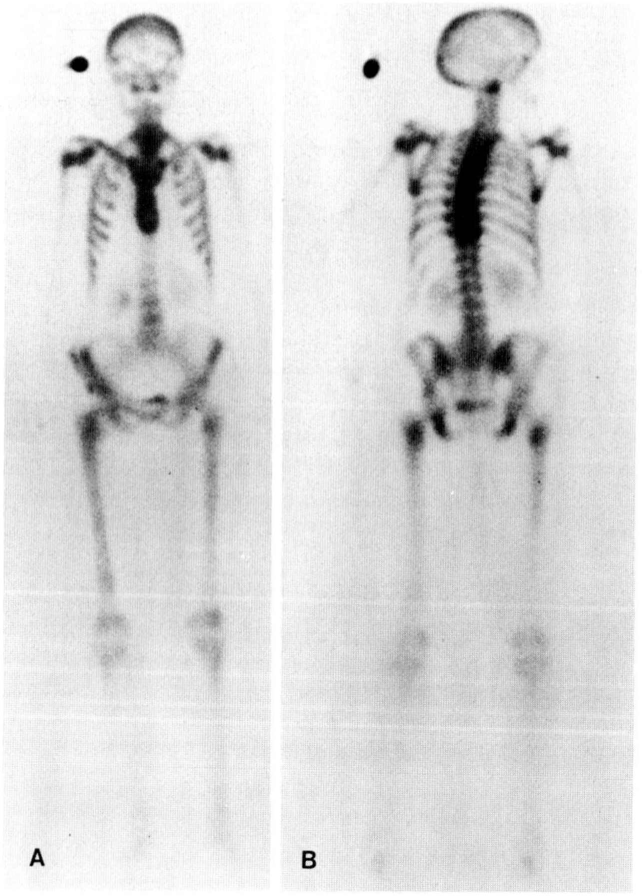

**Figure 38-1. (A)** Anterior and **(B)** posterior radionuclide bone scans that appear to be within normal limits.

on bone metabolism. Occasionally, an abnormality is manifested as a focal area of decreased labeling (photopenic lesion), caused by nearly complete replacement of normal bone by neoplastic tissue. In rare instances, widespread tumor infiltration of bone may result in diffusely increased labeling of the entire skeleton. This scan appearance can be erroneously interpreted as normal because of the uniform, symmetric uptake of isotope (Fig. 38-1). However, the clue to the proper diagnosis is that there is usually decreased or no labeling of the kidneys. In pa-

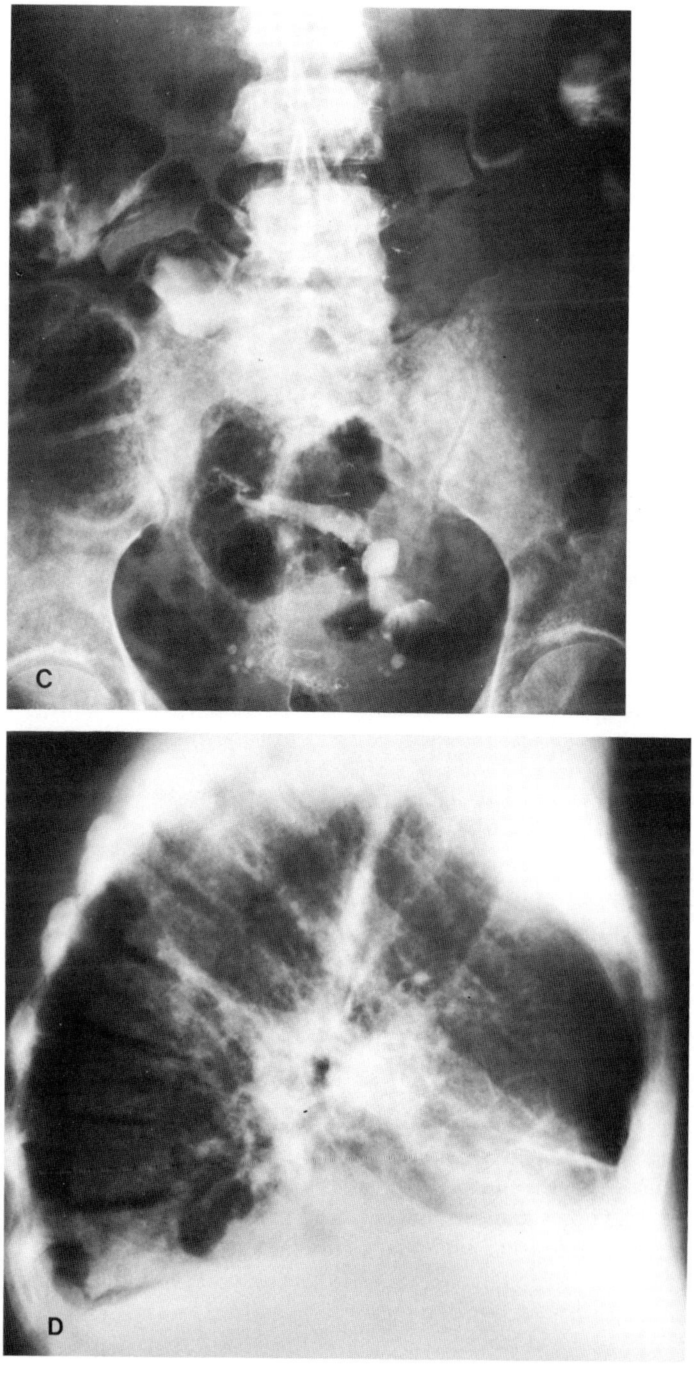

**Figure 38-1.** (*Continued*) **(C)** Anteroposterior view of the lumbar spine and **(D)** lateral view of the thoracic spine demonstrate diffuse blastic metastases secondary to carcinoma of the breast. This is an example of increased uniform and symmetric labeling due to diffuse metastatic disease. Of interest, the labeling of the kidneys is only minimally decreased in this patient.

tients with diffuse bony metastases, so much of the radionuclide is taken up by the skeletal structures that little or none remains to be excreted by the usual renal route.

False-negative radionuclide bone scans occasionally occur in certain clinical situations. Myeloma and metastases from certain anaplastic tumors sometimes stimulate little host response and therefore may produce no focal abnormality on the isotope scan. A similar lack of uptake with skeletal metastases may occasionally occur in severely debilitated patients with impaired host response. Radiation therapy may mask metastatic lesions because of alteration of local vascularity. Metastatic disease in the pelvis may also be obscured by excess activity in a distended urinary bladder; therefore, the patient should void before the examination. To eliminate many of these potential sources of false-negative examinations, a radiograph of the pelvis should be obtained when no abnormalities are detected on the radionuclide bone scan.

The adjunctive use of single photon emission computed tomography (SPECT) for radionuclide bone scanning holds the promise of increased diagnostic accuracy. Early experience with SPECT imaging of the skeleton suggests that this technique may improve the delineation of questionable areas of increased isotope uptake. It may also increase sensitivity and specificity by detecting alterations in normal morphology caused by less reactive processes (*e.g.*, multiple myeloma). Thus, further regional evaluation by SPECT scanning may be indicated when conventional radionuclide bone scans are negative or equivocal in the face of strong clinical symptoms or suspicion.

## Conventional Radiography

Conventional radiography, in the form of a "skeletal survey," should be largely abandoned as a screening examination for metastases because of its relative insensitivity. The radionuclide bone scan can detect early or very small metastatic lesions, whereas significant bone destruction or bone reaction must occur before a lesion can be recognized radiographically. This is especially true in the axial skeleton, which is composed of mostly trabecular rather than cortical bone. Experimental studies have demonstrated that approximately 30% to 50% of the bone in a vertebral body must be destroyed before it can be detected radiographically.

The only rational use of conventional radiography as a screening test for metastases is in the evaluation of patients with plasma cell dyscrasias, most commonly myeloma. These tumors elicit little host response, and studies have shown that 27% to 50% of radiographically demonstrable metastatic lesions of this type are missed by radionuclide bone scanning.

It is imperative that all symptomatic sites in patients with neoplastic disease be examined radiographically unless the radionuclide bone scan unequivocally demonstrates diffuse metastatic disease. This approach is required because of the possibility of a false-negative bone scan, as previously discussed.

Although the radionuclide bone scan is extremely sensitive, it is, unfortunately, not very specific. Many benign lesions may also cause an abnormality. Therefore it is essential to further evaluate most focal abnormalities with an imaging modality that permits a more specific diagnosis. Conventional radiography is the preferred technique because it is inexpensive, universally available, and has relatively high spatial resolution, which may permit the diagnosis of a precise pathologic entity. There are several exceptions to the theoretical "rule" requiring radiography of all focal scan abnormalities. The presence of multiple focal abnormalities involving the axial skeleton and, occasionally, the shafts of long bones is typical of metastatic disease; therefore, it is necessary only to examine radiographically a single lesion or area to confirm the diagnosis (Fig. 38-2). It is not necessary to repeat the radiographs when scans are performed for follow-up examinations to determine therapeutic response or progression of disease. Focal areas of increased labeling in joints, usually in the lower extremities (but sometimes also in upper extremities) in older patients is a pattern that is so characteristic of degenerative arthritis that radiographic confirmation need not be obtained (Fig. 38-3).

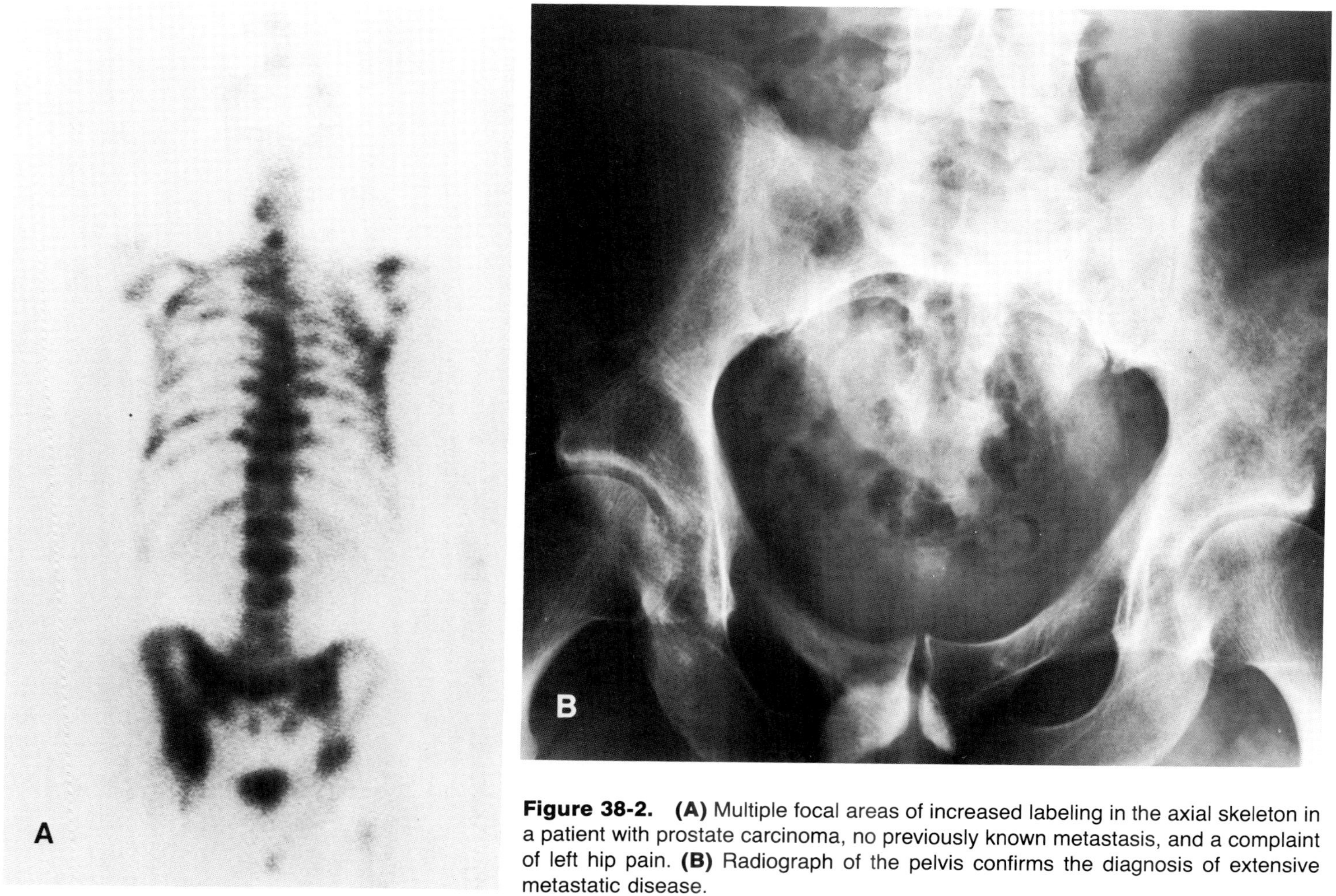


**Figure 38-2.** **(A)** Multiple focal areas of increased labeling in the axial skeleton in a patient with prostate carcinoma, no previously known metastasis, and a complaint of left hip pain. **(B)** Radiograph of the pelvis confirms the diagnosis of extensive metastatic disease.

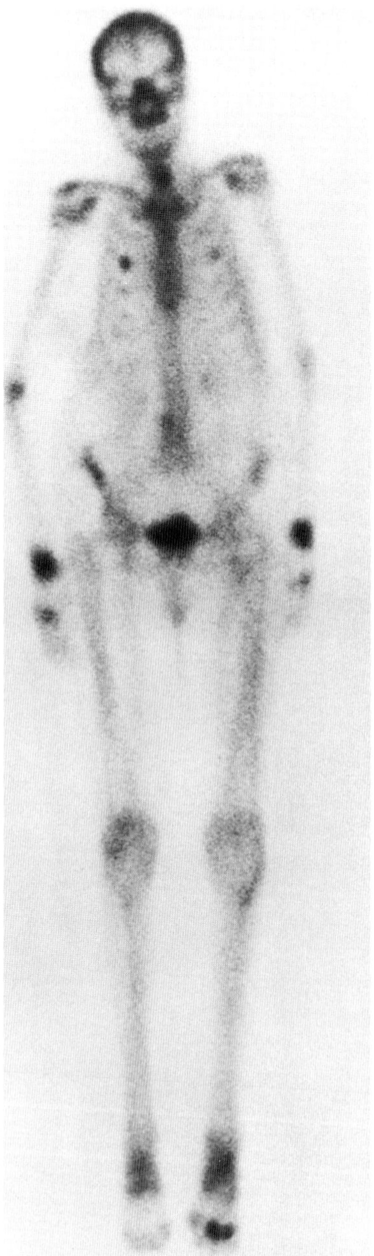

**Figure 38-3.** Radionuclide bone scan demonstrates focal areas of increased labeling around both knees, ankles, wrists, and several metacarpophalangeal joints of both hands and the metatarsophalangeal joints of the left foot, all of which are typical of degenerative arthritis. Increased labeling of the third anterior ribs bilaterally is due to rib fractures that were confirmed radiographically.

If radiographs demonstrate a typically benign process corresponding in location to the solitary focal abnormality detected on the radionuclide bone scan, it may be assumed that this benign lesion is the cause of the scan abnormality. Although not proven in controlled studies, experience has shown that it is exceedingly rare for a solitary metastatic lesion to be completely obscured by a radiographically demonstrable benign process. Occasionally, pathologic fractures may be difficult to distinguish radiographically from simple fractures, especially in the ribs. If doubt persists in a given case, further evaluation with the modalities discussed later in this chapter should resolve the question.

Focal bone scan abnormalities that are associated with normal radiographs generally represent metastatic lesions. In most instances, the lesions will become radiographically apparent within 3 to 18 months. False positives are extremely rare. In some circumstances, however, more specific confirmation than the inferential diagnosis of positive scan–negative radiograph is required. This is especially important when a solitary scan abnormality (normal radiographically) is the sole evidence for changing the patient's classification at the time of initial presentation from *in situ* or local disease to disseminated metastases (Fig. 38-4). A second example is the patient with known neoplastic disease who is being considered for palliative treatment with radiation therapy for focal pain (Fig. 38-5). In both cases, the inferential diagnosis is frequently considered inadequate proof because of tremendous therapeutic and prognostic implications in the former, and the potential risk of injury in the latter. Therefore, computed tomography (CT), magnetic resonance imaging (MRI), and even biopsy may be required.

## Computed Tomography

Computed tomography has replaced conventional tomography and fine-detail radiography for the evaluation of specific abnormalities identified on a screening radionuclide bone scan. In addition, CT is employed to evaluate specific areas that are symptomatic and clinically suspi-

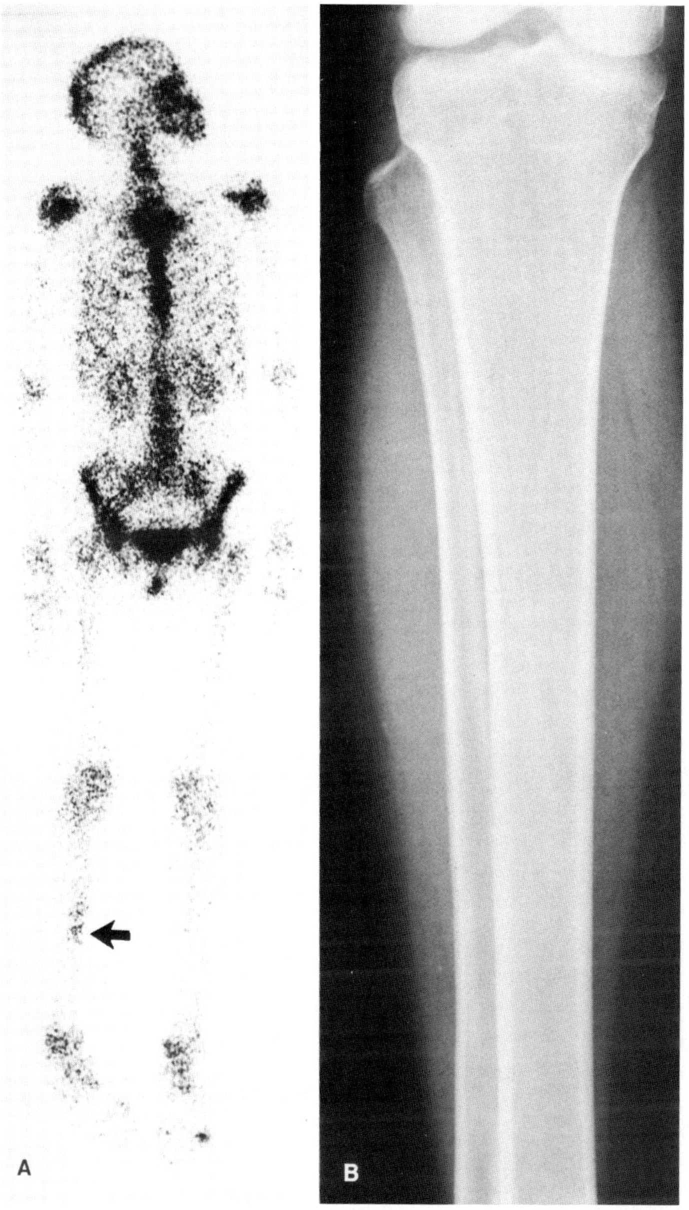

**Figure 38-4.** **(A)** Radionuclide bone scan demonstrates focal area of increased labeling (*arrow*) in the right tibia during initial staging of a patient with histiocytic lymphoma. **(B)** The radiograph was normal, and the lesion could not be identified by other modalities. Open biopsy confirmed the diagnosis of a lymphomatous lesion.

cious after conventional radiography has failed to demonstrate or adequately characterize a lesion (Figs. 38-5 and 38-6). It must be emphasized, however, that CT should never be considered as an initial screening examination for suspected skeletal metastases.

The superb inherent contrast resolution of CT (approximately tenfold greater than that of radiography) and the cross-sectional imaging display make this modality very sensitive for identifying skeletal lesions, especially in the flat bones and vertebrae. Destruction of trabecular bone or replacement of marrow fat by neoplastic tissue results in alteration of the attenuation value (CT number), which enables detection of small medullary lesions too subtle to be recognized with other radiographic modalities.

(*Text continues on p. 565.*)

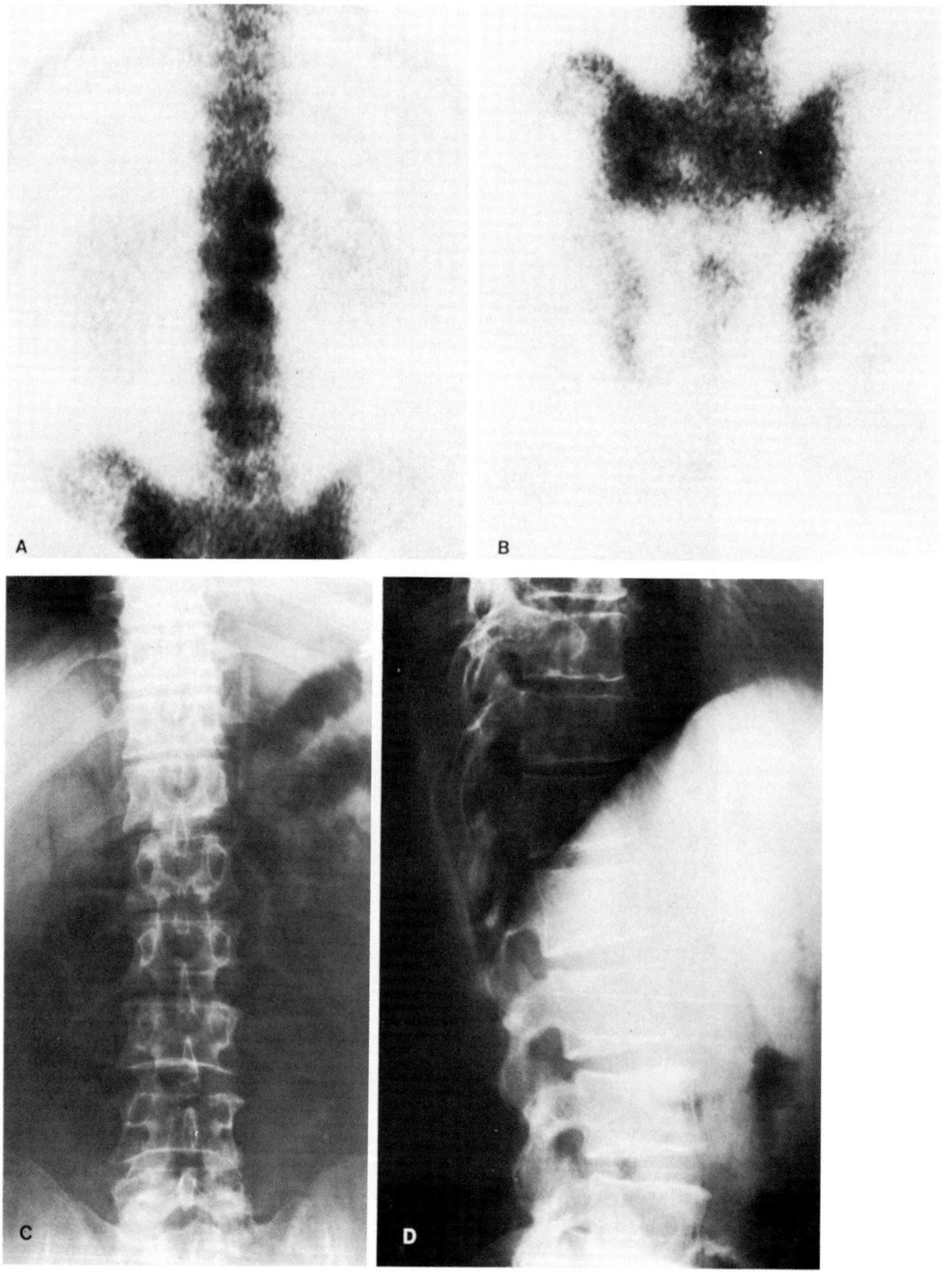
A
B
C
D

**Figure 38-5.** **(A)** Anterior and **(B)** posterior radionuclide bone scans demonstrate multiple focal areas of increased labeling in a patient with lung carcinoma who had no previously known metastatic disease but who developed severe back pain. **(C, D)** Plain radiographs of the lumbar spine were considered equivocal. Conventional tomograms were also equivocal. **(E, F, G)** CT scans confirm destructive lesions in several vertebrae and the sacrum (*arrows*), typical of metastatic disease.

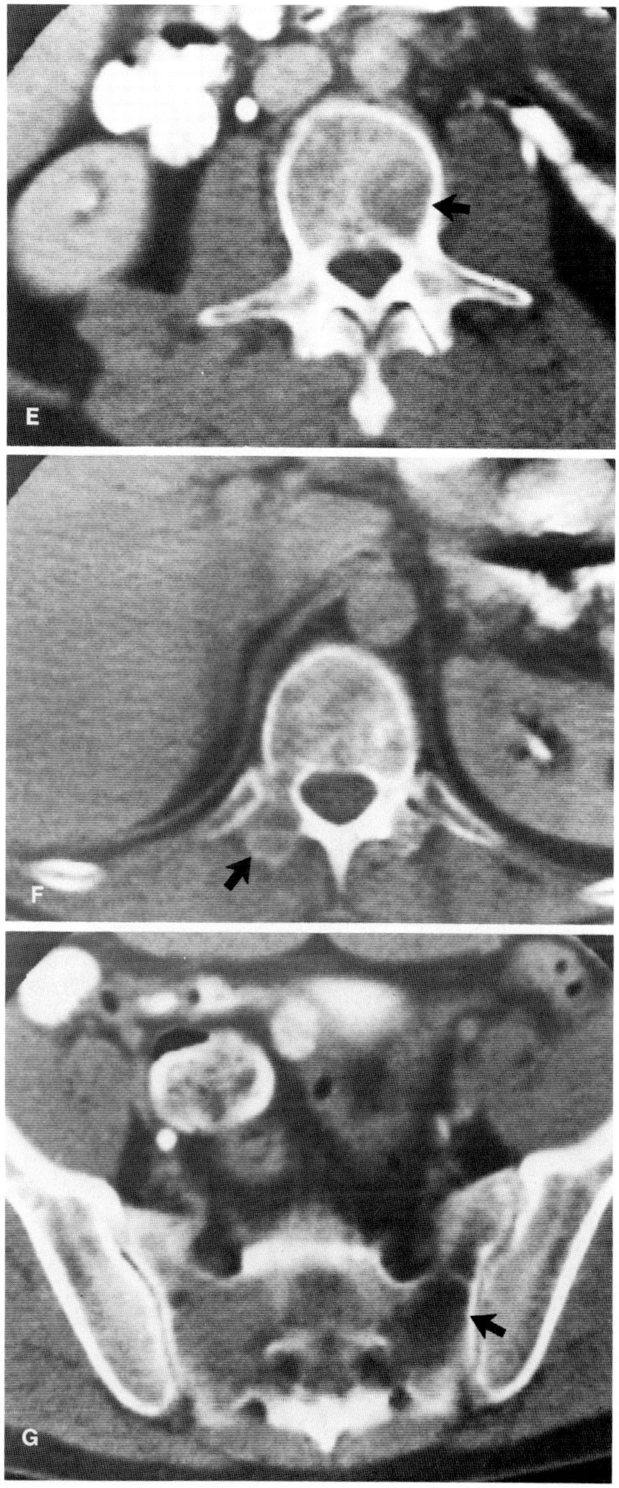

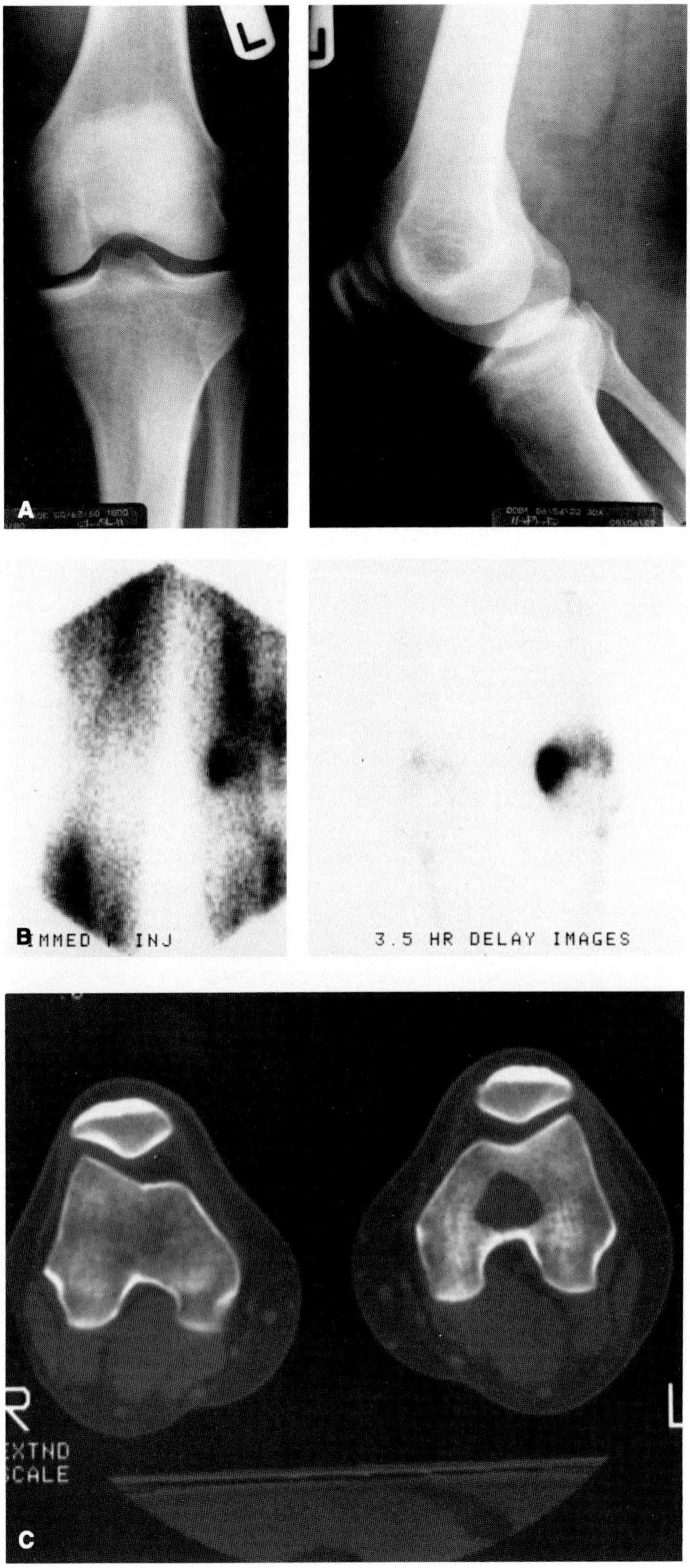


**Figure 38-6. (A)** Anteroposterior and lateral radiographs of the left knee in a 31-year-old man with a 1-month history of left knee pain. The examination was interpreted as normal. **(B)** Radionuclide bone scan demonstrates increased uptake in the region of the medial femoral condyle and in the vastus lateralis muscle group of the left knee on the blood-pool sequence (*left*) and markedly increased uptake in the epiphyseal portion of the left femur, especially the medial femoral condyle, on the delayed images (*right*). **(C)** CT scan shows a focal area of destruction primarily involving the intercondylar region of the left femur. Needle biopsy resulted in a diagnosis of large cell lymphoma.

In patients with known neoplastic disease who have a nonspecific focal abnormality on the radionuclide scan, demonstration of a characteristic lesion on CT may permit the institution of palliative radiotherapy even without a proven tissue diagnosis.

Computed tomography is noninvasive and is risk free except for the radiation dose.

### Magnetic Resonance Imaging

The role of MRI in the detection of skeletal metastases is not yet clearly defined. In the immediate future, MRI will be a secondary or tertiary diagnostic modality and serve as an alternative or, occasionally, as a complement to CT for further evaluation of specific radionuclide scan abnormalities that have a normal or indeterminate appearance on conventional radiography. Like CT, only a region of the skeleton can be evaluated by MRI, and thus this technique should be employed for further evaluation of a suspicious lesion rather than for whole body screening for "silent" metastases.

Normal bone appears on MRI as a moderate to high signal intensity (seen as gray to white) of the medullary bone, which is principally due to the contribution of marrow fat. This is surrounded by the very low signal intensity (seen as black) of cortical bone. A metastatic lesion in medullary bone appears on T1-weighted images as a focal area of variably decreased signal intensity compared with normal fat-containing marrow (Fig. 38-7). On T2-weighted images, a metastasis typically produces an area of relatively increased signal intensity compared with normal fat-containing marrow. Metastatic involvement of the cortex usually appears as a focal heterogeneous signal intensity in the normally very homogenous, low signal intensity of cortical bone. It may also cause an irregularity of the usually smooth cortical margin.

The superior soft-tissue contrast of MRI compared with CT permits better recognition of the extension of metastases beyond the confines of affected bone into adjacent soft-tissue structures. This depiction of extraosseous spread, combined with the capability of producing direct coronal and sagittal images, makes MRI extremely valuable for both surgical and radiation therapy planning.

Magnetic resonance imaging has no known complications and does not subject the patient to ionizing radiation. However, it is expensive and currently not as widely available as CT. In the near future, the choice between CT and MRI in assessing a suspected metastatic lesion will probably be determined by their relative availability.

### Needle Biopsy

Needle biopsy is the best method when a tissue diagnosis of a suspected metastatic lesion is required. The nature and location of the lesion govern the biopsy technique. Osteolytic lesions or those with a soft-tissue component can be successfully biopsied with a Vim or Tru-Cut needle (Travenol) or simply by fine-needle aspiration. Osteoblastic or medullary lesions with surrounding intact cortex require a large cutting needle, such as the Craig (Becton-Dickinson) or Ackerman (Sianco, Becton-Dickinson) needle. The procedure usually is performed under local anesthesia, although general anesthesia may be required for vertebral lesions. Fluoroscopic guidance is usually sufficient, but CT may be helpful, particularly when it is the only modality that can demonstrate the lesion. "Blind" needle biopsy, performed when a radionuclide scan abnormality is the only evidence of a lesion, is likely to be unrewarding and is rarely done, although risk versus benefit must be judged in each case. Several series have reported 80% to 90% accuracy rates for needle biopsies.

Complications of the fine-needle aspiration technique are virtually nonexistent. With the cutting technique, pain is the most frequent complication, although bleeding and infection have also been reported. When the biopsy is in the thoracic region, pneumothorax may occur with either technique, and meticulous care is mandatory. Tumor seeding of the needle tract is a theoretical complication, but it is of little practical significance in metastatic lesions because there has not been a reported case.

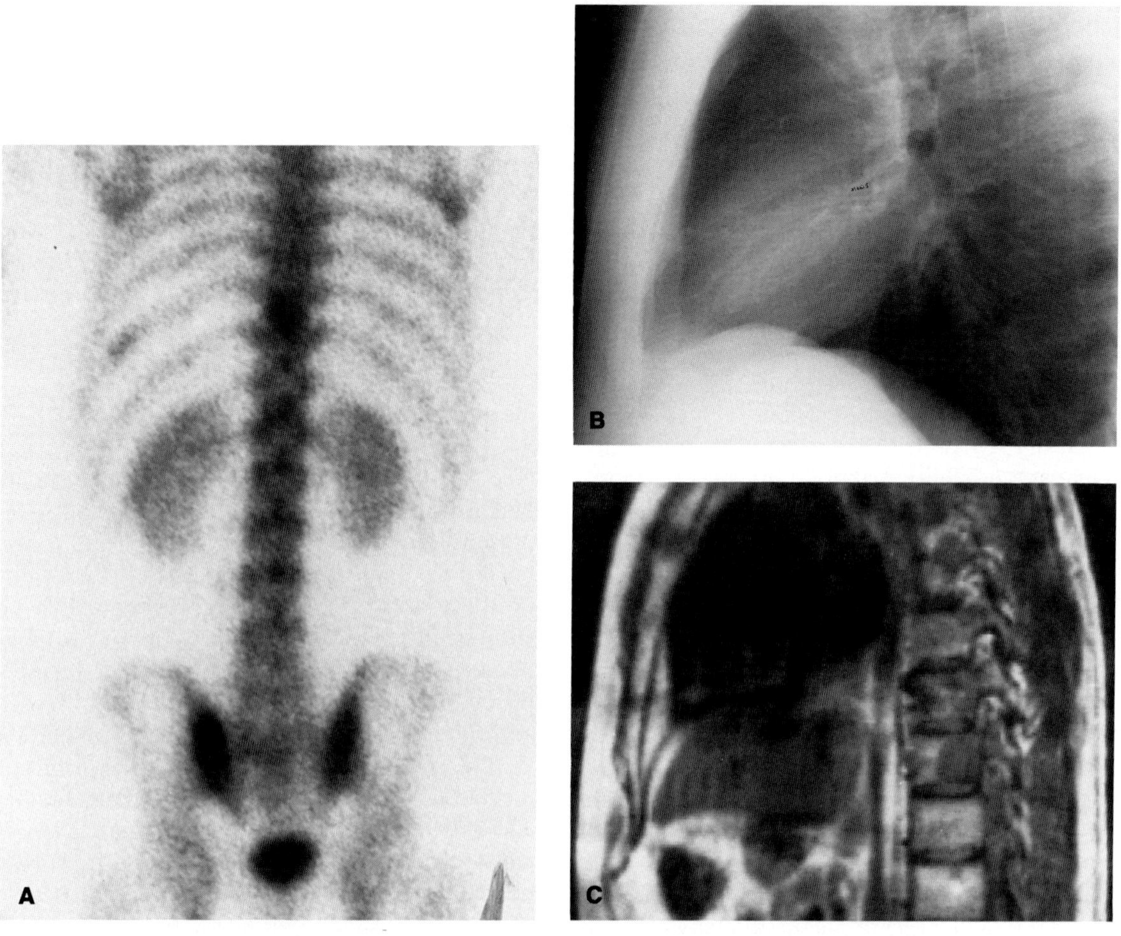

**Figure 38-7. (A)** Radionuclide scan demonstrates a focal area of increased labeling in the T9 vertebral body in this 26-year-old man with back pain and known rhabdomyosarcoma of the shoulder. **(B)** Lateral radiograph of the thoracic spine was considered normal and did not explain the abnormality on the bone scan. **(C)** T1-weighted sagittal MRI (TE, 30 msec; TR, 500 msec) demonstrates a focal area of decreased signal intensity in the T9 vertebral body corresponding to the abnormality on the bone scan. This was subsequently confirmed to be a metastatic lesion.

## Surgical Biopsy

Open surgical biopsy is the ultimate method for obtaining diagnostic proof of the presence of skeletal metastases. However, with the current wide availability of less invasive diagnostic modalities, open surgical biopsy should rarely be required for this purpose. When surgical biopsy is contemplated as a last recourse for diagnostic confirmation, a careful review of all previous imaging studies is necessary to avoid the pitfall of missing the lesion. Whenever possible, intraoperative radiographic localization of the biopsy site should be performed.

Although the risk of open surgical biopsy is obviously dependent on the location of the lesion, complications of the procedure are primarily those associated with anesthesia. Pathologic fracture, infection, or bleeding may occur following surgical biopsy, but they are uncommon.

## Bibliography

Adler O, Rosenberger A: Fine needle aspiration biopsy of osteolytic metastatic lesions. AJR 133: 15–18, 1979

Daffner RH, Lupetin AR, Dash N et al: MRI in the detection of malignant infiltration of bone marrow. AJR 146:353–358, 1986

deSantos LA, Lukeman JM, Wallace S et al: Percutaneous needle biopsy of bone in the cancer patient. AJR 130:641–649, 1978

Genant HK, Cann CE, Chafetz NI et al: Advances in computed tomography of the skeletal system. Radiol Clin North Am 19:645–674, 1981

Hardy DC, Murphy WA, Gilula LA: Computed tomography in planning percutaneous bone biopsy. Radiology 134:447–450, 1980

Mall JC, Beckerman C, Hoffer PB et al: A unified radiological approach to the detection of skeletal metastases. Radiology 118:323–328, 1976

McNeil BJ: Rationale for the use of bone scans in selected metastatic and primary bone tumors. Semin Nucl Med 8:336–345, 1978

Pistenna DA, McDougall R, Kriss JP: Screening for bone metastases—Are only scans necessary? JAMA 231:46–50, 1975

Wilson JS, Korobkin M, Genant HK et al: Computed tomography of musculoskeletal disorders. AJR 131:55–61, 1978

## SUSPECTED SKELETAL METASTASES

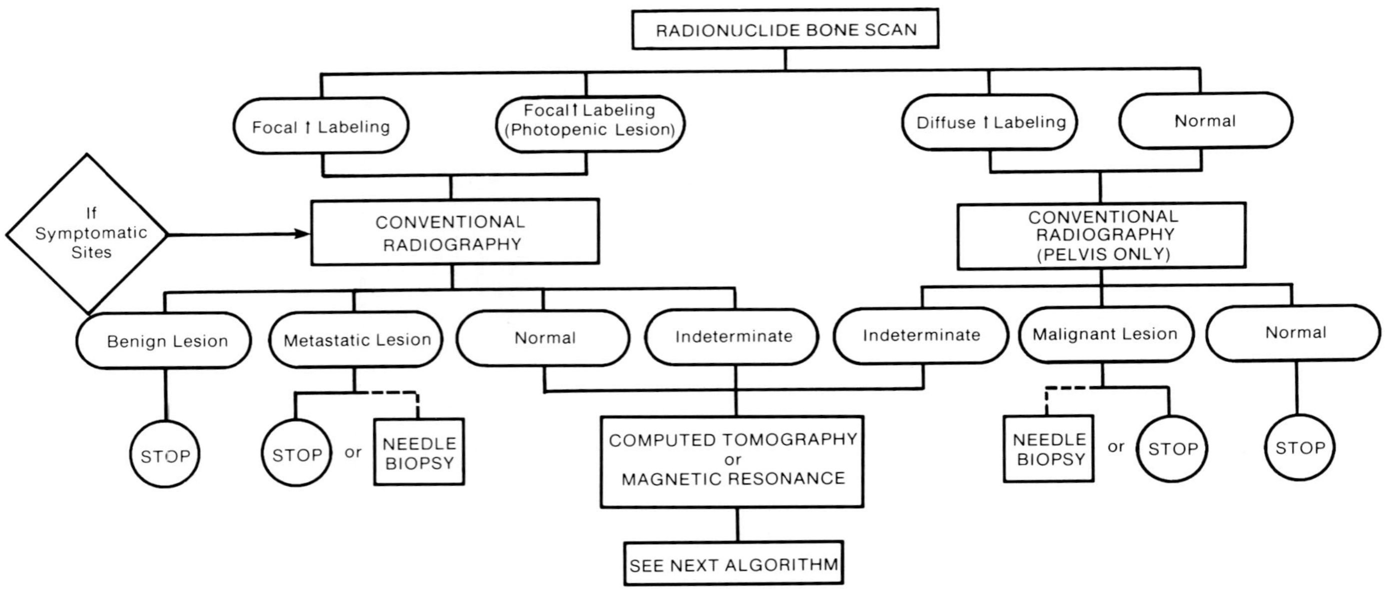

**SUSPECTED SKELETAL METASTASES**

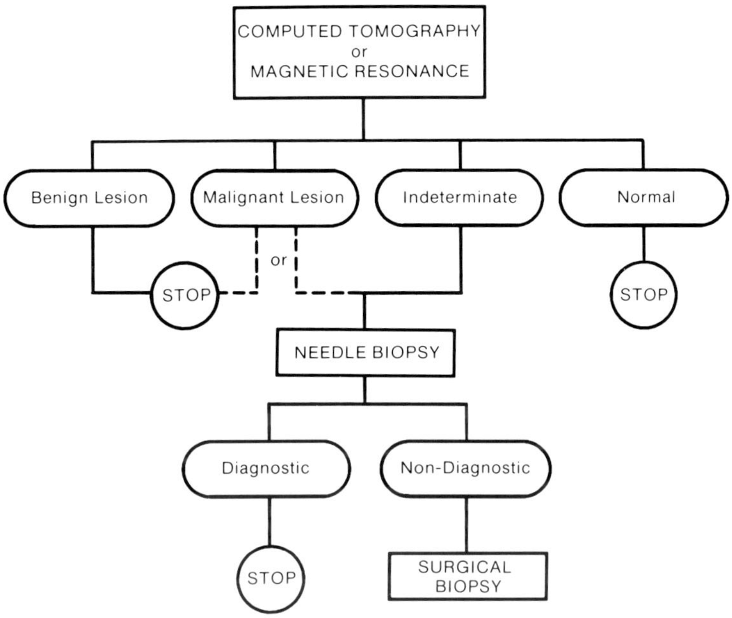

# Chapter 39

# Central Nervous System Metastases

*David B. Hackney*

Up to 20% of patients with systemic cancer develop significant neurologic symptoms, most of which are due to central nervous system metastases. Although cures are rare in this population, early diagnosis and appropriate treatment may significantly prolong survival and improve the quality of life. Current imaging techniques are highly sensitive and specific for detecting central nervous system metastases and have a very low procedure-related morbidity.

For the purposes of this chapter, metastases involving the central nervous system can be conveniently classified into four categories by the structures affected: intracerebral, spinal, leptomeningeal, and metastases involving other sites.

## INTRACEREBRAL METASTASES

Brain metastases occur in approximately 10% to 15% of patients dying of cancer, and up to three fourths of these patients have suffered neurologic symptoms during life. The most common primary tumor sites are lung, breast, skin (melanoma), gastrointestinal tract, and kidney. The high incidence of brain metastases from lung cancer (31%–53% of patients) reflects both the frequent occurrence of this neoplasm and the unique position of the lung in the circulatory system. Indeed, hematogenous metastases to the brain (regardless of the primary site) usually arise from tumor deposits in the lung. This "cascade" phenomenon implies that when brain metastases are detected, dissemination to other sites is likely. However, since brain metastases frequently become symptomatic when quite small, they may be detected earlier than metastases to other organs. In addition, asymptomatic brain metastases are often identified by computed tomography (CT).

Brain metastases primarily involve the cerebrum (81%); the cerebellum (16%) and brain stem (3%) are less common sites. Solitary metastases are reported to occur in 14% to 35% of patients and are especially common in metastases from breast and renal-cell carcinoma.

Metastatic tumor cells typically lodge at the gray matter–white matter junction and often produce gross edema of the white matter, which may be disproportionately great considering the size of the tumor. Large masses are often soft or liquefied and may reach the surface of the brain and infiltrate the leptomeninges.

Although the vessels in the center of a well-developed metastasis lack a blood–brain barrier (BBB), metastatic deposits are initially supplied by normal brain vessels with an intact BBB. Therefore, brain metastases may be isolated from systemic chemotherapy as well as from diagnostic imaging techniques that rely on detecting BBB defects.

Hemorrhage may be observed in intracerebral metastases, especially those from choriocarcinoma, melanoma, bronchogenic carcinoma, and renal-cell carcinoma. The hemorrhage tends to occur at the periphery of the tumor, rather than centrally. Brain metastases infrequently calcify. Initial reports indicated that calcification developed in 1% to 2% of intracranial metastases. A slightly higher calcification rate has been reported in more recent studies in the CT era.

Headache is the single most common presenting symptom in patients with brain metastases, although it occurs in only about half the cases. Other common complaints include focal weakness, behavorial or mental changes, gait ataxia, seizures (more commonly generalized than focal), and speech difficulty. A classic, although relatively infrequent, symptom of primary or secondary brain tumor is an early morning headache that disappears after rising, recurs the following night, and progresses with time. In most patients, the clinical signs and symptoms progress over a period of days to weeks. An acute presentation may result from seizures with or without hemorrhage into the neoplasm.

## DIAGNOSTIC IMAGING

### *DIAGNOSTIC MODALITIES*

1. Computed tomography without contrast enhancement
2. Contrast-enhanced computed tomography
3. Magnetic resonance imaging
4. Contrast-enhanced magnetic resonance imaging

#### Computed Tomography Without Contrast Enhancement

Most radiographically detectable brain metastases can be identified by plain CT. The dominant feature of the lesion on noncontrast scans is edema, the magnitude of which may be strikingly out of proportion to the size of the neoplasm. The attenuation characteristics of a metastasis are nonspecific, and the mass may have a value less than, equal to, or greater than that of surrounding brain parenchyma. Calcification is very rarely identified.

#### Contrast-Enhanced Computed Tomography

Computed tomography with intravenous contrast enhancement is the single most valuable imaging modality for detecting and characterizing intracerebral metastases (Fig. 39-1). The overwhelming majority of metastases detected by CT demonstrate contrast enhancement. Although it is not clear to what extent contrast enhancement increases the sensitivity of CT scanning for de-

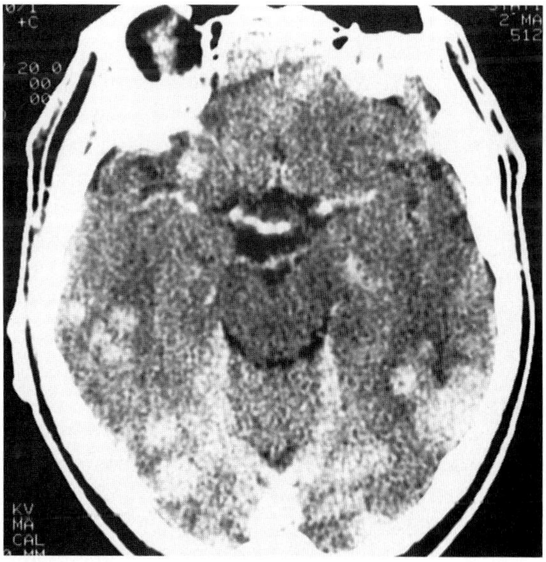

**Figure 39-1.** CT scan with intravenous contrast demonstrates multiple enhancing intracerebral metastases.

tecting abnormalities, enhanced scans are considerably more specific because they demonstrate disruption of the blood–brain barrier, which is extremely common in well-developed metastatic lesions. In patients with only mild disruption of the blood–brain barrier, prolonged exposure to high iodine concentrations may be required for a detectable amount of contrast material to accumulate in the lesion. Thus, delayed high-dose contrast scans may better demonstrate a lesion or detect additional lesions that cannot be identified on immediate postcontrast scans.

Intracerebral metastases are infrequent in patients with leukemia or lymphoma. In a review of 156 patients with leukemia and positive cerebrospinal fluid cytology, leukemic brain masses were identified in only eight (all with acute leukemia). No masses were identified in another 89 patients with leukemia and normal cerebrospinal fluid cytology. The leukemic masses were isodense or hypodense to normal brain on noncontrast scans and were associated with a variable degree of edema. After the administration of contrast material, these masses demonstrated homogeneous or peripheral enhancement. Of 160 patients with lymphoma in the same report, lymphomatous masses were identified in seven, all of whom were among the 22 patients with abnormal cerebrospinal fluid cytology. The masses were isodense to slightly hyperdense on noncontrast scans and showed homogeneous enhancement (Fig. 39-2).

The administration of contrast material in patients with intracerebral metastases entails a risk of precipitating iatrogenic seizures, especially if there is a pre-existing seizure history. Prophylaxis with diazepam is recommended for such patients.

## Magnetic Resonance Imaging

Magnetic resonance imaging (MRI) has proven to be far more sensitive than CT for detecting abnormalities of the brain parenchyma. Magnetic resonance imaging is of particular advantage when suitable CT scans cannot be obtained. Patients with renal failure or a history of severe contrast reaction are best evaluated by MRI to avoid the risks involved in contrast administration. In certain portions of the cranial cavity, especially the posterior and middle fossae, artifacts tend to degrade the CT image. Although thin-section CT and coronal scanning may partially overcome this limitation, these artifacts do not occur with MRI, and multiplanar imaging can be obtained more easily using MRI than with CT. Magnetic resonance imaging may be used to further evaluate equivocal findings on CT scans or to search for additional abnormalities. Small metastases with little or no contrast enhancement and minimal edema may be very difficult to detect by CT. The high sensitivity of MRI for identifying edema should provide an increased rate of detection of small lesions. This is especially important if the diagnosis of metastatic disease is in doubt, because in some cases the multiplicity of lesions alone may confirm the diagnosis. If a biopsy is required but the abnormality revealed by CT is relatively inaccessible, MRI may be useful in identifying a more suitable biopsy site.

Spin-echo pulse sequences with long repetition times (TR) and echo times (TE) provide the greatest contrast between most intraparenchymal lesions and normal brain. These parameters produce images that maximize contrast based on differences in T2 and spin density. Brain edema and most intraparenchymal lesions have slower spin–spin relaxation rates (longer T2) and higher spin densities than normal brain. Although a number of studies have attempted to identify the ideal screening pulse sequences for detecting intraparenchymal brain lesions, practical scanning continues to represent a compromise among sensitivity, specificity, scanning time, and patient cooperation.

The differentiation of edema from a true lesion may often be difficult if incorrect timing parameters (TR, TE) are employed. It is possible to select parameters that maximize or minimize contrast between normal and abnormal tissues and between edema and tumor. However, if inappropriate parameters are used, much information potentially obtainable from MR images may be lost. In most instances, the solution to

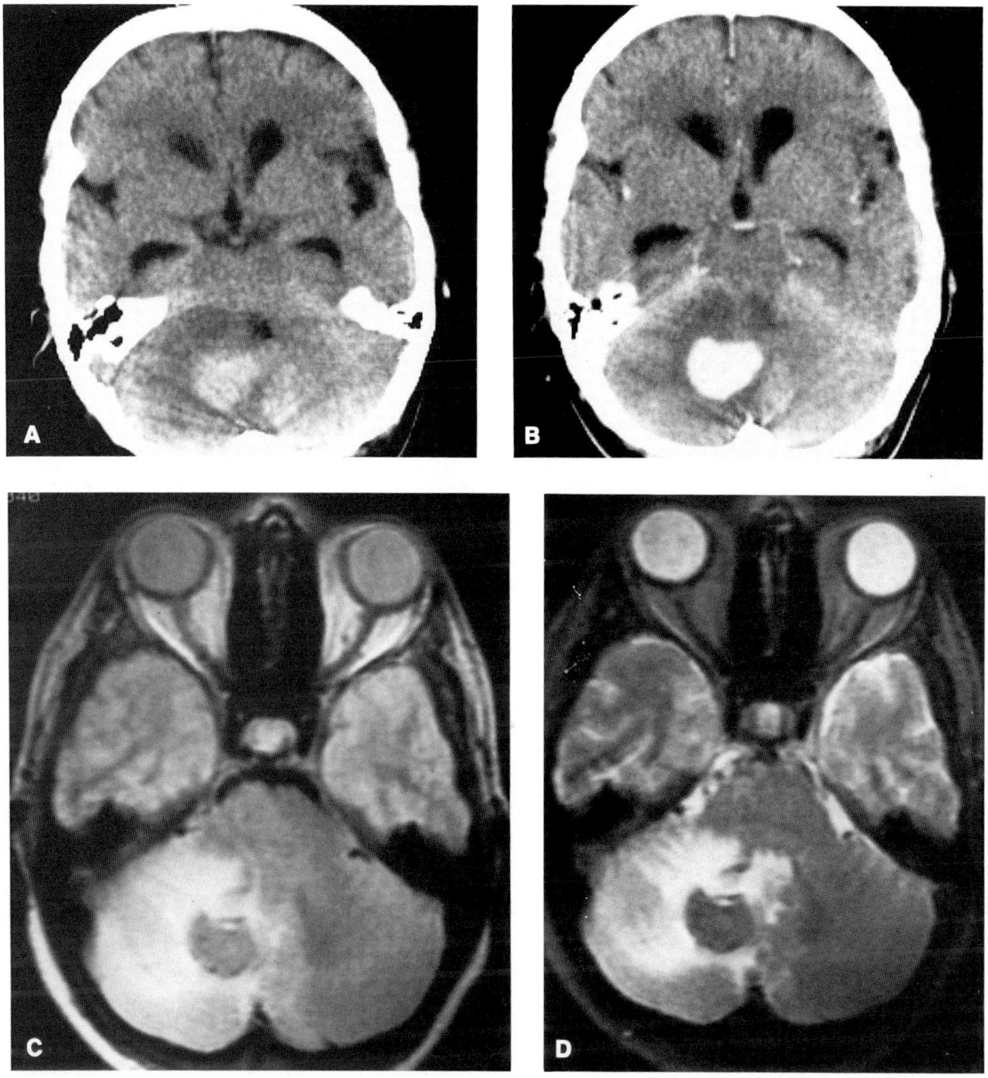

**Figure 39-2. (A)** Noncontrast and **(B)** contrast CT scans show a solitary cerebellar lesion that is initially isodense to slightly hyperdense and enhances uniformly. This pattern is typical of a metastasis from non-Hodgkin's lymphoma. Spin-echo MR images (TR, 2500 msec; TE, 30 msec **[C]**; and TE, 80 msec **[D]**) show the mass to be isointense to slightly hypointense to the cerebellum, very well-demarcated, and surrounded by considerable edema.

this problem includes performing a number of scans with different parameters or generating synthesized images based on calculated relaxation and density values. Both strategies are intended to produce sets of images in which the contributions of T1, T2, and spin density to signal intensity vary, so as to avoid the possibility that a lesion will have the same intensity as normal brain and thus be missed on images produced with a single set of parameters.

There have been reports of T1-weighted images having a success rate of 80% in differentiating tumor from edema. These tumors had longer T1 values than edema and thus appeared as areas of lower signal intensity on T1-weighted spin-echo or inversion-recovery images.

### Contrast-Enhanced Magnetic Resonance Imaging

Gadolinium diethylenetriaminepentaacetic acid (Gd-DTPA) is the most widely tested contrast agent for clinical MRI. After intravenous administration, the clearance of gadolinium from the blood and uptake in brain lesions appears to parallel the behavior of standard iodinated radiographic contrast media. At present, however, there is insufficient data to adequately compare contrast-enhanced MRI and CT examinations.

## SPINAL METASTASES

Spinal metastasis is a fundamentally different disease from intracerebral metastasis. Unlike intracerebral metastatic lesions that primarily involve the parenchyma of the central nervous system, spinal metastases affect the cord only secondarily due to compression by tumor masses. Intramedullary metastases are extremely rare.

The overwhelming majority (97%) of spinal metastases are epidural lesions, most of which reflect osseous metastases to the vertebral bodies. Approximately 20% to 35% of patients with extraskeletal primary malignancies develop skeletal metastases during the course of their disease, and approximately 5% of cancer patients develop symptomatic spinal epidural metastases. The most common primary malignancies causing skeletal metastases are cancers of the breast, prostate, lung, and kidney, as well as lymphoma and myeloma. Approximately one half of all spinal metastases arise in patients with lymphoma or carcinomas of the lung or breast.

As the life expectancy of cancer patients improves, the incidence of spinal metastases will increase. Similarly, the impact of prompt diagnosis and treatment on the subsequent quality of life will become greater as longevity increases. Except in cases of high cervical cord compression, spinal metastases themselves are rarely fatal, and 30% of patients with these lesions survive longer than 1 year. Indeed, only a minority of spinal metastases produce symptoms. In a study of 168 patients with breast carcinoma, 59% had spinal metastases but only 8.7% developed cord compression.

Vertebral metastases may occur at any level. The incidence of involvement of each portion of the canal is proportional to its length, so that the thoracic spine is most commonly affected. Cord compression usually occurs at a single level, although in approximately 17% of patients there may be involvement of two or more sites during the course of disease. Metastases to the epidural space generally arise by direct extension from the vertebral body. In contrast, lymphoma may grow through the neural foramen and cause spinal cord compression without bone destruction.

The spinal intervertebral disk and dura mater are significant barriers to tumor extension. Thus, metastases to the vertebral body rarely extend to adjacent vertebrae, and epidural masses rarely involve the subdural or subarachnoid space. Extradural soft-tissue masses may involve the epidural space anteriorly, laterally, or posteriorly. Determination of the precise position of the mass with respect to the thecal sac may be important in planning the surgical therapy.

Cord compression may be caused by the epidural tumor itself or may be secondary to pathologic fracture of a vertebral body with an associated hematoma or retropulsion of osseous fragments. Neurologic dysfunction is caused by vascular compromise (venous compression and congestion) that produces cord ischemia.

Pain is the most common presenting symptom of spinal cord compression due to metastases, occurring in 96% of patients. In most cases, the pain is initially localized to the back at the level of vertebral involvement, develops gradually, and tends to precede other symptoms by several weeks (range of 5 days to 2 years). Radicular pain appears later and is classically unilateral and worse at night. The next most common symptom is weakness, which is present in about 76% of cases by the time of diagnosis. Approximately half of patients have bowel and bladder dysfunction and a similar number have sensory symptoms (*e.g.*, numbness and paresthesias). The onset of motor symptoms usually heralds a period of rapid progression that may lead to paraplegia or quadriplegia within hours or days.

The prognosis for recovery of neurologic function in patients with spinal cord compression due to metastatic disease is related to the nature of the primary malignancy. Hematologic neoplasms have a much better response to therapy than do other lesions. The severity of the neurologic deficit, the rate of progression of dysfunction, and the duration of symptoms also have been related to the prognosis. Complete paraplegia with total loss of all motor and sensory function below the level of the lesion implies very little chance of improvement with treatment (only 2% of these patients regain the ability to walk). If there is some preservation of neurologic function at the time of presentation, the probability of the patient eventually becoming ambulatory rises to 25%. Slowly progressing lesions in which the neurologic deficit develops over several days have a more favorable prognosis than those that develop more rapidly. Patients with long-standing neurologic deficits are less likely to respond to treatment than are those with symptoms of short duration. This higher success rate for earlier and milder deficits emphasizes the need for rapid diagnosis and treatment. Approximately 28% of patients presenting with paraparesis become paraplegic within 24 hours. In some reports, up to 60% of patients presenting with paraparesis became paraplegic before surgical therapy was instituted. Therefore, the imaging evaluation of the patient with a suspected spinal metastasis must not only be specific and detailed, but also must be performed as rapidly as possible.

## DIAGNOSTIC IMAGING

### *DIAGNOSTIC MODALITIES*

1. Plain radiographs of the spine
2. Plain tomography of the spine
3. Radionuclide bone scanning
4. Myelography
5. Computed tomography
6. Magnetic resonance imaging

#### Plain Radiographs of the Spine

Plain radiographs of the spine are abnormal in 60% to 85% of patients with epidural metastases. The most common radiographic pattern is multiple lytic lesions, which usually must be at least 1 cm to 2 cm in diameter to be detected and imply destruction of at least 50% of cancellous bone in the region. Metastases from renal and thyroid primaries may produce bubbly, expansile, cystic-appearing metastases. Osteoblastic lesions arise from carcinomas of the prostate and stomach, medulloblastoma, carcinoid tumor, and osteosarcoma. Metastases from carcinoma of the breast are most commonly lytic, but may be blastic or mixed.

Frontal and lateral plain radiographs of the spine are generally the first imaging procedures obtained in the patient with a suspected epidural spinal metastases. This study can identify most significant osseous metastases and assist in planning the additional examinations that must be performed before appropriate treatment can be instituted. Pathologic collapse of vertebral bodies may produce bone fragments in the spinal canal that contribute to cord compression. Because compression of the spinal cord by bone usually can be relieved by surgery but not by radiotherapy, the identification of osseous fragments may have important therapeutic implications.

#### Plain Tomography of the Spine

Plain tomography of the spine may be of value in identifying and characterizing metastases as well as in determining the severity of encroachment upon the spinal canal by osseous fragments. However, CT is now preferred to plain tomography for making these assessments.

#### Radionuclide Bone Scanning

Radionuclide bone scanning is the most sensitive study for detecting osseous metastases. In 20% to 40% of cases, this modality can identify more skeletal abnormalities than are demonstrated on plain radiographs. Skeletal metastases typically produce multiple areas of increased isotope uptake. A solitary hot spot occurs in approximately 10% of patients. An uncommon pattern produced by some metastases from breast and prostate carcinomas is the "superscan," in which there is diffuse high isotope activity of the skeleton with little or no soft-tissue uptake. Thus, the radionuclide bone scan may be the best imaging modality for identifying skeletal lesions and confirming a diagnosis of metastatic disease. However, acute spinal cord compression requires urgent evaluation, and the findings on radionuclide bone scans are not sufficiently detailed or anatomically precise to assist in planning treatment. Therefore, radionuclide bone scanning usually does not play a role in the initial evaluation of the patient with suspected intraspinal metastases.

## Myelography

Myelography has long been the definitive procedure for evaluating epidural metastases causing compression of the spinal cord or cauda equina. Although CT and MRI are becoming increasingly important in this clinical setting, myelography remains the primary imaging study. In most cases, intrathecal contrast is initially administered via a lumbar puncture unless clinical or radiographic evidence suggests extensive involvement of this region. If it appears likely that a lumbar puncture would entail a significant risk of puncturing the tumor, the initial administration of contrast may be made by the cervical route.

Although analysis of the cerebrospinal fluid may be of value in assessing patients with malignancies, especially those with a tendency to seed the subarachnoid space, removing cerebrospinal fluid after lumbar puncture below a spinal block is potentially dangerous and may precipitate progression of neurologic dysfunction. In one study, the incidence of postmyelographic neurologic deterioration in patients evaluated for spinal block was far higher with lumbar puncture than with cervical puncture. It is assumed that suddenly lowering the pressure below a complete block results in more severe impaction of the spinal cord against the intruding mass, which may produce a more profound compression and ischemia with worsening of the neurologic status. To avoid such complications, it is standard procedure to perform lumbar myelography in these patients without removing any cerebrospinal fluid. If a complete block is encountered, it is clear that contrast material should not be aspirated at the conclusion of the study.

Pantopaque (iophendylate) has been the traditional contrast agent used for myelography in cancer patients. One to three milliliters of contrast are injected and manipulated to the level of the block. Frontal, lateral, and, if needed, oblique radiographs are obtained to document the obstruction and to confirm the epidural nature of the lesion. Water-soluble contrast agents have become increasingly popular for myelography in the patient with a suspected spinal block (Fig. 39-3). This material frequently bypasses areas that would completely obstruct the flow of oily Pantopaque. Although the dilute collection of contrast material above the block may not be detected on plain radiographs, it often can be identified on CT scans. If there is not sufficient contrast above the lesion for a satisfactory CT examination, a C1–C2 puncture is performed to outline the superior extent of the block.

An alternative approach is to force the oily or water-soluble contrast material beyond the block by injecting filtered air, metrizamide diluent, or sterile saline through the spinal puncture needle. Despite the documented risk inherent in changing the pressure around a spinal block, no significant complications have been described in several reports of variations of this technique. An advantage of this approach is the avoidance of a cervical puncture. In addition, if there are multiple blocks along the spinal canal, lumbar and cervical punctures in which contrast material is not pushed beyond the first obstruction do not provide information about the segment of the spinal canal between the lowest and highest blocks.

## Computed Tomography

Computed tomography without intrathecal contrast can define the osseous structure of a patho-

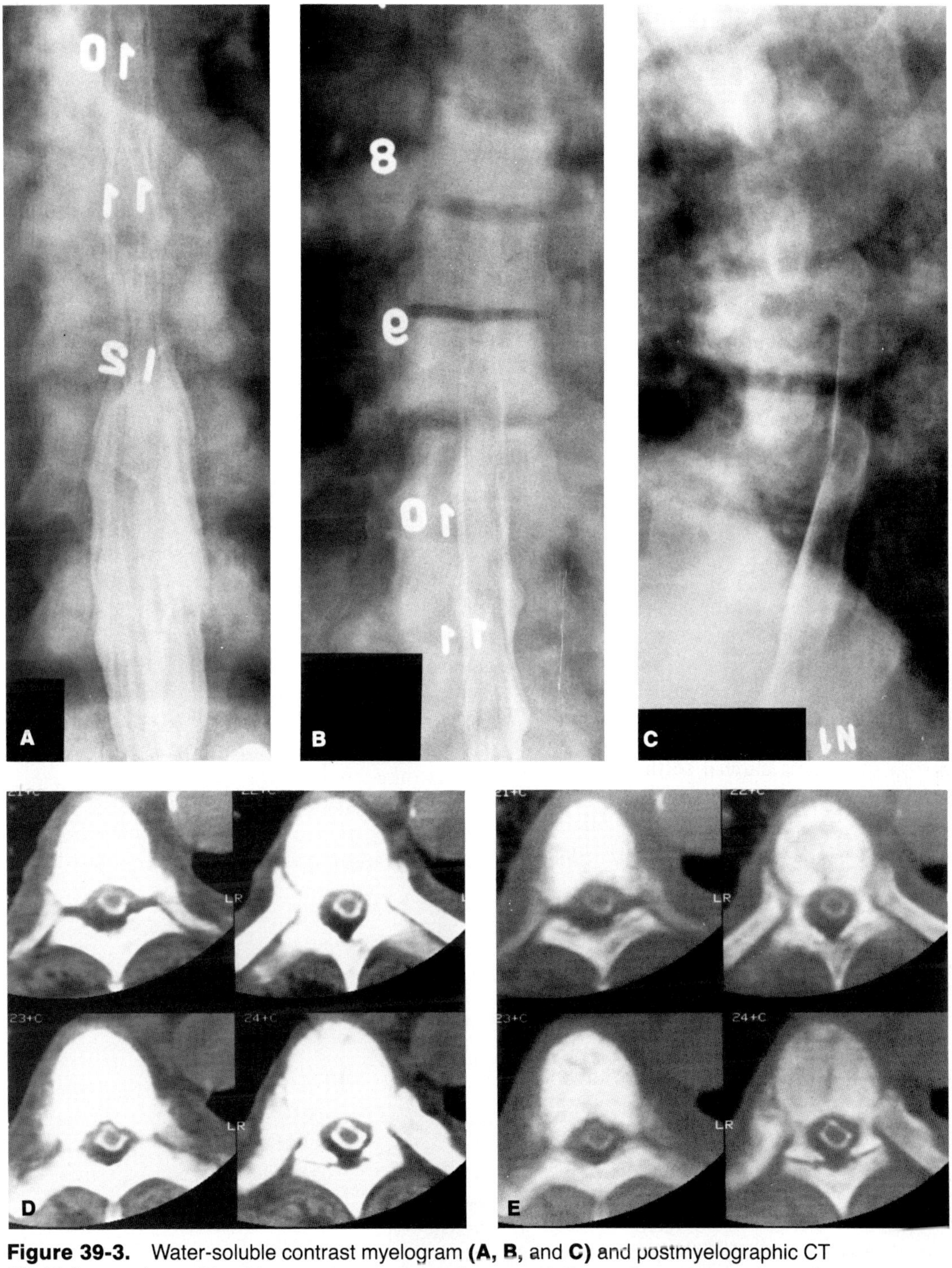


**Figure 39-3.** Water-soluble contrast myelogram **(A, B,** and **C)** and postmyelographic CT **(D, E)** in a patient with widespread metastases from prostatic carcinoma show dramatic obliteration of the intraspinal epidural space beginning at T11–12 and extending rostrally to a nearly complete block at T7 (between the "8" and "9" lead markers). There are osteoblastic lesions in all vertebral bodies. CT images demonstrate extensive encroachment on the thecal sac by the epidural tumor.

logically fractured vertebral body and is the best imaging modality available for determining the presence and severity of cord compression due to bony fragments in the spinal canal (Fig. 39-4). However, since a suspected epidural metastasis presenting with progressive neurologic deficit requires prompt treatment, CT is rarely performed before myelography. After myelography, CT continues to be the definitive study for detecting bone fragments in the spinal canal. In addition, CT may identify small amounts of water-soluble contrast that pass above a partial block at myelography and thus obviate the need for a cervical puncture. Computed tomography also can further characterize a lesion in which the relation of the mass to the thecal sac is unclear.

## Magnetic Resonance Imaging

Magnetic resonance imaging should become the primary modality for evaluating the patient with suspected spinal metastases. It is completely noninvasive and poses no risk of precipitating neurologic deterioration. Magnetic resonance imaging can simultaneously evaluate the spinal cord and the osseous elements of the canal. The sensitivity of MRI for identifying bone metastases should make it a valuable technique for assessing response to therapy.

Magnetic resonance imaging for the evaluation of spinal block is primarily performed in the sagittal plane. Short TR and TE images (*e.g.*, TR = 400–600 msec; TE, as short as the instrument will permit) provide high-quality anatomic detail, with the signal intensities determined largely by differences in T1 values. Thus, the cerebrospinal fluid appears dark and the spinal cord is the only structure normally identified within the spinal canal. Because cortical bone has a very low density of mobile protons and is thus of low intensity, on these short spin-echo sequences there is little or no contrast between cortical bone and the cerebrospinal fluid. Although MRI can clearly define skeletal metastases involving the medullary space and can identify distortions of the cord contour representing frank compression, significant bony encroachment on the thecal sac may occur without causing detectable abnormalities on these images. Therefore, the short spin-echo sequences are supplemented with long TR and longer TE sequences (*e.g.*, TR = 1500–2500 msec, TE = 40–80 msec), which exploit the very long T2 of liquids to obtain optimum contrast between bone and cerebrospinal fluid. These images can define deformities of the thecal sac caused by osseous fragments that are not large enough to indent the spinal cord.

As with myelography, the entire spinal column must be evaluated, because clinical findings and plain radiographs may not adequately local-

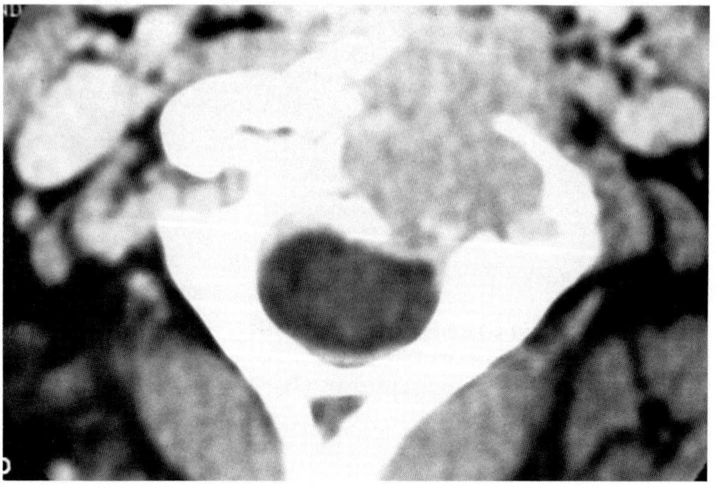

**Figure 39-4.** Contrast-enhanced axial CT scan demonstrates lytic metastases involving a cervical vertebral body with epidural encroachment on the spinal canal and thecal sac (lung primary).

ize the level of involvement and, in a small number of cases, multiple levels are affected. High-quality imaging of the spine requires the use of surface coils. However, the field of view of current surface coils is small and does not permit coverage of the entire spine with a single scan. Therefore, to obtain a complete study the coil must be repositioned once or several times, and this requires that the patient sit up or get off the scanning table in order to physically move the coil. If the patient has significant weakness or is immobile, it may be necessary to lift him above the scanning table while the coil is moved. This substantially prolongs the imaging time. Improved surface coils, which cover the full length of the spine without being moved, may be developed in the future. Although the avoidance of a lumbar puncture with MRI is desirable, cytologic examination of the cerebrospinal fluid is especially useful in patients with tumors that have a predilection for seeding the meninges. Magnetic resonance imaging offers the option of identifying the lesion, instituting therapy, and deferring spinal puncture until after cord compression has been relieved and the risk of precipitating neurologic deterioration is small.

## INTRADURAL–EXTRAMEDULLARY SPINAL METASTASES

Approximately 5% of symptomatic spinal metastases appear as intradural–extramedullary masses, which most commonly arise from primary tumors of the breast, lung, skin (melanoma), and uterus. The clinical presentation is similar to cord or cauda equina compression caused by an epidural metastasis and consists of local and radicular pain, back tenderness, bowel and bladder dysfunction, and a sensory level. However, patients with intradural–extramedullary masses tend to have a more rapid clinical deterioration, and surgical decompression is less effective than with epidural metastases. Approximately 90% of intradural–extramedullary masses are associated with brain parenchymal metastases, and in a similar number of cases the spinal metastasis involves the nerve roots of the cauda equina.

The radiographic imaging of intradural–extramedullary masses parallels the work-up of epidural metastases because the clinical presentation is similar. Plain radiographs of the spine are initially required and are followed by myelography with or without CT or MRI. Although MRI should demonstrate metastases large enough to cause significant cord or cauda equina compression, it may fail to detect smaller intradural nodules.

## INTRAMEDULLARY SPINAL METASTASES

Symptomatic intramedullary spinal metastases are extremely rare and tend to occur in patients with widespread metastatic disease, nearly all of whom have associated brain or lung metastases. The most common primary lesion is carcinoma of the lung; other tumors that may produce intramedullary spinal metastases include carcinoma of the breast, melanoma, and lymphoma. The clinical presentation resembles extradural lesions with cord compression and consists of pain (initially localized to the back but later becoming radicular), localized tenderness, weakness, spasticity, bowel or bladder dysfunction, and a sensory level.

The radiologic diagnosis of intraspinal metastases is challenging. Evidence of bone disease can be detected in less than one third of cases, and myelograms may be normal in over 40% of symptomatic patients. Although an intramedullary lesion classically produces uniform widening of the cord, myelography may demonstrate unusual characteristics, such as an exophytic growth producing the appearance of an extramedullary mass. Computed tomography following myelography or MRI may be of value in determining the relation of the lesion to the cord. Because most patients with intramedullary spinal metastases have widespread disease and frequently have been previously irradiated, paraneoplastic and radiation-induced myelopathy are usually differential considerations. At present, there are no imaging studies that can convincingly distinguish intramedullary spinal metastases from these other diagnostic possibilities.

## LEPTOMENINGEAL METASTASES

Leptomeningeal seeding has been described in patients with primary central nervous system malignancy, metastases from solid systemic tumors, and hematopoietic neoplasms. Among primary central nervous system tumors, primitive neural ectodermal tumors (PNET) and malignant gliomas have the greatest tendency to seed the meninges. Melanoma and cancers of the lung and breast are the solid systemic neoplasms that most often cause leptomeningeal metastases. The characteristic clinical feature is involvement of more than one site (brain, cranial nerves, spine) in the central nervous system. The spine is most commonly affected (80% of patients) with signs and symptoms including reflex asymmetry, weakness and sensory loss, paresthesias, and back or radicular pain. Cranial nerve findings are the next most frequent manifestation, with extraocular muscle paresis and facial weakness often described. Cerebral symptoms occur in about half of the patients and consist of headache, mental status changes, difficulty walking, and nausea or vomiting.

Analysis of the cerebrospinal fluid is the single most important test in diagnosing leptomeningeal metastases. Although the initial examination demonstrates some abnormality in almost all patients, the specific finding of malignant cells is present in only slightly more than 50%. Repeating the collection of cerebrospinal fluid up to seven times and occasionally obtaining fluid from more than one site (lumbar, cisternal, and ventricular sources) significantly raises the yield of cytologic examination. Although there often are associated interparenchymal or dural metastases, these lesions without leptomeningeal metastases rarely, if ever, cause positive cytologic findings. In a small percentage of patients, positive cytologic findings may reflect limited focal deposits rather than disseminated disease, and the cytologic findings may be positive in the absence of clinically or radiographically apparent leptomeningeal metastases.

Myelography has been reported to detect leptomeningeal metastases in up to 50% of patients with negative cerebrospinal fluid cytology. Manifestations include smooth or irregular thickening of nerve roots, solitary or multiple intradural nodules, and a variable degree of spinal block with an appearance suggesting arachnoiditis (Figs. 39-5 and 39-6). In the cervical and thoracic region, the spinal cord may have a nodular contour and, if these changes extend over a long segment, there is a "cloaking" effect. Myelography is especially indicated in children with central nervous system malignancies, who are prone to develop leptomeningeal metastases, and in patients in whom there is a clinical suspicion of disseminated meningeal disease.

Cranial CT shows leptomeningeal metastases as abnormal enhancement of the sulci, cisterns, or ependyma. Although identified in only 20% to 40% of cases, these findings are characteristic of leptomeningeal metastases. The basal cisterns are often obliterated, and nodules may be identified in the subarachnoid space (Figs.

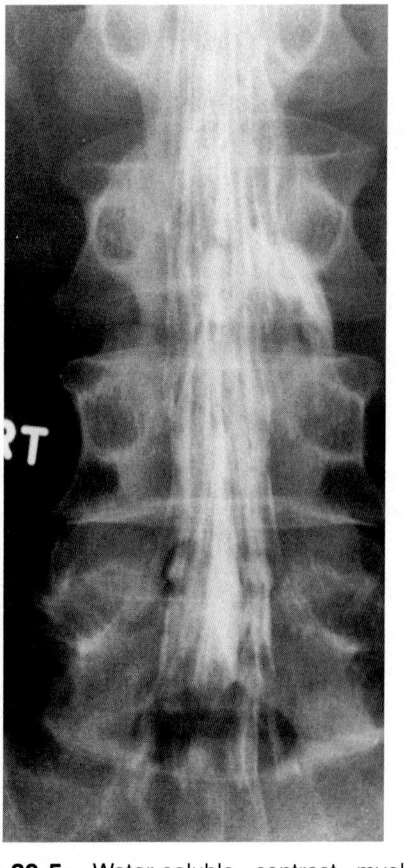


**Figure 39-5.** Water-soluble contrast myelogram demonstrates nodular seeding of cauda equina nerve roots (cerebellar primitive neuroectodermal tumor).

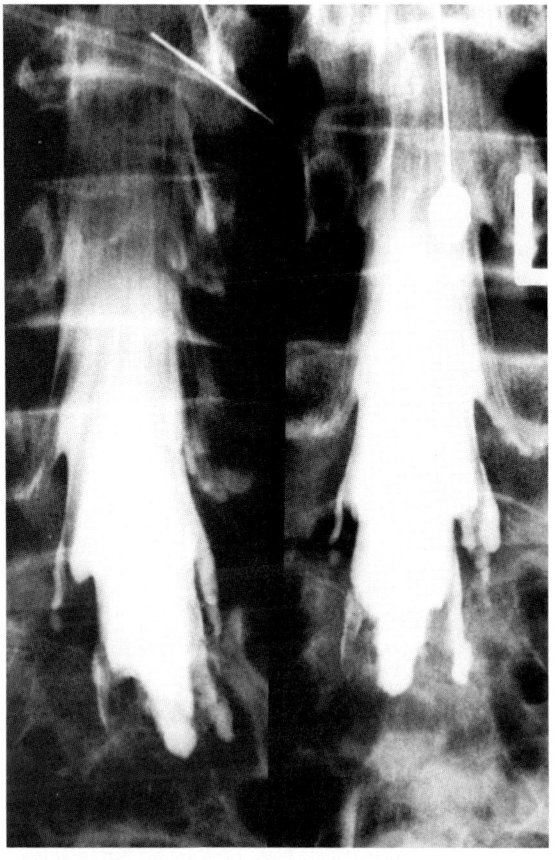

**Figure 39-6.** Water-soluble contrast lumbar myelogram shows a large intradural nodule at the termination of the thecal sac related to the right S2 nerve root (cerebellar primitive neuroectodermal tumor).

39-7 and 39-8). Ventricular dilatation, with or without pathologic enhancement, is by far the most common abnormality (60%) in patients with proven leptomeningeal metastases. This finding should be viewed with suspicion in the patient with a known malignancy and an appropriate clinical presentation even if more specific abnormalities are absent.

Although no detailed reports are available, MRI will probably prove to be of limited value in detecting leptomeningeal metastases. Magnetic resonance imaging can demonstrate the common ventricular enlargement and may detect large cisternal nodules, but its limited spatial resolution (as compared to myelography) should prevent detection of the small intradural nodules and nerve root thickening that are characteristic of this condition. In patients with massive infiltration of the meninges and extensive obliteration of the subarachnoid space, MRI may display the loss of normal contrast between the cerebrospinal fluid and the spinal cord. However, until major technical improvements are achieved, MRI will not replace myelography for identifying leptomeningeal metastases.

## OTHER METASTASES

In addition to compressing the spinal cord or cauda equina, osseous metastases may involve the central nervous system by invading the dura and producing epidural or subdural deposits

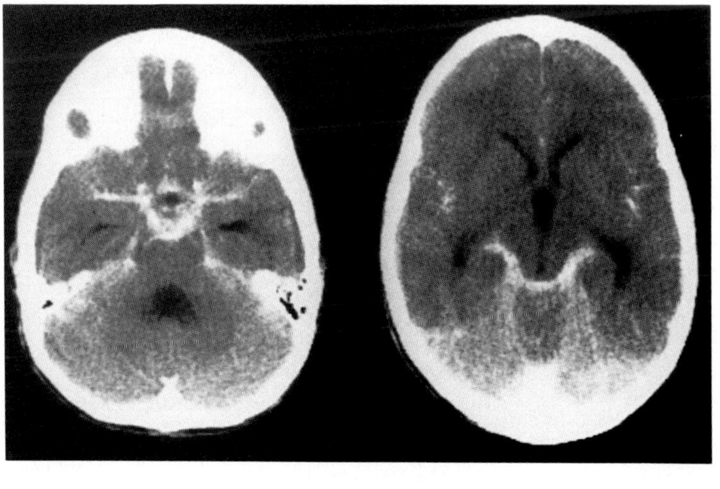

**Figure 39-7.** Intravenous contrast CT demonstrates extensive tumor seeding of the subarachnoid space. There is high-density material coating the tentorium; filling the suprasellar, quadrigeminal, and ambient cisterns; and entering the sylvian fissures (spinal cord astrocytoma).

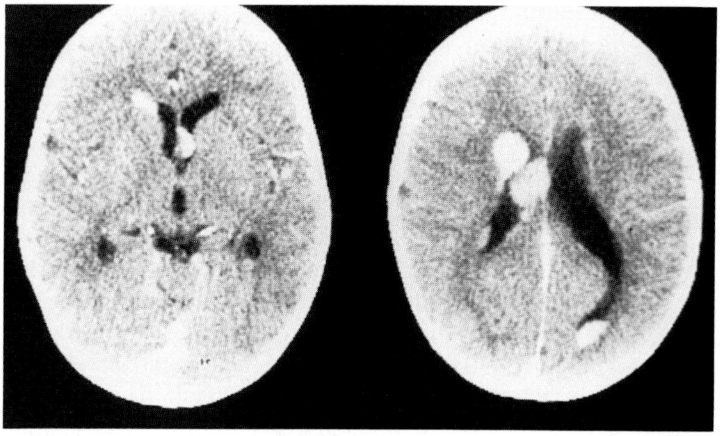

**Figure 39-8.** Intravenous contrast CT demonstrates multiple enhancing subependymal nodules (cerebellar primitive neuroectodermal tumor).

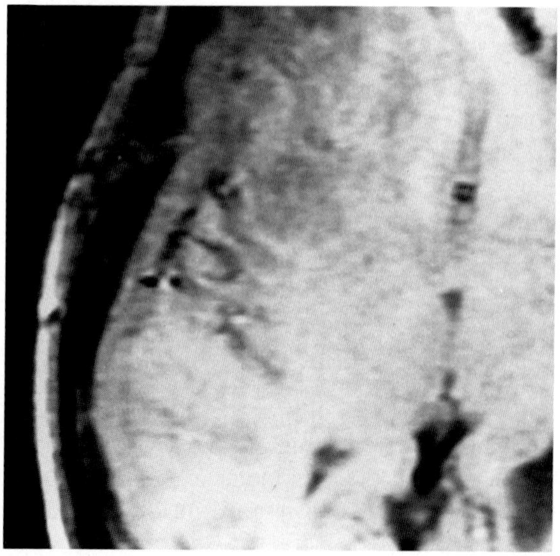

**Figure 39-9.** Axial MRI (TR, 600 msec; TE, 20 msec) demonstrates a thick rind of dural tumor (*arrows*) displacing cortical vessels medially (*arrowheads*) (breast primary).

(Fig. 39-9). Hemorrhagic subdural deposits may result in subdural hematomas, most commonly in patients with lymphoma or carcinomas of the breast or stomach. The dura appears thickened on MRI, and both thickened and enhanced on CT.

Tumors of the face, paranasal sinuses, and oral cavity may spread to the cranial cavity by infiltrating along cranial nerves (especially the maxillary division of the trigeminal nerve). The major CT manifestation is widening and obliteration of fat planes in the pterygopalatine fossa. The tumor (especially adenoid cystic carcinoma) enlarges the foramen rotundum and extends through it into Meckel's cave, where it presents as a mass in the gasserian ganglion or the middle cranial fossa.

## Bibliography


Anand AK, Potts DG: Calcified brain metastases: Demonstration by computed tomography. Am J Neuroradiol 3:527–529, 1982

Black P: Spinal metastases: Current status and recommended guidelines for management. Neurosurgery 5:726–746, 1979

Bradley WG: Magnetic resonance imaging in the central nervous system: Comparison with computed tomography. In Kressel HY (ed): Magnetic Resonance Annual, pp 81–122. New York, Raven Press, 1986

Brant–Zawadski M, Norman D, Newton TA et al: Magnetic resonance of the brain: The optical screening technique. Radiology 152:71–77, 1984

Cairncross JG, Posner JB: The management of brain metastases. In Walker MD (ed): Oncology of the Nervous System, pp 341–377, Boston, Martinus Nijhoff, 1985

Claussen C, Laniado M, Schoner W et al: Use of gadolinium-DTPA MR imaging of glioblastomas and intracranial metastases. Am J Neuroradiol 6:669–674, 1985

Costigan DA, Winkleman MD: Intramedullary spinal cord metastasis. A clinical pathological study of 13 cases. J Neurosurg 62:223–227, 1985

Curtin HD, Williams R, Johnson J: CT of perineural

tumor extension: Pterygopalatine fossa. Am J Neuroradiol 5:731–737, 1984

Edelson RN, Deck MDF, Posner JB: Intramedullary spinal cord metastasis. Clinical and radiographic findings in nine cases. Neurology 22:1222–1231, 1972

Felix R, Schorner W, Laniado M et al: Brain tumors: MR imaging with Gd-DTPA. Radiology 156: 681–688, 1985

Gilbert RW, Kim JG, Posner JB: Epidural spinal cord compression from metastatic tumor: Diagnosis and treatment. Ann Neurol 3:40–51, 1978

Glass JP, Melamed M, Chernick KL, Posner JB: Malignant cells in the cerebral spinal fluid (CSF): The meaning of a positive CSF cytology. Neurology 29:1369–1375, 1979

Graif M, Bydder GM, Stiener RE et al: Contrast enhanced MR imaging of malignant brain tumors. Am J Neuroradiol 6:855–862, 1985

Hackney DB, Wismer GL, Edelman R et al: Magnetic resonance imaging of the spine: Non-invasive evaluation of spinal block. Presented at the Annual Meeting American Society of Neuroradiology, New Orleans, February, 1985

Hashizume Y, Harino A: Intramedullary spinal cord metastasis: Pathological findings in five autopsy cases. Acta Neuropathol (Berl) 61:214–218, 1983

Hayman LA, Evans RA, Hinck VZ: Delayed high dose iodine contrast computed tomography—cranial neoplasms. Radiology 136:677–684, 1980

Hollis PH, Malis LI, Zappulla RA: Neurologic deterioration after lumbar puncture below complete spinal subarachnoid block. J Neurosurg 64: 253–256, 1986

Holtas S, Cronqvist S: Cranial computed tomography of patients with malignant myeloma. Neuroradiology 22:123–127, 1981

Lee BCP, Kneeland JB, Cahill PT, Deck MDF: MR recognition of supratentorial tumors. Am J Neuroradiol 6:871–878, 1985

Lee Y-Y, Glass JP, Geoffrey A, Wallace S: Cranial computed tomographic abnormalities in leptomeningioma metastases. Am J Neuroradiol 5: 559–563, 1984

Lee YY, Glass JP, Wallace S: Myelography in cancer patients: Modified technique. Am J Neuroradiol 6:617–621, 1985

Mandybur TI: Intracranial hemorrhage caused by metastatic tumors. Neurology 27:650–655, 1977

Packer RJ, Seigel KR, Sutton LN et al: Leptomeningeal dissemination of primary central nervous system tumors of childhood. Ann Neurol 18:217–221, 1985

Pagani JJ, Hayman LA, Bigelow RH et al: Diazepam prophylaxis of contrast media-induced seizures during computed tomography of patients with brain metastases. AJR 140:787–792, 1983

Pagani JJ, Libshitz HI, Wallace S, Hayman LA: Central nervous system leukemia and lymphoma: Computed tomographic manifestations. AJR 137:1195–1201, 1981

Perrin RG, Livingston KE, Aarabi B: Intradural extramedullary spinal metastasis. A report of ten cases. Acta Neuropathol (Berl) 61:214–218, 1983

Potts DG, Abbott GF, von Sneidern JV: National Cancer Institute study: Evaluation of computed tomography in the diagnosis of intracranial neoplasms. III. Metastatic tumors. Radiology 136: 657–664, 1980

Rorke L: The cerebellar medulloblastoma and its relationship to primitive neuroectodermal tumors. J Neuropathol Exp Neurol 42:1–15, 1983

Russell DS, Rubinstein LJ: Pathology of tumors of the central nervous system, pp 352–360. Baltimore, Williams & Wilkins, 1977

Shapiro R: Myelography. Chicago, Yearbook Medical Publishers, 1984

Shi M, Wallace S, Libshitz HI et al: Cranial computed tomography of breast carcinoma. J Comput Tomogr 6:77–88, 1982

Stanley P, Senac MO, Segall HD: Intraspinal seeding from intracranial tumors in children. Am J Neuroradiol 5:805–809, 1984

Sutton D: Tumours and tumour-like lesions of bone. In Sutton D (ed): A Textbook of Radiology and Imaging, 3rd ed, pp 89–93. Edinburgh, Churchill, Livingstone, 1980

Tarver RD, Richmond BD, Klatte EC: Cerebral metastases from lung carcinoma: Neurological and CT correlation. Work in Progress. Radiology 153:689–692, 1984

Wasserstrom WR, Glass JP, Posner JB: Diagnosis and treatment of leptomeningio and metastases from solid tumors: Experience with 90 patients. Cancer 49:759–772, 1982

Weiss L, Gilbert HA, Posner JB (eds): Brain Metastasis. Boston, GK Hall, 1980

Wilner D: Cancer metastases to bones. In Wilner D (ed): Radiology of Bone Tumors and Allied Disorders, pp 3641–3908. Philadelphia, WB Saunders, 1982

Zimmerman RA, Bilaniuk LT: Computed tomography of acute intratumoral hemorrhage. Radiology 135:355–359, 1980

## SUSPECTED INTRACEREBRAL METASTASES

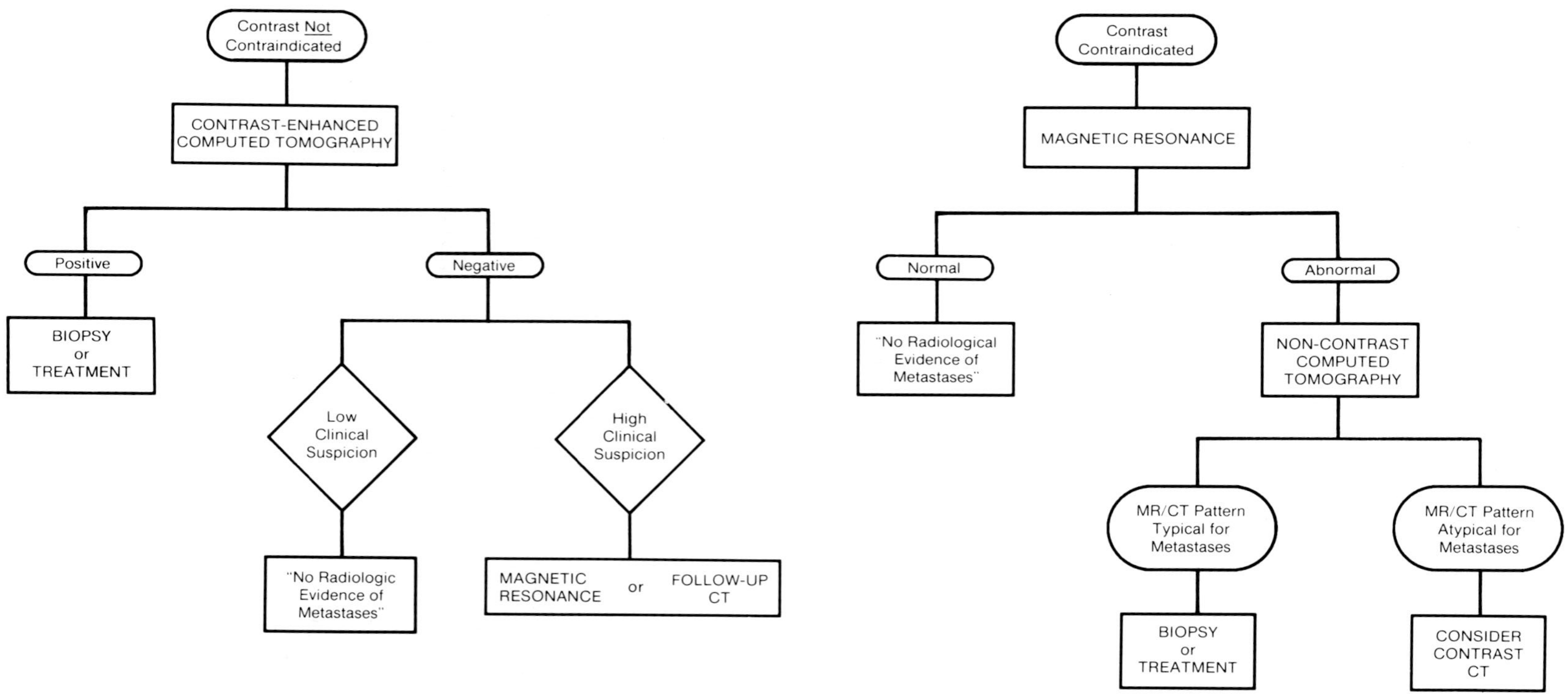


Note: This algorithm is constructed with the assumption that intravenous contrast enhancement with Gd-DTPA for MR imaging is not readily available. Although to date there has been very little documentation of the role of Gd-DTPA for evaluating cerebral metastases, preliminary results suggest that when Gd-DTPA becomes available it may replace contrast-enhanced CT scanning.

# SUSPECTED INTRASPINAL METASTASES

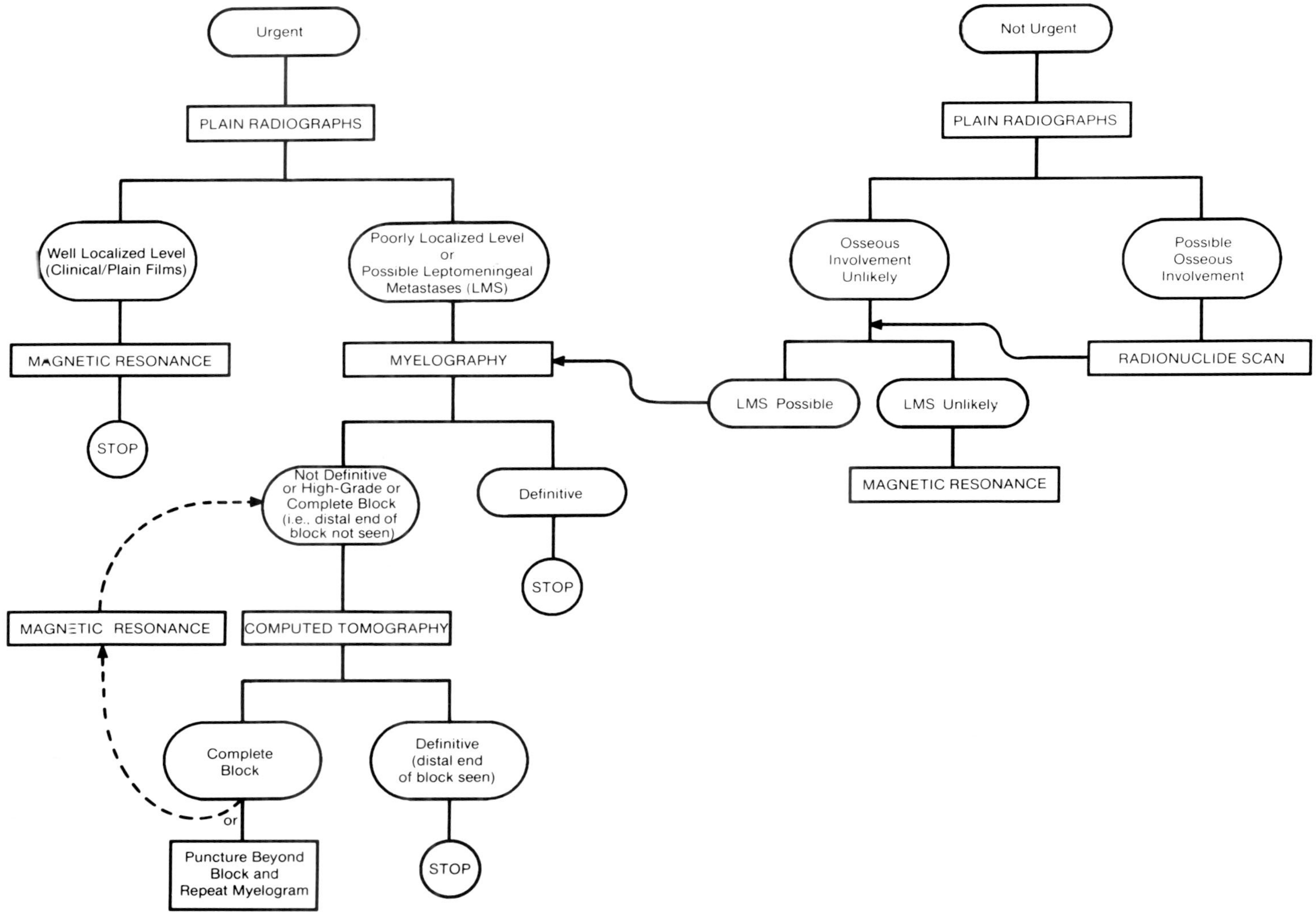

# Chapter 40

# Staging of Esophageal Carcinoma

*William M. Thompson*
*Robert A. Halvorsen*

Carcinoma of the esophagus accounts for 1.5% of all cancers and 7% of gastrointestinal cancers in the United States. Despite recent advances in surgery, radiation therapy, and chemotherapy, the survival of patients with carcinoma of the esophagus remains poor. The 5-year survival rate is less than 10% in most reports. Considerably better survival figures have been reported from Japan and China, probably because many of the patients in these countries have carcinoma *in situ* at the time of diagnosis.

For the purpose of this chapter, adenocarcinoma of the gastroesophageal junction is excluded, because of the differences between this tumor and the far more common squamous cell carcinoma of the esophagus.

## CLINICAL FINDINGS

Progressive dysphagia is the most common clinical presentation of carcinoma of the esophagus. Indeed, the development of dysphagia in a person over 40 years of age should always be assumed to be due to esophageal cancer until proven otherwise. The dysphagia usually is progressive, first being produced by solids and then advancing so that semisolid foods and even liquids cause difficulty in swallowing. Another manifestation of carcinoma of the esophagus is pain, which is usually steady and located substernally or in the back. This represents an unfavorable sign, because it usually indicates local invasion. Systemic symptoms, principally anorexia and weight loss, are usually present by the time the diagnosis is made. At times, it may be difficult to determine whether anorexia is caused directly by difficulty in swallowing or indirectly from the systemic effect of the tumor.

Significant acute upper gastrointestinal hemorrhage occurs in less than 5% of patients with esophageal cancer. Chronic blood loss is more common and produces symptoms of iron-deficiency anemia. Other rare symptoms are hoarseness, caused by involvement of the recurrent laryngeal nerve, and cough, due to either aspiration of retained material in the esophagus or the formation of a tracheoesophageal fistula.

Aspiration pneumonia resulting from esophageal obstruction is the most common complication of carcinoma of the esophagus. Tumor involvement of contiguous organs often occurs. Fistulas from the esophagus to the trachea or bronchi lead to recurrent pneumonia or pulmonary abscess. Erosion of the tumor into the aorta produces rapid exsanguination. Less common manifestations of esophageal carcinoma include hypercalcemia and the production of hormonally active substances (*e.g.*, gonadotropins and ACTH). Other than weight loss, the physical findings usually are not striking in the patient with carcinoma of the esophagus. Supraclavicular lymphadenopathy or an enlarged liver due to metastatic disease may develop.

## TUMOR BEHAVIOR

In order to design an imaging approach for investigating the patient with any cancer, it is essential to have a clear understanding of the behavior of the tumor. Before becoming widely disseminated, squamous cell carcinomas are characterized by extensive local growth and lymph node metastases. As the esophagus courses from the neck to the abdomen, it comes into close proximity with a number of vital structures, especially the heart, aorta, trachea, and lung. Because the esophagus has only mucosal and submucosal layers and no serosa, carcinomas typically penetrate through the esophageal wall into the mediastinum to invade contiguous structures early in the course of the disease. Because of this aggressive local extension, the location of the primary tumor has prognostic significance. Carcinomas in the distal esophagus have a significantly better prognosis than those in the upper esophagus.

An extensive interconnecting network of submucosal and muscular lymphatics course the entire length of the esophagus. Smaller lymphatics arise within the mucosa and external muscularis and drain into the more extensive network in the deeper layers of the esophageal wall. Because lymph can flow through many pathways in the wall of the esophagus before emerging from the lymphatic vessels to drain into lymph nodes, the spread of tumor cells to adjacent lymph nodes is unpredictable. Figure 40-1 shows the percentage of positive lymph nodes found at surgery for carcinomas in the upper, middle, and lower thirds of the esophagus. Note that almost one third of patients with cancers of the upper third of the esophagus have evidence of involvement of subdiaphragmatic lymph nodes. Another important example of the unpredictability of the lymphatic drainage is the phenomenon of skip areas of involvement. As much as 8 cm of normal esophagus may be interposed between the site of gross neoplasm and micrometastases within lymphatic vessels of the esophagus.

Because of the frequent local invasion and

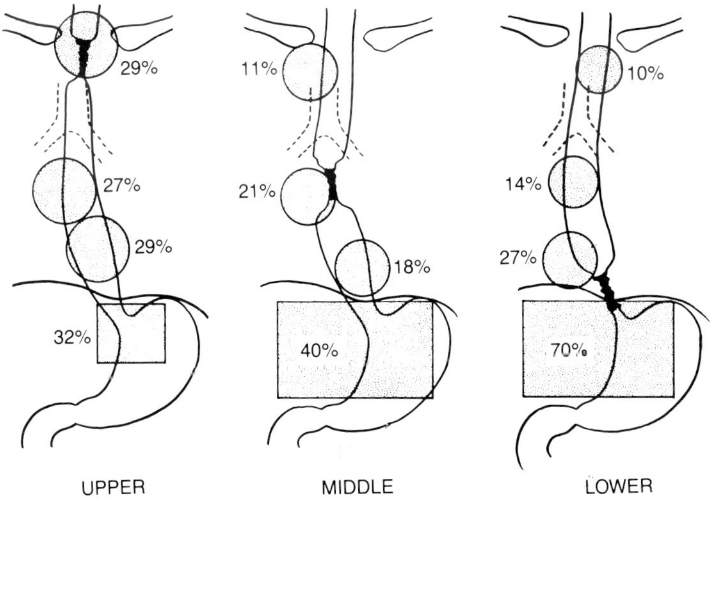


**Figure 40-1.** Percentage of positive lymph nodes found at surgery for carcinomas in the upper, middle, and lower thirds of the esophagus. (Thompson WM: Esophageal cancer. Int J Radiat Oncol Biol Phys 9:1533–1565, 1983; with permission)

lymph node involvement of carcinoma of the esophagus, distant metastases rarely dominate the clinical course. Nevertheless, distant metastases are reported in 90% of autopsy studies and most commonly involve the lung and liver.

## STAGING

Tumor staging is essential for treatment planning and to compare the effectiveness of different therapies on homogeneous populations. However, the classification and staging of carcinoma of the esophagus has been slow to evolve and no staging system has gained wide acceptance. A major difficulty with the preoperative staging systems is that the esophagus is a relatively inaccessible organ, so that the extent of the tumor cannot be clearly defined with available diagnostic imaging modalities. Because many patients with esophageal cancer are treated with preoperative radiation or chemotherapy, surgical findings often cannot be used to evaluate staging modalities obtained prior to therapy.

Of all the currently used imaging procedures, computed tomography (CT) provides the most specific staging information. However, additional studies are needed before CT can be accepted as an accurate, cost-effective preoperative staging method for carcinoma of the esophagus.

The most common method used to stage esophageal carcinoma is the clinical–diagnostic TNM system devised by the American Joint Committee. This staging system classifies esophageal cancer according to its anatomical extent. The differentiation between T1 and T2 primary lesions depends on the length of tumor as defined by an esophagogram. However, an esophagogram cannot precisely determine the length of the primary lesion (when compared with pathologic specimens) nor can it accurately determine local invasion (T3 lesions). Prior to the advent of CT, surgery was the only method available for determining local invasion, lymph node involvement, or distant metastases.

A relatively new system of classification has been developed that divides patients with esophageal cancer into four groups using CT criteria. Stage I refers to an intramural esophageal mass without wall thickening. In stage II, there is wall thickening greater than 5 mm. The combination of wall thickening (>5 mm) and spread to contiguous mediastinal structures defines stage III, and distant metastatic spread indicates stage IV.

## DIAGNOSTIC EVALUATION

### *DIAGNOSTIC MODALITIES*

1. Plain chest radiography
2. Esophagogram
3. Radionuclide studies
4. Ultrasound
5. Computed tomography
6. Magnetic resonance imaging
7. Percutaneous biopsy

### Plain Chest Radiography

Plain chest radiographs are a standard part of the workup of any patient with a known malignancy, including carcinoma of the esophagus. Patients with squamous cell carcinoma of the esophagus have an increased incidence of associated lung cancer (and head-neck cancer). In addition, the spread of esophageal cancer can produce specific radiographic abnormalities. The most common of these are an abnormal azygoesophageal line, a widened mediastinum, tracheal deviation, and widening (>4 mm) of the retrotracheal stripe (Fig. 40-2). Although some reports have suggested that these findings (especially a widened retrotracheal stripe) have prognostic significance, other studies have shown no significant difference in survival rates of patients with esophageal carcinoma regardless of whether chest film abnormalities were present. Occasionally, chest radiographs can demonstrate overt evidence of esophageal carcinoma invading the lung (Fig. 40-3).

### Esophagogram

The esophagogram is a sensitive technique for detecting advanced esophageal carcinoma. It

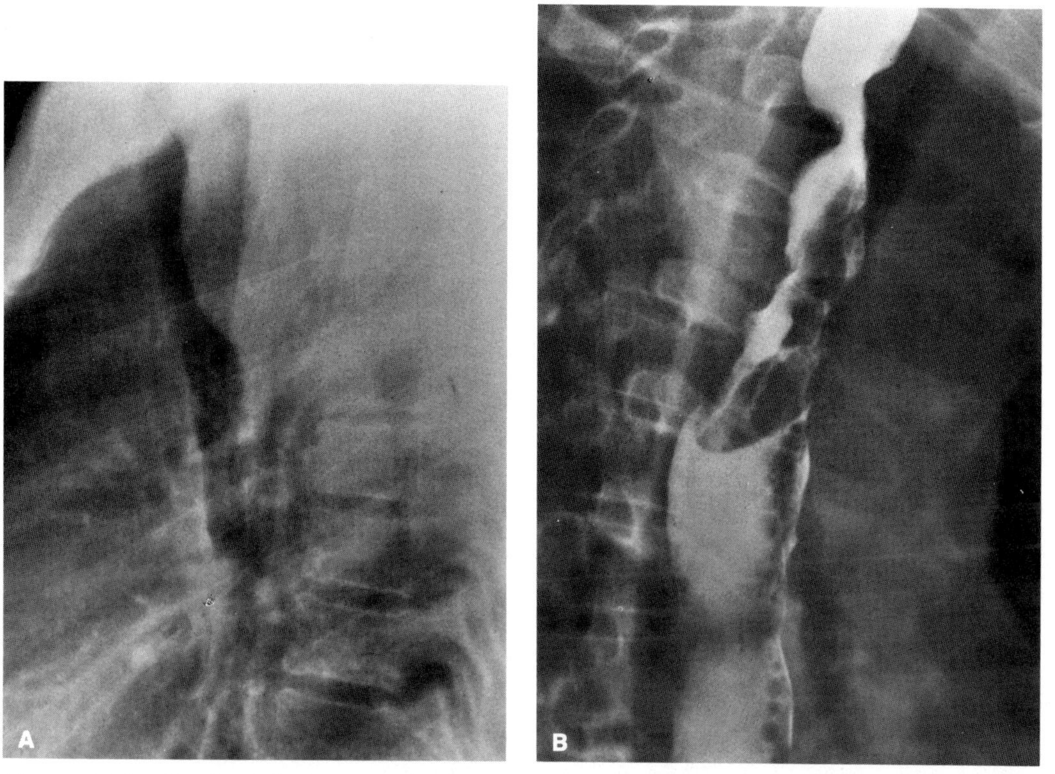


**Figure 40-2.** Tracheal displacement by large esophageal carcinoma. **(A)** Lateral chest radiograph shows anterior displacement of the trachea. **(B)** Esophagogram demonstrates the large esophageal malignancy. (Rubin P: Clinical Oncology for Medical Students and Physicians: A Multidisciplinary Approach, 6th ed. New York, American Cancer Society, 1983; with permission)

cannot identify carcinoma *in situ,* but it is effective in showing superficial and early (small) tumors if the double-contrast technique is employed (Fig. 40-4). Early, or small, carcinoma of the esophagus is not consistently defined but usually refers to tumors less than 3.5 cm in length; some reports have indicated better survival rates in patients with these small tumors, while others have not.

Despite some deficiencies, the esophagogram is an important modality for localizing and characterizing a known or suspected tumor. Most esophageal carcinomas are large and partially obstructing at the time of diagnosis and produce a characteristic appearance. Occasionally, an esophageal carcinoma may mimic a benign stricture (Fig. 40-5), varices, achalasia, or a local inflammatory lesion. The radiologist must be familiar with the various manifestations of esophageal cancer and must consider any asymmetric stricture malignant until it is proven benign.

The esophagogram has been used to separate T1 and T2 esophageal carcinomas based on whether the lesion is less than or greater than 5 cm in length. The double-contrast examination is recommended, because it provides better delineation of the tumor than does the single-contrast technique (Fig. 40-6). Even using double-contrast techniques the prognostic significance of tumor length as determined by an esophagogram is controversial, and most authors rely on CT for more complete staging.

Deviation of the esophageal axis on single-contrast examination has been described as evidence of mediastinal invasion and, therefore,

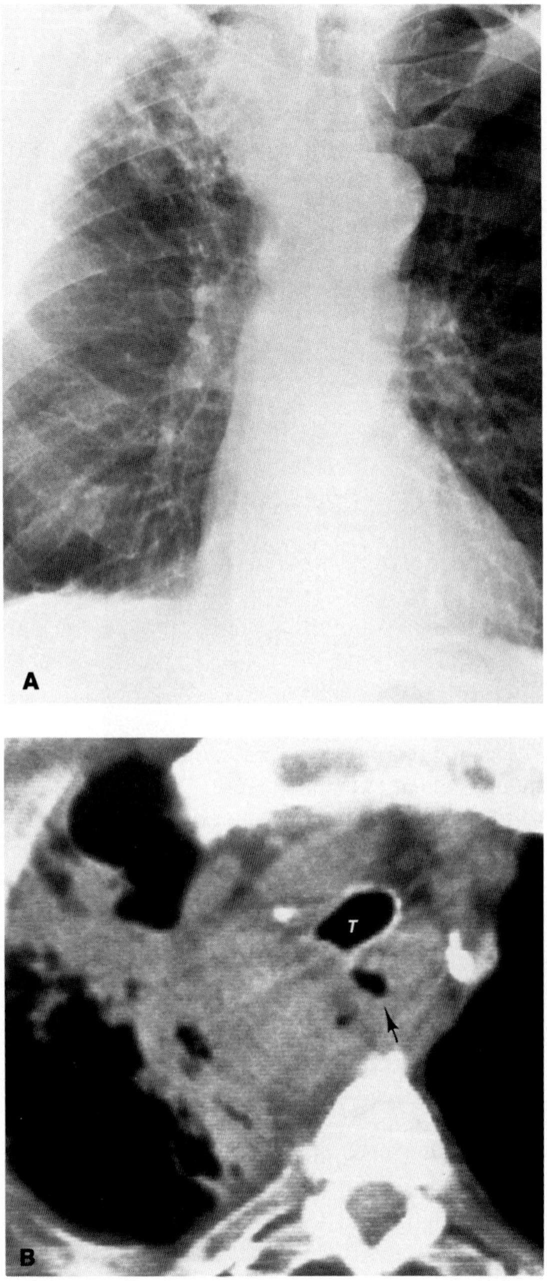

**Figure 40-3.** Invasion of the lung by esophageal carcinoma. **(A)** Frontal chest radiograph shows a mass in the right upper lobe. **(B)** CT scan through the upper chest shows the huge squamous cell carcinoma growing out into the lung and invading the trachea. The arrow points to the esophageal lumen. (*T*, tracheal lumen)

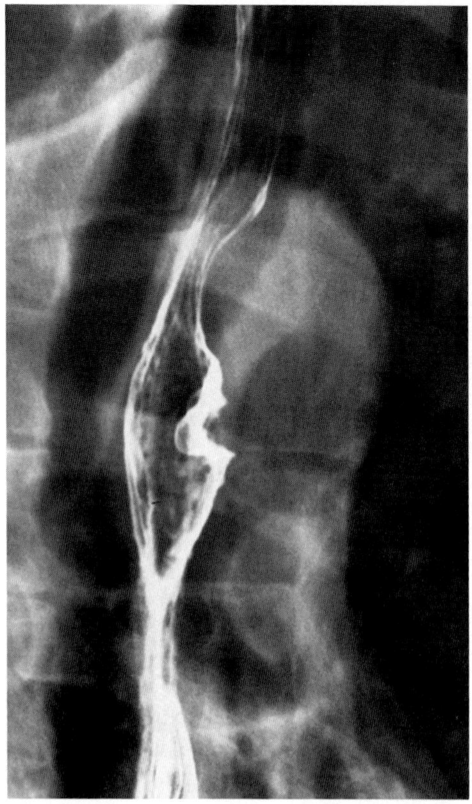

**Figure 40-4.** Double-contrast esophagogram shows a small polypoid squamous carcinoma. The single-contrast study was normal. (Thompson WM: Sychronous and metachronous squamous cell carcinomas of the head, neck and esophagus. Gastrointest Radiol 3:123–127, 1978; with permission)

unresectability for cure (Fig. 40-7). Tortuosity of the esophagus results from fixation of the tumor to surrounding mediastinal structures, with prestenotic dilatation and elongation. Angulation and displacement are caused by fixation or traction due to local invasion of mediastinal structures. To adequately evaluate its axis, radiographs of the esophagus must be taken in two perpendicular planes, because an abnormal esophageal axis cannot be excluded in only one plane. Even though some series have reported deformity of the esophageal axis in approximately 80% of locally invasive esophageal cancers, this technique is employed by only a few authors, and CT is generally considered a more accurate method for determining local invasion.

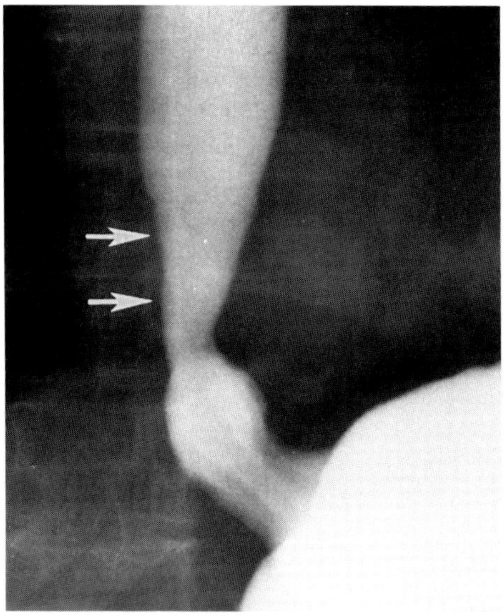

**Figure 40-5.** Esophagogram shows asymmetric stricture (*arrows*) due to distal esophageal carcinoma.

Despite its limitations, the double-contrast esophagogram will remain an important modality in evaluating the patient with a known or suspected esophageal cancer. It also complements endoscopy for defining the exact location and, in many cases, the precise mucosal extent of an esophageal cancer.

### Radionuclide Studies

Radionuclide studies can detect abnormalities in the liver, brain, or skeletal system in patients with suspected metastases from esophageal cancer. However, the results of radionuclide studies are usually nonspecific, and thus this modality is not used as a routine staging procedure. Gallium studies are not useful procedures, because they cannot accurately stage esophageal cancer.

### Ultrasound

Although ultrasound is not a routine procedure in staging patients with esophageal carcinoma, it can provide a noninvasive, relatively inexpensive technique for evaluating abnormalities suspicious for metastases on liver CT or radionuclide liver–spleen scans. Ultrasound also can be used to direct percutaneous biopsies of suspected metastases.

### Computed Tomography

Computed tomography is currently the single most accurate preoperative method for evaluating the patient with carcinoma of the esophagus. It can display the anatomy of the esophagus and demonstrate any extraesophageal spread of tumor to contiguous mediastinal structures in more than 95% of patients. Using the previously described CT-oriented staging system, more than 90% of patients with esophageal cancer can be accurately staged.

The apparent thickness of the esophageal wall on CT varies with the degree of distention of the esophageal lumen. In at least 60% of normal people, CT can show air in the esophageal lumen and thus permit measurement of the thickness of the esophageal wall (normally, 3 mm–5 mm). The use of contrast material in the esophagus can aid in identifying the lumen and permit measurement of wall thickness in almost all patients.

Computed tomography is currently the only imaging modality that allows detection of early mediastinal invasion (Table 40-1). To make this

**Table 40-1** CT Staging of Esophageal Cancer: Predicting Invasion or Metastases (Results from Three Series)

| Anatomic Area | Sensitivity $\frac{TP}{TP + FN}$ | Specificity $\frac{TN}{TN + FP}$ | Accuracy $\frac{TP + TN}{Total}$ |
|---|---|---|---|
| Tracheobronchial | 98% | 95% | 96% |
| Aorta | 88% | 92% | 92% |
| Pericardium | 100% | 95% | 96% |
| Periesophageal Nodes | 60% | 97% | 95% |
| Liver | 78% | 100% | 98% |
| Abdominal Nodes | 76% | 93% | 87% |

FP, false positive; FN, false negative; TP, true positive, TN, true negative

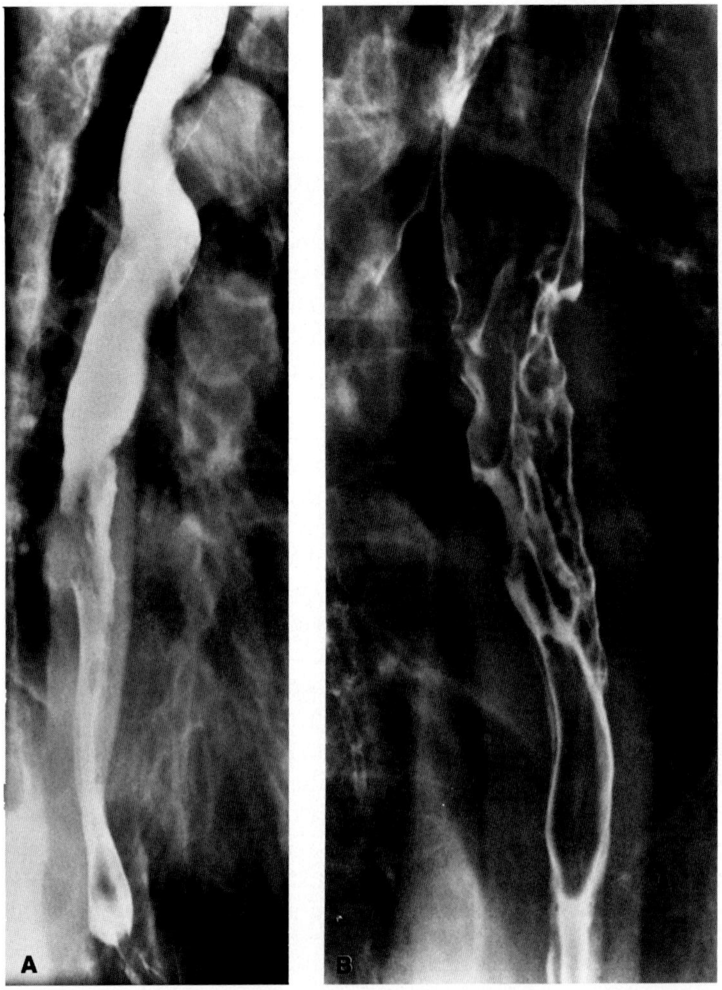

**Figure 40-6.** Staging of esophageal carcinoma by esophagography. **(A)** Single-contrast study demonstrates the midesophageal carcinoma. **(B)** Double-contrast study in the same patient more clearly defines the extent of the tumor.

diagnosis, the tumor mass must be shown to extend directly into adjacent structures without any separation by intervening fat planes. The presence of a normal fat plane between a neighboring structure and the esophageal tumor excludes invasion of the structure at that level. However, the absence of a fat plane does not necessarily imply invasion, because in some portions of the mediastinum the esophagus is in direct contact with normal contiguous structures without an intervening fat plane. In addition, the mediastinal fat planes are frequently absent in cachectic patients. Therefore, findings other than absence of fat planes must be utilized to determine whether there is local invasion by an esophageal cancer.

Computed tomography is extremely accurate in detecting involvement of the tracheobronchial tree, which is a frequent site of mediastinal invasion in patients with esophageal cancer. Normally, there is a 2-mm to 3-mm separation between the tracheal and esophageal lumens. Displacement and indentation of the tracheobronchial tree by an esophageal tumor (Figs. 40-8 and 40-9) has a very high predictability for local invasion of the tracheobronchial tree (see Table 40-1).

The middle third of the esophagus lies in direct contact with the aorta, and there often may be no visible fat planes separating the two structures. However, obliteration of the fat plane between the aorta and esophagus at the

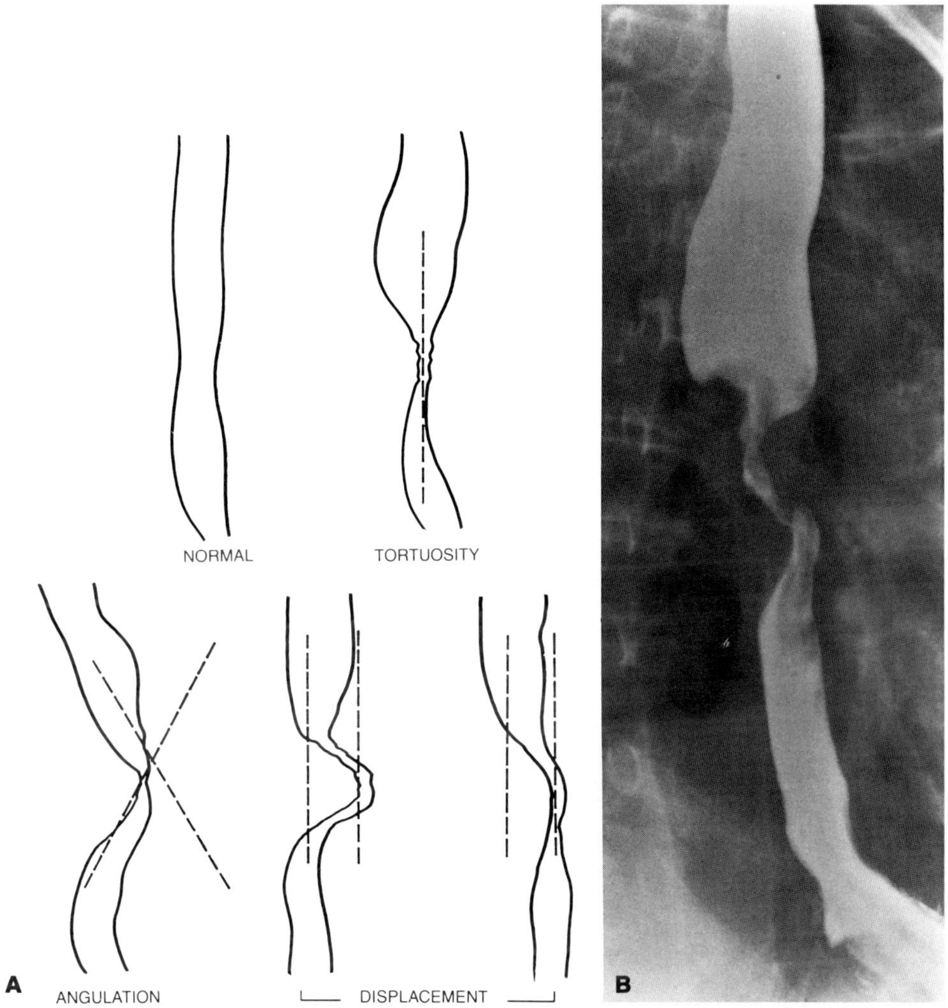


**Figure 40-7.** Deviation of esophageal axis. **(A)** Types of deformities of esophageal axis that may be produced by esophageal carcinoma. **(B)** Esophagogram shows an abnormal axis in a patient with invasive esophageal carcinoma. (Thompson WM: Esophageal cancer. Int J Radiat Oncol Biol Phys 9:1533–1565, 1983; with permission)

level of an esophageal tumor in the face of preserved fat planes above and below that level is considered a positive sign for invasion (Fig. 40-10). Similar criteria apply to tumor invasion of the pericardium. A system has been developed in which the amount of contact of a tumor with the aorta is used as an indicator of invasion. This system has an overall accuracy rate of 80%. Tumors involving less than one eighth (<45°) of the aortic circumference are considered noninvasive, while tumor contact with more than one fourth (>90°) of the aortic circumference is considered evidence of invasion. Contact between one eighth to one fourth (45°–90°) is considered indeterminate for invasion. Therefore, preservation of the para-aortic fat planes and tumor contact with less than one eighth (<45°) of the aortic circumference indicates that the tumor is not invading the aorta (Fig. 40-11).

The major limitation of CT in detecting

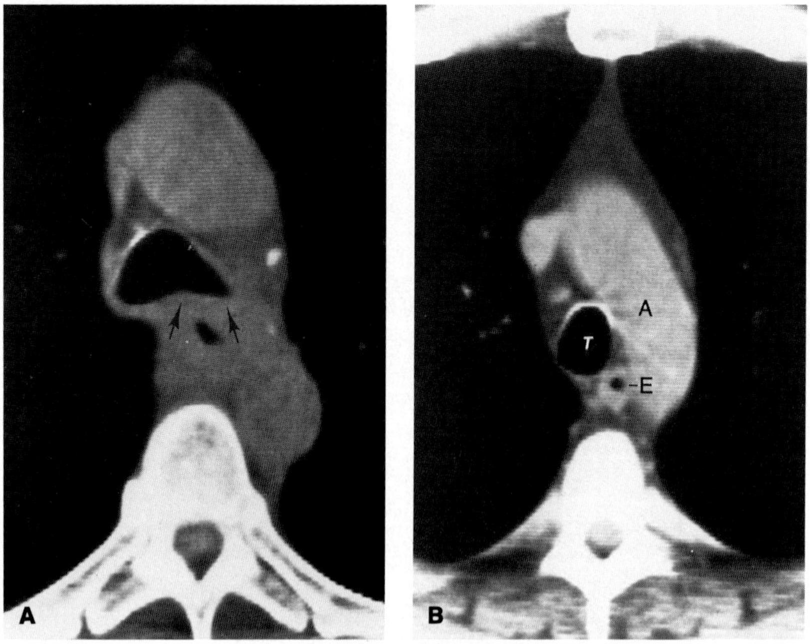


**Figure 40-8.** Tracheal invasion. **(A)** CT scan just below the aortic arch shows the esophageal tumor invading the trachea (*arrows*). Note also the aortic invasion. **(B)** CT scan from a different patient shows the normal relationships between the aorta (*A*), trachea (*T*), and esophagus (*E*).

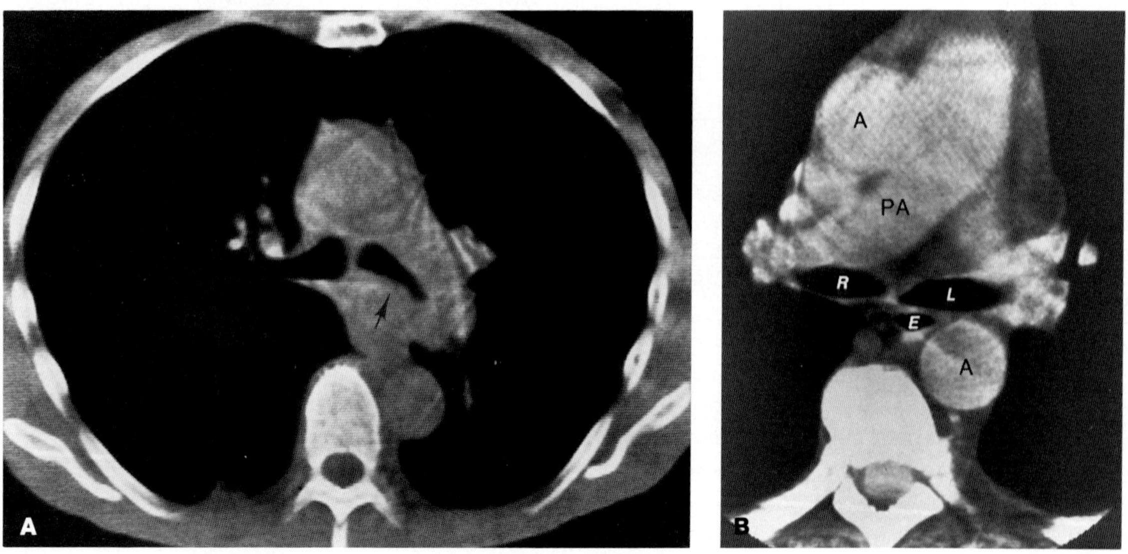


**Figure 40-9.** Bronchial invasion. **(A)** CT scan through the main stem bronchi shows direct invasion of the left main bronchus as a tumor mass indenting the posterior bronchial wall (*arrow*). **(B)** CT scan in a different patient shows the normal relationships. (*A,* aorta; *PA,* main pulmonary artery; *E,* esophagus; *L,* left main bronchus; *R,* right main bronchus)

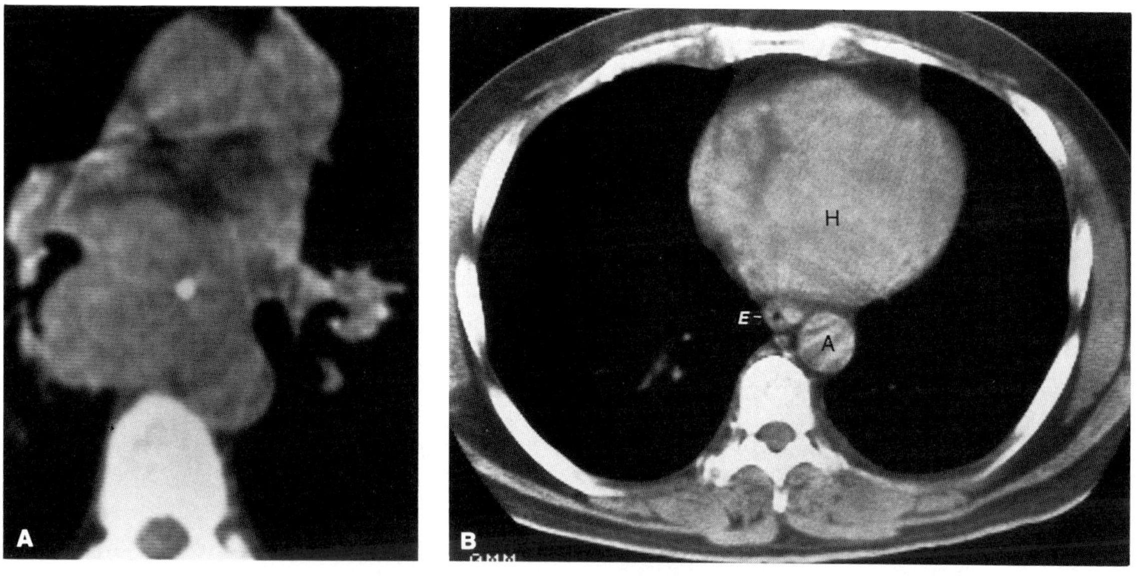


**Figure 40-10.** Aortic and pericardial invasion. **(A)** CT scan in a patient with a large esophageal cancer shows lack of fat planes between the esophagus and the pericardium and aorta. CT scans above and below this level demonstrated normal mediastinal fat planes. There is a feeding tube in the esophageal lumen. **(B)** CT scan in a different patient shows the normal relationships. (*H,* heart; *A,* aorta; *E,* esophagus)

tumor spread to mediastinal lymph nodes relates to the inability of CT to differentiate small, normal lymph nodes from small lymph nodes containing tumor. Computed tomography cannot distinguish benign from malignant causes of lymph node enlargement, nor can it separate lymph nodes adjacent to the tumor from the tumor itself. It is generally agreed that mediastinal lymph nodes must be larger than 1 cm in length along their short axis to be considered enlarged and to contain tumor.

Invasion of other paraesophageal structures can occasionally be detected by CT if there is obvious envelopment or destruction. For example, invasion of the spine can produce CT-detectable bone destruction and large esophageal tumors may be shown to extend into the lung (see Fig. 40-3). Vascular invasion can occasionally be detected if contrast-enhanced CT shows obstruction due to tumor involvement.

Because a significant portion of patients with esophageal cancer have subdiaphragmatic metastases at the time of diagnosis, it is important to also scan the upper abdomen to include the entire liver and the upper abdominal lymph nodes. Liver metastases generally appear as nonspecific low-density lesions (Fig. 40-12*A*). Equivocal or suspicious lesions can be confirmed by percutaneous biopsy. Subdiaphragmatic lymph nodes in the area of the gastrohepatic ligament or celiac axis that are larger than 1 cm (>8 mm according to one report) should be considered positive for lymph node metastases (Fig. 40-12*B*).

## Magnetic Resonance Imaging

Magnetic resonance imaging (MRI) has not yet been used to evaluate a large group of patients with esophageal cancer. One study reported that MRI was less accurate than CT for staging esophageal cancer. However, this study used an early-generation MRI system without the ad-

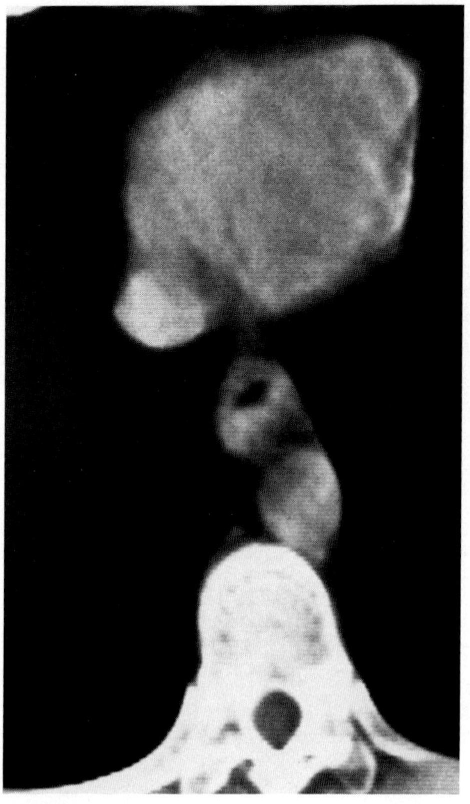

**Figure 40-11.** No invasion. CT scan shows an esophageal carcinoma with normal surrounding fat planes, consistent with a tumor limited to the wall of the esophagus.

vantages of newer modifications and pulse sequences. Thus, more extensive studies on state-of-the-art equipment are required to determine the precise role of MRI in the staging of patients with carcinoma of the esophagus.

### Percutaneous Biopsy

Percutaneous biopsy using small needles (20–22 gauge) has gained wide acceptance as a standard and safe technique for confirming both primary and secondary neoplastic lesions in almost every location in the body. It can be performed under either fluoroscopic, ultrasound, or CT guidance. In patients with esophageal cancer, percutaneous biopsy is primarily employed to obtain tissue samples from hepatic and adrenal masses and from enlarged lymph nodes suspected of containing metastases.

## OVERALL IMAGING APPROACH

Once the unequivocal diagnosis of esophageal cancer is made by esophagogram and endoscopy with biopsy, CT is the most effective procedure for staging. This modality can determine the potential surgical curability of an esophageal tumor in approximately 90% of patients. Findings on CT that unequivocally indicate that the patient has an incurable lesion are: (1) extension of tumor into the trachea or a bronchus producing an esophagorespiratory fistula; (2) evidence of distant metastatic disease to lymph nodes, liver or adrenal glands; and (3) obvious metastases to lung, pleura, bones, or other thoracic structures. The loss of fat planes between the tumor and surrounding structures does not have the same degree of accuracy for indicating incurability. If CT shows that the tumor is clearly separate from the surrounding structures, there is a more than 80% chance that the tumor is locally confined and that attempted curative resection is warranted. The false-negative rates of CT for predicting tumor invasion in the chest and distant abdominal metastases are 5% to 6% and 10% to 12%, respectively. A small number of patients are so cachectic that their CT scans are indeterminate and cannot be accurately evaluated; in such cases, other imaging studies or exploratory surgery is recommended.

Some patients with squamous cell carcinoma undergo chemotherapy and/or radiation therapy either prior to or in lieu of surgery. In the past, there was no accurate way to stage these patients. Computed tomography now provides an important method for evaluating tumor bulk and tumor extent, as well as for determining the response of the tumor to either radiation or chemotherapy. Even though most patients with carcinoma of the esophagus undergo palliative therapy, new protocols including combined preoperative radiation and chemotherapy are being used in an attempt to cure the tumor. The effective use of staging and follow-up CT will enable the radiologist to continue to play an important

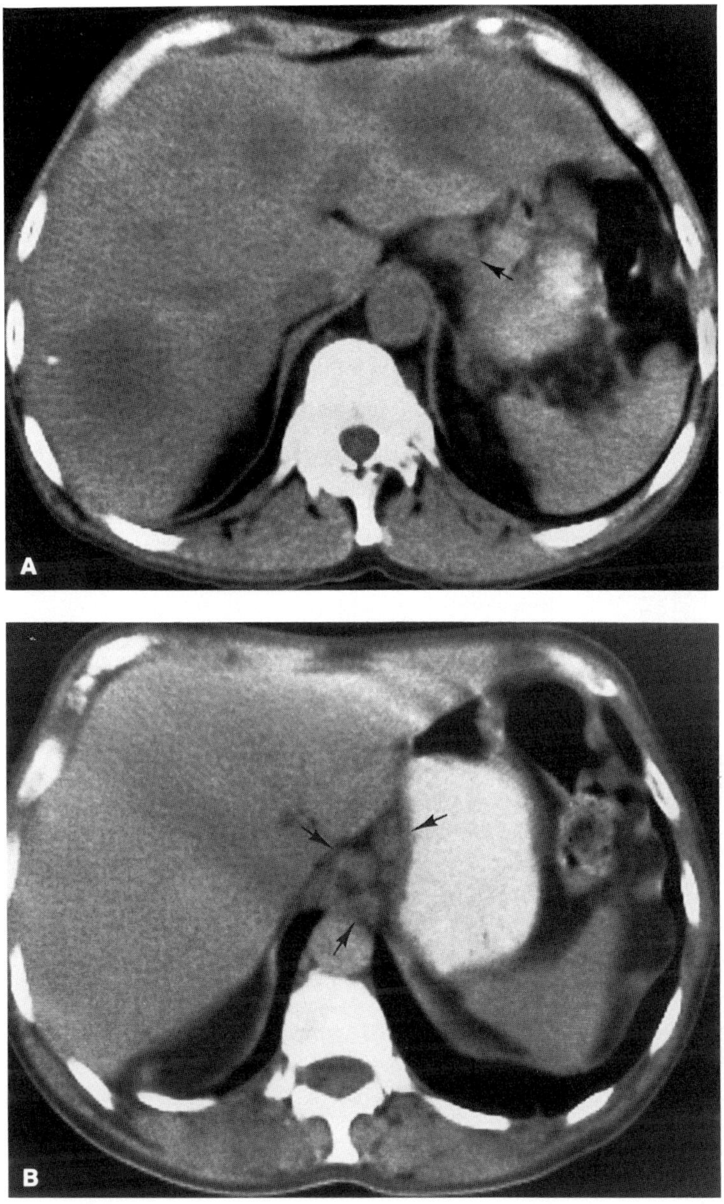


**Figure 40-12.** Metastases to lymph nodes and liver. **(A)** CT scan in a patient with carcinoma of the lower third of the esophagus demonstrates an enlarged lymph node (*arrow*) and multiple low-density lesions in the liver due to metastases. **(B)** CT scan through the upper abdomen in a different patient with a locally noninvading midesophageal cancer demonstrates enlarged (>1 cm) lymph nodes that contained tumor (*arrows*).

role in the management of patients with this devastating disease.

## Bibliography

Akiyama H: Surgery for carcinoma of the esophagus. Curr Probl Surg SVII:55–120, 1980

American Joint Committee: Staging of Cancer of the Esophagus. Manual for Staging of Cancer, pp 65–70, 1978

Balfe DM, Mauro MA, Koehler RE et al: Gastrohepatic ligament: Normal and pathologic CT anatomy. Radiology 150:485–490, 1984

Daffner RH, Halber MD, Postlethwait RW et al: CT of the esophagus. II. Carcinoma. AJR 133: 1051–1055, 1979

Earlam R, Cunha-Melo JR: Oesophageal squamous cell carcinoma. A critical review of surgery. Br J Surg 67:384–390, 1980

Earlam R, Cunha-Melo JR: Oesophageal squamous cell carcinoma. II. A critical review of radiotherapy. Br J Surg 67:457–461, 1980

Freeny PC, Marks WM: Adenocarcinoma of the gastroesophageal junction: Barium and CT examination. AJR 138:1077–1084, 1982

Halvorsen RA, Thompson WM: Computed tomographic evaluation of esophageal carcinoma. Semin Oncol 11:113–126, 1984

Halvorsen RA, Thompson WM: Critical review of esophageal carcinoma by Quint LE, Glaser GM, Orrager MB, Gross BH. Radiology 155:171–175, 1985. Invest Radiol 22:84–87, 1987

Heiken JP, Balfe DM, Roper CL: CT evaluation after esophagogastrectomy. AJR 143:550–560, 1984

Huang GJ: Early detection and surgical treatment of esophageal carcinoma. Jap J Surg 11:399–405, 1981

Kondo M, Ando N, Kosuda S et al: Ga-67 scan in patients with intrathoracic esophageal carcinoma planned for surgery. Cancer 49:1031–1034, 1982

Lawson TL, Dodds WJ: Infiltrating carcinoma simulating achalasia. Gastrointest Radiol 1:245–248, 1976

Lindell MM, Jr, Hill CA, Libshitz HI: Esophageal cancer: Radiographic chest findings and their prognostic significance. AJR 133:461–465, 1979

Moss AA, Schnyder P, Thoeni RF, Margulis AR: Esophageal carcinoma: Pretherapy staging by computed tomography. AJR 136:1051–1056, 1981

Norton GA, Postlethwait RW, Thompson WM: Esophageal carcinoma: A survey of populations at risk. South Med J 73:25–27, 1980

Picus D, Balfe DM, Koehler RE et al: Computed tomography in the staging of esophageal carcinoma. Radiology 146:433–438, 1983

Postlethwait RW: Squamous cell carcinoma of the esophagus. In Surgery of the Esophagus, 2nd ed, pp 369–442. New York, Appleton-Century-Crofts, 1986

Quint LE, Glazer GM, Orringer MB: Esophageal imaging by MR and CT: Study of normal anatomy and neoplasm. Radiology 156:727–731, 1985

Quint LE, Glazer GM, Orringer MB, Gross BH: Esophageal carcinoma: CT findings. Radiology 155:171–175, 1983

Rosenberg JC et al: Cancer of the esophagus. In Devita VT, Jr, Hellman S, Rosenberg SA (eds): Cancer: Principles and Practice of Oncology, 2nd ed, pp 621–657. Philadelphia, JB Lippincott, 1985

Rubin P: Cancer of the gastrointestinal tract. I. Esophagus: Detection and diagnosis. JAMA 226: 1544–1546, 1973

Rubin P: Clinical Oncology for Medical Students and Physicians: A Multidisciplinary Approach, 6th ed. New York, American Cancer Society, 1983

Steiger Z, Franklin R, Wilson RF et al: Eradication and palliation of squamous cell carcinoma of the esophagus with chemotherapy, radiotherapy and surgical therapy. J Thorac Cardiovasc Surg 82: 713–719, 1981

Suzuki H, Kobayashi S, Endo M, Nakayama K: Diagnosis of early esophageal cancer. Surgery 71: 99–103, 1972

Thompson WM: Esophageal cancer. Int J Radia Oncol Biol Phys 9:1533–1565, 1983

Thompson WM, Halvorsen RA, Foster WL et al: Computed tomography for staging esophageal and gastroesophageal cancer. A re-evaluation. AJR 141:951–958, 1983

Zornoza J, Lindell MM, Jr: Radiologic evaluation of small esophageal carcinoma. Gastrointest Radiol 5:107–111, 1980

**SUSPECTED ESOPHAGEAL CARCINOMA**

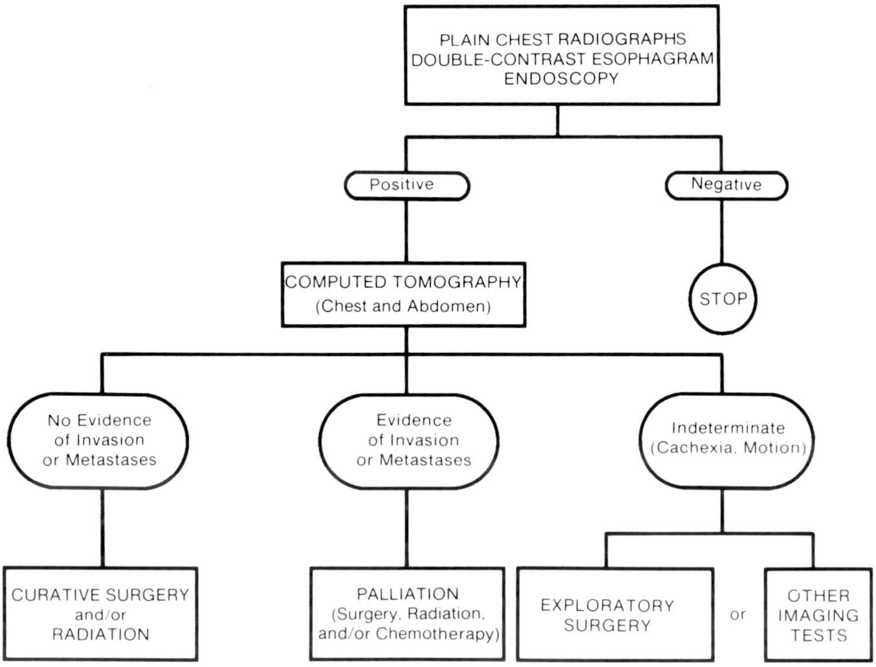

# Chapter 41

# Staging and Detection of Recurrence of Gastric and Colorectal Cancer

*Matthew A. Mauro*
*L. Alden Parker*

## GASTRIC CANCER

The death rate from gastric cancer in the United States has shown a steady decline from 30 per 100,000 in 1930 to 8 per 100,000 in 1980. Despite these encouraging statistics, gastric carcinoma is still a common cause of cancer deaths (the fifth leading cause of cancer deaths in men) and has a relatively dismal prognosis. The 5-year survival rate for patients with localized disease is less than 50% and only 5% to 15% for those with diffuse disease that has penetrated the serosa. Patients with unresectable tumors have a median survival of 4 to 9 months. Five-year survival rates of 95% have been reported for early and superficial spreading gastric carcinomas, but these lesions account for only 7% of the gastric carcinomas in the United States. In Japan, where the incidence of gastric cancer is far higher, approximately 30% of gastric cancer is of the early (tumor limited to the mucosa or submucosa) or superficial spreading (lesion without polypoid features or ulceration) types. This difference may be due in part to the greater attention given to the early diagnosis of gastric cancer in that country.

The demographics and etiologic factors related to the development of gastric cancer are beyond the scope of this chapter. However, it is worth noting that gastric cancer is more common in workers who are exposed to asbestos, a relatively common carcinogen in industrialized society. There appears to be no increased risk of gastric cancer due to the use of alcohol or tobacco, both of which are strongly associated with the development of esophageal cancer. There is an increased incidence of gastric cancer (5%–10%) in patients with pernicious anemia.

Approximately 95% of gastric malignancies are adenocarcinomas, and it is this histologic type that is generally referred to when the term *gastric cancer* is used. The remaining 5% of gastric malignancies are predominantly leiomyosarcomas and lymphomas.

The TNM classification (Table 41-1) is used to stage gastric cancer (Table 41-2), and provides a basis for comparing large groups, assessing the efficacy of treatment regimens, and offering prognostic data for both patients and clinicians. Most, if not all, of the information needed to accurately stage gastric cancer can be obtained at the time of surgery. Preoperative efforts at staging are primarily directed toward identifying those patients with unresectable disease who are not candidates for a palliative surgical procedure and to assist the surgeon in preoperative planning by accurately defining the extent of disease. In general, the presence of widespread metastatic disease, fixation of the stomach to adjacent organs, or ascites secondary to peritoneal carcinomatosis makes a patient incurable by surgery. A surgical procedure for palliation may be undertaken to debulk the tumor and to minimize complications such as hemorrhage, perforation, and further obstruction. It may also make the changes of chemotherapy more effective. Marking unresectable disease with surgical clips can aid the radiation therapist in defining the appropriate treatment portal. In patients with gastric outlet obstruction, the performance of a gastroenterostomy has not been recommended, because this procedure may not relieve the obstruction and may be associated with unwarranted risks.

**Table 41-1** Gastric Cancer: TNM Classification

| | |
|---|---|
| Primary Tumor (T) | |
| $T_{is}$ | Tumor limited to mucosa without penetration into the lamina propria |
| $T_1$ | Tumor limited to mucosa, or mucosa and submucosa |
| $T_2$ | Tumor involves the mucosa and the submucosa and extends to or into the serosa, but does not penetrate through the serosa |
| $T_3$ | Tumor penetrates through the serosa without invading contiguous structures |
| $T_{4a}$ | Tumor penetrates through the serosa and involves immediately adjacent tissues |
| $T_{4b}$ | Tumor penetrates through the serosa and involves other organs. |
| Nodal Involvement (N) | |
| $N_0$ | No metastases to regional lymph nodes |
| $N_1$ | Involvement of perigastric lymph nodes within 3 cm of the primary tumor along the lesser or greater curvature |
| $N_2$ | Involvement of regional lymph nodes that are situated more than 3 cm from the primary tumor and are removed or removable at operation |
| $N_3$ | Involvement of other intra-abdominal lymph nodes that are not removable at operation |
| Distant Metastasis (M) | |
| $M_0$ | No (known) distant metastasis |
| $M_1$ | Distant metastasis present |

**Table 41-2** Gastric Cancer: Stage Grouping

| | | | |
|---|---|---|---|
| Stage 0 | $T_{is}$ | $N_0$ | $M_0$ |
| Stage I | $T_1$ | $N_0$ | $M_0$ |
| Stage II | $T_2$, $T_3$ | $N_0$ | $M_0$ |
| Stage III | $T_1$–$T_3$ | $N_1$, $N_2$ | $M_0$ |
| | $T_{4a}$ | $N_0$–$N_2$ | $M_0$ |
| Stage IV | $T_1$–$T_3$ | $N_3$ | $M_0$ |
| | $T_{4b}$ | Any N | $M_0$ |
| | Any T | Any N | $M_1$ |

## CLINICAL AND LABORATORY FINDINGS

Unfortunately, the symptoms of gastric cancer are often vague and nonspecific and correlate poorly with the resectability of the lesion. When physical signs of the disease have become manifest, the patient is usually incurable. The carcinoembryonic antigen (CEA) and the urinary polyamine assays have not proven to be effective screening tests for diagnosis, although they may have some prognostic value in patients with advanced disease (stage III or stage IV), because they most likely reflect a large tumor burden. Liver function tests may be abnormal in patients with extensive hepatic metastases, but they are insensitive to small metastatic deposits and may be affected by benign conditions.

## DIAGNOSTIC EVALUATION

### *DIAGNOSTIC MODALITIES*

1. Computed tomography
2. Upper gastrointestinal radiography/ endoscopy
3. Arteriography
4. Nuclear medicine procedures
5. Ultrasound
6. Magnetic resonance imaging
7. Surgery

### Computed Tomography

Computed tomography (CT) is the imaging modality of choice for the preoperative staging of gastric carcinoma (Fig. 41-1) and all gastrointestinal tract malignancies. Because CT can provide staging information previously obtainable only by direct inspection at surgery, a uniform CT-based staging system for malignant neoplasms of the alimentary tract is now in general use (Table 41-3). Computed tomography can detect the extragastric extension of tumor to adjacent organs and lymph nodes (Fig. 41-2) as well as metastases to the liver, peritoneum, and omentum. Distant metastases to the lung and adrenal glands can be detected by CT, which can also be used to guide percutaneous thin-needle aspiration biopsy for confirmation of tumor spread.

Computed tomography has been shown to be a cost-effective method for identifying those patients with gastric carcinoma (up to one third of cases) who present with such extensive disease that they are not candidates for either curative or palliative resection. Such patients have a high operative mortality, and palliative procedures may not achieve their intended purpose. Computed tomography also can be used for designing treatment ports for postoperative radiation therapy. This therapeutic approach has been advocated by some as a means of treating microscopic residual tumor deposits that frequently remain following surgery and may lead to the relatively

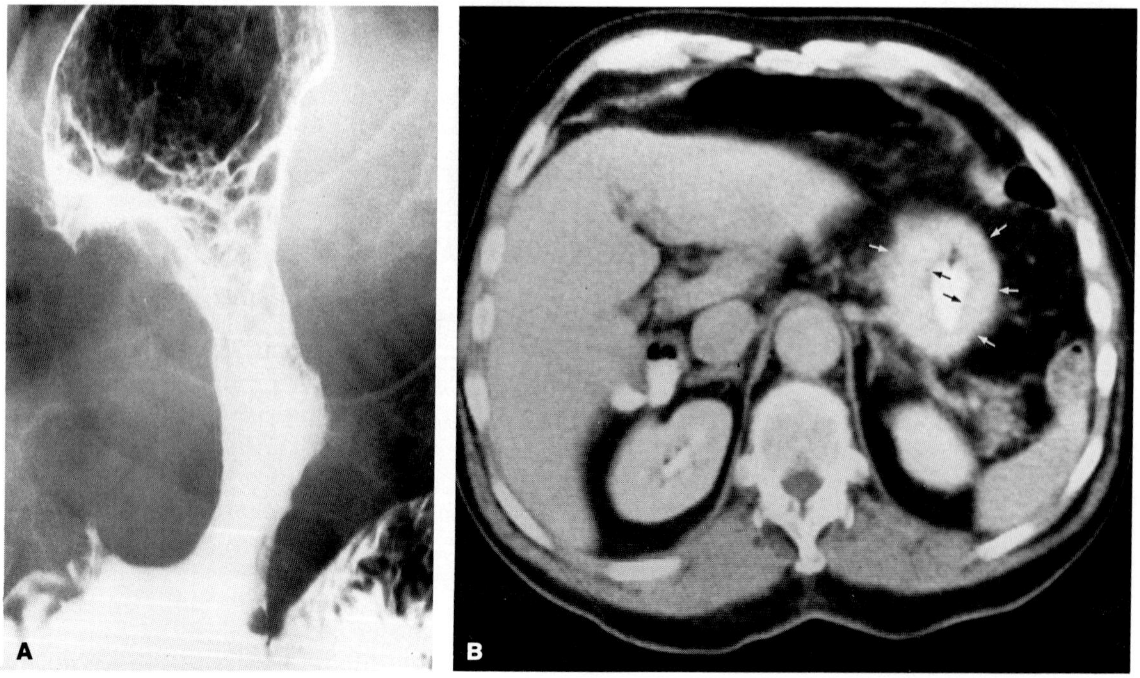


**Figure 41-1. (A)** Upper gastrointestinal series shows narrowing of the body of the stomach due to gastric adenocarcinoma. **(B)** CT scan demonstrates the thickened gastric wall (*arrows*).

**Table 41-3** CT-Based Staging System for Gastrointestinal Malignancy

| | |
|---|---|
| Stage I | Wall of the gut is of normal thickness and a polypoid lesion protrudes into the lumen |
| Stage II | Wall of the gut is thickened but there is no extension of tumor beyond the wall |
| Stage III | Wall of the gut is thickened and there is direct extension of tumor into surrounding tissue. There may be local or regional lymph node involvement, but no distant metastases.<br><br>For rectal lesions<br>(A) No spread to pelvic sidewall<br>(B) Spread to surrounding pelvic structures |
| Stage IV | Distant metastases |

high incidence of local or regional recurrence in the absence of distant metastases. In patients who have disseminated disease and are being treated with chemotherapy, CT provides a method for assessing the therapeutic response.

Computed tomography is of value in the detection of recurrent disease following gastric resection (Fig. 41-3). A baseline CT examination following surgery is recommended to aid in the subsequent differentiation between postoperative changes and recurrent tumor, both of which appear as soft-tissue masses in the operative field. Thin-needle aspiration under CT direction can be used to histologically confirm the presence of recurrent disease.

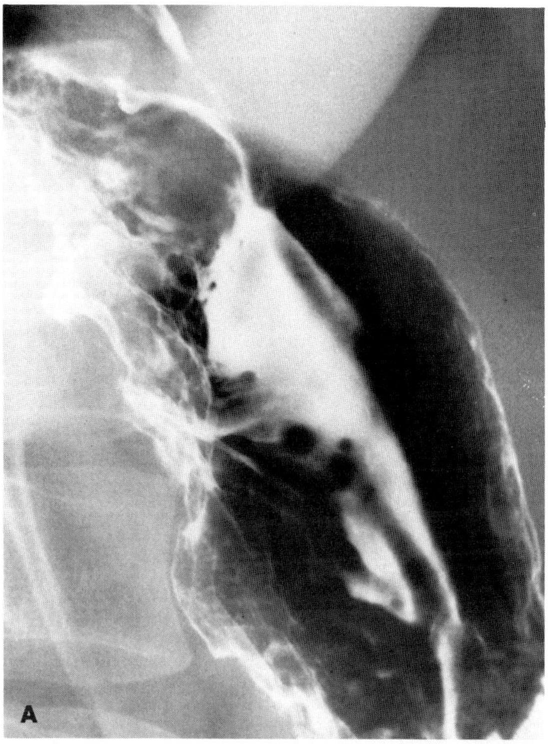

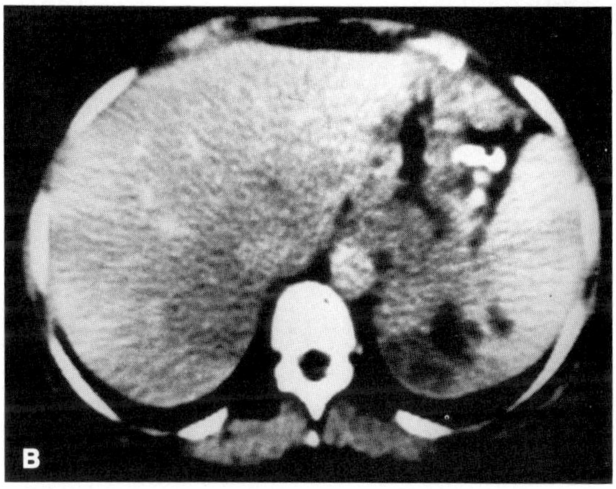

**Figure 41-2.** **(A)** Upper gastrointestinal series demonstrates a fundal mass representing gastric adenocarcinoma. **(B)** Contrast-enhanced CT scan shows the gastric mass extending to invade the spleen.

## Upper Gastrointestinal Radiography/Endoscopy

These modalities are primarily used in the detection of gastric cancer and are of limited value in staging. Accuracy rates as high as 86% have been reported for the detection of early gastric cancer using double-contrast techniques. Endoscopy can detect 90% to 95% of all gastric can-

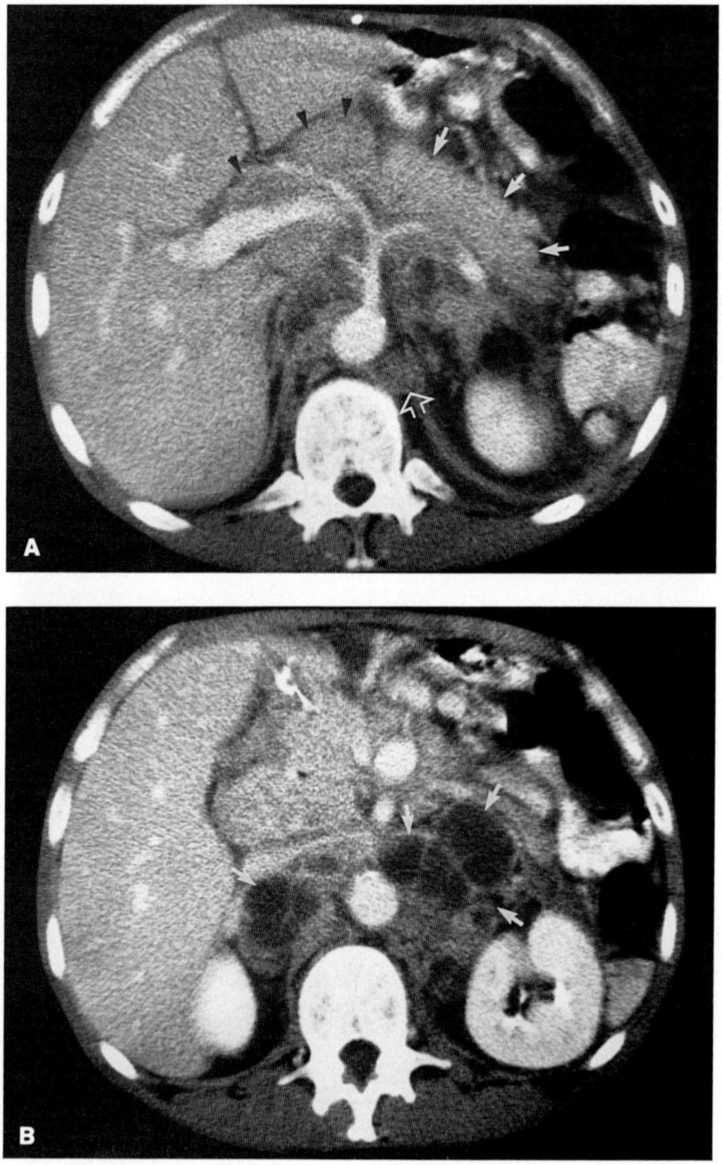


**Figure 41-3. (A)** CT scan shows recurrent gastric carcinoma in the surgical bed (*arrows*), nodes in the porta hepatis (*arrowheads*), and retrocrural adenopathy (*open arrow*). **(B)** At a lower level, a CT scan shows retroperitoneal extension of recurrent cancer with necrosis (*arrows*).

cers and almost 100% of lesions protruding into the gastric lumen.

## Arteriography

Although arteriography was formerly used to stage gastric cancer by demonstrating tumor vascularity, vascular invasion, and altered hepatic vascular architecture in the presence of metastates, the use of this expensive, invasive procedure has been eliminated by the availability of CT.

## Nuclear Medicine Procedures

Traditional radionuclide scintigraphy has been supplanted by CT in the evaluation of hepatic metastases from gastric carcinoma. However, in the future single photon emission computed tomography (SPECT) may provide a less expensive alternative to CT for assessing the regression of hepatic metastases in response to chemotherapeutic regimens. The use of isotopically labeled monoclonal antibodies to CEA is being evaluated as an imaging technique, although the elevation of CEA in patients with gastric cancer tends to be substantially lower than in patients with colorectal tumors.

### Ultrasound

Ultrasound may be used to detect a tumor in the distended stomach, ascites, or the presence of hepatic metastases. However, these abnormalities are better identified by CT, which also can detect lung metastases and can better define any exophytic extension of the tumor. The primary role of ultrasound in patients with gastric cancer is to provide an inexpensive modality for guiding percutaneous biopsy to confirm the presence of metastatic disease.

### Magnetic Resonance Imaging

The role of magnetic resonance imaging (MRI) is continually evolving, and this modality may prove to be as sensitive, if not more so, than CT for defining the extragastric extension of disease.

### Surgery

The final staging in the TNM classification is based on surgical–pathologic findings. In general, a radical subtotal gastrectomy and regional lymph node resection is the surgical procedure of choice for stages I to III. Patients with stage IV disease may also undergo resection of involved adjacent organs if this is technically possible. Experience with repeat laparotomy for resection of recurrent disease has been limited, and these procedures have been associated with relatively high operative mortality. At present, only palliative procedures are offered to patients with recurrent gastric cancer; in the future, repeat operations may be justified even if only a small additional cure rate can be achieved.

## COLORECTAL CANCER

Colorectal cancer, which ranks second only to lung cancer in incidence in the United States, accounts for approximately 15% of all cancer-related deaths. Of the more than 100,000 new cases of colorectal carcinoma diagnosed each year, more than half the patients will die of their disease. The need for routine preoperative staging of colorectal cancer remains controversial, with opinions varying not only among different institutions but also among surgeons in the same institution. The majority of colorectal cancers will be resected regardless of the extent of disease, so that these tumors can be staged at the time of operation. Nevertheless, staging of a tumor prior to surgery is particularly important when preoperative radiation is being considered, which may improve survival, decrease local recurrences, and permit a previously unresectable tumor to be surgically removed. Preoperative staging is also of value in patients with colorectal cancer in whom metastatic disease to the liver is to be treated by segmental resection (solitary metastasis) or by a surgically implanted hepatic artery chemotherapy infusion pump (diffuse metastatic disease). Most surgeons agree that patients with colorectal cancer who are poor surgical risks or are suspected of having advanced disease will benefit from pretreatment staging. The two clinical–pathological staging systems in common use for patients with colorectal carcinoma are the modified Dukes (Table 41-4) and TNM (Tables 41-5 and 41-6) systems.

**Table 41-4** Colorectal Cancer: Dukes Classification

| | |
|---|---|
| A | Tumor limited to mucosa |
| B1 | Tumor extends to muscularis propria but does not penetrate muscle layer |
| B2 | Tumor penetrates muscle layer |
| C1 | Tumor does not penetrate bowel wall, but positive regional lymph nodes are present |
| C2 | Tumor penetrates bowel wall, and positive regional lymph nodes are present |
| D | Metastases to liver, lung, bone, peritoneum, or bowel, or unresectability of tumor because of involvement of adjacent organs |

**Table 41-5** Colorectal Cancer: TNM Classification

| | |
|---|---|
| Primary Tumor (T) | |
| $T_0$ | Metastases present but no primary tumor found |
| $T_{is}$ | Carcinoma *in situ* (without invasion of lamina propria) |
| $T_1$ | Tumor limited to mucosa or submucosa |
| $T_{2a}$ | Tumor penetrates to muscularis propria |
| $T_{2b}$ | Tumor penetrates through muscularis propria |
| $T_3$ | Tumor penetration includes serosa |
| $T_4$ | Tumor extension to contiguous tissues/organs |
| Nodal Involvement (N) | |
| $N_0$ | No lymph node involvement |
| $N_1$ | Involvement of one to three regional lymph nodes |
| $N_2$ | Involvement of lymph nodes that extend to line of resection or ligature of vessels |
| $N_3$ | Involvement of lymph nodes, but number and site undetermined |
| Distant Metastasis (M) | |
| $M_0$ | No distant metastasis |
| $M_1$ | Distant metastasis |

**Table 41-6** Colorectal Cancer: Stage Grouping

| | | | |
|---|---|---|---|
| Stage 0 | Carcinoma *in situ* | | |
| | $T_{is}$ | $N_0$ | $M_0$ |
| Stage Ia | $T_1$ | $N_0$ | $M_0$ |
| Stage Ib | $T_2$ | $N_0$ | $M_0$ |
| Stage II | $T_3$ | $N_0$ | $M_0$ |
| Stage III | Any T | $N_1$ $N_2$ $N_3$ | $M_0$ |
| | $T_4$ | $N_0$ | $M_0$ |
| Stage IV | Any T | Any N | $M_1$ |

Approximately 30% to 50% of patients undergoing resections for colorectal cancer will develop recurrent disease. Half of the recurrences develop within 1 year of surgery, while 80% of recurrences occur by the end of the second postoperative year. Approximately 90% of recurrences develop contiguous to the area of surgical resection, and about 60% of the patients have no evidence of distant metastases at the time their local recurrence is detected. The early detection of local recurrence may permit surgical resection and prolong survival. The staging of recurrent disease is a major factor in determining whether to offer the patient further surgery (limited resectable disease) or radiation therapy and/or chemotherapy (extensive unresectable local disease or distant metastases).

## CLINICAL AND LABORATORY FINDINGS

Although liver function tests are often abnormal in patients with diffuse liver metastases from colorectal cancer, they are insensitive for detecting early liver metastases and are unreliable as a screening test for small metastatic deposits.

The CEA is a circulating glycoprotein produced in variable amounts by colorectal tumor cells. A new and persistently elevated CEA level following surgery, in the absence of a disease such as cirrhosis or pancreatitis that can elevate the CEA level, suggests the presence of recurrent malignant colorectal disease. Approximately 90% of patients undergoing laparotomy based on an elevated CEA level will be proven to have recurrent disease. However, only 65% to 70% of patients with recurrent disease have elevated CEA levels. In addition, CEA measurements are more reliable in detecting hepatic metastases than local recurrences (only 50% of patients with local recurrences have elevated CEA levels).

## DIAGNOSTIC EVALUATION

### *DIAGNOSTIC MODALITIES*

1. Computed tomography
2. Percutaneous aspiration biopsy
3. Arteriography
4. Ultrasound
5. Nuclear medicine studies
6. Magnetic resonance imaging
7. Barium enema examination
8. Endoscopy
9. Surgery

## Computed Tomography

### Pretreatment Staging

Although the need for preoperative staging of all patients with colorectal cancer remains controversial, the imaging modality of choice for this purpose is CT. Most portions of the colon are generally well seen on CT, because they are surrounded by fat. The primary colorectal tumor can be detected in at least 85% of cases and may appear as an intraluminal mass (Fig. 41-4), focal or circumferential wall thickening (Fig. 41-5), or a discrete extraluminal mass. Large tumors often demonstrate a central low-attenuation area representing tumor necrosis. Although CT cannot accurately determine the degree of infiltration of the bowel wall, it can show obliteration of pericolonic or perirectal fat, indicating extramural extension of tumor to surrounding structures (Fig. 41-6). Computed tomography can also identify extension of tumor to the bladder, prostate, seminal vesicles, ovaries, bowel, pelvic musculature, and bony pelvis (Fig. 41-7).

In addition to determining the local extent of the disease, CT can show regional and distant lymphadenopathy as well as hepatic metastases. Although the specificity is high, CT has a low sensitivity (25%) in detecting lymph node metastases from colorectal cancer, primarily due to the presence of metastatic deposits in normal-sized nodes. False-positive scans occur when lymph

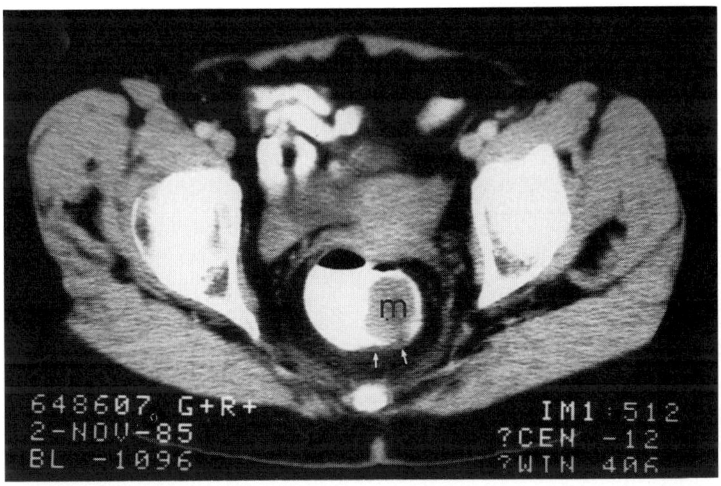


**Figure 41-4.** CT scan shows a large intraluminal rectal mass (*m*) associated with slight thickening of the posterior rectal wall (*arrows*). There was no extramural disease.

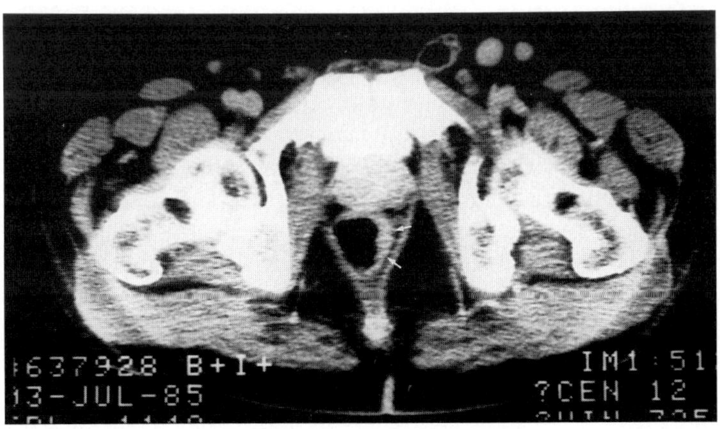


**Figure 41-5.** CT scan shows thickening of the rectal wall (*arrows*) representing the primary tumor (CT stage II). At surgery, the disease was confined to the rectum.

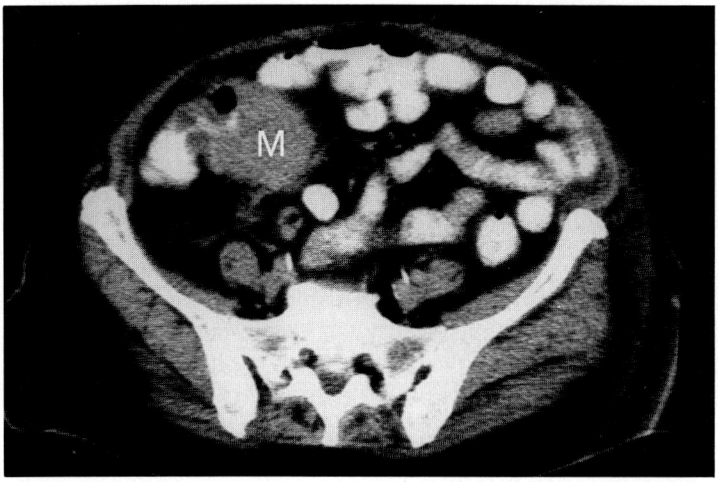


**Figure 41-6.** CT scan shows a stage III adenocarcinoma of the right colon (*M*) with extramural extension.

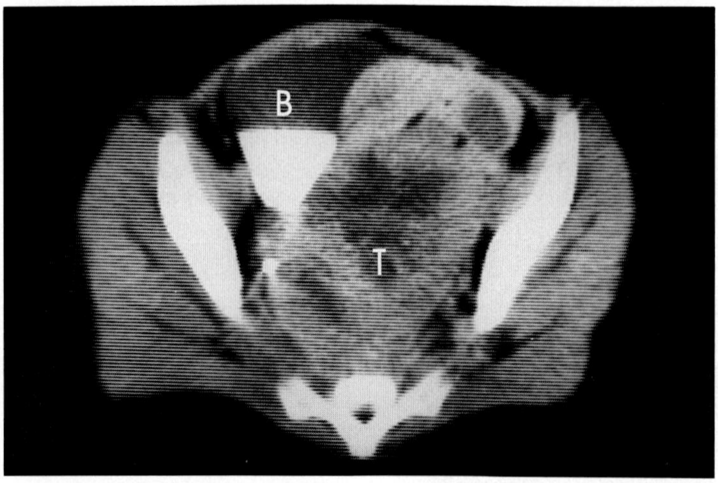


**Figure 41-7.** CT scan shows a large stage IIIB rectal or rectosigmoid tumor (*T*) with extension to the pelvic sidewalls. The patient underwent radiation therapy and a diverting colostomy. (*B*, bladder)

nodes are enlarged secondary to reactive or inflammatory changes. It is important to note, however, that this low accuracy for detection of subtle regional lymphadenopathy does not affect treatment, because all of these patients undergo surgical resection.

Bolus dynamic scanning with table incrementation is currently the preferred noninvasive CT method used for detecting and staging hepatic metastases (Figs. 41-8 and 41-9). Because it is reproducible, CT can be used to follow the course of liver lesions after therapy. An even more sensitive technique is CT angiography, in which dynamic CT sections with table incrementation are obtained during contrast infusion from a catheter placed within either the hepatic artery (CT arteriography) or the superior mesenteric artery (CT portography). In one study of patients with colorectal cancer, dynamic bolus incremental CT scanning of the liver had a sensitivity of 72%, a specificity of 98%, and an accuracy of 96%. Most of the hepatic metastases missed during this study were surface lesions that were less than or equal to 1 cm in diameter.

### Detection and Staging of Recurrent Tumor

Computed tomography is the imaging modality of choice for detecting and staging recurrent colorectal cancer. Although endoscopy is very sen-

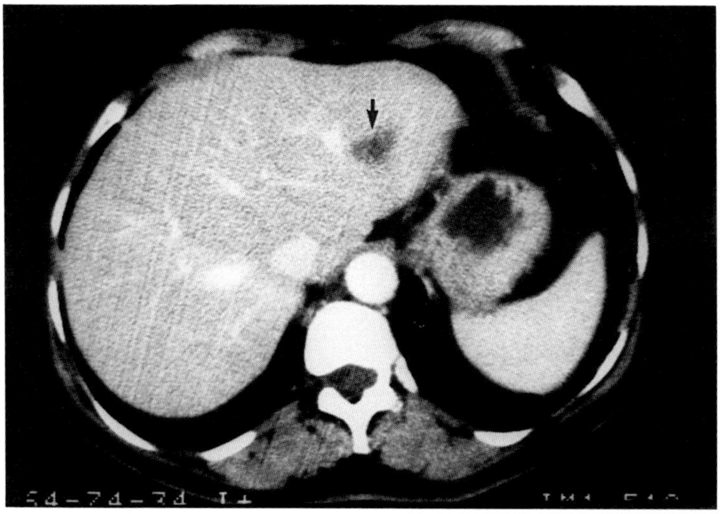

**Figure 41-8.** Dynamic incremental bolus CT scan shows a solitary liver metastasis (*arrow*). The patient underwent celiac arteriography followed by segmental hepatic resection.

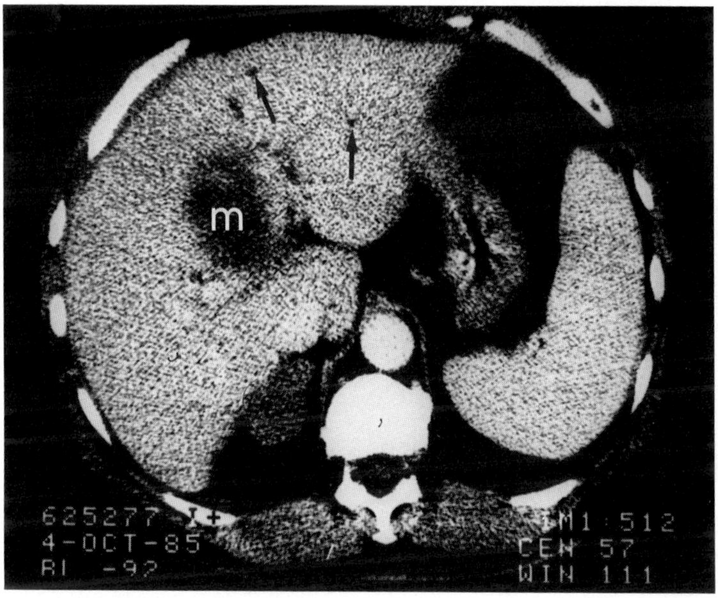


**Figure 41-9.** Dynamic incremental bolus CT scan viewed with narrow windows shows a dominant central liver metastasis (*m*) and several small (5 mm) scattered metastases (*arrows*). A celiac arteriogram was performed in preparation for placement of an intra-arterial chemotherapy infusion pump.

sitive in the detection of anastomotic recurrences and allows biopsy confirmation of recurrent tumor, this technique (unlike CT) provides no information about the extent of spread of the neoplastic mass. In patients with a primary anastomosis following bowel resection, the CT findings of recurrent tumor include bowel wall thickening (focal or circumferential), a discrete mass, extension of a mass into adjacent structures (visceral organs, pelvic musculature, bony skeleton), enlarged lymph nodes, and hepatic metastases (Fig. 41-10). The CT findings have direct implications for therapy. Local, resectable recurrences (no sidewall invasion) can be treated with a second surgical procedure. The presence of sidewall invasion (implying advanced local disease) or distant metastases indicates a need for radiation therapy and/or systemic chemotherapy.

Computed tomography is the method of

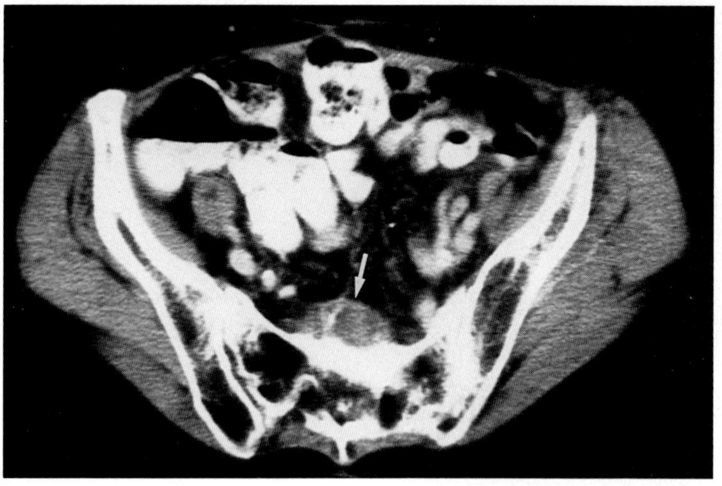

**Figure 41-10.** CT scan following segmental resection for a sigmoid carcinoma shows a local recurrence as a soft-tissue mass (*arrow*) anterior to the sacrum. Bony erosion was seen on bone window settings. Endoscopy failed to show any intraluminal tumor.

choice for detecting early recurrences in patients following abdominoperineal resection (Fig. 41-11). At times, it may be difficult to differentiate recurrent tumor from postoperative or postradiation changes. Postoperative changes generally decrease in prominence between 4 and 9 months following surgery, although minimal streaky densities or a thin, transverse crescentic density separate from the sacrum may remain. Tumor recurrences usually present as globular masses in the posterior portion of the pelvis, the presacral region in men and the posterior vaginal wall and rectovaginal pouch in women. Recurrent masses invading surrounding organs (bladder, seminal vesicles, prostate) or structures (pelvic musculature, bone) can be easily detected. False-positive interpretations may arise when relocated pelvic organs (uterus, seminal vesicles), small bowel loops, or postoperative fibrosis are mistaken for recurrent tumor.

Because the early detection and treatment of recurrent colorectal cancer can lead to increased survival, and because recurrences may occur in asymptomatic patients who have a normal CEA level, some physicians recommend routine postoperative CT scanning. According to this concept, a baseline scan should be obtained 2 to 4 months following surgery and then every 6 months for the first two postoperative years. The development of local symptoms or a newly and persistently elevated CEA level should prompt immediate CT scanning.

## Percutaneous Aspiration Biopsy

Percutaneous thin-needle aspiration biopsy under CT guidance is of value in the detection and histologic confirmation of recurrent colorectal tumor (Fig. 41-11*C*). This technique is particularly useful in patients with nonspecific soft-tissue pelvic masses in the area of a previous abdominoperineal resection. A transgluteal thin-needle biopsy under CT guidance offers a simple, quick, safe, and direct approach for obtaining specific histologic documentation of recurrent disease.

## Arteriography

The only use for arteriography in the staging of colorectal cancer is in the evaluation of patients with metastatic disease to the liver who are being considered for segmental resection or the surgical placement of a hepatic artery chemotherapy infusion catheter. Because of the variation of blood supply to the liver, an arterial "road map" is required for proper placement of the infusion catheter. The blood supply to the right lobe may arise totally or partially from the superior mesenteric artery; the blood supply to the left lobe may originate completely or in part from the left gastric artery. Knowledge of the precise vascular supply to the liver is required to determine the site of catheter placement and the number of

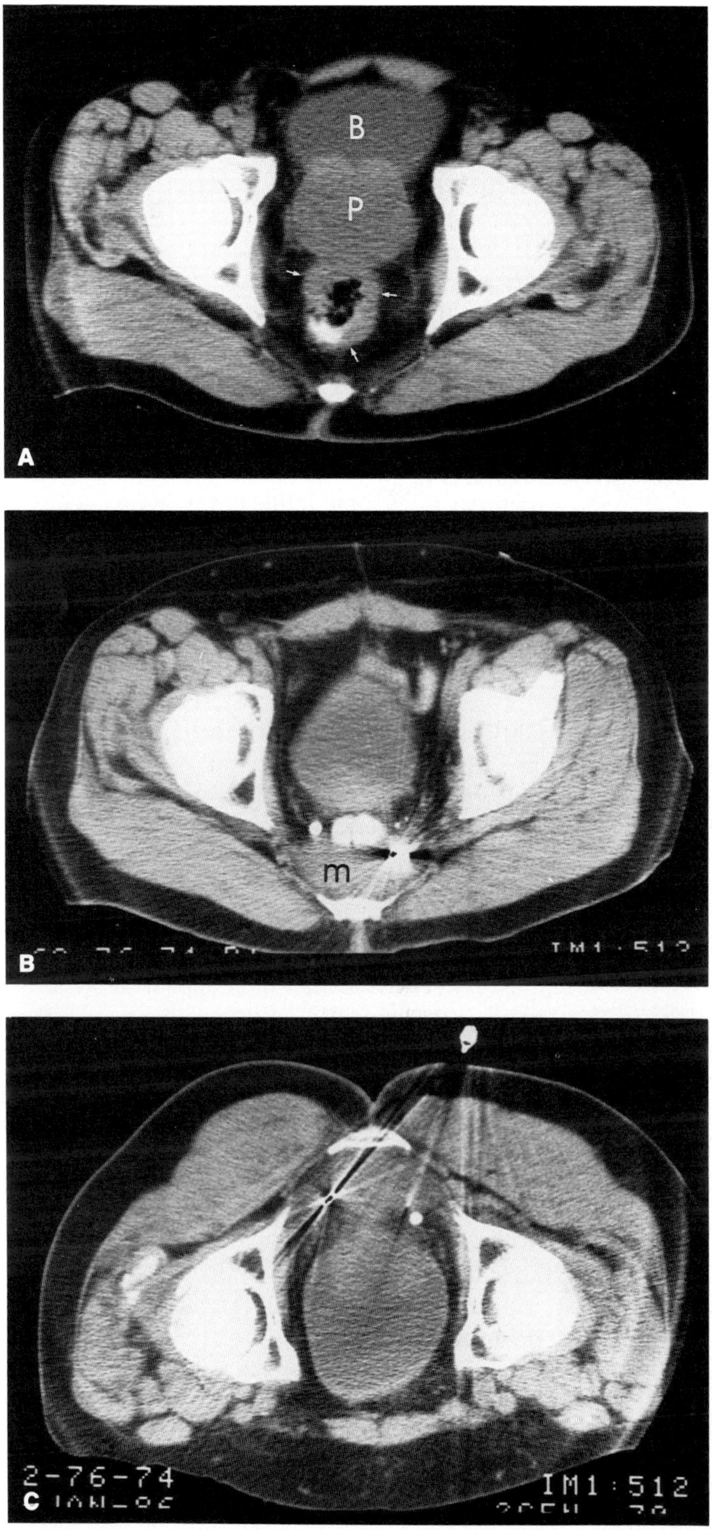


**Figure 41-11. (A)** Initial CT scan shows circumferential thickening of the rectal wall (*arrows*) caused by adenocarcinoma (*B,* bladder; *P,* prostate). **(B)** CT scan 1 year following abdominoperineal resection shows a presacral soft-tissue mass (*m*) in the operative bed. **(C)** Scan from CT-guided transgluteal needle aspiration of the presacral mass (*arrows* point to the needle) was conclusive for recurrent adenocarcinoma.

catheters required for complete hepatic perfusion. In cases in which the hepatic arterial supply originates from more than one location, the hepatic artery(ies) may be amenable to transcatheter embolization, so that only one surgically placed infusion catheter may need to be inserted.

The resection of solitary liver metastases has been shown to increase the survival rate of patients with colorectal cancer. Preoperative arteriography is used to provide a map of the hepatic vessels for surgical planning. In addition, the injection of a bolus of contrast material via a catheter placed within either the hepatic artery (CT arteriography) or the superior mesenteric artery (CT portography) can increase the sensitivity of dynamic incremental CT scanning in the detection of small hepatic metastases.

### Ultrasound

Transrectal ultrasound can identify three distinct layers of the bowel wall. The inner (musocal) and outer (serosal) layers appear echogenic and are separated by a larger hypoechoic layer representing the muscularis propria. Rectal tumors within the reach of the ultrasound probe appear hypoechoic and their depth of invasion within the wall can be assessed. Ultrasound can detect the extrarectal spread of disease and may be of some value in selecting patients suitable for local excision. However, this modality is much less useful than CT in the evaluation of lymphadenopathy and distant metastatic spread. Following a low anterior resection, ultrasound can be of value in the detection of local tumor recurrence.

### Nuclear Medicine Procedures

Isotopically labeled ($^{131}$I or $^{111}$In) monoclonal antibodies to CEA will localize to CEA-producing tumors, which can be subsequently imaged by scintillation scanning. This radioimmunodetection technique, which has been reported to be more sensitive than the simple measurement of circulating CEA, can be used both for preoperative staging of tumor or for the detection of recurrent disease. In addition, studies are under way to evaluate the use of monoclonal antibodies attached to a radiotherapeutic agent for tumor treatment.

### Magnetic Resonance Imaging

Although the utility of MRI in the evaluation of the gastrointestinal tract remains to be determined, the inherent ability of this modality to image the pelvis in multiple projections may allow more accurate evaluation of local pelvic tumors and better detection of recurrent disease. Magnetic resonance imaging already can detect metastatic disease to the liver with sensitivity and accuracy rates comparable to CT. With the introduction of phase-contrast liver imaging and very short repetition time/echo time (TR/TE) spin-echo sequences, MRI is likely to prove superior to CT for the detection of hepatic metastases.

### Barium Enema Examination

Barium enema examinations using the double-contrast technique for detailed mucosal evaluation can be used to detect recurrent colorectal cancer in the patient who has undergone a segmental bowel resection with a primary anastomosis. This modality primarily demonstrates mucosal recurrences, which appear as focal irregularity, nodularity, or plaquelike masses that tend to occur at or near the anastomotic site. Comparison with a postoperative baseline study aids in distinguishing tumor recurrence from postsurgical changes. The detection of a possible tumor recurrence on barium enema examination should be followed by endoscopic biopsy for histologic confirmation.

### Endoscopy

Endoscopy is a very sensitive technique for detecting anastomotic recurrences in patients with colorectal cancer who have undergone a primary tumor resection and retain continuity of their gastrointestinal tract. In addition, this technique allows biopsy confirmation of recurrent tumor.

Although endoscopy cannot demonstrate an extraluminal recurrence, many local recurrences that develop outside the bowel wall secondarily penetrate the anastomosis to permit endoscopic detection. Patients who have undergone abdominoperineal resections for rectal carcinoma are not candidates for endoscopic evaluation, and the detection of tumor recurrence in these patients requires radiographic imaging.

## Surgery

Surgical excision of the tumor is performed in virtually all patients with colorectal cancer. The involved segment of colon along with its mesentery and regional nodes are removed *en bloc.* Surgery is often performed in incurable patients to avoid potential colonic obstruction, perforation, or intestinal hemorrhage. Whenever technically possible, the operation of choice is a segmental resection with a primary intestinal anastomosis that maintains continuity of the gastrointestinal tract and sphincter control. For distal rectal lesions, an abdominoperineal resection is required. In patients with unresectable rectal lesions that are locally advanced and adherent to adjacent structures, a diverting colostomy is often performed. Preoperative radiation may be effective in shrinking the tumor mass and allowing subsequent surgical resection. A subsequent laparotomy (second-look procedure) with resection of residual tumor is often performed when recurrent disease is diagnosed or suspected.

## Bibliography


Alderson PO, Adams PF, McNeil BJ et al: Computed tomography, ultrasound, and scintigraphy of the liver in patients with colon or breast carcinoma: A prospective comparison. Radiology 149: 225–230, 1983

Astler VB, Caller FA: The prognostic significance of direct extension of carcinoma of the colon and rectum. Ann Surg 139:846–852, 1954

Beahrs OH, Myers MH (eds): Manual for Staging of Cancer, 2nd ed, pp 67–72. Philadelphia, JB Lippincott, 1983

Beart RW, Jr, O'Connell MJ: Postoperative follow-up of patients with carcinoma of the colon. Mayo Clin Proc 58:361–363, 1983

Butch RJ, Wittenberg J, Mueller RR et al: Presacral masses after abdominoperineal resection for colorectal carcinoma: The need for needle biopsy. AJR 144:309–312, 1985

Dehn TCB, Reznek RH, Nockler IB et al: The preoperative assessment of advanced gastric cancer by computed tomography. Br J Surg 71:413–417, 1984

Deland FH, Kim ED, Pumus FJ et al: In vivo radioimmunodetection of occult recurrent colonic carcinoma. AJR 138:145–148, 1982

Freeny PC, Marks WM, Ryan JA et al: Colorectal carcinoma evaluation with CT: Pre-operative staging and detection of postoperative recurrence. Radiology 158:347–353, 1986

Grabbe E, Winkler R: Local recurrence after sphincter-saving resection for rectal and rectosigmoid carcinoma. Radiology 155:305–310, 1985

Hildebrandt U, Feifel G: Pre-operative staging of rectal cancer by intrarectal ultrasound. Dis Colon Rectum 28:42–46, 1985

Kelvin FM, Korobkin M, Heaston DK et al: The pelvis after surgery for rectal carcinoma: Serial CT observations with emphasis on non-neoplastic features. AJR 141:959–964, 1983

Kubota S, Yamasaki Z, Yoshimoto M et al: The value of urinary polyamine assay in stomach cancer. Cancer 56:1630–1635, 1985

Lee JKT, Stanley RJ, Sagel SS et al: CT appearance of the pelvis after abdomino-perineal resection for rectal carcinoma. Radiology 141:737–741, 1981

Macdonald JS, Gunderson LL, Cohn I: Cancer of the stomach. In DeVita VT, Hellman S, Rosenberg SA (eds): Cancer—Principles and Practice of Oncology, pp 534–562. Philadelphia, JB Lippincott, 1982

Mayes GB, Zornoza J: Computed tomography of colon carcinoma. AJR 135:43–46, 1980

McCarthy SM, Barnes D, Deveney K: Detection of recurrent rectosigmoid carcinoma: Prospective evaluation of CT and clinical factors. AJR 144: 577–579, 1985

Moss AA, Margulis AR, Schnyder P: A uniform, CT-based staging system for malignant neoplasms of the alimentary tube. AJR 136:1251–1252, 1981

Moss AA, Schnyder P, Marks W et al: Gastric adenocarcinoma: A comparison of the accuracy and economics of staging by computed tomography and surgery. Gastroenterology 80:45–50, 1981

Moss AA, Thoeni RF, Schnyder P et al: Value of

computed tomography in the detection and staging of recurrent rectal carcinomas. J Comput Assist Tomogr 5:870–874, 1981

Oliver GC, Shorb PE, Jr: The totally implantable infusion pump in treatment of metastatic colorectal cancer. Dis Colon Rectum 28:18–23, 1985

Olson RM, Perencevich NP, Malcolm AW et al: Patterns of recurrence following curative resection of adenocarcinoma of the colon and rectum. Cancer 45:2969–2974, 1980

Roswit B, Higgins GA, Jr, Keehn RJ: Pre-operative irradiation for carcinoma of the rectum and rectosigmoid colon: Report of a National Veterans Administration study. Cancer 35:1597–1602, 1975

Shirkhoda A, Staab EV, Bunce LA: Computed tomography in recurrent or metastatic colon cancer: Relation to rising serum carcinoembrymic antigens. J Comput Assist Tomogr 8:704–708, 1984

Silverberg E, Lubera JA: A review of American Cancer Society estimates of cancer cases and deaths. Cancer 33:1–25, 1983

Staab HJ, Anderer FA, Brummendorf T et al: Prognostic value of pre-operative serum CEA level compared to clinical staging: II. Stomach Cancer. Br J Cancer 45:718–727, 1982

Stark DD, Wittenberg J, Middelton MS et al: Liver metastases: Detection by phase-contrast MR imaging. Radiology 158:327–332, 1986

Thoeni RF, Moss AA, Schnyder P et al: Detection and staging of primary rectal and rectosigmoid cancer by computed tomography. Radiology 141: 135–138, 1981

Van Waes PFGM, Koehler PR, Feldberg MAM: Management of rectal carcinoma: Impact of computed tomography. AJR 140:1137–1142, 1983

Welch JP, Donaldson GA: Detection and treatment of recurrent cancer of the colon and rectum. Am J Surg 135:505–511, 1978

Wong WS, Goldberg HI: Gastric, small bowel and colorectal cancer. In Bragg DG, Rubin P, Yonker JE (eds): Oncologic Imaging, pp 243–285. New York, Pergamon Press, 1985

**STAGING OF GASTRIC CANCER**

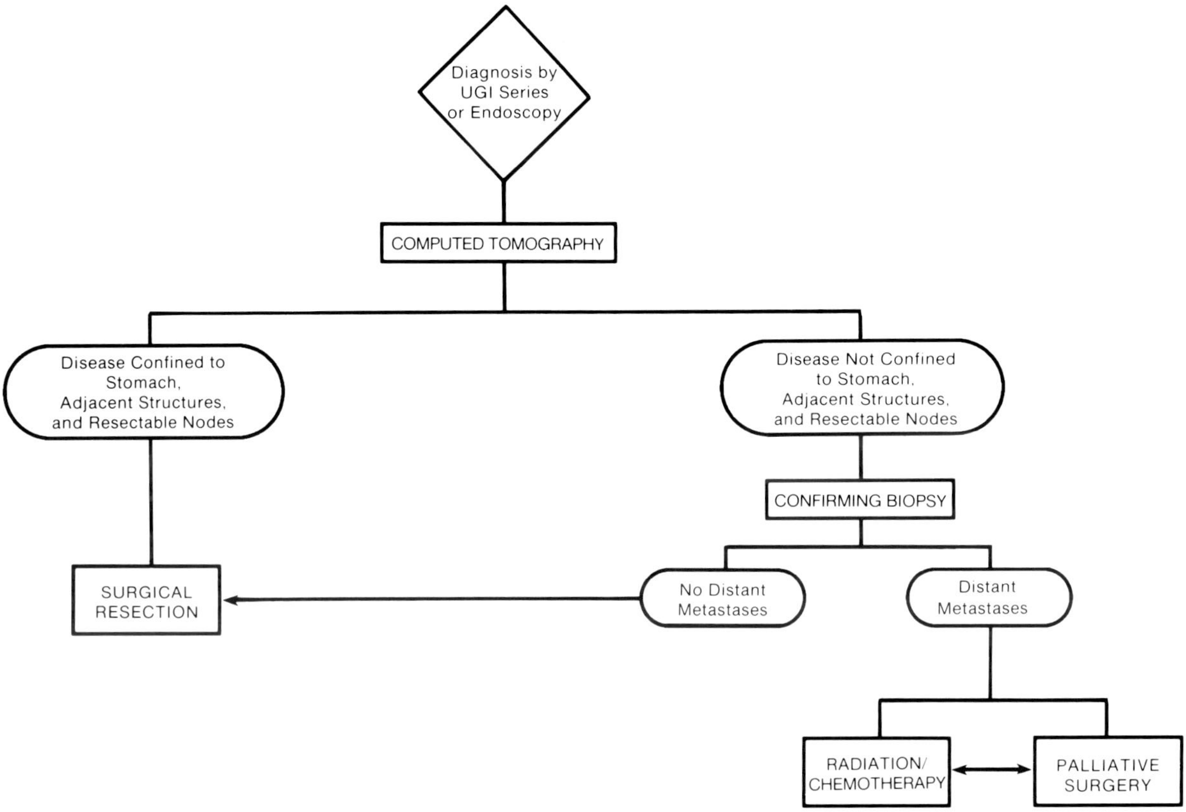

## COLORECTAL CANCER: DETECTION AND STAGING OF INITIAL AND RECURRENT DISEASE

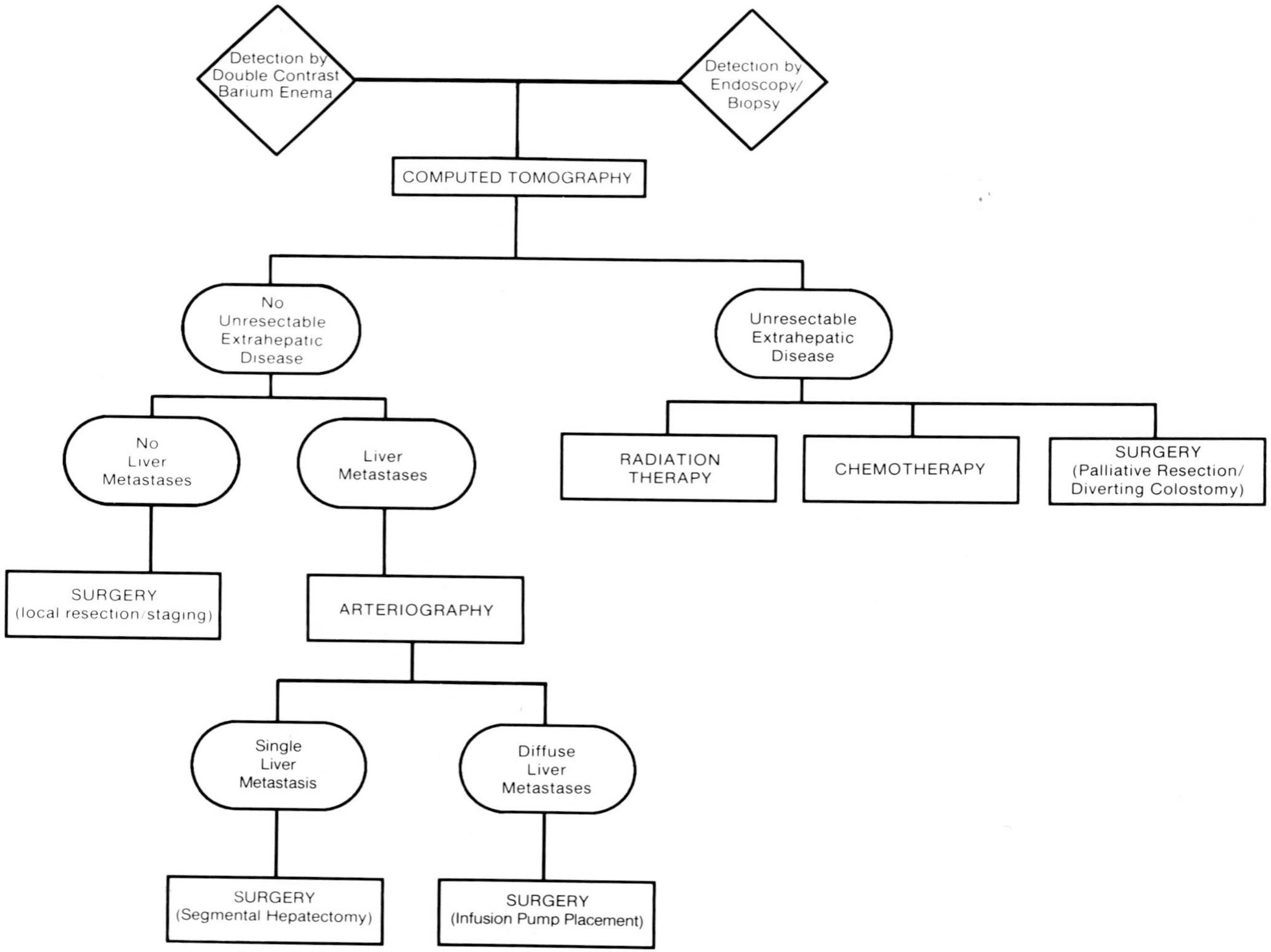

# Chapter 42

# Staging of Malignancies of the Female Genital Tract

*Vishan L. Giyanani*

Neoplasms of the uterus, cervix, and ovary are the most common malignant tumors of the female genital tract. Cancers of the vagina, vulva, and fallopian tubes are relatively infrequent. The primary goal of clinical, laboratory, and imaging studies is to accurately assess tumor staging, which is essential for the selection of definitive treatment and the determination of prognosis. In the early stages, the pelvic examination is the most accurate test for determining the origin and extent of a malignancy in the female genital tract. In the later stages of disease, however, clinical examination can determine only vaginal extension, and imaging studies are required to demonstrate pelvic and retroperitoneal lymphadenopathy, parametrial extension to the pelvic sidewalls, peritoneal seeding, and distant metastases to other organs.

## DIAGNOSTIC EVALUATION

### *DIAGNOSTIC MODALITIES*

1. Computed tomography
2. Magnetic resonance imaging
3. Ultrasound
4. Plain chest radiography and whole lung tomography
5. Excretory urography
6. Barium enema
7. Lymphangiography
8. Plain abdominal radiography
9. Surgery

### Computed Tomography

Computed tomography (CT) is an excellent modality for evaluating the pelvis because of the excellent inherent pelvic tissue contrast and the absence of peristaltic and respiratory motion artifacts in this region. In addition to identifying the site of origin, CT can determine the degree of tumor extension into the parametrium and elsewhere in the pelvis, show the effect of the tumor on the urinary tract, and document metastases to distant organs and retroperitoneal lymph nodes.

#### Carcinoma of the Cervix

The proper treatment and prognosis of cervical carcinoma is highly dependent on accurate staging (Table 42-1). In the early stages (carcinoma

**Table 42-1** International Federation of Gynecology and Obstetrics (FIGO) Classification and CT Criteria in Staging Cervical Carcinoma

| Stage | FIGO Classification | CT Criteria |
|---|---|---|
| 0 | *In situ* | |
| I | Tumor confined to cervix | Tumor confined to cervix |
| IA | Microinvasive | |
| IB | All other cases of stage I | Mild cervical enlargement with anteroposterior diameter > 3 cm<br>Smooth, well-defined lateral cervical margins<br>Normal periureteric fat planes, absence of soft-tissue density in parametrium |
| II | Tumor extends beyond the cervix but not to pelvic sidewalls or lower third of vagina | |
| IIA | No obvious parametrial involvement | |
| IIB | Obvious parametrial involvement | Moderate cervical enlargement with anteroposterior diameter of 3 cm to 6 cm (average 4 cm)<br>Irregular, interrupted, indistinct cervical outlines<br>Loss of periureteric fat planes<br>Soft-tissue mass or strands extend into the parametrium but are separated from pelvic sidewall by definite fat plane (3 mm–4 mm) |
| III | Tumor extends to pelvic sidewall or lower third of vagina or causes ureteral obstruction | |
| IIIA | No extension to pelvic sidewall | |
| IIIB | Extension to pelvic sidewall or ureteral obstruction | Severe cervical enlargement<br>Hydronephrosis (unilateral or bilateral)<br>Extension of tumor to pelvic sidewall<br>Solid tumor involving the obturator internus laterally and pyriformis muscle posterolaterally<br>Soft-tissue strands invade these muscles |

(*continued*)

**Table 42-1** (continued)

| Stage | FIGO Classification | CT Criteria |
|---|---|---|
| IV | Extends beyond the true pelvis or invades the mucosa of urinary bladder or rectum | |
| IVA | Spreads to adjacent organs | Focal obliteration of perivesical and/or perirectal fascial plane with asymmetric thickening of wall<br>Nodular depression or irregularity of rectal or urinary bladder wall<br>Intraluminal mass |
| IVB | Spreads to distant organs | Metastatic spread to inguinal lymph nodes, peritoneum, liver, and lungs |

Walsh JW: AJR 137:997, 1981

*in situ,* stages I and IIA), clinical examination is more accurate than CT. However, in advanced disease CT is superior to clinical staging because of its ability to detect parametrial extension and retroperitoneal lymph node involvement (Fig. 42-1). As in other parts of the body, the CT criterion for detecting nodal metastases is lymph node enlargement (>1.5 cm). Therefore, normal-sized nodes containing tumor cannot be detected by CT, while nodal enlargement due to reactive hyperplasia cannot be distinguished from that reflecting metastatic disease. Computed tomography can be used to guide aspiration biopsy of suspected abnormal nodes to permit a tissue diagnosis (Fig. 42-2).

Computed tomography can detect hydronephrosis and determine the cause, level, and degree of ureteral obstruction. It can also assess renal function following the intravenous injection of contrast material.

Computed tomography is often used for radiation treatment planning and in follow-up examinations after surgical or radiation treatment, because it is highly accurate in detecting tumor recurrence.

## Carcinoma of the Uterus

Computed tomography is extremely useful for accurately assessing the extent of a uterine malignancy. Intravenous contrast material is required for CT staging (Table 42-2), because the normal myometrium enhances (Fig. 42-3*A*) while endometrial carcinoma usually does not enhance to the same degree and is seen as an abnormal area of decreased attenuation (Fig. 42-3*B*). The degree of myometrial invasion is an important factor in determining lymphatic spread and the ultimate prognosis. If more than half the thickness of the myometrium is affected by tumor, there is a high likelihood of lymphatic spread and a poor prognosis. Prior to the advent of CT, the only way in which to demonstrate the degree of myometrial involvement was by pathologic examination following hysterectomy.

The CT manifestations of endometrial uterine carcinoma include (1) a mass of decreased density in the uterine cavity or myometrium, (2) a fluid-filled uterus secondary to tumor obstruction of the endocervical canal or vagina, (3) a contrast-enhancing lesion in the myometrium,

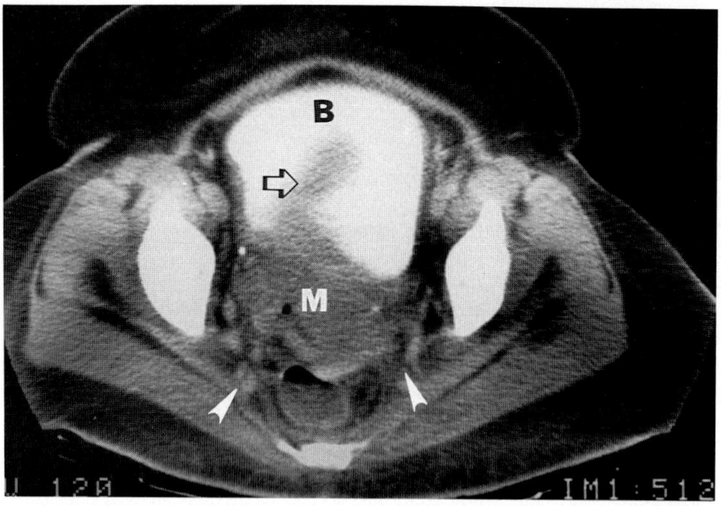


**Figure 42-1.** CT demonstration of stage IVA cervical carcinoma. The cervix is enlarged by the tumor (*M*), which extends (*open arrow*) into the urinary bladder (*B*). There is also loss of the fat plane between the tumor and the bladder, as well as tumor extension to the pelvic wall (*arrowheads*).

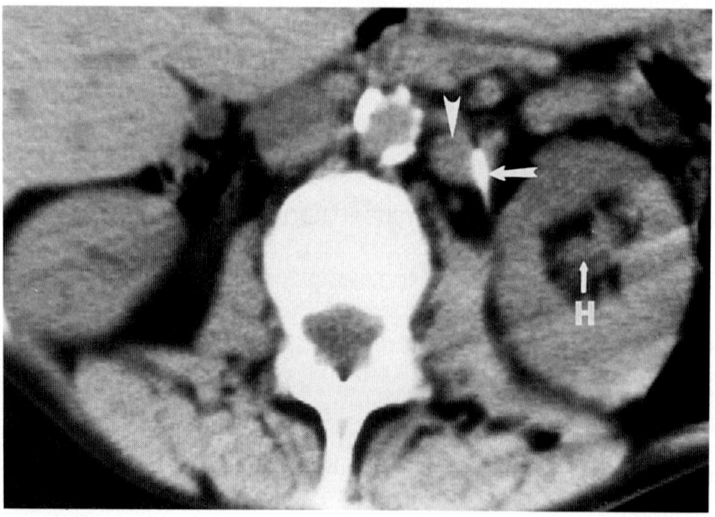


**Figure 42-2.** CT scan of stage IVB cervical carcinoma shows enlarged lymph nodes (*arrowhead*) with needle tip (*arrow*) for biopsy. Note the hydronephrosis (*H*) on the left.

(4) less dense fluid surrounding a uterine polypoid mass of decreased density, and (5) focal or diffuse enlargement of the uterus.

Computed tomography can detect cervical involvement of endometrial carcinoma by showing enlargement of the cervix and an abnormal area of decreased density within it. Although a carefully performed fractional curettage also may indicate cervical invasion, extreme care must be taken in interpreting the specimen. The curettage from the endometrium may contaminate the cervical specimen and lead to a misdiagnosis of cervical invasion.

Parametrial extension, invasion of the urinary bladder and/or rectum, pelvic and retroperitoneal lymph node involvement, and peritoneal seeding can all be easily detected by CT. In stage III and IV disease, CT has an accuracy rate of approximately 85% in predicting extrauterine tumor extension and often identifies nodal metastases and peritoneal seeding in tumors that were clinically staged as I and II. This modality has an accuracy rate of approximately 90% in showing that the tumor is confined to the uterus in stage I and II endometrial neoplasms.

**Table 42-2** FIGO Staging System: Endometrial Carcinoma

| Stages | FIGO Classification | CT Staging |
|---|---|---|
| I | Carcinoma confined to the corpus | Carcinoma confined to the corpus |
| IA | Length of uterine cavity 8 cm or less | Hypodense mass in uterine cavity or myometrium |
| IB | Length of uterine cavity >8 cm | Fluid-filled uterus<br>Contrast-enhancing lesions in myometrium<br>Hypodense polypoid mass in uterine cavity surrounded by less dense fluid |
| II | Carcinoma has involved corpus and cervix but has not extended outside uterus | Tumor involving corpus and cervix |
| III | Carcinoma has extended outside uterus but not outside true pelvis | Tumor extension outside uterus to involve parametrium, adnexa, pelvic sidewall, or pelvic nodes |
| IV | Tumor extends outside the true pelvis or involves the mucosa of bladder or rectum | |
| IVA | Spread to adjacent organs, bladder and/or rectum | Bladder or rectal involvement |
| IVB | Spread to distant organ | Para-aortic lymphadenopathy<br>Omental, serosal, and peritoneal metastases<br>Lung and liver involvement |

## Ovarian Carcinoma

The diagnosis of ovarian carcinoma is generally made by clinical examination and/or sonography, and then surgical exploration is usually performed without additional imaging studies. Computed tomography often does not play a primary role in the initial assessment of ovarian carcinoma, because it is less accurate than surgical staging (Table 42-3). Nevertheless, CT has an important complementary role, because it is more effective than clinical examination or surgery in detecting small amounts of ascites, liver metastases, and uterine involvement. Computed tomography is of special value in detecting small intrahepatic lesions, especially those located on the posterior aspect of the liver, which are difficult to palpate during physical examination or at surgical exploration. Biopsy of these intrahepatic lesions, guided by CT, is more accurate than random biopsy performed during an operative procedure.

The CT appearance of ovarian carcinoma varies from a cystic mass with multiple thick irregular septations (Fig. 42-4) to a mixed lesion containing both cystic and solid components to an entirely solid mass. Computed tomography is superior to ultrasound in detecting metastases to the peritoneum and bowel. Peritoneal metastases (>2 cm) usually appear as small nodular densities along the lateral surface of the abdomen, especially along the surface of the liver and spleen in a patient with ascites. Omental metastases produce characteristic soft-tissue masses anterior to bowel loops. Computed tomography is better than ultrasound for showing enlargement of retroperitoneal lymph nodes and can well evaluate the urinary tract for possible ureteral involvement.

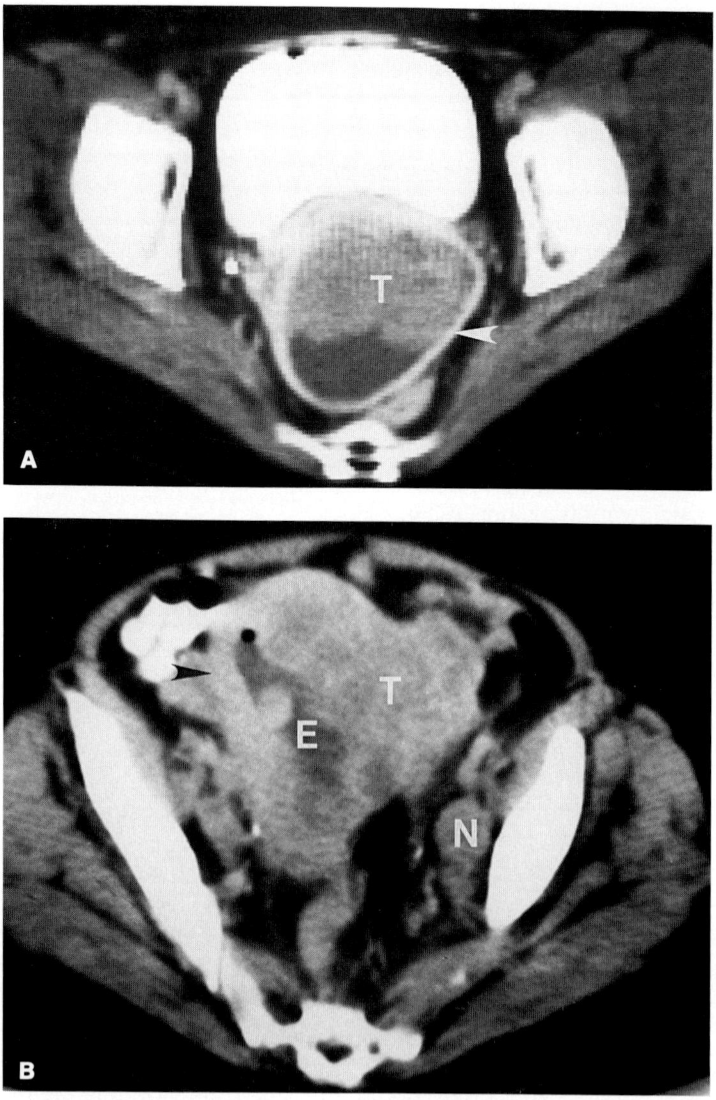


**Figure 42-3.** CT scan of stage II endometrial sarcoma. **(A)** The uterus shows a hypodense polypoid mass (*T*) anteriorly with endometrial fluid (*F*) posteriorly. Note the uniform enhancement of the normal myometrium (*arrowhead*). **(B)** Inhomogeneous mass (*T*) with thickening and expansion of the left myometrial wall. The endometrial cavity (*E*) is displaced to the right by the tumor. There is an enlarged pelvic lymph node (*N*) near the left pelvic wall. Note the normal right myometrial wall (*arrowhead*). (*A*, Walsh JW, Vick CW: Staging of female genital tract cancer. In Walsh JW (ed): Computed Tomography of the Pelvis. New York, Churchill Livingstone, 1985)

## Magnetic Resonance Imaging

Magnetic resonance imaging (MRI) is rapidly becoming a major modality for staging patients with malignancy of the female genital tract. Noninvasive and without ionizing radiation, MRI is not adversely affected by bowel gas and the patient's body habitus as is ultrasound. Images can be obtained in multiple planes with superior soft-tissue contrast resolution. Blood vessels are well delineated and can be distinguished from lymph nodes without the need for intravenous administration of contrast material. Magnetic resonance imaging can demonstrate the site of origin of a neoplasm as well as its extent, lymph node metastases, and involvement of adjacent and distant organs. The major disadvantages of MRI are its long scanning time and its inability to be performed in patients with vascular clips, cardiac pacemakers, and large metallic devices.

Magnetic resonance imaging examinations of the pelvis are generally performed with spin echo techniques using prolonged repetition time (TR) and echo time (TE).

**Table 42-3** International Federation of Gynecology and Obstetrics (FIGO) Classification of Ovarian Carcinoma

| Stage | FIGO Classification |
|---|---|
| I | Tumor limited to ovaries |
| IA | One ovary; no ascites |
| IB | Both ovaries; no ascites |
| IC | One or both ovaries; ascites present with malignant cells in fluid |
| II | Tumor involving one or both ovaries with pelvic extension |
| IIA | Extension and/or metastases to the uterus and/or tubes only |
| IIB | Extension to other pelvic tissue |
| III | Growth involving one or both ovaries with widespread intraperitoneal metastases (the omentum, the small intestine and its mesentery) limited to the abdomen |
| IV | Growth involving one or both ovaries with distant metastases outside peritoneal cavity |

## Carcinoma of the Cervix

Because the cervix varies in length and orientation, MR images in both axial and sagittal planes are necessary to completely delineate the cervical anatomy. T2-weighted images of the normal cervix show two separate zones. The cervical epithelium and mucus appear as a central area of high signal intensity surrounded by a zone of low signal intensity that may represent fibrous stroma. The outermost region of medium-high signal intensity represents the parametrium.

Cervical carcinoma appears as an irregular mass of high signal intensity (Fig. 42-5) that is well differentiated from surrounding normal cervical tissue. However, because MRI cannot distinguish a benign from a malignant neoplasm, the diagnosis of cervical carcinoma should be made prior to imaging. Once the diagnosis is established, the multiplaner imaging capability of MRI permits accurate staging of the lesion. Parametrial involvement produces an abnormal tumor intensity extending into the parametrium or an asymmetric appearance of the parametrium. Vaginal extension of tumor produces a mass of high signal intensity within the low signal intensity of the normal vagina.

As with CT, the MRI detection of pelvic and retroperitoneal lymphadenopathy requires demonstration of lymph node enlargement. Despite its superior soft-tissue discrimination, MRI cannot detect destruction of lymph node architecture and therefore cannot differentiate lymph node enlargement secondary to hyperplasia from that due to metastases.

## Carcinoma of the Uterus

The normal endometrium appears on T2-weighted images as a zone of high signal intensity that varies in width during the different phases of the menstrual cycle and in a woman receiving hormonal therapy. In postmenopausal women who are not receiving hormonal treatment, the normal endometrium usually measures less than 2 mm in width. Widening of the endometrium (>2 mm) or the presence of a decreased signal intensity mass indicates an endometrial malignancy.

The normal myometrium appears on T2-weighted images as a zone of high signal intensity that is separated from the high signal intensity of the endometrium by a band of low signal intensity termed the *junctional zone.* This junctional zone is well preserved in a patient whose uterine malignancy is localized to the endometrium. Myometrial invasion causes the junctional zone to be indistinct or segmentally visualized. However, it is important to remember that complete nonvisualization of the junctional zone may be a normal finding in postmenopausal women, in whom this appearance must be evaluated in conjunction with other criteria to diagnose myometrial invasion.

In addition to detecting myometrial invasion, MRI can demonstrate the extension of endometrial carcinoma to the cervix (Fig. 42-6), parametrium, and other pelvic structures as well as the involvement of retroperitoneal nodes.

A major disadvantage of MRI in the evaluation of patients with uterine carcinoma is the inability of this technique to differentiate adenomatous hyperplasia from an endometrial

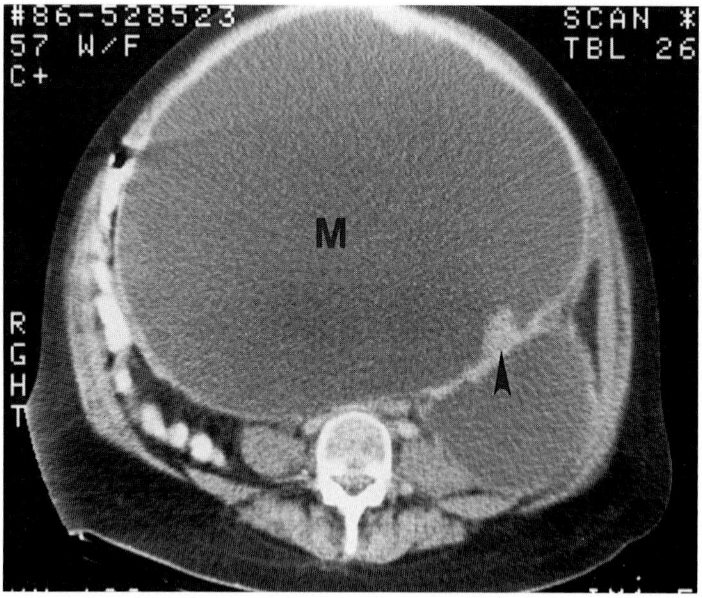


**Figure 42-4.** CT scan of ovarian carcinoma. Predominantly cystic mass (*M*) with nodular septation (*arrowhead*).

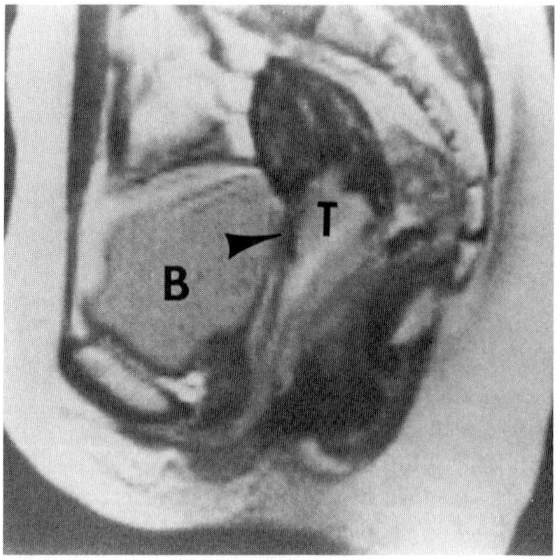


**Figure 42-5.** MRI of cervical carcinoma (TR, 2 sec; TE, 60 msec). The cervical canal is expanded by a tumor mass (*T*) of high signal intensity. The remaining cervical stroma (*arrowhead*) is of low signal intensity and is not involved by the tumor (*B,* urinary bladder). (Hricak H: MRI of the female pelvis: A review. AJR 146:1115–1122, © American Roentgen Ray Society, 1986)

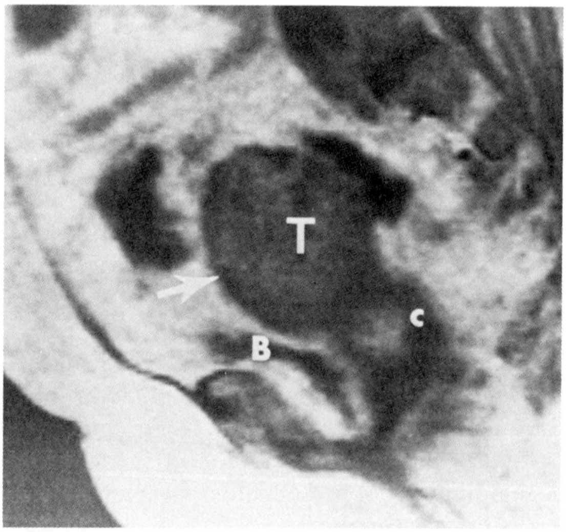


**Figure 42-6.** MRI of endometrial carcinoma (TR, 1 sec; TE, 28 msec). Sagittal scan in a postmenopausal patient demonstrates an expanded endometrial cavity containing a tumor (*T*) with medium signal intensity. The compressed myometrium (*arrow*) appears as an area of low signal intensity. The cervical canal (*C*) is expanded by an area of high signal intensity representing tumor extension (*B,* urinary bladder). (Hricak H: MRI of the female pelvis: A review. AJR 146:1115–1122, © American Roentgen Ray Society, 1986)

malignant neoplasm. Because both conditions produce high signal intensity in the endometrial zone, they can be distinguished only by histologic examination.

### Ovarian Neoplasm

Magnetic resonance imaging has not been extensively used in the staging of malignant tumors of the ovary. Unlike CT, the long scanning time of MRI precludes the detection of peritoneal seeding because of artifacts from bowel peristalsis and respiratory motion. Benign ovarian tumors may be indistinguishable from malignant lesions, because the solid component of hemorrhage within a mass can mimic a malignant process.

## Ultrasound

Before the advent of CT and MRI, ultrasound was the major imaging modality for staging of malignant tumors of the female genital tract. Noninvasive, relatively inexpensive, and without ionizing radiation, ultrasound can produce excellent cross-sectional images of the pelvis in multiple planes without the loss of resolution inherent in reconstruction techniques. Ultrasound can confirm the presence of a clinically suspected mass; determine the organ of origin; and show whether the lesion is cystic, solid, or complex. It can clearly show hydroureter and hydronephrosis due to ureteral involvement by the primary tumor or its extension. Ultrasound is less accurate than CT in defining the extent of tumor and nodal involvement because of the inability of sound waves to penetrate the bowel gas and bony structures of the pelvis. This modality is also difficult to use in obese patients, because excessive fatty tissue attenuates the sound beam and results in poor visualization of underlying structures. Therefore, once the diagnosis of malignancy is confirmed, CT (or MRI) is usually employed to accurately assess tumor staging.

### Carcinoma of the Cervix

Carcinoma of the cervix, even in its early stages, frequently appears as a solid mass posterior to the urinary bladder. The mass progressively enlarges when surrounding tissue is involved by tumor. However, cervical enlargement identical to that caused by carcinoma may be due to benign neoplasms (leiomyoma) or inflammation or may be a normal variant. Therefore, the diagnosis of cervical carcinoma should be made clinically, with ultrasound reserved for demonstrating the extent of the lesion.

Carcinoma of the cervix is most often hypoechoic, although it may demonstrate a mixed echo pattern (Fig. 42-7) due to tumor necrosis or hemorrhage. Extension of tumor to involve the parametrium produces an echogenic mass of varying texture adjacent to or contiguous with the uterus. Lymph node metastases appear as separate echogenic masses; invasion of the bladder or rectum also can be shown. Ultrasound can demonstrate hydroureter and hydronephrosis caused by the tumor, although it cannot assess renal function as excretory urography or contrast-enhanced CT can.

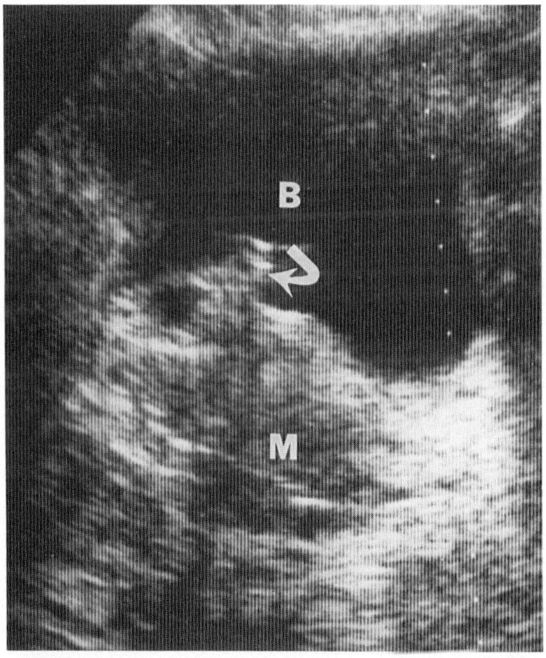


**Figure 42-7.** Ultrasound of cervical carcinoma. Transverse scan shows enlargement of the cervix by a nonhomogeneous malignant mass (*M*). There is extension of tumor (*curved arrow*) into the urinary bladder (*B*).

## Carcinoma of the Endometrium

Endometrial carcinoma usually produces abnormalities in uterine size, configuration, and echo texture. In most cases the uterus is enlarged, although it may be normal or even atrophied. The uterus has a bulbous or normal configuration in approximately 95% of patients of stage I or II disease, while it becomes globular in approximately 80% of patients with stage III or IV disease.

The echo pattern of the uterus involved by tumor varies widely. The trans-sonicity of the uterus is generally normal, although it may be decreased if the uterus is obstructed and filled with fluid. The endometrial layer may be irregular and abnormally thick (>6 mm), and the endometrial cavity may be hypoechoic due to hemorrhage.

Ultrasound is less accurate than contrast-enhanced CT for assessing myometrial invasion, tumor extension into adjacent pelvic structures, involvement of pelvic and retroperitoneal lymph nodes, and peritoneal seeding. However, ultrasound can determine the uterine length with greater accuracy than CT and as well as the far more expensive MRI.

## Ovarian Carcinoma

Ultrasound can reliably detect both solid and cystic ovarian neoplasms in more than 90% of cases, and it is the diagnostic study most frequently used for evaluating the woman with a palpable pelvoabdominal mass. This technique is highly accurate in differentiating benign from malignant ovarian tumors. A sonolucent mass devoid of solid components or septations, or with septations of normal thickness, is most frequently benign; tumors with solid components or multiple thick, irregular septations are usually malignant (Fig. 42-8).

Although ultrasound is accurate in assessing the organ of origin and nature of an ovarian mass, it is inferior to CT or surgical exploration in defining tumor extent. Small degrees of as-

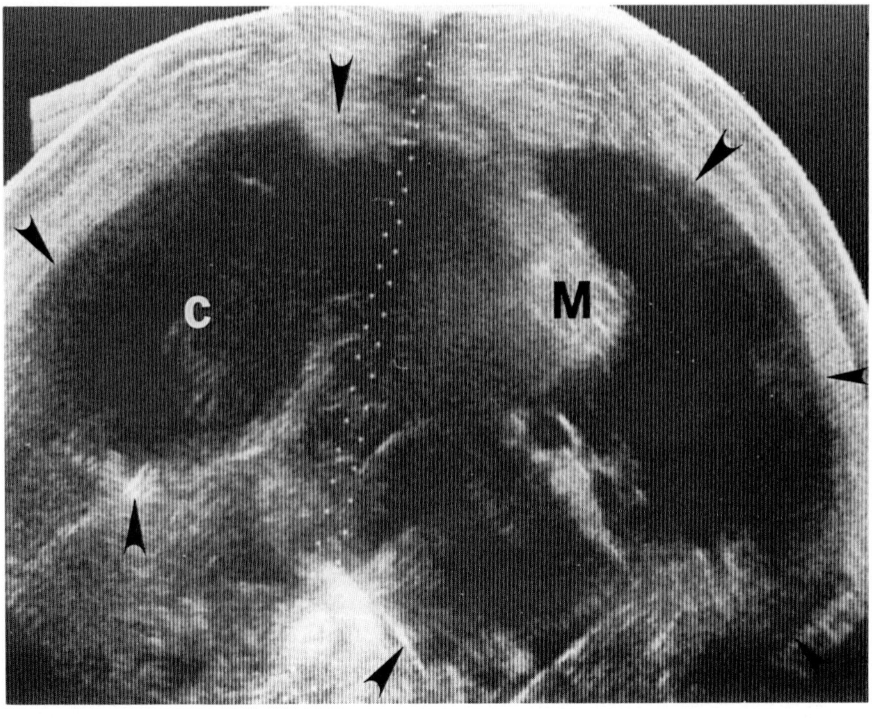


**Figure 42-8.** Ultrasound of ovarian carcinoma. Transverse scan demonstrates an ovarian mass (*arrowheads*) containing cystic (*C*) and solid (*M*) components.

cites are generally missed, while small omental and peritoneal implants can be detected in only about half the patients. Metastases to the urinary bladder, bowel, and lymph nodes are not easily demonstrated. Therefore, ultrasound has an overall accuracy rate of less than 50% in correctly staging ovarian malignancy.

## Plain Chest Radiography

The presence of pulmonary metastases is a poor prognostic sign in patients with malignant tumors of the female genital tract. Women with carcinoma of the cervix and endometrium who have lung metastases have a mortality rate of 80% within 1 year. Pulmonary metastases in ovarian carcinoma are often associated with extensively disseminated disease and imminent death. Hematogenous spread of cervical carcinoma leads to pulmonary involvement in approximately one fourth of patients. Initial plain chest radiographs show evidence of pulmonary metastases in 3% of patients with carcinoma of the cervix, in 5% of those with endometrial carcinoma, and in 15% of women with ovarian cancer.

Plain chest radiographs are an essential component of the initial evaluation of the patient with female genital tract malignancy (Fig. 42-9). Whole lung tomography is usually of little value, because there is excellent correlation between plain chest films and conventional tomography in 95% of cases. Whole lung tomography is primarily of value in accurately determining the size and number of metastatic nodules detected on plain chest radiographs, so that the response to therapy can be more precisely evaluated. Whole lung tomography is less sensitive than plain films for detecting the presence of pleural fluid.

Although CT is both more accurate and more sensitive for detecting lung metastases and assessing the presence of pleural fluid than plain chest radiographs or whole lung tomography, it is far more expensive and may miss a single small lung nodule due to partial-volume averaging and different degrees of respiration, especially in an uncooperative patient.

In summary, plain chest radiographs should be performed for staging of female genital tract malignancy and should be supplemented by either whole lung or computed tomography to determine the response to therapy.

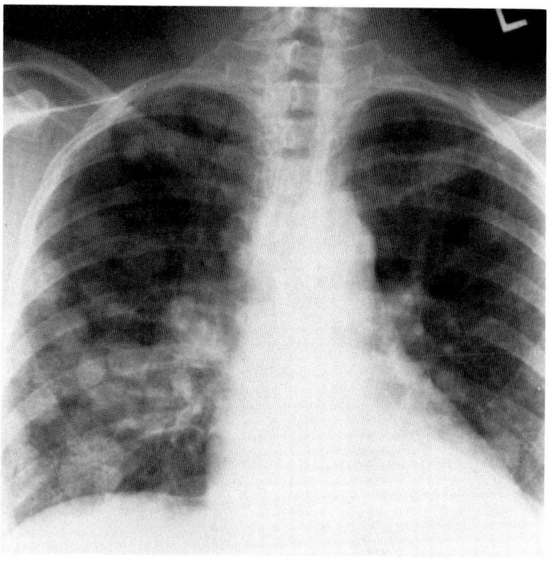

**Figure 42-9.** Pulmonary metastases secondary to cervical carcinoma. Frontal view of the chest shows multiple metastatic pulmonary nodules that are located predominantly in the lower lobes.

## Excretory Urography

Because the urinary tract is often affected secondarily by malignant tumors of the female genital tract, an excretory urogram traditionally has been a routine part of the staging process. Large pelvic masses may displace and impress the ureters and urinary bladder, although this is a nonspecific appearance that may also be due to benign genitourinary lesions, pelvic infection, hematoma, and lymphadenopathy.

The distal ureters course through the parametrium to enter the base of the urinary bladder. Therefore, a female genital tract tumor extending to involve the parametrium and bladder may compress the ureters and lead to unilateral or bilateral obstruction. An excretory urogram can detect an obstruction as well as assess its degree and level, although it cannot determine the exact cause of obstruction because the underlying tumor cannot be directly visualized as with ultrasound, CT, and MRI. As with excretory urography, contrast-enhanced CT can assess the degree of renal function.

The selection of diagnostic studies in patients with symptoms related to the urinary tract depends on the clinical presentation. If a patient has renal failure and a pelvic mass, ultrasound is the initial diagnostic modality of choice to determine the nature of the mass and the cause of the renal failure. An excretory urogram is preferred if the patient presents with primary urinary tract symptoms, while CT should be performed for tumor staging in the patient with a definite pelvic malignancy.

### Barium Enema

Prior to the availability of the newer imaging modalities, the barium enema examination was used to provide indirect evidence of spread of gynecologic malignancy. However, small tumors frequently produce no effect on the barium-filled colon, while large benign neoplasms, hematomas, and inflammatory disease may cause displacement and stretching of bowel loops indistinguishable from that caused by malignant neoplasms. The barium enema examination is inaccurate in staging of malignancies of the female genital tract and only extremely rarely shows an abnormality that is not detected by other techniques. Therefore, its routine use in staging cannot be justified, and the barium enema should be reserved only for those situations in which bowel symptoms or colonic obstruction are suspected. Because colon carcinoma frequently metastasizes to the ovary, a barium enema examination occasionally may be helpful in differentiating a primary from a secondary ovarian tumor.

### Lymphangiography

Lymphangiography can detect metastatic deposits to pelvic and para-aortic lymph nodes from malignancies of the female genital tract. Carcinomas of the cervix and uterus commonly spread primarily by the lymphatic system, while ovarian carcinoma much less frequently metastasizes via this route.

Unlike CT and MRI, which rely on changes in the size of the lymph nodes to detect metastatic disease, lymphangiography can demonstrate alterations in internal nodal architecture and thus detect metastatic deposits in normal-sized lymph nodes. If the primary lesion is extensive and there is strong clinical suspicion of pelvic or retroperitoneal nodal involvement but normal-sized nodes on CT, a lymphangiogram may be indicated. However, lymphangiography does not fill all the potential sites of metastatic nodal spread and fails to show tumor in nodes that are not opacified because of total neoplastic destruction.

### Plain Abdominal Radiography

Although plain films of the abdomen are routinely obtained in patients presenting with pelvic symptoms or a pelvic mass, they have such low sensitivity and specificity as to be of no practical value. Therefore, there is no justification for the routine use of plain abdominal radiographs in the diagnosis or staging of a patient with a malignant tumor of the female genital tract.

### Surgical Exploration

Surgical exploration is essential for the proper management of women with genital tract carcinoma, particularly of the ovary. It confirms the clinical diagnosis and permits the acquisition of tissue required for grading the tumor and defining its histologic type. Surgery also allows accurate staging and tissue biopsy of tumor that has spread to the peritoneum, omentum, bowel surface, diaphragm, and parametrium, as well as metastases to the liver and pelvic and para-aortic lymph nodes. The primary tumor and its extension into other tissues can be excised at the same time, thus reducing the tumor mass and improving the therapy.

## Bibliography


Amendola MA, Walsh JW, Amendola BE et al: Computed tomography in the evaluation of carcinoma of the ovary. J Comput Assist Tomogr 5:179–186, 1981

Deland M, Fried A, Nagell, Jr et al: Ultrasonography in the diagnosis of tumors of the ovary. Surg Gynecol Obstet 148:346–348, 1979

Dooms GC, Hrick H, Tscholakoff D: Adnexal structures: MR Imaging. Radiology 158:693–646, 1986

Fleischer AC, Entman SS, Porrah SA et al: Sonographic evaluation of uterine malformation and disorders. In Sancers RC, Everette J, Jr (eds): The Principles and Practice of Ultrasonography in Obstetrics and Gynecology. Norwalk, CT, Appleton-Century-Crofts, 1985

Ginaldi S, Wallace S, Jing BS et al: Carcinoma of the cervix: Lymphangiography and computed tomography. AJR 136:1087–1091, 1981

Gordon RE, Mettler RA, Wicks JD et al: Chest x-ray and full lung tomograms in gynecologic malignancy. Cancer 52:559–562, 1983

Hricak H: MRI of the female pelvis: A review. AJR 146:1115–1122, 1986

Johnson RJ, Blackledge G, Eddleston B et al: Abdomino-pelvic computed tomography in the management of ovarian carcinoma. Radiology 146:447–452, 1983

Reguard CK, Wicks JD, Mettler FA, Jr: Ultrasonography in the staging of endometrial adenocarcinoma. Radiology 140:781–785, 1981

Severini A, Petrillo R, Kenda R et al: The value of double contrast enema in the assessment of ovarian carcinoma's diffusion. Gynecol Oncol 11: 17–22, 1981

Walsh JW, Goplerud DR: Prospective comparison between clinical and CT staging in primary cervical carcinoma. AJR 137:997–1003, 1981

Walsh JW, Vick CW: Staging of female genital tract cancer. In Walsh JW (ed): Computed Tomography of the Pelvis. New York, Churchill Livingstone, 1985

## CARCINOMA OF CERVIX OR UTERUS

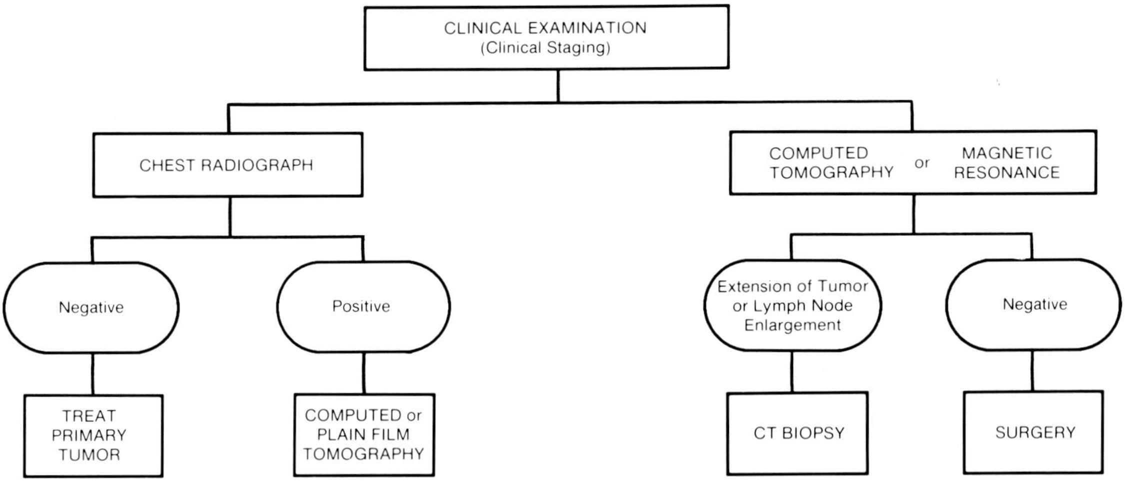


Note: Ultrasound, excretory urography, barium enema, and plain abdominal radiographs are not necessary

## OVARIAN CARCINOMA

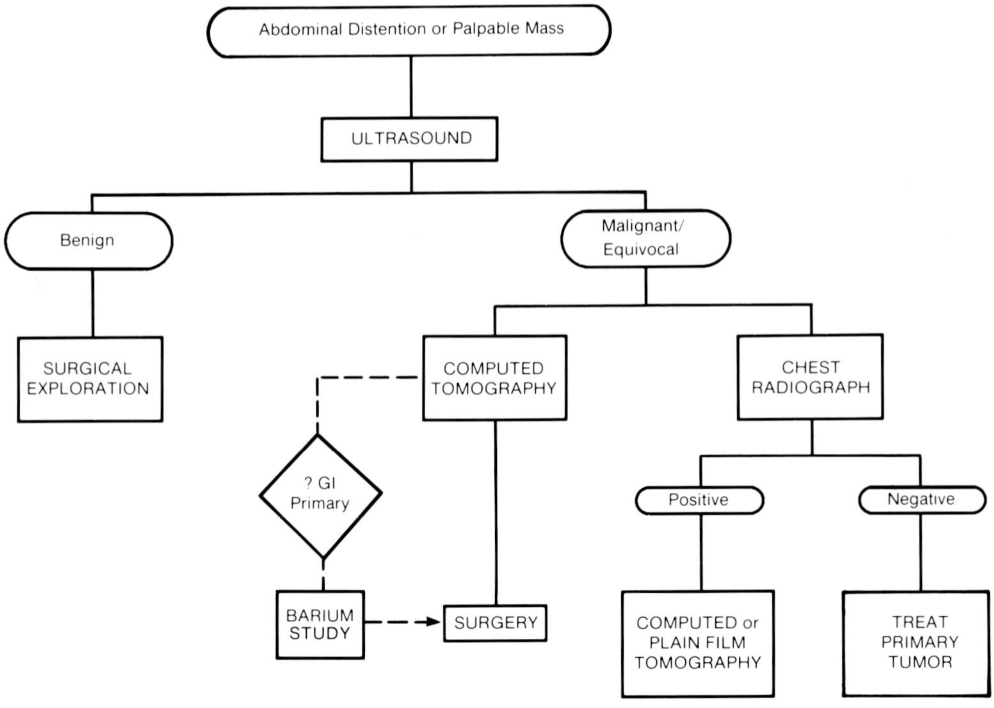


Note: Excretory urography and plain abdominal radiographs are not necessary; role of MRI is still to be explored.

# Chapter 43

# Diagnosis and Staging of Carcinoma of the Prostate

*Erich K. Lang*

Carcinoma of the prostate is the second most common malignancy in men. The disease is rare before the age of 50 years, and the incidence increases with advancing age. The tumor can be slow-growing and asymptomatic for long periods or can behave aggressively with extensive metastases.

Screening for asymptomatic carcinoma of the prostate has traditionally relied on digital rectal examination. In the past few years, however, transrectal, transvesical, and urethral ultrasound have assumed increasing importance in the early detection of prostate cancer, especially in evaluating suspicious areas in patients with prostatic hypertrophy. Ultrasound-guided biopsy can identify small foci of prostatic carcinoma undetectable by digital examination.

## LABORATORY STUDIES

The measurement of serum acid phosphatase (prostatic fraction) is the most valuable screening test for indicating the presence of advanced carcinoma of the prostate. In one study, 38% of patients with stage A prostatic carcinoma undetectable by digital examination had elevated levels of serum acid phosphatase, which is indicative of advanced disease.

## DIAGNOSTIC EVALUATION

### *DIAGNOSTIC MODALITIES*

1. Excretory urography
2. Ultrasound
3. Computed tomography
4. Magnetic resonance imaging
5. Lymphangiography
6. Radionuclide bone scanning
7. Surgery (staging lymphadenectomy)

### Excretory Urography

Excretory urography may be the imaging procedure that indicates the presence of prostatic enlargement. Although this study can document ureteral obstruction and associated compromise of renal function, it is of virtually no value in the staging of patients with carcinoma of the prostate.

## Ultrasound

Transrectal, transvesical, and transurethral ultrasound are the screening procedures of choice for identifying focal areas of altered echogenicity in the patient with suspected prostatic carcinoma. Technically satisfactory transrectal and transvesical sonograms can demonstrate tumor extension through the prostate capsule and can even document enlargement of pelvic lymph nodes. Histologic verification of primary tumor, metastatic implants, and neoplastic lymphadenopathy can be obtained by ultrasound-guided biopsy.

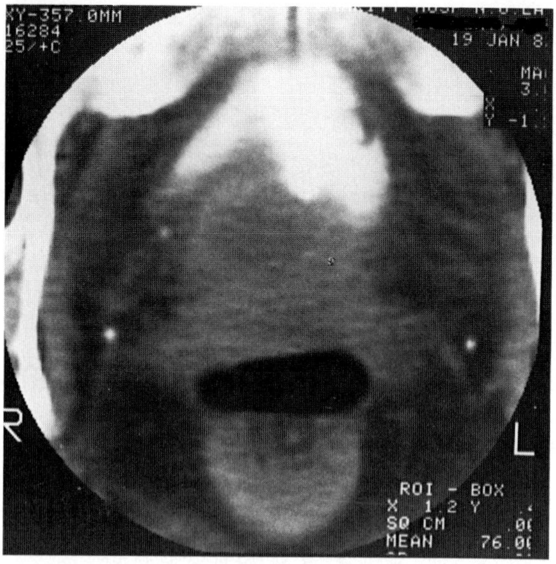

**Figure 43-1.** CT scan shows nodular components of a significantly enlarged prostate protruding into the base of the bladder. Note the total obliteration of the fat pad separating the prostate from the seminal vesicles. Invasion by carcinoma of the prostate into the seminal vesicles and floor of the bladder was proven on subsequent surgical exploration.

## Computed Tomography

Computed tomography (CT) is the imaging modality of choice for demonstrating extension of carcinoma of the prostate through the capsule into the periprostatic space and lateral pelvic wall (Fig. 43-1). This technique also can show contiguous involvement of the rectum, bladder, and seminal vesicles, although recent studies question whether obliteration of the fat pad between the prostate and seminal vesicles always indicates tumor extension. The CT demonstration of enlarged lymph nodes (>1.5 cm) suggests metastatic involvement, and histologic confirmation may be obtained using CT-guided biopsy (Fig. 43-2). Histologic confirmation of a suspected pulmonary metastasis is required if its presence would influence the decision between radical prostatectomy and radiation therapy and/or adjunctive hormone therapy.

## Magnetic Resonance Imaging

The initially claimed ability of magnetic resonance imaging (MRI) to differentiate between benign and malignant prostatic tissue is now in serious question. However, the MRI demonstration of displacement of the readily identifiable periprostatic venous plexus is an indication of tumor extension through the capsule of the prostate into the periprostatic space. Magnetic resonance imaging can provide direct sagittal and coronal reconstructions that are of value in demonstrating direct contiguous extension of tumor as well as metastases to regional and para-aortic lymph nodes. Like CT, the MRI criterion for nodal metastases is based on the demonstration of lymph node enlargement. Ultrasound- or CT-guided biopsy is required for histologic confirmation.

## Lymphangiography

Lymphangiography is the only imaging modality that can suggest the presence of metastases from prostatic carcinoma in normal-sized nodes on the basis of intrinsic changes in nodal architecture. Nevertheless, ultrasound- or CT-guided biopsy is often necessary to eliminate false-positive re-

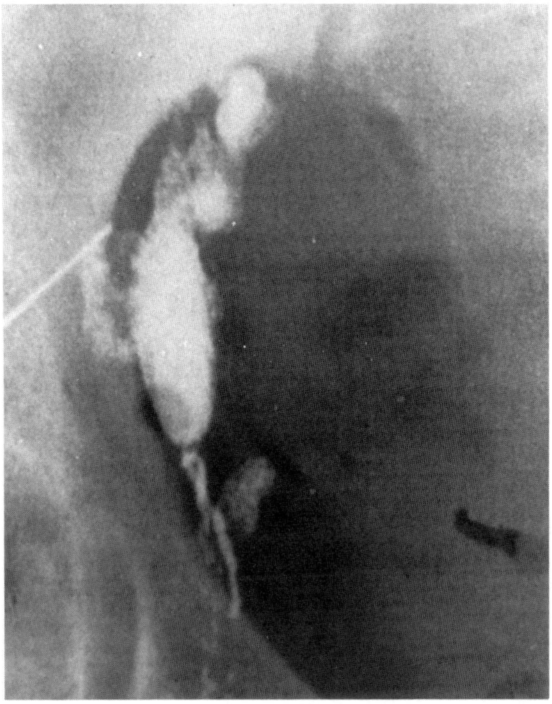

**Figure 43-2.** Percutaneous thin-needle biopsy of a lymph node, a segment of which shows architectural changes suggestive of tumor implants. Positive cytology proved the presence of metastatic disease in a normal-sized node. (Lang EK: Bladder and pelvic arteriography. In Abrams HL (ed): Abrams' Angiography. Boston, Little, Brown & Co, 1983)

sults caused by fibrotic or fatty nodal implants or by sinus histiocytosis. The major disadvantage of pedal lymphangiography is the frequent inability to opacify the obturator, internal iliac, and presacral nodes, the most common primary sites of prostatic metastases. Because of its relatively low yield, high cost, and technical complexity, as well as the almost universal availability of relatively noninvasive CT, lymphangiography now is rarely used for the detection of lymphatic metastases from carcinoma of the prostate.

### Radionuclide Bone Scanning

Radionuclide bone scanning is a highly sensitive (although not specific) imaging technique for detecting the frequent skeletal metastases from carcinoma of the prostate. Indeed, skeletal metastases may be detected in patients who present with bone pain but are still asymptomatic with regard to their primary prostatic neoplasm. A positive radionuclide bone scan is generally followed by plain skeletal radiographs to validate the findings and to eliminate false-positive results caused by degenerative disease, inflammation, or trauma.

Experimental studies are under way to investigate the use of tumor-specific isotopically labeled antibodies for detection of lymph node metastases from carcinoma of the prostate.

### Surgery (Staging Lymphadenectomy)

Staging lymphadenectomy remains the "gold standard" for determining the degree of involvement of pelvic lymph nodes by metastatic carcinoma of the prostate. In approximately 50% of patients, the initial clinical and imaging staging must be elevated based on the results of staging pelvic lymphadenectomy. Although metastases to lymph nodes is an early manifestation of spread of carcinoma of the prostate, it is typically the most difficult to detect by currently available imaging techniques. For example, up to 45% of patients with clinical stage B tumors and up to 85% of those with clinical stage C tumors are found to have pelvic lymph node metastases on staging lymphadenectomy. Approximately 25% of lymph node metastases are deposits less than 2 mm in diameter (micrometastases), which cannot be detected by current imaging techniques.

## SCREENING FOR PROSTATIC CARCINOMA

Digital rectal examination and ultrasound (transrectal or transvesical) are recommended as the initial screening approach to the patient with suspected carcinoma of the prostate. If both of these examinations are negative, further diagnostic workup is not required. If either of these examinations is positive, ultrasound-guided biopsy can be performed to confirm the diagnosis. The demonstration of a large, unequivocal prostatic lesion is an indication to begin appropriate staging procedures.

The patient with an elevated serum acid phosphatase requires a more intensive workup. If the digital rectal examination or ultrasound study is negative, radionuclide bone scanning is indicated to identify those patients with skeletal metastases who have a small and still undetectable primary carcinoma of the prostate.

## APPROACH TO STAGING OF PROSTATIC CARCINOMA

The imaging procedures for staging of carcinoma of the prostate are designed to identify local extension, lymphadenopathy, or distant metastases, because their presence greatly influences the choice of treatment as well as potential curability and survival.

**Table 43-1** Staging of Prostatic Carcinoma

| | |
|---|---|
| $A_1$ | Three or fewer microscopic foci, accidental finding on TUR section chips |
| $A_2$ | Multifocal or diffuse carcinoma |
| $B_1N$ | Solitary nodule <1.5 cm in diameter |
| $B_1$ | Nodule involving most of one lobe |
| $B_2$ | Diffuse nodular involvement of both lobes |
| C | Extension through the prostatic capsule |
| $D_1$ | Metastases to lymph nodes below the aortic bifurcation |
| $D_2$ | Metastases to lymph nodes above the aortic bifurcation |

Computed tomography or ultrasound (transrectal or transvesical) are the imaging procedures of choice for assessing local tumor extension and lymph node metastases, which can be confirmed by guided biopsy. A positive biopsy obviates the need for further imaging, because it is evidence of at least D1 disease. If the guided biopsy is negative, staging lymphadenectomy is recommended for all patients other than those staged clinically as A1 lesions (currently followed without any further specific therapy).

Skeletal metastases are best detected by radionuclide bone scanning. A negative scan excludes skeletal metastases, and thus there is no indication for obtaining a plain radiographic "metastatic survey." Positive findings on a radionuclide bone scan should be confirmed by plain radiographs of the affected region.

Liver metastases can be detected by radionuclide scanning, ultrasound, CT, or MRI and confirmed by ultrasound- or CT-guided biopsy. It is important to remember that abnormal liver function studies alone do not confirm the diagnosis of metastatic disease to the liver.

Plain chest radiography generally is considered the imaging procedure of choice for detecting lung metastases. Some authors prefer to obtain five randomized CT sections through the lung as the primary modality for excluding pulmonary metastases. This limited study has proven to be highly sensitive and, because of its limited survey nature, relatively cost effective. Biopsy guided by CT may be performed to confirm the histologic nature of a possibly metastatic lesion demonstrated on chest radiography or CT.

At present, MRI and lymphangiography do not have a substantial impact on the staging of prostatic carcinoma and thus are relegated to investigational use.

## Bibliography

Arduino LJ, Glucksman MA: Lymph node metastases in early carcinoma of the prostate. J Urol 88:91, 1962

Bisson J, Vichers M, Fagen WT, Jr: Bone scan in clinical perspective. J Urol 111:665–669, 1974

Bruce W, O'Cleirea CH, Ain F et al: Carcinoma of the prostate: A clinical look at staging. J Urol 117:319, 1977

Buonocore E, Hesemann C, Pavlicek W et al: Clinical and in vitro magnetic resonance imaging of prostatic carcinoma. AJR 143:1267, 1984

Efriemidis SC, Dan SJ, Neiburgs H et al: Carcinoma of the prostate: Lymph node aspiration for staging. AJR 136:489–492, 1981

Emory TH, Reinke DB, Hill AL et al: Use of CT to reduce understaging in prostatic cancer: Comparison with conventional staging techniques. AJR 141:351, 1983

Fujino A, Scardino PT: Transrectal ultrasonography

for prostatic cancer: Its value in staging and monitoring the response to radiotherapy and chemotherapy. J Urol 133:806–810, 1985

Goldenberg DM, DeLand FH, Bennett SJ et al: Radioimmunodetection of prostatic cancer. In vivo use of radioactive antibodies against prostatic acid phosphatase for diagnosis and detection of prostatic cancer by nuclear imaging. JAMA 250: 630–635, 1983

Grossman IC, Carpiniello V, Greenberg SH et al: Staging pelvic lymphadenectomy for carcinoma of the prostate: Review of 91 cases. J Urol 124: 632–634, 1980

Hastak SM, Gammelgaard J, Holm HH: Ultrasonically guided transperoneal biopsy in the diagnosis of prostatic carcinoma. J Urol 128:69, 1982

Hricak H, Williams RD: Magnetic resonance imaging and its application in urology. Urology 23: 442–454, 1984

Jewett HJ: Editorial: Prostatic cancer. J Urol 108:829, 1972

Levins MS, Arger PH, Coleman PJ et al: Detecting lymphatic metastases from prostatic carcinoma: Superiority of CT. AJR 137:207–211, 1981

Loening SA, Schmidt JD, Brown RC et al: A comparison between lymphangiography and pelvic node dissection in staging of prostatic cancer. J Urol 117:752–756, 1977

McLaughlin AP, Saltzstein SL, McCullough DL et al: Prostatic carcinoma incidence in location of unsuspected lymphatic metastases. J Urol 115:89, 1976

Merrin C, Wajsman Z, Baumgartner G et al: The clinical value of lymphangiography: Are the nodes surrounding the nerve visualized? J Urol 117:762–764, 1977

Morgan CL, Calkins RR, Cavalcanti EJ: Computed tomography in the evaluation, staging and therapy of carcinoma of the bladder and prostate. Radiology 140:751–761, 1981

Okafor PIS, Wild SR, Beynon LL et al: Progress in transrectal ultrasonography for prostatic disease. Br J Urol 55:721, 1983

Peeling WB, Griffiths GJ: Imaging of the prostate by ultrasound. J Urol 132:217–224, 1984

Poon PY, McCallum RW, Henkelman RM et al: Magnetic resonance imaging of the prostate. Radiology 154:143, 1985

Ray P, Feinstein C, Ray V et al: Staging errors in prostatic cancer. J Urol 132:125–126, 1984

Resnick MI: Use of transrectal ultrasound in evaluating prostatic cancer. J Urol 134:314, 1985

Resnick MI, Willard JW, Boyce WH: Transrectal ultrasonography in the evaluation of patients with prostatic carcinoma. J Urol 124:482, 1980

Styles RA, Seltzer SE: CT staging of prostatic cancer. Radiology 157:838, 1985

Weinerman PM, Arger PH, Pollack HM: CT evaluation of bladder and prostate neoplasms. Urol Radiol 4:105–115, 1982

Whitehead ED, Leiter E: Prostatic carcinoma clinical and surgical staging of. NY State J Med 81: 184–193, 1981

Wilson CS, Dahl DS, Middleton RG: Pelvic lymphadenectomy for staging of apparently localized prostatic cancer. J Urol 117:197, 1977

**DIAGNOSIS OF CARCINOMA OF PROSTATE**

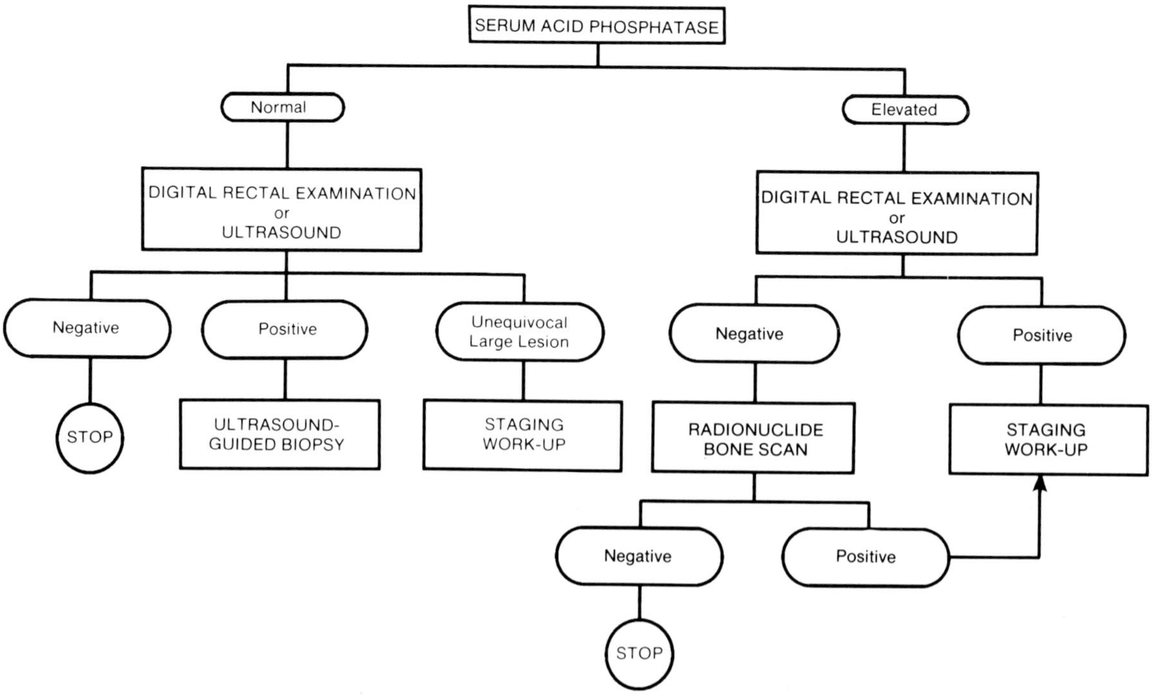


**STAGING OF CARCINOMA OF PROSTATE**
**(For Local Extension/Lymph Node Metastases)**

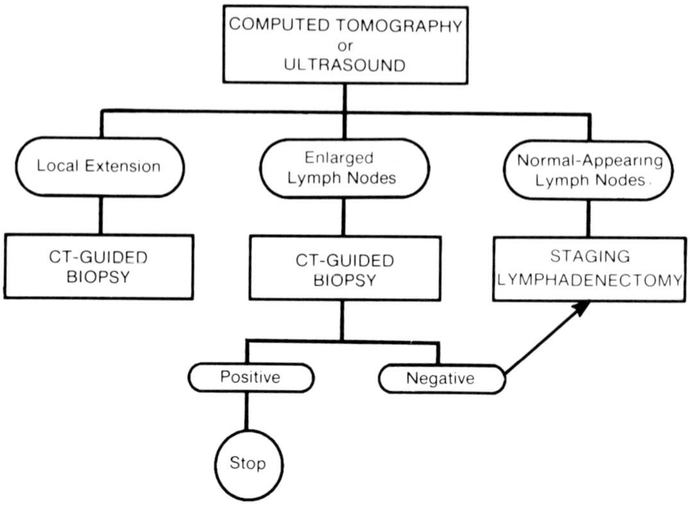

## STAGING OF CARCINOMA OF PROSTATE
(For Distant Metastases)

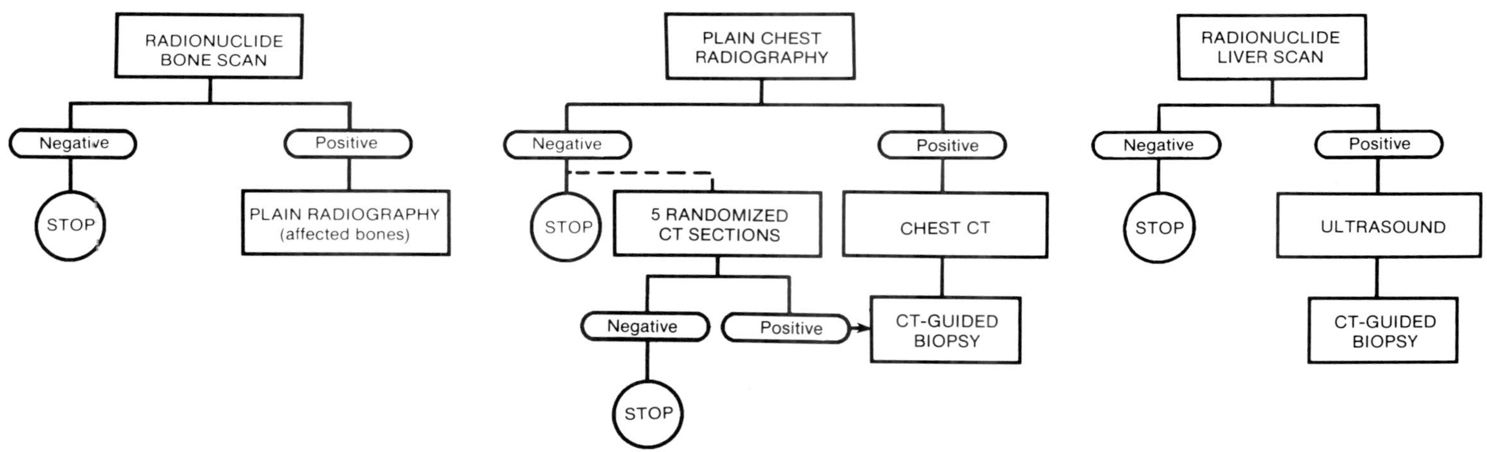

# Chapter 44

# Carcinoma of the Bladder

*Erich K. Lang*

The floor of the urinary bladder is the most common site of involvement by transitional-cell carcinoma. There is convincing evidence that the stage (depth of infiltration) of bladder carcinoma greatly influences curability and patient survival. The presence of regional lymph node metastases is a particularly ominous finding, because only 7% of patients with regional lymphatic metastases survive 5 years after radical cystectomy.

**Table 44-1** Jewett's Clinical Classification of Bladder Tumors

| Stage | Tumor Extension |
|---|---|
| A | Submucosal |
| $B_1$ | Inner one third of muscularis |
| $B_2$ | Outer two thirds of muscularis |
| C | Perivesical fat |
| $D_1$ | Pelvic nodes |
| $D_2$ | Para-aortic nodes—distant metastases |

## CLINICAL AND LABORATORY FINDINGS

As with all malignancies of uroepithelial origin, urine cytology is an effective screening examination for detecting lesions in asymptomatic patients. Examination under anesthesia traditionally has been used to stage the local invasiveness and extent of bladder neoplasms. Unfortunately, clinical staging often significantly under- or overestimates the spread of disease (particularly in understaging the consequential D1 lesion), indicating a major staging role for imaging modalities.

## DIAGNOSTIC EVALUATION

### *DIAGNOSTIC MODALITIES*

1. Excretory urography
2. Computed tomography
3. Lymphangiography
4. Ultrasound
5. Magnetic resonance imaging
6. Guided biopsy and staging lymphadenectomy

## Excretory Urography

Excretory urography is an imaging procedure that detects the presence of a neoplasm of the bladder. Lack of distensibility of a segment of the involved bladder wall and mass effect displacing the perivesical fat plane indicate permeation of the muscularis and extension of tumor into the perivesical fat. At times, the presence of a bladder neoplasm near the ureter of a nonfunctioning renal unit may suggest total obstruction and thus permeation of the muscular wall by the neoplasm. In general, however, excretory urography is of minimal value in staging carcinoma of the bladder.

## Computed Tomography

Computed tomography (CT) is the imaging modality of choice for identifying contiguous extension of a bladder neoplasm into perivesical fat, invasion of local tissue, and the presence of lymph node metastases (Fig. 44-1). The major criteria indicating neoplastic extension into the perivesical fat are haziness and loss of definition of the perivesical fat plane. At times, the inflammation and edema that often accompany bulky B2 lesions may mimic extension of the neoplasm into the perivesical fat. Dynamic CT following the administration of intravenous contrast material can improve the detection and characterization of these usually hypervascular tumors. The densely enhancing neoplasm can be further highlighted by distending the bladder with low-attenuation contrast (emulsified oil). Image reconstruction in sagittal and coronal planes also is of value in defining the extent of tumor penetration into the perivesical space or extension to the lateral pelvic wall (Fig. 44-2).

The use of dynamic CT has largely eliminated the substantial number of over- and understaging errors that occur with unenhanced CT scanning (Fig. 44-3). Plain CT has been shown to overstage proven B lesions in more than 33% of patients and to understage proven C tumors in up to 75% of cases. In contrast, dynamic CT has an accuracy of 80% to 85% for staging B and C lesions.

The identification of D1 lesions by CT requires the demonstration of enlarged lymph nodes. Unlike lymphangiography, CT can detect lymph node enlargement in all locations, including the obturator and internal iliac groups that are especially prone to harbor metastatic implants. However, CT cannot depict the internal architecture of lymph nodes and thus cannot detect tumor involvement that does not cause nodal enlargement.

## Lymphangiography

Lymphangiography is the only imaging modality that can diagnose metastases in normal-sized lymph nodes on the basis of intrinsic changes in nodal architecture. However, ultrasound- or CT-guided biopsy is often required to eliminate false-positive studies caused by fibrotic or fatty implants or by sinus histiocytosis. The major limitation of pedal lymphangiography is its frequent inability to opacify obturator and internal iliac nodes, major sites of metastases from carcinoma of the bladder. Because of its relatively low yield, high cost, and technical complexity, as well as the general availability of relatively noninvasive CT, lymphangiography now is rarely used as a primary modality for detecting lymphatic metastases from bladder carcinoma.

## Ultrasound

It is still unclear whether intravesical, transrectal, or standard transabdominal ultrasound can provide staging information equal to that afforded by CT. Initial studies have suggested that intravesical ultrasound has a high accuracy in assessing the primary neoplasm as well as metastatic spread to regional lymph nodes.

## Magnetic Resonance Imaging

Magnetic resonance imaging (MRI) can provide direct sagittal and coronal reconstructions that offer valuable information about the extent of a bladder carcinoma and any metastatic spread to

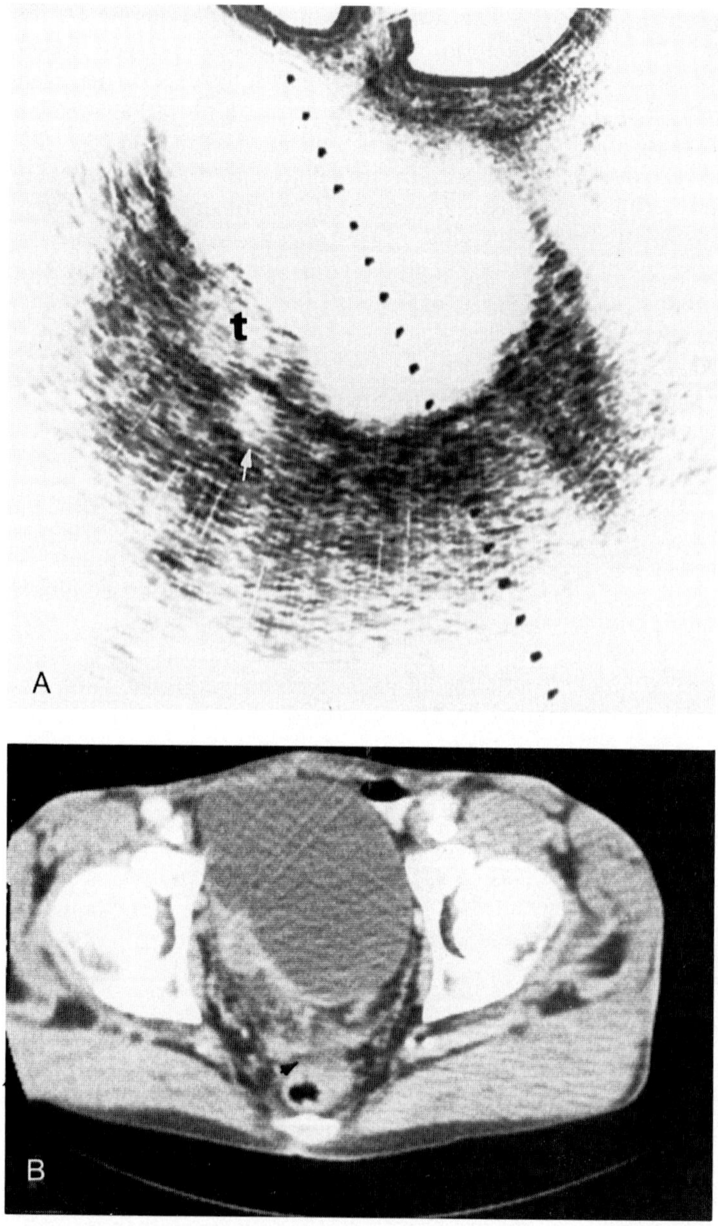


**e 4 -1.** **(A)** Ultrasound sector through the bladder shows a ..or (*t*) involving the right posterolateral wall and penetrating through the muscularis into the perivesical fat plane. Note an enlarged node (*arrow*) of the internal iliac chain. **(B)** Dynamic CT scan demonstrates dense enhancement and staining of the tumor involving and penetrating the left posterolateral wall of the bladder. There is contiguous extension into the perivesical fat. The enlarged hypogastric lymph node shown in *A* (*arrow*) is also demonstrated by CT. (Lang EK: Bladder and pelvic arteriography. In Abrams HL (ed): Abrams' Angiography. Boston, Little, Brown & Co, 1983)

enlarged regional or abdominal lymph nodes. Major limitations of MRI include its limited availability and high cost.

## Guided Biopsy and Staging Lymphadenectomy

The staging of bladder carcinoma is usually accomplished by the demonstration of local extension (Fig. 44-4), lymphadenopathy, and distant metastases on noninvasive imaging techniques (CT, ultrasound, MRI). Ultrasound- or CT-guided biopsy can confirm or sometimes exclude metastases as the cause of enlarged nodes on an imaging study. However, the magnitude of the operative intervention for curative radical cystectomy mandates that lymph node metastases to nonenlarged nodes be excluded with a

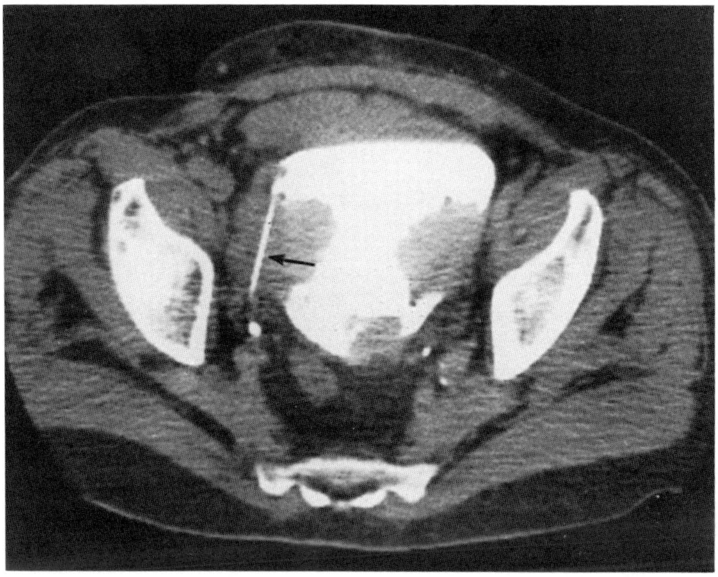

**Figure 44-2.** Coronal CT reconstructions through the pelvis demonstrate the lateral extension of a bladder neoplasm. This information is most useful for determining the feasibility of *en bloc* resection. (Lang EK: Neoplasms of the bladder, prostate and urethra. Semin Roentgenol 18: 288–289, 1983)

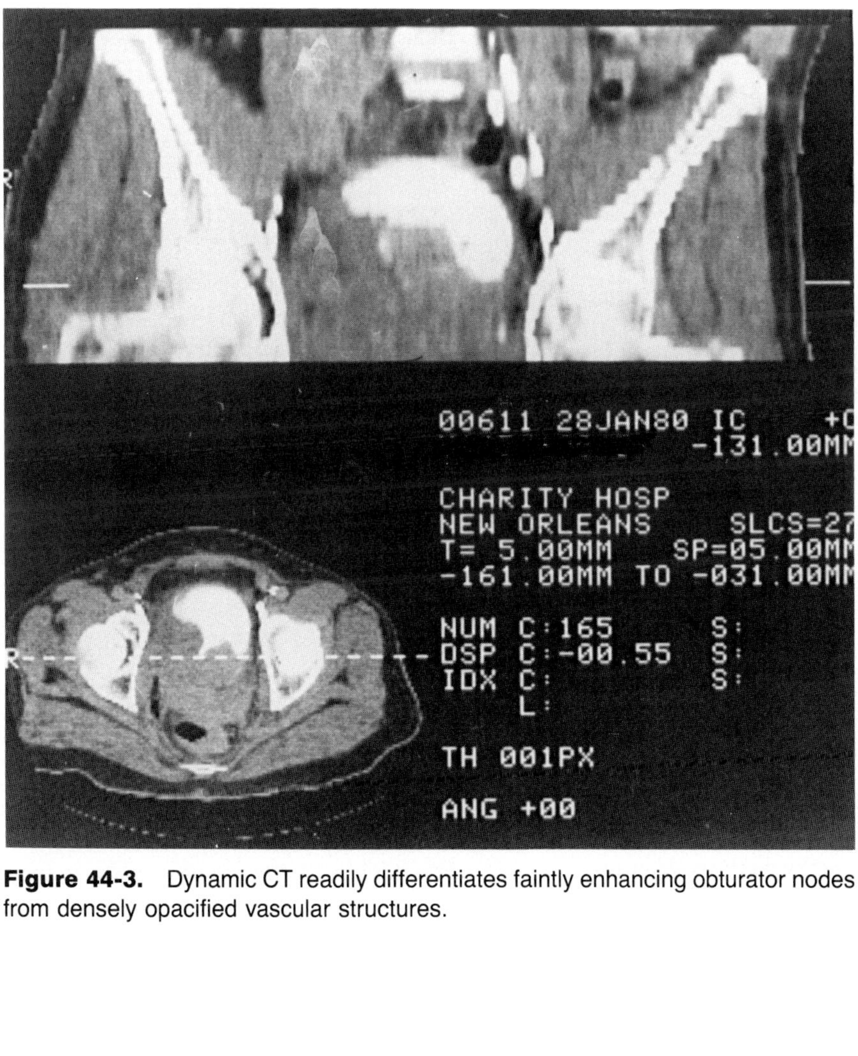


**Figure 44-3.** Dynamic CT readily differentiates faintly enhancing obturator nodes from densely opacified vascular structures.

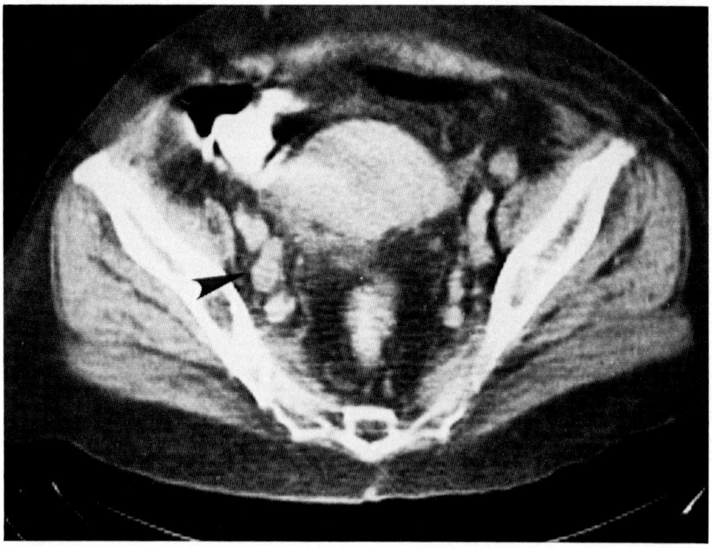

**Figure 44-4.** CT-guided thin-needle biopsy (*arrowhead*) confirms the presence of a bladder neoplasm extending to the perivesical space.

high degree of accuracy by surgical staging lymphadenectomy.

## APPROACH TO STAGING OF BLADDER CARCINOMA

Following the diagnosis of carcinoma of the bladder and examination under anesthesia to clinically determine the local extent of disease, plain chest radiography and radionuclide bone scanning are usually employed to detect distant pulmonary and skeletal metastases that would place the patient in stage D2. If there is no evidence of distant metastases, dynamic CT or ultrasound (transrectal or transvesical) is the next imaging modality. If both imaging studies and clinical examination under anesthesia show that the lesion is stage B2 or less, cystectomy can be considered after a staging lymphadenectomy has excluded lymph node metastases. Even stage C lesions, in which there is tumor extension into perivesical fat, can be considered for radical cystectomy if imaging studies and staging lymphadenectomy have indicated the absence of nodal metastases. The presence of nodal or distant metastases excludes potentially curative surgery and requires a different therapeutic approach (usually chemotherapy and/or radiation therapy).

Arteriography, lymphangiography, and cystography are no longer used for staging of bladder carcinoma, because the information they supply can be better obtained using CT or ultrasound.

## Bibliography

Ahlberg NE, Calisserndorff B, Wijkstrom H: Computed tomography in staging of bladder carcinoma. Acta Radiol (Diagn) 23:47–53, 1982

Bree RL, Silva TM: Pictorial essay—Sonography of bladder and perivesical abnormalities. AJR 136:1101–1104, 1981

Frodin L, Hemmingsson A, Johansson A et al: Computed tomography in staging of bladder carcinoma. Acta Radiol (Diag) 21:763–767, 1980

Gibod LB, Katz M, Cochand B et al: Lymphography and percutaneous fine needle node aspiration biopsy in staging of bladder carcinoma. J Urol 132:24–26, 1984

Hamlin DJ, Cockett ATK, Burgener FA: Computed tomography of the pelvis: Sagittal and coronal imagery reconstruction in the evaluation of infiltrative bladder carcinoma. J Comput Assist Tomogr 5:27–33, 1981

Harada K, Igari D, Tanahashi Y et al: Staging of bladder tumors by means of transrectal ultrasonography. J Clin Ultrasound 5:388–392, 1977

Hodson NJ, Husband JE, McDonald JS: The role of computed tomography in staging of bladder carcinoma. Clin Radiol 30:389–395, 1979

Hricak H, Williams RD: Magnetic resonance imaging and its application in urology. Urology 23: 442–454, 1984

Jeffrey RB, Palubinskas AJ, Federle MP: CT evaluation of invasive lesions of the bladder. J Comput Assist Tomogr 5:22–26, 1981

Jewett HJ, Strong GH: Infiltrating carcinoma of the bladder: Relation of depth of penetration of the bladder wall to incidence of local extension of metastases. J Urol 55:366–372, 1946

Koss JC, Arger PH, Coleman PG et al: CT staging of bladder carcinoma. AJR 137:359–362, 1981

Lang EK: Neoplasms of the bladder, prostate and urethra. Semin Roentgenol 18:288–289, 1983

Lang EK: Triple cystogram and selective arteriography. JAMA 207:342–344, 1969

Murphy GP: Developments in preoperative staging of the bladder tumors. Urology 11:109–115, 1978

Resnick MI: Ultrasonic evaluation of prostate and bladder. Semin Ultrasound 1:69, 1980

Sager EM, Talle K, Fossa S et al: Role of Ct in demonstrating perivesical tumor growth in the preoperative staging of carcinoma of the urinary bladder. Radiology 146:443–446, 1983

Smith JA, Whitmore WF, Jr: Regional lymph node metastases from bladder cancer. J Urol 126: 591–593, 1981

Strijk SP, Debruyne FMJ, Herman CJ: Lymphography in the management of urologic tumors: Radiological-pathological correlation. Radiology 146:39–45, 1983

Whitmore WJ, Jr, Batata MA, Hilaris BS et al: A comparative study of two preoperative regimens with cystostomy for bladder cancer. Cancer 40:1077–1086, 1977

## STAGING OF CARCINOMA OF BLADDER

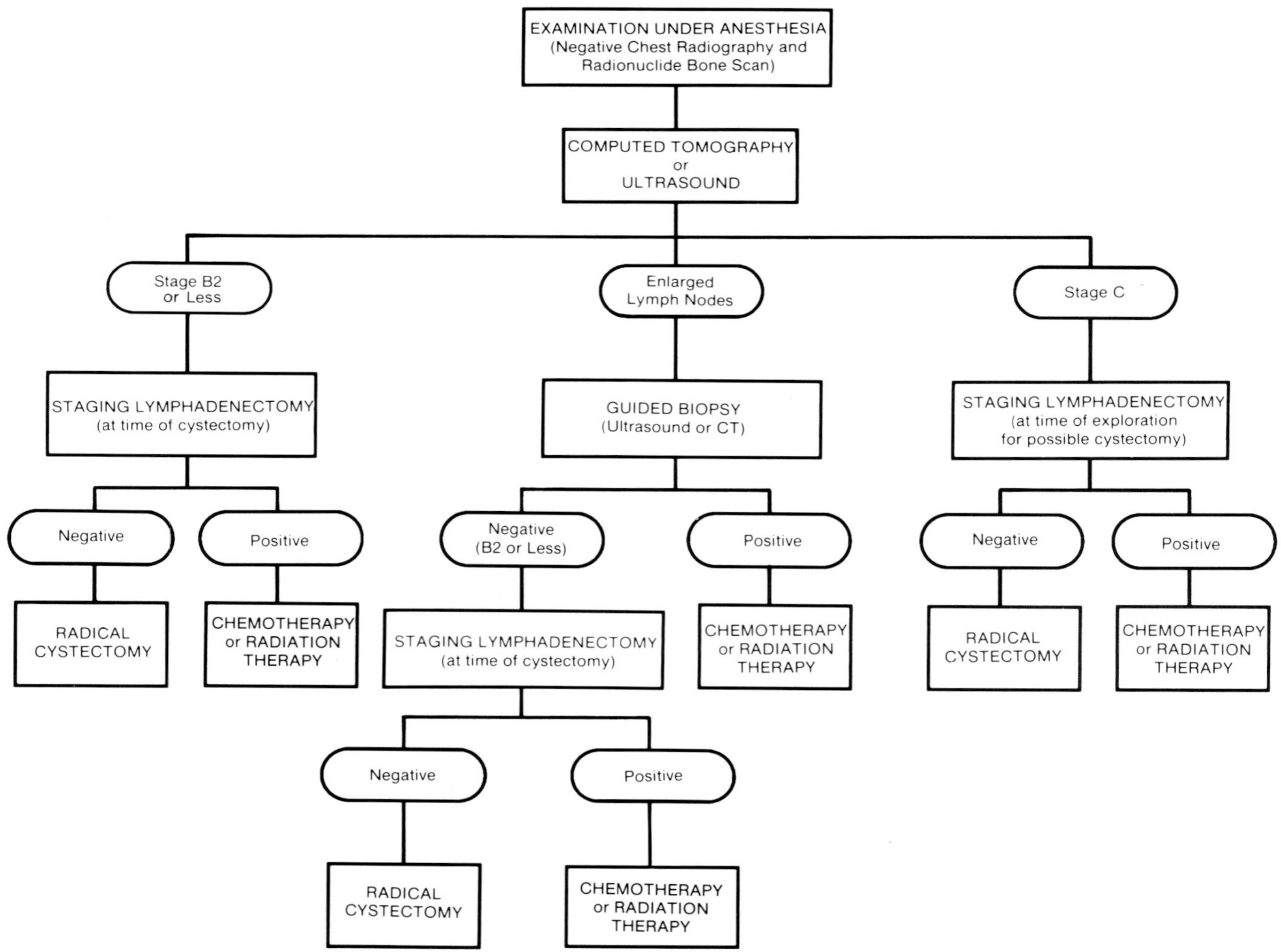

# Chapter 45

# Staging of Malignant Lymphomas

*Stephen I. Marglin*
*Ronald A. Castellino*

When confronted by a patient with the recently established diagnosis of either Hodgkin's disease or non-Hodgkin's lymphoma, clinicians and radiologists alike often appear bewildered by the multiplicity of potentially relevant imaging procedures (*e.g.*, radionuclide scanning, lymphography, computed tomography, ultrasound and, most recently, magnetic resonance imaging). Unfortunately, there is still no unequivocal consensus about which of these imaging studies are required or their proper sequencing. Despite this, the primary objective of this chapter is to formulate specific recommendations with the understanding that they will undoubtedly need to be modified as additional data become available.

## THE NATURE OF THE TWO DISEASES

Because of the numerous similarities between Hodgkin's disease and the heterogeneous group of diseases known as the non-Hodgkin's lymphomas (diffuse nodal enlargement and a well-defined measurable potential for extending beyond nodal structures to involve major thoracic and abdominal viscera), it is tempting to assume that the same imaging strategy is appropriate for patients in both groups. Unfortunately, important differences between Hodgkin's disease and non-Hodgkin's lymphoma make this "singular" approach to imaging somewhat less than completely satisfactory.

The prevalence of disease in specific anatomic sites (mediastinum, mesenteric nodes, bone marrow) at the time of initial presentation are substantially different (Table 45-1). The anticipated biologic behavior of the two diseases also differs markedly. Hodgkin's disease, more than many other tumors, behaves in a highly predictable fashion. This predictability (in conjunction with a high rate of response to both chemotherapy and radiation therapy) probably accounts for the gratifyingly high cure rate. Hodgkin's disease appears to spread through directly connected lymphatic pathways. Thus, for example, a patient with disease involving the supraclavicular region might be expected, by virtue

**Table 45-1** Prevalence of Disease Involvement in Specific Anatomic Sites in Previously Untreated Patients

| | Hodgkin's Disease | | | Non-Hodgkin's Lymphoma | | |
|---|---|---|---|---|---|---|
| | Adult | | Child | Adult | | Child |
| Thoracic nodes | | 65% | | | 25% | |
| Lung parenchyma | | 10% | | | 4% | |
| Pleural effusion | 10% | | 4% | 7% | | 14% |
| Para-aortic nodes | 34% | | 19% | 55% | | 30% |
| Mesenteric nodes | | 4% | | | 51% | |
| Spleen | | 34% | | | 33% | |
| Liver | | 6% | | | 14% | |
| Bone marrow | | 3% | | | 20% | |
| Gastrointestinal tract | | 0% | | 8% | | 18% |
| Urinary tract | | 0% | | | 3% | |

(Data from Kadin et al, Goffinet et al, Castellino et al, and Castellino et al)

of presumed retrograde flow in the thoracic duct, to have an increased likelihood of disease in the high para-aortic and paracaval lymph nodes, as well as within the spleen. Low retroperitoneal or pelvic involvement with sparing of these upper abdominal nodes would be highly unusual and should call into question the diagnosis of Hodgkin's disease. Non-Hodgkin's lymphoma disseminates in a considerably less predictable manner, and this may partially explain why localized or regional forms of therapy so rarely result in cure. Another factor influencing the poorer prognosis of non-Hodgkin's lymphoma relative to that of Hodgkin's disease is that a considerably higher percentage of patients with non-Hodgkin's lymphoma present with far advanced stages of disease. Thus, it is generally agreed that local forms of therapy (*e.g.*, surgery or irradiation) are unlikely to be curative for patients with non-Hodgkin's lymphoma, except for the small group of patients with bona fide stage I disease. The other 90% of patients with non-Hodgkin's lymphoma therefore undergo a systemic form of treatment (chemotherapy, total body irradiation, or possibly bone marrow transplantation). If these regimens are used, it can be effectively argued that precise anatomic information regarding the spread of the disease may not be mandatory (although such information is helpful in assessing the prognosis).

## REASONS FOR DIAGNOSTIC IMAGING PROCEDURES

For both Hodgkin's disease and non-Hodgkin's lymphoma, imaging procedures may be performed for any of the following reasons:

1. To determine the stage of the disease
2. As an adjunct to biopsy (especially staging laparotomy)
3. To assist in treatment planning
4. To help in formulating a prognosis
5. To evaluate response to therapy
6. To assist in detecting a relapse
7. For research and epidemiologic reasons

The Ann Arbor staging system (Table 45-2) is employed for both Hodgkin's disease and non-Hodgkin's lymphoma. The goal of the system is to amalgamate patients with similar anatomic distributions of disease into categories that permit a reasonable estimate of prognosis and provide a basis for treatment planning. It is important to remember that, in this system, involvement of the spleen is treated conceptually as the equivalent of lymph node involvement.

Even a casual perusal of the Ann Arbor system suggests that there is a considerable difference between the process of staging and the process whereby a determination is made about the actual extent of disease. For example, the detec-

**Table 45-2** Ann Arbor Staging Classification of the Malignant Lymphomas

| | |
|---|---|
| Stage I: | Involvement of a single lymph node region (I) or of a single extra-lymphatic organ or site (IE) |
| Stage II: | Involvement of two or more lymph node regions on the same side of the diaphragm (II) or localized involvement of an extralymphatic organ or site, and of one or more lymph node regions on the same side of the diaphragm (IIE). |
| Stage III: | Involvement of lymph node regions on both sides of the diaphragm (III), which may also be accompanied by involvement of the spleen (IIIS) or by localized involvement of an extra-lymphatic organ or site (IIIE) or both (IIISE). |
| Stage IV: | Disseminated involvement of one or more extralymphatic organs or tissues, with or without associated lymph node involvement. |

For all stages, substage A = Asymptomatic patients and substage B = Patients with history of fever, sweats, or weight loss of greater than 10% body weight

tion of a single abnormal abdominal lymph node (by whatever noninvasive means) in a patient with previously demonstrable disease above the level of the diaphragm is sufficient to categorize the patient as being (at least) stage III. More complete imaging evaluation of this patient, perhaps including surgical exploration, might reveal unexpected extensive nodal or splenic involvement. Even though this information might conceivably be germane to treatment planning and/or prognosis, it would not alter the stage of the patient's disease.

After the patient has been staged and initially treated, a new set of issues often emerges. At the time of initial presentation, an energetic quest for the most comprehensive information can easily be justified because of the potential for cure and the need to choose among a variety of therapeutic options. Cost containment, although important, is not the overriding issue at this time. Later in the course of the patient's disease, however, serious questions could be raised regarding the justification for extensive periodic imaging surveillance. Similarly, if there is a suspicion of recurrent disease, the anatomic extent of involvement may be greater than it was at the time of initial presentation. Therefore, if the primary purpose is to document relapse, a less sensitive imaging modality may suffice.

## DIAGNOSTIC EVALUATION

Reports describing the accuracy of various imaging modalities in Hodgkin's disease or non-Hodgkin's lymphoma are often difficult to evaluate, because the patients are at various stages in the natural evolution of their diseases. Therefore, much of the analysis that follows is based on information derived from patients at the time of their initial presentations and prior to receiving any therapy. At this stage the detection of disease may be most difficult, thus placing the maximum demand on a given imaging modality.

### *DIAGNOSTIC MODALITIES*

1. Supradiaphragmatic disease
   a. Standard chest radiography
   b. Conventional tomography
   c. Computed tomography
   d. Magnetic resonance imaging
   e. Radionuclide scanning
2. Infradiaphragmatic disease
   a. Plain abdominal radiography
   b. Opacification of adjacent structures
      Excretory urography
      Inferior vena cavography
      Barium studies of the GI tract
   c. Lymphangiography
   d. Computed tomography
   e. Ultrasound
   f. Radionuclide scanning
   g. Magnetic resonance imaging

### Supradiaphragmatic Disease

Standard frontal and lateral chest radiographs can demonstrate most significant intrathoracic abnormalities, especially those involving the pulmonary parenchyma. If lymphoma only involves the mediastinum, both plain chest radiography and conventional tomography are limited by their inability to assess more than the outer contour of the mediastinum. Modestly enlarged lymph nodes remain undetectable until the mediastinal contour is sufficiently stretched and distorted to indicate their presence. Although it is clear that conventional tomography can provide diagnostic information that is not evident on standard chest radiographs, in the case of the malignant lymphomas these additional findings have been shown to result in a change in staging in only 1.2% of patients and a change in contemplated therapy in only 3.3%. Therefore, the incremental yield from conventional tomography is low if the initial standard chest radiographs (carefully interpreted) appear normal.

Although cross-sectional imaging techniques (computed tomography, magnetic resonance imaging) are more sensitive than standard chest radiographs or conventional tomography because of their ability to look within the mediastinum, the additional information provided by these modalities would appear to infrequently change either the patient's stage or the contemplated therapy. In a recent series of 203 patients with newly diagnosed Hodgkin's disease who were studied with both conventional chest radiographs and chest computed tomography (CT), the incremental information derived from CT prompted a change in therapy in only 9.4% of cases. This rate was highest (13.8%) for patients whose contemplated form of therapy was irradiation, intermediate (8.2%) for those whose therapy was to involve both irradiation and chemotherapy, and lowest (0%) for those whose intended therapy involved chemotherapy alone.

## Infradiaphragmatic Disease

Comprehensive pretreatment protocols for patients with one of the malignant lymphomas, especially those that have included staging laparotomy, have strongly indicated that there is no valid justification for performing examinations such as excretory urography, barium studies of the gastrointestinal tract, radionuclide liver–spleen scans, radionuclide bone scans, or skeletal surveys as part of the staging evaluation.

Intrinsic lymphomatous involvement of the gastrointestinal tract is extremely rare in patients with Hodgkin's disease. In the non-Hodgkin's lymphomas, gastrointestinal involvement is almost invariably associated with symptoms that would have indicated the need for barium studies. The possibility of urinary tract obstruction can be effectively evaluated by CT or ultrasound. Asymptomatic osseous involvement at the time of presentation also is uncommon and usually can be detected by a careful review of routine plain chest and abdominal radiographs. At present, therefore, it appears that the assessment of lymphomatous involvement of the abdomen realistically involves a choice among lymphography, CT, and ultrasound. Although MRI may ultimately prove to play a significant role, its precise impact has yet to be determined.

### Lymphangiography

Bipedal lymphangiography (infusion of contrast material into lymphatic channels on the dorsum of the feet) routinely opacifies those lymph nodes that lie adjacent to the external and common iliac arteries and veins, the inferior vena cava, and the aorta (approximately to the level of the renal vessels). Retroperitoneal lymph nodes cephalad to this level, or those situated more anteriorly or laterally, are not consistently opacified. Intra-abdominal lymph nodes, as well as those situated deep in the bony pelvis, are also generally not opacified and thus are not amenable to investigation by this technique.

Unlike other procedures for lymph node imaging, lymphangiography possesses excellent spatial resolution. The infused contrast material is largely trapped within the sinusoidal network of the nodes; little, if any, actually penetrates the follicular tissue. The resulting radiographic image is a remarkably precise depiction of the nodal architecture. Normal nodes are characterized by the uniform distribution of contrast material in the sinusoids and by the small size of the negative filling defects (*i.e.*, the follicles). If the lymph node contains tumor, the diffuse "filling defects" commonly produce a lacelike or bubbly appearance. Although typical of lymphomatous involvement, this appearance is not pathognomonic nor is it the only manifestation of nodal lymphoma. Lymphomatous nodes may become focally enlarged (especially in Hodgkin's disease) and may display solitary, discrete filling defects similar to those produced by solid epithelial tumors.

Lymphangiography is the only imaging technique that demonstrates the internal architecture of lymph nodes well enough to permit the detection of macroscopic tumor within nodes that are still normal in size. In addition, lymphangiography is the sole imaging modality that can allow discrimination of nodes that are enlarged as a result of benign conditions (*e.g.*, benign reactive hyperplasia) from those that are enlarged due to tumor. If there is need for surgical confirmation of a lymphangiographic abnormality, a plain abdominal radiograph at the time of laparotomy can ensure that the relevant nodes have been sampled or, alternatively, fluoroscopy can permit percutaneous aspiration of cells from the suspect nodes. Because contrast material can be visualized within opacified nodes for 12 months or longer following lymphangiography, periodic appraisal of nodal size can be made using a simple and relatively inexpensive abdominal radiograph.

A major limitation of lymphangiography is the conviction of many radiologists that the technique is tedious, difficult to master, and excessively time-consuming. From the patient's perspective, the minor discomfort and occasionally protracted nature of the examination may be significant disadvantages. In addition, lymphangiography does involve "minor surgery" and the attendant small risks associated with local anesthesia, a cutdown, and the use of vital dyes and contrast agents. Although complications of lymphangiography are uncommon, the radiologist must fully understand that this examination is contraindicated in patients with right-to-left intracardiac shunts or severe pulmonary disease.

In a study of 632 consecutive, unselected, and newly diagnosed patients with Hodgkin's disease and non-Hodgkin's lymphoma (Table 45-3), lymphangiography achieved an overall accuracy of 91% based on the histopathologic interpretation of nodes obtained at staging laparotomy. Even more impressive, 98% of patients with Hodgkin's disease whose lymphograms were interpreted as negative had no evidence of nodal involvement by tumor at staging laparotomy.

### Computed Tomography

During the past decade, CT of the abdomen has transformed the practice of diagnostic oncology. The extraordinary contrast resolution of CT permits evaluation of areas of the abdomen previously regarded as "opaque." Computed tomography can visualize not only those retroperitoneal and pelvic nodes routinely opacified by lymphangiography but also those nodes in the upper retroperitoneum, mesentery, and hila of the kidney, spleen, and liver. This modality also allows direct assessment of the abdominal viscera. The technique of a CT examination is relatively straightforward and requires neither the skill, patience, nor dexterity of a standard bipedal lymphogram. The interpretation of a CT

**Table 45-3** Accuracy of Lymphangiography in 632 Patients with Hodgkin's Disease and Non-Hodgkin's Lymphoma

| | Hodgkin's Disease | Non-Hodgkin's Lymphoma | Total |
|---|---|---|---|
| Sensitivity | 93% (100/107) | 89% (101/114) | 91% |
| Specificity | 92% (284/309) | 86% (88/102) | 91% |
| Accuracy of positive LAG | 80% (100/125) | 88% (101/115) | 84% |
| Accuracy of negative LAG | 98% (284/291) | 87% (88/101) | 95% |
| Overall accuracy | 92% (384/411) | 88% (189/216) | 91% |

(Data from Marglin and Castellino)

examination often appears less intimidating than that of a lymphangiogram, especially to those whose experience in use of the latter modality is limited.

In this age of intense cost consciousness, it should be noted that the cumulative cost of sequential CT examinations far exceeds that of periodic surveillance with plain abdominal radiographs following lymphangiography.

Comparing the results of CT and lymphangiography (Table 45-4), lymphangiography has a statistically significant advantage in evaluating retroperitoneal lymphadenopathy in patients with Hodgkin's disease and a probable advantage in patients with non-Hodgkin's lymphoma. The sensitivity of CT in detecting mesenteric lymph node involvement in patients with non-Hodgkin's lymphoma is a disappointing 67% (Table 45-4), despite the fact that mesenteric involvement is known to be common in these patients. Splenic involvement is also fairly common in both Hodgkin's disease and non-Hodgkin's lymphoma (see Table 45-1). Unfortunately, CT has proven relatively insensitive for detecting the presence of splenic lymphoma (Tables 45-5 and 45-6). This failure of detection should not come as a surprise, considering that splenic involvement commonly occurs as small foci (often <1 cm) in spleens that are normal in size. In both Hodgkin's and non-Hodgkin's lymphoma, initial involvement of the liver is uncommon. For this reason, the reported high overall accuracy in the detection of hepatic lymphoma (Tables 45-5 and 45-6) should more appropriately be considered a reflection of low prevalence than an indication of the inherent sensitivity of CT in this region.

### Ultrasound

A discussion of the relative utility of the various abdominal imaging modalities would be incomplete without at least a brief consideration of the role of diagnostic ultrasound. Ultrasound is noninvasive, relatively inexpensive, well tolerated and accepted by patients, and devoid of side-effects. Along with CT, ultrasound can evaluate the entire abdomen, rather than merely the retroperitoneal nodes. Whereas CT is occasionally difficult to interpret in thin patients with a paucity of retroperitoneal fat, these are precisely the patients in whom ultrasound performs best. Unfortunately, many abdominal ultrasound examinations are technically suboptimal and incomplete due to the presence of intervening bowel gas. This problem can sometimes be circumvented by maneuvers such as judicious delay, changing the patient's position, or having the patient drink copious amounts of water, but these techniques are not uniformly successful. Of major clinical importance, most clinicians who treat patients with malignant lymphomas appear to feel more comfortable with CT images than with the narrow-field images obtained from real-time ultrasound, presumably because of the lack of easily identifiable landmarks in ultra-

**Table 45-4** Histopathologic Correlation of CT and LAG in Newly Diagnosed, Previously Untreated Patients

| | Retroperitoneal Nodes | | | |
|---|---|---|---|---|
| | Hodgkin's Disease | | Non-Hodgkin's Lymphoma | |
| | CT | LAG | CT | LAG |
| Sensitivity | 65% (13/20) | 85% (17/20) | 86% (12/14) | 100% (14/14) |
| Specificity | 92% (80/87) | 98% (85/87) | 75% (6/8) | 75% (6/8) |
| Accuracy of positive diagnosis | 65% (13/20) | 89% (17/19) | 86% (12/14) | 88% (14/16) |
| Accuracy of negative diagnosis | 92% (80/87) | 97% (85/88) | 75% (6/8) | 100% (6/6) |
| Overall accuracy | 87% (93/107) | 95% (102/107) | 82% (18/22) | 91% (20/22) |

(Data from Castellino et al)

**Table 45-5** Accuracy of CT in Newly Diagnosed, Previously Untreated Patients with Hodgkin's Disease

| | Mesenteric Nodes | Spleen | Liver |
|---|---|---|---|
| Sensitivity | 0% (0/1) | 33% (17/51) | 25% (1/4) |
| Specificity | 99% (90/91) | 76% (53/70) | 100% (117/117) |
| Accuracy of positive diagnosis | 0% (0/1) | 50% (17/34) | 100% (1/1) |
| Accuracy of negative diagnosis | 99% (90/91) | 61% (53/87) | 98% (117/120) |
| Overall accuracy | 98% (90/92) | 58% (70/121) | 98% (118/121) |

(Data from Castellino et al)

**Table 45-6** Accuracy of CT in Newly Diagnosed, Previously Untreated Patients with Non-Hodgkin's Lymphoma

| | Mesenteric Nodes | Spleen | Liver |
|---|---|---|---|
| Sensitivity | 67% (10/15) | 45% (6/11) | 67% (2/3) |
| Specificity | 75% (6/8) | 83% (10/12) | 100% (21/21) |
| Accuracy of positive diagnosis | 83% (10/12) | 71% (5/7) | 100% (2/2) |
| Accuracy of negative diagnosis | 55% (6/11) | 63% (10/16) | 95% (21/22) |
| Overall accuracy | 70% (16/23) | 65% (15/23) | 96% (23/24) |

(Data from Castellino)

sound. It would seem that the role of ultrasound is largely adjunctive in the staging of patients with malignant lymphomas.

## Radionuclide Scanning

Radionuclide scanning with $^{67}$Ga citrate can detect lymphomatous involvement in a variety of sites. The accuracy of this technique within the abdomen is less than that in the thorax, presumably because of the "interference" caused by the accumulation of isotope within bowel and liver. When data from a large cooperative study are compared with that in Tables 45-3 and 45-4, $^{67}$Ga scanning is seen to be less accurate than either lymphangiography or CT in evaluating the retroperitoneal nodes. It has been suggested that the accuracy of gallium scanning may be improved by increasing the dose and by the use of triple-peak Anger cameras, but to date the evidence for this contention is still incomplete. Although some have found gallium scanning to be helpful in the initial evaluation of patients with malignant lymphomas, this has not been our experience, and thus we cannot recommend the routine utilization of this imaging modality for staging purposes.

## Magnetic Resonance Imaging

Current reports do not yet permit well-reasoned judgments about the role that MRI will eventually play in the evaluation of patients with Hodgkin's disease or non-Hodgkin's lymphoma. There is reason to believe that the current low spatial resolution of MRI will make it difficult to detect tumor within normal-sized lymph nodes. It is uncertain whether MRI will eventually be able to distinguish enlarged, tumor-containing lymph nodes from those that are enlarged as a result of benign conditions such as reactive hyperplasia. Upcoming technical advances and newer imaging sequences (*e.g.*, short TI inversion recovery, or STIR) may eventually overcome these current limitations.

## SELECTION AND SEQUENCING OF IMAGING EXAMINATIONS

The selection of appropriate imaging procedures for a patient with either Hodgkin's disease or one of the non-Hodgkin's lymphomas involves more than a simple comparison of the "accuracies" of the competing modalities. Consideration must also be given to the expected "behavior" of the disease (*i.e.*, its unique patterns of metastatic spread) and to the anticipated impact of the information obtained on patient management. For example, there may be no indication for routine use of a test that is accurate when assessing a site of infrequent disease. Similarly, there may be no indication for a test if the information obtained is unlikely to alter either the staging of disease or the contemplated therapy. In addition, the subjective desires of the patient must also be taken into consideration. No imaging procedure can provide as much information as can direct surgical visualization and biopsy, yet few patients would willingly opt for this means of monitoring response to therapy or detecting tumor recurrence.

### The Thorax

For patients with Hodgkin's disease, the results of thoracic CT can be anticipated to influence therapy (especially radiation therapy) in approximately 10% of patients. For patients who will undergo chemotherapy, a frequent clinical dilemma is whether the therapy is adequate. This question is easier to answer if a detailed "baseline" thoracic CT scan is available for comparison. For both of these reasons we recommend that a thoracic CT scan be obtained on newly diagnosed, previously untreated patients. Standard plain chest radiographs are generally sufficient for following a patient's intrathoracic disease. Follow-up CT examinations are reserved for the patient whose symptoms are suggestive of recurrence but in whom conventional chest radiographs are either normal, ambiguous, or unchanged.

For patients with one of the non-Hodgkin's lymphomas, the decision of whether to obtain chest CT depends on the specific clinical situation. Since enormous prognostic and therapeutic significance is attendant on distinguishing stage I disease from all other stages of non-Hodgkin's lymphoma, CT is routinely employed if there is any ambiguity. For the vast majority of patients with more advanced disease, the issue is far more difficult. Patients in this category almost invariably will be treated with some form of systemic therapy (chemotherapy, total body radiation, and/or bone marrow transplantation). Thus, the detection of subtle mediastinal adenopathy has no influence on treatment. Nevertheless, as in patients with Hodgkin's disease, questions often arise regarding whether a given therapeutic regimen has induced a complete remission. To provide the most complete pre- and post-treatment information to address these questions, we still are inclined to obtain chest CT in almost all newly presenting patients with non-Hodgkin's lymphoma (except, perhaps, in those with obvious bulky lymphadenopathy). In this group of patients, it may potentially be useful to obtain a "baseline" CT examination when standard plain chest radiographs revert to a normal or near-normal appearance.

### The Abdomen

In patients with Hodgkin's disease, the decisions about performance of a staging laprarotomy and/or the form(s) of therapy to employ generally depend on accurate assessments of the degree of abdominal involvement. Many medical oncologists and radiotherapists have routinely recommended a staging laparotomy prior to making these decisions. Although staging laparotomy has greatly enhanced our understanding of Hodgkin's disease, it is important to recognize that staging laparotomy is not a requisite part of the pretreatment evaluation for all patients. Currently, staging laparotomy is largely reserved for those institutions actively involved in clinical investigation and for those patients whose therapy would be significantly altered by information obtained in this manner. Because laparotomy is neither an absolute nor general requirement, it is essential that clinical determinations be based on the most accurate imaging information available.

We have found lymphangiography to have a statistically significant advantage over CT in the assessment of lymphomatous involvement of retroperitoneal nodes. This greater sensitivity may be crucial in the selection of appropriate therapy by determining whether the disease is restricted to the supradiaphragmatic region (stages I or II), or is present on both sides of the diaphragm (stage III). Even if it has been decided to perform a staging laparotomy, lymphangiography can be of value to the surgeon in ensuring that those nodes that appear most abnormal are appropriately sampled. Because contrast material remains within opacified nodes for 12 to 18 months, it is convenient and inexpensive to follow patients with periodic postlymphangiography abdominal radiographs.

It must be acknowledged that our excellent results with lymphangiography may be directly related to our extensive personal interest and experience in this field of imaging. Thus, clinicians with less interest and less time to devote to this modality may experience a smaller or no statistical advantage of lymphangiography over CT. Nevertheless, we would still recommend that consideration be given to referring a patient for lymphangiography if (for whatever reason) the decision has been made not to perform this examination locally.

Because splenic involvement in Hodgkin's disease can occur in the absence of lymphographically overt retroperitoneal node involvement, this might suggest a substantial role for CT in assessing the spleen. Unfortunately, 65% of patients with pathologically proven splenic involvement can be expected to have a false-negative CT examination, presumably because splenic involvement commonly occurs as small foci that are usually less than 1 cm in diameter in spleens that are normal in overall size. Nevertheless, we still recommend obtaining an abdominal and pelvic CT scan for patients with Hodgkin's disease, both for the immediate value of the information provided and for use as a baseline for any subsequent examinations.

Although the majority of patients with non-Hodgkin's lymphoma present with extensive, widespread disease, the detection of retroperitoneal lymphadenopathy is still of considerable value. The status of the retroperitoneal nodes will be closely followed during and after treatment, and the information obtained will be consciously integrated into decisions about the need for additional therapy. In these patients, however, tumor can commonly be found in sites other than the retroperitoneal nodes (*e.g.*, mesenteric lymph nodes, nodes in the splenic and hepatic hila), as well as in a multiplicity of extranodal locations. Because of this propensity of non-Hodgkin's lymphoma to disseminate widely, the importance or advantages of lymphangiography's increased ability to detect retroperitoneal lymphadenopathy probably should not be overemphasized. Computed tomography, although far from perfect in its assessment of the mesentery, spleen, and liver, is still the most accurate modality currently available. Because of its ability to provide an excellent noninvasive overview of the entire abdomen, CT should be regarded as the single best imaging modality for the pretreatment evaluation of a patient with non-Hodgkin's lymphoma. In actual practice, we also continue to recommend lymphangiography because of its ability to economically assess the status of disease and the adequacy of therapy on postlymphangiography abdominal radiographs. If this option is selected, there should be no reluctance to perform an abdominal CT examination whenever there is a clinical suspicion of recurrent disease that is unconfirmed by the result of the postlymphangiography abdominal radiograph. This is especially important if only scanty amounts of contrast material remain within the retroperitoneal lymph nodes.

## POST-TREATMENT EVALUATION

Plain chest and abdominal radiographs are usually obtained at the following time intervals after the conclusion of therapy (so long as sufficient post-lymphangiographic nodal contrast remains):

- First year: every 2 months
- Second year: every 3 months
- Fourth and fifth years: every 6 months
- After five years: every 12 months

This approach is based on an analysis of the periods during which patients appear to be at the greatest risk of relapsing, as well as on data describing the contributions of imaging to the documentation of tumor recurrence.

The process of restaging a patient with a malignant lymphoma (*i.e.*, re-evaluating the extent of disease following a period of aggressive therapy) is similar to the initial staging process. Presuming that the patient's bone marrow biopsy contains no evidence of tumor, a CT examination of the chest probably should be performed. If abundant retroperitoneal contrast material remains (often not the case), a routine plain abdominal radiograph is sufficient. If there is inadequate residual contrast or, in patients with non-Hodgkin's lymphoma, if the option of obtaining a lymphangiogram was not initially selected, a CT examination of the abdomen should be performed. Depending on the disease in question and the result of the CT examination, a repeat lymphangiogram may be required. In most cases, a repeat lymphangiogram is no more difficult to perform than the initial lymphangiogram.

## COMMENT

As mentioned in the introduction to this chapter, there currently is no clear-cut consensus regarding which imaging modalities should be used in the staging or post-treatment follow-up of patients with newly diagnosed Hodgkin's disease or non-Hodgkin's lymphoma. The recommendations made are based on our personal analysis of the data and seem to work well in our hands. We have attempted to indicate those factors that may make these recommendations inapplicable for radiologists who practice in an environment different from our own. Because of the rapid changes in the field of oncology, it is important to stress that those physicians who deal with patients suffering from lymphoma have an obligation to remain current not only with the new advances in imaging but also with the implications these advances may have on the field of oncologic therapy. Only then can we be certain that the advice we offer will be truly helpful to the patient.

## Bibliography

Anderson KC, Leonard RCF, Canellos GP et al: High dose gallium imaging in lymphoma. Am J Med 75:327–331, 1983

Blackledge G, Best JJK, Crowther D et al: Computed tomography in the staging of patients with Hodgkin's disease: A report on 136 patients. Clin Radiol 31:143–147, 1980

Bydder GM, Yound IR: MR imaging: Clinical use of the inversion recovery sequence. J Comput Assist Tomogr 9:659–675, 1985

Castellino RA: Observations on "reactive (follicular) hyperplasia" as encountered in repeat lymphography in the lymphomas. Cancer 34:2042–2050, 1974

Castellino RA, Blank N, Cassady JR et al: Roentgenologic aspects of Hodgkin's disease. II. Role of routine radiographs in detecting initial relapse. Cancer 31:316–323, 1973

Castellino RA, Bellani FF, Gasparini M et al: Radiographic findings in previously untreated children with non-Hodgkin's lymphoma. Radiology 117:657–663, 1975

Castellino RA, Blank N, Hoppe RT et al: Contributions of chest CT scanning in the initial staging evaluation of newly diagnosed Hodgkin's disease. Radiology 160:603–605, 1986

Castellino RA, Filly R, Blank N: Routine full-lung tomography in the initial staging and treatment planning of patients with Hodgkin's disease and non-Hodgkin's lymphoma. Cancer 38:1130–1136, 1976

Castellino RA, Goffinet DR, Bland N et al: The role of radiography in the staging of non-Hodgkin's lymphoma with laparotomy correlation. Radiology 110:329–338, 1973

Castellino RA, Hoppe RT, Blank N et al: Computed tomography, lymphography, and staging laparotomy: Correlations in initial staging of Hodgkin disease. AJR 143:37–41, 1984

Dooms GC, Hricak H: Radiologic imaging modalities, including magnetic resonance, for evaluating lymph nodes. West J Med 144:49–57, 1986

Fabian CE, Nudelman EJ, Abrams HL: Post-lymphangiogram films as an indication of tumor activity in lymphoma. Invest Radiol 1:386–393, 1966

Glatstein E, Trueblood HW, Enright IP et al: Surgical staging of abdominal involvement in unselected patients with Hodgkin's disease. Radiology 97: 425–432, 1970

Goffinet DR, Castellino RA, Dorfman L et al: Staging laparotomies in unselected patients with non-Hodgkin's lymphomas. Cancer 32:672–681, 1977

Goffinet DR, Warnke R, Dunnick NR et al: Clinical and surgical evaluation of patients with non-Hodgkin's lymphomas. Cancer Treat Rep 61: 981–992, 1977

Johnston GS, Go MT, Benua RS et al: Gallium-67 citrate imaging in Hodgkin's disease: Final report of cooperative group. J Nucl Med 18:692–698, 1977

Kademian M, Wirtanen G: Accuracy of bipedal lymphography in Hodgkin's disease. AJR 129: 1041–1042, 1977

Kadin ME, Glatstein EJ, Dorfman RE: Clinicopathologic studies in 117 untreated patients subjected to laparotomy for the staging of Hodgkin's disease. Cancer 27:1277–1294, 1971

Kaplan HS: Hodgkin's Disease, 2nd ed. Cambridge, MA, Harvard University Press, 1980

Kinmonth JB: Lymphangiography in man. Clin Sci 11:13–20, 1952

Marglin SI, Castellino R: Lymphographic accuracy in 632 consecutive, previously untreated cases of Hodgkin's disease and non-Hodgkin's lymphoma. Radiology 140:351–353, 1981

Marglin SI, Castellino RA: Selection of imaging studies for the initial staging of patients with Hodgkin's disease. Semin Ultrasound CT MR 6:380–393, 1985

Marglin SI, Castellino RA: Selection of imaging studies for newly presenting patients with non-Hodgkin's lymphoma. Semin Ultrasound CT MR 7:2–8, 1986

Parker BR, Blank N, Castellino RA: Lymphographic appearance of benign conditions simulating lymphoma. Radiology 111:267–274, 1974

Wallace S, Jackson L, Schaffer B: Lymphangiograms: Their diagnostic and therapeutic potential. Radiology 76:179–199, 1961

Zornoza J, Ginaldi S: Computed tomography in hepatic lymphoma. Radiology 138:405–410, 1981

# PART SEVEN

# Miscellaneous

# Chapter 46

# Deep Venous Thrombosis

*Robert W. Holden*
*John T. Mail*
*Gary J. Becker*

Lower extremity pain, swelling, tenderness, and erythema suggest the presence of deep venous thrombosis (DVT). However, it is currently accepted that a clinical evaluation by a qualified examiner has only a 50% sensitivity for detecting this condition. The limb with typical signs and symptoms of DVT may have an entirely normal venous system; conversely, thrombus may be present without clinical symptoms or objective physical findings. The accurate diagnosis of DVT is critical, because of both its therapy (extensive and inconvenient hospitalization plus potentially dangerous anticoagulants) and complications (life-threatening pulmonary emboli and deep venous insufficiency).

## RISK FACTORS

The most common risk factors predisposing to DVT include birth control pills, prolonged bedrest, recent surgery, infection, trauma, malignancy, obesity, pregnancy, congestive heart failure, and advanced age. There is increasing evidence of biochemical risk factors (deficiencies in antithrombin III, protein C, protein S), and these should be investigated if DVT develops in a patient under 40 years of age who has none of the traditional risk factors.

## PATHOPHYSIOLOGY OF THROMBOSIS

Virchow's classic triad of mural abnormality, stasis, and hypercoagulability continues to encompass our understanding of venous thrombosis. Despite the frequently used term "thrombophlebitis," the inflammatory component in DVT is minimal or absent; indeed, thrombosis commonly begins without an identifiable anatomic mural lesion. The earliest stage of thrombus formation is the accumulation of platelet and fibrin deposits in the apex of the valve pocket of a vein. The thrombus then extends out of the valve pocket into the main venous channel, producing turbulence that promotes further fibrin formation and red cell entrapment (Fig. 46-1). Continued growth of the thrombus leads to obstructive stasis (Fig. 46-2), with resultant rapid and extensive retrograde and proximal thrombus formation.

The sequence of thrombus growth is important in understanding the patient's presenting symptoms and physical findings, which are determined by the site and degree of venous obstruction (and resulting distal venous distention and edema formation). Occlusive thrombi involving the major draining veins of the upper leg usually produce clinically apparent edema, whereas occlusive thrombi in one of the veins of the lower leg are generally asymptomatic. The pain and tenderness associated with DVT reflect a combination of edema, venous distention, and local inflammation. Thus, extensive DVT can occur without significant symptoms and physical findings if there is no inflammation and if the collateral venous pathways are adequate to compensate for the degree of venous obstruction, thereby avoiding edema formation.

Most DVT originates in the lower leg. Although the large, valveless soleal veins traditionally have been considered the primary site of origin, it is now clear that clot also may originate in any of the many valve pockets of the lower leg. In a recent prospective study of symptomatic patients, venographically documented DVT involved the deep veins of the calf in almost 95% of patients and there was extension of the thrombus into the popliteal and superficial femoral veins in almost 60%. Isotopically labeled fibrinogen studies of postoperative patients suggest that DVT originates in the calf and is initially asymptomatic. Clinically apparent venous and embolic complications of DVT occur when the thrombus extends into the larger deep veins of

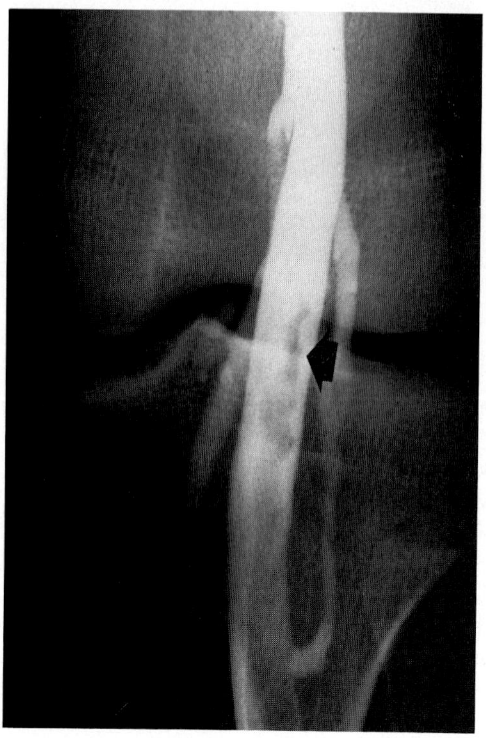

**Figure 46-1.** Contrast venogram demonstrates early nonocclusive thrombus extending from a valve cusp. The arrow points to the thrombus tail, the portion most likely to embolize.

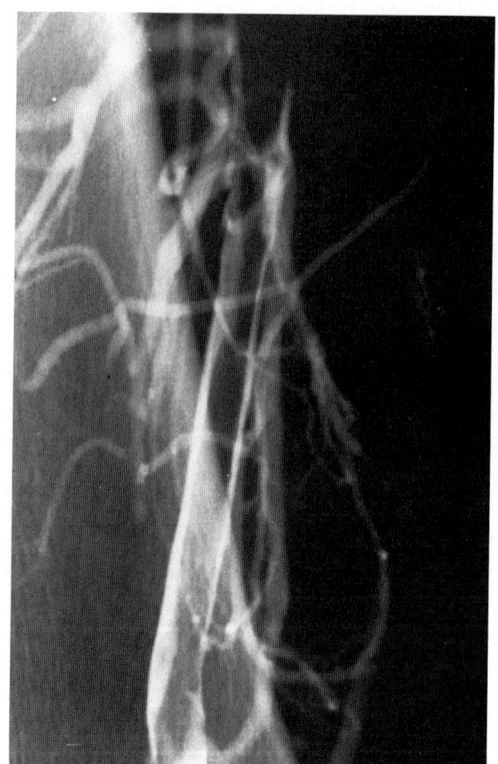

**Figure 46-2.** Contrast venogram demonstrates growth and proximal extension of thrombus, which has resulted in occlusion of the popliteal vein at the adductor hiatus.

the thigh and pelvis, or when the thrombus develops *de novo* in these areas. The risk of symptomatic pulmonary embolism from asymptomatic calf DVT is small.

## COMPLICATIONS

The two major complications of DVT are pulmonary embolism and the chronic postphlebitic syndrome. The two features of DVT that correlate with the life-threatening complication of pulmonary embolism are the degree of venous obstruction and the size of the emboli. The tail of a fresh, nonocclusive thrombus bathed in a flowing venous system is more likely to embolize than the tail of thrombus in a completely occluded vein. Larger emboli arising from more proximal veins of the thigh and pelvis are more likely to cause right-heart outflow obstruction and a fatal result than are smaller emboli arising from more distal veins in the lower extremity.

Occlusive distention of involved veins promotes physiologic fibrinolysis and recanalization of the occlusion that may destroy the valves and produce insufficiency (Fig. 46-3). Valvular incompetence may be manifested by venous hypertension with upright posture, reversal of blood flow through incompetent communicating (perforating) veins, and collateral circulation through the superficial venous system. Increased superficial flow may produce increased pressure in these vessels, with complicating varicose veins and cutaneous ulceration.

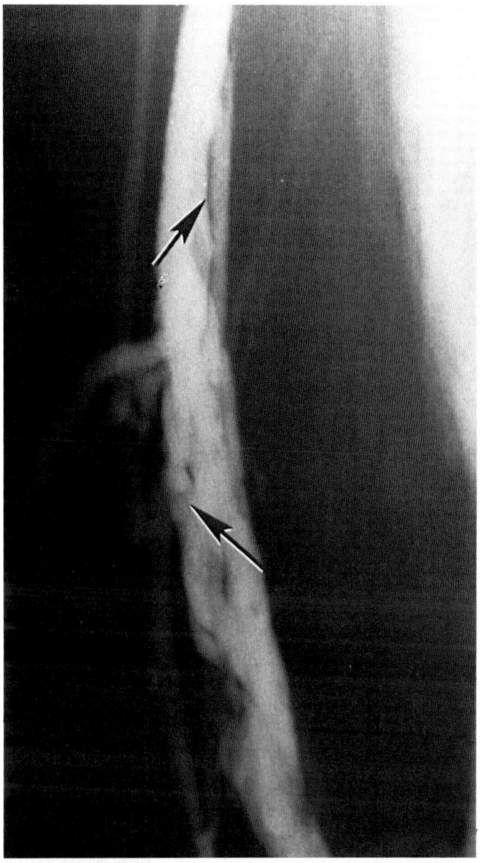

**Figure 46-3.** Contrast venogram shows linear scarring seen *en face* (*arrows*) in a recanalized superficial femoral vein. The accompanying valve destruction results in the chronic postphlebotic syndrome.

## THERAPY

Pulmonary embolism complicates approximately 15% to 25% of cases of untreated DVT. Continuous infusion heparin therapy (partial thromboplastin maintained at twice normal) reduces this risk about fivefold but does not prevent the development of the postphlebitic syndrome. After 7 to 10 days, heparin therapy is switched to secondary prophylaxis with oral Coumadin (warfarin). Relatively low doses of Coumadin have been shown to substantially reduce bleeding complications without increasing the number of recurrent thrombotic episodes. High-dose intravenous thrombolytic therapy is effective in accelerating clearance of thrombus from the deep venous system but carries a significant risk of hemorrhagic complications. At present, there is no convincing evidence that fibrinolytic therapy is any better than heparin anticoagulation for prophylaxis against the postphlebitic syndrome.

## DIAGNOSTIC EVALUATION

### *DIAGNOSTIC MODALITIES*

1. Phlebography
2. Doppler ultrasound

3. Radionuclide studies
   a. Fibrinogen scanning
   b. Radiolabeled platelets
   c. Radionuclide venography
   d. Sulfur colloid scanning
   e. Monoclonal antibodies
4. Impedance plethysmography
5. Computed tomography
6. Magnetic resonance imaging

## Phlebography

Phlebography has been widely accepted as the most definitive test for the diagnosis of DVT and is currently the "gold standard" against which all other examinations are compared. Despite this acceptance and efficacy, numerous complications are associated with this invasive technique. Ionic contrast material is irritating to the venous endothelium; indeed, it can actually induce thrombosis, the very condition one is trying to diagnose. Other well-known complications that result from ionic contrast material include cutaneous ulceration, renal toxicity, shock, and death. The recent introduction of nonionic contrast material should dramatically reduce most of these complications (still insufficient data to determine the nephrotoxic potential of nonionic contrast agents). Although nonionic agents decrease patient discomfort, they have no effect on the radiation exposure and even increase the relatively high cost. The undesirable characteristics make frequent re-examination impractical for following the course of DVT or monitoring the efficacy of treatment with heparin or fibrinolytic agents.

If properly performed and interpreted, phlebography is extremely accurate in documenting the presence or absence of DVT from the foot to the inferior vena cava in all but two anatomic areas. It is inconsistent in demonstrating the profunda femoral vein and rarely provides diagnostic information about the hypogastric and pelvic veins. Venography is the only examination that provides intraluminal visualization of all the veins of the lower extremity, and thus defines an anatomic and physiologic road map of the venous drainage of the limb. It allows assessment of the degree of venous obstruction; the extent of thrombosis; and the presence of collateral flow, chronic venous changes, and varices.

In summary, phlebography is an extremely reliable technique for diagnosing DVT and is now associated with minimal risk if nonionic contrast agents are used. Although some studies have suggested that phlebography should now be used only to confirm DVT in patients with positive noninvasive examinations, the substantial incidence of false-negative noninvasive studies would result in missing cases of DVT that would have been detected by venography.

## Doppler Ultrasound

Doppler ultrasound is the simplest and fastest method of evaluating the veins of the lower extremity. The technique depends on sound pattern recognition of phasic venous velocity signals and the response of flow velocity signals to various limb compression maneuvers. The examination's simplicity and portability make it ideal for low-cost screening of large numbers of patients. However, since the interpretation is subjective and no objective recording is possible, Doppler ultrasound is highly dependent on the examiner's skill, experience, and attention to detail.

One large study showed Doppler ultrasound to have an 84% agreement with phlebographically demonstrated DVT above the knee. The examination is much less specific in the calf, where it is compromised by the multiplicity of veins in both the superficial and deep systems. Most series report a 25% agreement with phlebographically demonstrated DVT below the knee. Doppler ultrasound is very insensitive to nonocclusive thrombus, because the sound flow signals require complete occlusion for alteration. Although Doppler ultrasound is very specific in defining venous valvular insufficiency, intraluminal venous scarring occasionally can produce flow-signal aberrations consistent with acute DVT.

Doppler ultrasound is superior to impedance plethysmography for diagnosing DVT in patients with elevated central venous pressure or arterial insufficiency. It is also of value in the examination of patients whose legs are in traction.

## Radionuclide Studies

### Fibrinogen Scanning

Isotopically labeled fibrinogen is the most sensitive noninvasive examination for the detection of early calf DVT and is the only noninvasive study that can demonstrate nonocclusive DVT in this region. Traditionally, fibrinogen has been labeled with relatively low-energy $^{125}$I. The use of higher energy $^{123}$I permits gamma camera imaging. Fibrinogen scanning has about a 95% correlation with venographically demonstrated acute calf thrombus. Thus, this technique has enabled investigators to determine the prevalence and natural history of DVT as well as to identify risk factors and evaluating prophylactic regimens. A positive examination depends on the incorporation of circulating labeled fibrinogen into a developing or existing thrombus. Incorporated fibrogen is then detected by an increase in surface radioactivity, as measured by a scintillation probe connected to a digital counter display. Asymmetric or segmental areas of increased counts document the presence of DVT.

Fibrinogen scanning is unique in that it can be prospectively administered to a high-risk patient prior to an insult that may result in the development of DVT. Approximately 10% to 20% of these prospective screening examinations show increased counts in the calf region even though the patients have normal venograms. While venography may miss small thrombi in muscular veins, these patients have an extremely low danger of thrombus propagation or pulmonary embolism. False-positive fibrinogren scanning may result from inflammation, infection, hematoma, or minimal hemorrhage accompanying trauma or wound healing.

In the evaluation of an acutely symptomatic limb, a delay of 12 hours is required for the fibrinogen scan to become positive; 48-hour follow-up studies are needed to confidently exclude DVT. False-negative examinations are frequently reported in patients on anticoagulant therapy. Less commonly, false-negative results reflect a chronic thrombus that is not actively incorporating fibrinogen.

The most significant limitation of fibrinogen scanning is the increased background radiation from the trunk, bladder, and femoral vessels that obscures the detection of DVT in the groin or pelvis. Deep venous thrombosis in the proximal iliofemoral region is common following hip surgery and is frequently isolated to the femoral vein near the operative site. Thrombi in this region, which occasionally can arise *de novo,* have a substantial potential for causing large, life-threatening pulmonary emboli. Because of its inability to effectively evaluate the proximal portion of the lower extremity, fibrinogen scanning is often used in combination with impedance plethysmography or Doppler ultrasound of the upper leg.

### Radiolabeled Platelets

Indium-111–labeled platelet scanning has shown encouraging preliminary results for detecting DVT. The radiolabeled platelets are incorporated into propagating thrombus, and the high energy of indium permits imaging of the upper leg and pelvis. Current limitations of this method include the inability to label adequate numbers of platelets and the inconsistency of the isotopic label. Radiolabeled platelet scanning is theoretically superior to fibrinogen scanning, because experimental studies have shown higher thrombus-to-blood ratios for platelets in fresh clots, and pathologic studies have confirmed that platelets are more plentiful than fibrin in the early formative stages of venous thrombosis.

### Radionuclide Venography

Radionuclide venography refers to the gamma camera monitoring of venous injections of isotope to produce flow studies similar to contrast phlebography. Both $^{99m}$Tc-labeled macroaggregated albumin and microspheres have been used. The isotope solution is injected into a dorsal pedal vein; by splitting the dose, both legs can be imaged simultaneously. The isotope solution is nonirritatintg and causes minimal radiation exposure. Radionuclide venography can easily be integrated with conventional perfusion lung scanning; the perfusion lung images are obtained after the flow study. The diagnosis of DVT by radionuclide venography is based on lack of visualization of the deep venous system, segmental nonfilling, collateral veins, and post-transit accumulation of isotope "hot spots." Because the gamma camera is unable to resolve intraluminal filling defects in the flowing mixture of isotope and blood, a thrombus must cause venous occlusion for the diagnosis of DVT to be made (Fig. 46-4).

Radionuclide venography can detect approximately 80% of DVT involving the thigh, pelvis, and inferior vena cava. It is unreliable for demonstrating calf DVT because of the multiplicity of superficial and deep veins in the calf region. In patients with previous documented DVT, the radionuclide venogram is often abnormal because of altered flow due to incomplete recanalization of the previously thrombosed veins. Therefore, radionuclide venography should not be used in such patients to diagnose acute DVT; it can be used to define venous blood flow. Radionuclide venography is an excellent procedure for following the degree of patency of the inferior vena cava following filter placement.

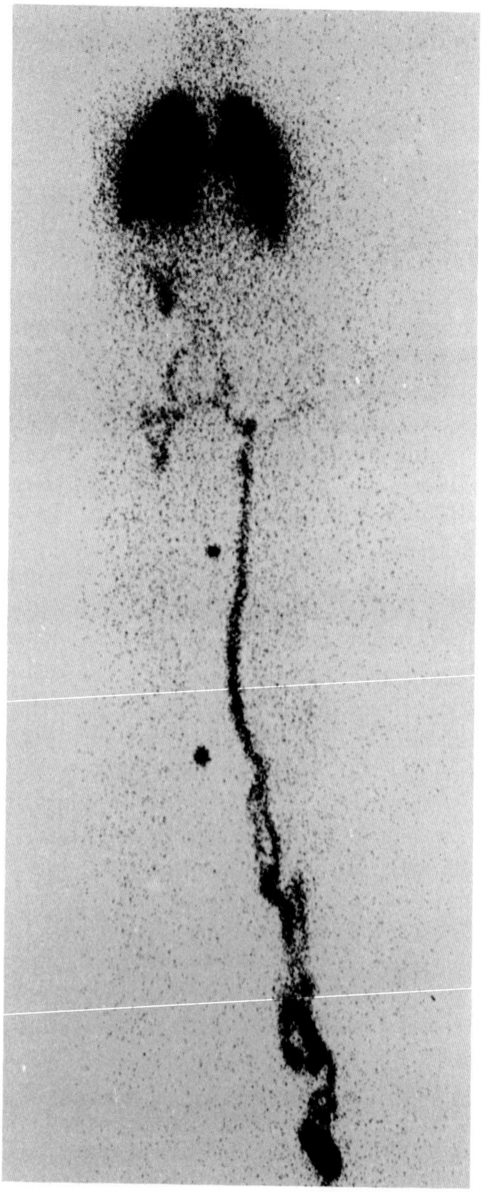

**Figure 46-4.** Radionuclide venogram using $^{99m}$Tc-MAA injected into a dorsal pedal vein. Because of DVT, there is isotope only in the greater saphenous vein (located superficially and medially). Collateral flow in the abdomen reflects obstruction of the iliac vein and inferior vena cava.

### Sulfur Colloid Scanning

Initial studies have reported "hot spots" that represent the active aggregation of $^{99m}$Tc-sulfur colloid on venous thrombi. At present, we have not found this examination to be of value.

### Monoclonal Antibodies

Previous efforts to develop an antibody to fibrin have been complicated by cross-reactivity to fibrinogen. Recently, however, a murine monoclonal antibody (Mab) has been developed that is reactive with human fibrin but has no cross-reactivity to fibrinogen. Previous experience with Mab radioimmunoimaging of tumors has shown that the target substrate may be very small (pico–nanogram range). In DVT, a far greater amount (milligrams) of fibrin is present and permits Mab detection. Early experimental work suggests that an interval of 24 to 48 hours is required for Mab antifibrin studies to be diagnostic; however, some studies have been positive in as little as 3 hours. In very limited experience, we have found antifibrin Mab to be diagnostic in establishing the presence of pulmonary emboli (human clot) in a rabbit pulmonary embolism model.

Murine monoclonal antibodies are composed of antigenic foreign protein (currently, mouse hybridoma clone cultures). Therefore, the injection of even small amounts of the protein may sensitize the host so that future repeat injections of the diagnostic agent may result in severe and perhaps life-threatening hypersensitivity reactions.

## Impedance Plethysmography

Occlusive cuff impedance plethysmography (IPG) is the most sensitive noninvasive examination for detecting occlusive DVT in the popliteal, femoral, and iliac veins. However, it is relatively insensitive for detecting DVT in the calf. The principle of this examination is based on the observation that the variation in calf blood volume produced by inflation and deflation of a pneumatic thigh cuff results in changes in electrical resistance (impedance). Because blood is a good conductor of electricity, the impedance to an electrical current (measured between two electrodes wrapped around the calf) decreases as the volume of blood increases. A patient with proximal obstructive DVT has an increased calf blood volume and thus decreased electrical impedance. At present, IPG is designed to quantitate both the capacity of the venous system to distend in response to proximal temporary venous obstruction (pneumatic cuff) and the rate of venous outflow following rapid release of the cuff. Three technical modifications have substantially improved the sensitivity and specificity of the examination: (1) 2-minute cuff insufflation ensures maximal venous filling; (2) confirmation of an abnormal result by repetitive testing avoids technical false positives; (3) sequential examinations over a 5- to 10-day period allow the disease process to extend into the proximal veins and become occlusive, thereby avoiding false-negative examinations that might otherwise occur with nonocclusive thrombus. Impedance plethysmography is simple and easily performed in normal limbs. However, the technique is impossible to use in patients with flexion contractures, plaster casts, traction apparatus, or certain congenital deformities. The examination is extremely operator dependent and should be performed by experienced technicians.

Impedance plethysmography can detect proximal occlusive thrombi that increase the venous capacitance of the calf. However, DVT with nonocclusive thrombi may lead to false-negative examinations. Impedance plethysmography fails to detect most calf vein thrombi, because DVT in this location does not significantly alter calf venous volume due to the multiplicity of veins. Proximal venous thrombi with well-developed collaterals also may be missed by IPG. False-positive examinations usually are caused by the inability of IPG to differentiate between thrombotic and nonthrombotic obstruction to venous outflow. In addition, inadequate arterial inflow secondary to atherosclerotic disease also may decrease occlusive venous volume and thereby produce a false-positive result. Other conditions known to cause false-positive IPG examiantions include pelvic hematoma with venous compression, Baker's cyst, congestive heart failure with raised central venous pressure and impaired venous outflow, previous DVT with inadequate collateral drainage, inadequate calf muscle relaxation, and improper patient positioning.

A recent prospective study of serial IPGs on outpatients with clinically suspected DVT reported a 92% agreement with confirmatory phlebography performed at the time of the established abnormal IPG. Of all abnormal studies, 85%, 9%, 4%, and 2% became abnormal on days 1, 2, 5, and 10, respectively. This study demonstrates that a positive IPG generally requires proximal extension of DVT and venous occlusion. Of those patients with an abnormal IPG, 89% had proximal thrombi with or without calf DVT; only 11% had calf thrombi alone. In ambulatory outpatients who develop DVT, the vast majority have initial calf disease, which then extends into the proximal veins. Because of the inability of IPG to detect early calf involvement, serial IPG examinations or radio-labeled fibrinogen scanning is required to noninvasively establish the diagnosis of calf DVT prior to proximal extension. At present, there is considerable debate about the therapy of DVT that is confined to the calf. The study described previously suggests a low incidence of clinically manifest pulmonary emboli from early calf DVT, thus seeming to justify the reservation of anticoagulation for patients with more advanced proximal disease. The study did not address the anticipated increase in the postphlebitic syndrome resulting from the proximal progression and late initiation of anticoagulant therapy.

### Computed Tomography

Although there has been no report of a prospective study of the efficacy of computed tomography (CT) in the diagnosis of DVT, numerous case reports have demonstrated the value of this modality in venous disease of the chest, abdomen, and pelvis. Computed tomographic findings of venous thrombosis include enlargement of a thrombosed vein, an intraluminal filling defect, peripheral ringlike contrast enhancement (doughnut sign), and collateral venous channels. Although direct intravenous injection of contrast material distal to the area of DVT provides optimal visualization, peripheral intravenous contrast injection may permit adequate imaging. Computed tomography provides a three-dimensional image of an affected vein and surrounding structures, unlike venography, which shows luminal abnormalities but can only provide indirect information about the venous wall and perivascular spaces. Contrast-enhanced CT can demonstrate extrinsic masses compressing veins, and thus this modality has been advocated for the initial evaluation of patients with superior vena cava obstruction. Numerous studies have reported CT detection of thrombi in intra-abdominal veins (renal, ovarian, superior mesenteric, splenic, and portal veins) (Fig. 46-5).

### Magnetic Resonance Imaging

Unlike rapidly flowing arterial blood, which appears as a signal void (black) on spin-echo magnetic resonance images, slower flowing venous blood may produce a signal and appear white. Thus, it is currently difficult on magnetic resonance imaging (MRI) to differentiate the signal of slowly flowing blood from that of intraluminal thrombus. The simplest method to determine the cause of an intraluminal signal is to repeat the scan with increased repetition time. This results in an increased interval that allows time-of-flight effect to produce a signal void within an unobstructed vessel. More sophisticated techniques involve the detection of flow-dependent

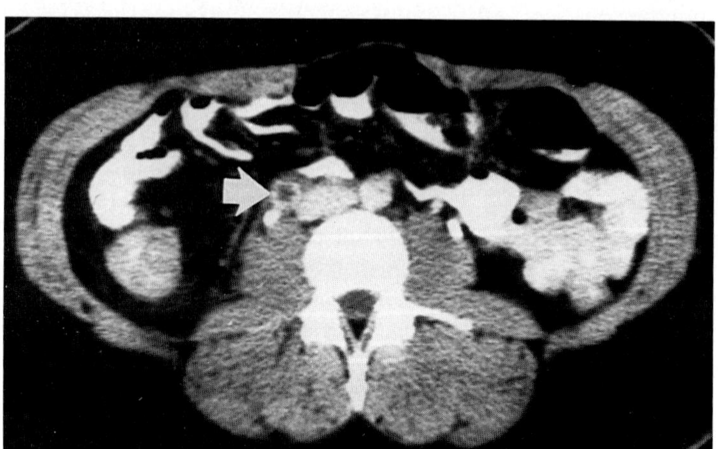

**Figure 46-5.** CT examination shows the typical "doughnut sign" (*arrow*) of acute thrombophlebitis in the right ovarian vein.

changes of phase between precessing protons. For example, if a second-echo image demonstrates even-echo rephasing (*i.e.*, an absolute signal intensity increase), the intraluminal signal represents flowing blood. Thrombus produces an intravascular signal that is slightly less intense in absolute magnitude on second-echo images. Other phase-dependent techniques include specialized pulse sequences, reconstruction methods, and image subtraction to selectively enhance motion on the final image.

Currently, MRI is in its infancy with respect to intravascular imaging. Nevertheless, the potential of this modality to quantitate flow seems far more promising than other diagnostic techniques. In the future, an improved ability to image flow with computer assistance should provide MRI "flow casts" of the extremities that can clearly demonstrate nonobstructive thrombi, unlike other noninvasive modalities that require complete venous obstruction to confidently detect DVT. Indeed, MRI may evantually eliminate the need for invasive contrast studies in the diagnosis of DVT. The major limitations of MRI are the availability of the equipment and the high cost of the examination. However, the noninvasive character of MRI makes it the ideal modality for serial examinations and clinical investigation of DVT.

## Bibliography

Bernstein EF (ed): Noninvasive Diagnostic Techniques in Vascular Disease, 3rd ed. St Louis, CV Mosby, 1985

Bettman MA, Paulin S: Leg phlebography: The incidence, nature and modification of undesirable side effects. Radiology 122:101–104, 1977

Canley JJ, Canos AJ, Sull WJ: The diagnosis of deep venous thrombosis. Arch Surg 111:34–36, 1976

Engel IA, Auh YH, Rubenstein WA et al: CT diagnosis of mediastinal and thoracic inlet venous obstruction. AJR 141:521–526, 1983

Havig O: Deep vein thrombosis and pulmonary embolism: An autopsy study with multiple regression analysis of possible risk factors. Acta Chir Scand (Suppl) 478:1–120, 1977

Holden RW, Becker GJ, Kriepke DL et al: Pathophysiology of thrombosis and fibrinolysis. Semin Intervent Radiol 2:315–320, 1985

Holden RW, Klatte EC, Park HM et al: Efficacy of noninvasive modalities for diagnosis of thrombophlebitis. Radiology 141:63–66, 1981

Holden RW, Wass JL: Phlebography in the diagnosis of peripheral venous disease. In Bang NU, Glover JL, Holden RW, Triplett DA (eds): Thrombosis and Atherosclerosis, pp 43–56. Chicago, Year Book Medical Publishers, 1982

Hricak H, Amparo E, Fisher MR et al: Abdominal venous system: Assessment using MR Radiology 156:415–422, 1985

Huisman MV, Buller HR, ten Cate JW et al: Serial impedance plethysmography for suspected deep venous thrombosis in outpatients. N Engl J Med 314:823–828, 1986

Hull R, Delmore T, Genton E et al: Warfarin sodium versus low-dose heparin in the long-term treatment of venous thrombosis. N Engl J Med 301: 855–858, 1979

Hull R, Hirsh J, Sackett DL et al: Clinical validity of a negative venogram in patients with clinically suspected venous thrombosis. Circulation 3: 622–625, 1981

Hull R, Hirsh J, Sackett DL et al: Cost effectiveness of clinical diagnosis, venography and noninvasive testing in patients with symptomatic deep-vein thrombosis. N Engl J Med 304:1561–1567, 1981

Hull R, Hirsh J, Sackett DL et al: Replacement of venography in suspected venous thrombosis by impedance plethysmography and 125 I-fibrinogen leg scanning. Ann Int Med 94:12–15, 1981

Hull R, Taylor DW, Hirsh J et al: Impedance plethysmography: The relationship between venous filling and sensitivity and specificity for proximal vein thrombosis. Circulation 58:898–902, 1978

Kakkar VV, Howe, CT, Flanc C et al: Natural history of postoperative deep-vein thrombosis. Lancet 2:230–233, 1969

Kistner RL, Ball JJ, Nordyke RA et al: Incidence of pulmonary embolism in the course of thrombophlebitis of the lower extremities. Am J Surg 124: 169–76, 1972

Moser KM, LeMoine JR: Is embolic risk conditioned by location of deep venous thrombosis? Ann Intern Med 94:439–444, 1981

O'Donnell TF, Jr, Abbott WM, Athanasoulis CA et al: Diagnosis of deep venous thrombosis in the outpatient by venography. Surg Gynecol Obstet 150:69–74, 1980

Rabinov K, Paulin S: Roentgen diagnosis of venous

thrombosis in the leg. Arch Surg 104:134–144, 1972

Ramchandani P, Soulen RL, Fedullo LM et al: Deep vein thrombosis: Significant limitations of noninvasive tests. Radiology 156:47–49, 1985

Rosebrough SF, Kudryk B, Grossman ZD et al: Radioimmunoimaging of venous thrombi using iodine-131 monoclonal antibody. Radiology 156: 515–517, 1985

Salzman EW: Venous thrombosis made easy. N Engl J Med 314:847–848, 1986

Wheeler HB, Pearson D, O'Connell D et al: Impedance phlebography. Arch Surg 104:164–169, 1972

## DEEP VENOUS THROMBOSIS

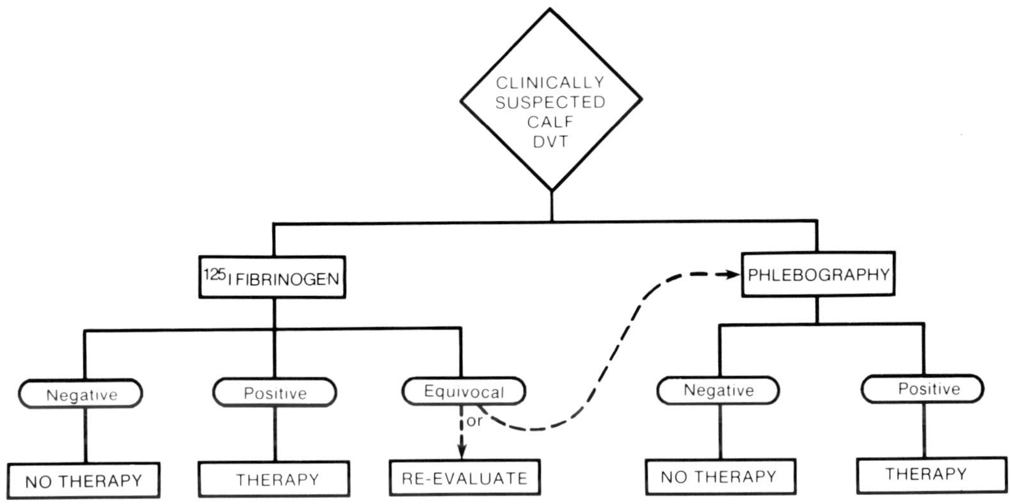


## DEEP VENOUS THROMBOSIS

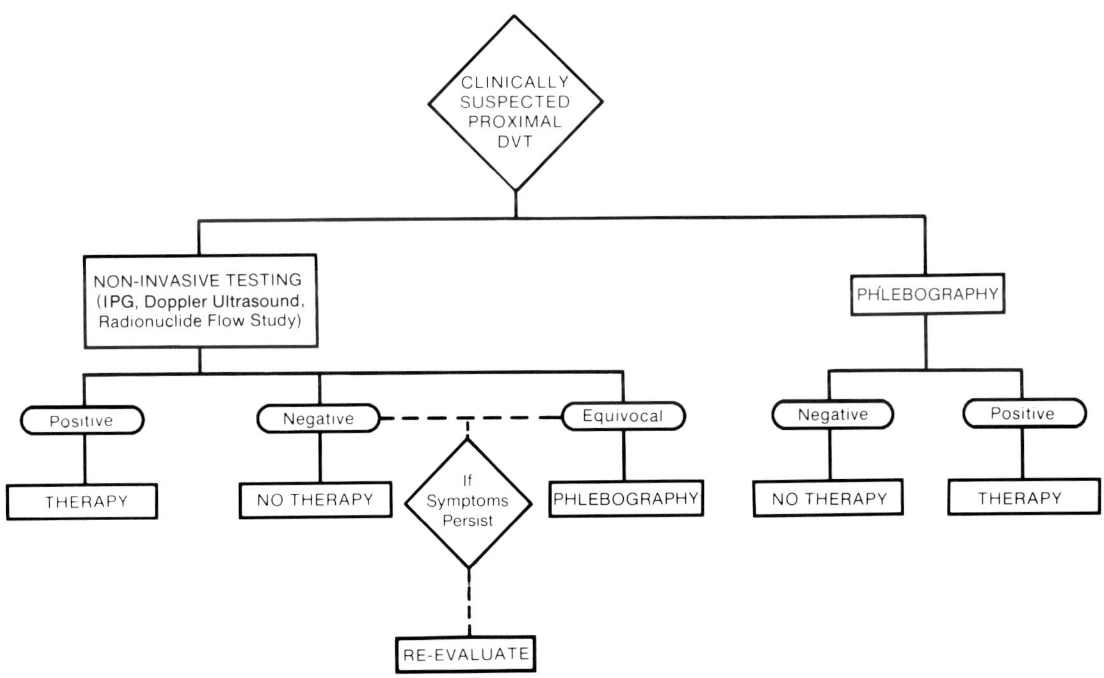

# Chapter 47

# Soft-Tissue Tumors of the Extremity

*Marvin M. Lindell, Jr.*
*Bao-shan Jing*

The radiologic imaging procedures employed for the evaluation and staging of soft-tissue tumors of the extremity are designed to ascertain the location, nature, and extent of disease. This permits the selection of appropriate therapy to attempt complete eradication of the tumor while maintaining maximum function. The advent of ultrasound, computed tomography (CT), and magnetic resonance imaging (MRI) has permitted the identification of tumors too small to be detected by conventional radiography. In addition to earlier diagnosis, these newer modalities also permit improved staging of extremity lesions as well as earlier detection of metastases.

The most common soft-tissue tumors of the extremities are lipoma, melanoma, liposarcoma, malignant fibrous histiocytoma, clear cell sarcoma, and epithelioid sarcoma. Additional malignant lesions include metastases and various types of soft-tissue sarcoma (Ewing's sarcoma, osteosarcoma, chondrosarcoma, fibrosarcoma, rhabdomyosarcoma, alveolar soft-parts sarcoma). Nontumoral conditions include Baker's cysts, rheumatoid cysts, joint effusions, pigmented villonodular synovitis, vascular neoplasms, aneurysms, and abscesses.

## DIAGNOSTIC EVALUATION

### *DIAGNOSTIC MODALITIES*

1. Conventional radiography and tomography
2. Soft-tissue radiography and xeroradiography
3. Ultrasound
4. Computed tomography
5. Magnetic resonance imaging
6. Angiography
7. Lymphangiography
8. Percutaneous needle biopsy

### Chest Radiography and Tomography

Chest radiography and whole-lung tomography have traditionally been routine procedures in the search for lung metastases in the patient suspected of having a soft-tissue malignancy. The frequency of pulmonary metastases varies widely depending on the size and nature of the primary tumor and its propensity to metastasize. For example, 50% of alveolar soft-parts sarcomas and more than 60% of synovial sarcomas metastasize to the lung, whereas pulmonary metastases occur in less than 0.5% of patients with desmoplastic sarcoma.

Whole-lung tomography is usually performed with the patient standing and generally requires high kilovoltage (125 kVp–150 kVp) technique. The primary examination consists of 1-cm sections that include the entire lungs from posterior to anterior ribs. Thinner cuts (0.3 cm–0.5 cm) may be obtained as required. A thoracoabdominal or diaphragm radiograph also is obtained to better visualize the lung bases.

At present, CT is considered the imaging modality of choice in the search for pulmonary metastases from a suspected soft-tissue malignancy. Scans at 1-cm intervals are made throughout the thorax; if necessary, thinner sections are obtained. Although the degree of specificity is not yet clear, the sensitivity rates of CT, whole-lung tomography, and chest radiography for detecting pulmonary metastases are about 90%, 60%, and 45% respectively.

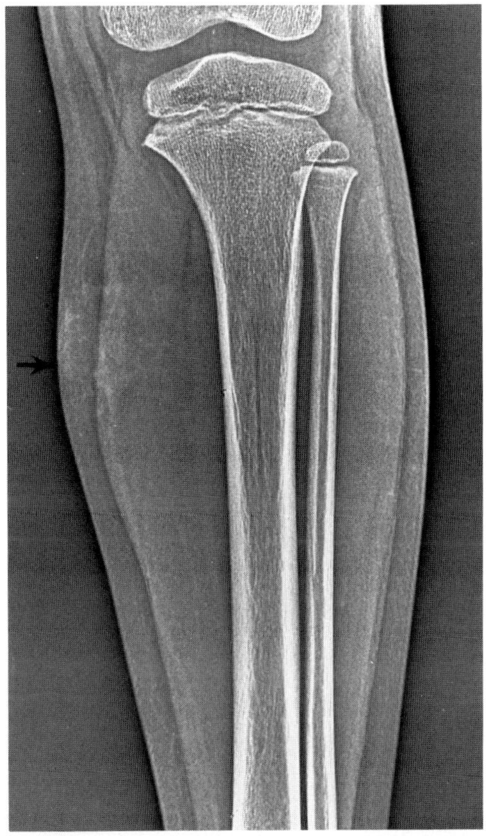

**Figure 47-1.** Soft-tissue hemangioma. Frontal xeroradiograph of the leg shows amorphous calcification (*arrow*) within the mass.

## Soft-Tissue Radiography and Xeroradiography

Soft-tissue tumors containing fat, air, or calcification, or those that distort the fascial fat planes, may be well demonstrated on soft-tissue radiographs and/or xeroradiographs (Fig. 47-1). Pigmented villonodular synovitis, rheumatoid cysts, Baker's cysts, aneurysms, and synovial sarcomas are most frequently situated adjacent to large joints, especially the knee (Fig. 47-2). The presence of low-density areas of fat within a tumor suggests a lipoma or liposarcoma (Fig. 47-3). Nonspecific calcifications are seen in synovial sarcomas (30%), liposarcomas (15%), and malignant fibrous histiocytomas (10%–15%). Specific types of calcification in soft-tissue sarcomas include ringlet calcifications in chondrosarcoma and amorphous calcifications in soft-tissue osteosarcomas. However, the majority of soft-tissue neoplasms present similar radiographic features regardless of histology, and distinguishing between malignant and benign tumors is often impossible.

Because of its inherent property of edge-enhancement, xeroradiography shows the fascial planes and borders of a tumor to better advantage. Benign or slow-growing neoplasms, cysts, and aneurysms usually have a sharp, well-defined outline, while malignant or rapidly progressing tumors and abscesses are poorly defined because of loss of the fascial-fat planes (Fig. 47-4). Xeroradiography is superior to soft-tissue radiography for demonstrating calcification or fat within a tumor, as well as the periosteal reaction and bone destruction that may indicate the extent and nature of disease (Fig. 47-5).

## Ultrasound

Ultrasound is a rapid and highly accurate method for demonstrating the exact size and shape of a soft-tissue neoplasm of the extremity.

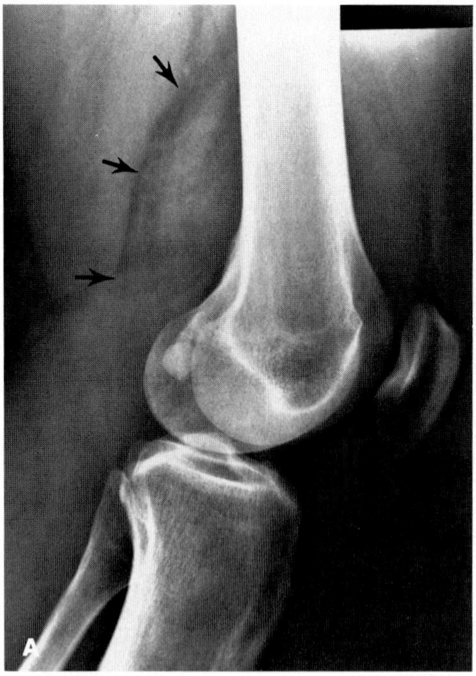

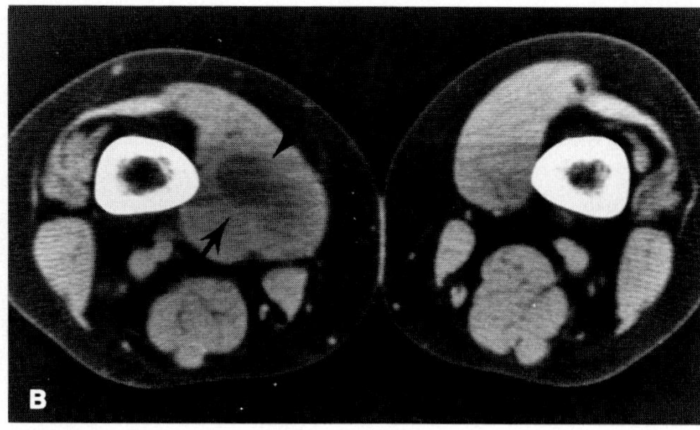

**Figure 47-2.** Synovial sarcoma. **(A)** Lateral radiograph of the knee shows the mass (*arrows*) in the posterior aspect of the distal thigh. **(B)** CT scan shows the low-attenuation mass (*arrows*).

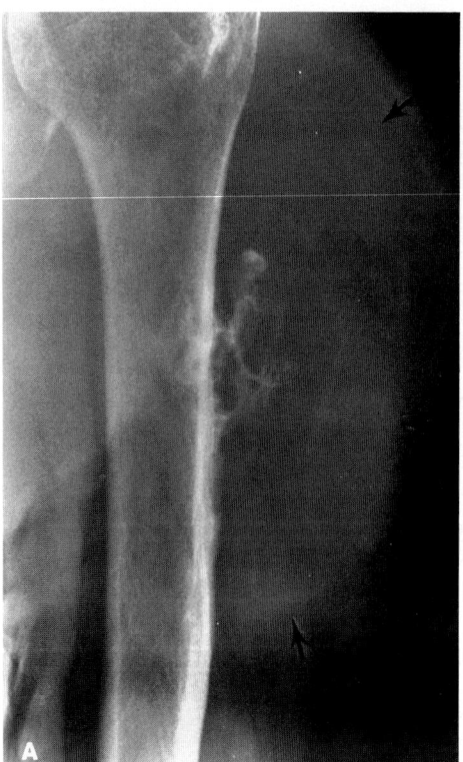

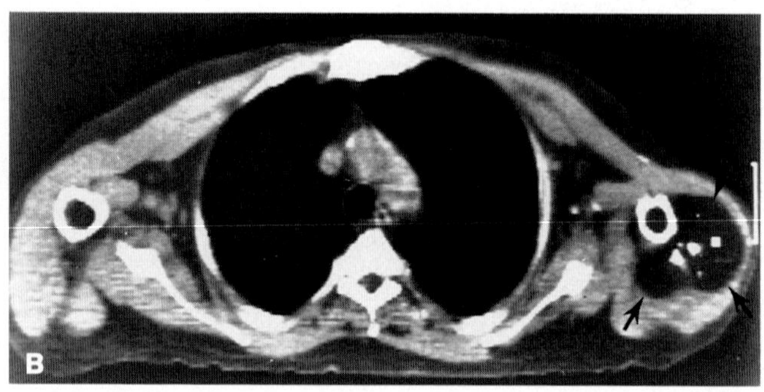

**Figure 47-3.** Lipoma. **(A)** Frontal radiograph of the proximal humerus shows a mass containing calcification and fat (*arrows*). **(B)** CT scan shows the low density of the lipoma (*arrows*). Note the calcification within the mass.

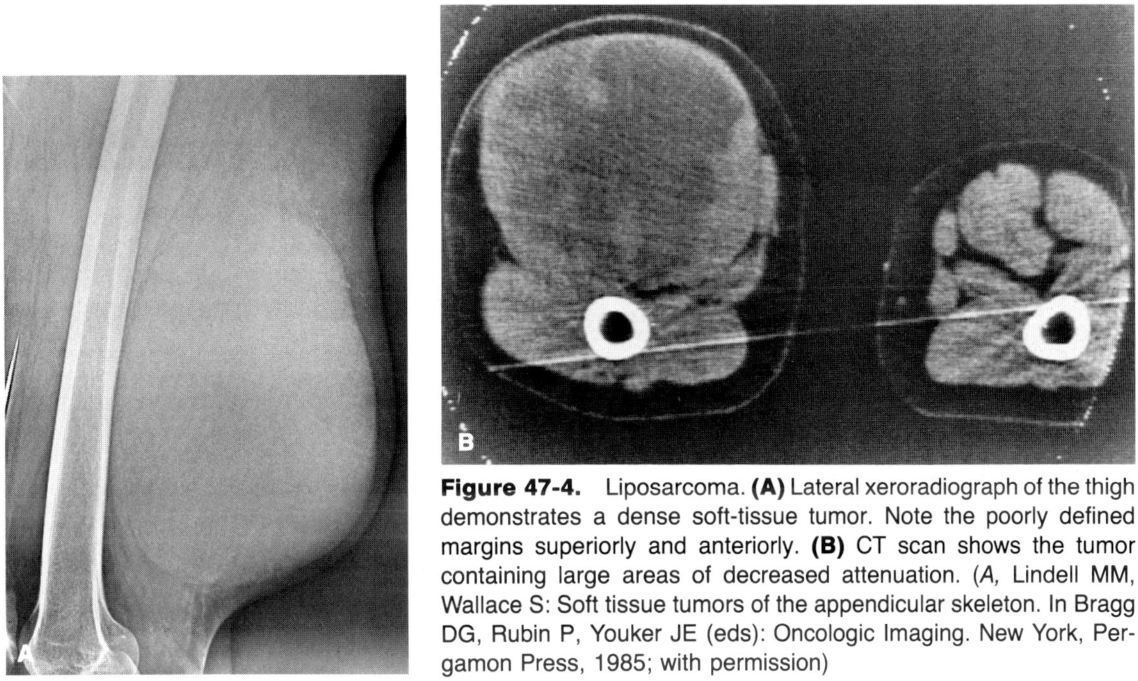

**Figure 47-4.** Liposarcoma. **(A)** Lateral xeroradiograph of the thigh demonstrates a dense soft-tissue tumor. Note the poorly defined margins superiorly and anteriorly. **(B)** CT scan shows the tumor containing large areas of decreased attenuation. (*A,* Lindell MM, Wallace S: Soft tissue tumors of the appendicular skeleton. In Bragg DG, Rubin P, Youker JE (eds): Oncologic Imaging. New York, Pergamon Press, 1985; with permission)

The differentiation among cystic, solid, and complex masses can usually be made, although benign and malignant tumors may have identical sonographic appearances (Fig. 47-6). An inability to clearly define acoustic interfaces, even with scanning in multiple planes, usually indicates invasion of adjacent fascial planes. Radiation or surgical fields can be quickly and accurately mapped on the patient's skin at the time of the ultrasound examination. This is an important consideration in follow-up examinations and for detection of recurrences in patients with soft-tissue tumors of the extremities treated by surgery, radiation therapy, or chemotherapy (Fig. 47-7*A, B*). Ultrasound guidance of percutaneous biopsies is very accurate and is being increasingly used, especially intraoperatively.

Soft-tissue lesions of the extremities can be studied by both static B-mode and real-time scanning, using 7.5 MHz to 10 MHz internally focused transducers. Real-time scanning shows better detail and is more accurate in detecting small soft-tissue lesions; static B-mode scans are more useful for follow-up evaluation after treatment. Multiple sections are made through the lesion at intervals of 0.5 cm to 1 cm. The electronic calipers of the sonographic unit can define the exact measurements of the length, width, and depth of the tumor.

## Computed Tomography

Computed tomography is a very useful imaging procedure for evaluating soft-tissue tumors of the extremity. Its ability to discriminate small differences in density permits recognition of anatomic structures as well as alterations of intrinsic architecture. The size and configuration of a soft-tissue tumor can be estimated with fairly high accuracy by the latest generation machines. Smaller lesions may escape detection because of volume averaging. Computed tomography can demonstrate involvement of adjacent bones and is the most accurate modality for detecting tumor extension into the vascular bundle (Fig. 47-7*C, D*). Drip infusion or bolus injection of contrast material into a vein distal to the lesion can clearly demonstrate the vascular anatomy and any enhancement of the tumor. At times, however, intravenous contrast may render a neoplasm isodense, thereby obscuring the lesion.

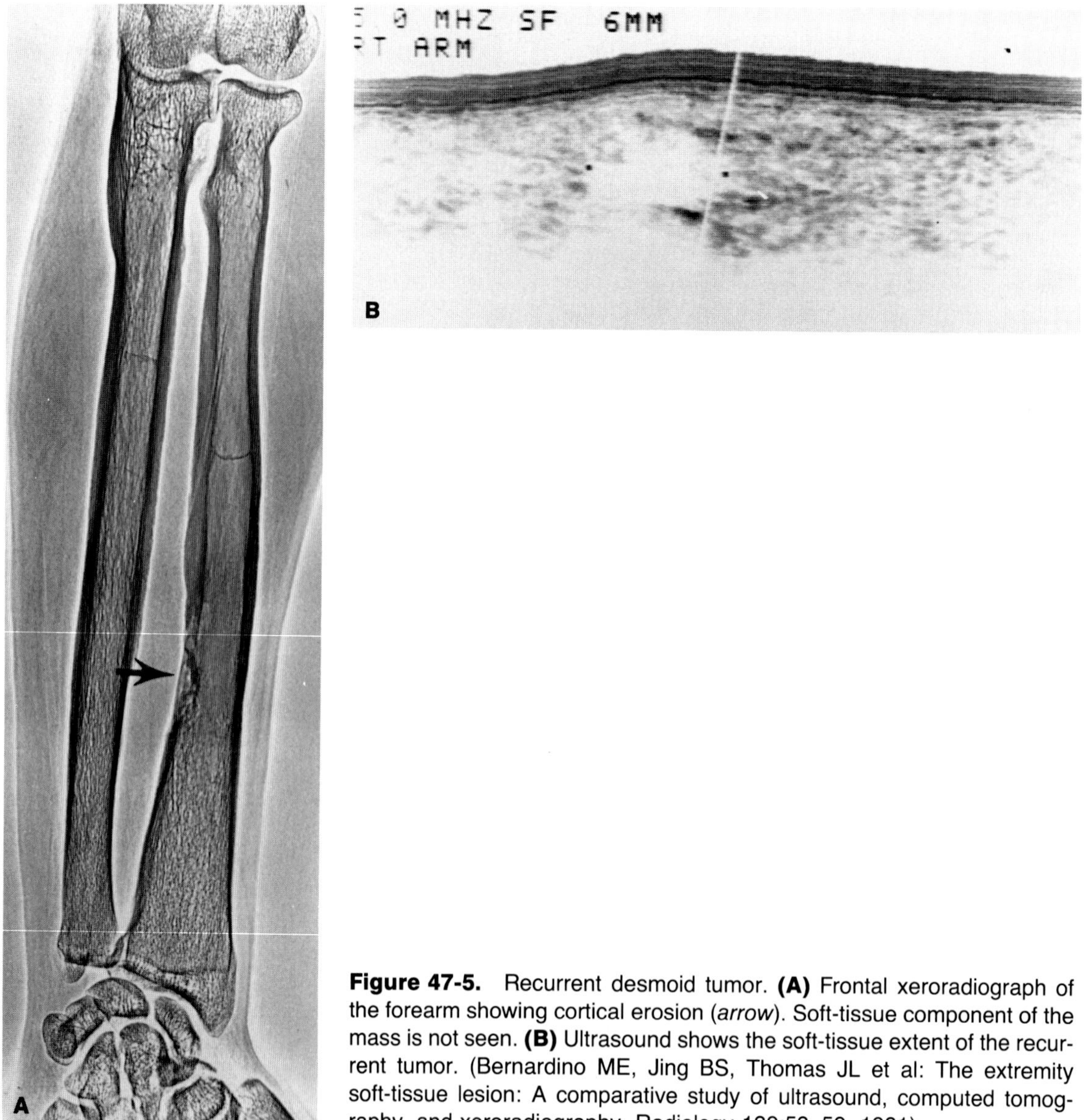


**Figure 47-5.** Recurrent desmoid tumor. **(A)** Frontal xeroradiograph of the forearm showing cortical erosion (*arrow*). Soft-tissue component of the mass is not seen. **(B)** Ultrasound shows the soft-tissue extent of the recurrent tumor. (Bernardino ME, Jing BS, Thomas JL et al: The extremity soft-tissue lesion: A comparative study of ultrasound, computed tomography, and xeroradiography. Radiology 139:53–59, 1981)

The presence of fat, air, or calcium within a tumor may suggest its histologic diagnosis (See Fig. 47-3*B*). Lipomas almost always appear as well-circumscribed masses of low attentuation (Fig. 47-8), whereas liposarcomas present a nonspecific pattern ranging from well to poorly defined margins and have varying attenuation values depending on tissue content (see Fig. 47-4*B*). When sufficient fat is present, the very low attenuation is easily detectable. However, it may be impossible to differentiate a fatty tumor from tissue necrosis.

For comparative purposes, CT scans should include both extremities. Sections are obtained at 8-mm to 10-mm levels, using a 10-mm or 8-mm collimator. Lesions as small as 1 mm to 3 mm may be detected by using thin slices and tight collimation. The use of overlapping sections provides even greater resolution.

Computed tomography has also proven to

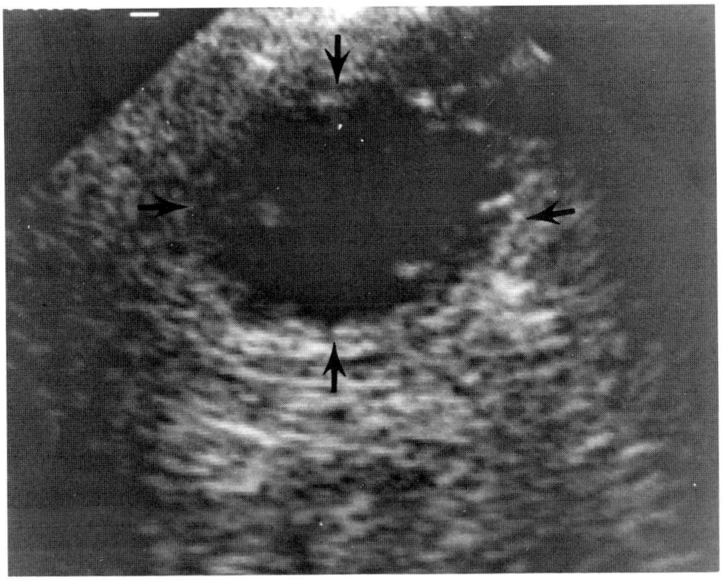

**Figure 47-6.** Abscess. Real-time ultrasound shows a large cystic lesion of the thigh (*arrows*) containing internal echoes.

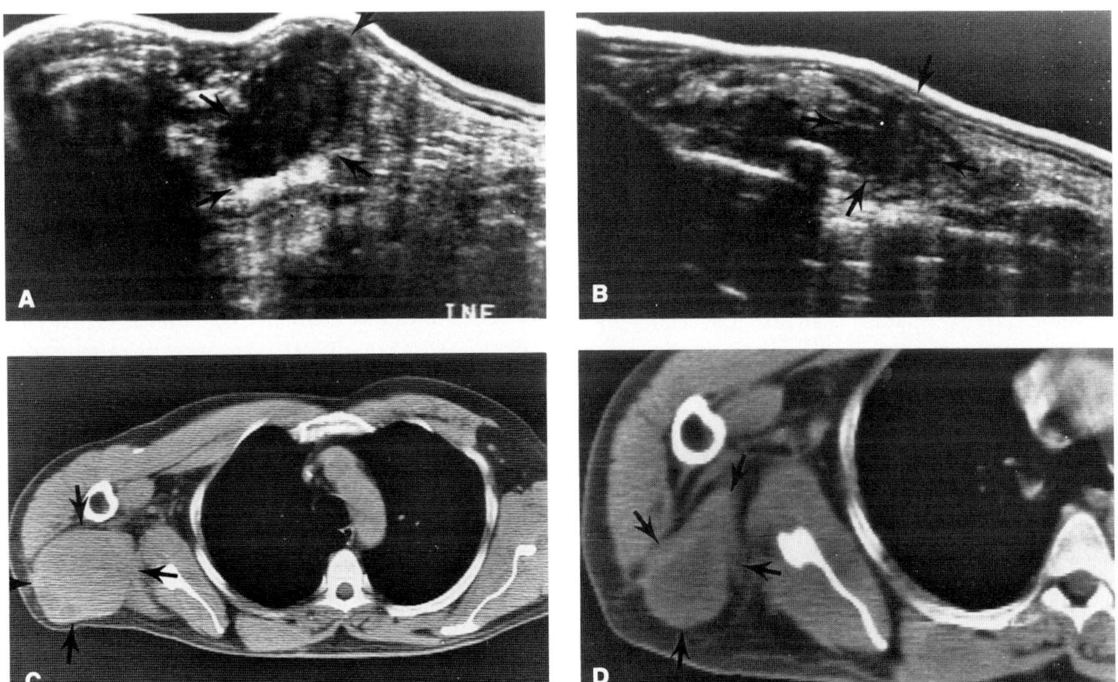


**Figure 47-7.** Malignant fibrous histiocytoma. **(A)** Longitudinal static ultrasound of the shoulder shows the soft-tissue tumor (*arrows*). **(B)** Repeat examination 3 months later shows regression of the tumor (*arrows*) following chemotherapy. **(C)** CT scan prior to therapy shows the soft-tissue mass (*arrows*). **(D)** Repeat CT scan 3 months later shows regression of the tumor (*arrows*) following chemotherapy.

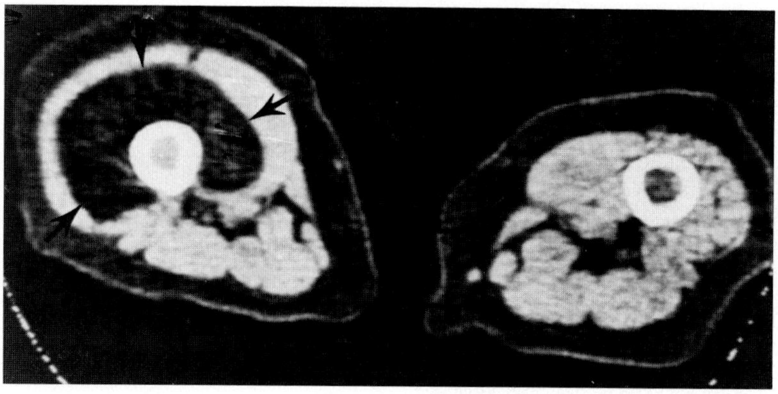

**Figure 47-8.** Lipoma. CT scan shows the low-attenuation mass (*arrows*) of the thigh.

be highly accurate in localizing lesions for percutaneous needle biopsy, especially those not demonstrated by other imaging procedures.

Although CT may provide important diagnostic information, at present ultrasound remains the best single modality for evaluating both benign and malignant soft-tissue lesions of the extremity.

## Magnetic Resonance Imaging

Magnetic resonance imaging produces high-quality tomographic images similar to CT but with a unique set of parameters for tissue characterization. It utilizes no ionizing radiation and does not require opaque contrast material. Unlike CT, imaging planes are not limited to the axial section. Any required plane can be imaged and individual planes can be extracted from the computer memory without repeating the scanning process. The entire three-dimensional volume of the mass may be imaged. In addition, MRI data obtained from several nuclei may provide more specific metabolic information.

Magnetic resonance imaging demonstrates excellent detail of the soft tissues of an extremity because it includes the fascial-fat planes about muscle groups. The signal intensity of normal muscle is intermediate between the intensities of fat and cortical bone. The high-intensity signal of the osseous marrow cavity and the low signal of cortical bone provide accurate evaluation of cortical and/or marrow cavity invasion by tumor or other pathologic processes. Because of the low signal intensity of flowing blood, MRI usually demonstrates any compromise or displacement of the vascular bundle.

Coronal and transaxial images generated with T1-weighted spin-echo (SE) pulse sequences with short repetition times (TR) and short echo times (TE) have been reported to show excellent contrast between fat (high signal intensity), muscle (intermediate signal), and cortical bone (low signal). Both T1- and T2-weighted images should be obtained for optimal display of the overall anatomy and specific detail of the soft-tissue lesion, respectively.

Multiplanar MRI may prove to be more accurate than CT and ultrasound for the evaluation of soft-tissue lesions of the extremity, as well as for assessment of cortical bone and marrow cavity disease (Fig. 47-9). At present, the major disadvantages of this modality include the high initial cost and operating expense of the equipment, the higher cost to the patient, and the longer time required to obtain MR images.

## Angiography

Although angiography (arteriography and venography) was previously the major modality for demonstrating the extent, nature, and operability of soft-tissue tumors, at present it plays a secondary role when less invasive procedures provide equivocal results. Angiography can determine the extent of the mass and its relation to major vessels and septal and fascial planes; delineate the nature of a tumor by analysis of

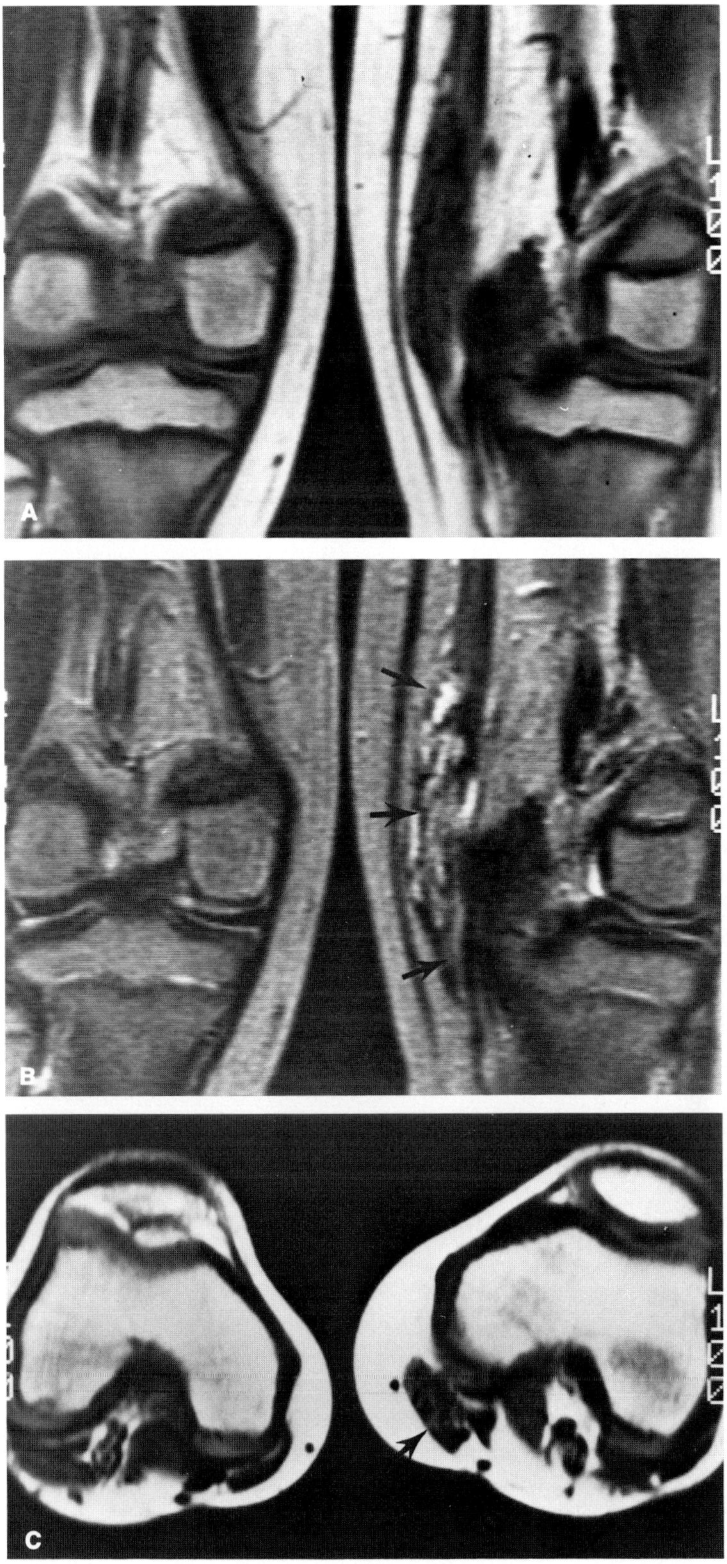

**Figure 47-9.** Hemangioma. **(A)** T1-weighted coronal MRI of the distal thigh (TR, 800 msec; TE, 25 msec) shows the general anatomy. **(B)** T2-weighted image (TR, 2000 msec; TE, 80 msec) shows the hemangioma (*arrows*) that could not be demonstrated by any other imaging procedure. **(C)** Transaxial T1-weighted image (TR, 800 msec; TE, 25 msec) shows the tumor (*arrow*) and the asymmetry of soft tissues.

neoplastic vascularity; and provide therapeutic alternatives such as tumor embolization, occlusive therapy, and transcatheter infusion of chemotherapeutic agents.

There are no pathognomonic criteria for the angiographic diagnosis of malignant neoplasms. Neovascularity (bizarre conglomerate of vessels with pooling of contrast material) and vascular encasement (abrupt and irregular change in caliber) are the most consistent and reliable findings of malignancy. However, a similar appearance of wildly distorted vascularity can be seen with benign conditions such as angiomatous lesions and myositis ossificans (Fig. 47-10). Hypervascular masses as small as 5 mm may be detectable. However, hypovascular lesions must be at least 2 cm in diameter to cause sufficient distortion and displacement of adjacent major vessels to be detected.

Angiography can accurately demonstrate the extent of disease if residual or recurrent tumor is suspected. The degree of vascularity of the recurrence is usually similar to that of the primary lesion. At least 2 to 3 months should elapse prior to postoperative angiography, because apparent tumor staining and neovascularity may be the result of surgery. Angiography also can show the presence of intravascular extension of tumor.

An extremely promising use of angiography in the treatment of soft-tissue neoplasms is intra-arterial chemotherapy (Fig. 47-11). Whenever possible, this is followed by surgical resection in an attempt to control local disease without an

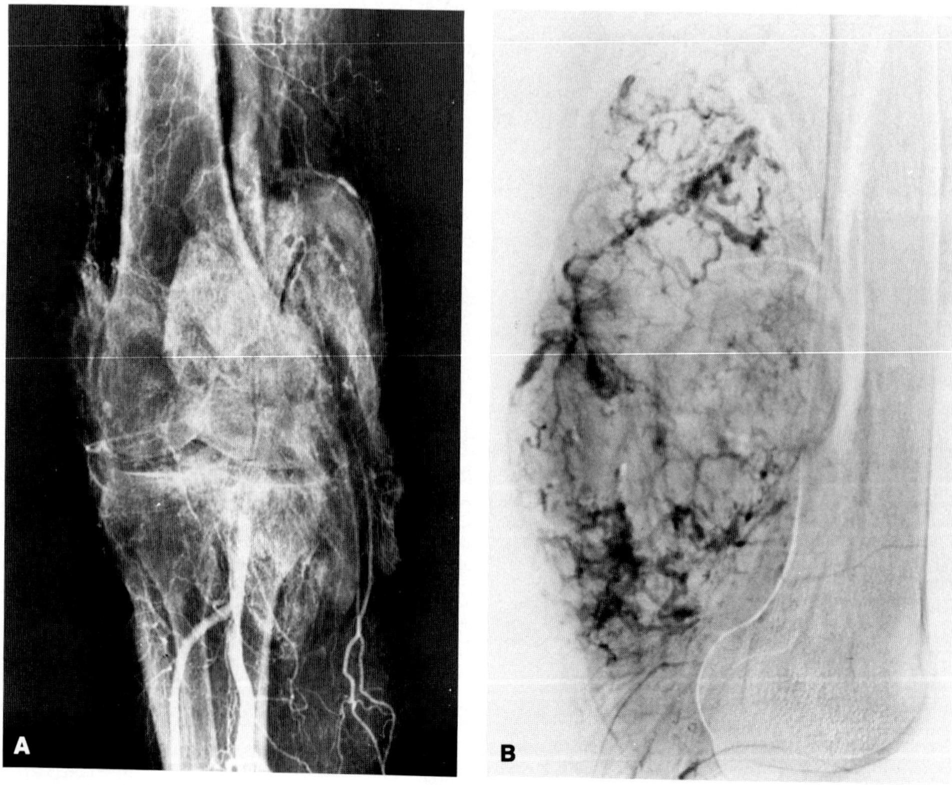


**Figure 47-10.** Angiography of soft-tissue masses. **(A)** Pronounced neovascularity of pigmented villonodular synovitis about the knee. **(B)** Distorted vasculature about the distal lateral thigh caused by a hamartoma. (*B,* Bernardino ME, Jing BS, Thomas JL et al: The extremity soft-tissue lesion: A comparative study of ultrasound, computed tomography, and xeroradiography. Radiology 139:53–59, 1981)

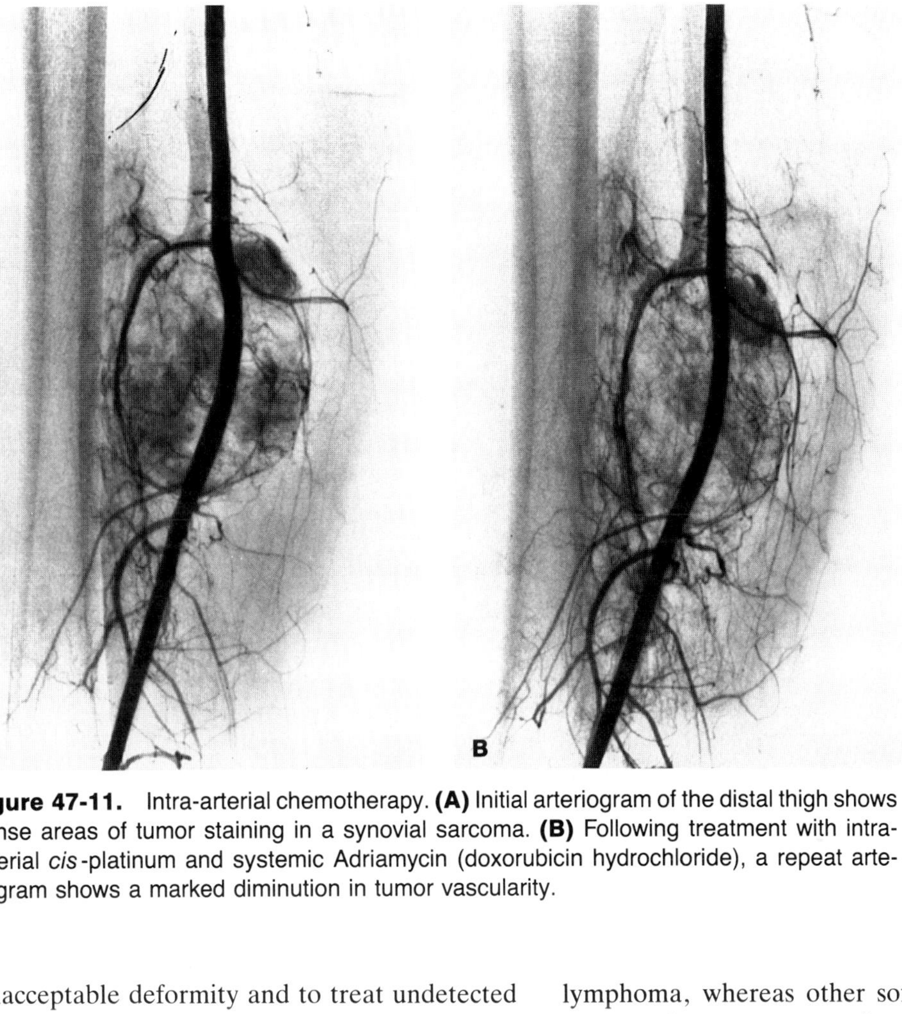

**Figure 47-11.** Intra-arterial chemotherapy. **(A)** Initial arteriogram of the distal thigh shows dense areas of tumor staining in a synovial sarcoma. **(B)** Following treatment with intra-arterial *cis*-platinum and systemic Adriamycin (doxorubicin hydrochloride), a repeat arteriogram shows a marked diminution in tumor vascularity.

unacceptable deformity and to treat undetected metastases.

## Lymphangiography

Lymphangiography can be of value in staging soft-tissue malignancies of the extremity by providing additional information about the extent of disease. Rigid criteria are essential if the lymphangiographic diagnosis of metastases is to correlate closely with the pathologic findings. The most accurate indication of metastases from carcinoma and most types of soft-tissue sarcomas is a filling defect in a node not traversed by lymphatic channels (Fig. 47-12A). Rhabdomyosarcomas may produce a pattern of multiple irregular filling defects (Fig. 47-13) similar to lymphoma, whereas other soft-tissue sarcomas may produce a pattern of crescent-shaped defects that are usually situated at the upper or lower end of the node (Fig. 47-12*B*) as with carcinoma. Obstruction of lymphatic channels may occur when the nodes are partially or completely replaced by tumor. This often leads to opacification of collateral channels (lymphatic to lymphatic, lymphatic to prelymphatic, lymphatic to venous). If there is total replacement of a node, disruption of the lymphatic pathways is secondary evidence of nodal disease. Appropriate confirmatory studies (angiography, ultrasound, CT, needle biopsy) should then be performed. Computed tomography provides the most information of any single study. Ultrasound is very accurate in assessing the retroperitoneum and the presence of vascular occlusion. Angiography is

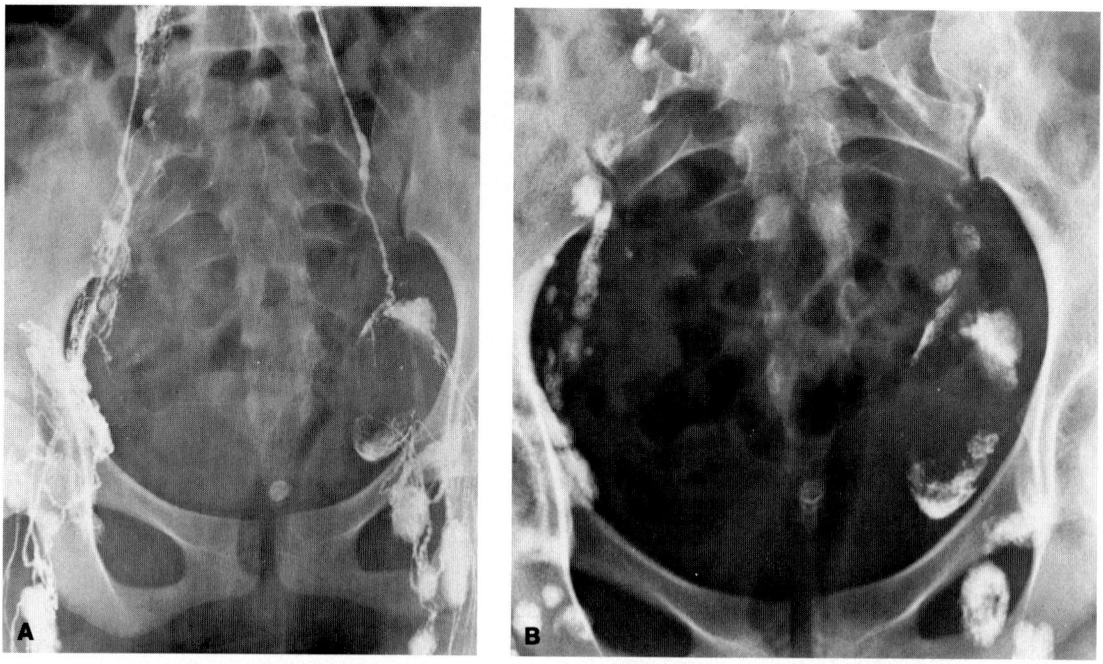

**Figure 47-12.** Lymphatic metastases. **(A)** Lymphatic phase of a lymphangiogram shows a filling defect in a pelvic node not traversed by lymphatic channels. **(B)** In the nodal phase, there are characteristic crescent-shaped defects. (*A,* de Santos LA et al: Angiography and lymphangiography in peripheral soft tissue sarcomas. In Clark RL: Management of Primary Bone and Soft Tissue Tumors. Chicago, Year Book Medical Publishers, 1977; *B,* Lindell MM, Wallace S: Soft tissue tumors of the appendicular skeleton. In Bragg DG, Rubin P, Youker JE (eds): Oncologic Imaging. New York, Pergamon Press, 1985; with permission)

specific in demonstrating the location and nature of normal vascular channels and any abnormal vessels.

Soft-tissue sarcomas metastasize to lymph nodes in approximately 20% to 35% of cases. Those soft-tissue sarcomas that most commonly metastasize to lymph nodes include malignant fibrohistiocytoma, synovial sarcoma, rhabdomyosarcoma, and clear cell sarcoma of the tendon sheath and aponeurosis. Fibrosarcomas and liposarcomas infrequently metastasize to lymph nodes.

## Percutaneous Needle Biopsy

A precise identification of the histologic nature (neoplastic, cystic, inflammatory, vascular) of a soft-tissue tumor of the extremity is necessary before it is possible to plan the appropriate therapy (surgery, radiation therapy, chemotherapy, or any combination). After the position and contours of the mass are identified radiographically, needle biopsy is performed in the most accessible area. This is rarely the epicenter of the tumor, a region that may be necrotic and should not be used for tissue specimens, because it may contain no recognizable tumor cells.

Biopsies of soft-tissue neoplasms of the extremity can be easily obtained with slotted cutting needles that provide a core of tissue adequate for obtaining histopathologic and electron microscopic analyses. Although frequently performed, percutaneous needle aspiration (18–23 gauge) often results in a cytologic specimen that is inadequate for precise histologic identification. Percutaneous needle aspiration is useful for evaluating possible tumor recurrence, be-

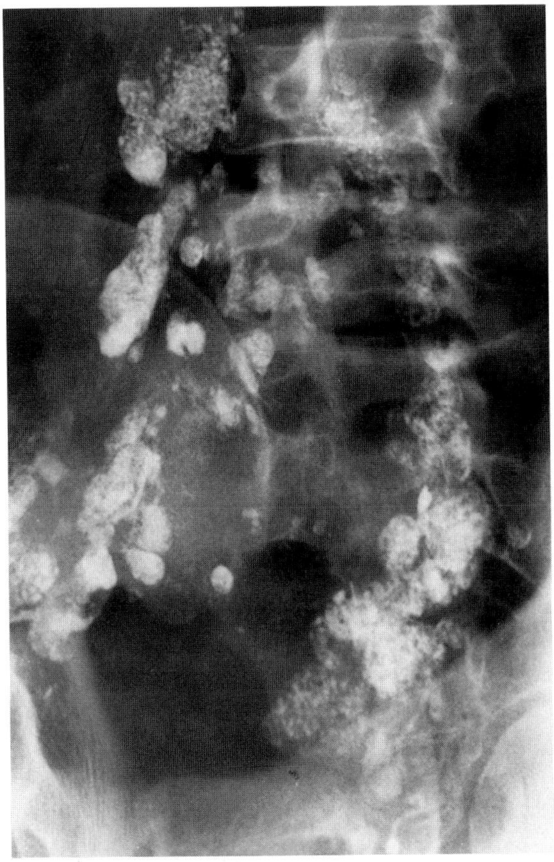

**Figure 47-13.** Rhabdomyosarcoma of the leg. Lymphangiogram shows multiple irregular filling defects typical of the lymphomas.

cause there are usually enough neoplastic cells obtained to compare to the initial diagnostic material. As the needle enters the neoplastic tissue, there is usually a feeling of resistance, and the needle can then be firmly advanced into the tumor. One to four needle aspirations are usually sufficient to ensure adequate material for cytologic diagnosis.

Lymph nodes suspected of containing metastatic deposits can be easily biopsied percutaneously using a 23-gauge needle under fluoroscopic guidance. The needle is placed within the post-lymphangiographic lucent nodal defect that is caused by tumor replacement. The procedure may be performed on an outpatient basis, and the patient requires no special medication or orders. Laboratory evidence of abnormal bleeding parameters is generally considered a contraindication to performing percutaneous needle biopsy. The seeding of tumor cells along the needle tract is an uncommon complication and represents a minimal risk compared with the diagnostic reward.

## SUMMARY OF TUMOR IMAGING STRATEGIES AND PROCEDURES

A soft-tissue tumor of the extremity may be detected by one or several of the diagnostic modalities previously described. If the tumor is small and situated so that removal is feasible without unacceptable deformity and dysfunction, surgical resection is performed. Ultrasound is the imaging modality of choice for demonstrating the location and size of a mass; other modalities (CT and angiography) may be required. Angiography is of special value in providing the surgeon with a vascular map as well as for assessing the integrity of adjacent vessels and their relation to the neoplasm.

Neoplasms of larger size, as well as those involving the vascular bundle, require a different therapeutic approach. Intra-arterial chemotherapy is administered at intervals of 1 month and continued as long as there is evidence of tumor response (decrease in size and tumor vascularity of the mass, or sharper delineation of its contours). Conventional soft-tissue radiography or xeroradiography, ultrasound, CT, MRI, angiography, and percutaneous needle biopsy can all be utilized as follow-up procedures to evaluate tumor response. These procedures are selected on the basis of the clinical situation and progress from less to more invasive, depending on the information required. When there is evidence of no further tumor response, the residual mass is evaluated by percutaneous biopsy. Past experience has shown that the residual mass may be stable with or without viable tumor cells. If chemotherapy results in enough shrinkage of tumor that resection is considered feasible, angiography should be performed prior to surgery.

Computed tomography of the chest is the most sensitive modality for excluding pulmonary metastases in the patient with a soft-tissue tumor of the extremity. Because of the relatively high cost of CT, conventional chest radiography at 3-month intervals during the first year is an alternative screening test for metastases. However, if any change in management of the patient is planned, chest CT should be obtained.

## Bibliography

Bernardino ME, Jing BS, Thomas JL et al: The extremity soft tissue lesion: A comparative study of ultrasound, computed tomography, and xeroradiography. Radiology 139:53–59, 1981

Bien ME: Plain film diaphragm view as adjunct to full lung tomography. AJR 133:215, 1979

Cavanagh RC: Tumors of the soft tissues of the extremities. Semin Roentgenol 3:73–89, 1973

Chuang VP, Wallace S: Arterial infusion and occlusion in cancer patients. Semin Roentgenol 16: 13–25, 1981

Damadian R, Zaner K, Hor D et al: Human tumors detected by nuclear magnetic resonance. Proc Natl Acad Sci USA 71:1471–1473, 1974

de Santos LA, Ginaldi S, Wallace S: Computed tomography in liposarcoma. Cancer 47:46–54, 1981

Goldberg BB: Ultrasonic evaluation of superficial masses. J Clin Ultrasound 3:91–94, 1975

Gothlin JH: Post-lymphographic percutaneous fine needle biopsy of lymph node guided by fluoroscopy. Radiology 120:205–207, 1976

Harms SE: Current status of nuclear magnetic resonance imaging. In Hamilton B: Medical Diagnostic Imaging Systems: Technology and Applications. pp 169–191. New York. Frost and Sullivan Press, 1982

Hawkins IF, Jr, Hudson T: Priscoline in bone and soft tissue angiography. Radiology 110:541–546, 1974

Heiken JP, Lee JKT, Smathers RL et al: CT of benign soft-tissue masses of the extremities. AJR 142: 575–580, 1984

Jing BS, Wallace S: Lymphatic imaging of solid tumors. In Clouse M, Wallace S (eds): Lymphatic Imaging: Lymphangiography, Computed Tomography and Scintigraphy. Baltimore, Williams & Wilkins, 1985

Levin DC, Gordon DH, McSweeney I: Arteriography of peripheral hemangiomas. Radiology 121: 625–630, 1976

Libshitz HI, North LB: Pulmonary metastases. Radiol Clin North Am 20:437–451, 1982

Lindell MM, Wallace S, deSantos LA et al: Diagnostic technique for the evaluation of the soft tissue sarcoma. Semin Oncol 8:160–171, 1981

Martel W, Abell MR: Radiologic evaluation of soft tissue tumors. A retrospective study. Cancer 32: 352–366, 1973

Murphy WA, Totty WG, Carrol JE: MRI of normal and pathologic skeletal muscle. AJR 146: 565–574, 1986

Ney FG, Feist JH, Altemus L et al: The characteristic angiographic criteria of malignancy. Radiology 104:567–570, 1972

Shuman LS, Chuang VP, Wallace S et al: Intraarterial chemotherapy of malignant fibrous histiocytoma of the pelvis. Radiology 142:343–346, 1982

Simon MA, Enneking WF: The management of soft tissue tumors of the extremities. J Bone Joint Surg 58A:317–327, 1976

Suit HD, Russell WO, Martin RG: Management of patients with sarcoma of soft tissue in an extremity. Cancer 31:1247–1255, 1973

Viamonte M, Jr, Roen S, LaPage J: Nonspecificity of abnormal vascularity in the angiographic diagnosis of malignant neoplasms. Radiology 106: 59–63, 1973

Wallace S, Charnsangavej C, Carrasco CH: Transcatheter management of the cancer patient. In DeVita VT, Jr, Hellman S, Rosenberg SA (eds): Cancer: Principles and Practice of Oncology. Philadelphia, JB Lippincott, 1985

Wallace S, Chuang VP: Transcatheter management of musculoskeletal neoplasms. In Wilkins RA, Viamonte M, Jr (eds): Interventional Radiology. London, Blackwell Scientific Publications, 1982

Wallace S, Chuang VP, Anderson JH et al: Steel coil embolus and its therapeutic applications. In Abrams HL (ed): Abrams' Angiography. Boston, Little, Brown & Co, 1983

Wallace S, Jackson L, Dodd GD et al: Lymphangiographic interpretation. Radiol Clin North Am 3:467–485, 1965

Zornoza J, Wallace S, Goldstein HM et al: Transperitoneal percutaneous retroperitoneal lymph node aspiration biopsy. Radiology 122:111–115, 1977

**SOFT-TISSUE TUMOR OF THE EXTREMITIES**

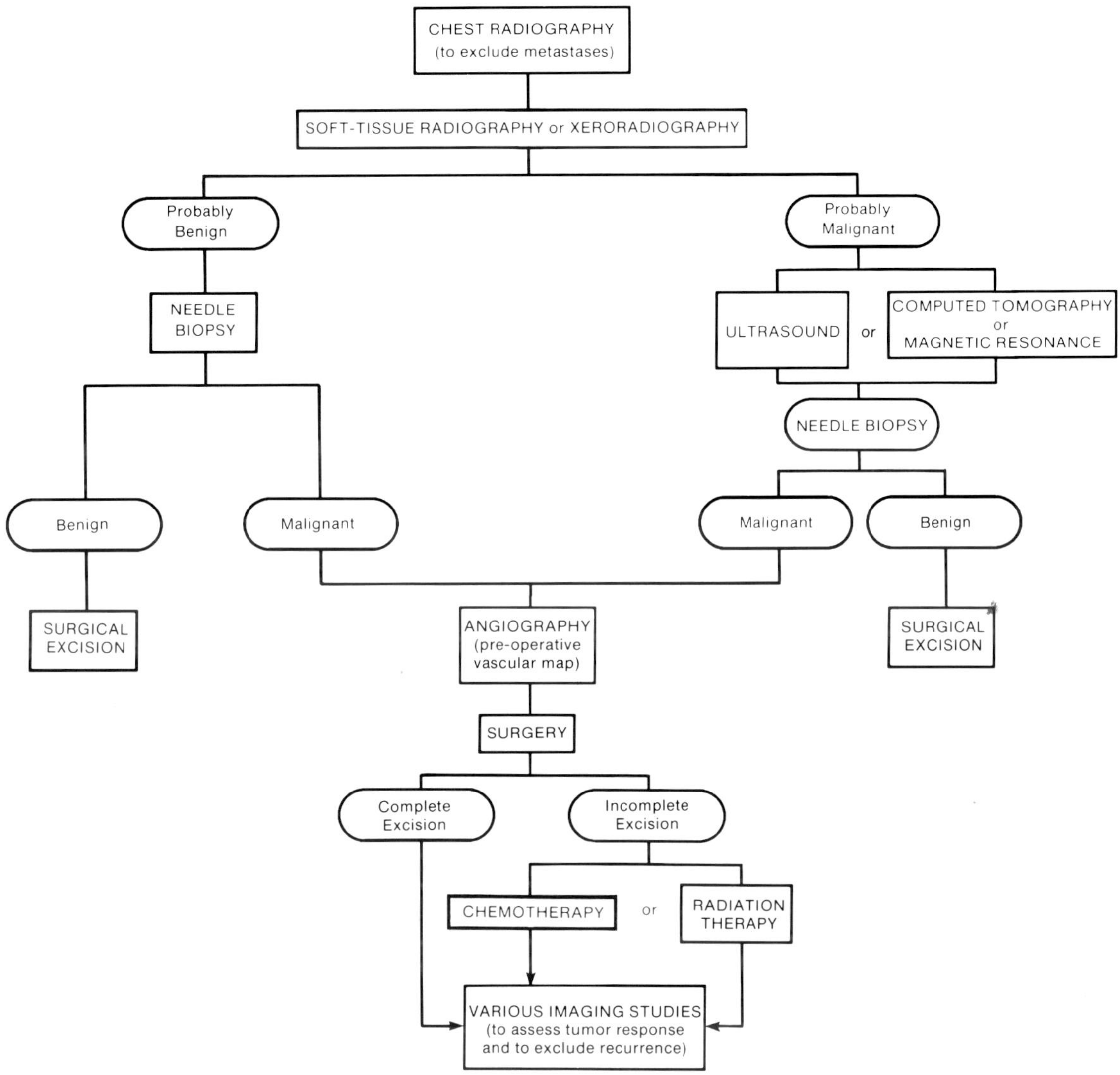

## SUSPECTED LOCAL RECURRENCE

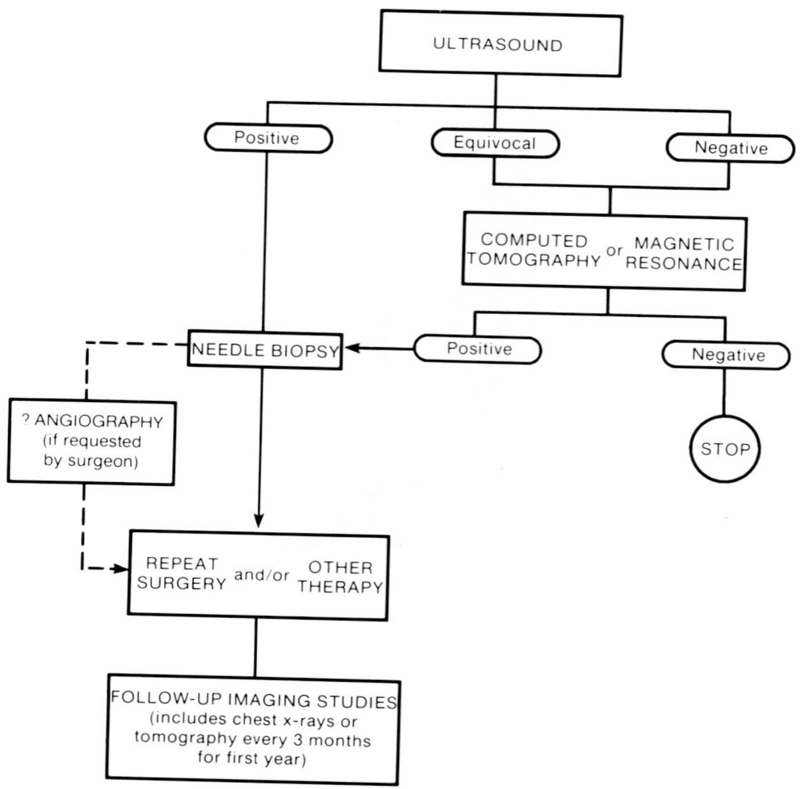


## SUSPECTED PULMONARY METASTASES

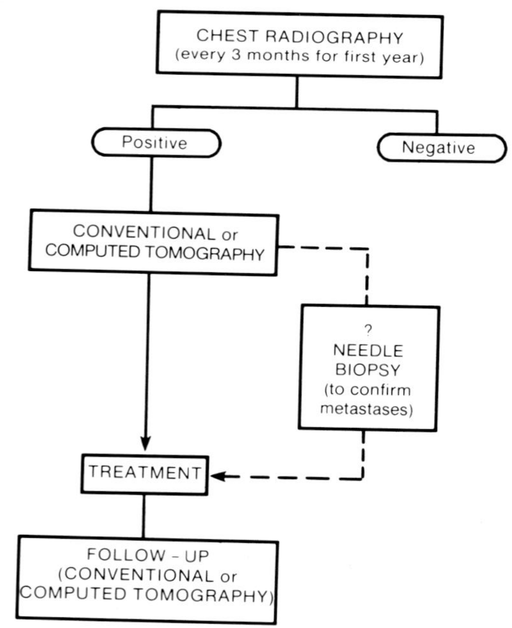

# Appendix

**Table A-1** Pulmonary and Cardiac Procedures

| Procedure | Relative Cost | Patient Status | Complications | Patient Discomfort |
|---|---|---|---|---|
| Electrocardiography | .75× | out | none | none |
| Chest radiography | × | out | none | none |
| Chest fluoroscopy | 1.5× | out | none | none |
| Chest tomography | 2× | out | none | none |
| Radionuclide perfusion scan | 3× | out | rare | mild |
| Radionuclide ventilation scan | 3× | out | rare | mild |
| Radionuclide myocardial scan | 3× | out | rare | mild |
| Lung biopsy (percutaneous) | 4× | out | moderate | moderate |
| Echocardiography | 4–5× | out | none | none |
| Computed tomography | 7–10× | out | rare | mild |
| Thoracic aortography | 7–10× | in (1 day) | moderate | moderate |
| Stress test | 7–15× | out | moderate | moderate |
| Pulmonary arteriography | 9–15× | in (1 day) | marked | moderate |
| Mediastinoscopy | 10× | in (1 day) | moderate | marked |
| Magnetic resonance imaging | 12–20× | out | none | none |
| Coronary arteriography | 15–30× | in (1 day) | moderate | moderate |
| Surgery | >40× | in | marked | marked |

**Table A-2** Gastrointestinal Tract Procedures

| Procedure | Relative Cost | Patient Status | Complications | Patient Discomfort |
|---|---|---|---|---|
| Plain abdominal radiography | × | out | none | none |
| Oral cholecystography | 2× | out | rare | mild |
| Esophagography | 2× | out | rare | mild |
| Upper GI Series | 2.5× | out | rare | mild |
| Barium enema | 2.5× | out | rare | mild |
| Abdominal or pelvic ultrasound | 3× | out | none | none |
| Intravenous cholangiography | 3× | out | moderate | mild |
| Radionuclide liver–spleen scan | 3× | out | rare | mild |
| Radionuclide biliary scan | 3× | out | rare | mild |
| Radionuclide gallium scan | 4× | out (3 days) | rare | mild |
| Endoscopy/colonoscopy | 6–8× | out | few | moderate |
| Computed tomography | 7–10× | out | rare | mild |
| PTHC | 8–10× | in (1 day) | moderate | moderate |
| ERCP | 9–12× | in (1 day) | mild | moderate |
| Abdominal arteriography | 9–15× | in (1 day) | moderate | moderate |
| Magnetic resonance imaging | 12–15× | out | none | none |
| Surgery | >40× | in | marked | marked |

**Table A-3** Renal Procedures

| Procedure | Relative Cost | Patient Status | Complications | Patient Discomfort |
|---|---|---|---|---|
| Plain abdominal radiography | × | out | none | none |
| Excretory urography | 3× | out | few | mild |
| Ultrasound | 3× | out | none | none |
| Radionuclide renal scan | 3× | out | rare | mild |
| Renal cyst puncture | 4× | out | rare | mild |
| Split renal functions | 6× | out | moderate | mild |
| Computed tomography | 7–10× | out | rare | mild |
| Renal arteriography | 9–15× | in (1 day) | moderate | moderate |
| Renal/IVC venography | 9–15× | in (1 day) | rare | moderate |
| Surgery | 40× | in | marked | marked |

**Table A-4** Skeletal Procedures

| Procedure | Relative Cost | Patient Status | Complications | Patient Discomfort |
|---|---|---|---|---|
| Cervical or lumbar spine radiography | 1.5× | out | none | none |
| Conventional tomography | 2× | out | none | none |
| Radiographic bone survey | 3× | out | none | none |
| Radionuclide bone scan | 3–4× | out | rare | mild |
| Bone biopsy | 4× | out | rare | mild |
| Facet block/epidural block | 4× | out | rare | mild–moderate |
| Myelography | 5–9× | in (1 day) | moderate | moderate |
| Skeletal computed tomography | 7–10× | out | rare | mild |
| Magnetic resonance imaging | 10–12× | out | none | none |
| Epidural venography | 12× | in (1 day) | moderate | moderate |

**Table A-5** Central Nervous System Procedures

| Procedure | Relative Cost | Patient Status | Complications | Patient Discomfort |
|---|---|---|---|---|
| Plain skull radiography | 2× | out | none | none |
| Sellar tomography | 3× | out | none | none |
| Radionuclide brain scan | 4× | out | rare | mild |
| Computed tomography of head | 5–7× | out | rare | mild |
| Cerebral arteriography | 9–15× | in (1 day) | moderate | moderate |
| Magnetic resonance imaging | 10–12× | out | none | none |

**Table A-6** Miscellaneous Procedures

| Procedure | Relative Cost | Patient Status | Complications | Patient Discomfort |
|---|---|---|---|---|
| Soft-tissue radiographs of neck | × | out | none | none |
| Radioactive iodine uptake | × | out | rare | mild |
| Radionuclide thyroid imaging | 2× | out | rare | mild |
| Ultrasound of the thyroid | 2× | out | none | none |
| Sialography | 2.5× | out | rare | moderate |
| Laryngography | 3× | out | moderate | moderate |
| Lymphangiography | 7× | out | moderate | moderate |

# INDEX

# INDEX

Page numbers in italics indicate figures; page numbers followed by t indicate tabular material.